The complete, annotated contents for the DVDs is found on page xxi, following the contents. ... chapter, before references, is a boxed listing of the videos that demonstrate the techniques described in that chapter. See inside back cover for DVDs 3 and 4 and their contents.

Surgical Treatment of Orthopaedic Trauma

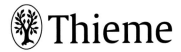

Surgical Treatment of Orthopaedic Trauma

James P. Stannard, M.D.
Professor
Department of Orthopaedic Surgery
Chief, Division of Orthopaedic Trauma
University of Alabama School of Medicine
Birmingham, Alabama

Andrew H. Schmidt, M.D.
Associate Professor
Department of Orthopaedic Surgery
University of Minnesota Medical School
Division of Orthopaedics
Hennepin County Medical Center
Minneapolis, Minnesota

Philip J. Kregor, M.D.
Associate Professor
Department of Orthopaedics and Rehabilitation
Vanderbilt University School of Medicine
Chief, Division of Orthopaedic Trauma
Vanderbilt Orthopaedic Institute
Nashville, Tennessee

Thieme
New York • Stuttgart

Thieme Medical Publishers, Inc.
333 Seventh Ave.
New York, NY 10001

Consulting Medical Editor: Esther Gumpert
Associate Editor: J. Owen Zurhellen
Editorial Assistants: Judith Tomat, Janet Rogers, and Cristina Baptista
Vice President, Production and Electronic Publishing: Anne T. Vinnicombe
Production Editor: Print Matters, Inc.
Sales Director: Ross Lumpkin
Associate Marketing Manager: Verena Diem
Chief Financial Officer: Peter van Woerden
President: Brian D. Scanlan
Compositor: Compset, Inc.
Printer: Grammlich, Pliezhausen

Medical Illustrators: Anthony M. Pazos and Birck Cox

Cover Illustrator: Karl Wesker

Library of Congress Cataloging-in-Publication Data

Surgical treatment of orthopaedic trauma/[edited by] James P. Stannard, Andrew H. Schmidt, Philip J. Kregor.
    p.; cm.
    Includes bibliographical references and index.
    ISBN 1-58890-307-9 (hc) — ISBN 3-13-136941-8 (gtv)
    1. Orthopaedic surgery. 2. Wounds and injuries—Surgery. I. Stannard, James P. II. Schmidt, Andrew H. III. Kregor, Philip J.
    [DNLM: 1. Orthopaedic Procedures. 2. Wounds and injuries—Surgery. 3. Musculoskeletal system—Surgery. WE 190 S961 2007]
    RD732.8.S872 2007
    617.4'7—dc22   2006045679

Important note: Medical knowledge is ever-changing. As new research and clinical experience broaden our knowledge, changes in treatment and drug therapy may be required. The authors and editors of the material herein have consulted sources believed to be reliable in their efforts to provide information that is complete and in accord with the standards accepted at the time of publication. However, in view of the possibility of human error by the authors, editors, or publisher of the work herein or changes in medical knowledge, neither the authors, editors, or publisher, nor any other party who has been involved in the preparation of this work, warrants that the information contained herein is in every respect accurate or complete, and they are not responsible for any errors or omissions or for the results obtained from use of such information. Readers are encouraged to confirm the information contained herein with other sources. For example, readers are advised to check the product information sheet included in the package of each drug they plan to administer to be certain that the information contained in this publication is accurate and that changes have not been made in the recommended dose or in the contraindications for administration. This recommendation is of particular importance in connection with new or infrequently used drugs.

Some of the product names, patents, and registered designs referred to in this book are in fact registered trademarks or proprietary names even though specific reference to this fact is not always made in the text. Therefore, the appearance of a name without designation as proprietary is not to be construed as a representation by the publisher that it is in the public domain.

Printed in Germany

5 4 3 2 1

The Americas	1-58890-307-9
	978-1-58890-307-5
Rest of World	3-13-136941-8
	978-3-13-136941-3

To members of my family who inspired and supported this effort: Carolyn, Jennifer, Luke, James, Michael, Rebecca, Sarah, John, and Gladys Stannard

—James P. Stannard

To the many mentors whom I have been privileged to learn from and who have inspired me throughout my career, as well as to my wife, Jamie Lohr, and my children, Michael and Katherine Schmidt

—Andrew H. Schmidt

To my parents, Philip and Bernadine Kregor; to my sisters, Jani and Kathy; to my brothers, Mark and Mike; to my early and consistent orthopaedic mentor, Marc F. Swiontkowski; to my hip and pelvic surgery mentors, Joel Matta, Jeff Mast, Keith Mayo, and Chip Routt; to all my other orthopaedic friends and teachers from whom I have learned so much. Importantly and individually, to my son, Chase Kregor, for showing me the beauty and joy of life.

—Philip J. Kregor

Contents

DVD Contents

24. Subtrochanteric Femur Fractures

25. Femoral Shaft Fractures

26. Distal Femur Fractures

30. Tibial Shaft Fractures

Video 30–1 **Intramedullary Nailing of a Tibia Fracture.** Intramedullary nailing of the tibia is shown using a nail that allows nailing in extension. Placement of the starting point is emphasized.

Video 30–2 **Anterolateral Percutaneous Plating of a Spiral Distal Tibial Shaft Fracture.** This video shows reduction and percutaneous plate fixation of a displaced spiral fracture of the distal tibial metaphysis. The video emphasizes the use of imaging and percutaneous reduction techniques

Video 30–3 **External Fixation of the Tibia.** This video shows the application of a uniplanar external fixator to the tibia of a 12-year-old child with an unstable tibia fracture and compartment syndrome. The fixator was applied after fasciotomies and wound VAC application. The stepwise construction of the frame is shown.

31. Distal Tibia Fractures

Video 31–1 **Application of an Ankle-Spanning External Fixator.** This video shows the application of a spanning fixator across the ankle for the initial management of a distal tibia fracture.

Video 31–2 **ORIF of a Partial Articular (Type B) Pilon Fracture.** This video shows the delayed reduction and internal fixation of a partial articular tibial plafond fracture in a patient that had been initially managed in an ankle-spanning external fixator. A medial periarticular plate (ACE-DePuy, Warsaw, Indiana) was applied through an anteromedial incision with percutaneous screw fixation of the distal fibula.

Video 31–3 **ORIF of a Pilon Fracture with a Periarticular Nonlocking Plate.** This video demonstrates the use of a periarticular plate through minimal incisions to treat a type 43B fracture. We review the approaches for treating pilon fractures, as well as key principles used in the successful treatment of these difficult fractures.

Video 31–4 **Locked Plating of a Pilon Fracture.** This video demonstrates ORIF of a pilon fracture using locked plating. The benefits of stabilization of the fibula as part of the treatment strategy are reviewed. We also discuss the importance of planning the location of incisions to keep all options open. **See Video 4–6, Disk 1.**

Video 31–5 **ORIF of a Pilon Fracture Using a Posterior Approach.** This video demonstrates ORIF of a pilon fracture with a severe soft tissue injury anteriorly. The posteromedial approach is used to avoid the damaged soft tissue envelope. Potential posterior approaches and the intervals the surgeon utilizes are discussed.

32. Ankle Fractures and Dislocations

Video 32–1 **ORIF of an Open Ankle Fracture.** This video demonstrates ORIF of a Weber B ankle fracture with an open medial malleolus fracture. Soft tissue handling, extension of the fibula fracture proximally, and fixation of the medial malleolus are discussed.

33. Foot Fractures

Video 33–1 **ORIF of a Talus Fracture.** This video demonstrates open reduction and internal fixation of a talus fracture using a lag screw combined with a small plate. The two-incision technique is used to allow full visualization of the reduction.

Video 33–2 **ORIF of a Calcaneus Fracture.** This video demonstrates open reduction and internal fixation of a comminuted intra-articular calcaneus fracture with the addition of Norion cement to supplement the fixation.

Video 33–3 **Closed Reduction and External Fixation of a Cuboid (Lateral Column) Fracture.** This patient sustained a "nutcracker" comminuted cuboid fracture. He was treated with external fixation to maintain the length of the lateral column and allow healing.

Video 33–4 **ORIF of a Lisfranc Fracture Dislocation.** This video demonstrates ORIF of a Lisfranc fracture, taking care to obtain a reduction of the keystone of the base of the second metatarsal against the middle and medial cuneiforms.

34. The Polytrauma Patient

Video 34–1 **Unreamed Femoral Nailing To Treat Bilateral Femur Fractures in a Multitrauma Patient.** This video shows the use of unreamed nails in a multitrauma patient with a pulmonary injury and bilateral femur fractures. Decision-making and the steps to treat this patient are reviewed. **See Video 24–1, Disk 3.**

Video 34–2 **Application of an Ankle-Spanning External Fixator.** This video shows the application of a spanning fixator across the ankle for the initial management of a distal tibia fracture. **See Video 31–1, Disk 4.**

Video 34–3 **The Use of a Reamer-Irrigator-Aspirator in a Multitrauma Patient.** This video demonstrates a new reamer that reams long bones in a single pass while aspirating the medullary contents. Animal data and transesophageal echocardiography demonstrate that this system decreases the volume of pulmonary emboli during reaming of long bones. **See Video 5–3, Disk 1.**

Foreword

The authors of *Surgical Treatment of Orthopaedic Trauma* have created a welcome addition to the teaching armamentarium of orthopaedic traumatologists and to the library of community hospitals everywhere. James Stannard, Andrew Schmidt, and Philip Kregor set out to create a different type of textbook on the surgical management of orthopaedic trauma by adding high-quality, well-edited surgical technique videos to a comprehensive set of chapters covering the breath and depth of surgery for musculoskeletal injuries. Contributors to this book include surgeons in mid-career who have substantial hands-on experience in conducting the surgical procedures and teaching them to colleagues and to residents and fellows. The chapters are comprehensively written and include bibliographies that are useful to the practicing surgeon and resident in training, but are not exhaustive to the point that key references are difficult to find. The line drawings are of very high quality and not under- or over-finished.

The unique contribution of this work is, of course, the surgical technique videos. Their quality is high and the edit-ing skillful. Although Drs. Stannard, Schmidt, and Kregor chose not to use professional voice-over, the accompanying audio descriptions of the techniques are useful and not overdone.

I believe these experienced and skillful mid-career orthopaedic trauma surgeons have hit the mark creating something for residents and fellows everywhere, and to the practicing orthopaedic surgeons in the community setting who need help with the management of common musculoskeletal injuries. The authors are to be congratulated on the end product, but more importantly on having the vision and, even more critically, the drive to see the project through. Patients with musculoskeletal injuries everywhere will be the benefactors.

Marc F. Swiontkowski, M.D.
Professor and Chair of Orthopaedic Surgery
University of Minnesota
Minneapolis, Minnesota

Foreword

The stated aim of James P. Stannard, Andrew H. Schmidt, and Philip J. Kregor has been to produce a book on up-to-date surgical treatment of orthopaedic trauma with a concise text, clear illustrations, and a section with "tips and tricks" in each chapter for quick orientation, as well as a box with "pearls." The three editors have achieved that. Emphasis is given to the outcomes with a special section on published outcome data. Finally, the text is supplemented by four DVDs with videos of the most common surgical procedures.

Besides five general chapters on soft tissues, compartment syndrome, infection, mal- and nonunion as well as the evolving concepts of plating, we find twenty-nine chapters on fractures and dislocations of all long bones and anatomical regions of the human body, including hand and foot as well as the pelvis. Four chapters are dedicated to fractures and injuries of the spine, while three others cover the injuries of the shoulder girdle and knee with special emphasis on ligamentous and other soft tissue lesions of these joints. Besides the management and treatment of the acute trauma, we also find detailed descriptions of corrective and reconstructive procedures. Ending the book is a chapter on the management and priorities of the polytrauma patient.

The text is brief and easy to understand and is a useful adjunct to the surgical videos. The many hours of DVD footage are a unique and attractive feature for the reader, as entire operative procedures from the planning and patient positioning to the suturing of the skin are shown. Oral comments of the surgeons, highlighting hazards and pitfalls, as well as graphics and anatomical models, provide helpful additional information. The videos also demonstrate that even experts may sometimes struggle with a difficult reduction maneuver and that only a perfect reconstruction of a joint is acceptable.

Anatomical line drawings, clinical photographs, and of course x-rays nicely illustrate the different steps of a procedure. Some 60 experienced surgeons have contributed to this new book, which was a monumental task for the editors, as it is extremely difficult to collect and edit all the manuscripts and videos in a given time frame. The three editors are therefore to be complimented and congratulated for this great and innovative textbook, which will certainly find a large audience worldwide.

Thomas P. Rüedi, M.D., F.A.C.S.
Founding member of the AO Foundation
Davos, Switzerland

Preface

Orthopaedic trauma is a complex, rapidly evolving, technique- and implant-oriented field with a very rich history. Successful management of skeletal injuries requires that one be able to synthesize a huge amount of data regarding specific aspects of the diagnosis, classification, and multiple treatment options for a given injury. Furthermore, decisions must often be made in an expedient manner and under some duress, since many of these injuries are limb- or life-threatening. Even for less severe injuries, improper initial management of the injury may compromise later reconstructive options. When faced with a patient with a complex fracture or multiple injuries, it is imperative that one be able to quickly make correct decisions. In order to do this, a single reference text containing "everything that you need to know" would be an ideal resource for the orthopaedic resident, fellow, or practicing surgeon that is involved in the care of trauma patients.

When we initially considered writing and editing a completely new book on skeletal trauma, we realized it would be a huge job and that there are already several excellent books on the market. However, when we looked more critically at the existing texts, we felt that there were a number of missing features that would be helpful to an orthopaedic surgeon preparing for a case. At that point, we decided to embark on a journey to create our vision of an "ideal" book on orthopaedic trauma.

First and foremost, we have set out to create a succinct text that concentrates on the surgical treatment of orthopaedic trauma. We have intentionally minimized the discussion of nonoperative treatment methods. This was not done because nonoperative treatment is unimportant, but rather to allow us to focus clearly on surgical issues. We have attempted to limit the length of the book, recognizing the tremendous time constraints that limit the reading time of most orthopaedic surgeons—especially when faced with an urgent decision about an injured patient. The goal was to produce a text that provides concise surgical detail about currently accepted treatment options without forcing the reader to wade through pages of less pertinent material. Decisions about which surgical method or approach to use are just as important as the details of how to perform the surgery; we asked each contributor to cover thoroughly the indications for surgery as well as to describe currently used techniques in detail. Additionally, we have included a number of sections in most chapters that are intended to aid the reader and decrease study time. The first of these is the "Tips and Tricks" section. We asked our contributors to summarize key points that expedite the successful treatment of skeletal injuries. Another important section is the outcomes section, which provides a summary of published outcome studies in one concise section. The "Pearls" section is a bulleted list of information that is frequently found on examinations. This should be a help to all orthopaedic surgeons, whether taking the in-training exam, studying for the boards, or recertifying later in their career. Finally, we have included a discussion of new techniques where it is appropriate. This section is designed to provide information on techniques that are currently being employed at trauma centers, but that are not yet completely validated by peer-reviewed studies. This section attempts to provide very current information, but the reader must be aware that these techniques are not completely proven yet.

Another unique feature of this book is the accompanying set of four DVDs. Featuring 105 high-quality surgical videos, these DVDs provide more than a mere supplement to the book's discussion of surgical treatments for skeletal trauma. With these videos, the reader gains the valuable opportunity to learn what to expect in the operating room prior to performing each procedure. Together with the book's descriptions, technical details, illustrations, and tips and tricks, these videos show the reader how to incorporate the latest techniques into everyday practice.

We have integrated the video and text in a number of ways. First, a separate contents of the videos following the text contents is provided to help the reader quickly locate surgical cases of interest. Second, a shaded text box at the end of each chapter directs the reader to relevant videos on the DVDs that demonstrate techniques described in the chapter. Third, there are citations within the text to indicate corresponding videos.

The surgical videos represent a wide variety of procedures, from the relatively straightforward to the highly complex. Several procedures are new and have yet to be completely validated by prospective outcome studies in the peer reviewed literature. Examples of these cases include the use of negative pressure wound therapy with skin grafts, the double bundle ACL reconstruction, use of the reamer-irrigator-aspirator to harvest bone grafts, and ORIF of the proximal femur with the locking proximal femur plate. All of the procedures featured on the DVDs are being performed at major teaching centers in the United States and elsewhere.

We filmed most of the cases with at least two cameras, enhancing the quality of the viewer's experience, and have included a number of special effects that serve to make teaching points at key steps in a procedure. In many cases, errors or complications that occurred during the procedures were not edited out; we thus highlighted not only the difficulties likely to be encountered, but also offered guidance on how to avoid them. As was done in the text, tips and tricks are included in the videos.

We trust that you find *Surgical Treatment of Orthopaedic Trauma* to be a useful addition to your library. It is intended to be a comprehensive educational resource, combining a succinct text with instructional video. We hope this book and its accompanying videos will help you succeed as we all work to help patients recover from skeletal trauma.

Acknowledgments

We thank the contributors of each of the chapters. They were all selected because of their expertise in the fields of orthopaedic trauma which they wrote about. In addition, they have an active role in the treatment of a large number of injuries, and we trust readers will benefit from this. We are grateful for their hard work, expertise, and attention to detail.

The video portion of this project has been a huge undertaking, and we are very grateful to a number of people who helped turn our vision into a reality. First and foremost, we thank the video authors who contributed cases, as well as untold hours of time editing, providing voice and special effects, and editing again to create the final product. We thank the crew at Erwin Brothers Motion Pictures for putting up with surgeons' hours and for putting this project together at our convenience rather than theirs. Finally, we wish to acknowledge the work of Stephen Preston, Jason Schuck, Jack Smith, and Jon Erwin. You all are very talented and we appreciate your work. We also thank Joan Stephens for donating countless hours to the organization and review of this project—her help was greatly appreciated.

We are deeply appreciative of support of corporations who manufacture products used in surgery and who, understanding the vision behind our project, generously provided the necessary funding to complete the videos. We did not want this project to be exclusively funded by any one company, nor did we want to use the products of a single manufacturer. In fact, the reader will notice that the implants and techniques featured in the book and on the videos draw from the complete spectrum of equipment currently available to manage orthopaedic trauma. All of the companies that provided funding agreed to do so with "no strings attached." The decision to use specific implants was left to the sole discretion of the individual who created the video, without regard to the companies providing funding.

We extend special thanks to Synthes USA; Zimmer; Smith & Nephew Orthopaedics; Kinetic Concepts Inc.; and Mitek. This project would not have been completed without their generous financial support.

Special Thanks

This project demanded a large time commitment from all of us. We thank our families for putting up with us and encouraging us during some of the difficult moments along the journey to production of this book. Jim Stannard thanks Carolyn, Jennifer, Luke, James, Michael, Rebecca, Sarah, and John Stannard for their love, patience, and support during this project. Andy Schmidt recognizes Jamie Lohr, M.D., and Michael and Katherine Schmidt for tolerating countless evenings and weekends without their husband/father because he was holed up in his office writing and editing. Phil Kregor thanks his parents (Philip and Bernadine Kregor), brothers (Mark and Mike) and sisters (Jani and Kathy) for their support and encouragement throughout the years. His son, Chase Kregor, has been understanding and supportive while his dad completed this book.

James P. Stannard

Andrew H. Schmidt

Philip J. Kregor

Contributors

Jorge Alonso, M.D.
Department of Orthopaedic Surgery
University of Alabama School of Medicine
Birmingham, Alabama

Jeffrey O. Anglen, M.D.
Boone Orthopaedic Associates LLC
Columbia, Missouri

Carlos Bellabarba, M.D.
Assistant Professor
Department of Orthopaedics and Sports Medicine
University of Washington
Seattle, Washington

Martin I. Boyer, M.D., M.Sc., F.R.C.S.C.
Associate Professor
Department of Orthopaedic Surgery
Director
Orthopaedic Hand Surgery Service
Washington University School of Medicine
St. Louis, Missouri

J. Scott Broderick, M.D.
Assistant Professor
Department of Orthopaedics
Greenville University Medical Center
Director of Orthopaedic Trauma
Greenville Hospital System
Greenville, South Carolina

David S. Brokaw, M.D.
Orthopaedic Trauma Surgeon
OrthoIndy
Clinical Assistant Professor
Department of Orthopaedic
Surgery Indiana University
Indianapolis, Indiana

Lisa Cannada, M.D.
Assistant Professor
Department of Orthopaedic Surgery
University of Texas–Southwestern
Dallas, Texas

Jens R. Chapman, M.D.
Division of Orthopedics
Harborview Medical Center
Seattle, Washington

Peter Alexander Cole, M.D.
Professor
University of Minnesota
Chief, Orthopaedic Surgery
Regions Hospital
St. Paul, Minnesota

Cory A. Collinge, M.D.
John Peter Smith Orthopaedic Surgery Residency Program
Harris Methodist Fort Worth Hospital
Fort Worth, Texas

Kyle F. Dickson, M.D.
Professor
Department of Orthopaedic Surgery
Director of Orthopaedic Trauma
University of Texas–Houston Medical Center
Houston, Texas

John Charles France, M.D.
Robert C. Byrd Health Science Center
Morgantown, West Virginia

Jeffrey A. Geller, M.D.
Assistant Professor
Department of Orthopaedic Surgery
Columbia University College of Physicians and Surgeons

New York-Presbyterian/Columbia University
 Medical Center
New York, New York

Thomas J. Graham, M.D.
Clinical Associate Professor
Departments of Orthopaedic and Plastic Surgery
Johns Hopkins University Hospital
Chief
The Curtis National Hand Center
Vice-Chairman
Department of Orthopaedic Surgery
Decker Orthopaedic Institute
Director
MedStar Sports Health
Union Memorial Hospital
Baltimore, Maryland

George J. Haidukewych, M.D.
Florida Orthopaedic Institute
Tampa, Florida

Neil Harness, M.D.
Southern California Permanente Medical Group
Orange County Orthopaedics
Kaiser Anaheim Medical Center
Yorba Linda, California

Mitchel B. Harris, M.D.
Associate Professor
Department of Orthopaedic Surgery
Harvard Medical School
Chief of Orthopaedic Trauma
Brigham and Women's Hospital
Boston, Massachusetts

Keith Heier, M.D.
Metrocrest Orthopedics and Sports Medicine
Chairman
Department of Orthopedics
Presbyterian Hospital of Plano
Dallas, Texas

James P. Higgins, M.D.
Faculty Member
The Curtis National Hand Center
Union Memorial Hospital
Baltimore, Maryland

Philip J. Kregor, M.D.
Associate Professor
Department of Orthopaedics and Rehabilitation
Vanderbilt University School of Medicine
Chief, Division of Orthopaedic Trauma
Vanderbilt Orthopaedic Institute
Nashville, Tennessee

Christian Krettek, M.D.
Professor and Chairman
Orthopaedic Trauma Department
Hannover Medical School (MHH)
Hannover, Germany

Daniel Joseph Marek, M.D.
Orthopaedic Surgery Resident
Department of Orthopaedic Surgery
University of Minnesota
Minneapolis, Minnesota

Steven L. Martin, M.D.
Blue Ridge Orthopaedic Associates
Clemson, South Carolina

Amir Matityahu, M.D.
Assistant Clinical Professor
Department of Orthopaedics
University of California–San Francisco
Director
Division of Pelvis and Acetabular Trauma
 Reconstruction
San Francisco General Hospital
San Francisco, California

Robert K. Mehrle, M.D.
Assistant Professor
Department of Orthopedics and Rehabilitation
University of Mississippi Medical Center
Jackson, Mississippi

Theodore Miclau III, M.D.
Division of Orthopaedics
San Francisco General Hospital
San Francisco, California

Michael A. Miranda, M.D.
Orthopaedic Associates of Hartford PC
Hartford, Connectitut

Sohail K. Mirza, M.D.
Division of Orthopedics
Harborview Medical Center
Seattle, Washington

Erika J. Mitchell, M.D.
Assistant Professor
Department of Orthopaedics
Division of Orthopaedic Trauma
Vanderbilt University
Nashville, Tennessee

Mary S. Moon, PA-C
Private Practice
South Windsor, Connecticut

Sean E. Nork, M.D.
Associate Professor
Division of Orthopaedics
Harborview Medical Center
Seattle, Washington

Brent L. Norris, M.D.
University of Tennessee College of Medicine
Chattanooga, Tennessee

Peter J. Nowatarski, M.D.
Associate Professor
Co-Director
Department of Orthopaedic Traumatology
The University of Tennessee Health Science Center
Erlanger Medical Center and T. C. Thompson Children's
   Hospital
Chattanooga, Tennessee

William T. Obremskey, M.D., M.P.H.
Associate Professor
Vanderbilt Orthopaedic Institute
Nashville, Tennessee

Jeffrey D. Placzek, M.D.
Department of Orthopaedic Surgery
Detroit Medical Center/Wayne State University
Novi, Michigan

Mark Cameron Reilly, M.D.
Associate Professor
Department of Orthopaedic Surgery
University of Medicine and Dentistry of New Jersey
Newark, New Jersey

David Ring, M.D.
Assistant Professor
Department of Orthopaedic Surgery
Harvard Medical School
Director of Research
Hand and Upper Extremity Service
Department of Orthopaedic Surgery
Massachusetts General Hospital
Boston, Massachusetts

George V. Russell, M.D.
Associate Professor
Department of Orthopedics and Rehabilitation
University of Mississippi Medical Center
Jackson, Mississippi

Angela Scharfenberger, B.Sc. P.T., M.D., F.R.C.S.C.
Orthopaedic Surgeon
Department of Medicine and Dentistry
Division of Orthopaedic Surgery
University of Alberta
Edmonton, Alberta

Robert C. Schenck Jr., M.D.
Department of Orthopaedics
University of New Mexico
Albuquerque, New Mexico

Andrew H. Schmidt, M.D.
Associate Professor
Department of Orthopaedic Surgery
University of Minnesota Medical School
Division of Orthopaedics
Hennepin County Medical Center
Minneapolis, Minnesota

Stephen Andrew Sems, M.D.
Clinical Instructor
Department of Orthopaedic Surgery
Mayo Clinic
Rochester, Minnesota

Rajiv K. Sethi
Chief Resident
Harvard Combined Orthopaedic
   Surgery
Massachusetts General Hospital
Brigham and Women's Hospital
Boston, Massachusetts

Franklin D. Shuler, M.D., Ph.D.
Associate Professor
Department of Orthopaedics and
   Rehabilitation
Vanderbilt University Medical Center
Nashville, Tennessee

Paul M. Simic, M.D.
Southern California Orthopaedic
   Institute
Van Nuys, California

Stephen H. Sims, M.D.
Chief of Fracture Service
Carolinas Medical Center
Charlotte, North Carolina

James P. Stannard, M.D.
Professor
Department of Orthopaedic Surgery
Chief, Division of Orthopaedic Trauma
University of Alabama School of Medicine
Birmingham, Alabama

Rena L. Stewart, M.D., F.R.S.C.
Assistant Professor
Department of Orthopaedic Surgery
University of Alabama School of Medicine
Birmingham, Alabama

Michael Stover, M.D.
Associate Professor
Director of Orthopaedic Trauma
Department of Orthopaedic Surgery
Loyola University Medical Center
Maywood, Illinois

David C. Templeman, M.D.
Division of Orthopaedics
Hennepin County Medical Center
Minneapolis, Minnesota

Gregory Tennant, D.O.
Clinical Fellow
Division of Orthopaedic Trauma
Vanderbilt Orthopaedic Institute
Nashville, Tennessee

Steven M. Theiss, M.D.
Associate Professor
Department of Orthopaedic Surgery
University of Alabama School of Medicine
Birmingham, Alabama

David A. Volgas, M.D.
Department of Orthopaedic Surgery
University of Alabama School of Medicine
Birmingham, Alabama

J. Tracy Watson, M.D.
Professor
Department of Orthopaedic Surgery
Saint Louis University School of Medicine
Saint Louis, Missouri

Jeffrey Todd Watson, M.D.
Assistant Professor
Department of Orthopaedics and Rehabilitation
Vanderbilt University Medical Center
Nashville, Tennessee

Timothy G. Weber, M.D.
Orthopaedic Trauma Surgeon
OrthoIndy
Indianapolis, Indiana

Kirkham B. Wood, M.D.
Associate Professor
Department of Orthopaedic Surgery
Harvard Medical School
Division of Orthopaedic Surgery
Massachusetts General Hospital
Boston, Massachusetts

Michael Zlowodzki, M.D.
Resident
Department of Orthopaedic Surgery
University of Minnesota Medical School
Minneapolis, Minnesota

Video Contributors

Jeffrey O. Anglen, M.D.
Boone Orthopaedic Associates LLC
Columbia, Missouri

Peter Alexander Cole, M.D.
Professor
University of Minnesota
Chief, Orthopaedic Surgery
Regions Hospital
St. Paul, Minnesota

Thomas R. Hunt III, M.D.
John D. Sherrill Professor of Surgery
Department of Orthopaedic Surgery
University of Alabama School of Medicine
Birmingham, Alabama

Philip J. Kregor, M.D.
Associate Professor
Department of Orthopaedics and
    Rehabilitation
Vanderbilt University School of Medicine
Chief, Division of Orthopaedic Trauma
Vanderbilt Orthopaedic Institute
Nashville, Tennessee

Christian Krettek, M.D.
Professor and Chairman
Orthopaedic Trauma Department
Hannover Medical School (MHH)
Hannover, Germany

Peter J. Nowatarski, M.D.
Associate Professor
Co-Director
Department of Orthopaedic Traumatology
The University of Tennessee Health
    Science Center
Erlanger Medical Center and T. C. Thompson
    Children's Hospital
Chattanooga, Tennessee

Andrew H. Schmidt, M.D.
Associate Professor
Department of Orthopaedic Surgery
University of Minnesota Medical School
Division of Orthopaedics
Hennepin County Medical Center
Minneapolis, Minnesota

James P. Stannard, M.D.
Associate Professor
Department of Orthopaedic Surgery
Chief, Division of Orthopaedic Trauma
University of Alabama School of Medicine
Birmingham, Alabama

Steven M. Theiss, M.D.
Associate Professor
Department of Orthopaedic Surgery
University of Alabama School of Medicine
Birmingham, Alabama

James L. Thomas, D.P.M.
Associate Professor
Department of Orthopaedic Surgery
University of Alabama School of Medicine
Birmingham, Alabama

Dan Tunmire Jr., R.N., C.N.O.R., C.R.N.F.A.
Department of Orthopaedic Surgery
University of Alabama School of Medicine
Birmingham, Alabama

David A. Volgas, M.D.
Department of Orthopaedic Surgery
University of Alabama School of Medicine
Birmingham, Alabama

J. Tracy Watson, M.D.
Professor
Department of Orthopaedic Surgery
Saint Louis University School of Medicine
Saint Louis, Missouri

Jeffry Todd Watson
Assistant Professor
Department of Orthopaedics and Rehabiliation
Vanderbilt University Medical Center
Nashville, Tennessee

1 Care of the Soft Tissue Envelope

David A. Volgas

The care and handling of the soft tissue is often the most crucial aspect of fracture management. In the decades since the development of the concept of early rigid skeletal fixation and functional use of the extremity following fractures, surgeons have shifted their focus from the care of the fracture to the care of the soft tissues surrounding the fracture. Innovative concepts such as the Less Invasive Stabilization System (LISS [Synthes USA, Paoli, Pennsylvania])[1–6] and Minimally Invasive Percutaneous Plate Osteosynthesis (MIPPO)[7,8] techniques have been developed and are being refined, allowing surgeons to address the requirement for stable internal fixation without causing additional surgical trauma to the surrounding soft tissues.

The majority of complications that are persistent and problematic for surgeons and patients are those associated with soft tissue injury. Indeed, the number of wound problems and deep infections far exceeds the number of nonunions. Furthermore, orthopaedic surgeons often feel inadequate to address these issues definitively because of inadequate training in the art of soft tissue handling. This chapter discusses the anatomy of skin, soft tissue, and bone; demonstrates handling techniques that can help protect the injured but viable soft tissue envelope; and describes how to manage problems that inevitably arise.

Classification

There are two classification systems used to describe soft tissue injury. The Tscherne classification of closed fractures was developed in 1982.[9] This classification system relies on a relatively subjective description of the general condition of the soft tissues based on observation, mechanism of injury, and severity of the fracture. It is only applied to closed fractures. **Table 1–1** describes the Tscherne classification.

This classification system is inherently subjective, and moderate interobserver variability exists, but it is nevertheless widely used.

This classification was expanded by the AO[10] to provide a more objective system of classification, which incorporates injury grading of each component of soft tissue. In this system, wounds are classified by the extent of injury to the integument, muscle and tendon, and neurovascular tissue **(Table 1–2)**. This classification system is very complicated and difficult to use in practice, but it does encourage the surgeon to think systematically about the injury to soft tissue.

In the management of a patient with soft tissue trauma, it is less important to appropriately classify the wound than to critically examine all aspects of the soft tissues and plan surgical treatment appropriately. The surgeon should consider the injury to each component of the soft tissue and the implication of that injury in terms of healing the fracture.

Nonoperative Treatment

The nonoperative treatment of soft tissue injury is centered on controlling swelling and preventing further injury to the soft tissue. Most commonly, this involves immobilization followed by elevation. For closed fractures with mild soft tissue injuries, this is frequently all that is required. However, the surgeon must consider the *wound trajectory,* that is, what is expected to happen to the wound over time. This is largely a judgment based on experience. It incorporates the mechanism and energy of injury, the patient (smoker, elderly, diabetes, compliance, etc.), and the fracture. A wound that was caused by a high-energy mechanism such as a motor vehicle accident or bumper injury

Table 1—1 Tscherne Grade (Closed Fractures)

Grade 0	Grade I	Grade II	Grade III
No or minor soft tissue injury	Superficial abrasion or contusion	Deep contaminated wounds or deep contusions; imminent compartment syndrome	Extensive soft tissue contusion, abrasion, destruction of muscle, Morel-Lavallée lesion, compartment syndrome, vascular injuries
Indirect fracture, simple pattern	Pressure from fracture fragments on skin		
		Medium to severe fracture patterns	
	Simple or medium-energy fracture		Severe comminution, high-energy mechanism of injury

Table 1—2 AO Soft Tissue Classification

Closed Skin Lesions (IC)		Open Skin Lesions (IO)		Muscle/Tendon Injury (MT)		Neurovascular Injury (NV)	
IC1	No skin lesion	IO 1	Skin breakage from inside out	MT 1	No muscle injury	NV 1	No neurovascular injury
IC 2	No skin laceration but contusion	IO 2	Skin breakage from outside in < 5 cm, contused edges	MT 2	Circumscribed muscle injury, one compartment only	NV 2	Isolated nerve injury
IC 3	Circumscribed degloving	IO 3	Skin breakage from outside in 5 cm, increased contusion, devitalized edges	MT 3	Considerable muscle injury, two compartments	NV 3	Localized vascular injury
IC 4	Extensive, closed degloving	IO 4	Considerable, full-thickness contusion, abrasion, extensive abrasion, extensive open degloving, skin loss	MT 4	Muscle defect, tendon laceration, extensive muscle contusion	NV 4	Extensive segmental vascular injury
IC 5	Necrosis from contusion			MT 5	Compartment syndrome/ crush syndrome with wide injury zone	NV 5	Combined neurovascular injury, including subtotal or even total amputation

will swell immediately, but the edema may increase for 3 to 5 days before beginning to resolve. Likewise, a patient with a relatively low-energy injury, such as a closed ankle fracture, may swell and develop fracture blisters over the course of the following week simply because the patient does not elevate the extremity.

Pneumatic compression devices such as the PlexiPulse device (NuTech, San Antonio, Texas) have been shown to reduce the time for swelling in lower extremity fractures.[11-15] These devices seem to work by stimulating venous return from the lower extremity. In our experience, however, despite the gains in edema reduction, the devices are not well tolerated by patients because of pain and the constant noise associated with inflation and deflation of the device. They are also not well suited for use in an outpatient setting.

The treatment of fracture blisters is as much tradition as science. Fracture blisters represent separation of the dermis from the epidermis. Blood blisters imply slightly deeper tissue damage. Giordano et al studied the histology of fracture blisters and found that there was little difference between the histology of serous blisters and blood blisters except that there were more epithelial cells present in the clear blisters.[16] Furthermore, there did not seem to be any dermal injury in the blister bed or surrounding tissue for either type of blister. Although many surgeons have their own treatment protocol for managing fracture blisters, Giordano and Koval, in a prospective study, reported no difference in infection rate or wound healing between unroofing the blister and applying Silvadene and simply leaving the blister intact.[17]

Surgical Treatment

Indications

The indications for surgical treatment of fractures are well established. Some variation exists in the treatment of fractures that have little soft tissue damage such as type I ankle fractures. Some surgeons feel that a good superficial debridement in the emergency department (ED) is adequate. Others feel that all open fractures must be debrided in the operating room. There is little literature support for ED treatment of these injuries. However, if there is gross contamination, prolonged delay before initial cleaning of the skin, or evidence of debris in the wound, debridement should be done in the operating room if possible.

The role of topical antibiotics on open wounds has been the subject of some study in the military. During warfare or other times of mass casualties, IV and topical antibiotics may be of some benefit. However, this should not take the place of an adequate debridement and stabilization of the fracture at the earliest possible opportunity.

Anatomy

The blood supply to the skin is supplied though a variety of vascular patterns. However, common to all patterns is that skin in the extremities is dependent on blood flow through vessels oriented perpendicular to the arterial blood flow.[18,19] Unlike muscles, which derive their blood supply from arteries that travel down the length of the muscle,

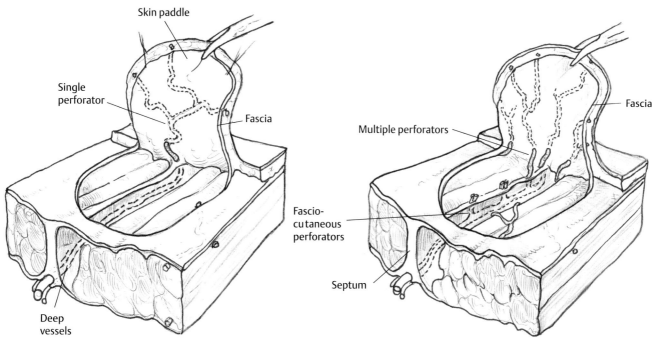

Figure 1–1 Fasciocutaneous flap demonstrating perforating vessels.

skin depends on perforating arterioles arising from longitudinally oriented arteries that lie within the muscular septae or in deep fascia (**Fig. 1–1**). The terminal ends of these skin vessels then may run for short distances in the dermal layer of skin. This pattern implies that any injury that causes the dermis to become separated from the underlying fascia may compromise the vascularity to that skin, explaining why Morel-Lavallée lesions often lead to skin necrosis. As a rule, skin that has little underlying muscle is dependent on longitudinal blood flow, whereas skin that has good underlying musculature is supplied by numerous perforating vessels.

Vascular territories have been described for the lower extremities. Haertsch[18] performed injection studies of cadaveric lower extremities. He found discrete patterns of vasculature supply to the skin based on the saphenous artery and the peroneal artery (**Fig. 1–2**).

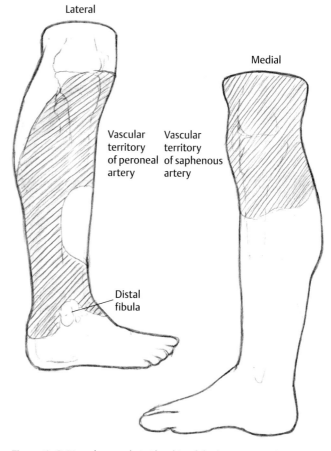

Figure 1–2 Vascular supply to the skin of the lower extremity.

Initial Wound Management

The use of high-pressure pulsatile lavage has been well documented to reduce bacterial load and infection rates following open fractures.[20–22] The effect of high-pressure lavage on bone healing, however, has only recently been studied. Adili et al[23] found that pulsatile lavage had a significant adverse effect on the strength of fracture callous during the first 3 weeks but negligible effect at 6 weeks in rats. Similarly, Dirschl et al[24] found that pulsatile lavage was more likely to impair early healing in a rabbit model. The adverse impact on initial callus formation disappeared by 2 weeks following the injury. Because the efficacy of high-pressure pulsatile lavage in reducing bacterial load is greater than that of bulb syringe, most surgeons continue to use it to irrigate acute open fractures.

The timing of irrigation and the irrigation solution used may impact fracture healing. Park et al[25] found that rabbits that underwent lavage of an osteotomy on 3 consecutive days failed to form callus. The rabbits that underwent lavage on the third and fourth day following osteotomy formed less callus compared with those rabbits that did not undergo lavage. Bhandari et al[26] reported that low-pressure pulsatile lavage caused less bone damage than high-pressure lavage and was effective at removing bacteria 3 hours after inoculation. However, they noted that by 6 hours following bacterial inoculation, low-pressure lavage was not effective at removing bacteria from bone. In another study[20] it was determined that soap solution with low-pressure pulsatile lavage was more effective at removing bacteria in contaminated wounds and had less adverse impact on bone healing than povidone-iodine or chlorhexadine-gluconate solutions.

Although many surgeons consider irrigation and debridement of a wound a simple surgical procedure, there are two errors frequently made during the procedure. First, surgeons, especially less experienced surgeons, take a laissez-faire attitude toward this procedure. Simply placing a curet in the wound and then running several liters of fluid through it does not result in an adequate irrigation and debridement. The surgeon must aggressively seek out and remove all necrotic tissue and foreign matter. This should be done in a thorough manner while avoiding additional trauma to the tissues as a result of excessively aggressive dissection. Once the wound is thoroughly cleansed of all nonviable tissue, the wound should be irrigated. The second error is to inadequately debride nonviable or questionably viable tissue for fear of an inability to close the wound as a result. This error is also more common with less experienced trauma surgeons. The appropriate approach is to adequately debride the wound irrespective of how it will be covered, and then find someone to obtain wound coverage.

Preoperative Considerations

Preoperative planning is essential to the success of soft tissue coverage procedures. The thought processes involve (1) assessment of the characteristics of the defect, including size, location, and condition of the adjacent tissue; (2) assessment of the viability of the proposed graft material; (3) the design of the flap; (4) intraoperative equipment needs; and (5) the postoperative care of the flap. Other patient factors such as age, smoking history, presence of chronic or acute osteomyelitis, and systemic illnesses may impact the selection of wound coverage.

Assessment of the Defect

The wound should be examined with the patient under anesthesia to fully assess the extent of the defect. The surgeon should attempt to define the "wound trajectory."[27] The wound trajectory is determined by serial examinations of the soft tissues and making a prediction of the natural history of the wound based on what has happened in the past. For example, a wound that shows a small laceration but deep ecchymosis of the surrounding skin and bruising of the underlying muscle on the first day may progress to a full-thickness skin loss by day 3 and then to muscle necrosis by day 5. Likewise, a wound that initially starts to heal and then stalls out suggests that the wound has reached its capacity to heal. When a wound is changing rapidly with regard to the extent of tissue viability, the surgeon should delay definitive coverage until final tissue viability within the wound has been determined.

A systematic approach to the wound should be used, beginning with an assessment of the skin. Viable skin has a good subcutaneous layer firmly attached to the dermis. Skin that shows significant ecchymosis within the subcutaneous fat is at risk. Skin that has been avulsed from the subcutaneous fat will likely become nonviable and may be debrided initially. Deeply contaminated skin should be removed because the contamination cannot be thoroughly removed without significant compromise of the skin's integrity. Eschar can occasionally be left as a "biological dressing" when it is very small and overlies viable muscle. The deeper tissue should support granulation tissue and a reepithelialization from under the eschar. Areas larger than approximately 5 cm^2 will take longer to heal unless excised. Often, the subcutaneous layer may be avulsed from the underlying fascia. If the subcutaneous fat does not have ecchymosis, it may be left, but larger areas of avulsion will often slough.

Muscle may be assessed by using the four Cs. This is a time-honored (though very subjective) method of assessing muscle viability. Muscle should be red in *color*. Look carefully for areas of bruising within the muscle. Dark red muscle indicates rupture of muscular capillaries. This muscle may survive but is very risky to use for a rotational flap. Gray muscle is necrotic and should be removed if there is continued risk of contamination because it may serve as a nidus of infection. Muscle *contractility* is judged most commonly by touching the muscle with the electrocautery pencil, but it often will respond to tapping or pinching with forceps. Viable muscle should contract with direct stimulation even when a depolarizing anesthesia agent is used or spinal cord injury has denervated the muscle. Muscle contractility may be decreased in the initial time period following blunt trauma. Therefore, great care should be exercised when assessing muscle viability by assessing contractility. The *consistency* of viable muscle should be familiar to most surgeons. The muscle should have good turgor and should not pull apart with gentle teasing. Consistency remains good until muscle is clearly necrotic and therefore is a late sign. The *capacity to bleed* is also a less reliable sign because muscle with extensive rupture of capillaries may bleed initially as a result of release of an intramuscular hematoma. Other methods to assess muscle viability such as laser Doppler have some value in research settings but have not proven reliable for general clinical use.[28–30]

The periosteum should be carefully assessed. Ecchymosis within the periosteum indicates more severe injury but does not necessarily require excision. If there is good continuity with the remainder of the periosteum, the damaged periosteum will likely survive. However, periosteum that is separated from its overlying muscle and from the rest of the periosteal sleeve is not likely to provide much support for bone and may be removed.

Tendon sheaths will support a split-thickness skin graft, especially if granulation tissue is allowed to grow over it initially. However, split-thickness skin grafts will not survive well when placed directly on tendon due to the relative avascularity of the tendon.

The size and location of the soft tissue defect are important factors when considering coverage options. Split-thickness skin grafts will contract with time, making them less attractive for use around major joints, especially those that have a large range of motion. Likewise, free flaps used for the foot and ankle may preclude the use of standard shoes because of their bulk. In our experience, areas of exposed bone up to 2 cm in diameter may be closed using topical negative pressure with a Vacuum Assisted Closure (VAC) (Kinetic Concepts Inc., San Antonio, Texas) to promote granulation tissue.

A careful assessment of the health of surrounding tissue should be performed. Often, it is better to excise marginal tissue around the defect and use a larger flap or graft than to attempt to use marginal tissue to support the skin graft or flap.

Assessment of the Donor Site

If a skin graft or flap is selected for coverage of a soft tissue defect, the potential donor site must be assessed prior to surgery. Especially in the case of rotational flaps, the donor tissue is often in the zone of injury and trauma may compromise the viability of the flap. Likewise, abrasions over the proposed donor site may preclude use of the ipsilateral thigh for skin graft. It is recommended that gastrocnemius and soleus flaps not be used when there is marked comminution of the tibia.[31]

Choice of Coverage

The choice of coverage for soft tissue injuries is dependent on the location, and severity of soft tissue damage; the condition of the patient; and the capabilities of the individual surgeon and hospital.

Timing of Coverage

The timing of coverage of soft tissue defects is dependent upon a number of factors. An excellent review of the literature regarding timing is found in an article by Weitz-Marshall and Bosse.[32] Ideally, the initial traumatic wound should be converted to a clean wound that has viable tissue at its base. Often, this will be achieved at the initial surgical debridement, but definitive wound closure should be delayed until this condition is attained. Wounds that have gross contamination, farm injuries, high-energy gunshot wounds, electrical injuries, and water injuries should generally undergo an initial debridement followed by delayed primary closure in no less than 48 to 72 hours.

Surgical Techniques

Vertical Dissection

When dissecting, remember that skin receives its blood supply largely through perforating vessels, rather than by longitudinal vessels. Therefore, dissection should be done by orienting scissors in the plane of the skin incision, rather than developing a plane between the subcutaneous tissue on the underlying fascia **(Fig. 1–3)**. Preserving connections between the fascia and skin will help preserve these vessels and improve the ability of skin to heal. The surgeon should avoid exposing anything that doesn't directly aid the treatment of the fracture. Most contemporary plates are designed to be placed directly over the periosteum; therefore, the periosteum should be preserved whenever possible.

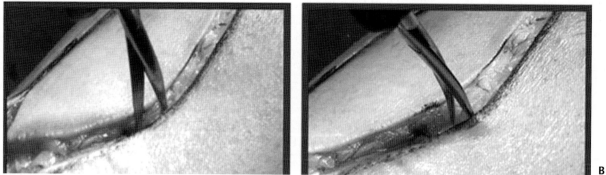

Figure 1–3 (A) Vertical dissection along the line of the incision should be carried out. **(B)** Avoid horizontal dissection that separates the skin from the underlying fascia.

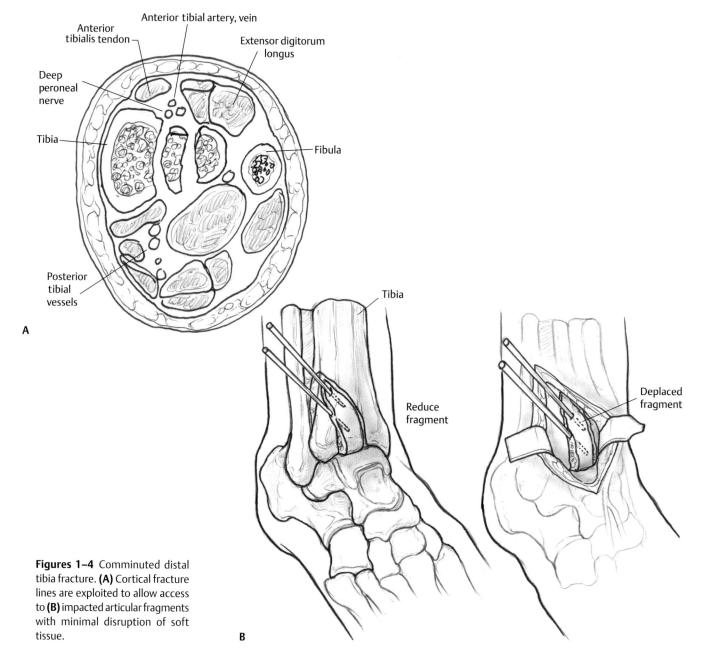

A

B

Figures 1–4 Comminuted distal tibia fracture. **(A)** Cortical fracture lines are exploited to allow access to **(B)** impacted articular fragments with minimal disruption of soft tissue.

Internal Fracture Reduction

Periarticular fractures can be reduced from within the fracture itself. **Fig. 1–4A,B** shows an approach to central depression of an articular fracture that allows fixation and bone grafting with minimal soft tissue dissection. This is accomplished by planning the skin incision over a cortical fracture line that would allow access to the depression fracture. The cortical wall fragment is displaced with a lamina spreader, and the depressed fragment is reduced. Bone graft is placed in the metaphysis. The cortical fragment is then closed and stabilized with a percutaneous screw, or a plate is placed using a percutaneous technique.

"No Touch" Technique

The "no touch" technique for the treatment of calcaneus fractures is widely accepted. Using this technique, the surgeon exposes the calcaneus through a lateral approach and then places a K-wire in the fibula and the talar neck as retractors for the remainder of the case. This technique reduces injury to the flap by maintaining constant, firm retraction on the soft tissue flap **(Fig. 1–5)**. This same technique can be used elsewhere, such as the distal tibia. Retractors are used on the skin only until K-wires can be inserted to provide retraction. Avoid the use of forceps with teeth on thin skin flaps. Pay close attention to the strength and length of retraction. Often, the assistant will increase pressure on the retractor during the case, giving

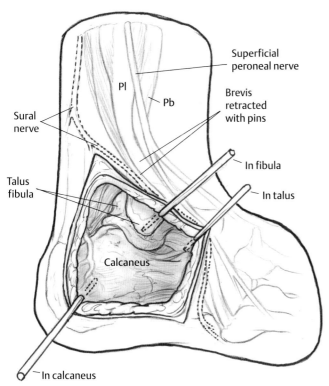

Figure 1–5 No touch technique of soft tissue retraction in calcaneus fractures. Pb, peroneus brevis; Pl, peroneus longus.

excellent exposure at the cost of later wound complications. The old surgical adage "The key is exposure" may be contrary to current concepts of minimal soft tissue dissection. There is a balance between not dissecting soft tissue and the overuse of retractors to improve exposure. When retractors are used, retraction should be relaxed when awaiting equipment for the next stage of the procedure.

Despite careful attention to tissue handling, problems can and do arise. The next section addresses operative approaches to soft tissue defects.

Free Muscle Flaps

Free muscle transfers remain the mainstay of treatment for large or distal wounds. They require experience and training in microvascular techniques and thus are beyond the scope of this book.

Gastrocnemius Flap (see Video 1–1, Disk 1)

Indications

The gastrocnemius flap may be used to cover soft tissue defects over the medial, lateral, and anterior borders of the proximal tibia. When taken from the medial side, the flap can provide coverage from the superior border of the patella to approximately 2 cm distal to the tibial tubercle. When taken from the lateral side, coverage provided is somewhat smaller because the flap must travel around the fibula. There may be significant variation between individuals regarding the length of the muscle belly. Similarly, the tendon may begin much higher in some patients. Often the surgeon can palpate the musculotendinous junction on the well leg.

Contraindications

Fractures of the tibia with severe comminution, electrical burns, or extensive soft tissue damage to the popliteal area or calf

Blood Supply

Each head of the gastrocnemius is supplied by a sural artery that enters the muscle proximal to the knee joint.

Surgical Technique

The patient is placed supine. A debridement of the defect should be carried out, removing all necrotic and purulent material prior to attempting coverage. In cases involving infection or gross contamination, antibiotic beads may be left under the flap. A tourniquet should be inflated at the start of the case. A longitudinal incision is made from 2 cm proximal to the knee joint to the musculotendinous junction of the Achilles tendon **(Fig. 1–6)**. This incision is midway between the posterior aspect of the tibia and

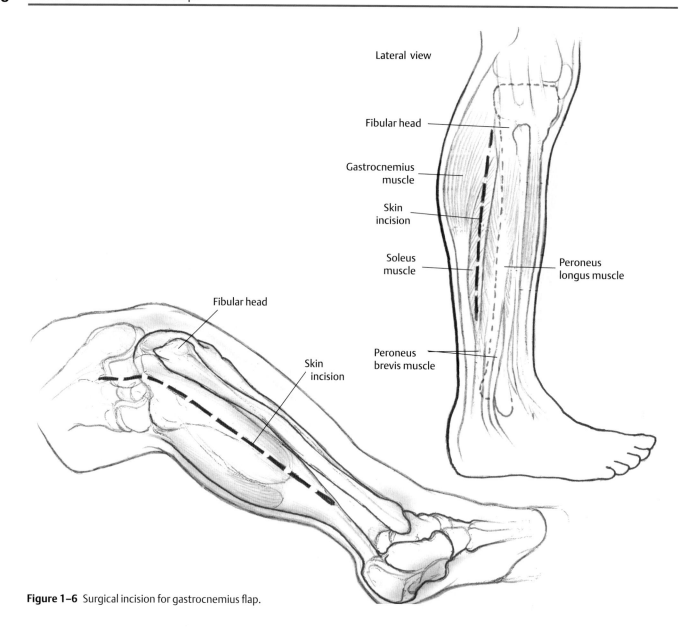

Figure 1–6 Surgical incision for gastrocnemius flap.

the posterior aspect of the calf. The subcutaneous tissue is divided using Metzenbaum scissors, preserving the saphenous vein and nerve. The muscular fascia is identified and incised. The plane between the soleus and gastrocnemius can now be identified easily. Blunt dissection will free the gastrocnemius from the soleus and the overlying fascia. There are perforating arteries that penetrate the soleus and secondarily supply the gastrocnemius. These vessels mark the separation between the medial and lateral halves of the gastrocnemius and should be preserved.

The plane between the gastrocnemius and soleus is developed down to their coalescence in the Achilles' tendon. Here, the medial half of the gastrocnemius is divided transversely with a knife **(Fig. 1–7).** Blunt dissection can continue splitting the gastrocnemius in line with its fibers as far proximally as the knee joint. The nerve that accom-

panies the sural artery proximally into the muscle is divided to reduce the incidence and severity of muscle cramps postoperatively. A transverse incision is made from the proximal end of the longitudinal incision to the defect to allow the muscle to be rotated into the defect with tunneling under the skin bridge. It is sutured into the defect with an absorbable suture. The incision is closed over a drain. The muscle flap is covered with a split-thickness skin graft.

When a gastrocnemius flap is taken from the lateral side, a similar technique is used. On the lateral side, however, extreme care must be taken to avoid injury to the peroneal nerve. Additionally, the flap must go around the fibular head. These factors limit the usefulness of the lateral gastrocnemius flap to some extent. The flap may be passed deep to the peroneal nerve to increase its reach, but if the flap is bulky, this may create a nerve palsy.

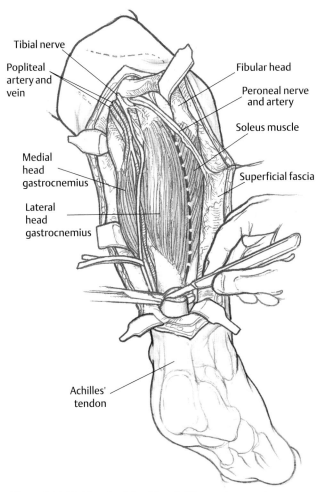

Figure 1–7 Dividing the lateral head of the gastrocnemius.

Postoperative Care

Avoid pressure on the flap by padding posteriorly proximal and distal to the flap. Patients frequently have muscle spasm following rotational flaps, and a muscle relaxer such as diazepam is often prescribed for the initial 2 to 3 days. The extremity should be elevated for the first 2 weeks after surgery, and care must be taken to avoid constrictive dressings or splints that put pressure on the flap. After 6 weeks, the flap may be elevated from the side opposite the muscle pedicle to allow for bead removal or bone grafting, if necessary. After a year, there is presumed to be adequate collateral flow to the flap to allow it to be raised from either side, if necessary, but if possible, it should still be raised on the side opposite the muscle pedicle.

Soleus Flap (see Video 1–2, Disk 1)

Indications

The soleus flap may be used to cover soft tissue defects over the middle third of the tibia.

Contraindications

Severely comminuted fractures of the tibia, electrical burns

Blood Supply

The soleus is supplied by a major branch proximally from the posterior tibial and peroneal arteries, and by smaller branches that perforate more distally. It can survive with only the proximal branch intact.

Surgical Technique

Following exsanguination of the leg, the tourniquet is inflated. A longitudinal incision is made from 2 cm proximal to the knee joint to the musculotendinous junction of the Achilles' tendon. This incision is midway between the posterior aspect of the tibia and the posterior aspect of the calf (**Fig. 1–8**). The subcutaneous tissue is divided using Metzenbaum scissors, preserving the saphenous vein and nerve. The muscular fascia is identified and incised. The plane between the soleus and gastrocnemius can now be identified easily. Blunt dissection will free the soleus from the gastrocnemius and the overlying fascia. There are perforating arteries that penetrate and supply the soleus. These vessels mark the separation between the medial and lateral halves of the soleus and should be preserved. The plane between the soleus and gastrocnemius is developed down to their coalescence in the Achilles' tendon (**Fig. 1–9**). Here, the medial half of the soleus is divided transversely with a knife. Blunt dissection can continue splitting the soleus in line with its fibers all the way to the knee joint. The muscle belly is then rotated forward into the defect. It is sutured into the defect with an absorbable suture. The incision is closed over a drain. The muscle flap is covered with a split-thickness skin graft.

Postoperative Care

Avoid pressure on the flap by padding proximal and distal to the flap. Patients frequently have muscle spasm following rotational flaps, and a muscle relaxer such as diazepam is often prescribed for the initial 2 to 3 days.

Reverse-Flow Sural Artery Flap (see Video 1–3, Disk 1)

Indications

Lesions up to 10 × 15 cm in size in the distal third of the lower extremity. The flap may be used to cover defects as far distally as the metatarsals.

Contraindications

Absent sural artery based on Doppler assessment

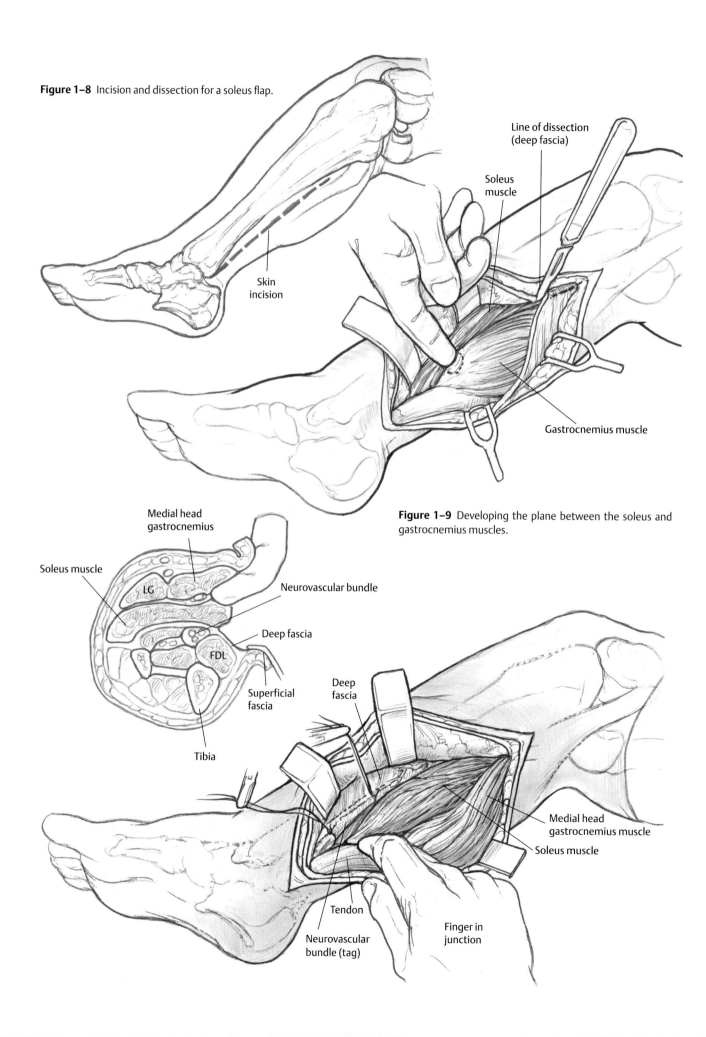

Figure 1–8 Incision and dissection for a soleus flap.

Line of dissection (deep fascia)

Soleus muscle

Skin incision

Gastrocnemius muscle

Figure 1–9 Developing the plane between the soleus and gastrocnemius muscles.

Medial head gastrocnemius

Soleus muscle

LG

Neurovascular bundle

Deep fascia

FDL

Superficial fascia

Tibia

Deep fascia

Medial head gastrocnemius muscle

Soleus muscle

Tendon

Neurovascular bundle (tag)

Finger in junction

Surgical Technique

The wound is thoroughly debrided and irrigated. A Doppler probe is used to identify the perforating arteries that supply the sural artery. The most distal, which is usually located 4 to 5 cm superior to and 2 cm posterior to the tip of the lateral malleolus, is the pivot point for the flap. Other segmental perforating vessels are located with Doppler and are generally spaced about 5 to 7 cm apart. The location of the segmental perforating vessels will help locate the sural artery as it continues proximally. Beginning 2 cm proximal to the most distal perforator, a ruler is bent to the beginning of the soft tissue defect. This is the length of the pedicle that will be necessary to accomplish the procedure. A line is drawn from a point 2 cm superior to the most distal perforator along the course of the sural artery for a distance equal to the length determined above for the pedicle. The length and width of the pedicle are measured, and a skin paddle is drawn that is roughly 25% larger than the size of the defect to account for shrinkage of the flap.

The skin is incised over the pedicle. The patient is placed in the prone position. Care must be taken to ensure that the bony prominences are padded, the arm is not abducted more than 90 degrees, and there is no pressure on the genitals or nipples. The lower extremity is exsanguinated, and the tourniquet is inflated. The soft tissue defect is irrigated and debrided of any nonviable tissue and any frank pus. The skin is excised over the skin pedicle that was previously drawn. The subcutaneous tissue may be divided using a pair of small Metzenbaum scissors. The neurovascular bundle should be evident lying on top of the fascia between the subcutaneous tissue and the muscle (**Fig. 1–10**).

Care must be taken to preserve this pedicle throughout the case. A 2 cm cuff of fascia is taken as this pedicle is raised (**Fig. 1–11**). Small scissors are used to dissect laterally approximately 2 cm from the vascular pedicle on both sides. Next, a Kelly clamp is placed underneath the fascia, and a vessel loop is passed under the fascia. There may be three or four segmental arteries coming from the deep muscular septum or the fascia that join the sural artery. These may be ligated and then cut, taking care to preserve the last feeder, which is approximately 4 cm above the malleolus. As the fascial incisions 2 cm lateral and medial to the skin pedicle are raised, the entire pedicle may be raised. A knife is used to circumscribe the skin paddle. A knife may be used down to the deep fascia. There are normally one or two veins that join the sural vein within the skin paddle. These veins may be ligated if necessary. If at all possible the saphenous vein and its connection to the sural system should be preserved. The knife is used to go down to the deep fascia. The deep fascia is divided using scissors.

The neurovascular bundle should be located at the very top of this skin paddle. The neurovascular bundle should be in the center of the skin island proximally. There are occasions when the sural nerve separates from the sural ar-

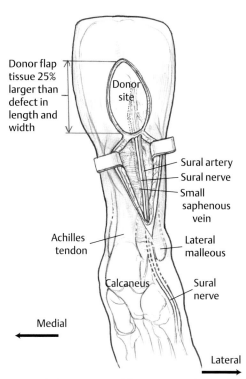

Figure 1–10 Exposure of the neurovascular bundle during sural flap.

Labels on figure: Donor flap tissue 25% larger than defect in length and width; Donor site; Sural artery; Sural nerve; Small saphenous vein; Achilles tendon; Lateral malleous; Calcaneus; Sural nerve; Medial; Lateral

tery and runs deep. This should not be a major concern to the surgeon because it represents a normal anatomical variant. Once the skin paddle is free from all underlying soft tissue, it may be rotated into the graft site. A transverse or oblique incision is made to connect the donor site with the graft site. Although the incision does not necessarily have to go down to the deep fascia, it is often advantageous if it does. The flap should not be tunneled underneath the skin. There is often a septum that connects the deep fascia that is part of this graft with the Achilles' tendon and the Achilles' tendon sheath. The septae must be carefully divided in the distal aspect of the pedicle incision because they will tether this flap and put tension on the vascular supply. Again, care must be taken not to divide the most distal perforating artery. 3–0 Monocril suture (Ethicon, Inc., Somerville, New Jersey) can be used to sew the fascia of this flap down to the base of the defect covering the bone. It is uncommon for the thickness of this flap to match the thickness of the defect, and therefore it is very common not to sew the skin edges down. Nevertheless, with a deep fascia covering the wound, this becomes a watertight seal very quickly. If the skin is forcefully reapproximated, it will often necrose. The pedicle incision is then closed using 2–0 Vicryl sutures and staples. The skin paddle defect is covered with a split-thickness skin graft.

The most important aspect of this flap is to avoid all pressure on the vascular pedicle. This may be accomplished by constructing a splint as follows: (1) the pedicle, which may or may not be covered by skin graft, is covered with a nonadherent dressing, such as Adaptic; (2) the pedi-

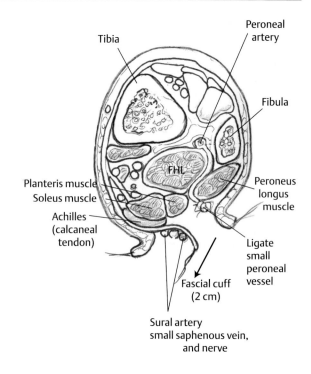

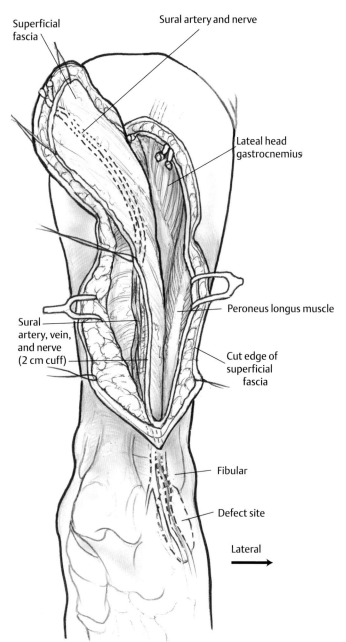

Figure 1–11 Dissection raising the pedicle for a sural flap.

cle incision; and (3) the skin graft which may be covered with Adaptic Non-Adhering Dressing (Ethicon, Boston, Massachusetts) and a VAC dressing or with a bolster padding consistent with 4 × 8 dressings, ABD padding should be used to build in the area proximal to the vascular pedicle and distal to the vascular pedicle so that when the patient is lying supine there is no pressure on the pedicle itself. Sheet cotton is used to keep these dressings in place. A bulky Jones dressing is then applied over the previously described dressings and followed by a plaster splint. Alternatively, a light dressing may be placed over these wounds, and then an external fixator may be constructed bridging the flap with a kickstand built off the back of the fixator to elevate the foot completely off the ground.

An alternative technique to taking a full-thickness fasciocutaneous graft is to take only the fascia with the sural artery. In other words, this is exactly like a fasciocutaneous flap, but instead of having skin coverage, this procedure yields simply fascia coverage over the defect. A VAC device (Kinetic Concepts Inc., San Antonio, Texas) may then be placed over the fascia to promote granulation tissue, and then a skin graft may be placed either primarily or after the granulation tissue has developed. Again, care must be taken to keep pressure off the vascular pedicle.

Postoperative Care

The leg should be elevated for approximately 2 weeks, and weight bearing should be avoided during that time period. It is very common to have some vascular congestion of this flap because the venous drainage is often somewhat compromised. However, in almost all cases this will still yield a viable flap. As the patient is followed postoperatively, the edges of the flap should be checked to be sure that they are sealed and that there is no drainage from those areas. It will take 2 to 3 months for the adipose tissue to reepithelialize unless it is covered with skin graft primarily. Over time, this graft will thin down and allow the use of standard shoe wear. Eventually it will shrink as much as 50% in terms of thickness, width, and length, making it an ideal flap for use around the foot and ankle.

Split-Thickness Skin Graft (see Video 1–4, Disk 1)

Split-thickness skin grafts are the workhorse of soft tissue coverage. They are relatively easy to master, and it is very worthwhile taking the time to learn the details of the harvesting and application of split-thickness skin grafts.

Indications

Any soft tissue defects that have a viable muscle base or granulation tissue over the wound bed

Contraindications

Wounds with exposed bone or tendon without peritenon

Surgical Technique

The wound defect is thoroughly debrided of all necrotic tissue. Any defects that have split-thickness skin graft will not adhere readily to bone, and the graft generally sloughs when applied directly to bone. Split-thickness skin grafts will adhere to tendon with or without peritenon, however. When placed over a tendon without peritenon, the graft may slough because of poor vascularity or may so tightly adhere to the tendon that it restricts motion across the joint. Therefore, split-thickness skin grafts should be used with caution in these circumstances. The wound bed should be prepared by thoroughly debriding the wound; if there is granulation tissue present, it should be "freshened" by gently scraping with a curet to stimulate some bleeding, and more importantly to remove the superficial bacterial colonization. Pulse lavage should be used to clean the wound.

The thigh is the most common donor site for split-thickness skin grafts. The donor site should be shaved prior to harvesting the skin graft. The graft is preferentially taken from the lateral aspect of the thigh but may be taken from the posterior or anterior thigh as well. The donor site should be free of any abrasions. The size of the defect is measured with a ruler. Graft and skin grafts are usually meshed at $1\frac{1}{2}$, which means that a 10×5 cm defect could be covered by a segment of skin that is approximately 11×3 cm, accounting for a slight loss of length when the width is expanded by about $1\frac{1}{2}$ times the width of the harvested graft. Mineral oil should be placed on the donor site. Tension should be pulled across the skin as the graft is taken, using either tongue blades proximally and distally or towel clips, with an assistant holding tension during harvest. The dermatome should be set for 0.0015 in., and its depth can be confirmed by passing a no. 15 scalpel blade between the blade of the dermatome and the guide. The no. 15 blade should pass easily between the blade of the dermatome and the guide. The rib on the back of the blade will not pass through.

The appropriate width of the cutting guide is selected. Frequently, a 2 in. guide is what is used, which will allow coverage of approximately 3 in. of the wound. Expect some shortening of the graft when it is meshed. Generally, the graft should be harvested approximately 10% longer than the actual length of the wound to be covered.

The dermatome is started with the blade on the skin. Firm downward pressure should be applied as a general forward motion is carried out. Forceps may be used to bring the skin graft out of the dermatome to keep it from bunching up. Once the graft is taken, it is placed on a dermal carrier and taken to the mesher. The graft is then meshed generally at a $1:1\frac{1}{2}$ ratio. It is applied with the epidermal side up. There are many ways to secure it. Frequently, simply stapling the edges of the skin graft to the edge of skin is adequate. Alternatively, suture may be used to suture the edges of the graft to skin. Excess skin graft may be trimmed using small scissors. It is very important, then, to apply a dressing that eliminates all dead space under the skin graft and absorb any fluid collections underneath the graft. This may be accomplished either with a bolster or negative pressure wound therapy (NPWT) using a VAC device. The VAC device has been evaluated as an adjunct for use with skin grafts and found to be more effective at eliminating dead space and increasing the percentage of graft take, lessening the need for repeat surgery. For this procedure, the foam dressing may be applied either directly to the graft or over a nonocclusive dressing such as Adaptic (Ethicon, Inc., Somerville, New Jersey) or Xeroform (The Kindall Company, Mansfield, Massachusetts). Our preference is to cover the skin graft with a nonocclusive dressing and then apply the NPWT. NPWT is particularly effective when used over irregular surfaces that can be subject to muscle movement and therefore shearing under the graft. Alternatively, a bolster may be used, especially in areas that do not have a great deal of topographic irregularity and therefore few dead spaces. In this technique, a nonocclusive dressing is applied to the top of the wound and stapled around the edges. Cotton balls that are soaked in mineral oil are applied uniformly over the skin graft on top of the dressing, which is then folded over the top and stapled under some tension. The cotton balls function to hold gentle and uniform pressure on the skin graft, increasing the take.

The donor site may be dressed in a number of ways following harvest of the skin graft: fine meshed gauze soaked with lidocaine or bupivacaine with epinephrine is very effective at controlling bleeding and relieving initial pain. Alternatively, Xeroform may be applied directly over the donor site. A sterile 4×4 bandage and Ace pad are applied over the initial dressing. As a rule, the skin grafts dressed with a bolster are left 5 days with the initial dressing in place, whereas those treated with NPWT require only 3 days. The donor site may be undressed after 2 days, and patients may use a heat lamp or hair dryer to dry the wound each day. The nonadherent dressing is cut away when it peels up as the skin reepithelializes underneath the dressing.

Skin Traction (rubber bands and staples)

- A very effective technique for achieving wound closure is the use of vessel loops and staples. This technique is applicable when wounds cannot be closed as a result of swelling of the soft tissues. This is commonly the case with fasciotomies done for compartment releases, but it may be applied to other injuries where a wound cannot be closed simply because of the soft tissue swelling. It is not successful for wounds where there is tissue missing. Using this technique, a vessel loop is stapled to the apex of a wound near the wound edge. Then, in a fashion somewhat similar to shoelaces, the vessel loop and staples are alternated back and forth across the wound. This will produce constant pressure on the skin edges, and as the swelling decreases, the skin edges may be brought close enough to reapproximate using suture at a second surgery. This technique may also be used in cases where one wishes to avoid wound retraction while awaiting definitive skin grafting.

Soft Tissue Handling

- Perhaps the most difficult thing to teach in a book or even in practice is soft tissue handling. The trauma surgeon frequently deals with tissue that is poorly vascularized before injury and is quite tenuous when injured. Perhaps the best method for teaching these techniques is by observation. The DVD accompanying this book demonstrates some of the more important tenets of soft tissue handling.

New Techniques

Skin Graft Substitutes

There has been substantial recent work[33-36] on skin graft substitutes, and they are becoming more widely available. However, they remain an expensive alternative to split-thickness skin grafting. Substitutes may have a role when split-thickness skin graft is not available. One type of a skin graft substitute is cultured keratinocytes that require harvesting followed by incubation and then transfer to a living host. This requirement makes the use of cultured keratinocytes somewhat limited in terms of coverage for acute wounds. Allograft skin may be rendered immunologically inert by removing the cells, freeze drying it, but preserving the acellular matrix. It may then be covered by a very thin split-thickness skin graft. One negative feature of allograft skin is that it does have the potential to harbor viruses from the donor. Skin graft substitutes are primarily used in burn patients rather than acute trauma patients.

Negative Pressure Wound Therapy (Vacuum-Assisted Closure)

Vacuum-assisted closure, or negative pressure wound therapy, is a relatively new concept. It is a concept that enjoys widespread clinical success,[37-39] but there is limited published basic science data. Nevertheless, clinically it has been very successfully used for complex traumatic wounds. NPWT is postulated to work by a combination of three different mechanisms: increased angiogenesis,[40-44] edema reduction,[45,46] and the mechanical stretching of soft tissue leading to tissue genesis.[38,45-48] Clinically, it is evident that NPWT can produce a tremendous amount of granulation tissue in a very short time when applied to a viable wound bed. It can also produce granulation tissue covering approximately 2 cm defects without vascularized tissue in the wound bed,[49] relying on ingrowth from adjacent tissue. However, it is not as successful when applied to larger areas of exposed bone and may actually dessicate and compromise the vascularity of the bone. There is some animal evidence that the VAC can decrease bacterial counts in wounds,[40] but clinical studies have not been published that confirm the findings.

Currently, there are few published studies regarding the use of NPWT in orthopaedic patients. Herscovici et al published a consecutive nonrandomized study using the VAC to provide negative pressure wound therapy for orthopaedic trauma patients. They concluded that it was cost-effective and remarkably decreased the number of patients requiring flap coverage of their wounds.[50] There have also been case reports published using NPWT as an adjunct to treat infected total knee arthroplasties,[51] as well as to obtain wound closure over exposed hardware and tendons.[52-54] Prospective randomized clinical trials are under way to assess the role of VAC in closed wounds that are at high risk for wound breakdown, such as distal tibia and calcaneus, as well as for treatment of postsurgical hematomas. An additional prospective randomized trial is under way regarding the use of NPWT in patients with severe open fractures. Although it is clear that NPWT has a major role to play in severe wounds following skeletal trauma, the results of these ongoing studies will clarify the precise indications for use of the VAC.

Antibiotic Bead Pouch (see Video 1–5, Disk 1)

Antibiotic bead pouches[55-61] are commonly used for open contaminated wounds and are used widely for any open fracture where immediate closure is not possible or desired. Antibiotic beads are constructed by taking one package of polymethyl methacrylate (PMMA) cement and mixing with it antibiotics that are heat stable, such as vancomycin or tobramycin. Commonly, with wounds that are grossly contaminated, 2 g of vancomycin and 2.4 g of tobramycin are mixed with one package of cement. Before the cement hardens, the surgeon creates small pellets that are usually 5 to 10 mm in diameter. These pellets are then placed like beads on a stout suture, usually a no. 5 nonabsorbable suture. Once the beads harden, they are placed in the wound bed. Benzoin is then painted around the edges of the wound to help seal the very abundant exudate into the wound. A nonpermeable drape is then placed over the entire wound, sealing the edges and retaining the antibiotic-laden exudate within the wound. Over the next few days, a tremendous exudate will be produced, which will have extremely high antibiotic concentrations and will coat and bathe the local tissues with an antibiotic-rich solution that is many times higher than what can be obtained using intravenous antibiotics. This may be left in place for an interval ranging from several days up to approximately 6 weeks, until the patient can be brought back to the operating room for definitive coverage.

Basic Science Research

A great deal of basic science research has been done recently on the role of cytokines in wound healing, and much more is understood now than was understood 10 years ago.[62–70] However, there is still no thorough understanding of the interaction of the various inflammatory mediators on wound healing, and there are no commercially available medications that are effective to enhance acute wound healing.

Gene therapy designed to promote the production of certain wound healing mediators at the correct time is on the horizon.[71] The technical aspects of gene manipulation are being refined and will probably facilitate widespread clinical application of gene manipulation in the near future. It will also provide a significant basic science research tool for investigating the inflammatory cascade and the effect of specific mediators on cells during the wound healing process.

Outcomes

Results of soft tissue coverage techniques have improved dramatically over the past 2 decades as understanding of basic microvascular principles, anatomy, and wound physiology has improved. However, to obtain results similar to the reported results requires the availability of individuals within the institution who are able to perform coverage procedures in a timely manner.

Rotational flaps have traditionally been used to cover exposed bone in the proximal and middle third of the

tibia. However, the recent Lower Extremity Assessment Program (LEAP) study,[31] a multicenter study sponsored by the Orthopaedic Trauma Association, suggests that free flaps may be more appropriate for certain wounds. In this study, 190 patients with 195 injuries requiring flap coverage were studied. Complications occurred in 27% of these cases. This was not a randomized study; patients with more severe damage to the calf musculature tended to receive a free flap rather than a rotational flap. Although the overall success of flaps was the same between free flaps and rotational flaps, the study concluded that rotational flaps have a significantly higher complication rate in patients with severe osseous injuries (AO type C).

Many studies that address the success of free flap transfer for acute traumatic wounds use flap survival as the end point.[72–82] Even in these studies, a wide range of outcomes is reported. Complete flap necrosis as low as 0% is reported, but most authors report a 5 to 10% failure rate. These outcomes seem to reflect the experience of the authors because most small series accumulated over a long time tend to have worse results than those from surgeons with a higher volume. Most of these studies tend to view success as survival of the flap. However, most of the studies also report significant complication rates with these procedures that do not lead to flap necrosis. Furthermore, most studies do not address the issue of operative time required to perform a free flap, which can be considerable in less experienced hands.

Fasciocutaneous flaps appear to have an increasingly important role in trauma patients.[83] Robotti et al[84] reported a single failure in 12 patients. Price et al[85] similarly reported success in 11 patients with a traumatic injury. Fraccalvieri et al[86] reported successful use of sural artery flaps in 16 trauma patients. In our institution, these flaps have been used in 18 acute trauma patients with only a single failure.

Complications

Open fractures and high-energy injuries are fraught with potential complications. Certainly, the current trend toward very early coverage of soft tissue defects and less invasive surgical techniques is driven by the idea that complications of these injuries can be reduced. However, these techniques themselves have a new set of complications.

Free Flap Complications

Flap viability is dependent upon an adequate blood supply. Free flap survivability is very dependent on surgeon experience. **Table 1–3** summarizes recent reports of flap

Table 1—3 Free Flap Complications

Authors	Flap Type	Number	Reoperations (%)	Infections (%)	Flap Failure (%)
Ozkan et al[87]	Anterolateral thigh flap	32	15.6	0	3.1
Vranckx et al[88]	Gracilis	60	?	?	1.7
Yildririm et al[89]	Anterolateral thigh flap	21	4.7	?	0
Fasano et al[90]	Various	100	?	?	13
Muramatsu et al[90]	Various	70	20	?	8
Pollak et al[91]	Various	107	20.6	18.7	8.4
Redett et al[92]	Gracilis	22	13.6	7	4.5

Table 1—4 Rotational Flap Complications

Author	Flap Type	Number	Reoperations (%)	Infections (%)	Flap Failure (%)
Pollak et al[31]	Gastrocnemius/soleus	82	27	22	8

Table 1—5 Fasciocutaneous Flap Complications

Authors	Flap Type	Number	Reoperations (%)	Infections (%)	Flap Failure (%)
Baumeister et al[93]	Sural	70	2.9	7.1	18.6
Meyer et al[94]	Sural	21	0	0	4.7
Hollier et al[95]	Sural	11	0	0	

complications. Some failures are due to inadequate planning. Surgeons may attempt to use a damaged vessel for anastomosis caused by early thrombosis and flap death. Surgeons may attempt to use a damaged vessel for anastomosis leading to vessel thrombosis and flap death. Preoperative arteriography may help prevent this. Other failures are due to inadequate postoperative care. Surgeons must be aware of patient compliance issues, smoking history, and other systemic problems that may compromise results. For flaps that required revascularization, about 70% were successful.

Rotational Flap Complications

As with free flaps, rotational flaps such as gastrocnemius and soleus flaps may fail. The most common reason for failure is unrecognized injury to the most proximal arteries. This risk may be increased in patients with severe bone injury to the proximal tibia. It is difficult to quantify complications of rotational flaps based on the literature. The most recent large series is that of Pollak et al.[92] There have been three additional series published regarding sural flaps. **Tables 1–4** and **1–5** document the reported complications in these series.

Pearls

- Debridement is not a "wash out." It is a thorough, critical assessment of the soft tissues and removal of all nonviable tissue.
- Debridement should not be limited by availability of soft tissue coverage. Don't compromise, temporize, if necessary.
- Malunion can be cured, infection is much more difficult. Don't take unnecessary risks with the soft tissue envelope.
- Wound breakdown happens often enough as a result of injury. Don't add to the incidence by poor soft tissue handling.

On the DVDs

Video 1–1 (Disk 1) Gastrocnemius Flap This video demonstrates a gastrocnemius flap, which is a simple, rotational flap that may be used to cover soft-tissue defects in the upper third of the tibia.

Video 1–2 (Disk 1) Soleus Flap This video is a soleus flap, which is a simple, rotational flap which may be used to cover defects in the middle third of the tibia.

Video 1–3 (Disk 1) Reverse-Flow Sural Artery Flap The reverse-flow sural artery flap is a rotational and hindfoot.

Video 1–4 (Disk 1) Split Thickness Skin Grafting This video demonstrates wound coverage using a split thickness skin graft with the use of a VAC as the post-operative dressing.

Video 1–5 (Disk 1) Antibiotic Bead Pouch This video shows how to make antibiotic beads and create a bead pouch to treat an infection or severely contaminated wound.

References

1. Cole PA, Zlowodzki M, Kregor PJ. Less Invasive Stabilization System (LISS) for fractures of the proximal tibia: indications, surgical technique and preliminary results of the UMC Clinical Trial. Injury 2003;34(Suppl 1):A16–A29
2. Goesling T, Frenk A, Appenzeller A, Garapati R, Marti A, Krettek C. LISS PLT: design, mechanical and biomechanical characteristics. Injury 2003;34(Suppl 1):A11–A15
3. Frigg R, Appenzeller A, Christensen R, Frenk A, Gilbert S, Schavan R. The development of the distal femur Less Invasive Stabilization System (LISS). Injury 2001;32(Suppl 3):SC24–SC31
4. Schandelmaier P, Partenheimer A, Koenemann B, Grun OA, Krettek C. Distal femoral fractures and LISS stabilization. Injury 2001;32 (Suppl 3):SC55–SC63
5. Schutz M, Kaab MJ, Haas N. Stabilization of proximal tibial fractures with the LIS-System: early clinical experience in Berlin. Injury 2003;34(Suppl 1):A30–A35
6. Stannard JP, Wilson TC, Volgas DA, Alonso JE. Fracture stabilization of proximal tibial fractures with the proximal tibial LISS: early experience in Birmingham, Alabama (USA). Injury 2003;34(Suppl 1): A36–A42
7. Krettek C, Schandelmaier P, Miclau T, Tscherne H. Minimally invasive percutaneous plate osteosynthesis (MIPPO) using the DCS in proximal and distal femoral fractures. Injury 1997;28(Suppl 1): A20–A30
8. Krettek C, Gerich T, Miclau T. A minimally invasive medial approach for proximal tibial fractures. Injury 2001;32(Suppl 1):SA4–13
9. Tscherne H, Ouster HJ. A new classification of soft-tissue damage in open and closed fractures. Unfallheilkunde 1982;85:111–115
10. Müller ME, Allgöwer M, Schneider R. Manual of Internal Fixation. New York: Springer-Verlag; 1991
11. Caschman J, Blagg S, Bishay M. The efficacy of the A-V impulse system in the treatment of posttraumatic swelling following ankle fracture. J Orthop Trauma 2004;18:596–601
12. Myerson MS, Henderson MR. Clinical applications of a pneumatic-intermittent impulse compression device after trauma and major surgery to the foot and ankle. Foot Ankle 1993;14:198–203
13. Stockle U, Hoffmann R, Schutz M, von Fournier C, Sudkamp NP, Haas N. Fastest reduction of posttraumatic edema: continuous cryotherapy or intermittent impulse compression? Foot Ankle Int 1997;18:432–438
14. Thordarson DB, Ghalambor N, Perlman M. Intermittent pneumatic pedal compression and edema resolution after acute ankle fracture: a prospective, randomized study. Foot Ankle Int 1997;18: 347–350
15. Myerson MS, Juliano PJ, Koman JD. The use of a pneumatic intermittent impulse compression device in the treatment of calcaneus fractures. Mil Med 2000;165:721–725
16. Giordano CP, Koval KJ, Zuckerman JD, Desai P. Fracture blisters. Clin Orthop Relat Res 1994;307:214–221
17. Giordano CP, Koval KJ. Treatment of fracture blisters: a prospective study of 53 cases. J Orthop Trauma 1995;9:171–176
18. Haertsch PA. The blood supply to the skin of the leg: a postmortem investigation. Br J Plast Surg 1981;34:470–477
19. Nakajima H, Fujino T, Adachi S. A new concept of vascular supply to the skin and classification of skin flaps according to their vascularization. Ann Plast Surg 1986;16:1–19
20. Bhandari M, Adili A, Schemitsch EH. The efficacy of low-pressure lavage with different irrigating solutions to remove adherent bacteria from bone. J Bone Joint Surg Am. 2001;83-A: 412–419
21. Lee EW, Dirschl DR, Duff G, Dahners LE, Miclau T. High-pressure pulsatile lavage irrigation of fresh intraarticular fractures: effectiveness at removing particulate matter from bone. J Orthop Trauma 2002;16:162–165
22. Anglen JO. Wound irrigation in musculoskeletal injury. J Am Acad Orthop Surg 2001;9:219–226
23. Adili A, Bhandari M, Schemitsch EH. The biomechanical effect of high-pressure irrigation on diaphyseal fracture healing in vivo. J Orthop Trauma 2002;16:413–417
24. Dirschl DR, Duff GP, Dahners LE, Edin M, Rahn BA, Miclau T. High pressure pulsatile lavage irrigation of intraarticular fractures: effects on fracture healing. J Orthop Trauma 1998;12:460–463

25. Park S-H, Silva M, Bahk W-J, McKellop H, Lieberman JR. Effect of repeated irrigation and debridement on fracture healing in an animal model. J Orthop Res 2002;20:1197–1204

26. Bhandari M, Schemitsch EH, Adili A, Lachowski RJ, Shaughnessy SG. High and low pressure pulsatile lavage of contaminated tibial fractures: an in vitro study of bacterial adherence and bone damage. J Orthop Trauma 1999;13:526–533

27. Steed DL. Wound-healing trajectories. Surg Clin North Am 2003; 83:547–555

28. De Backer D, Dubois M-J. Assessment of the microcirculatory flow in patients in the intensive care unit. Curr Opin Crit Care 2001; 7:200–203

29. Heller L, Levin LS, Klitzman B. Laser Doppler flowmeter monitoring of free-tissue transfers: blood flow in normal and complicated cases. Plast Reconstr Surg 2001;107:1739–1745

30. Hupel TM, Schemitsch EH, Kowalski MJ, Swiontkowski MF. In vitro evaluation of a laser Doppler flowmetry implantable fibre system: the effect of flow velocity and concentration on perfusion assessment. Int J Surg Investig 1999;1:29–37

31. Pollak AN, McCarthy ML, Burgess AR. Short-term wound complications after application of flaps for coverage of traumatic soft-tissue defects about the tibia. J Bone Joint Surg Am 2000; 82:1681–1691

32. Weitz-Marshall AD, Bosse MJ. Timing of closure of open fractures. J Am Acad Orthop Surg 2002;10:379–384

33. van den Bogaerdt AJ, van Zuijlen PP, van Galen M, Lamme EN, Middelkoop E. The suitability of cells from different tissues for use in tissue-engineered skin substitutes. Arch Dermatol Res 2002; 294:135–142

34. Boyce ST, Warden GD. Principles and practices for treatment of cutaneous wounds with cultured skin substitutes. Am J Surg 2002; 183:445–456

35. Hodde J. Naturally occurring scaffolds for soft tissue repair and regeneration. Tissue Eng 2002;8:295–308

36. Kuroyanagi Y, Yamada N, Yamashita R, Uchinuma E. Tissue-engineered products: allogeneic cultured dermal substitute composed of spongy collagen with fibroblasts. Artif Organs 2001;25: 180–186

37. Scherer LA, Shiver S, Chang M, Meredith JW, Owings JT. The vacuum assisted closure device: a method of securing skin grafts and improving graft survival. Arch Surg 2002;137:930–934

38. Webb LX. New techniques in wound management: vacuum-assisted wound closure. J Am Acad Orthop Surg 2002;10:303–311

39. Wongworawat MD, Schnall SB, Holtom PD, Moon C, Schiller F. Negative pressure dressings as an alternative technique for the treatment of infected wounds. Clin Orthop Relat Res 2003;414:45–48

40. Morykwas MJ, Argenta LC, Shelton-Brown EI, McGuirt W. Vacuum-assisted closure: a new method for wound control and treatment: animal studies and basic foundation. Ann Plast Surg 1997;38: 553–562

41. Fabian TS, Kaufman HJ, Lett ED, et al. The evaluation of subatmospheric pressure and hyperbaric oxygen in ischemic full-thickness wound healing. Am Surg 2000;66:1136–1143

42. Genecov DG, Schneider AM, Morykwas MJ, Parker D, White WWL, Argenta LC. A controlled sub-atmospheric pressure dressing increases the rate of skin graft donor site reepithelialization. Ann Plast Surg 1998;40:219–225

43. Morykwas MJ, Faler BJ, Pearce DJ, Argenta LC. Effects of varying levels of subatmospheric pressure on the rate of granulation tissue formation in experimental wounds in swine. Ann Plast Surg 2001;47:547–551

44. Morykwas MJ, Howell H, Bleyer AJ, Molnar JA, Argenta LC. The effect of externally applied subatmospheric pressure on serum myoglobin levels after a prolonged crush/ischemia injury. J Trauma 2002;53: 537–540

45. Banwell PE, Teot L. Topical negative pressure (TNP): the evolution of a novel wound therapy. J Wound Care 2003;12:22–28

46. Morykwas MJ. External application of sub-atmospheric pressure and healing: mechanisms of action. Wound Healing Society Newsletter 1998;8:4–5

47. Harvey EJ, Grujic L, Early JS, Benirschke SK, Sangeorzan BJ. Morbidity associated with ORIF of intra-articular calcaneus fractures using a lateral approach. Foot Ankle Int 2001;22:868–873

48. Morykwas MJ, Argenta LC. Non-surgical modalities to enhance healing and care of soft tissue wounds. J South Orthop Assoc 1997;6:279–288

49. Attinger C, Cooper P. Soft tissue reconstruction for calcaneal fractures or osteomyelitis. Orthop Clin North Am 2001;32: 135–170

50. Herscovici D Jr, Sanders RW, Scaduto JM, Infante A, DiPasquale T. Vacuum-assisted wound closure (VAC therapy) for the management of patients with high-energy soft tissue injuries. J Orthop Trauma 2003;17:683–688

51. Fox MP, Fazal MA, Ware HE. Vacuum assisted wound closure a new method for control of wound problems in total knee arthroplasty. J Bone Joint Surg Br 2000;83-B:19

52. de la Torre JI, Martin SA, Oberheu AM, Vasconez LO. Healing a wound with an exposed Herrington rod: a case study. Ostomy Wound Manage 2002;48:18–19

53. Heugel JR, Parks KS, Christie SS, Pulito JR, Zegzula DH, Kamalyan NA. Treatment of the exposed Achilles' tendon using negative pressure wound therapy: a case report. J Burn Care Rehabil 2002; 23:167–171

54. Yuan-Innes MJ, Temple CL, Lacey MS. Vacuum-assisted wound closure: a new approach to spinal wounds with exposed hardware. Spine 2001;26:E30–E33

55. Burd TA, Anglen JO, Lowry KJ, Hendricks KJ, Day D. In vitro elution of tobramycin from bioabsorbable polycaprolactone beads. J Orthop Trauma 2001;15:424–428

56. Eckman JB Jr, Henry SL, Mangino PD, Seligson D. Wound and serum levels of tobramycin with the prophylactic use of tobramycin-impregnated polymethylmethacrylate beads in compound fractures. Clin Orthop Relat Res 1988;237:213–215

57. Henry SL, Ostermann PA, Seligson D. The prophylactic use of antibiotic impregnated beads in open fractures. J Trauma 1990;30: 1231–1238

58. Moehring HD, Gravel C, Chapman MW, Olson SA. Comparison of antibiotic beads and intravenous antibiotics in open fractures. Clin Orthop Relat Res 2000;372:254–261

59. Ostermann PA, Henry SL, Seligson D. The role of local antibiotic therapy in the management of compound fractures. Clin Orthop Relat Res 1993;295:102–111

60. Ostermann PA, Seligson D, Henry SL. Local antibiotic therapy for severe open fractures: a review of 1085 consecutive cases. J Bone Joint Surg Br 1995;77:93–97

61. Wichelhaus TA, Dingeldein E, Rauschmann M, et al. Elution characteristics of vancomycin, teicoplanin, gentamicin and clindamycin from calcium sulphate beads. J Antimicrob Chemother 2001;48: 117–119

62. Cross KJ, Mustoe TA. Growth factors in wound healing. Surg Clin North Am 2003;83:531–545

63. Henry G, Garner WL. Inflammatory mediators in wound healing. Surg Clin North Am 2003;83:483–507

64. Kälicke T, Schlegel U, Printzen G, Schneider E, Muhr G, Arens S. Influence of a standardized closed soft tissue trauma on resistance

to local infection: an experimental study in rats. J Orthop Res 2003;21:373–378

65. Schaser K-D, Vollmar B, Menger MD, et al. In vivo analysis of microcirculation following closed soft-tissue injury. J Orthop Res 1999; 17:678–685

66. Schwentker A, Billiar TR. Nitric oxide and wound repair. Surg Clin North Am 2003;83:521–530

67. Van de Berg JS, Robson MC. Arresting cell cycles and the effect on wound healing. Surg Clin North Am 2003;83:509–520

68. Wagner S, Coerper S, Fricke J, et al. Comparison of inflammatory and systemic sources of growth factors in acute and chronic human wounds. Wound Repair Regen 2003;11:253–260

69. Williams JZ, Barbul A. Nutrition and wound healing. Surg Clin North Am 2003;83:571–596

70. Zhang L, Bail H, Mittlmeier T, Haas NP, Schaser K-D. Immediate microcirculatory derangements in skeletal muscle and periosteum after closed tibial fracture. J Trauma 2003;54:979–985

71. Petrie NC, Yao F, Eriksson E. Gene therapy in wound healing. Surg Clin North Am 2003;83:597–616

72. Dennis RH II, McCampbell BL. Outcome of microvascular freetissue transfer in lower extremity fractures. J Natl Med Assoc 1996;88:705–708

73. Francel TJ, Vander KCA, Hoopes JE, Manson PN, Yaremchuk MJ. Microvascular soft-tissue transplantation for reconstruction of acute open tibial fractures: timing of coverage and long-term functional results. Plast Reconstr Surg 1992;89:478–487

74. Gonzalez MH, Tarandy DI, Troy D, Phillips D, Weinzweig N. Free tissue coverage of chronic traumatic wounds of the lower leg. Plast Reconstr Surg 2002;109:592–600

75. Gould JS, Shi SM. Free vascularized soft tissue flaps for coverage of the foot and ankle. Clin Orthop Relat Res 1995;314:26–36

76. Hammert WC, Minarchek J, Trzeciak MA. Free-flap reconstruction of traumatic lower extremity wounds. Am J Orthop 2000;29(Suppl 9): 22–26

77. Kolker AR, Kasabian AK, Karp NS, Gottlieb JJ. Fate of free flap microanastomosis distal to the zone of injury in lower extremity trauma. Plast Reconstr Surg 1997;99:1068–1073

78. Ninkovi M, Schoeller T, Wechselberger G, Otto A, Sperner G, Anderl H. Primary flap closure in complex limb injuries. J Reconstr Microsurg 1997;13:575–583

79. Peat BG, Liggins DF. Microvascular soft tissue reconstruction for acute tibial fractures: late complications and the role of bone grafting. Ann Plast Surg 1990;24:517–520

80. Redett RJ, Robertson BC, Chang B, Girotto J, Vaughan T. Limb salvage of lower-extremity wounds using free gracilis muscle reconstruction. Plast Reconstr Surg 2000;106:1507–1513

81. Trabulsy PP, Kerley SM, Hoffman WY. A prospective study of early soft tissue coverage of grade IIIB tibial fractures. J Trauma 1994;36: 661–668

82. Zukowski M, Lord J, Ash K, Shouse B, Getz S, Robb G. The gracilis free flap revisited: a review of 25 cases of transfer to traumatic extremity wounds. Ann Plast Surg 1998;40:141–144

83. Lamberty BG, Cormack GC. Fasciocutaneous flaps. Clin Plast Surg 1990;17:713–726

84. Robotti E, Verna G, Fraccalvieri M, Bocchiotti MA. Distally based fasciocutaneous flaps: a versatile option for coverage of difficult war wounds of the foot and ankle. Plast Reconstr Surg 1998;101: 1014–1021

85. Price MF, Capizzi PJ, Waterson PA, Lettieri S. Reverse sural artery flap: caveats for success. Ann Plast Surg 2002;48:496–504

86. Fraccalvieri M, Verna G, Dolcet M, et al. The distally based superficial sural flap: our experience in reconstructing the lower leg and foot. Ann Plast Surg 2000;45:132–139

87. Ozkan O, Coskunfirat OK, Ozgentas HE. The use of free anterolateral thigh flap for reconstructing soft tissue defects of the lower extremities. Ann Plast Surg 2004;53:455–461

88. Vrancky JJ, Misselyn D, Fabre G, Verhelle N, Heymans O, Van den hof B. The gracilis free muscle flap is more than just a "graceful" flap for lower-leg reconstruction. J Reconstr Microsurg 2004;20:143–148

89. Yildirim S, Gideroglu K, Akoz T. Anterolateral thigh flap: ideal free flap choice for lower extremity soft-tissue reconstruction. J Reconstr Microsurg 2003;19:225–233

90. Fasano D, Montanari FM, Zarabini AG, Merelli S, Mingozzi M. Considerations on 100 cases of free microsurgical flaps in the reconstruction of the soft tissues of the lower limb. Chir Organi Mov 2002;87:79–86

91. Muramatsu K, Shigetomi M, Ihara K, Kawaj S, Doi K. Vascular complication in free tissue transfer to the leg. Microsurgery 2001; 21:362–365

92. Redett RJ, Robertson B, Chang B, Girotto J, Vaughan T. Limb salvage of lower extremity wounds using free gracilis muscle reconstruction. Plast Reconstr Surg 2000:106:1507–1513.

93. Baumeister SP, Spierer R, Erdmann D, Sweis R, Levin LS, Germann GK. A Realistic Complication analysis of 70 sural artery flaps in a multimorbid patient group. Plast Reconstr Surg 2003;112: 129–140

94. Meyer C, Hartmann B, Horas U, Kilian O, Heiss C, Schnettler R. Reconstruction of the lower leg with the sural artery flap. Langenbecks Arch Surg 2002;387:320–325

95. Hollier L, Sharma S, Babigumira E, Klebuc M. Verstaility of the sural fasciicutaneous flap in the coverage of lower extremity wounds. Plast Reconstr Surg 2002;110:1673–1679

2 Musculoskeletal Infection Associated with Skeletal Trauma

Jeffrey O. Anglen and J. Tracy Watson

Infection is a dreaded complication of musculoskeletal trauma. It occurs most commonly after open fractures but can also develop after surgical treatment of closed fractures. The reported incidence ranges from 10 per 1000 (0.1%) for Gustilo type I open fractures to 25 to 50% of Gustilo type III open fractures. When it occurs, treatment becomes more difficult and prolonged, management options are restricted, and patient outcomes are compromised. If infection complicates treatment of a long bone fracture, the cost of care is increased by an average of 20.5% per patient, and the length of hospital stay is increased by an average of 36.2%. These numbers and other calculations from the late 1980s indicated an annual national cost of over $270 million from infection in the treatment of long bone fractures.[1]

Prevention of Infection

Because of the difficulty in treating musculoskeletal infection, prevention is of paramount importance. Measures should be taken to optimize the host's defensive capabilities. Nutrition should be assessed and supported. Malnutrition is common in injured or hospitalized orthopaedic patients and leads to immune compromise.[2,3] Protein malnutrition adversely affects both humoral and cell-mediated immune mechanisms. History or physical findings suggestive of malnutrition can be evaluated with laboratory tests such as serum albumin and total lymphocyte count, which should be above 3.5 mg/mL and 1500 cells/mL, respectively. In cases of obvious malnutrition or diagnostic laboratory values, nutritional support and supplementation should be instituted. Tobacco use can lead to wound healing failure with resultant infection. Medical conditions that impair immune function should be aggressively treated.

Prevention of infection in open fractures has been discussed in the previous chapter. Some of the factors contributing to the development of infection in open fractures are under at least partial control of the surgeon. Of these, the adequacy of the initial debridement and irrigation as well as antibiotic treatment is the most important. The initial debridement procedure must be thorough, careful, and systematic. Traumatic wounds should be extended longitudinally. The ends of the bone should be exposed and examined in high-energy open fractures. All foreign material as well as obviously devascularized tissue must be identified and removed, using sharp dissection. The tourniquet should be used sparingly and briefly because tissue bleeding is one of the best indicators of viability, and marginal tissue should not be subjected to additional ischemia. Exploration and debridement should be done using a systematic layer-by-layer approach. Skin that has questionable viability but is in an essential area (hands, feet, pretibial area) should be preserved if possible. Repeat debridement at 24 to 48 hour intervals is performed until a clean, viable wound is obtained. Irrigation with high volumes (8 to 10 L) of fluid is performed. Use of higher irrigation pressure increases the effectiveness of particle removal, but animal studies have suggested it could delay bone healing. The use of antibiotic additives is of no proven value in open fractures, and antiseptics such as Betadine or hydrogen peroxide should be avoided because they are potentially harmful to host defenses. Detergent irrigation additives have shown some promise in laboratory studies.[4] Between debridement procedures prior to definitive wound closure or coverage, the wound should be prevented from desiccating by the use of appropriate dressing techniques (e.g., an antibiotic bead pouch[5]) or by use of negative pressure wound therapy using the Vacuum Assisted Closure (VAC) system (Kinetic Concepts Inc., San Antonio, Texas).[6]

Systemic antibiotic treatment for open fractures is considered the standard of care, although the details of the selection of agents and duration of use are controversial. First-generation cephalosporin coverage for 2 to 3 days is adequate for low-grade open fractures, whereas higher-grade (III) open fractures may benefit from the addition of an aminoglycoside and coverage for a longer period (5 days). Specific injury settings, such as agricultural or aquatic settings, may dictate additional antibiotic coverage. Penicillin should be added for soil contamination to cover anaerobic organisms.

Stabilizing the fracture is a key component of preventing infection. For unstable fractures, this may be done with internal or external fixation. The use of internal fixation is acceptable in open fractures once the wound is adequately debrided and irrigated.[7] It is critical to avoid additional surgical trauma to the vascularity of the bone or soft tissues by use of gentle, minimally invasive techniques.

Prevention of infection in the surgical treatment of closed fractures follows the same principles as other orthopaedic operations, except that these should be considered high-risk operations due to the implantation of hardware and the immune compromise that go along with trauma. Strict adherence to "aseptic technique" has been shown historically to dramatically reduce infection rates.[2] This includes limitation of traffic through the operating room (OR), shaving the affected area at the time of surgery (not before), careful thorough preparation of the skin with antiseptic, gentle handling of tissues, and awareness of sterile technique on the part of everyone involved in the operation. Preoperative antibiotics have been shown to reduce infection rates in the surgery of closed fractures in a prospective randomized, blinded, and placebo-controlled trial.[8] Prophylactic antibiotics should be given within the 2 hours preceding incision, at least 10 minutes before tourniquet inflation.[9] There is no documented benefit to continuing antibiotics beyond 24 hours postoperatively, and one study showed successful prophylaxis with a single preoperative dose of ceftriaxone.[8] Cefazolin has been commonly chosen because of its activity against the most common pathogens (gram-positive skin flora), coverage of common gram-negative aerobes, high peak concentrations, long half-life, and a tendency to concentrate in the hematoma.[9]

One key aspect of avoiding infection in trauma surgery is appropriate timing. Many closed fractures are surrounded by significantly damaged soft tissues with impaired ability to heal incisions or perform the defensive barrier functions of normal skin. In this situation, one must wait until the soft tissues have healed before performing definitive fracture surgery. Contrary to previous opinion, there is no safe early window in which one can operate on damaged tissues. A commonly used indicator of when the skin is ready is the "wrinkle test," performed by gently pinching the skin together between two fingers. If it is soft, mobile, and forms normal wrinkles, it may be able to tolerate a surgical incision **(Fig. 2–1)**. While awaiting the resolution

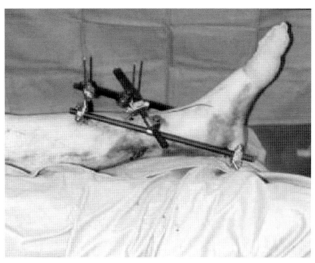

Figure 2–2 Temporary external fixation. An ankle-spanning external fixator with half pins in the femur and/or tibia and a transfixion pin in the calcaneus allows elevation of the extremity and maintenance of length and alignment. The fixator provides an approximate reduction of the major fragments through ligamentotaxis.

of blisters, ecchymosis, and swelling, temporary external fixation may be used to maintain the length and alignment of the extremity and to provide some stability for the healing of the tissues. This technique has been called "traveling traction" and can span joints without adverse effect[10] **(Fig. 2–2)**. This technique allows elevation of the extremity by suspending the frame and application of pneumatic devices such as foot pumps to aid in the resolution of swelling. Soft tissue healing may take several weeks. This staged treatment strategy for complex injuries has been shown in several studies to reduce infection rates compared with acute open reduction and internal fixation (ORIF).[11]

At the time of conversion to definitive fixation, the frame should be partially disassembled to the minimum required for maintenance of stability intraoperatively. The fixator can be prepped and draped into the operative field and used to maintain reduction during internal fixation.[12] The infection rate for intramedullary nailing after external fixation has been reported to be unacceptably high if there has been pin site infection,[13] but this complication seems to be less common if the pin sites are clean and the duration of fixation is short. Although performing the conversion to intramedullary (IM) fixation within 2 weeks is best, we have used temporary external fixation for up to 4 weeks without a problem.

Diagnosis

Established posttraumatic osteomyelitis often presents with pain, instability, chronic skin changes, and purulent drainage through fistulas **(Fig. 2–3)**. When this occurs,

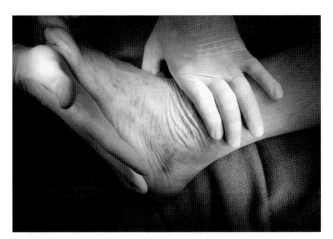

Figure 2–1 The wrinkle test for soft tissue swelling. The skin should be soft and mobile and should easily form wrinkles with gentle pinching. This calcaneus is ready for surgery.

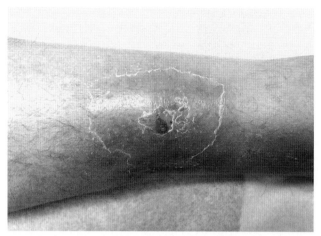

Figure 2–3 This patient presented with pain, swelling, erythema, warmth, tenderness, and skin changes 6 weeks after open tibia fracture. Note the marginal flaking of the skin around the point of drainage, which is common.

diagnosis is easy, but treatment can be much more difficult than when infection is found early. Local infection at the site of surgical intervention that manifests itself within 14 days of internal fixation is usually confined to the soft tissues only.[14] However, the classic clinical signs and symptoms of wound infection may be difficult to interpret in the setting of fracture surgery. The traditional signs of pain, fever, swelling, tenderness, warmth, and erythema may be attributed to the injury or surgical treatment. Damage to the soft tissue envelope in the proximity of the fracture is frequently underestimated during the initial evaluation and management.[15] Marginal skin necrosis or superficial wound breakdown with erythema or minimal serous drainage may not represent bacterial infection but rather a process related to the soft tissue trauma itself.

Patients who present more than 2 weeks following their surgery more commonly display the classic signs of infection. These findings occur beyond the time frame attributable to the surgery, and may be worsening rather than improving.[14,16–19] Patients may have a "low-grade" or indolent infection in which the clinical signs and symptoms are absent or subtle. One should have a high level of suspicion regarding infection throughout the course of fracture treatment, particularly when confronted with delayed or nonunion.

Diagnostic Laboratory Studies

Preliminary studies that should be obtained when one suspects an early postoperative infection usually include white blood cell count (WBC), erythrocyte sedimentation rate (ESR), and the C-reactive protein (CRP). An elevated WBC may be seen with acute infection but is often normal with chronic osteomyelitis. The ESR is a sensitive but nonspecific measure of inflammation and is elevated in 90% of

patients who present with a serious orthopaedic infection. It can be influenced by numerous factors such as age, fluid balance, nutritional status, smoking status, and hormonal changes. After major surgical interventions or extensive trauma, the ESR often increases to high levels but should return to normal within 6 months. As a result of high sensitivity, the ESR is utilized as a screening tool. Because of the lack of specificity, care must be taken in the interpretation of a persistently elevated or even rising sedimentation rate as an isolated clinical finding. The sedimentation rate in combination with the patient's age and immune status has predicted the success of antibiotic treatment; however, the sedimentation rate's response alone is not a clear predictor of success.

CRP is an "acute phase reactant," a substance that rises in concentration in the bloodstream as a response to inflammation or tissue damage. The concentration of CRP increases several hundredfold within 6 hours after a triggering infectious inflammatory stimulus. There is a constant clearance rate of CRP from the bloodstream with a half-life of approximately 24 to 28 hours. A return of CRP levels to baseline indicates effectiveness of treatment. However, if high levels of CRP persist or a second spike is noted, this may be a warning sign of a new process or exacerbation of the previous inflammatory or infectious process.[20] A transient rise in CRP is demonstrated following uncomplicated fracture surgery, which peaks at about 2 days and should decline rapidly over the next few days. Baseline levels are achieved by 3 weeks after uncomplicated surgery. Infected fractures will demonstrate a rapid rise and will not normalize unless specific therapy is undertaken. Normalization of CRP is rapid after control of the infection, and declining levels can be seen within 8 hours of instituting effective treatment. Measurement of both ESR and CRP is helpful in differentiating septic and mechanical loosening with failing hardware, detecting complications, and monitoring the effects of treatment. CRP is more sensitive than ESR for these purposes.[21]

Imaging

Radiographic Imaging

Conventional radiographs remain the initial imaging modality in the diagnosis of subacute or chronic infection. Patients seen with a deep infection may present with classic x-ray findings, such as periosteal elevation, endosteal scalloping, areas of hardware failure or loosening, radiolucencies around implants, and endosteal and periosteal scalloping (**Fig. 2–4A,B**). These radiographic changes occur later in the course of the infectious process and require actual bone destruction or reactive changes. Posttraumatic changes and hardware may obscure findings on radiographs and make interpretation difficult, yielding a low sensitivity (< 20%).

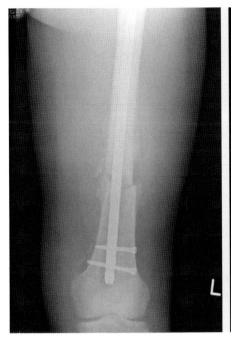 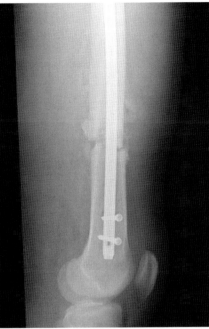

A,B

Figure 2–4 Plain radiographic signs of infection. Four weeks following intramedullary (IM) nailing of an open femur fracture, this patient presented with pain, swelling of the thigh, fever, and erythrocyte sedimentation rate > 70. **(A)** Anteroposterior view. **(B)** Lateral view demonstrating hallmarks of acute infection: endosteal scalloping, circumferential lucencies surrounding the nail and locking screws, periosteal elevation, and reactive bone formation.

Computed Tomographic Scanning

Computed tomographic (CT) scanning can be a useful method to detect osseous destruction and the presence of a sequestrum, foreign body, or gas formation. However, it is generally less sensitive than other modalities in the detection of early bone formation or erosion. CT is valuable in the determination of osseous continuity. CT scanning will give valuable information regarding the three-dimensional architecture of regions of bone loss or defects. This information is crucial to plan the reconstructive procedures necessary following the eradication of an infection.[22,23]

Nuclear Medicine

Bone scintigraphy is much more sensitive than conventional radiographs. A variety of radiopharmaceuticals are available for use in scintigraphy. Traditional bone scanning uses technetium polyphosphate (^{99m}Tc), which accumulates in areas of reactive new bone formation and increased bone blood flow. However, it does not specifically diagnose the increased uptake as osteomyelitis.[22] The specificity of this test for infection following trauma may be below 20%.[24] To overcome this limitation, ^{99m}Tc scans are often combined with other types of scanning, such as gallium 67 or indium-labeled leukocyte scans.

The use of indium-111–labeled leukocytes for scanning increases the specificity for infection. This technique involves removal of blood by venipuncture, in vitro radiolabeling of the leukocytes, reinjection into the patient, and delayed (16 to 24 h) scanning. Indium scans are much less sensitive in the detection of *chronic* infections and are not indicated for this purpose. Similar information can be obtained more rapidly, with better images, accuracy, and specificity and without the need for handling patient blood by use of immunoscintigraphy, using radiolabeled monoclonal antibodies that bind leukocytes in vivo.[25]

The combination of ^{99m}Tc and ^{111}In-labeled leukocytes may increase the sensitivity and specificity to over 80% for diagnosis of infection in united fractures. Labeled leukocyte localization returns to a normal pattern faster than magnetic resonance imaging (MRI) after bone trauma, surgical procedures, and treatment of osteomyelitis; thus the incidence of false-positive exams is significantly less.[26]

Magnetic Resonance Imaging

MRI provides more accurate information on the local extent of the soft tissue involvement in patients with musculoskeletal infection. The superior anatomical resolution compared with nuclear imaging helps differentiate bone and soft tissue infection and the extent of each. MRI has become critical in the delineation of many types of musculoskeletal infection, in particular the evaluation of soft tissue infections, including cellulitis, myositis, fasciitis, abscesses, and septic arthritis. In several comparative studies MRI has been superior to scintigraphy, CT scan, and conventional radiography in detecting the presence and determining the extent of osteomyelitis. MRI visualization of the bone marrow allows for highly sensitive detection of early osteomyelitis, although specificity for the diagnosis is aided by other findings, including cortical destruction, which may be best seen with CT scanning. The overall sensitivity of MRI for bone infection approaches 100%, whereas specificity is 60 to 75%.[24,27] Use of gadolinium enhancement with MRI improves the ability to distinguish abscess from cellulitis or myositis. MRI may facilitate differentiation of acute from chronic osteomyelitis and may help to detect reactivation of old infection in the presence of chronic inflammation or other posttraumatic lesions.[28]

Retrospective review of MRI studies has revealed that overall specificity regarding the diagnosis of bone involvement can be improved to over 80% without significant loss of sensitivity if increased marrow signal intensity on T2-weighted images is included as an additional criterion in the diagnosis of bone infection. As now practiced, evidence of osteomyelitis on MRI consists of abnormalities of the bone marrow with decreased signal intensity on the T1-weighted images and increased image sensitivity and enhancement as seen with the T2-weighted or short T1 inversion recovery (STIR) images[22] **(Fig. 2–5A,B).** Acute activity in a chronic osteomyelitis can be excluded with a high probability if the MRI findings are negative.[29]

Many prospective studies have compared MRI versus three-phase bone scanning versus indium-labeled WBC scanning (^{111}In-WBC scanning) to diagnosis *acute* infection. Patients were evaluated at presentation with all three modalities; sensitivity of each modality was calculated using additional biopsy as the gold standard. The sensitivity for MRI is consistently 90% or greater, compared with 70% for bone scan and 45% for indium scan. MRI should be used to evaluate patients with positive bone scintigraphy to improve the specificity and accuracy of diagnosis for osteomyelitis.[30] It permits the differentiation of septic arthritis or cellulitis from osteomyelitis.

Positron Emission Tomography

Positron emission tomographic (PET) scanning with the use of fluorine 18–labeled fluorodeoxyglucose (FDG-PET) is becoming more frequently used in the diagnosis of infection. It has high sensitivity and specificity but is not widely available.

Cultures

Specific bacteriological diagnosis requires positive culture of pathogens from biopsy material. Swabs of drainage from cutaneous fistulas or open wounds are not adequate, nor are specimens obtained by needle biopsy.[31] Multiple specimens from different sites and tissues should be obtained in surgery and sent for aerobic and anaerobic culture. Selected patients, such as those with compromised immune status, should have specimens analyzed for fungi or mycobacterium. It is useful to obtain a stat Gram stain of the culture material, both for the early institution of therapy and to ensure prompt processing of the specimen, which will result in better recovery of organisms.

Staging and Classification

Cierny et al developed a useful classification for the staging of chronic osteomyelitis according to the anatomy of the involved bone and physiological status of the host.[32] They identified four anatomical types:

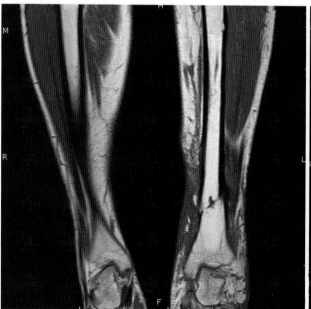
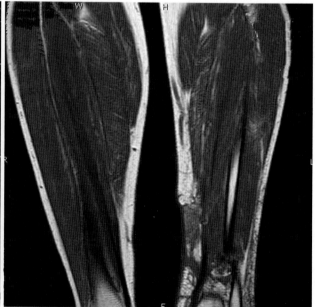

Figure 2–5 Magnetic resonance imaging findings in skeletal infection. This patient had an open tibia fracture treated with irrigation, debridement, delayed primary closure, and casting. When the cast was removed at initial follow-up, the limb was noted to be swollen and tender. **(A)** T1-weighted images reveal decreased signal intensity at the midportion of the fracture site. **(B)** T2 images show increased image signal and marrow enhancement at the region just below the fracture site, with edema indicated in the soft tissues.

- *Type 1* is a medullary osteomyelitis and is primarily an endosteal process. It denotes infection confined to the intramedullary surface of the bone.
- *Type 2* is a superficial infection, which involves only the outer portion of the cortex. This occurs when a contiguous focus of infection exposes bone.
- *Type 3* is a localized osteomyelitis involving cortical sequestration, with cavitation extending into the medullary cavity, and combines features of types 1 and 2.
- *Type 4* is a diffuse osteomyelitis with a permeating, circumferential, and through-and-through lesion with extensive involvement of the medullary cavity and often involves an entire segment of bone. All infected fractures and nonunions are considered type 4 osteomyelitis.

Physiologically, patients are classified as types A, B, or C hosts. Type A hosts have a competent immune system, with normal physiology and metabolism and good vascular supply to the affected area. A type B host is compromised either locally or systemically or both. Examples of a type B host would include those patients taking corticosteroids and patients with peripheral vascular disease. A type C host is one that would not benefit from treatment.

The clinical stage of osteomyelitis is determined by considering the anatomical type and the physiological host status. Most patients with posttraumatic osteomyelitis are classified as having Cierny stages 3 and 4 disease. A chronic wound infection can lead to stage 2 osteomyelitis. Patients with infected medullary rods or nails and an intact, healed, stable tibia have stage 1 osteomyelitis.

A variety of other characteristics can be used to classify musculoskeletal infection following trauma, for the purposes of making treatment decisions or prognostic estimations. Fracture healing versus nonunion can be very important with regard to treatment options. If the patient has undergone internal fixation, the hardware construct may be stable or unstable. The temporal relationship from surgical intervention to the development of symptoms helps to define the etiology and severity of the infection. The infection can be described as acute (within the first 2 to 3 weeks), subacute, or chronic. Local infection at the site of surgical intervention that manifests itself within 14 days of internal fixation is usually confined to the soft tissues only.[14,18]

Treatment

Pin or Wire Site Infection

The most common complication associated with the use of external fixation is pin tract infection. The etiology of pin tract infection is multifactorial and includes soft tissue impingement or tethering, poor insertion technique, inadequate site care, and loosening of fixation. Multiple studies have documented the relationship between pin loosening and pin sepsis. Stabilizing the pin–bone interface can reduce the prevalence of pin-related complications. Pins in cancellous bone frequently loosen over time, whereas fixation pins in cortical bone can remain intact and infection free for extended periods of time. Each pin in a fixation construct should be continually evaluated for these potential problems to avoid an unstable fixator.[33,34]

Radiographic evidence of pin loosening includes cortical rarefaction and lucency, which typically occur initially at the near cortex (**Fig. 2–6A,B**). The occurrence of pin tract lucency is reduced by hydroxyapatite coating or by use of titanium pins, which have demonstrated a marked improvement in their holding power (torque on removal) when compared with stainless steel pins.[34] Histological examinations of multiple retrieved pin specimens reveal that tight pin tracts are characterized by a lack of bone remodeling, whereas loose pin tracts are characterized by extensive bone resorption and inflammatory infiltrates. However, it should be noted that pin tract infection can occur without mechanical pin loosening.

Pin insertion technique is important to improve the initial pin torque resistance and minimize loosening. Correct technique begins with a generous skin incision directly at the site of pin insertion. This is followed by gentle blunt dissection to the periosteum, which is incised as well. A small Penfield-type elevator is used to gently reflect the periosteum off the bone at the site of insertion. With this technique, extraneous soft tissue tethering and necrosis are avoided. A trocar/drill sleeve assembly is advanced directly to the bone. A pilot hole is predrilled, and the pin is inserted by hand to the correct depth. Any soft tissue tethering should be released with a small scalpel following pin insertion.

The use of self-drilling, self-tapping pins results in less purchase in the bone compared with the purchase achieved with the predrilled pin technique. Frequently, there is a tendency to increase the depth of insertion when using self-drilling pins to achieve comparable pin purchase. This can lead to more soft tissue invagination into the pin tract.[33] Excessive heat generation during insertion can lead to bone necrosis ("ring sequestrum") and early loosening. Temperatures in excess of 55°C can occur during the insertion of self-drilling pins. Self-drilling pins have shown increased microfracture of both cortices with increased bone absorption, decreased pullout strengths, and insertion torque.[35,36]

Pin and wire site complications are now graded by the classification as described by Dahl et al.[37] A Grade 0 pin site appears normal and requires only weekly pin care. Grade 1 infections show marginal inflammation; however,

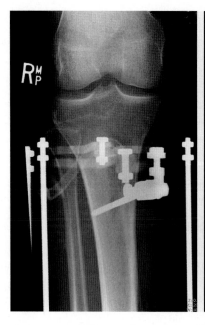
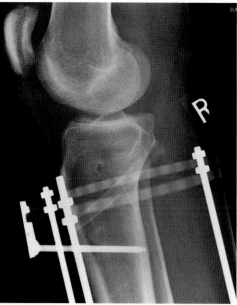

A,B

Figure 2–6 Radiographic signs of pin tract infection. **(A)** Schanz pin tract with lucency around the near cortex, indicating some degree of potential pin loosening. The far cortex is intact, and therefore this pin should be monitored closely for signs of infection. **(B)** Lateral view of the same Schanz pin. A previously removed proximal pin tract remains, with evidence of chronic sequestrum in the depths of the pin tract. Note the radiodensity within the lucency. At the time of Schanz pin removal, the proximal pin tract should also be vigorously curetted to remove the offending sequestrum.

no drainage is apparent, and treatment requires more frequent pin care consisting of daily cleansing with mild soap or half-strength peroxide and saline solution **(Fig. 2–7)**. Grade 2 pin tract infections consist of an inflamed pin site with serous discharge. Grade 3 pin tract infection consists of an inflamed pin site with purulent discharge. Both grade 2 and grade 3 pin tract infections require oral antibiotics and continuing daily pin care. Grade 4 pin tract infection consists of serous or seropurulent drainage in concert with erythema, inflammation, and radiographs demonstrating osteolysis at both the near and far cortices. Once osteolysis is visible, demonstrating bicortical involvement, removal of the offending pin should be performed immediately, with reinsertion at another site if the pin is required for frame stability. Local soft tissue debridement of the pin tract with peroxide or other astringent irrigant may be performed. Formal surgical management is unnecessary as long as there are no obvious radiodensities noted on the plain x-rays at the site of osteolysis. Grade 5 pin tract infection consists of inflammation, purulent drainage, and osteolysis, as well as sequestrum noted or a Brodie's abscess within the medullary canal. At this point deep-seated infection is present and requires formal irrigation and debridement procedures in concert with culture-specific antibiotics. Pin exchange should be performed in conjunction with the pin removal process **(Fig. 2–6A,B)**.[38,39]

There is no universal standard for pin care. Pin site care recommendations are based more often on local preference and individual experience than on strict research findings. If appropriate insertion technique is utilized, the pin sites will heal completely around each individual pin. Once healed, showering without any other

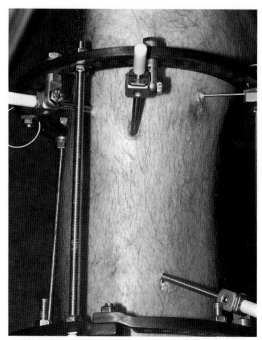

Figure 2–7 Multiple pin sites with minimal redness and slight drainage. Pin sites have completely healed with a stable pin–skin interface. These are examples of grade 1 and 2 pin sites. Continued cleaning routine is the only treatment recommended because of the lack of inflammation and purulent drainage. No antibiotics are necessary.

pin cleaning procedures is all that is necessary, with the exception of the occasional removal of crust using dilute hydrogen peroxide and saline.[40] One should avoid ointments for postcleansing care because these tend to inhibit the normal skin flora and alter the normal skin bacteria and thus can lead to a superinfection or pin site colonization. It is important to remove the buildup of crusting material, which will tend to stiffen the pin–skin interface and increase shear forces at the pin–bone interface, leading to the development of additional necrotic tissues and fluid buildup around the pin. Immediate postoperative compressive dressings should be applied to the pin sites to stabilize the pin–skin interface. These compressive dressings can be removed within 10 days to 2 weeks. If pin drainage does develop (a grade 1, 2, or 3 pin tract infection), pin care three times per day should be initiated. This may also involve rewrapping and compressing the offending pin site in an effort to minimize the abnormal pin–skin motion.

Acute or Subacute Infection with Stable Hardware

The knee-jerk recommendation of nonsurgical consultants is often to remove all hardware, obtain deep cultures, and administer antibiotics. This is partially correct. Cultures are helpful, antibiotics are essential, but removal of stable, functioning hardware in the setting of the acutely infected fracture should be resisted resolutely. Although it is well known that the presence of inanimate material surfaces increases the risk of infection, lowers the inoculum necessary to cause infection, and reduces the chances of successful treatment, longstanding clinical experience teaches that skeletal stability reduces the infection rate.[7,41] This reduction is supported by the results of animal studies.[42,43] The mechanism by which instability promotes infection is not clear but may have to do with interference with revascularization of injured tissues, ongoing tissue damage, or increased micro–dead space. Although instability seems to interfere with the resolution of infection, the presence of infection does not necessarily prohibit bone healing. A logical strategy is to maintain stable internal fixation, which will facilitate union, and plan for hardware removal later if infection persists after the bone is healed **(Fig. 2–8A–F)**.

If a collection of pus exists around an implant or under a flap or incision, it must be thoroughly drained. Incisions made for irrigation and debridement of infection should rarely be closed and should be placed carefully to avoid exposing hardware, bone, tendon, or neurovascular structures. If these are unavoidably exposed, consideration should be given to flap coverage of the wound. The VAC (Kinetic Concepts Inc.) dressing can be used while awaiting definitive coverage **(Fig. 2–9)**.

Antibiotics

Empirical antibiotic coverage is begun after obtaining samples for culture, utilizing a broad-spectrum drug such as cefazolin. Culture results should be used to guide definitive antibiotic therapy. *Staphylococcus aureus* is the most common pathogen,[44] although *Staphylococcus epidermidis* and gram-negative organisms are increasing in frequency. Antibiotic resistance to penicillin is common, and resistance to the antipenicillinase penicillins (methicillin, oxacillin) is increasing. Vancomycin resistance has been reported in *Staphylococcus* but is rare to this point. To preserve the efficacy of vancomycin, it should only be used in documented cases of methicillin resistance, and combination drug regimens should be considered to increase efficacy. Rifampin is a commonly used supplementary drug that can be given orally, but when used alone can lead to rapid development of resistance.[44,45] Quinolone antibiotics have become popular for oral treatment of osteomyelitis due to gram-negative enteric organisms in adult patients,[44] but failure is more common in cases caused by *Pseudomonas aeruginosa* or *S. aureus*. For *S. aureus* associated with orthopaedic implants, combination with oral rifampin is promising.[46] It is important to be aware that there is experimental evidence from a rat model that fluoroquinolones, specifically ciprofloxacin, inhibit bone healing.[47] In cases of unusual, multiple, or resistant organisms, infectious disease consultation may be useful.

The traditional duration of antibiotic treatment for musculoskeletal infection is 4 to 6 weeks. Intravenous antibiotics can be administered as an outpatient or at home via a peripherally inserted central catheter (PICC) line. Recently, a shorter-term course (< 2 weeks) of IV antibiotics followed by oral administration for 4 to 6 weeks has been proposed as an equally efficacious regimen in adult osteomyelitis.[48]

The treatment of infection following stable osteosynthesis using irrigation/drainage and antibiotics can be successful in a high percentage of patients. One study of 20 osteomyelitis patients treated with IV teicoplanin with and without oral ciprofloxacin or rifampin, followed by oral antibiotic therapy for an average of 28 weeks (range: 12 to 64), was successful in 100%.[49] In another study of treatment of infected orthopaedic implants (joint replacements as well as fracture fixations), only oral antibiotics consisting of rifampin and ofloxacin were used. A successful outcome was achieved in 74% of the 47 patients.[46]

Acute or Subacute Postoperative Infection with Unstable Hardware

Debridement

The presence of excessive motion, the displacement of hardware position on radiographs, or the visualization of radiolucencies around screws, rods, or fixator pins denotes

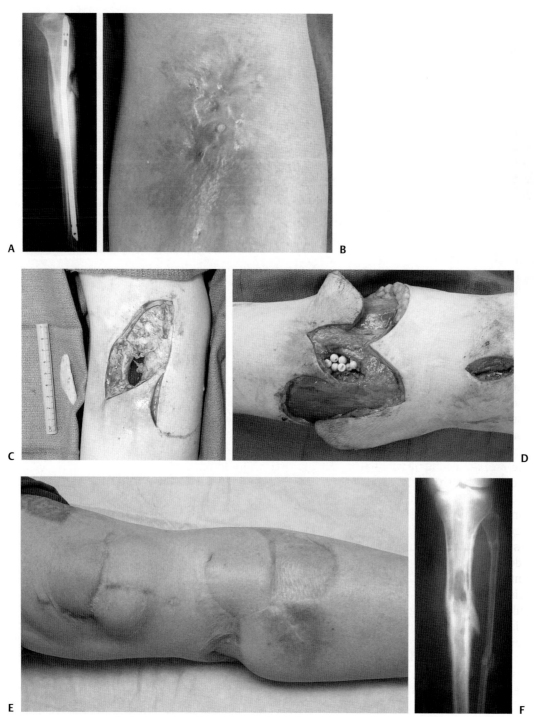

Figure 2–8 Treatment of infection with stable internal fixation. This patient had an open tibia fracture treated with irrigation, debridement, and reamed IM nailing. By 8 weeks postoperatively, swelling, erythema, and drainage occurred through the open wound. Irrigation, debridement, and biopsy for culture were performed, followed by wound care and antibiotics. **(A)** The nail providing stability was maintained until the fracture was healed. **(B)** Appearance of the anterior tibial wound after fracture healing, with continued intermittent wound drainage. The patient was taken to the operating room for excision of scarred soft tissues, nail removal, intramedullary debridement, and implantation of absorbable antibiotic beads. **(C)** Appearance after debridement and sequestrectomy. **(D)** Bead implantation followed by fasciocutaneous rotation flaps performed for coverage. **(E,F)** Clinical picture and anteroposterior radiograph after healing with no recurrence of infection at 1 year.

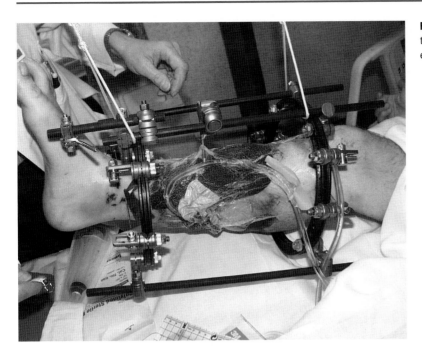

Figure 2–9 VAC dressing applied to an open tibial fracture wound after debridement and stabilization with an external fixator.

an unstable situation. This instability compromises the ability to overcome infection and to heal the fracture. Bacteria that are attached to surfaces such as metallic fixation devices or dead bone become resistant to the action of antibiotics through the production of a biofilm that forms a protective covering. In the face of unstable hardware or fracture malalignment, the hardware should be removed **(Fig. 2–10A-G)**.

Devascularized fragments of bone, missed at the original debridement or created during internal fixation, may be present in the fracture site. In most instances, this dead fragment cannot be extruded, and antibiotics will not penetrate it **(Fig. 2–8C)**. The infection will never be eradicated unless the fragment is excised.[32,38,50]

Thin, scarred skin should be removed along with sinus tracts and avascular soft tissues. The dense fibrous sheath around infected hardware should be completely excised, with care taken not to strip periosteum from living bone with elevators or retractors **(Fig. 2–8B,C)**. During debridement the bone should be constantly visualized for evidence of punctate bleeding, which indicates adequate vascular inflow. This "paprika sign" is characteristic of living bone and is useful for establishing the limits of debridement.[50] The use of a high-speed bur with the tourniquet down to remove cortical bone gently allows the surgeon to watch for this sign. The bur should be kept cool with irrigation.

Infection restricted to the medullary canal is debrided adequately by reaming. After removal of infected intramedullary nails, avascular material in the nail tract can be debrided by passing a flexible intramedullary reamer 1 to 2 mm larger in diameter than the nail down the tract. If this technique is used, the surgeon should avoid devital-

izing cortical bone by stripping the periosteum and then reaming the endosteal vessels. This is commonly done when an unstable plate construct is converted to a nailing. There is substantial risk of creating a long sequestrum. Staging the procedures with a 6 week interval will reduce the risk.[50,51] To decrease the potential thermal effects of reaming, the tourniquet should not be inflated, progress should be slow, and irrigation should be used. A distal tibial medullary portal, or "blowhole," is useful to provide lavage throughout the canal to create a constant outflow.[51,52] The ability to achieve a culture-negative wound may require at least two sequential debridements.[32,53]

Defect Management

Removal of bone and hardware creates "dead" space, which will need to be filled with living tissue. Elimination of dead space and provision of durable soft tissue coverage are both essential for the control of infection. In acute or subacute wound infections, closure is desirable; however, the wounds must frequently be left open. Coverage with free or rotational tissue transfer will be necessary. Bone defects may be temporarily treated with local antibiotic delivery using antibiotic-impregnated beads. Local antibiotic delivery systems are discussed in detail below.

External Fixation

After hardware removal, the bone is most commonly stabilized with external fixation. Once stability is achieved, the inflammatory phase of fracture healing and infection becomes markedly reduced, decreasing the complexity of the problem. The type of external fixator depends on

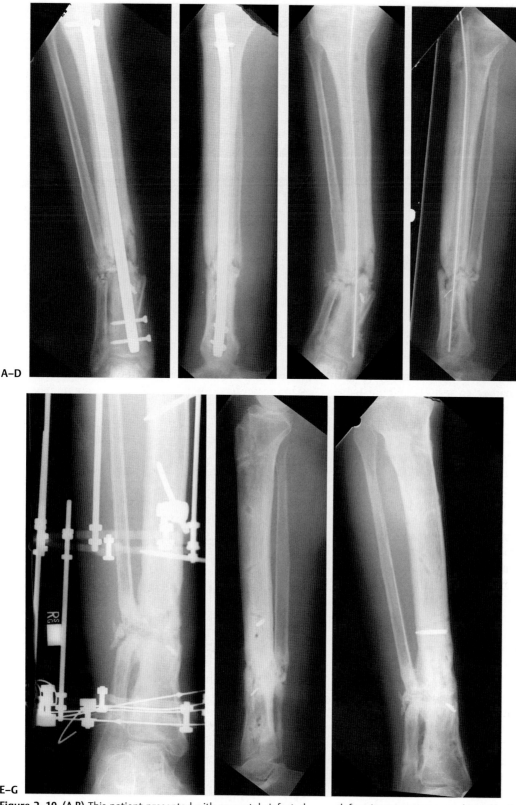

A–D

E–G

Figure 2–10 (A,B) This patient presented with an acutely infected tibial nail following an open tibial shaft fracture. Circumferential radiolucencies are present around the rod and locking screws. Malalignment is also present. **(C,D)** Following rod removal and medullary debridement, dead space management was provided for with an antibiotic-impregnated polymethyl methacrylate IM nail. **(E,F)** After 6 weeks of appropriate antibiotics, the rod was removed, and gradual deformity correction was achieved by the use of a circular ring fixator. Multiple deformities were corrected, including angulation, length, and rotation. **(G)** Closed distraction was able to achieve distraction regenerate bone, and an additional bone graft was unnecessary. After 15 weeks total treatment time, closed distraction had achieved a healed, infection-free tibial shaft.

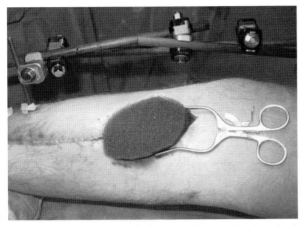

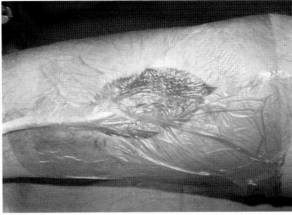

Figure 2–11 A patient with a tibial plateau fracture developed sub-acute infection at 5 weeks postop open reduction and internal fixation with compartment syndrome. A knee-spanning fixator provided temporary stabilization during multiple debridements, hardware removal, and antibiotic beads placement. Following eradication of infection and recovery of soft tissues (rotational flap required), formal plating and bone grafting achieved a stable plateau. **(A)** After debridement in the spanning external fixator (pins in the femur and tibia), a VAC sponge is used because the wound could not be closed. **(B)** After application of suction to the VAC.

wound location and fracture complexity. Less stable fractures require more complex frames to control motion at the bone ends. Weight bearing should be allowed if possible because intermittent loading prevents additional bone loss from disuse atrophy. In the presence of periarticular infection, spanning external fixation provides satisfactory stability for the hard and soft tissues. This would allow for debridement and subsequent soft tissue reconstruction because the pins are placed on either side of the joint out of the zone of soft tissue reconstruction **(Fig. 2–11A,B).**

Applying an Ilizarov circular fixator (Smith & Nephew, Memphis, Tennessee) is advantageous for extra-articular locations because it allows weight bearing and correction of deformity or malalignment **(Fig. 2–12).** Additionally, it can achieve compression or distraction at potential nonunion sites. The Ilizarov technique allows reconstruction of segmental skeletal defects and difficult infected fractures.[37,54-56]

Chronic Osteomyelitis

Debridement

Chronic infection after injury is largely a surgical disease and is rarely successfully treated by antibiotics alone. If infection persists after fracture union, hardware must be removed and avascular bone and soft tissue debrided. In general, previous incisions should be used, and all necrotic soft tissue should be removed. In the case of structures important to function and with questionable viability (tendons and ligaments), a staged approach can be taken. Care should be taken not to strip viable periosteum from bone. Sclerotic or sequestered bone should be removed until all the remaining bone appears healthy and bleeds well. A high-speed bur, as described earlier, is a gentle way to accomplish bone removal.

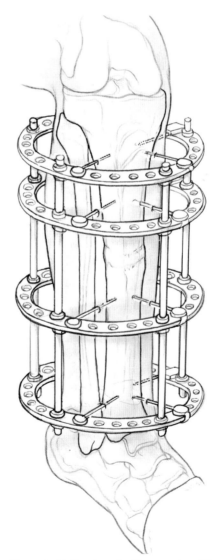

Figure 2–12 Drawing of an Ilizarov external fixator used for deformity correction and distraction osteogenesis. The fixator can use tensioned small wires (as shown) or combine the small wires with half pins.

Local Antibiotic Delivery (see Video 2–1, Disk 1)

To prepare defects for grafting or coverage following debridement, antibiotic-impregnated polymethyl methacrylate (PMMA) beads, rods, or blocks are often placed to deliver a high concentration of antibiotics locally while avoiding systemic toxicity. Antibiotic elutes from the PMMA by diffusion from the surface. Although most of the drug comes out in the first 24 hours, therapeutic levels of drugs have been detected in some cases for as long as 90 days. Tissue concentrations may be higher and persist longer than those seen in elution experiments. Local gentamicin concentrations around beads may be up to 200 times achievable tissue levels with systemic administration of the drug.[57] Serum and urine concentrations are at least 5 to 10 times less than tissue concentrations and are undetectable in many studies.

Animal studies have suggested that treatment with antibiotic-impregnated PMMA beads for osteomyelitis is as good as or better than systemic antibiotic treatment.[58,59] The use of beads combined with systemic antibiotics significantly improved eradication of infection from rabbit wounds containing contaminated necrotic bone when compared with systemic antibiotics alone.[60] Necrotic bone gets no exposure to systemic antibiotics, whereas locally delivered antibiotics can achieve high concentrations.

In clinical studies of antibiotic bead treatment for chronic osteomyelitis, results have generally shown improved efficacy when the beads are used in conjunction with systemic antibiotics. Although many surgeons believe that antibiotic beads used to treat osteomyelitis should be removed, one retrospective study suggested that improved outcomes followed leaving the beads in situ.[61]

Many antibiotics have been used in beads. The antibiotic chosen must be water soluble, wide spectrum, well tolerated, heat stable, bactericidal in low concentrations, and available in powder form. Antibiotics can be mixed together. A common example in clinical use is tobramycin plus vancomycin. Palacos Bone Cement (Biomet Orthopedic Inc., Warsaw, Indiana) is reported to elute antibiotics better than other cement types. We commonly use 2.4 g (two vials) of tobramycin powder added to a 40 g pouch of PMMA. More antibiotic can be added, but the volumetric ratio of 24 mL antibiotic to 120 mL Palacos cement is the limit for successful hardening. The mixture is made into beads in a commercially available mold or rolled by hand and strung on wire or suture **(Fig. 2–13)**. Beads can be stored in sterile containers at room temperature for long periods of time. When using antibiotic bead treatment, the wound should be closed, covered with a tissue flap, or covered with a semipermeable membrane (the antibiotic bead pouch technique) **(Fig. 2–14)**.

After removal of an intramedullary rod, placement of antibiotic beads offers no mechanical support. Beads within the intramedullary canal must be removed within 10 to 14 days or subsequent removal may be extremely difficult.[17,50,52] Antibiotic cement rods can be custom-made at the time of surgery using varying chest tubes as molds.[56] Chest

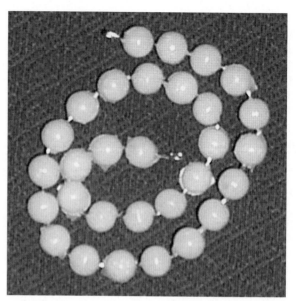

Figure 2–13 Mold-made polymethyl methacrylate antibiotic beads on a wire.

tubes are selected based on their inner diameter using the extracted nail as a template for the length and diameter of the fabricated rod. A 3 mm guidewire is prebent and placed down the center of the chest tube mold to provide overall contour and dimensions of the fabricated rod. The liquid cement/antibiotic mixture is then poured into a cement gun and injected down the chest tube to surround the metal guide rod. Once the cement begins to cure, the chest tube is incised longitudinally and peeled off the intact cement rod. Following thorough medullary canal debridement, the antibiotic rod is inserted and does provide some mechanical

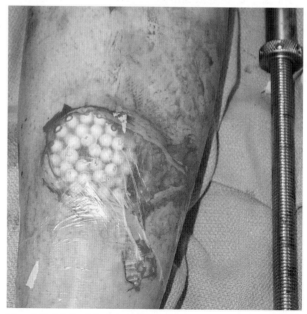

Figure 2–14 Antibiotic bead pouch covering an open tibia fracture wound after initial debridement.

stability **(Fig. 2–10A–G)**. If additional debridements are necessary, the antibiotic rod is exchanged. At the time of definitive closure, the antibiotic rod is left intact in the canal, and the wound is closed directly over it. After a 6 to 8 week interval, bony reconstruction can be undertaken.

A variety of bioabsorbable carrier materials have been investigated to deliver antibiotics locally with an improved drug release and without a requirement for removal. These materials include demineralized bone matrix, bone graft,[62] lyophilized human fibrin, polyglycolic acid (PGA),[63] and polycaprolactone.[64] The material that has achieved the most clinical utility is calcium sulfate beads. The substance is osteoconductive and can also function as a bone graft substitute. Because the body absorbs it, calcium sulfate beads should release the entire load of antibiotic, whereas PMMA will only release ~20% of the impregnated drug. In a study of 25 patients with posttraumatic infected long bone defects, treatment with antibiotic-impregnated calcium sulfate beads eradicated the infection in 23 (92%) and healed 14 of 16 nonunions (nine required bone graft).[65] It has been noted that some patients have a sterile drainage that resolves when the pellets are absorbed.

Soft Tissue Coverage

Coverage of soft tissue defects improves blood flow and provides an intact protective barrier. Coverage may be accomplished with primary closure but frequently requires some type of flap. Local rotation flaps or distant free flaps may be utilized. Muscle flaps are highly vascular and improve the local resistance to infection by increasing the blood flow to the area, thus delivering cellular and humoral immune elements as well as systemic antibiotics.[66,67] The coverage method and timing should be planned before the first operation. These techniques are discussed in more detail in Chapter 1. Flap coverage may be performed over antibiotic bead spacers with delayed bone grafting,[52] or the procedures may be performed concurrently.[68] A free flap will not be mature enough to tolerate flap reelevation for approximately 6 to 8 weeks following surgery. When adequate debridement is combined with immediate muscle flap coverage, the course of intravenous antibiotic coverage can be shortened to 2 weeks, with a success as high as 90% in one series of 27 patients with lower extremity osteomyelitis.[69] Free tissue transfer is a technically demanding procedure and has a high rate of complications and donor site morbidity and a risk of flap failure. Patients with segmental defects and instability have a higher rate of recurrent sepsis despite successful coverage, indicating the importance of skeletal stability to the control of infection.[67]

Achieving Union: Reconstruction of Bone Defects after Debridement

Occasionally, the tissue remaining after adequate debridement has osteogenic potential, but union is prevented by excessive motion. Intervening fibrocartilaginous tissue has osteogenic potential, which can be exploited once torsional and axial instabilities are eliminated. The pluripotential cells that are present at the fracture site will selectively divide into the osteogenic precursor lineage in an environment of coupled stability and vascularity.[54] In this case, healing may be achieved by revision surgery with a variety of internal fixation devices. The stability afforded by nailing along with suppressive antibiotic therapy has been shown to produce excellent results. Select plating techniques often work well in metaphyseal infections once the soft tissues have been reconstructed and the wounds are under control **(Fig. 2–15A–C)**.

Frequently, debridement will result in extensive gaps in the bone, which are beyond the healing capacity of the patient. If debridement includes significant portions of an articular surface, the reconstructive options are limited. Occasionally, resection of an infected joint can be treated with antibiotic-impregnated cement spacer, systemic antibiotics, and eventually prosthetic total joint arthroplasty. Often, however, it will require arthrodesis, resectional arthroplasty, or amputation, particularly in compromised hosts or those infected with multiple or resistant organisms. When the resected bone involves mostly diaphysis or metaphysis, there are multiple reconstructive options to restore skeletal integrity. These include shortening, autogenous or allogeneic bone grafting, or distraction osteogenesis.

Autogenous bone graft heals quickest and most reliably but is limited in quantity and involves donor site morbidity. Allograft bone can be cancellous or cortical, or processed into components of bone such as demineralized bone matrix. Distraction osteogenesis is a technique for generating new bone by applying tension to healing mesenchymal tissues using external fixation techniques. In certain situations, other approaches such as primary shortening may be appropriate.

Bone grafts have three potential functions: osteogenesis, osteoconduction, and structural support. Osteogenesis can occur in two ways. Surface osteoblasts can survive the transplantation by receiving nutrition through diffusion, and then proliferate to form more living bone tissue. There is more surface area in cancellous graft, and thus it has more potential for surviving cells than cortical graft. The other method of osteogenesis is by osteoinduction, which is the process of recruitment and stimulation of osteoprogenitor mesenchymal cells from the host tissue. This process is stimulated by graft-derived growth factors such as bone morphogenetic proteins, transforming growth factor β, insulin-like growth factors 1 and 2, platelet-derived growth factor, and others.

The second function of a bone graft is osteoconduction, or serving as a scaffold for the growth of host bone. This three-dimensional process involves vascular proliferation and ingrowth of capillaries along the open spaces in the

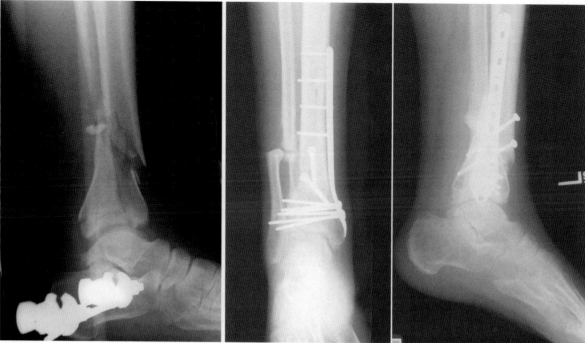

A–C

Figure 2–15 An open distal tibial fracture was initially treated with local wound care and cast. The patient developed acute infection with otherwise good soft tissues. **(A)** A spanning external fixator was applied with irrigation and debridement procedures to eradicate in- fection. Following soft tissue healing, the fixator was removed to al- low for pin site healing prior to definitive reconstruction. **(B,C)** Suc- cessful metaphyseal plating with bone graft achieved healed, infection-free limb.

graft, followed by the differentiation of cells and the pro- duction and remodeling of bone. The third function of the graft is to provide structural support. In the diaphysis, this requires cortical graft. In filling-contained metaphyseal voids to support articular surfaces (e.g., tibial plateau), cancellous graft can be used.

Graft incorporation proceeds in five stages of host re- sponse, with the duration of each phase depending on the type of graft. Hemorrhage and inflammation are the initial two phases, and many active cytokines are produced, which help initiate later stages. The third stage is vascular proliferation and ingrowth. The invading capillaries bring perivascular tissue with mesenchymal cells that can differ- entiate into osteoprogenitor cell lines. The fourth stage consists of osteoclastic resorption of the avascular bone graft lamellae and simultaneous production of new bone matrix by osteoblasts. In the final stage, the newly formed bone is remodeled and reoriented based on the mechani- cal environment of the host site.[70]

Graft incorporates fastest in autogenous cancellous bone and slowest in avascular cortical bone. In a canine model, the same phases occurred with allograft as with autograft, but the rate was about half as fast with the allo- graft. In humans, the process seems to be slower than in dogs, and avascular cortical strut allografts may take years to incorporate by "creeping substitution" through the haversian system of the graft. In many cases, complete substitution will never occur.

Cancellous Autograft

Fresh cancellous autograft provides the quickest and most reliable type of bone graft. Its trabecular structure provides for rapid revascularization—a 5 mm graft may be totally revascularized in 20 to 25 days. The large surface area al- lows for survival of numerous graft cells. Graft handling is important to optimize survival; it should be kept in chilled saline or blood and not allowed to dry out after harvesting. It does not provide structural support, except in the case of a contained metaphyseal defect such as a depressed tibial plateau fracture, in which it can support an articular sur- face if packed firmly. These grafts depend on ingrowth of host vessels and perform best in well-vascularized beds **(Fig. 2–16A–C)**.

Harvesting cancellous bone from the iliac crest begins with a surgical approach to the ilium **(Fig. 2–17)**. Bone can be obtained from the anterior crest in the supine posi- tion, or from the posterior crest in the prone position. To approach the posterior crest, an incision is made along the palpable curve of the crest, using the posterior superior iliac spine as the guide to position. Soft tissues are divided in line and held with self-retaining retractors. The "white line" of muscular attachment to the lateral crest is identified. The abductor muscles are detached from the crest using the Bovie, retaining a cuff of tissue for repair. The lateral ilium is exposed at the subperiosteal plane. Sharp acetabular ream- ers are used to harvest graft from the ilium, staying caudad

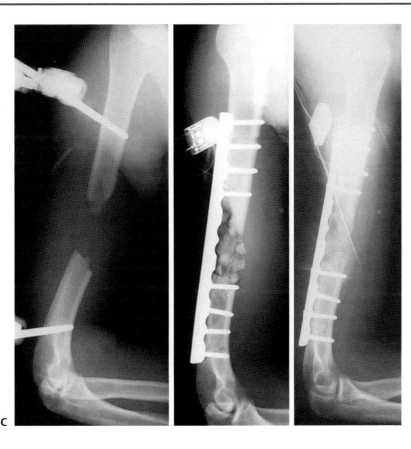

Figure 2–16 A young male patient suffered an open humeral fracture with segmental bone loss in a motor vehicle accident. **(A)** After irrigation and debridement, external fixation was applied. A large diaphyseal defect remained. **(B)** When the soft tissue wound was healed, plating and cancellous bone grafting of the defect were performed. An implantable bone stimulator was used. **(C)** By 5 months postoperatively, the defect was solidly healed.

A–C

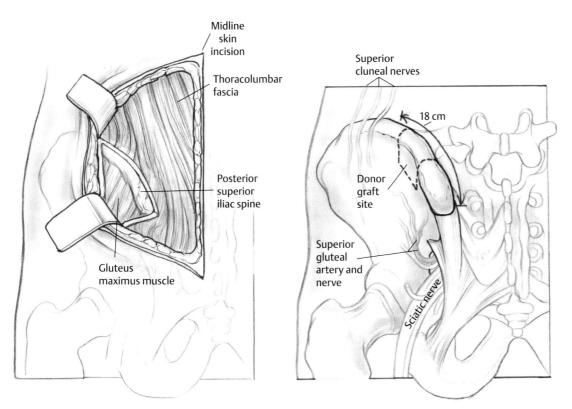

Figure 2–17 Surgical approach for harvesting autograft from the posterior iliac crest.

to the crest and moving to a new area when the inner table is contacted. Curets are used to collect cancellous bone from between the tables at the edges of the reamed area. The graft is kept moist under a wet laporotomy sponge until needed. The defect in the ilium is filled with a piece of Gelfoam containing thrombin and Marcaine with epinephrine. The abductor muscle origin is repaired, and the wound is closed in layers. Additional Marcaine is injected in the site.

Donor site morbidity is one problem associated with autologous cancellous bone graft harvesting. Iliac donor site complications include pain, neurovascular injury (lateral femoral cutaneous, iliohypogastric, ilioinguinal, cluneal, superior gluteal), fracture including avulsion of the anterior superior iliac spine (ASIS) infection, hematoma, herniation of abdominal contents, gait disturbance, violation of the sacroiliac (SI) joint, and ureteral injury.[71] Due to the limited quantity of bone available, some advocate limiting this technique to defects under 6 cm. However, one study reported eight large tibial defects averaging 10 cm that were successfully reconstructed using autogenous cancellous bone.[72]

Use of antibiotic-impregnated autogenous cancellous bone graft improves the eradication of infection and had no effect upon the rate of graft maturation and incorporation.[73] Expanders can be added to autogenous bone graft to increase the volume available. Most function in osteoconduction, with variable and rather unpredictable degrees of osteoinduction. Examples include ceramics such as calcium phosphate, hydroxyapatite, tricalcium phosphates, or calcium sulfate. Bovine collagen composites with calcium phosphate (e.g., collagraft) and demineralized bone matrix products function the same way. Alone, they are not able to stimulate sufficient bone to fill major gaps, but they may have a role when mixed with autograft. The exact indications and efficacy have not been clearly documented in the literature.

Cancellous graft is usually placed in spaces where the soft tissues can be closed, as in the posterolateral approach to tibial nonunions. In some cases of infected nonunion, however, the open or Papineau technique can be used. After adequate debridement of soft tissue and bone, the limb is stabilized with external fixation, allowing access to the defect, which is left open. It is treated with dressing changes or a VAC device until the cavity is completely lined with granulation tissue. The defect is then packed with cancellous graft, which is covered with dressings kept moist with physiological solution. Granulation grows slowly around and through the graft. Once covered with granulation, a split-thickness skin graft is applied. The average time in the external fixator is 7.5 months. With wider availability of microvascular and bone transport technology, open bone grafting is done less frequently.

Allograft

Frozen or freeze-dried allograft can be used to reconstruct large bone defects. These grafts incorporate by the same mechanisms and stages as autograft but much more slowly. In humans, large cortical allografts may never be completely replaced with living host bone. No bone cells survive the preparation process, so the graft cannot form bone directly. Allograft may be weakly osteoinductive. Corticocancellous chips may be used to support and fill contained metaphyseal defects. Cortical segments or strips can be used as structural elements. They will frequently require supplemental autogenous cancellous graft to heal to the host, and virtually always require support by internal fixation **(Fig. 2–18)**. One long-term study of intercalary allografts after tumor resection showed a success rate of 84%. Of the 15 that failed, half were ultimately salvaged with another graft or procedure. Thirty-one failed to unite at one or the other end, requiring 81 additional procedures to achieve union.[74]

The advantages of allograft are unlimited quantity, no size restriction, and the potential to include joint surfaces. The disadvantages include incomplete incorporation, healing problems, high cost, and the risk of disease transmission. The risk of viral transmission from allograft

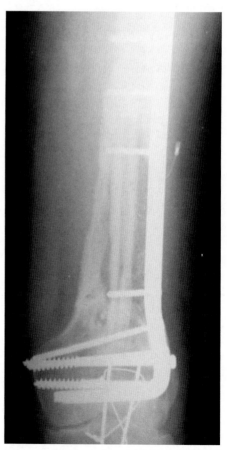

Figure 2–18 A large femoral defect resulting from an open femoral fracture was treated with wound care, external fixation, and eventually reconstructed with a blade plate and a fibular strut allograft. This anteroposterior view is 8 months postoperative when the patient had returned to full weight bearing and work as a deliveryman.

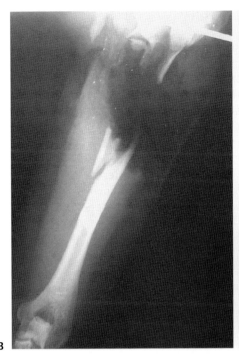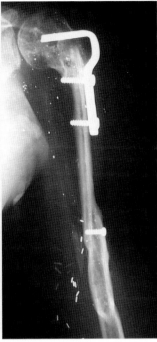

Figure 2–19 (A) A large humeral defect resulting from a gunshot wound. Neurological function in the hand was intact. **(B)** Seventy-two months after free fibular reconstruction of the defect, with a subsequent procedure for proximal nonunion, the patient has a stable union and uses the hand for activities of daily living.

A,B

is ~1 in 600,000. The biggest risk with the use of allograft is infection. Consequently, they are rarely used to fill bone defects that result from osteomyelitis. In a setting of bone loss from tumor, the risk of infection is 5 to 12%, and with a previous history of infection it is likely to be higher.

Vascularized Bone Grafts

Vascularized grafts consist of corticocancellous bone segments that are transferred with their vascular attachments. These can be either pedicled grafts (blood vessels left intact while the bone is rotated) or free vascularized grafts (vessels divided and reattached in the new location using microvascular technique). Most commonly, these techniques involve the fibula. Alternatives include iliac crest transfer with attached deep circumflex iliac artery, or rib transfer with posterior intercostal vessels. In some cases, either or both skin and muscle can be transferred at the same time as a composite flap. Vascularized bone grafts offer rapid incorporation, independence from host bed vascularity, and structural support. They will hypertrophy with time to handle increased loads. Rib is rarely used due to high donor site morbidity. Iliac crest is limited to a 5 to 6 cm straight segment, incorporates slowly, and up to 50% require supplemental cancellous grafting. Iliac crest vascularized graft harvest has a high morbidity rate, including hernia of abdominal contents.

The free fibula is the real workhorse for reconstructing diaphyseal defects. It provides up to 20 cm of bone, and in some cases, a growing epiphysis can be transplanted as part of the free fibula. Donor site morbidity is minimal. If handled correctly, up to 90% of cells in the graft will survive.[75,76] The vascularized fibula graft was initially used

to restore integrity in tibial defects. Subsequently, it has become the most commonly used free bone flap for diaphyseal defects due to its length and minimal donor site morbidity. In cases of large defects (> 6 cm), many authors consider it the treatment of choice, particularly in sites with poor host bed vascularity **(Fig. 2–19A,B)**. Nutrition for the graft comes from the branches of the peroneal vessels that run along with it, and from periosteal vessels. Because the graft has its own blood supply, it is relatively independent of the vascularity of the host bed.

It can be transferred with some soleus muscle and/or some skin (osteoseptocutaneous graft) to reconstruct both bone loss and soft tissue defects with a single graft.[75] The skin paddle allows monitoring of the vascular supply to the graft. Jupiter et al reported on the use of this graft for reconstruction of segmental radius defects in nine patients, with successful healing in eight of those nine.[77] Heitmann et al reported on the use of this graft in eight segmental humerus defects. Seven of the eight had early fixation failure or fracture of the graft, but were resolved with open reduction and internal fixation with cancellous grafting. One infected case required a second free fibula.[78]

Donor site problems are generally mild and include moderate gait disturbance for the first 18 months (particularly difficulty with stairs), minor gait problems thereafter, slight decrease in calf strength and ankle eversion, FHL contracture, and paresthesias of the peroneal nerve.[76]

Distraction Osteogenesis (see Video 2–2, Disk 1)

Ilizarov discovered distraction osteogenesis in the late 1940s or early 1950s in the Soviet Union, and the technique now bears his name. It involved an entirely new aspect of the biological behavior of bone. Ilizarov discovered that new bone formation could be induced by very slowly pulling apart two well-vascularized bone segments using external fixation. The concepts of distraction osteogenesis allow the dynamic correction of stiff axial, rotation, and translational deformities while also providing the capabilities of addressing limb length discrepancy or bone gaps during the course of treatment.[54,55] When torsional and shear forces are eliminated by applying a circular fixator, distraction forces applied lead to new bone formation and healing of the fracture site A critical factor in promoting the metaplastic conversion of fibro-cartilaginous tissue at the fracture site is the ability to provide microenvironmental stabilization. Under these stabilized conditions pluripotential cells from local mesenchymal sources preferentially divide along the osteoblast/osteocyte line. This process involves local neovascularization and increased biosynthetic activity and results in intramembranous bone formation in the gap between the segments.[79]

The first step is application of an external fixator. The classic Ilizarov fixator uses tensioned transfixion wires and rings linked with threaded rods (**Fig. 2–12**). Half-pin monolateral fixators can be used in a similar fashion for many applications of the technique. The bone is cut with a percutaneous corticotomy, usually in the metaphysis, preserving as much as possible of the intramedullary and periosteal blood supply. After corticotomy, there is a latency period of 5 to 14 days before distraction is begun. Once the distraction process is initiated, the cut bone surfaces are slowly pulled apart at a rate of ~0.25 mm every 6 hours. Increments of distraction too large (e.g., 1 mm once a day) inhibit osteogenesis. If the rate of distraction is too slow, the gap may close by normal fracture healing. Any instability producing shear stress inhibits osteogenesis. The tissue between the cut bone surfaces develops into a bipolar fibrovascular zone with collagen fibers oriented parallel to the direction of pull. Bone begins to form by intramembranous ossification arising from the full width of the cut bone surface. This bone forms in a highly uniform, ordered fashion of columns or cones ~200 μ in diameter, surrounded by microvascular channels. Mineralization proceeds in proximity to the vessels, which grow parallel to the distraction force.[79]

There are two strategies for use of distraction osteogenesis in the face of bone deficits. The first involves acute shortening and compression at the fracture site after contouring the bone ends for stability, followed by corticotomy and lengthening at a separate metaphyseal location. This allows for reduction of the size of the soft tissue defect and will often allow delayed primary closure or skin grafting of a defect that otherwise would require a soft tissue flap.[80] A frame can be constructed to simultaneously compress at the fracture site and distract at a separate location. The second strategy involves putting on the frame

with the limb at the correct length and alignment, and then using an internal lengthening of one or both segments to fill the gap. This is called bone transport, and the advantage is that the limb can be functional, even weight bearing, during the process.

Bone transport has a high rate of ultimate success, with many series reporting upward of 90% eventually healing with arrest of infection.[80,81] Unfortunately, most reports are small series, usually fewer than 20 patients, without comparison groups or controls. There is no donor site morbidity associated with transport because all the new bone comes from the injured leg. In addition, the leg can be functional and weight bearing during treatment (**Fig. 2–20A–E**). However, the treatment does require prolonged time in the external fixator, in some series up to 2 months per centimeter of gap filled. Substantial time is due to delayed healing of the docking site, which frequently requires bone grafting. Docking site healing problems occur in up to half the cases in some series. The prolonged time in the frame contributes to a high rate of complications, such as pin site infections, cellulitis, contracture, and edema.

Technique modifications to shorten the time in the frame include double-segment transport, pregrafting the docking site, or transport over an unreamed IM nail. Called the "monorail technique," transport of a segment over a nail minimizes malalignment, and once the docking occurs and is compressed, the nail can be interlocked and the frame removed.[82] A similar approach uses transport under a minimally invasive bridge plate, which provides stability after the segment is transported and allows earlier frame removal.

There are three studies that compare Ilizarov techniques for handling bone gaps with "conventional" techniques.[38,83,84] They each use separate outcome measures and define things differently in terms of treatment success and complications. Two of the studies are retrospective, whereas one reports on a "prospective protocol" compared with historical controls. None compare concurrently treated patients randomized to different groups. Conventional treatment consisted of Papineau grafting in one paper,[38] cancellous bone grafting in another,[84] and cancellous grafting or free fibula transplant in the third.[83] Combining all three studies, there are 101 total patients, 48 of which were treated with bone transport. The average defect was 5.2 cm for transport patients, and 5.7 cm for conventional technique patients. The rate of successful healing with infection arrest ranged from 71 to 90%, with no significant differences found between the comparison groups. The conventionally treated patients needed more secondary procedures (112 vs 35). One study showed that conventional treatment resulted in many more transfusions, longer hospitalizations, and more total OR hours.[83] Marsh et al found a distinct advantage for Ilizarov treatment in terms of ultimate leg length discrepancy, but they included patients in the conventional group who had been treated with intentional shortening.[84] Many of the Ilizarov patients needed bone

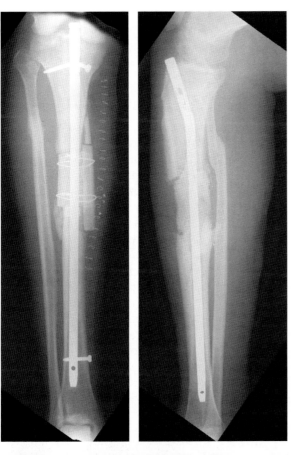

A,B

Figure 2–20 Bone transport for segmental defect in the tibia. **(A)** An open tibial fracture was treated with IM nailing and allograft with cerclage wires. Infection developed. **(B)** After segmental resection of infected bone and soft tissues, placement of antibiotic-impregnated cement spacer was done. **(C)** A circular frame was applied for distal to proximal bone transport. **(D)** Bone grafting was required at the docking site. **(E)** Eventual healing occurred with full weight bearing and resolution of infection.

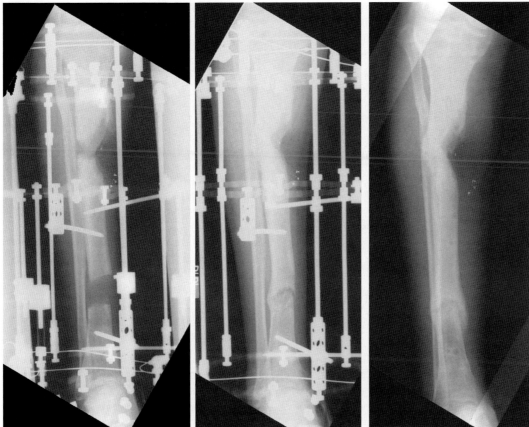

C–E

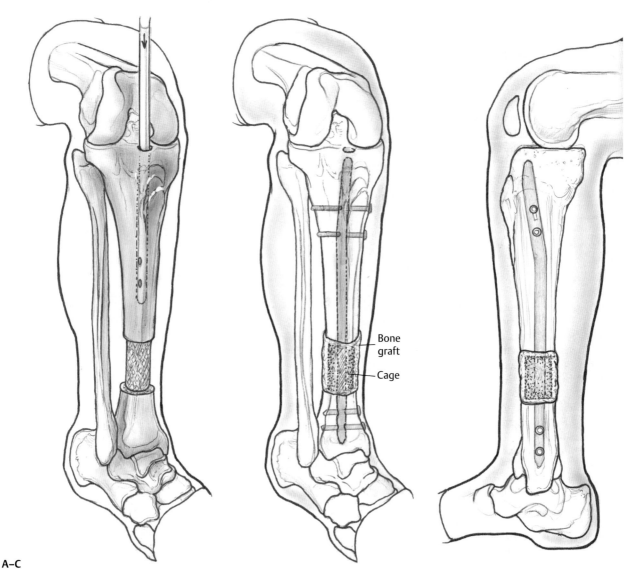

A–C

Figure 2–21 Drawing of intramedullary nailing through a titanium cage. This technique allows early weight bearing as a result of the stability from the nail and the cage. Bone graft is packed around the outside of the cage to allow filling of the diaphyseal defect. **(A)** Demonstrates the nail going into the tibia with the cage in place in the tibial defect. **(B)** Bone graft is packed around the cage. **(C)** Demonstrates union of the tibia.

grafting for problems at the docking site, but the authors noted that those bone grafts were much less extensive and required less volume than the grafts in the conventional group.

New Technique

Intramedullary Nailing of the Tibia with a Titanium Cage

A recently described technique from Europe to treat chronic osteomyelitis of the tibia employs aggressive excision of necrotic and infected bone, followed by intramedullary nailing through a titanium cage with cancellous bone grafting **(Fig. 2–21).** The initial step is excision of all necrotic

and sequestered bone. The next step is selecting a titanium cage of appropriate height to reestablish normal leg length. An intramedullary nail is then introduced into the tibia to the level of the bone defect. The titanium cage is then placed in the defect, and the nail is driven through the middle of the nail, followed by distal interlocking. The final step is cancellous bone grafting around (not in the middle of) the cage. There are no published data on this technique, but early results are quite promising. A major advantage is early stability and weight bearing.

Pearl

- The overall sensitivity of MRI for bone infection approaches 100%, specificity is 60–75%.

On the DVDs

Video 2–1 (Same as Video 1–5, Disk 1) Antibiotic Bead Pouch This video shows how to make antibiotic beads and create a bead pouch to treat an infection or severely contaminated wound.

Video 2–2 (Disk 1) Circular External Fixation of the Lower Extremity This video demonstrates placement of a circular external fixator on a proximal tibia fracture. The principles of application are very similar for deformity correction to reconstruct following infection.

Video 2–3 (Disk 1) Arthrodesis of the Knee Arthrodesis of the knee is accomplished using compression plating following a sep-

tic knee that led to severe damage to the articular cartilage and periarticular bone. The technique demonstrated uses cutting jigs designed for a total knee arthroplasty to obtain good alignment and stable bone surfaces in order to achieve arthrodesis.

Video 2–4 (Disk 1) Above-Knee Amputation This video demonstrates treatment of a mangled lower extremity with an above-knee amputation. The technique includes myodesis of the adductor and hamstring muscles.

References

1. Bloom BS, Esterhai JL Jr. Musculoskeletal infection: impact, morbidity, and cost to society, medicine and government. In: Esterhai JL Jr, Gristina AG, Poss R, eds. Musculoskeletal Infection. Rosemont IL: American Academy of Orthopaedic Surgeons;1992:5–11

2. Nelson CL. Prevention of infection. In: McCollister Evarts C, ed. Surgery of the Musculoskeletal System. 2nd ed. New York: Churchill Livingstone; 1990

3. Pratt WB, Veitch JM, McRoberts RL. Nutritional status of orthopaedic patients with surgical complications. Clin Orthop Relat Res 1981;155:81–84

4. Anglen JO. Wound irrigation in musculoskeletal injury. J Am Acad Orthop Surg 2001;9:219–226

5. Henry SL, Osterman PA, Seligson D. The antibiotic bead pouch technique. Clin Orthop Relat Res 1993;295:54–62

6. Webb LX. New techniques in wound management: vacuum-assisted wound closure. J Am Acad Orthop Surg 2002;10:303–311

7. Schmidt AH, Swiontkowski MF. Pathophysiology of infections after internal fixation of fractures. J Am Acad Orthop Surg 2000;8: 285–291

8. Boxma H, Broekhuizen T, Patka P, Oosting H. Randomized, controlled trial of single dose antibiotic prophylaxis in surgical treatment of closed fractures: The Dutch Trauma Trial. Lancet 1996;347:1133–1137

9. Oishi CS, Carrion WV, Hoaglund FT. Use of parenteral prophylactic antibiotics in clean orthopaedic surgery. Clin Orthop Relat Res 1993;296:249–255

10. Anglen JO, Aleto T. Temporary transarticular external fixation of the knee and ankle. J Orthop Trauma 1998;12:431–434

11. Haidukewych GJ. Temporary external fixation for the management of complex intra- and periarticular fractures of the lower extremity. J Orthop Trauma 2002;16:678–685

12. Watson JT, Occhietti MJ, Moed BR, Karges DE, Cramer KE, Parmar VS. Perioperative external fixator management during secondary surgical procedures. Presented at the OTA annual meeting, Charlotte, NC, October 24, 1999. Abstract available online accessed 8/26/03: http://www.hwbf.org/ota/am/ota99/otapa/OTA99902.htm

13. Maurer DJ, Merkow RL, Gustilo RB. Infection after intramedullary nailing of severe open tibial fractures initially treated with external fixation. J Bone Joint Surg Am. 1989;71:835–838

14. Hofmann GO, Bar T, Buhren V. The osteosynthesis implant and early postoperative infection: healing with or without removal of material? [in German] Chirurg 1997;68:1175–1180

15. Hoch RC, Rodriquez R, Manning T. Effects of accidental trauma on cytokine and endotoxin production. Crit Care Med 1993;21:839–845

16. Court-Brown CM, Keating JF, McQueen MM. Infection after intramedullary nailing of the tibia: incidence and protocol for management. J Bone Joint Surg Br1992;74:770–774

17. Keating JF, Blachut PA, O'Brien PJ, Meek RN, Broekhuyse H. Reamed nailing of open tibial fractures: does the antibiotic bead pouch reduce the deep infection rate? J Orthop Trauma 1996;10: 298–303

18. Leutenegger AF. Acute infection following osteosynthesis. Ther Umsch 1990;47:593–596

19. Zych GA, Hutson JJ Jr. Diagnosis and management of infection after tibial medullary nailing. Clin Orthop Relat Res 1995;315: 153–162

20. Foglar C, Lindsey RW. C-reactive protein in orthopaedics. Orthopedics 1998;21:687–691

21. Unkila-Kallio L, Kallio MJ, Eskola J, Petola H. Serum C-reactive protein, erythrocyte sedimentation rate, and white blood cell count in acute hematogenous osteomyelitis of children. Pediatrics 1994; 93:59–62

22. Santiago Restrepo C, Gimenez CR, McCarthy K. Imaging of osteomyelitis and musculoskeletal soft tissue infections: current concepts. Rheum Dis Clin North Am 2003;29:89–109

23. Gross T, Kaim AH, Regazzoni P, Widmer AF. Current concepts in posttraumatic osteomyelitis: a diagnostic challenge with new imaging options. J Trauma 2002;52:1210–1219

24. Kaim A, Ledermann HP, Bongartz G, Messmer P, Muller-Brand J, Steinbrich W. Chronic post-traumatic osteomyelitis of the lower extremity: comparison of magnetic resonance imaging and combined bone scintigraphy/immunoscintigraphy with radiolabelled monoclonal antigranulocyte antibodies. Skeletal Radiology 2000; 29:378–386

25. Hakki S, Harwood SJ, Morrissey MA, Camblin JG, Laven DL, Webster WB Jr. Comparative study of monoclonal antibody scan in diagnosing orthopaedic infection. Clin Orthop Relat Res 1997;335: 275–285

26. Seabold JE, Nepola JV. Imaging techniques for evaluation of postoperative orthopedic infections. Q J Nucl Med 1999;43:21–28

27. Erdman WA, Tamburro F, Jayson HT, Weatherall PT, Ferry KB, Peshock RM. Osteomyelitis: characteristics and pitfalls of diagnosis with MR imaging. Radiology 1991;180:533–539

28. Umans H, Haramati N, Flusser G. The diagnostic role of gadolinium enhanced MRI in distinguishing between acute medullary

bone infarct and osteomyelitis. Magn Reson Imaging 2000;18: 255–262

29. Hovi I, Valtonen M, Korhola O, Hekali P. Low-field MR imaging for the assessment of therapy response in musculoskeletal infections. Acta Radiol 1995;36:220–227

30. Williamson MR, Quenzer RW, Rosenberg RD, et al. Osteomyelitis: sensitivity of 0.064 T MRI, three-phase bone scanning and indium scanning with biopsy proof. Magn Reson Imaging 1991;9: 945–948

31. Perry CR, Pearson RL, Miller GA. Accuracy of cultures of material from swabbing of the superficial aspect of the wound and needle biopsy in the preoperative assessment of osteomyelitis. J Bone Joint Surg Am 1991;73:745–749

32. Cierny G 3rd, Mader JT, Penninck JJ. A clinical staging system for adult osteomyelitis. Clin Orthop Rel Res 2003;414:7–24

33. Moroni A, Vannini F, Mosca M, Giannini S. State of the art review: techniques to avoid pin loosening and infection in external fixation. J Orthop Trauma 2002;16:189–195

34. Pommer A, Muhr G, David A. Hydroxyapatite-coated Schanz pins in the external fixators used for distraction osteogenesis: a randomized, controlled trial. J Bone Joint Surg Am 2002;84-A: 1162–1166

35. Halsey D, Fleming B, Pope MH, Krag M, Kristiansen T. External fixator pin design. Clin Orthop Relat Res 1992;278:305–312

36. Seitz WH Jr, Froimson AI, Brooks DB, Postak P, Polando G, Greenwald AS. External fixator pin insertion techniques: biomechanical analysis and clinical relevance. J Hand Surg [Am] 1991;16:560–563

37. Dahl MT, Gulli B, Berg T. Complications of limb lengthening a learning curve. Clin Orthop Relat Res 1994;301:10–18

38. Green SA. Skeletal defects: a comparison of bone grafting and bone transport for skeletal defects. Clin Orthop Relat Res 1994;301: 111–117

39. Seguin B, Harari J, Wood RD, Tillson DM. Bone fracture and sequestration as complications of external skeletal fixation. J Small Anim Pract 1997;38:81–84

40. Gordon JE, Kelly-Hahn J, Carpenter CJ, Schoenecker PL. Pin site care during external fixation in children: results of nihilistic approach. J Pediatr Orthop 2000;20:163–165

41. McClinton MA, Helgemo SL Jr. Infection in the presence of skeletal fixation in the upper extremity. Hand Clin 1997;13:745–760

42. Merritt K, Dowd JD. Role of internal fixation in infection of open fractures: studies with *Staphylococcus aureus* and *Proteus mirabilis*. J Orthop Res 1987;5:23–28

43. Worlock P, Slack R, Harvey L, Mawhinney R. The prevention of infection in open fractures: an experimental study of the effect of fracture stability. Injury 1994;25:31–38

44. Lew DP, Waldvogel FA. Osteomyelitis. N Engl J Med 1997;336: 999–1007

45. Norden CW, Bryant R, Palmer D, Montgomerie JZ, Wheat J. Chronic osteomyelitis caused by *Staphylococcus aureus*: controlled trial of nafcillin therapy and nafcillin-rifampin therapy. South Med J 1986;79:947–951

46. Drancourt M, Stein A, Argensen JN, Zannier A, Curvale G, Raoult D. Oral rifampin plus ofloxacin for treatment of *Staphylococcus* infected orthopaedic implants. Antimicrob Agents Chemother 1993;37:1214–1218

47. Huddleston PM, Steckelberg JM, Hanssen AD, Rouse MS, Bolander ME, Patel R. Ciprofloxacin inhibition of experimental fracture healing. J Bone Joint Surg Am. 2000;82:161–173

48. Swiontkowski MF, Hanel DP, Vedder NB, Schwappach JR. A comparison of short and long-term intravenous antibiotic therapy in

the post-operative management of adult osteomyelitis. J Bone Joint Surg Br. 1999;81:1046–1051

49. Pavoni GL, Falcone M, Baiocchi P, et al. Conservative medical therapy of infections following osteosynthesis: a retrospective analysis of a 6-year experience. J Chemother 2002;14:378–383

50. Mader JT, Cripps MW, Calhoun JH. Adult posttraumatic osteomyelitis of the tibia. Clin Orthop Relat Res 1999;360:14–21

51. Tetsworth K, Cierny G. Osteomyelitis debridement techniques. Clin Orthop Relat Res 1999;360:87–96

52. Ueng SW, Wei FC, Shih CH. Management of femoral diaphyseal infected nonunions with antibiotic bead local therapy, external skeletal fixation and staged bone grafting. J Trauma 1999;46:97–103

53. Patzakis MJ, Greene N, Holtom P, Sheperd L, Bravos P, Sherman R. Culture results in open wound treatment with muscle transfer for tibial osteomyelitis. Clin Orthop Relat Res 1999;360:66–70

54. Catagni MA, Guerreschi F, Holman JA, Catanneo R. Distraction osteogenesis in the treatment of stiff hypertrophic nonunions using the Ilizarov apparatus. Clin Orthop Relat Res 1994;301:159–163

55. Tetsworth K, Paley D. Accuracy of correction of complex lower extremity deformities by the Ilizarov method. Clin Orthop Relat Res 1994;301:102–110

56. Paley D, Herzenberg JE. Intramedullary infections treated with antibiotic cement rods: preliminary results in nine cases. J Orthop Trauma 2002;16:723–729

57. Wahlig H, Dingeldein E, Bergmann R, Reuss K. The release of gentamicin from polymethylmethacrylate beads: an experimental and pharmacokinetic study. J Bone Joint Surg Br 1978;60-B:270–275

58. Evans RP, Nelson CL. Gentamicin-impregnated PMMA beads compared with systemic antibiotic therapy in the treatment of chronic osteomyelitis. Clin Orthop Relat Res 1993;295:37–42

59. Seligson D, Mehta S, Voos K, Henry SL, Johnson JR. The use of antibiotic impregnated PMMA beads to prevent the evolution of localized infection. J Orthop Trauma 1992;6:401–406

60. Chen NT, Hong HZ, Hooper DC, May JW Jr. The effect of systemic antibiotic and antibiotic-impregnated PMMA beads on the bacterial clearance in wounds containing contaminated dead bone. Plast Reconstr Surg 1993;92:1305–1311

61. Henry SL, Hood GA. Seligson D. Long-term implantation of gentamicin-polymethylmethacrylate antibiotic beads. Clin Orthop Relat Res 1993;295:47–53

62. Miclau T, Dahners LE, Lindsey RW. In vitro pharmacokinetics of antibiotic release from locally implantable materials. J Orthop Res 1993;11:627–632

63. Galandiuk S, Wrightson WR, Young S, Myers S, Polk HC Jr. Absorbable, delayed release antibiotic beads reduce surgical wound infection. Am Surg 1997;63:831–835

64. Rutledge B, Huyette D, Day D, Anglen J. Treatment of osteomyelitis with local antibiotics delivered via bioabsorbable polymer. Clin Orthop Relat Res 2003;411:280–287

65. McKee MD, Wild LM, Schemitsch EH, Waddell JP. The use of an antibiotic-impregnated, osteoconductive, bioabsorbable bone substitute in the treatment of infected long bone defects: early results of a prospective trial. J Orthop Trauma 2002;16:622–627

66. Russell RC, Graham DR, Feller AM, Zook EG, Mathur A. Experimental evaluation of the antibiotic carrying capacity of a muscle flap into a fibrotic cavity. Plast Reconstr Surg 1988;81:162–170

67. Weiland AJ, Moore JR, Daniel RK. The efficacy of free tissue transfer in the treatment of osteomyelitis. J Bone Joint Surg Am 1984;66: 181–193

68. Monsivais JJ. Effective management of osteomyelitis after grade III open fractures. J South Orthop Assoc 1996;5:30–36

69. Anthony JP, Mathes SJ, Alpert BS. The muscle flap in the treatment of chronic lower extremity osteomyelitis: results in patients over 5 years after treatment. Plast Reconstr Surg 1991;88:311–318

70. Schemitsch EH, Bhandari M. Bone healing and grafting. In: Koval K, ed. Orthopedic Knowledge Update 7. Rosemont, IL: American Academy of Orthopaedic Surgeons; 2002:19–29

71. Ebraheim NA, Elgafy H, Xu R. Bone-graft harvesting from iliac and fibular donor sites: techniques and complications. J Am Acad Orthop Surg 2001;9:210–218

72. Christian EP, Bosse MJ, Robb G. Reconstruction of large diaphyseal defects, without free fibular transfer, in grade-IIIB tibial fractures. J Bone Joint Surg Am 1989;71:994–1004

73. Chan YS, Ueng SW, Wang CJ, Lee SS, Chen CY, Shin CH. Antibiotic-impregnated autogenic cancellous bone grafting is an effective and safe method for the management of small infected tibial defects: a comparison study. J Trauma 2000;48:246–255

74. Ortiz-Cruz E, Gebhardt MC, Jennings LC, Springfield DS, Mankin HJ. The results of transplantation of intercalary allografts after resection of tumors: a long term follow-up study. J Bone Joint Surg Am 1997;79:97–105

75. Yaremchuk MJ, Brumback RJ, Manson PN, Burgess AR, Poka A, Weiland AJ. Acute and definitive management of traumatic osteocutaneous defects of the lower extremity. Plast Reconstr Surg 1987; 80:1–14

76. Minami A, Kasashima T, Iwasaki N, Kato H, Kaneda K. Vascularized fibular grafts: an experience of 102 patients. J Bone Joint Surg Br 2000;82:1022–1025

77. Jupiter JB, Gerhard HJ, Guerrero J, Nunley JA, Levin LS. Treatment of segmental defects of the radius with use of the vascularized osteoseptocutaneous fibula autogenous graft. J Bone Joint Surg Am 1997;79:542–550

78. Heitmann C, Erdmann D, Levin LS. Treatment of segmental defects of the humerus with an osteoseptocutaneous fibular transplant. J Bone Joint Surg Am 2002;84-A:2216–2223

79. de Pablos J, Barrias C, Alfaro C, et al. Large experimental segmental bone defects treated by bone transportation with monolateral external distractors. Clin Orthop Relat Res 1994;298:259–265

80. Prokuski LJ, Marsh LJ. Segmental bone deficiency after acute trauma: the role of bone transport. Orthop Clin North Am. 1994;25:753–763

81. Dendrinos GK, Kontos S, Lyritsis E. Use of the Ilizarov technique for treatment of nonunion of the tibia associated with infection. J Bone Joint Surg Am 1995;77:835–846

82. Raschke MJ, Mann JW, Oedekoven G, Claudi BF. Segmental transport after unreamed intramedullary nailing: preliminary report of a "Monorail" system. Clin Orthop Relat Res 1992;282:233–240

83. Cierny G III, Zorn KE. Segmental tibial defects: comparing conventional and Ilizarov methodologies. Clin Orthop Relat Res 1994;301:118–123

84. Marsh JL, Prokuski LJ, Biermann JS. Chronic infected tibial nonunions with bone loss: conventional techniques vs. bone transport. Clin Orthop Relat Res 1994;301:139–146

3 Acute Compartment Syndrome

Andrew H. Schmidt

The term *compartment syndrome* refers to acute myoneural ischemia caused by elevated intramuscular pressures. Simplistically, compartment syndrome may be considered to result either from swelling within the minimally compliant muscle fascia or from external compression. Although the pathophysiological mechanisms are very complex and incompletely understood, either circumstance leads to increased pressure within the compartment. At some point, microcirculatory function within the involved compartment ceases, and the tissues traversing the compartment (muscle and nerve) are threatened. The tissue ischemia produces further edema, muscle excitability and rigidity, intracellular swelling, and ultimately further increases in pressure, initiating the self-perpetuating cycle of compartment syndrome. With increasing duration of ischemia, the tissue damage becomes irreversible. Reversal of the process by fasciotomy restores perfusion to the injured tissues, but additional reperfusion injury may result from the release of activated leukocytes and other by-products released by the damaged muscle. The sequelae of untreated compartment syndrome include prolonged or permanent hypoesthesia, dysesthesia, contractures, muscle weakness, renal failure from rhabdomyolysis and myoglobinuria, cardiac arrhythmias, sepsis, gangrene, amputation, or even death.[1]

Compartment syndrome may be initiated by many conditions, including fractures, crushing injury, vascular injury, burns, overexertion, hypothermia, prolonged limb compression, or contusions. In orthopedics, it is most common in association with both closed and open tibia fractures but also occurs with other fractures, soft tissue trauma, and after extrinsic compression such as from a cast or medical antishock trousers. Postischemic swelling due to reperfusion is associated with compartment syndrome that develops following repair of vascular injury, with ischemia due to prolonged pressure, and following surgery in the hemilithotomy position. Although initially intended to refer to the muscle compartments of the extremities, the so-called abdominal compartment syndrome is now commonly recognized in which there is abdominal visceral dysfunction (bowel ischemia, renal failure, etc.) resulting from elevated intra-abdominal pressures. Compartment syndrome has been described in most every location, including the deltoid, arm, forearm, hand, gluteal compartments, thigh, leg, and foot.

Diagnosis

It has been stated that the greatest difficulty in managing compartment syndrome is determining when a fasciotomy is indicated.[2] In North America, failure to correctly diagnose compartment syndrome is one of the most common causes of litigation against the medical profession.[3] A 1993 study of the malpractice costs found that an average indemnity of nearly $280,000 was awarded in cases of missed compartment syndrome.[3] More recently, 19 closed claims regarding compartment syndrome were discussed.[4] These claims were associated with a total liability of $3.8 million ($200,000 per claim). Ten of the claims (53%) were resolved in favor of the physician and required an average of 5.5 years to resolve. Three claims went to trial and resulted in a verdict for the physician. Poor physician–patient communication was found in six cases, all of which resulted in an indemnity payment ($p > .01$). Increasing time from the onset of symptoms to the fasciotomy was linearly associated with an increased indemnity payment ($p < .05$). In contrast, a fasciotomy performed within 8 hours of presentation of symptoms was always associated with a successful defense.[4]

The key to making a timely diagnosis of compartment syndrome is thinking about it in the first place. Hope and McQueen evaluated a series of 164 cases of compartment syndrome and found that cases occurring after a fracture were diagnosed sooner and were associated with less tissue necrosis at the time of fasciotomy than the cases that occurred without a fracture.[5] This suggests that the presence of a fracture heightens one's awareness of compartment syndrome. It is critical to consider that any patient with a swollen, painful limb might have compartment syndrome, even without obvious skeletal trauma. One must therefore be aware of circumstances in which compartment syndrome is possible. In large series of patients with tibia fractures, the overall incidence is low. McQueen et al reported an incidence of 1.5% in 67 tibia fractures and found that there were no differences in pressures between low- and high-energy fractures, open or closed fractures, or those treated before or after 24 hours from the time of injury.[6] More recent work from the same institution has shown that compartment syndromes are more common in young men with either or both tibial shaft and forearm fractures.[7] Compartment syndrome may be seen following fractures of the forearm in children; a recent report found the incidence to be greater following intramedullary fixation compared with closed reduction and casting.[8] One must not forget that compartment syndrome may also occur in open fractures, with a reported incidence of 2.7[9] to 33.3%.[10] Woll and Duwelius found that 48% of patients with segmental tibial fractures needed fasciotomy for acute compartment syndrome.[11] Although the leg is most frequently involved (80%), compartment syndromes have been reported in most every muscle compartment in the upper extremities, lower extremities, and trunk.[7]

The classic symptoms for the diagnosis of compartment syndrome are known as the five Ps: pain, pallor, pulselessness, paresthesia, and paralysis. However, these criteria are subjective, are not uniformly present, are often difficult to assess, and when present are indicative of an advanced stage of injury that may be irreversible. The most reliable symptom of acute compartment syndrome is pain out of proportion to the injury and pain with passive stretching of the involved muscles. One should avoid the use of regional anesthetic blockade in patients with compartment syndrome, and even the use of standard patient-controlled anesthesia can completely mask the increases in pain that occur with compartment syndrome.[12] The involved compartment is usually quite tense when palpated. Because of the sensitivity of peripheral nerves to ischemia, dysesthesias in a specific nerve located in the involved compartment are a very sensitive early finding (**Table 3–1**).[13,14] Gross neural dysfunction manifested by complete sensory loss represents a later finding, and when present is indicative of an advanced degree of pathology. One should remember that certain subsets of patients, such as schizophrenic patients,[15] patients receiving parenteral narcotics or regional anesthesia, or those who are obtunded or intoxicated might not demonstrate significant pain despite compartment syndrome.

The inconsistency and variability in signs and symptoms make the diagnosis of compartment syndrome largely one of clinical judgment. Although acute compartment syndrome is related to elevated intramuscular pressure, there is no specific, reliable, and reproducible test that confirms the diagnosis.[16–25] Ulmer reviewed the literature regarding compartment syndromes of the lower leg and found that the sensitivity of clinical findings for diagnosing

compartment syndrome was very low (13–19%).[23] Similarly, the positive predictive value of the clinical findings was only 11 to 15%. In contrast, the specificity and negative predictive value were each 97 to 98%. These findings indicate that the clinical findings associated with compartment syndrome of the lower leg are more useful in excluding the diagnosis by their absence than they are in confirming the diagnosis when present.[23] Given these problems with ascertaining when compartment syndrome is present, a high index of suspicion must be maintained for patients at risk, and the surgeon must err on the side of performing too many fasciotomies in order not to miss one.

To make the diagnosis of compartment syndrome less subjective and to relate the diagnosis to the underlying pathophysiology, techniques to measure intramuscular pressure have been developed and utilized clinically.[6,26–28] Both a commercially available device for measuring intramuscular pressure (Stryker Quick Pressure Monitor, Stryker Surgical, Kalamazoo, Michigan) and an intravenous manometric pump (Alaris Medical Systems, San Diego, California) have been shown to be accurate and to provide reproducible measurements.[26] However, controversy exists regarding what pressure criteria support the diagnosis of compartment syndrome,[20,29] and the level of tissue pressure at which fasciotomy is recommended varies considerably between authors. Fasciotomy has been recommended if pressures are above 45 mm Hg,[30] 30 mm Hg,[31] or within 30 mm Hg of the patient's diastolic blood pressure.[19,32,33] Although intramuscular pressure is readily measured, the significance of a given pressure for a given patient is not certain.[30,34] It has been shown that pressures vary within a single compartment, with statistically significant differences at distances as close as 5 cm from the site at which the highest pressure was recorded.[35] Intramuscular pressures have been shown to vary depending on the position of the adjacent joints.[36] Multiple intramuscular pressure measurements taken at different locations may be necessary, but there is no certainty as to which measurement is most predictive of the underlying pathophysiology. Janzing and Broos examined several different putative definitions for compartment syndrome based on either absolute intramuscular pressures or perfusion pressures, and showed that a consistent pressure threshold for compartment syndrome does not seem to exist.[29] Presently, a differential pressure (diastolic or mean-arterial pressure minus compartment pressure) of less than 30 to 40 mm Hg is considered more specific than an absolute pressure for the diagnosis of compartment syndrome.[33] The use of intramuscular pressure greater than 30 mm Hg as a fixed, absolute definition of compartment syndrome led to a 29% incidence of fasciotomy in one series.[20] This is higher than the expected rate and indicates that this definition is not specific enough, although one is not likely to miss a compartment syndrome with this definition.

Because of the problems with the clinical diagnosis of compartment syndrome as well as the inconvenience of

Table 3—1   Physical Findings of Hypoesthesia Are Related to Specific Peripheral Nerve Involvement in Patients with Compartment Syndrome of the Leg

Compartment	Specific Peripheral Nerve	Area of Hypoesthesia
Anterior	Deep peroneal nerve	First web space
Lateral	Superficial peroneal nerve	Dorsum of foot
Superficial posterior	Sural nerve	Lateral foot
Deep posterior	Tibial nerve	Plantar aspect of foot

performing multiple intramuscular pressure measurements, some investigators advocate continuous intramuscular pressure monitoring.[6,32] McQueen et al have demonstrated that the continuous monitoring of a cohort of patients with tibia fractures led to a marked reduction in the incidence of fasciotomy without any apparently missed compartment syndromes.[32] Moreover, when compartment syndrome occurred, it was diagnosed earlier, and those patients that underwent continuous monitoring also had improved clinical outcomes with fewer healing complications.[32] However, Ulmer et al recently showed that even intramuscular pressure measurements are not completely reliable for the diagnosis of compartment syndrome.[23] There are several possible reasons why even measurement of intramuscular pressure may be misleading for diagnosing compartment syndrome. Most importantly, intramuscular pressure is really a surrogate outcome and does not directly measure muscle or nerve ischemia. The development of muscle ischemia is dependent on both magnitude and duration of elevated pressure.[37,38] The tolerance of muscle to ischemia varies among patients because of shock, compensating hypertension, altered tone in vessel resistance, and degree of preexisting muscle injury.[18,39] Furthermore, inherent inconsistencies and inaccuracies of pressure measurement systems and techniques lead to diagnostic uncertainties, and measured pressures vary considerably at different sites within the same compartment.[17]

Technique for Measurement of Intramuscular Pressure

There are many methods of measuring intramuscular pressure. Whitesides et al initially presented a technique that utilizes a needle manometer and saline injection;[27] the method is cumbersome, and there are better alternatives today.

There are several commercially available devices that are designed specifically for the purpose of measuring intramuscular pressure (**Fig. 3–1**). The devices are handheld, have a digital display, and utilize specially designed sideport needles or slit catheters for continuous monitoring.

The following steps relate to the Stryker Quick Pressure Monitor (Stryker Surgical) (**Fig. 3–1**). The device is

assembled according to the manufacturer's directions. This requires the attachment of a small syringe filled with sterile saline. A sideport needle is attached to the opposite end of the device, and the system is flushed with saline to establish a fluid column. The needle is held at the level of the compartment to be measured and zeroed. The needle is inserted into the compartment of interest, and 0.3 mL of fluid is injected. This is enough to cause a transient increase in the intramuscular pressure, which then decreases to a steady-state value in 30 to 60 seconds. Repeated measurements are taken, both within and among the different compartments. For continuous monitoring, a slit catheter is recommended.[6] This may be attached to the same handheld unit described or to a blood pressure transducer.

Heckman et al found that tissue pressures are highest with 5 cm of the fracture in patients with tibia fractures.[35] It is probably best to take multiple measurements of tissue pressure both near and farther from the compartment. However, it is impractical to make multiple measurements of all compartments in a given extremity. Because the anterior compartment of the leg and the volar compartment of the forearm are typically the compartments with the highest pressures and are always involved when compartment syndrome occurs, they may considered to be "sentinel" compartments and should be the compartments most closely monitored.

Traditional imaging has only a minor role in the management of compartment syndrome; it is used primarily to diagnose the primary injury and assess possible fracture or dislocation. However, it has been recently demonstrated that magnetic resonance imaging (MRI) may have a role in the management of acute compartment syndrome. Rominger et al performed serial MRI in 15 patients (10 established, five "imminent") with compartment syndrome.[40] The MR images revealed swollen compartments with loss of normal muscle architecture. T2-weighted spin-echo and magnetization transfer images showed bright areas that enhanced after intravenous injection of gadolinium. Early follow-up images demonstrated changes in enhancement patterns, whereas late follow-up images showed fibrosis and cystic and fatty degenerations of the

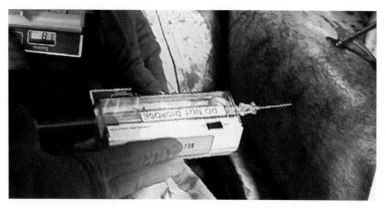

Figure 3–1 Photo of a handheld device (Quick Pressure Monitor device, Stryker Surgical, Kalamazoo, Michigan) as it is used to measure intramuscular pressure. The device is assembled, a fluid column is established, and the unit is held at the level of the limb to zero the pressure before insertion. The insert in the upper left of the photo shows the digital readout, in this case indicating a pressure of 81 mm Hg.

affected compartments.[40] These authors conclude that MRI can assist in the diagnosis of compartment syndrome in clinically ambiguous cases, points out the affected compartments, and allows the surgeon to selectively split the fascial spaces.[40]

There are several new, less invasive techniques that are currently being assessed for their efficacy in diagnosing compartment syndrome. These include measurements of the surface hardness of the compartment,[41] transcutaneous oxygen measurements, measurement of mechanical impedance,[42] near-infrared spectroscopy,[43] and thallium stress testing.[44] These are mostly research methods, and none have proven useful in diagnosing acute compartment syndrome. In a comparative study, Dickson et al found that the specificity of the noninvasive measurement of hardness compared with traditional invasive pressure measurement (0.82 vs 0.96) was too poor to support the use of the hardness monitor in the diagnosis of compartment syndrome.[45] Improved methods for the accurate diagnosis of acute compartment syndrome are needed.

Pearl

- The diagnosis of compartment syndrome depends upon a high degree of suspicion and careful, repeated, documented clinical examination. Decreased sensation in the first web space is often the earliest sign of compartment syndrome in the leg, indicating dysfunction of the deep peroneal nerve due to elevated pressure in the anterior compartment. However, pain is the most obvious symptom of compartment syndrome. Because pain is not easily assessed in the sedated, intoxicated, or head-injured patient, routine pressure monitoring is indicated in these conditions. The safest "threshold" for diagnosing compartment syndrome based on intramuscular pressures seems to be the perfusion pressure, calculated as ΔP = diastolic blood pressure minus intramuscular pressure. Using this definition, fasciotomy should be considered whenever $\Delta P \leq 30$ mm Hg.

Nonoperative Treatment

Several nonsurgical techniques for the treatment of compartment syndrome have been studied, but none are routinely successful, and the recommended treatment for acute compartment syndrome is surgical fasciotomy. Successful nonoperative management of compartment syndrome following rattlesnake envenomation has been reported; this indication in particular may be one of the few circumstances in which nonoperative treatment of recognized compartment syndrome may be initially considered.[46] Hutton et al demonstrated in dogs that compartment pressures returned to 0 after 2 hours of treatment with intravenous hypertonic mannitol.[47] Gershuni et al used intramuscular injections of hyaluronidase to decrease intracompartmental pressures in a canine model of compartment syndrome.[48] Christenson and Wulff demonstrated that diuretics seem to lower anterior leg compartment pressures after injury and/or surgery and recommended diuretic treatment in patients with injuries to the lower limb.[49] In an animal model, Odland et al were able to use tissue ultrafiltration to reduce intramuscular pressure; the removed tissue fluid had dramatically elevated levels of creatine phosphokinase and lactate dehydrogenase, suggesting that measurement of muscle enzymes may have diagnostic implications.[50] Finally, hyperbaric oxygen may have a role in the treatment of compartment syndrome by maintaining cellular adenosine triphosphate (ATP) levels,[51] but its practical application may be limited. Pneumatic foot compression stockings have also been shown to have some utility in preventing compartment syndrome in high-risk patients.[52]

Surgical Treatment

Once identified, compartment syndrome is treated by prompt fasciotomy **(Fig. 3–2A,B)**. A longitudinal incision of the fascia that spans the length of the involved muscle allows the muscle to swell out of the restricting fascial

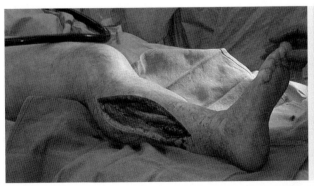
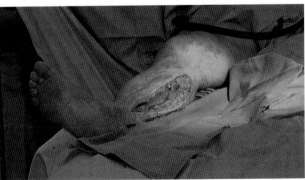

A   B

Figure 3–2 Clinical photos of the same right leg after **(A)** medial and **(B)** lateral fasciotomies were performed.

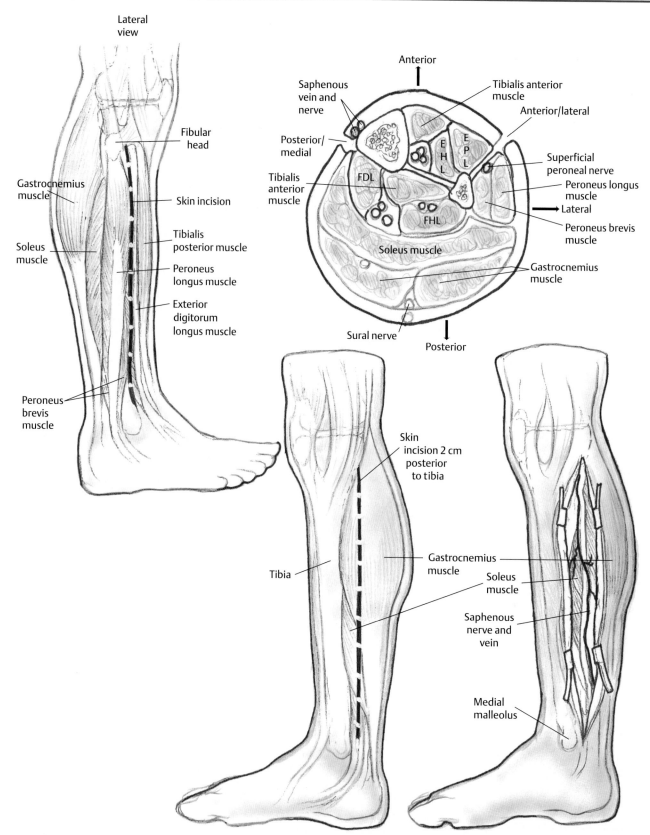

Figure 3–3 Illustration of the two-incision technique of fasciotomy in the lower extremity for management of compartment syndrome. Long lateral and medial incisions are required, with care to avoid neurovascular structures at risk. The upper right panel shows a cross section of the leg depicting the release of two compartments from each incision. Through the lateral incision, the anterior and lateral compartments may be released on each side of the intermuscular septum. On the medial side, the superficial and deep posterior compartments are readily released as shown. EDL, exterior digitorum longus; G, gastrocnemius muscle; T, tibia; PRM, peroneus brevis muscle.

envelope, resulting in decompression of the muscular compartment. The outcomes for early fasciotomy have been satisfactory.[53] Some authors recommend the liberal use of fasciotomy as a prophylaxis against compartment syndrome.[54] However, there are several potential complications that are associated with fasciotomy. If fasciotomy is done, the patient will receive one or two 20 to 30 cm scars, a prolonged hospital stay, further surgery to close the wound, increased risk of infection, measurable impairment of calf muscle function, and possibly chronic venous insufficiency.[31,55–57]

The success of a fasciotomy in preventing tissue and nerve damage is highly dependent upon a proper and timely diagnosis. Early diagnosis of compartment syndrome and prompt fasciotomy have been shown to lead to more rapid union and improved function in patients with tibial fractures.[19,32] In contrast, if fasciotomy is done late, there may be little benefit of the procedure, and delayed fasciotomy may actually be harmful.[58] Fasciotomy that is performed after myonecrosis has occurred only serves to expose necrotic tissue to potential bacterial colonization and possibly infection. Finkelstein et al reviewed five patients with compartment syndrome that had fasciotomy performed more than 35 hours after their injury and who, in retrospect, had a missed diagnosis of compartment syndrome or didn't arrive at their center until long after clinical symptoms of compartment syndrome were present. Of these five patients, one died of multiorgan failure, and the other four all had to have their limbs amputated because of localized wound sepsis (three cases) or an insensate, functionless foot (one case).[58]

> **Pearl**
>
> • There are no clear alternatives to fasciotomy, even in early or borderline cases. Fasciotomies must include an adequate skin incision in addition to the fascial release.

Fasciotomy

Wherever performed, fasciotomy must be done through one or more generous skin incisions with release of all constricting tissues. The specific incisions to be made and the structures that require release vary depending on the involved limb. Subcutaneous fasciotomy is not appropriate for acute compartment syndrome.[59] Because compartment syndrome must be treated promptly, fasciotomy may be performed even when the diagnosis is uncertain. Despite the complications of performing fasciotomy, surgeons will appropriately choose to perform a fasciotomy that may be unnecessary rather than miss a potential compartment syndrome.[41]

Two-Incision Leg Fasciotomy

Fasciotomy of the leg is often performed with two incisions, one medial and one lateral **(Figs. 3–2A,B; 3–3)** (see **Video 3–1, Disk 1**). Two incisions are used because it is simpler to release the deep posterior compartment of the leg from the medial side **(Fig. 3–4).** The lateral incision is used to decompress the anterior and lateral compartments **(Fig. 3–5)** (see **Video 3–2, Disk 1**). The superficial posterior compartment may be released from either incision. At least one of the two incisions—typically the lateral one—must span the length of the compartment to ensure that an adequate release of the skin has been done. Inadequate skin incision may lead to persistent elevation of the intramuscular pressure.[60] When the two-incision technique is used, the intervening skin flap may be at jeopardy if there has been damage to the anterior tibial artery. If anterior tibial artery injury is recognized before surgery, a single-incision four-compartment release may be more appropriate (see next section).

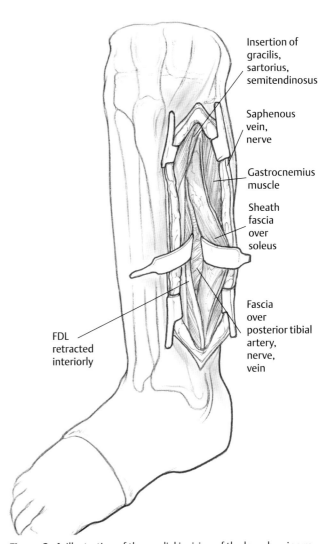

Insertion of gracilis, sartorius, semitendinosus

Saphenous vein, nerve

Gastrocnemius muscle

Sheath fascia over soleus

Fascia over posterior tibial artery, nerve, vein

FDL retracted interiorly

Figure 3–4 Illustration of the medial incision of the leg, showing release of the superficial and deep posterior compartments.

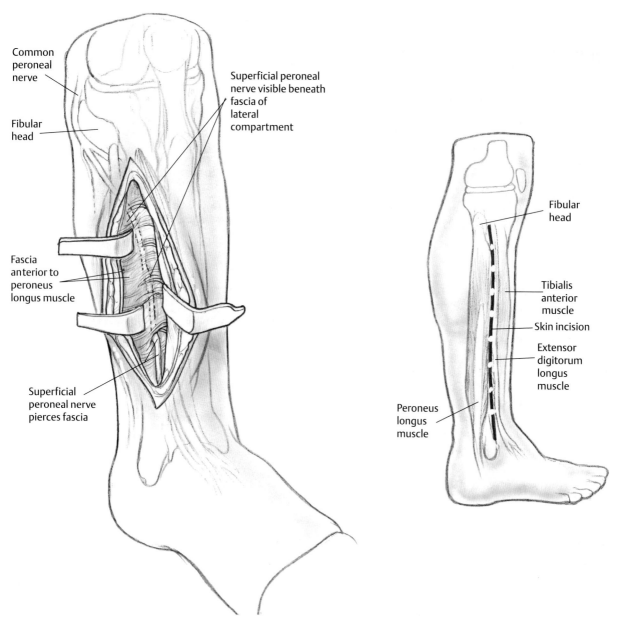

Figure 3–5 Illustration of the lateral incision of the leg, showing release of the anterior and lateral compartments.

The lateral incision is made at or anterior to the midlateral axis of the leg, midway between the fibula and anterior crest of the tibia (**Fig. 3–5**). The skin flaps are elevated by sharp dissection anteriorly and posteriorly, exposing the fascia of the anterior and lateral compartments. The fascia over the peroneal muscles is released (**Fig. 3–6**). The lateral intermuscular septum that divides the anterior and lateral compartments and the superficial peroneal nerve are identified (**Fig. 3–7**). Finally, the fascia over the anterior compartment is completely released (**Fig. 3–8**). Alternatively, the fascia overlying one compartment can be released followed by division of the intermuscular septum to decompress the other compartment. However, iatrogenic injury to the superficial peroneal nerve may be more likely with this technique.[34]

Next, a medial incision is made one fingerbreadth behind the posteromedial border of the tibia (**Fig. 3–4**). The saphenous nerve and vein should be identified. The fascia of the gastrocnemius–soleus complex should be completely released. Proximally, the soleus bridge should be released to identify and decompress the proximal portions of the flexor digitorum longus and posterior tibialis muscles. These components of the deep compartment should also be completely released.

Single-Incision Leg Fasciotomy (see Video 3–2, Disk 1)

Fasciotomy of the leg may also be performed with a single lateral incision, which should extend from the neck of the

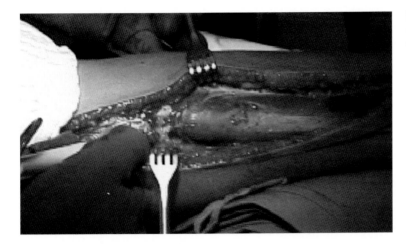

Figure 3–6 Intraoperative photo as the lateral compartment release is performed from distal to proximal. Note the typical bulging appearance of the muscle.

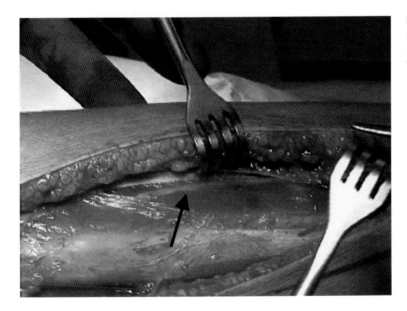

Figure 3–7 Photo after release of the lateral compartment, showing the superficial peroneal nerve (arrow). The nerve is vulnerable, and care must be taken to avoid injury to it.

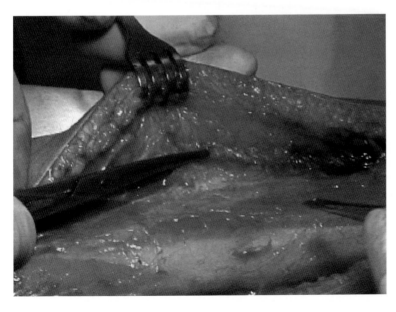

Figure 3–8 Clinical photo of the same leg showing release of the anterior compartment by a separate fasciotomy performed anterior to the intermuscular septum.

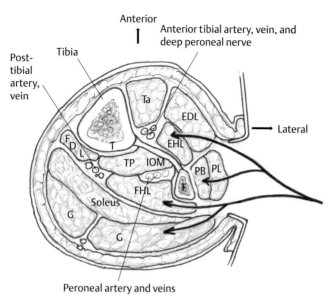

Figure 3–9 Illustration of the cross-sectional anatomy of the parafibular approach for single-incision, four-compartment release in the leg.

fibula to the lateral malleolus **(Fig. 3–5)**. Fibulectomy has been advocated in the past but is not necessary.[34] The anterior and lateral compartments are released in the same manner already described. The superficial posterior compartment, consisting of the gastrocnemius–soleus muscle complex, is easily released by elevating the skin posteriorly. Finally, a parafibular approach **(Fig. 3–9)** is used to decompress the deep posterior leg compartments. The peroneal muscles are retracted anteriorly, and the dissection is carried posterior to the fibula. With the lateral head of the gastrocnemius and soleus retracted posteriorly, the septum dividing the superficial and deep posterior compartments can be identified and released. If access to the deep posterior compartment is difficult, a medial incision can always be made as described earlier.

Pearl

- Although a single-incision fasciotomy can be a little more difficult, it is especially valuable in cases of compartment syndrome that are associated with a tibial plateau or tibial plafond fracture. These injuries are often associated with significant soft tissue injury and are often treated with plating techniques. In these circumstances, avoiding a second incision is very helpful in limiting further soft tissue injury. Finally, in these cases fasciotomy incisions should be planned with the later incisions that are needed for fracture fixation in mind.

Thigh Fasciotomy

A lateral thigh incision is made beginning just distal to the greater trochanter and extending to the lateral epicondyle. With subcutaneous dissection, the iliotibial band is exposed and divided longitudinally. The vastus lateralis is identified and its investing fascia opened. With a Cobb elevator, the muscle fibers of the vastus lateralis are teased off the lateral intermuscular septum, making sure to cauterize the perforating vessels as they are encountered. Make a 1 to 2 cm incision in the lateral intermuscular septum, and using Metzenbaum scissors, extend it proximally and distally the length of the incision to decompress the posterior (hamstring) compartment. After the anterior and posterior compartments have been released from the lateral side, palpate or measure the pressure of the medial (adductor) compartment. If elevated, make a separate medial incision to release the adductor compartment.

Upper Extremity Fasciotomy

Compartment syndrome in the upper extremity can involve the upper arm, the forearm, and/or the hand. All involved compartments should be released. When needed, the anterior release of the biceps/brachialis can be extended across the elbow and incorporated into a volar fasciotomy of the forearm. If necessary, the volar forearm release can also be extended into the palm of the hand to release the median (carpal tunnel) and ulnar nerves (Guyon's canal) **(Fig. 3–10)**.

To decompress the upper arm, an anterior incision is made along the medial side of the biceps. The fascia of the biceps and underlying brachialis are easily released. At the elbow, the incision should be carried across the flexor crease of the elbow in a zigzag fashion to avoid later contracture. The incision is then carried distally over the volar aspect of the forearm as needed. If necessary, the triceps are decompressed from a separate posterior incision.

To decompress the forearm adequately, numerous potential sites of constriction need to be released, including the lacertus fibrosus, the muscle fascia, and the flexor retinaculum. The incision should be carried along the medial border of the "mobile wad" toward the wrist. The mobile wad, consisting of the brachioradialis and radial wrist extensors, is released. The fascia of the finger flexors, supinator, and pronator quadratus are all released as needed. A separate dorsal fasciotomy can be performed if needed. Ronel et al evaluated four different approaches to release of the deep muscles of the forearm in 10 cadavers and attempted to define the approach that would cause the least damage to surrounding vessels, nerves, and muscles.[61] According to their findings, an ulnar approach to the deep space of the volar forearm is simple, results in the least iatrogenic surgical injury, and provides adequate access to the deep volar forearm structures.[61] The plane of dissection is between the flexor carpi ulnaris and the flexor

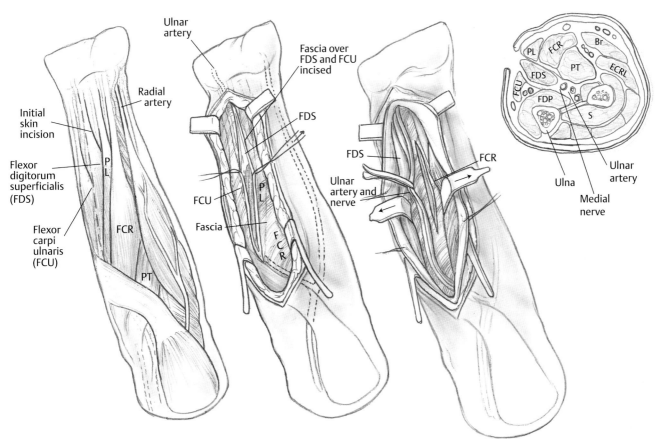

Figure 3–10 Illustration of sequential releases during volar fasciotomy of the forearm.

digitorum superficialis. It is necessary to divide one or two distal branches of the ulnar artery to the distal flexor digitorum superficialis in order expose the pronator quadratus. In the middle third of the forearm, the ulnar neurovascular bundle is elevated with the flexor digitorum superficialis to expose the flexor digitorum profundus and the flexor pollicis longus. This approach to the deep space requires no sharp dissection. In the dorsal forearm, a mid-line approach between the extensor digitorum communis and the extensor carpi radialis brevis is simple and safe.[61]

At the wrist, a standard carpal tunnel release is per-formed. If the forearm is also released, the incisions are carried across the wrist flexion crease in a zigzag fashion to avoid contracture. Injury to the palmar cutaneous branch of the median nerve must be avoided.

Finally, release of the thenar, hypothenar, and in-terosseous muscles of the hand are performed via short longitudinal incisions. Two dorsal hand incisions made between the second to third and fourth to fifth metacarpals are sufficient.

Foot Fasciotomy

The need for fasciotomy of the foot is debated, with some experts saying that compartment syndrome of the foot is often missed, whereas others feel that the morbidity of foot fasciotomy exceeds that of the sequelae of untreated foot compartment syndrome, namely clawing of the toes.

The foot has numerous functional compartments, but it seems that the abductor hallucis, interosseus muscles, and quadrator plantae (calcaneal compartment) are worthy of specific fasciotomy when compartment syndrome of the foot is diagnosed. As in the hand, the interosseous muscles are easily released with two dorsal longitudinal incisions. The abductor hallucis is released via a medial incision along the first ray, along with the quadratus plantae.

Management of Fasciotomy Wounds

There are many possible methods to manage a wound fol-lowing fasciotomy. Traditionally, such wounds are covered with sterile, moist gauze until they are ready for delayed closure or skin grafting (**Fig. 3–11**). Fasciotomy closure be-fore 5 days is not recommended and can be associated with recurrent compartment syndrome.[62] Fasciotomy closure with skin grafting is associated with fewer wound compli-cations than either primary or delayed wound closure.[63] Dermatotraction with simple vessel loops, prepositioned sutures, or commercially available skin closure devices may allow delayed wound closure without surgery or risk of

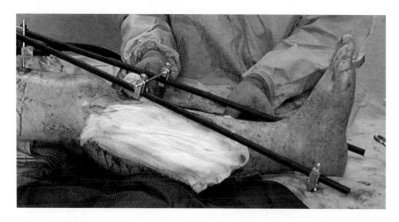

Figure 3–11 Clinical photograph of a leg fasciotomy covered with sterile, moist gauze.

recurrent compartment syndrome.[56,64] A recent advance in the management of fasciotomy wounds is the Vacuum Assisted Wound Closure (V.A.C. Therapy, Kinetic Concepts Inc., San Antonio, Texas). This is applied at the time of fasciotomy and may allow earlier fasciotomy closure and decreased need for skin grafting **(Fig. 3–12).** Clinical results of fasciotomy management with the Wound V.A.C. have not yet been published.

Outcomes

The outcome of compartment syndrome is difficult to determine because the associated injury may itself contribute to adverse outcomes.[65] There has been very little published that specifically addresses the influence of fasciotomy on patient outcomes. After fasciotomy, mortality rates of 11 to 15% and amputations in 11 to 21% of patients have been reported.[66] The outcome of patients with tibia fractures has been related to the timing of fasciotomy.[32,67] In a study of 25 patients with tibia fractures, one group that underwent continuous pressure monitoring had fas-

ciotomies performed at a mean of 16 hours after injury compared with 32 hours in those that weren't monitored. Ten of 11 patients in the delayed group had either or both muscle weakness and contractures at follow-up, as well as a higher risk of fracture healing complications.[32]

Mullett et al reviewed 17 cases of compartment syndrome associated with tibial shaft fractures at an average of 24 months' follow-up.[67] All patients had undergone reamed intramedullary nail using skeletal traction, and fasciotomies were performed at an average interval of 11 hours after nailing. Results were good in 10 cases, fair in four cases, and poor in the remaining three cases. Patients who had decompression within 12 hours had a good functional outcome. Patients with poor results were all treated at an interval greater than 24 hours. In another series of five patients that had markedly delayed fasciotomy (average ischemic time of 56 hours), the result was uniformly poor with one death and four amputations.[58]

Giannoudis et al performed a comprehensive outcomes analysis of 30 patients with compartment syndrome related to tibial shaft fractures.[68] All of these patients completed a standardized general outcomes score (the Euro-Qol), at a minimum of 1 year following injury. Patients were compared with age- and gender-related normative values obtained from a random cohort of patients with isolated closed tibial shaft fractures. Patients bothered by the appearance of the incision reported significantly poorer health-related quality of life than did other patients. Patients with skin grafts had more problems with pain and discomfort than those without skin grafts. Patients that had earlier wound closure demonstrated significantly better self-rated health status than did patients whose wounds were closed later. The authors felt that compartment syndrome may be associated with long-term impact on health-related quality of life.[68]

Heemskerk and Kitslaar reviewed 40 successive cases of lower extremity fasciotomy.[66] The mortality in this series was 15%, and patients had serious overall morbidity. The only factor that was predictive of a poor outcome was patient age greater than 50 years; the underlying diagnosis did not contribute to the results after fasciotomy.[66] In this series, 45% of the patients had good limb function, 28% had

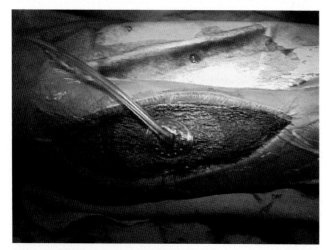

Figure 3–12 Clinical photograph of a leg fasciotomy covered with a Vacuum Assisted Wound Closure (V.A.C. Therapy, Kinetic Concepts Inc., San Antonio, Texas).

successfully salvaged limbs with diminished function, 12% underwent amputation, and 15% died.[66]

Complications

Complications of compartment syndrome are common, especially if the diagnosis is delayed or missed. Once irreversible myoneural ischemia occurs, patients have some degree of permanent neurological deficit and muscle dysfunction. Depending on the degree of muscle involvement, outcomes can range from mild weakness to ischemic contractures. Clawing of the toes is the frequent result of an untreated deep posterior compartment syndrome of the leg. If there is a sufficient volume of ischemic muscle, a so-called crush syndrome may result, with rhabdomyolysis, acute renal failure, and shock. In this circumstance, medical management with alkalinization of the urine and mannitol therapy are usually sufficient to avoid renal complications; rarely amputation of the involved extremity may be life saving.

When the diagnosis of compartment syndrome following a closed injury is delayed more than 12 to 24 hours, surgical treatment is contraindicated unless crush syndrome occurs that is unresponsive to medical management. The likely sequelae of severe sepsis that ensues following such surgery is a potentially life- and limb-threatening complication that is worse than the late muscle fibrosis that would occur with nonoperative management.[58]

Unfortunately, patients with compartment syndrome who have undergone appropriate fasciotomy may have complications as well. Some patients develop chronic venous insufficiency after leg fasciotomy.[55] Fasciotomy is also associated with wound healing complications, neurological or vascular injury, and infection. In one series, nerve damage occurred in 15%, excessive bleeding in 35%, and wound infection in 25%.[66] In another series of fasciotomies performed primarily following repairs of vascular trauma, wound-healing complications occurred in 29 of 73 (40%) fasciotomy cases.[63] Wound complications were especially common in patients that had postoperative arterial or venous thrombosis.[63]

New Techniques

There are several technologies that may soon improve the diagnosis of compartment syndrome. First, improved understanding of the pathophysiology of tissue ischemia may lead to the development of methods to lessen or even prevent tissue damage from occurring as a result of elevated intramuscular pressure. For example, Kearns et al recently demonstrated that pretreatment with vitamin C before fasciotomy reduced the expression of intercellular adhesion molecule-1, reduced infiltration of neutrophils, lessened tissue edema, and preserved muscle function in an animal model.[69]

As discussed earlier, imaging currently has no real role in the diagnosis of compartment syndrome. Several different imaging modalities may become more useful in the future. MRI is capable of demonstrating abnormal changes in muscle architecture in patients with impending or existing compartment syndrome.[40] Real-time measurement of microcirculatory function with a thermodiffusion probe demonstrates abnormalities that resolve with fasciotomy.[70]

Currently, the diagnosis depends on clinical assessment often supplemented by measurement of intramuscular pressure. Two technologies are available that may allow noninvasive assessment of impending tissue compromise. First, it is possible to measure muscle hypoxemia with use of transcutaneous near-infrared spectroscopy. A small clinical series demonstrated low muscle oxygen saturation that recovered following fasciotomy.[71] Second, an ultrasonic device that uses a pulsed phase-locked loop to measure submicron displacements of the fascia wall can detect changes in compartment diameter resulting from intramuscular pressure (IMP) changes of as little as 1 mm Hg in cadaveric tests.[72] Such devices have the potential to become inexpensive, noninvasive, and portable options to current methods for diagnosing acute compartment syndrome.

At present, fasciotomy remains the only available method to treat acute compartment syndrome. Tissue ultrafiltration has shown promise in animal models,[50] and human clinical trials of this are under way in patients with tibial fractures. So-called small-volume resuscitation with hypertonic saline improves microcirculatory function and lessens the inflammatory response in models of crush syndrome.[73] In the future, a combination of pharmacological interventions (ascorbate, superoxide dismutase), small-volume resuscitation, tissue ultrafiltration, intermittent plantar compression, and other modalities may allow for nonoperative management of many cases of impending or early compartment syndrome. Improved methods of diagnosis will allow the surgeon to identify those patients that need immediate fasciotomy and those that might be salvaged nonoperatively.

On the DVDs

Video 3–1   (Disk 1)   Two-Incision Leg Fasciotomy   This video shows the dual-incision technique for four-compartment release of the leg.

Video 3–2   (Disk 1)   Single-Incision Leg Fasciotomy   This video shows a four-compartment release of the leg from a single lateral incision, followed by application of a wound VAC to the wound.

References

1. Hayden JW. Compartment syndromes: early recognition and treatment. Postgrad Med 1983;74:191–202
2. Field CK, SenKowsky J, Hollier LH, et al. Fasciotomy in vascular trauma: it is too much, too often? Am Surg 1994; 60:409–411
3. Templeman D, Varecka T, Schmidt R. Economic costs of missed compartment syndromes. Paper 212, 60th Annual Meeting, American Academy of Orthopaedic Surgeons, San Francisco, CA. Feb. 1993
4. Bhattacharyya T, Vrahas MS. The medical-legal aspects of compartment syndrome. J Bone Joint Surg Am 2004;86-A:864–868
5. Hope MJ, McQueen MM. Acute compartment syndrome in the absence of fracture. J Orthop Trauma 2004;18:220–224
6. McQueen MM, Christie J, Court-Brown CM. Compartment pressures after intramedullary nailing of the tibia. J Bone Joint Surg Br 1990;72:395–397
7. McQueen MM, Gaston P, Court-Brown CM. Acute compartment syndrome: who is at risk? J Bone Joint Surg Br 2000;82:200–203
8. Yuan PS, Pring ME, Gaynor TP, Mubarak SJ, Newton PO. Compartment syndrome following intramedullary fixation of pediatric forearm fractures. J Pediatr Orthop 2004;24:370–375
9. Bonatus T, Olson SA, Lee S, Chapman MW. Nonreamed locking intramedullary nailing for open fractures of the tibia. Clin Orthop Relat Res 1997;339:58–64
10. Moehring HD, Voigtlander JP. Compartment pressure monitoring during intramedullary nailing of tibial fractures. Orthopedics 1995;18:631–635
11. Woll TS, Duwelius PJ. The segmental tibial fracture. Clin Orthop Relat Res 1992;281:204–207
12. Richards H, Langston A, Kulkarni R, Downes EM. Does patient controlled analgesia delay the diagnosis of compartment syndrome following intramedullary nailing of the tibia? Injury 2004;35:296–298
13. Mubarak SJ, Hargens AR. Acute compartment syndromes. Surg Clin North Am 1983;63:539–565
14. Rorabeck CH. The treatment of compartment syndromes of the leg. J Bone Joint Surg Br 1984;66:93–97
15. Murthy BV, Narayan B, Nayagam S. Reduced perception of pain in schizophrenia: its relevance to the clinical diagnosis of compartment syndrome. Injury 2004;35:1192–1193
16. Hargens AR, Mubarak SJ. Current concepts in the pathophysiology, evaluation and diagnosis of compartment syndrome. Hand Clin 1998;14:371–383
17. Heckman MM, Whitesides TE, Grewe SR, Judd RL, Miller M, Lawrence JH. Histologic determination of the ischemic threshold of muscle in the canine compartment syndrome model. J Orthop Trauma 1993;7:199–210
18. Mars M, Hadley GP. Raised intracompartmental pressure and compartment syndrome. Injury 1998;29:403–411
19. McQueen MM, Court-Brown CM. Compartment monitoring in tibial fractures: the pressure threshold for decompression. J Bone Joint Surg Br 1996;78:99–104
20. Ovre S, Hvaal K, Holm I, Stromsoe K, Nordsletten L, Skjeldal S. Compartment pressure in nailed tibial fractures: a threshold of 30 mm Hg for decompression gives 29% fasciotomies. Arch Orthop Trauma Surg 1998;118:29–31
21. Pearse MF, Harry L, Nanchahal J. Acute compartment syndrome of the leg. BMJ 2002;325:557–558
22. Sterk J, Schierlinger M, Gerngross H, Willy C. Intracompartmental pressure measurement in acute compartment syndrome: results of a survey of indications, measuring technique and critical pressure value [in German]. Unfallchirurg 2001;104:119–126

23. Ulmer T. The clinical diagnosis of compartment syndrome of the lower leg: are clinical findings predictive of the disorder? J Orthop Trauma 2002;16:572–577
24. Williams PR, Russell ID, Mintowt-Cyzy WJ. Compartment pressure monitoring: current UK orthopaedic practice. Injury 1998;29:229–232
25. Willy C, Sterk J, Volker HU, et al. Acute compartment syndrome: results of a clinico-experimental study of pressure and time limits for emergency fasciotomy [in German]. Unfallchirurg 2001; 104:381–391
26. Uliasz A, Ishida JT, Fleming JK, Yamamoto LG. Comparing the methods of measuring compartment pressures in acute compartment syndrome. Am J Emerg Med 2003;21:143–145
27. Whitesides TE, Haney TC, Morimoto K, Harada H. Tissue pressure measurements as a determinant for the need for fasciotomy. Clin Orthop Relat Res 1975;113:43–51
28. Wilson SC, Vrahas MS, Berson L, Paul EM. A simple method to measure compartment pressures in using an intravenous catheter. Orthopedics 1997;20:403–406
29. Janzing HM, Broos PLO. Routine monitoring of compartment pressure in patients with tibial fractures: beware of overtreatment! Injury 2001;32:415–421
30. Matsen FA 3rd, Winquist RA, Krugmire RB Jr. Diagnosis and management of compartment syndromes. J Bone Joint Surg Am 1980; 62:286–291
31. Mubarak SJ, Owen CA. Double-incision fasciotomy of the leg for decompression in compartment syndromes. J Bone Joint Surg Am 1977;59:184–187
32. McQueen MM, Christie J, Court-Brown CM. Acute compartment syndrome in tibial diaphyseal fractures. J Bone Joint Surg Br 1996;78:95–98
33. White TO, Howell GED, Will EM, Court-Brown CM, McQueen MM. Elevated intramuscular compartment pressures do not influence outcome after tibial fracture. J Trauma 2003;55:1133–1138
34. Tornetta P III, Templeman D. Instructional Course Lectures, The American Academy of Orthopaedic Surgeons—Compartment syndrome associated with tibial fracture. J Bone Joint Surg Am 1996;78A:1438–1444
35. Heckman MM, Whitesides TE Jr, Grewe SR, Rooks MD. Compartment pressure in association with closed tibia fractures: the relationship between tissue pressure, compartment, and the distance from the site of the fracture. J Bone Joint Surg Am 1994;76: 1285–1292
36. Kumar P, Salil B, Bhaskara KG, Agrawal A. Compartment syndrome: effect of limb position on pressure measurement. Burns 2003;29:626
37. Heppenstall RB, Scott R, Sapega A, et al. Comparative study of the study of the tolerance of skeletal muscle to ischemia: tourniquet application compared with acute compartment syndrome. J Bone Joint Surg Am 1986;68:820–828
38. Gulli B, Templeman D. Compartment syndrome of the lower extremity. Orthop Clin North Am 1994;25:677–684
39. Meyer RS, White KK, Smith JM, Groppo ER, Mubarak SJ, Hargens AR. Intramuscular and blood pressures in legs positioned in the hemilithotomy position: clarification of risk factors for well-leg acute compartment syndrome. J Bone Joint Surg Am 2002;84-A:1829–1835
40. Rominger MB, Lukosch CJ, Bachmann GF. MR imaging of compartment syndrome of the lower leg: a case control study. Eur Radiol 2004;14:1432–1439
41. Steinberg BD, Gelberman RH. Evaluation of limb compartment with suspected increased interstitial pressure: a noninvasive method for determining quantitative hardness. Clin Orthop Relat Res 1994;300:248–253

42. Winckler S, Reder U, Ruland O, Lunkenheimer PP. Mechanical impedance: a new noninvasive method for measuring tissue pressure in anterior compartment syndrome. II. Results of clinical measurements in patients with tibial trauma [in German]. Unfallchirurg 1991;94:28–32

43. Garr JL, Gentilello LM, Cole PA, Mock CN, Matsen FA. Monitoring for compartmental syndrome using near-infrared spectroscopy: a noninvasive continuous transcutaneous monitoring technique. J Trauma 1999;46:613–618

44. Trease L, van Every B, Bennell K, et al. A prospective blinded evaluation of exercise thallium-201 SPET in patients with suspected chronic exertional compartment syndrome of the leg. Eur J Nucl Med 2001;28:688–695

45. Dickson KF, Sullivan MJ, Steinberg B, Myers L, Anderson ER, Harris M. Noninvasive measurement of compartment syndrome. Orthopedics 2003;26:1215–1218

46. Gold BS, Barish RA, Dart RC, Silverman RP, Bochicchio GV. Resolution of compartment syndrome after rattlesnake envenomation utilizing non-invasive measures. J Emerg Med 2003;24:285–288

47. Hutton M, Rhodes RS, Chapman G. The lowering of postischemic compartment pressures with mannitol. J Surg Res 1982;32:239–242

48. Gershuni DH, Hargens AR, Lieber RL. Decompression of an experimental compartment syndrome in dogs with hyaluronidase. Clin Orthop Relat Res 1985;197:295–300

49. Christenson JT, Wulff K. Compartment pressure following leg injury: the effect of diuretic treatment. Injury 1985;16:591–594

50. Odland R, Schmidt AH, Hunter B, et al. Use of tissue ultrafiltration for treatment of compartment syndrome: a pilot study using porcine hindlimbs. J Orthop Trauma 2005;19:267–275

51. Kindwall EP, Gottlieb LJ, Larson DL. Hyperbaric oxygen therapy in plastic surgery: a review article. Plast Reconstr Surg 1991;88:898–908

52. Gardner AM, Fox RH, Lawrence C, Bunker TD, Ling RS, MacEachern AG. Reduction of post-traumatic swelling and compartment pressure by impulse compression of the foot. J Bone Joint Surg Br 1990;72:810–815

53. Lagerstrom CF, Reed RL II, Rowlands BJ, Fischer RP. Early fasciotomy for acute clinically evident posttraumatic compartment syndrome. Am J Surg 1989;158:36–39

54. Ernst CB. Fasciotomy-in perspective. J Vasc Surg 1989;9:829–830

55. Bermudez K, Knudson MM, Morabito D, Kessel O. Fasciotomy, chronic venous insufficiency, and the calf muscle pump. Arch Surg 1998;133:1356–1361

56. Janzing HM, Broos PL. Dermatotraction: an effective technique for the closure of fasciotomy wounds: a preliminary report of fifteen patients. J Orthop Trauma 2001;15:438–441

57. Mubarak SJ. Etiologies of compartment syndromes. In: Mubarak SJ, Hargens AR, Akeson WH, eds. Compartment Syndromes and Volkmann's Contracture, Vol. 3. Saunders Monographs in Clinical Orthopedics. Philadelphia: WB Saunders; 1981:71–97

58. Finkelstein JA, Hunter GA, Hu RW. Lower limb compartment syndrome: course after delayed fasciotomy. J Trauma 1996;40:342–344

59. Illig KA, Ouriel K, DeWeese JA, Shortell CK, Green RM. A condemnation of subcutaneous fasciotomy. Mil Med 1998;163:794–796

60. Cohen MS, Garfin SR, Hargens AR, Mubarak SJ. Acute compartment syndrome: effect of dermotomy on fascial decompression in the leg. J Bone Joint Surg Br 1991;73:287–290

61. Ronel DN, Mtui E, Nolan WB. Forearm compartment syndrome: anatomical analysis of surgical approaches to the deep space. Plast Reconstr Surg 2004;114:697–705

62. Wiger P, Tkaczuk P, Styf J. Secondary wound closure following fasciotomy for acute compartment syndrome increases intramuscular pressure. J Orthop Trauma 1998;12:117–121

63. Johnson SB, Weaver FA, Yellin AE, Kelly R, Bauer M. Clinical results of dermotomy–fasciotomy. Am J Surg 1992;164:286–290

64. Wiger P, Blomqvist G, Styf J. Wound closure by dermatotraction after fasciotomy for acute compartment syndrome. Scand J Plast Reconstr Surg Hand Surg 2000;34:315–320

65. Ellis H. Disabilities after tibial shaft fractures with special reference to Volkmann's ischemic contracture. J Bone Joint Surg Br 1958;40:190–197

66. Heemskerk J, Kitslaar P. Acute compartment syndrome of the lower leg: retrospective study on prevalence, technique, and outcome of fasciotomies. World J Surg 2003;27:744–747

67. Mullett H, Al-Abed K, Prasad CVR, O'Sullivan M. Outcome of compartment syndrome following intramedullary nailing of tibial diaphyseal fractures. Injury 2001;32:411–413

68. Giannoudis PV, Nicolopoulos C, Dinopoulos H, Ng A, Adedapo S, Kind P. The impact of lower leg compartment syndrome on health related quality of life. Injury 2002;33:117–121

69. Kearns SR, Daly AF, Sheehan K, Murray P, Kelly C, Bouchier-Hayes D. Oral vitamin C reduces the injury to skeletal muscle caused by compartment syndrome. J Bone Joint Surg Br 2004;86:906–911

70. Zapletal Ch, Herzog L, Martin G, Klar E, Meeder PJ, Buchholz J. Thermodiffusion for the quantification of tissue perfusion in skeletal muscle-clinical evaluation in standardized traumatological procedures with tourniquet and potential application in the diagnosis of compartment syndrome. Microvasc Res 2003;66:164–172

71. Giannotti G, Cohn SM, Brown M, Varela JE, McKenney MG, Wiseberg JA. Utility of near-infrared spectroscopy in the diagnosis of lower extremity compartment syndrome. J Trauma 2000;48:396–399

72. Lynch JE, Heyman JS, Hargens AR. Ultrasonic device for the noninvasive diagnosis of compartment syndrome. Physiol Meas 2004;25:N1–N9

73. Mittlmeier T, Vollmar B, Menger MD, Schewior L, Raschke M, Schaser KD. Small volume hypertonic hydroxyethyl starch reduces acute microvascular dysfunction after closed soft-tissue trauma. J Bone Joint Surg Br 2003;85:126–132

4 Evolving Concepts in Plate Fixation

Amir Matityahu, Christian Krettek, and Theodore Miclau III

"It is questionable if surgery should not ever be done except by highly trained men, with highly trained assistance, and highly trained hospitals; otherwise disaster is likely to result." This is a quote from a medical referee from the Aetna Insurance Company in 1928[1] after reviewing 34,753 compensation fracture files from Northern California. Plate osteosynthesis is still recognized as the treatment of choice for most articular and metaphyseal fractures and certain diaphyseal fractures. This chapter outlines evolving concepts in plate fixation with attention to mechanics and biological fixation of fractures.

History and Evolution of Plating

The first dynamic compression plate (the modified Collison plate) was introduced by George Bagby in 1956. This plate had oval holes with the distal end of the hole having a vertical slot allowing for motion of the plate relative to the conical screw head.[2] In 1958, 15 Swiss general and orthopedic surgeons met to discuss the status of the poor results obtained with both nonoperative and operative methods of fracture treatment in their country. This meeting led to the formation of the Arbeitsgemeinschaft für Osteosynthesefragen/Association for the Study of Internal Fixation (AO/ASIF). The meeting was initiated by Maurice Müller, who had spent time with Danis and was impressed by his concept of compression and rigid fixation. Four principles seemed clearly instrumental for obtaining optimal results and were accepted as a "working hypothesis." These were anatomical reduction, rigid internal fixation, atraumatic technique on the soft tissue and bone, and early pain-free active mobilization during the first 10 postoperative days.[3] Three years later, E. Müller described the outboard compression plate device.[4] A round-hole bone plate was screwed into the bone on one side of the fracture. On the other side of the fracture, a tension/compression device was screwed into the bone and hooked onto the plate. A nut was then tightened on the device, causing compression across the fracture (**Fig. 4–1**).

Since the inception of the AO/ASIF, plates and plating have evolved significantly with the aim of providing for improved healing. The first self-compression plate devised by the AO was reported in 1963[5] (**Fig. 4–2**). In 1969, the Dynamic Compression Plate (DCP) was designed and introduced for fracture treatment. The plate was similar in design to the Bagby plate, but with several marked improvements.[6-8] These features allowed the use of the DCP as a tension band, neutralization, compression, and buttress plate. Other techniques such as prebending and lag screw fixation were introduced to improve fracture compression and load contact sharing. These methods resulted in rigid fixation, and healing

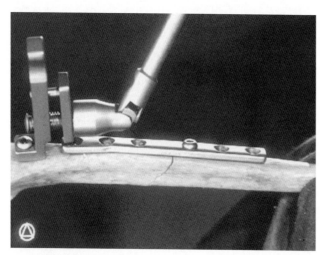

Figure 4–1 Use of a tension/compression device to obtain compression across a fracture. Reproduced with permission from AO International (Publishing).

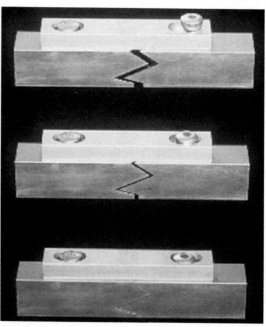

Figure 4–2 Wood blocks used to demonstrate compression achieved by a self-compressing dynamic compression plate. Reproduced with permission from AO International (Publishing).

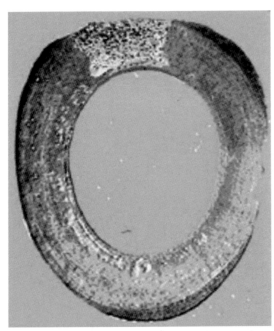

Figure 4–3 Cortical bone necrosis and porosis after removal of a dynamic compression plate. Reproduced with permission from JBJSB 2002:84B:1093–1110.

occurred by direct bone formation, with scarce radiographic callus formation.

The lack of callus in rigidly fixed fractures was described by Bagby and others[9] in animal experiments.[2] At that time, callus was most often viewed as a direct sign of instability, implant overload, and/or fretting corrosion.[10] Using the principles of exact anatomical reduction and absolute stabilization, a wide surgical exposure was necessary. Fracture fragments were often stripped of their soft tissues to achieve precise reconstruction of the bone. Furthermore, the stability of the plate–fracture construct using bicortical screws depends on the friction between the undersurface of the plate and the cortical surface of the underlying bone.[11] This friction increases as the torque of the screw increases.

A common observation after plate osteosynthesis is radiographic bone loss under the plate. Although this phenomenon has been attributed to implant-related stress protection, it has also been linked to transient bone necrosis and internal remodeling beneath the plates. Perren et al showed that porosis is present in areas of disturbed circulation between the plate and the bone (**Fig. 4–3**).[12] They hypothesized that improved circulation beneath the plate would decrease osteoporosis. During the early 1970s, investigators began to study the pressures exerted by plates on bones following compression plate osteosynthesis.[13] They found that the plate exerts an average pressure to the bone of ~7000 N/cm^2. Some postulated that that these findings would be useful in the development of more optimal systems for osteosynthesis.

Subsequent to this work, the Zespol system was developed in Poland and reported on by Ramotowski and Granowski.[14] This system represented the first internal fixator for stabilizing long bones. It used screw heads that

locked into a plate, which offset from the bone and could be used as either an internal or external fixator. The plate did not apply any direct pressure to the underlying bone, thereby preserving the vascularity and avoiding porosis.

In the early 1980s, Brunner and Weber introduced the wave plate[15] (**Figs. 4–4, 4–5**), and Heitemeyer and Hierholzer developed the bridge plate.[16] These plates were designed to span the fracture site, with a plate fixed proximally and distally to the fracture. The wave plate provided the theoretical advantage of avoiding vascular disruption to the injured bone, allowing for the placement of corticocancellous bone graft at the fracture site, and altering the load of the plate to provide pure tension forces. These findings led to the development of plates with more limited plate–bone contact.[17]

The Limited Contact Dynamic Compression Plate (LC-DCP) (Synthes, Paoli, Pennyslvania), introduced by Perren in 1990, was designed to provide less than 50% contact between the plate and the bone (**Fig. 4–6**). Through this decreased contact, it was postulated that the blood supply to the underlying bone would be better preserved, thereby improving rates of fracture healing, decreasing the need for bone grafting, decreasing the incidence of infection and refracture, and decreasing implant-related stress risers following plate removal (**Fig. 4–7**). The design of the plate also has other features, including uniform spacing of the screw holes, a trapezoidal cross section, and symmetric plate holes. These modifications of the dynamic compression plate allow for a more evenly distributed force along the plate, a 40 degree tilt of each screw within the hole, and an ability to change more easily to a plate of different length.[17] Further, the plate was constructed of titanium to improve its tissue tolerance.[18]

Most recently, plating methods have focused on the principles of "biological fixation."[19] The Point Contact Fixator (PC-Fix) (Synthes, Paoli, Pennsylvania) was introduced in 1994. The plate was designed to contact the bone on pointed areas of its undersurface, with significantly less plate–bone contact than the LC-DCP (**Fig. 4–8**). The plate also utilized unicortical screws that locked into the plate and were less disruptive of the intramedullary blood supply than bicortical screws.[11,20,21] Clinical trials using the PC-Fix titanium plates have suggested that the plates are associated with decreased rates of infection.[22–24] PC-Fix–stabilized sheep tibia fractures have been shown to heal faster and with similar strengths to those treated with a DCP.[21] Other mechanical studies have shown that the fixation achieved with the PC-Fix (locked screw–plate–bone construct) is stronger than the DCP (nonlocked conventional screw– plate–bone construct) when applied to cadaveric human femurs.[25]

Fracture Stabilization and Vascularity

Over the past decade, stabilization techniques have evolved to provide for more biologically friendly approaches. Although articular fractures require anatomical

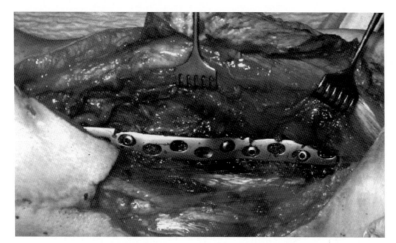

Figure 4–5 Clinical photograph demonstrating surgical application of a wave plate.

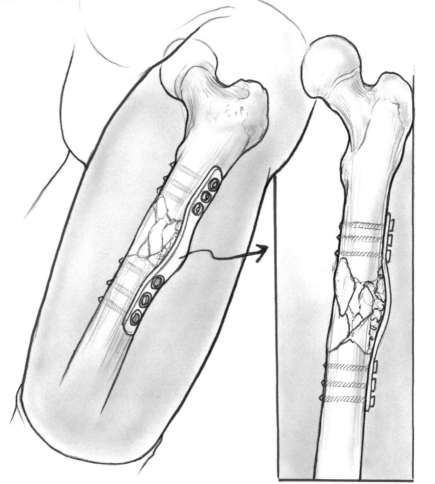

Figure 4–4 Diagram of a wave plate demonstrating spanning the fracture site and avoiding vascular disruption to the injured segment of the bone.

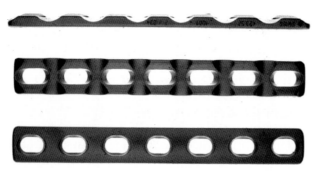

Figure 4–6 The Limited Contact Dynamic Compression Plate provides less than 50% contact between the plate and the injured bone.

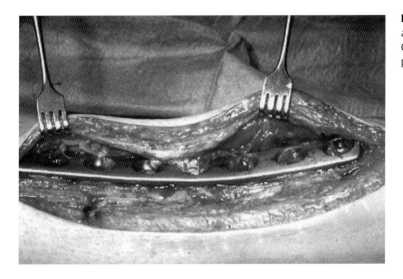

Figure 4–7 Clinical photograph demonstrating healthy and well-perfused bone following removal of a Limited Contact Dynamic Compression Plate. Reproduced with permission from AO International (Publishing).

reduction and stabilization, the extra-articular segments of bone do not require precise positioning and absolutely rigid stabilization. Overall limb alignment, rather than extra-articular fracture fragment position, should be the priority to maximize limb return to function. The wide dissection of multiple metaphyseal and diaphyseal fragments adds to the devitalization of the bone and should be avoided. Successful fracture healing depends on having a blood supply to the injured tissues. Ideally, the design of the implant should facilitate the blood supply to the bone, and the method of fixation should minimize the additional injury caused by surgical stabilization of the fracture.

Locking Plating (see Video 4–1, Disk 1)

There are clear differences between traditional compression plating and stabilization with a locked screw–plate construct. The stability of traditional bicortical screws

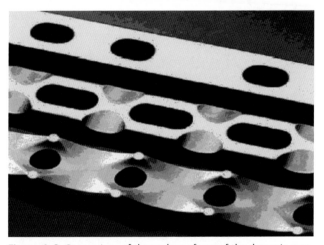

Figure 4–8 Comparison of the undersurfaces of the dynamic compression plate, the Limited Contact Dynamic Compression Plate, and the Point Contact Fixator. Reproduced with permission from JBJSB 2002:84B:1093–1116.

relies on obtaining compression between opposing cortices with the development of friction between the plate and underlying bone and tension along the axis of the screw. As the screw is tightened, there is an increase in compressive force between the plate and the bone, which generates friction between the two and allows for applied force to be transferred along the plate. A tight frictional interface and, ultimately, the pull-out strength of the screws are paramount for successful load transmission. This construct relies on the shear strength of the bone at the screw–thread interface. In patients with high-density bone, higher forces can be generated than in patients with osteopenic bone. When a patient applies a load that exceeds the fixation capacity of the construct, collapse occurs across the fracture site. This collapse is due to the lack of angular stability and subsequent motion between the plate and the screw. With conventional plates, unicortical screws have a significantly lower load-carrying capacity than bicortical screws.

Unlike traditional plating systems utilizing bicortical screws, however, locked screw-plating systems have angular stability, increasing their load-carrying capacity **(Fig. 4–9A,B)**. The angular stability results from the threaded screw head locked into the threaded plate hole, forming a fixed-angle construct. Functionally, each locked screw behaves like a miniature blade plate. The locked screw–plate construct allows for load transmission from the screw to the plate and relies on frictional forces applied from the threaded screw head to the threaded screw hole in the plate. Although the loads applied to conventional and locking plates are the same, the preloads necessary for construct stability are by necessity higher in the conventional plates and screws.

Mechanical studies showed the mechanical advantage of angular stability between a locking plate and screws.[13,26] Miclau et al evaluated the mechanical properties of PC-Fix–stabilized fractures with unicortical locking screws

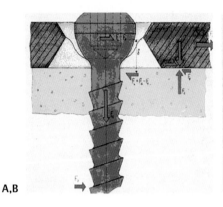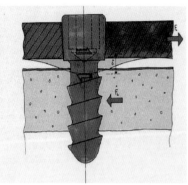

A,B

Figure 4–9 Diagram demonstrating the differences between **(A)** bicortical conventional and **(B)** unicortical locked screws. The bicortical conventional screw depends on the shear strength of the bone at the screw–thread interface for stability. The stability of the unicortical locked screw depends on frictional forces applied from the threaded screw head to the threaded screw hole in the plate. Reproduced with permission from JBJSB 2002:84B:1093–1110.

and compared them with those obtained with conventional bicortical plating in cadaveric sheep tibia.[21] They found no differences in torsional or bending strengths of the constructs. However, it was noted that the PC-Fix–stabilized fractures failed by pull-out of the entire construct compared with the bicortical screw plates that showed individual screw pull-out.[21]

The biomechanical properties of the Less Invasive Stabilization System (LISS) (Synthes, Paoli, Pennsylvania) locking plate have been a subject of recent interest. Marti et al compared the LISS with two conventional plating systems, the Condylar Buttress Plate (CBP) (Synthes, Paoli, Pennsylvania) and Dynamic Condylar Screw (DCS) (Synthes, Paoli, Pennsylvania), for the stabilization of distal femur fractures. They found that the LISS plates had a higher elastic deformation compared with the conventional plating systems, which is likely secondary to the different designs and material properties. However, the LISS plating system demonstrated an improved ability to withstand higher loads than conventional plates.[27] In a later study, lateral plating with the tibia LISS was compared with bilateral plating with conventional plates. Mechanical tests revealed that the LISS plates and bilateral plating constructs showed similar resistance to subsidence of the medial condyle during cyclic loading.[28]

Several investigators have shown that there are specific configurations of locking plates that increase the overall rigidity of the constructs. A study analyzing the configuration of screws with both in vitro and finite element models showed that the near-near, far-far concept of pin placement in external fixators also applies to screw placement in locking plates, which are also commonly referred to as internal fixators.[29] Using 12-hole locking plates with a gap and standardized homogeneous composite cylinders, Stoffel and colleagues were able to elucidate the extent to which an internal fixator can provide stability. The gap size, working length, number and position of screws, plate length, and material properties of the implants were tested for fatigue, axial stiffness, and torsional rigidity. The authors found that using a 12-hole plate with locking screws in the 1, 2, and 6 positions on either side of the fracture gap provided the most significant rigidity. Additional stability is conferred with decreasing distances from the plate to the bone and with increasing lengths of the plate (increased working distances).

Evolution of Minimally Invasive Plating (See Video 4–2, Disk 1)

The concept of indirect reduction evolved from the observation that the bone fragments can successfully heal if they are well vascularized and held out to length. By avoiding the fracture site and minimizing local trauma, the blood supply to the bone is better maintained[30] (**Fig. 4–10A,B**). Indirect reduction and "biological plating" were first performed with the goal of achieving compression across the fracture,[31,32] and later, without compression as an "internal splint."[16] The shift away from absolute stability to other forms of treatment was supported by the observation that fast, successful, and uncomplicated bone healing could be achieved with intramedullary "splinting," as seen with nails.

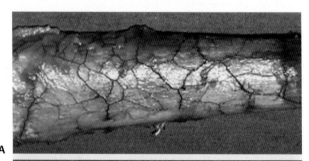

A

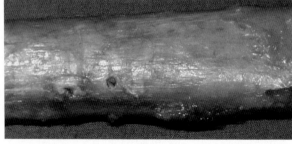

B

Figure 4–10 Blood supply following **(A)** minimally invasive percutaneous plate osteosynthesis compared with **(B)** conventional lateral plating technique demonstrated by a cadaver injection study. Reproduced with permission from Elsevier (Injury 28,S.1:7–12.)

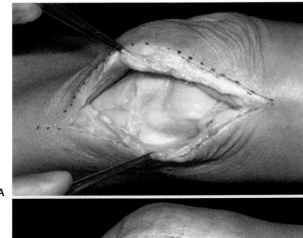

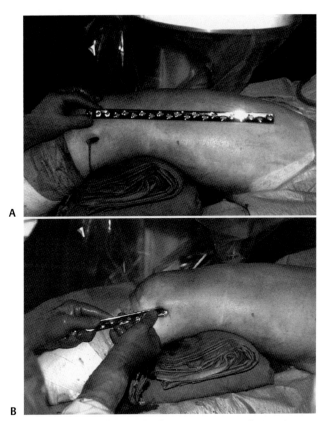

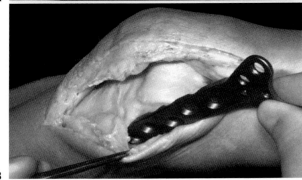

Figure 4–11 Minimally invasive plating using transarticular percutaneous plate osteosynthesis. **(A)** Shows incision and **(B)** submuscular passage. Reproduced with permission from Elsevier (Injury 28,S.1:31–41).

Figure 4–12 Minimally invasive plating using minimally invasive percutaneous plate osteosynthesis. **(A)** Minimal incision, **(B)** shows the submuscular insertion of the plate. Reproduced with permission from Elsevier (Injury 28,S.1:20–30.)

Subsequently, surgeons began to develop more limited approaches to plating fractures, particularly of the femur.[33,34] Krettek and colleagues described several surgical approaches and "minimally invasive" plating techniques for the placement of submuscular plates to treat proximal and distal femur fractures: transarticular retrograde plate osteosynthesis (TARPO)[35] **(Fig. 4–11A,B)** and minimally invasive percutaneous plate osteosynthesis (MIPPO)[36] **(Fig. 4–12A,B)** (see **Video 4–2, Disk 1**). Since that time, a variety of minimally invasive approaches have been described to treat fractures, including the proximal and distal tibia.[37,38] These approaches were designed to introduce conventional bicortical plates (i.e., the dynamic compression, dynamic condylar plate, and condylar buttress plates), through the limited approaches. Because the instrumentation was designed to place these implants through larger incisions, the equipment made the procedures significantly more challenging. With the advent of the locking screws and angularly stable plating systems, implants can be placed on a single column of the femur or tibia and provide sufficient stabilization to the contralateral, unexposed side. More importantly, equipment and systems, such as the LISS, have been designed to facilitate the placement of these locking implants.

Locking Plates and Plating Systems

There are multiple types of plating systems available, ranging from traditional dynamic compression plates to locking-

periarticular plates. Because much has been written already about traditional bicortical plate insertion, this section will focus on some of the more recently introduced locking plates, including the LISS and periarticular locking plates for the distal femur, proximal tibia, distal tibia, and distal radius.

Indications for Locked Plating

The indications for locked plating continue to evolve. For simple metaphyseal fractures that require buttressing, metaphyseal fractures with good opposition, osteotomies, and articular fractures, standard plates with bicortical screws can provide excellent fixation and reliable healing. For comminuted diaphyseal or metaphyseal fractures, however, or in patients with poor bone stock, locking plates are indicated. The distal femur LISS is also useful in the treatment of periprosthetic fractures.

Surgical Technique for the Less-Invasive Stabilization System (see Video 4–3, Disk 1)

The LISS plating system was introduced as a precontoured plate for the distal femur and proximal tibia **(Fig. 4–13)**. The plate was designed for submuscular lateral insertion using an insertion handle and aiming device for the placement of the screws. The plate accommodates multiple angled

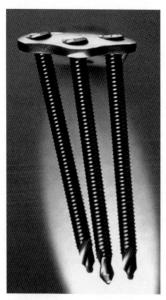

Figure 4–13 Locked plating with divergent screws provides improved stability when compared with conventional plate–screw constructs. The difference is most pronounced in poor quality bone. Reproduced with permission from AO International (Publishing).

self-drilling and self-tapping locked screws in the metaphysis and 5 mm locked unicortical screws in the diaphysis (**Fig. 4–14**). The plate and screws are constructed from a titanium alloy. The LISS is a relatively flexible plate and allows for micromotion at the fracture site, leading to greater callus formation than with rigidly fixed fractures. This motion and callus formation may confer healing benefits. Whether applying the LISS plate to the distal femur or proximal tibia, four major steps are performed: (1) exposure and

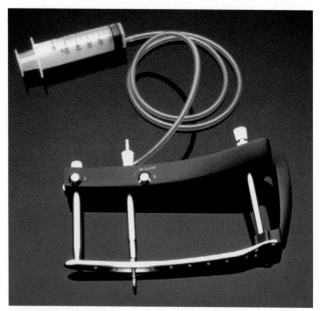

Figure 4–14 The Less Invasive Stabilization System was the initial minimally invasive locked plating system. Reproduced with permission from AO International (Publishing).

reconstruction of the articular fragment, (2) submuscular plate insertion, (3) fixation of the plate to the distal fragment, and (4) percutaneous plate fixation of the plate to the shaft.[39] Advantages of the LISS include decreased vascular disruption of the periosteum; higher elastic deformation of the system, allowing for micromotion and callus formation; increased rigidity in osteopenic bone; anatomical plate contour; and avoidance of a medial buttress plate to prevent varus collapse. Disadvantages of the LISS include a need for technically demanding surgical technique, required fluoroscopic imaging, and the expense of the system.

Less Invasive Stabilization System Femur (see Videos 4–4, 4–5, Disk 1)

The procedure begins with the patient positioned on a radiolucent table with a bump under the ipsilateral buttock. The leg is prepped and draped free. Anteroposterior (AP) and lateral fluoroscopic images are taken before prepping and draping to ensure that there is no impedance to the x-ray beam. A bump is placed under the knee to flex the joint ~40 degrees to relax the calf musculature and assist with reduction. AP and lateral fluoroscopic images should be obtained with the bump in place to assess the effect of varying the placement and size of the bump. Small changes in location and size of the bump can change the reduction of the fracture. The surgeon should also apply manual traction at this time and carefully evaluate the fracture prior to making any incisions.

Once the fracture has been evaluated, an incision is made. A lateral peripatellar incision is used when there is a multifragment intra-articular fracture (**Fig. 4–15A**). A lateral incision is used when the fracture is simple and extra-articular (**Fig. 4–15B**). The iliotibial band is split in line with its fibers. The dissection is carried deeply in line with the incision.

If there is an articular fracture, reduction must be performed first. The articular surface can be visualized through the lateral parapatellar approach with medial reflection of the patella. This approach allows for the visualization of the medial condyle, while avoiding extensive soft tissue retraction near the metaphysis. The articular reduction must be anatomical and performed with rigid lag screw compression of the major fragments. Care must be taken to place the screws so that they do not interfere with the placement of the plate. Once the articular reduction is achieved, the LISS is then inserted in a submuscular fashion along the lateral aspect of the femur with the guide handle (**Fig. 4–16A**). Sliding a Cobb elevator in the submuscular plane prior to inserting the implant may ease the passage. The position of the plate and the reduction are then assessed fluoroscopically. Limb alignment, including length, rotation, varus/valgus alignment, and recurvatum/procarvatum, are evaluated. Once the desired reduction is achieved, the plate is held in place with threaded K-wires distally and proximally through the aiming handle. It is critical to obtain correct length, rotation, and

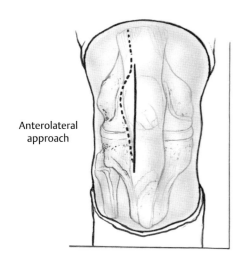

Anterolateral
approach

A

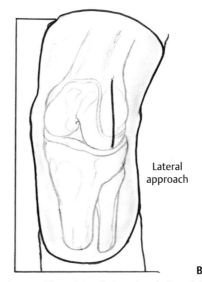

Lateral
approach

B

Figure 4–15 Drawing of the **(A)** anterolateral and **(B)** lateral approaches used for minimally invasive plating of the distal femur.

sagittal plane alignment prior to drilling the threaded wires. Prior to securing the plate to the bone, care must be taken to ensure that the plate position and reduction are satisfactory. Unlike with conventional plates that utilize bicortical screws, the LISS plate is locked into place with the placement of the first screw and is not reduced to the bone with locking screw placement. The pull-reduction device, or "whirlybird," can also be useful to pull fracture fragments to the plate and make adjustments to the varus/valgus alignment prior to screw placement **(Fig. 4–17A,B)**. The whirlybird device can also serve to keep the plate reduced to the bone, can be used in conjunction with another whirlybird device (proximal and distal to the fracture), and can prevent the bone from being pushed away from the plate with screw placement. Only minor adjustments to the construct are possible after the initial screws are placed; major changes will require removal of the entire implant.

Locking screws are then used to secure the articular block to the plate and fasten the plate to the diaphysis **(Fig. 4–16B)**. At least four unicortical 5 mm screws are placed in the diaphysis proximal to the fracture. Bicortical locking screws are not necessary but may be considered for osteoporotic bone. Ideal screw placement would include at least two screws adjacent to the fracture proximally and distally and two screws near each end of the implant. Care must be taken to ensure that the plate is aligned in the center of the bone; the unicortical locking screw will lock into the plate regardless of the screw's purchase **(Fig. 4–18A,B)**.

Minimally invasive techniques do not allow for direct open anatomical reduction of extra-articular fracture fragments, making the intraoperative assessment of correct frontal and sagittal plane axial alignment, length, and rotation difficult. When using minimally invasive techniques, it is essential to determine proper limb alignment intraoperatively and to recognize and correct deformities during the initial procedure. Several radiographically based techniques can be used to determine limb alignment, including the cable technique (frontal plane), Blumensaat's line and the recurvatum sign (sagittal plane alignment), meter stick technique (leg length); and the lesser trochanteric shape sign (rotational alignment).[40] For the intraoperative determination of frontal plane alignment, the cable technique is useful **(Fig. 4–19)**. This technique is based on data that demonstrate that the normal mechanical axis passes 10 mm medial to the center of the knee joint in the region of the medial tibial spine. The procedure is performed with the knee extended and the patella facing anteriorly. The image intensifier is used to identify the center of the femoral head and tibial plafond. The electrocautery cable is then placed over the two marks, and the knee is imaged. The position of the cable relative to the center of the knee joint indicates the frontal plane alignment. For sagittal plane alignment, Blumensaat's line is an intraoperative guide for sagittal plane alignment **(Fig. 4–20A–C)**. The angle formed between this line and the femoral shaft can be compared radiographically with that of the contralateral normal side. The notch sign can also be used for a rough judgment of sagittal plane alignment. The primary principal of this technique is that the AP radiographic projection of the intercondylar notch increases in depth with greater degrees of recurvatum. An AP fluoroscopic view can be taken to determine the appearance of the notch intraoperatively, which can be compared with the image from the uninjured contralateral side.

The meter stick technique involves the measurement of the femoral length from the top of the femoral head to the distal margin of the lateral femoral condyles using a radiographic ruler or meter stick and fluoroscopic guidance

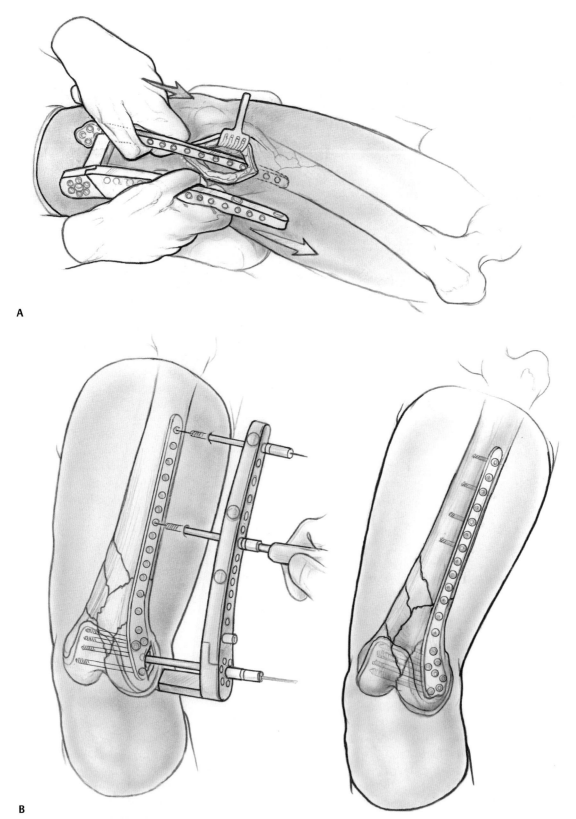

A

B

Figure 4–16 Drawings demonstrating **(A)** sliding the locked plate under the submuscular plane, **(B)** attaching the handle to the plate proximally, and final fixation with unicortical screws.

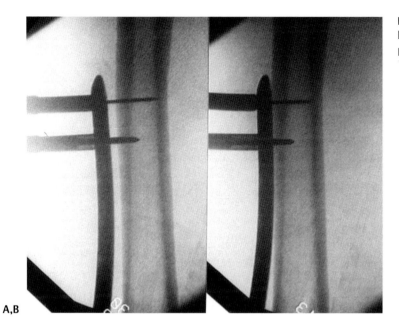

A,B

Figure 4–17 Use of the **(A)** "whirlybird" to reduce **(B)** the bone to the plate during a locked plating. Reproduced with permission from Springer (Operat Orthop Traumatol 2001; 13:178–197).

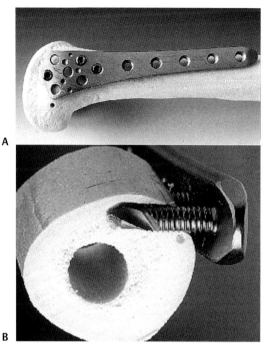

A

B

Figure 4–18 **(A)** Placement of a locked plate that is not centered in the midlateral plane. **(B)** This causes very poor purchase in the proximal screws due to the transcortical location of the screws. Reproduced with permission from Springer (Unfallchirurg 2000:103; 428–436).

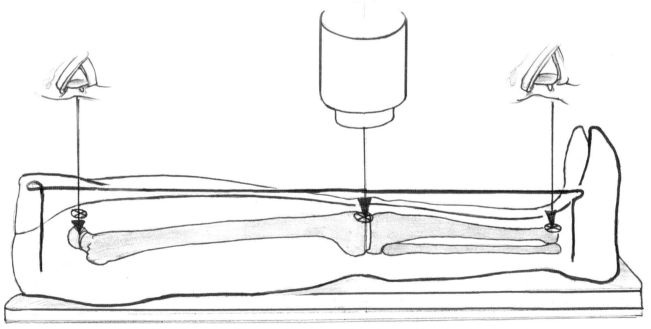

Figure 4–19 Diagram of the cable technique to determine frontal plane alignment. The patella is directed anteriorly, and the image intensifier is used to locate the center of the femoral head and the tibial plafond. The cable is then placed over the two sites, and the knee is imaged. The position of the cable relative to the center of the knee joint indicates the frontal plane alignment.

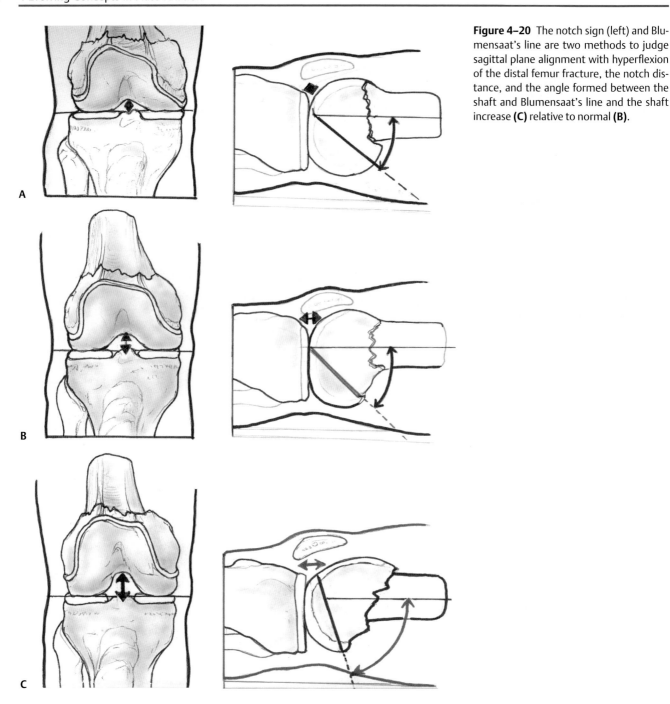

Figure 4–20 The notch sign (left) and Blumensaat's line are two methods to judge sagittal plane alignment with hyperflexion of the distal femur fracture, the notch distance, and the angle formed between the shaft and Blumensaat's line and the shaft increase **(C)** relative to normal **(B)**.

(Fig. 4–21). This measurement can be compared with the uninjured contralateral limb to determine proper length. Rotational alignment can be difficult to determine radiographically intraoperatively. Because rotational deformities are often not obvious on plain radiographs, these deformities have traditionally received less attention than deformities in other planes. The lesser trochanteric shape sign can be useful to determine femoral rotation intraoperatively **(Fig. 4–22A–D).** Because the lesser trochanter has an asymmetric shape, with external rotation, the lesser trochanter appears more prominent as it becomes less secured by the proximal femoral shaft. In internal rotation, the lesser trochanter appears smaller as it disappears behind the proximal femoral shaft. With the patella positioned directly anteriorly, the hip can be imaged to visualize the lesser trochanter. The trochanteric shape needs to be compared with that of the uninjured contralateral side.

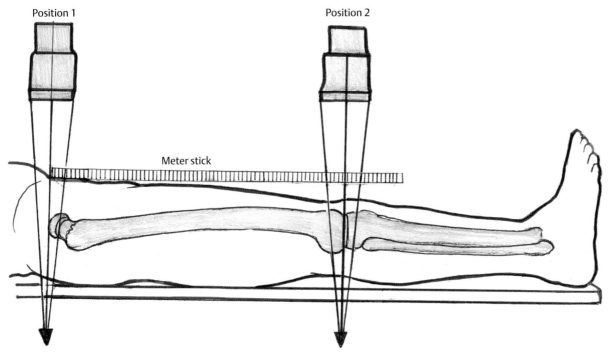

Figure 4–21 Drawing of the meter stick technique used to determine femoral length.

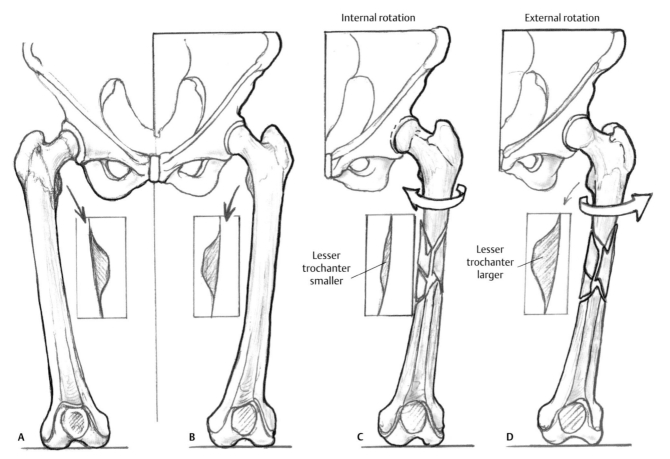

Figure 4–22 (A) The lesser trochanteric shape sign can help determine rotational alignment when compared with **(B)** the contralateral side. **(C)** The lesser trochanter is smaller with internal rotation of the proximal fragment and **(D)** larger with external rotation of the proximal fragment.

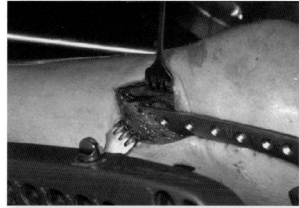

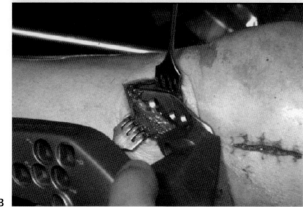

Figure 4–23 Submuscular minimally invasive plating of the proximal tibia. **(A)** Demonstrates minimal incision. **(B)** Shows the plate inserted in the submuscular plane.

Less-Invasive Stabilization System Tibia (see Video 4–5, Disk 1)

Many of the techniques used for application of the LISS to the femur also apply to the tibia (**Fig. 4–23A,B**). The patient is positioned on a radiolucent table with a bump under the ipsilateral buttock. The leg is prepped and draped free. AP and lateral fluoroscopic images are taken prior to prepping and draping to ensure that there is no impedance to the x-ray beam. A bump is placed under the knee bent to ~40 degrees of flexion, which serves to relax the calf musculature and aid in reduction. Similar to the technique with the femoral LISS, the fracture is reduced with traction, and fracture pattern and reduction are closely evaluated. Once the fracture is evaluated, a lateral curved or straight incision is performed beginning at the joint line and extending toward Gerdy's tubercle. In patients with intra-articular multifragmentary fractures, the incision may be extended proximally as needed. The dissection is carried deeply in line with the incision.

If there is an articular fracture, reduction must be performed first. The articular reduction must be anatomical and performed with rigid lag screw compression of the major fragments. Care must be taken to place the screws so that they do not interfere with the placement of the plate. Once the articular reduction is achieved, the LISS is

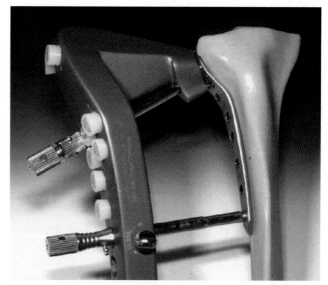

Figure 4–24 The use of a "whirlybird" to reduce the bone to the plate prior to placing locked screws.

inserted in a submuscular fashion along the lateral aspect of the femur with the guide handle. Sliding a Cobb elevator in the submuscular plane prior to inserting the implant may ease the passage. Limb alignment, including length, rotation, varus/valgus alignment, and recurvatum/procurvatum are evaluated. Once the desired reduction is achieved, the plate is held in place with threaded K-wires. Fluoroscopic imaging is undertaken to assess reduction and plate placement. The whirlybird is used in a manner similar to the femoral LISS technique. It allows correction of some coronal plane deformity, as well as the ability to pull the tibia to the plate. In many cases it is helpful to use at least one and sometimes two (proximal and distal to the fracture) whirlybird devices (**Fig. 4–24**). The plate can also be secured to the bone using a large clamp through a small hole in the proximal aspect of the plate. If the plate is not sitting snugly on the proximal tibia, it can be useful to clamp it to the bone using a large clamp.

Prior to securing the plate to the bone, care must be taken to ensure that the plate position and reduction are satisfactory. Locking screws are then used to secure the plate to the articular block. At least four 5 mm unicortical screws are placed in the diaphysis distal to the fracture, preferably adjacent to the fracture proximally and distally and two screws near each end of the implant. Care must be taken when placing the screws in the distal third of the tibia to avoid injury to the at-risk structures (i.e., the anterior tibial artery and superficial peroneal nerve), and ensure proper alignment of the plate centrally along the lateral surface of the tibia (P. Kregor, personal communication).

As described earlier, the intraoperative determination of limb alignment is essential with closed techniques.[40] Although tibial alignment is easier to determine on physical examination, and direct AP and lateral radiographs are useful to determine varus/valgus and antecurvatum/recurvatum deformities, fluoroscopic techniques can assist in the overall determination of tibial alignment. The meter-stick technique is useful to determine length, which is measured from the lateral tibial plateau to the upper margin of the body of the talus. Tibial rotation can be determined based on the angle formed between the femoral condyle and the medial malleolus. The image is compared with the intact contralateral side for both measurements.

Surgical Technique for Condylar Locking Compression Plate

Recently, the 4.5 mm Condylar Locking Compression Plate (Synthes, Paoli, Pennsylvania) has become available **(Fig. 4–25).** The system allows for either locking or nonlocking screw insertion in the diaphysis and metaphysis. The indications for its use include distal femur fractures with comminution of the medial column, supracondylar fractures, intra- and extra-articular condylar fractures, and malunions and nonunions of the distal femur. The fixed-angle design of the device resists varus collapse. The plate is less flexible than the LISS and it is constructed from stainless steel rather than a titanium alloy. The holes in the shaft of the plate combine a dynamic compression hole with a locking screw hole, providing for both axial compression and locking capability throughout the length of the plate. Locking screws engaged in the plate create a fixed-angle construct that improves fixation in osteopenic bone and multifragmentary fractures. Multiple screw fixation in the femoral condyle allows for improved fixation of many intra-articular fractures. The plate is low profile, anatomically shaped, and designed for left and right distal femurs. The distal aspect of the plate is contoured to match the lateral condyle of the distal femur, eliminating the need for intraoperative plate bending. The locking screws are self-drilling and self-tapping. The proximal aspect of the plate accepts an articulated tension device for compression and distraction if needed. Screws in the shaft can be either 4.0 mm locking or 4.5 mm cortical screws.

The percutaneous technique for fixation of distal femur fractures with the condylar locking compression plate is similar to that used for LISS insertion. A targeting device for plate and screw insertion is not yet commercially available, however. The plate can be placed using either a percutaneous or an open technique. Once the exposure is accomplished and the articular surface has been reconstructed using standard techniques, the plate is placed on the lateral surface of the femur. The plate can be pinned distally with three K-wires prior to screw placement. In contrast to the LISS, it is not critical to have the diaphyseal portion of the fracture reduced and pinned at this point in the surgery. Once the plate has been provisionally pinned to the femur with three wires, screws can be placed in the articular block.

There are several technique points that are important to remember when using a plate that allows both locking and conventional screw placement. The screw is selected based on the intended effect. If either interfragmentary or plate-to-bone compression is necessary, then conventional bicortical screws should be employed. If additional stability is needed due to poor bone quality (osteopenia or comminution), then locking screws should be selected. Care should be taken to lag the fragments prior to locking. If locked screws are used prior to the placement of a lag screw, the lag screw will either not achieve a lag effect, or it will cause the bone to fail around the locked screws. It should also be remembered that the most distal and posterior hole on the plate is frequently distal to Blumensaat's line when the plate is affixed to the distal femur. If that hole (or any other hole) is distal to Blumensaat's line, the selected screw should be short enough so that it does not enter the notch and damage the anterior or posterior cruciate ligament **(Fig. 4–26).** This is an ideal indication for a unicortical locked screw.

When the articular block has been adequately affixed to the plate with the desired combination of locked and conventional screws, the reduction of the shaft to the articular block should be checked and revised as necessary. Again, if lag or conventional screws are desired in the diaphyseal segment of bone, it is essential to lag prior to locking the fracture to the plate. A minimum of four screws proximal to the fracture is recommended. If unicortical screws are going to be used, it is essential to confirm that the plate will be centered over the lateral aspect of the femur. Because the current plate is straight and the femur is curved, the tendency is for the long condylar locking compression plate to be located eccentrically on the proximal femur. An eccentric location of the plate will result in intracortical locking screws that have poor pullout strength **(Fig. 4–18A,B).**

Surgical Technique for 4.5 mm Proximal Tibial Locking Compression Plate

Similar to the 4.5 mm condylar locking compression plate, the 4.5 mm tibial locking compression plate was designed to allow for either locking or nonlocking screw insertion in the diaphysis. The indications for its use are intra-articular bicolumnar tibial plateau fractures,

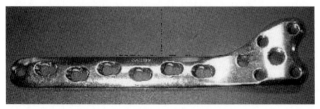

Figure 4–25 The locking condylar compression plate allows the use of both conventional and locked screws in supracondylar femur fractures. Reproduced with permission from Synthes.

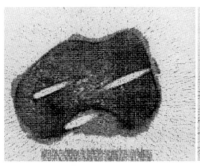
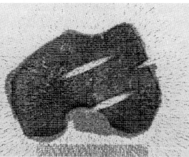

Figure 4–26 Screw placement into the femoral notch with the condylar locking compression plate. Reproduced with permission from AO International (Publishing).

proximal metaphyseal fractures, and malunions and nonunions of the proximal tibia. The proximal aspect of the plate is anatomically contoured to match the proximal tibia. The proximal three locking screws allow for a raft-type construct that supports the articular surface of the tibial plateau, obviating the need for a second plate placed medially or external fixation. Two 2 mm holes are also incorporated on the proximal plate for K-wire fixation or meniscal repair sutures. The plate has three 5 mm convergent locking screw holes that accept either 5 mm locking screws or 5 mm cortical screws. The distal aspect of the plate accepts the Articulated Tension Device for compression and distraction if necessary. Screws in the shaft can be either 4.0 mm locking or 4.5 mm cortical screws. The principles that govern the use of the condylar locking compression plate also apply to the tibial locking compression plate. If fragment or plate–bone compression is desired, nonlocking cortical screws should be selected. If the bone quality is poor due to osteopenia or comminution, then locking screws are indicated. If both screw types will be used, compression must be achieved prior to lagging.

Surgical Technique for Distal Tibia Locking Plates (see Video 4–6, Disk 1)

The medial distal tibia locking plate was designed to address tibial plafond fracture fixation. Like other plates designed for the medial aspect of the distal tibia, this plate is prominent and may cause skin irritation. The distal tibia locking plate can be placed percutaneously or through an open incision (**Fig. 4–27**). The indications for its use are evolving and may include tibial plafond fractures with metaphyseal comminution and diaphyseal extension. Before insertion, attention must be paid to the condition of the soft tissues. If there is marked swelling, blistering, or other parameters of soft tissue instability, a temporizing procedure, such as a spanning external fixator, must be used to decrease the rate of wound dehiscence and deep infection. After wrinkling has occurred and the soft tissues have stabilized, plating can be performed. The procedure begins with open or closed anatomical reduction of the ankle joint surface. Once the articular surface is reduced, fixation of the articular surface should be accom-

plished using the standard principles of articular fracture stabilization. This may require screw placement outside the distal tibial plate, or temporary fixation with K-wires followed by definitive stabilization using the plate. The articular block is then attached to the diaphysis. This can be done percutaneously with fluoroscopic control to avoid the need for large devitalizing incisions. The same principles discussed previously also apply to the selection of locking versus conventional screws in this plate, as well as the order in which they should be inserted. Stabilization should be accomplished using the smallest incisions possible. Gentle soft tissue handling is critical to decrease the rate of complications.

Surgical Technique for Distal Radius Plates

Palmar distal radius locking plates were developed to stabilize unstable, dorsally comminuted fractures. Although these fractures historically have been stabilized by dorsally applied plates to avoid collapse, their use was associated with a high prevalence of hardware-associated complications, including decreased extensor tendon gliding and rupture.[41–46] Due to these complications, the palmar approach has been used in conjunction with volarly placed locking plates to treat dorsally comminuted distal

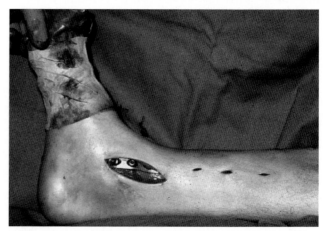

Figure 4–27 Percutaneous placement of the distal tibia locking plate.

radius fractures. Mechanical studies on this technique demonstrate that, although some of the plates are less stiff than dorsally applied buttress plates, others are stiffer, depending on the manufacturer.[47] Palmar locking plates provide length and rotational stability to dorsally comminuted, unstable fractures and are indicated for the treatment of these fractures through a volar approach. The locking features are particularly useful in patients who have significant osteopenia and/or comminution. The plates are contoured to the volar surface of the distal radius. The locking screws in these plates also allow for a raft-type construct to support the distal radial articular surface. Fractures requiring volar buttress plating do not specifically require locking plates.

A volar incision is made along the flexor carpi radialis tendon and carried deeply to the pronator quadratus muscle. The radial artery and vein are retracted radially. The pronator quadratus muscle is incised sharply along the border of the distal radius and reflected ulnarly. The fracture site is visualized and reduced. Articular reduction is performed first and can be held temporarily with K-wires. Once the proper alignment of the fracture is obtained, an appropriate-length plate is selected and positioned over the distal radius. Fluoroscopy can be used to aid with the proper alignment of the fracture and placement of the plate. With the plate held in place and the reduction obtained, a single bicortical screw can be placed distally through the oblong hole to maintain alignment of the plate and secure the plate against the bone. The plate can be rotated or moved proximally or distally as necessary. Once the plate is secured in place, then the distal fracture is reduced to the plate and fixed with locking screws. Care should be taken to ensure that the plate is positioned properly relative to the fracture (**Fig. 4–28A,B**) as well as being reduced against the bone because the locking screws will stabilize the distal fragment in the position in which it is held. In general, three or four screws should be placed both proximally and distally to the fracture, depending on the fracture pattern and the type of plate. Locking screws should be placed distally in a raft-type construct that supports the articular surface of the distal radius (**Fig. 4–28B**). Bicortical screws can then be placed in the remaining open screw holes proximal to the fracture.

Rehabilitation

Because of the stability achieved using locked plating, most patients can begin range of motion of the stabilized joint within the first week. The patients may be kept toe-touch or non–weight bearing, depending on the joint injured, concomitant injuries, and the patient. The sutures are removed at 10 days postoperatively. Radiographs are obtained at 6, 12, 16, and 20 weeks and 6-month follow-up visits to assess alignment and healing. Activity and weight bearing are advanced to partial weight bearing depending on the clinical and radiographic findings.

Tips and Tricks

The performance of locking plates is distinct to that of traditional bicortical plates. Surgeons should be aware of these differences and familiar with the implants. Of particular difficulty are the approaches that require closed reductions and locked plating. These technically demanding cases rely on fluoroscopic evaluations rather than open visualization for fracture reduction and implant placement. Below are tips and tricks for successful use of locking plates:

- Maintain the four steps in minimally invasive approaches: (1) articular reconstruction, (2) submuscular plate insertion, (3) fixation of plate to articular block, and (4) percutaneous fixation of proximal screws.
- The first screw in each main fragment determines alignment. Do not place locked screws through the plate until a satisfactory reduction is achieved in all planes.
- Use lag screws prior to locking screws in most situations when using a combination of both types of screws.
- Locking screws will not reduce fragments to the plate. Use a whirlybird device (or one proximally and distally) to reduce the fracture and/or the bone to the plate. The device will also prevent the screw from pushing the bone away from the plate. Reduction forceps are also useful for reducing the bone to the LISS plate.
- Avoid eccentric placement of screws (or screws out of the bone entirely) that will weaken the pull-out strength of the locking construct proximally. Proper alignment of the locking plate proximally and distally is necessary.
- Alignment may be improved by varying distance between implant and bone. However, if this distance is too great, it can impede joint mobility.
- Pay close attention to detail, particularly in the intraoperative radiographic analysis, to ensure proper alignment of the fracture and position of the hardware. Use intraoperative radiographic techniques to ensure proper limb length and frontal, sagittal, and rotational alignment.
- Following the placement of locking screws, small angular changes are possible by loosening the locking screws. Major alignment changes require implant removal.
- If unfamiliar with the implants and techniques, start with a "less invasive" approach and evolve to a "minimally invasive" technique.

Outcomes

Percutaneous plating techniques, which have gradually evolved to include the use of locked plates, were created to minimize the surgical trauma to the injured tissue. By better preserving the soft tissues and vascular supply about the fracture, as well as perhaps the fracture hematoma, surgeons hoped that the healing response would be enhanced and complications minimized. Krettek et al reviewed their early experience with percutaneous plating of 15 intra-articular distal femur fractures

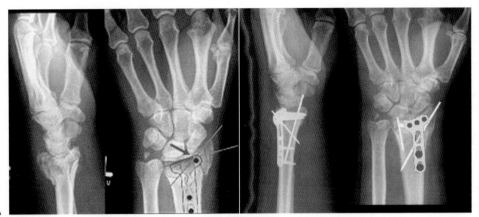

Figure 4–28 Volar plating of the distal radius. **(A)** Preoperative assessment is critical to ensure proper hardware position. **(B)** Stable fixation can be achieved, even in poor quality bone, by the placement of subchondral locking screws.

and compared it with the historical institutional results from 112 traditional open plating techniques.[48] They reported improvements in the rates for mean healing time (12.0 ± 3.0 vs 21.6 ± 13.9), primary bone grafting procedures (2 vs 61), secondary bone grafting (0 vs 24), infection (1 vs 7), refracture (0 vs 4), pseudarthrosis (0 vs 7), and revision surgery (0 vs 12). They concluded that the minimally invasive technique had biological benefits for healing. Subsequent to this report, several investigators began to publish their results using the LISS plating technique. As part of an AO prospective multicenter study, Schutz et al presented their results from 96 patients with 99 distal femur fractures that were followed up for a mean of 13.7 months.[49] They noted 23 revision surgeries in 21 patients, which they attributed to the severity of the trauma and a lack of experience with the implant. There were two cases of implant failure related to pseudarthrosis. They did not routinely perform bone grafting. This experience was consistent with that reported by other authors.[50–52] Schutz et al reported success using LISS for distal femur fractures with high Neer scores (73.9 to 77.2 points), and low rates of infection (0 to 4%), delayed union (2.4 to 6.1%), bone grafting (0 to 1.6% for primary and 0 to 5% for secondary grafting), screw loosening (0%), and implant failure (7.4%).

The results for tibial LISS have also been published and have been comparable to those for LISS plating of distal femur fractures.[53] Stannard et al reported results from 35 fractures and 32 patients of the tibial plateau and proximal tibia. Thirty-four fractures healed, with one nonunion.[54] Two of the 17 patients who had open fractures developed an infection. There was no loss of reduction, and range of motion averaged from 2 to 116 degrees. Schutz et al reported on patients with 20 to fractures treated with the proximal tibia LISS. With a follow-up rate of 91%, 19 out of 20 patients had healed fractures.[55] In the one ununited fracture, secondary bone grafting was performed. There was one soft tissue infection that healed uneventfully after repeat surgery.

Most recently, early reports on the use of the condylar locking compression plate have also been published.[56,57]

Sommer et al reported the results of a prospective multicenter study to treat 144 patients with 169 fractures of the tibia (57), femur (18), humerus (45), and radius (19). In 130 fractures healing was uncomplicated (86%). In 19 patients, there were 27 unexpected complications, with 13 patients needing 18 revision surgeries (five plate failures, one nonunion, two infections, and five fractures adjacent to the implant).[58]

Complications

The minimally invasive plating has been clinically successful as outlined here. Compared with the traditional plating methods, the rates of infection, delayed union, nonunion, need for secondary bone grafting, and implant loosening are more favorable with minimally invasive plating. The minimally invasive plating methods are technically de-

---

Pearls

- The four principal steps in a minimally invasive approach are (1) articular reconstruction, (2) submuscular plate insertion, (3) fixation of the plate to the articular block, and (4) percutaneous fixation of the proximal screws.
- Locked plates are indicated for comminuted diaphyseal or metaphyseal fractures, and in patients with poor bone stock secondary to osteoporosis or trauma. Conventional plates using bicortical screws are indicated for simple metaphyseal fractures that require buttressing, simple metaphyseal fractures with good opposition, osteotomies, and articular fractures.
- Locking screw–plate constructs fail as a unit. In contrast, bicortical screw–plate constructs fail by individual screw pull-out.
- When using both lag screws and bicortical screws through the same plate, the desired lag screw effect must be achieved prior to locking screw placement.

manding, however. A common theme in the literature is that these techniques are associated with malalignment. Despite favorable healing outcomes in the percutaneous plating group (15 intra-articular distal femur fractures) relative to the historical group that received traditional open plating (112 fractures), Krettek et al cited high rates of varus/valgus malalignment > 10 degrees (2 vs 4), shorten-

ing greater than 1 cm (3 vs 1), and malrotation > 15 degrees (2 vs 2) in the former group. This experience is similar to that of others in the use of the LISS for the distal femur and proximal tibia, as well as the locking condylar plate.[49,58] These results outlined the need for meticulous technique, careful intraoperative evaluation for alignment, and understanding that there is a learning curve to these procedures.

On the DVDs

Video 4–1 (Disk 1) Rules of Locked Plating This presentation reviews the "rules" that should be applied by surgeons employing locked plating. Included in this presentation is unicortical locked plating systems designed for minimally invasive submuscular application, as well as hybrid plating that includes mixing locked and unlocked screws. The appropriate order of application of screws is stressed.

Video 4–2 (Disk 1) Minimally Invasive Percutaneous Plate Osteosynthesis of the Distal Femur The patient in this case is treated with a DCS plate applied using MIPPO techniques and bridge plating. The surgeon demonstrates tricks for success with MIPPO, including judgement of length and rotation.

Video 4–3 (Disk 1) ORIF of a Periprosthetic Distal Femur Fracture with Submuscular Locked Plating LISS fixation of a distal femur fracture is performed in an osteoporotic distal femur fracture above a total knee arthroplasty. Minimal exposure of the fracture and closed reduction techniques are emphasized.

Video 4–4 (Disk 1) ORIF of a C2 Distal Femur Fracture with Submuscular Locked Plating Submuscular locked fixation is performed for a ballistic C2 distal femur fracture in a 34-year-old male. Delayed reconstruction is carried out following placement of a spanning external fixator, originally placed after repair of a vascular injury.

Video 4–5 (Disk 1) ORIF of a Comminuted Tibial Plateau Fracture with Locked Plating This case demonstrates techniques for handling a markedly comminuted bicondylar fracture. The video stresses the importance of centering the plate on the bone and the recommended screw placement proximally.

Video 4–6 (Disk 1) ORIF of a Distal Tibia Fracture with Locked Plating This video demonstrates the use of locked plating and minimally invasive approaches in a patient who has sustained a distal tibia fracture.

References

1. Gray RN. Disability and cost of industrial fractures. J Bone Joint Surg 1928;10:27–38
2. Bagby GW, Janes JW. The effect of compression on rate of fracture healing using a special plate. Am J Surg 1958;95:761–771
3. Muller M, Allgower M, Willenegger H. Manual of Internal Fixation. 3rd ed. Berlin: Springer-Verlag; 1991
4. Muller ME. Principes d'osteosynthese. Helv Chir Acta 1961;28:196–206
5. Muller ME, Allgower M, Willenegger H. Tecknik der operativen Frakturenbehandlung. Berlin: Springer; 1963
6. Perren SM, Russenberger M, Steinemann S, Muller ME, Allgower M. A dynamic compression plate. Acta Orthop Scand Suppl 1969;125:31–41
7. Allgower M, Ehrsam R, Ganz R, Matter P, Perren SM. Clinical experience would add new compression plate 'DCP'. Acta Orthop Scand Suppl 1969;125:45–61
8. Wagner M. General principles for the clinical use of the LCP. Injury 2003;34 (Suppl 2):B31–B42
9. Eggers GW. The influence of the contact-compression factor on osteogenesis in surgical fractures. J Bone Joint Surg Am 1949;31A:693–716
10. Perren SM. The concept of biological plate using a limited contact-dynamic compression plate (LC-DCP): scientific background, design and application. Injury 1991;22(Suppl 1):1–41
11. Teptic S, Perren SM. The biomechanics of the PC-Fix internal fixator. Injury 1995; (Suppl 2):5–10
12. Perren SM, Cordey J, Rahn BA, Gautier E, Schneider E. Early temporary porosis of bone induced by internal fixation implants: a reaction to necrosis, not to stress protection? Clin Orthop Relat Res 1988;232:139–151
13. Granowski R, Ramotowski W, Kaminski E, Pilawski K. "Zespol"–a new type of osteosynthesis, I: An internal self-compressing stabilizer of bone fragments [in Polish]. Chir Narzadow Ruchu Ortop Pol 1984;49:301–305
14. Ramotowski W, Granowski R. Zespol. An original method of stable osteosynthesis. Clin Orthop Relat Res 1991;272:67–75
15. Brunner C, Weber B. Besondere Osteosynthesetechniken. New York: Springer; 1981
16. Heitemeyer U, Hierholzer G. Die uberbruckende Osteosynthese bei geschlossennen Stuckfrakturen des Femurschftes. Aktuelle Tramotol 1985;15:205–209
17. Perren SM, Klaue K, Pohler O, Predieri M, Steinemann S, Gautier E. The limited contact dynamic compression plate (LC-DCP). Arch Orthop Trauma Surg 1990;109:304–310
18. Perren SM. The concept of biological plating using the limited contact-dynamic compression plate (LC-DCP): scientific background, design and application. Injury 1991;22:1–41
19. Perren SM. Evolution of the internal fixation of long bone fractures: the scientific basis of biological internal fixation: choosing a new balance between stability and biology. J Bone Joint Surg Br 2002;84:1093–1110
20. Tepic S, Remiger AR, Morikawa K, Predieri M, Perren SM. Strength recovery in fractured sheep tibia treated with a plate or an internal fixator: an experimental study with a two-year follow-up. J Orthop Trauma 1997;11:14–23
21. Miclau T, Remiger A, Tepic S, Lindsey R, McIff T. A mechanical comparison of the dynamic compression plate, limited contact-dynamic compression plate, and point contact fixator. J Orthop Trauma 1995;9:17–22

22. Eijer H, Hauke C, Arens S, Printzen G, Schlegel U, Perren SM. PC-Fix and local infection resistance: influence of implant design on postoperative infection development, clinical and experimental results. Injury 2001;32(Suppl 2):B38–B43

23. Fernandez Dell' Oca AA, Galante RM. Osteosynthesis of diaphyseal fractures of the radius and ulna using an internal fixator (PC-Fix): a prospective study. Injury 2001;32(Suppl 2):B44–B50

24. Johansson A, Lindgren JU, Nord CE, Svensson O. Material and design in haematogenous implant-associated infections in a rabbit model. Injury 1999;30:651–657

25. Borgeaud M, Cordey J, Leyvraz PE, Perren SM. Mechanical analysis of the bone to plate interface of the LC-DCP and of the PC-FIX on human femora. Injury 2000;31(Suppl 3):C29–C36

26. Koval KJ, Hoehl JJ, Kummer FJ, Simon JA. Distal femoral fixation: a biomechanical comparison of the standard condylar buttress plate, a locked buttress plate, and the 95-degree blade plate. J Orthop Trauma 1997;11:521–524

27. Marti A, Fankhauser C, Frenk A, Cordey J, Gasser B. Biomechanical evaluation of the less invasive stabilization system for the internal fixation of distal femur fractures. J Orthop Trauma 2001;15: 482–487

28. Goesling T, Frenk A, Appenzeller A, Garapati R, Marti A, Krettek C. LISS PLT: design, mechanical and biomechanical characteristics. Injury 2003;34(Suppl 1):A11–A15

29. Stoffel K, Dieter U, Stachowiak G, Gachter A, Kuster MS. Biomechanical testing of the LCP: how can stability in locked internal fixators be controlled? Injury 2003;34(Suppl 2):B11–B19

30. Farouk O, Krettek C, Miclau T, Schandelmaier P, Tscherne H. Effects of percutaneous and conventional plating techniques on the blood supply to the femur. Arch Orthop Trauma Surg 1998;117: 438–441

31. Mast J, Jakob R, Ganz R. Planning and reduction technique in fracture surgery. New York: Springer; 1989

32. Gerber C, Mast JW, Ganz R. Biological internal fixation of fractures. Arch Orthop Trauma Surg 1990;109:295–303

33. Bolhofner BR, Carmen B, Clifford P. The results of open reduction and internal fixation of distal femur fractures using a biologic (indirect) reduction technique. J Orthop Trauma 1996;10: 372–377

34. Ostrum R, Geel C. Indirect reduction and internal fixation of supracondylar femur fractures without bone graft. J Orthop Trauma 1995;9:278–284

35. Krettek C, Schandelmaier P, Miclau T, Bertram R, Holmes W, Tscherne H. Transarticular joint reconstruction and indirect plate osteosynthesis for complex distal supracondylar femur fractures. Injury 1997;28(Suppl 1):A31–A41

36. Krettek C, Schandelmaier P, Miclau T, Tscherne H. Minimally invasive percutaneous plate osteosynthesis (MIPPO) using the DCS in proximal and distal femoral fractures. Injury 1997;28(Suppl 1):A20–A30

37. Krettek C, Gerich T, Miclau T. A minimally invasive medial approach for proximal tibial fractures. Injury 2001;32(Suppl1):SA4–13

38. Helfet DL, Shonnard PY, Levine D, Borrelli J Jr. Minimally invasive plate osteosynthesis of distal fractures of the tibia. Injury 1997;28(Suppl 1):A42–A48

39. Schandelmaier P, et al. Stabilization of distal femoral fractures using the LISS. Tech Orthop 1999;14:230–246

40. Osada D, Viegas SF, Shah MA, Morris RP, Patterson RM. Comparison of different distal radius dorsal and volar fracture fixation plates: a biomechanical study. J Hand Surg [Am] 2003;28:94–104

41. Krettek C, et al. Techniques for assessing limb alignment during closed reduction and internal fixation of lower extremity fractures. Tech Orthop 1999;14:247–256

42. Herron M, Faraj A, Craigen MA. Dorsal plating for displaced intra-articular fractures of the distal radius. Injury 2003;34:497–502

43. Hahnloser D, Platz A, Amgwerd M, Trentz O. Internal fixation of distal radius fractures with dorsal dislocation: pi-plate or two 1/4 tube plates? A prospective randomized study. J Trauma 1999;47: 760–765

44. Rozental TD, Beredjiklian PK, Bozentka DJ. Functional outcome and complications following two types of dorsal plating for unstable fractures of the distal part of the radius. J Bone Joint Surg Am 2003;85-A:1956–1960

45. Jupiter JB, Lipton H. The operative treatment of intraarticular fractures of the distal radius. Clin Orthop Relat Res 1993;292:48–61

46. Leibovic SJ, Geissler WB. Treatment of complex intra-articular distal radius fractures. Orthop Clin North Am 1994;25:685–706

47. Fitoussi F, Ip WY, Chow SP. Treatment of displaced intra-articular fractures of the distal end of the radius with plates. J Bone Joint Surg Am 1997;79:1303–1312

48. Krettek C, Schandelmaier P, Richter M, Tscherne H. Distal femoral fractures [in German]. Swiss Surg 1998;6:263–278

49. Schutz M, Muller M, Krettek C, et al. Minimally invasive fracture stabilization of distal femoral fractures with the LISS: a prospective multicenter study: results of a clinical study with special emphasis on difficult cases. Injury 2001;32(Suppl 3):SC48–SC54

50. Schandelmaier P, Partenheimer A, Koenemann B, Grun OA, Krettek C. Distal femoral fractures and LISS stabilization. Injury 2001; 32(Suppl 3):SC55–SC63

51. Kregor PJ, Stannard J, Zlowodzki M, Cole PA, Alonso J. Distal femoral fracture fixation utilizing the Less Invasive Stabilization System (L.I.S.S.): the technique and early results. Injury 2001;32(Suppl 3):SC32–SC47

52. Kregor PJ. Distal femur fractures with complex articular involvement: management by articular exposure and submuscular fixation. Orthop Clin North Am 2002;33:153–175

53. Cole PA, Zlowodzki M, Kregor PJ. Less Invasive Stabilization System (LISS) for fractures of the proximal tibia: indications, surgical technique and preliminary results of the UMC Clinical Trial. Injury 2003;34(Suppl 1):A16–29

54. Stannard JP, Wilson TC, Volgas DA, Alonso JE. Fracture stabilization of proximal tibial fractures with the proximal tibial LISS: early experience in Birmingham, Alabama (USA). Injury 2003;34(Suppl 1):A36–A42

55. Schutz M, Kaab MJ, Haas N. Stabilization of proximal tibial fractures with the LIS System: early clinical experience in Berlin. Injury 2003;34(Suppl 1):A30–35

56. Sommer C, Gautier E. Relevance and advantage of new angular stable screw-plate systems for diaphyseal fractures (locking compression plate versus intramedullary nail). Ther Umsch 2003;60:751–756

57. Wagner M. General principles for the clinical use of the LCP. Injury 2003;34(Suppl 2):B31–42

58. Sommer C, Gautier E, Muller M, Helfet DL, Wagner M. First clinical results of the Locking Compression Plate (LCP). Injury 2003;34 (Suppl 2):B43–B54

5 Treatment Strategy for Nonunions and Malunions

Michael A. Miranda and Mary S. Moon

Surgical management of nonunions and malunions requires a sound understanding of the principles and biomechanics of internal fixation, the biology of fracture union, and the limits of the specific implants employed. Due to the unique nature of each patient's problem, patients with a nonunion or malunion require an individualized treatment plan with specific goals. This chapter focuses on general principles and strategies, allowing the reader to individualize management. Using these principles, the reader should be able to develop an individualized treatment plan. The initial evaluation of malunions and nonunions is generally similar, but the management is discussed separately because they require different treatment algorithms.

Evaluation

The evaluation of a patient with a malunion initially focuses on identifying if the perceived problem is a deformity of functional or future pathomechanical significance.[1,2] Nonunion evaluation, on the other hand, focuses on the potential etiologies for the nonunion and the degree of dysfunction caused by the nonunion. Both require a complete history and review of the initial treatment, as well as any complications of that treatment. One should document the pain severity and frequency as well as any pain medication taken on a daily basis. A thorough review of systems is necessary, including a list of medications the patient uses, taking particular note of steroids, tobacco, nonsteroidal anti-inflammatory drugs (NSAIDs), anticoagulants, and antiseizure medications.

Complaints of pain in the extremity with nonunion or malunion should be thoroughly considered and potential etiologies assessed. There are several potential etiologies for pain after a fracture other than the non- or malunion of the bone. Local pain factors can often be determined on physical exam by focusing on reproducing the symptoms and additionally by selective injection of local anesthetic. As Mast has noted (personal communication), more remote causes of pain may lie in adjacent or ipsilateral joints **(Table 5–1)**. Around the knee, for example, possibilities include arthrosis, joint instability, or mechanical symptoms due to an associated meniscal tear. As a result of the anatomy of the peripheral nerves and the possibility of referred pain, the hip should always be carefully evaluated for synovitis in patients complaining of knee pain.

Table 5—1 Potential Etiologies for Pain Following Fracture

Local	Remote
Neuroma	Ipsilateral joint or back
Hardware	Adjacent
Heterotopic ossification	Distant but referring

Physical examination should start with an evaluation of gait. Gross alignment in the frontal and sagittal planes should be determined. Joint motion, including the rigidity of the end point, as well as excessive mobility, is important to document. Ipsilateral joint contractures should be carefully assessed and considered as part of the patient's problem list. Motion at the site of the nonunion should be noted and differentiated from local joint motion. Rotational alignment should be determined compared with the normal side. Leg length discrepancy should be evaluated with note of apparent and true limb lengths.

Radiographic evaluation should include anteroposterior and lateral views of the involved extremity. Oblique radiographs of the involved side are also important for planning purposes[3] because most malunions occur out of the standard orthogonal planes. Stress views are helpful in determining mobility of the nonunion. Special views, such as tibial plateau views, may be necessary as well. Standing hip-knee-ankle views[4] are necessary to determine alignment with malunions. Anteroposterior and lateral views of the contralateral uninvolved extremity are necessary for preoperative planning purposes. Two-dimensional computed tomographic (CT) scans are helpful when evaluating rotational deformities,[5] degree of fracture consolidation, and leg length discrepancies. High-quality three-dimensional (3-D) CT scans often provide a summary image that plain radiographs cannot. However seductive 3-D CT scans may appear, a thorough study of the plain radiographs is necessary for decision making when using plain and fluoroscopic images intraoperatively. Magnetic resonance imaging (MRI) is a helpful adjunct to diagnose other potential etiologies of pain and dysfunction **(Fig. 5–1)** such as ligamentous or meniscal injuries as well as avascular necrosis.

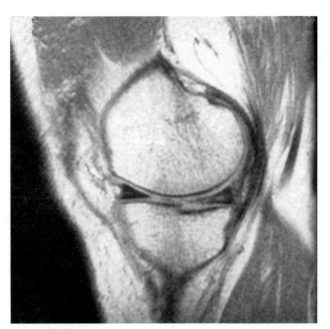

Figure 5–1 Magnetic resonance imaging demonstrating an intra-articular step-off as well as a meniscal tear in a patient with persistent knee pain after fracture.

Surgical Treatment for Malunions

Indications

Unfortunately, there are no scientifically based parameters regarding the need for surgical intervention for malunions. Therefore, functional limitations are the most consistently cited indication for surgical intervention in patients with a malunion. The indications for surgical correction of malunions in the upper extremity focus on the patient's ability to position the hand in space. A primary indication for surgical treatment of an upper extremity malunion is inability to perform activities of daily living because of the malunion. A relative indication would be a patient-specific desire to perform an activity impaired by the malunion. The primary concerns regarding malalignment in weight-bearing joints are quite different. The long-term implications of joint overload are significant in lower extremity malunions, due to impact on both articular cartilage health and the capsular and ligamentous tissues.[6,7]

In addition to malalignment, the treatment decision in extremity malunions must be made considering the patient's age, activity level, functional demands, and medical status. Clearly the risk:benefit ratio must be evaluated. For example, malrotation in the lower extremity after intramedullary nailing is a frequent complication; however, symptoms do not correlate with the degree of deformity.[8] This is likely due to the spherical shape of the femoral head allowing for rotational compensation during gait. Although Muller et al[6] have recommended derotation for asymmetry of 10 to 15 degrees or more, there are no clear

data to support that conclusion. Therefore, the surgical indications for malrotation should be made on an individual basis and, in clinical practice, often reflect the patient's ability to compensate for the malrotation during gait.

Patients will often present with concerns regarding cosmesis after malalignment of a fracture. The principle issues in these circumstances are whether there are functional limitations and reconciling this with the patient's perception of the deformity. Potential indications to consider deformity correction following a malunion include (1) mechanical overload,[8] (2) dysfunction, (3) capsuloligamentous strain, (4) subjective complaints, and (5) cosmesis.

Preoperative Planning

Preoperative planning is a tool used to improve outcomes while caring for these patients with complex problems. Although drawings are a key element to preoperative planning, they are only the final stage in a thought process. This process should state the goal of the procedure; document all issues in a patient problem list; define the surgical tactic, including the planned technique of reduction; and then ultimately include the radiographic tracings.

While seeming oversimplified, the first step of the preoperative plan is to state the problem and goals of surgery. This aids in determining the principles of treatment and also increases the likelihood that the procedure will address the concerns of the treating surgeon and the patient.

The patient's problem list should record the explicit problem (e.g., diaphyseal malunion), as well as implicit problems (e.g., impending joint degeneration). Confounding factors include the previous incision; the presence of hardware and its sequelae (e.g., screw holes or bony defects); systemic factors (e.g., diabetes mellitus); and then, in a separate column, how each issue will be addressed. The key principles employed in lower extremity correction are outlined in **Table 5–2.**

The surgical tactic is a stepwise algorithm outlining the procedure and should address each issue identified in the problem list. The surgical tactic should be divided into stages, each with a limited goal. Success in these difficult

---

Table 5—2   Principles for Lower Extremity Correction (Hierholzer)

1. Restore normal axial alignment.

   Mechanical axis bisects ankle/knee/center of femoral head.[12–14]

2. Restore ankle and knee joints parallel to floor.[16]

3. For hip, need concentric coverage and containment of femoral head.

   Tip greater trochanter at center of femoral head for lever arm and efficient gait.[2,17]

4. Equalize leg lengths within 2 cm to avoid problems with gait or spine.

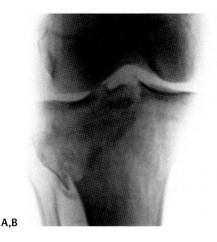
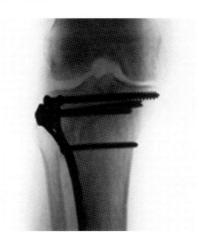

Figure 5–2 (A) An example of an intra-articular malunion and **(B)** its correction with an osteotomy.

cases is more certainly achieved if one can break the procedure down into a series of steps, each with limited goals, leading to the desired end result.

The surgeon should strongly consider performing the proposed surgical correction with cutouts of paper tracings of the fragments prior to the surgery to ensure the desired result will be achieved. In very complex malunions it is sometimes helpful to obtain a plastic bone model of the deformity to aid in planning for the correction. It is important to recognize that measured lengths on nondigitalized radiographs have an approximate magnification of 20%. The magnification on digitalized radiographs is variable but can often be found at the bottom of the film. Further reading on preoperative planning is available from other sources.[9]

Patients with poor soft tissue coverage require additional consideration. First, incisions should be planned so that hardware, tendon, or bone will not be exposed should wound problems occur. For example, in the distal tibia with a preexisting anteromedial wound, a posteromedial approach[10] for reconstruction will minimize damage to the blood supply of the soft tissues.[11] Second, a paucity of soft tissue usually means a limited blood supply will be available for union. Consideration should be given to improving vascular supply via vascularized bone graft or soft tissue transfer. Finally, in patients with poor soft tissue coverage, the surgeon should give consideration to gradual correction via distraction osteogenesis (Ilizarov) techniques.

Anatomy

Epiphyseal or intra-articular malunions will require intervention if there is a residual articular cartilage step-off or joint line obliquity of the knee or ankle based on standing radiographs.[12] The goals of treatment as outlined by Schatzker[12] are an accurate reduction of the joint surface with stable internal fixation, and the use of continuous passive motion (CPM) postoperatively. Early motion is advantageous because it promotes articular cartilage healing while also minimizing postoperative joint stiffness. Schatzker's goals may be accomplished by performing an intra-articular osteotomy with reduction or by osteotomy of the metaphysis to normalize the alignment or, in the case of degenerative arthritis, overcorrecting the alignment to unload the joint **(Fig. 5–2A,B).**

Metaphyseal malunions require intervention when there is residual joint line obliquity or malalignment on the standing hip-knee-ankle radiographs. Deformity correction is most easily evaluated by superimposing tracings of the abnormal side on the normal side **(Fig. 5–3A,B).** This technique will make evident the change necessary to normalize the limb. In the lower extremity, each plan must be superimposed on hip-knee-ankle tracings so as to avoid a translation, which can affect mechanical alignment. This problem is most commonly seen around the hip, where valgus osteotomy without lateralization of the shaft will predictably lead to valgus malalignment **(Fig. 5–4A,B).** Although the type of osteotomy required will be determined by the tracing, the choices are limited to oblique, opening, and closing wedges. Osteotomy choice should create the desired change as well as create intrinsic stability.[13] **Fig. 5–5A–D** shows two preoperative plans for the same patient. **Fig. 5–5A,B** shows adequate deformity correction with a 120 degree angled blade plate, but inadequate stability with a medial open area. **Fig. 5–5C,D** shows the preferred preoperative plan employing an adult 90 degree osteotomy plate with minimal residual opening medially thus improving stability in the final construct.

Hierholzer[7] states that opening wedge osteotomy in the lower extremity is to be avoided because it is intrinsically unstable. We believe this to be true in the absence of structural bone graft. In contrast, closing wedge and oblique osteotomies are easily made stable. Whenever possible the surgeon should create an osteotomy that leaves a residual obliquity, thus allowing an increased surface area for healing and for application of a lag screw. The technique of osteotomy should be performed as demonstrated in **Fig. 5–5C,D.** However, fragment mobilization should be done

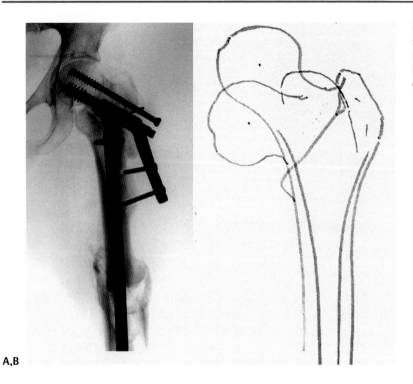

Figure 5–3 (A) An ipsilateral pertrochanteric and shaft fracture with failed internal fixation. **(B)** Superimposition of the involved side on the reversed tracing of the uninvolved side (from a sketch made by operating physician).

A,B

using tools with broad surfaces to minimize crushing of the bone. Manipulation of the diaphysis is also helpful in realigning the fragments (e.g., valgus intertrochanteric osteotomy).[14]

Fixation of a metaphyseal osteotomy must account for the limited capacity of cancellous bone to hold a cortical screw when compared with cortical bone.[15] In cancellous bone, therefore, it is wise to use fixed-angle devices such as blade plates or locking plates because these provide larger surface areas to avoid cutout **(Fig. 5–6)**. Locking screws and plates fail by forcing the bone to cut around the screw to have failure rather than the screws sequentially

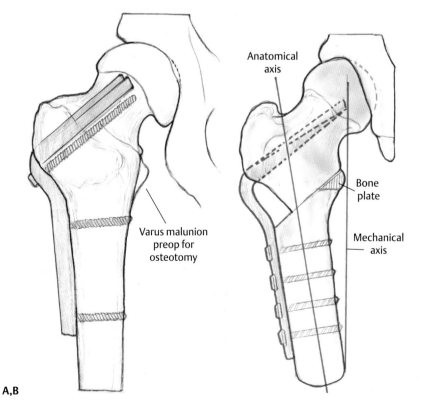

Figure 5–4 (A) Varus malformation of the proximal femur. **(B)** valgus osteotomy of the proximal femur with lateralization of the shaft, reestablishing a normal anatomical and mechanical axis.

Anatomical axis

Bone plate

Mechanical axis

Varus malunion preop for osteotomy

A,B

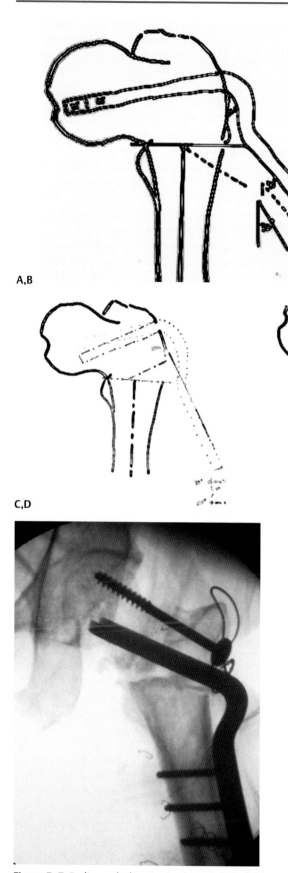

A,B

C,D

Figure 5–7 Radiograph showing inadequate bony bridge under the shoulder of the blade plate leading to loss of fixation in the proximal fragment.

Figure 5–5 Sketches drawn by the operating physician that demonstrate two different plans for the same deformity. **(A)** Varus malunion and **(B)** correction of the deformity with poor stability, yielding a suboptimal plan. **(C)** Varus malunion and **(D)** a plan that yields both adequate deformity correction and stability.

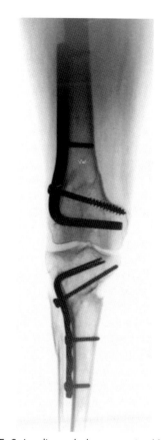

Figure 5–6 A radiograph demonstrating blade plate fixation in the metaphysis of the distal femur and tibia.

pulling out, as occurs with conventional plates. Once a blade plate or locked plate is seated in the metaphysis, compression will maximize construct stiffness and resist failure. The surgeon should take care to ensure that the blade or locked plate has an adequate bony bridge (e.g., 1.5 cm for valgus osteotomy) to resist failure based on pull-out of the implant from the metaphysis **(Fig. 5–7)** during compression.[7,16]

Diaphyseal malunions require thorough evaluation because they often have multiplanar involvement. In his evaluation of long-bone malunions, Milch[3,17] has determined that long bones can be considered straight or curved based on whether the mechanical axis is collinear with the anatomical axis. Examples of straight bones include the tibia, ulna, and humerus. This is of importance because a malunion or a curved bone such as the femur is more difficult to fully correct in all planes and may require a mathematically generated oblique osteotomy.[16]

Diaphyseal deformities often involve shortening in addition to the recognized coronal or sagittal plane abnormality. Therefore, length must be evaluated prior to creating a preoperative plan. If shortening is present, it is important to recognize that a closing wedge osteotomy will further shorten the limb, and therefore an oblique osteotomy may be a better choice to allow correction of both the shortening and the malalignment. If an oblique osteotomy is used, it will be necessary to prebend the plate[19] and add a lag screw.

General Principles of Internal Fixation for Malunions

The conventional wisdom in fracture fixation is that one should stabilize the epiphysis with screws, the metaphysis with plates, and the diaphysis with a rod. Although this holds true for acute fractures, compression is the fundamental tool for successful treatment of mal- and nonunions. Fixation after osteotomy or after nonunion treatment should focus on generating compression across the bony defect. Exceptions include femoral and some tibial nonunions where a reamed intramedullary nailing will trigger increased periosteal blood flow,[20] and the increased rod size will create a construct stiff enough to generate union. However, most nonunions and malunions require fixation in compression using either a lag screw through the plate[20] or an external fixator in the case of the proximal or distal tibial.[21] Internal fixation for malunion or nonunion has the advantage of being definitive, biomechanically predictable, and cosmetic, and it requires limited patient or surgeon aftercare. The disadvantage of open reduction and internal fixation (ORIF) is that imprecise correction, if not recognized intraoperatively, will require revision surgery.[20]

Successful internal fixation requires a mechanically sound construct able to resist cyclic muscular contraction generated during early functional activity.[14] For internal fixation, this requires a plate with sufficient length to resist torsional forces. Ring et al[22] found that, with humeral nonunions in osteoporotic bone, successful constructs used plates with lengths 80% of the length of the bone. The modern trend in choosing a longer plate length for reconstruction mimics the current trend in fracture treatment.[23] The use of the Articulating Tensioning Device (Synthes, Paoli, Pennsylvania) is helpful in generating compression in osteoporotic bone or in the femur where greater than 100 kPa is required.[25] Successful internal fixation requires bony surfaces with satisfactory cortical contact to achieve bony stability to protect the implant. If a defect is present, bone grafting is required at the osteotomy or nonunion site.

Types of Deformity

Rotational Deformities

Rotational malalignment is common after intramedullary nailing. Unfortunately, there are no scientifically supported criteria available in the literature to establish the degree of malrotation in the lower extremity that represents pathological significance. Once the decision has been made to correct malrotation, a transverse osteotomy is the ideal surgical intervention. In the case of shortened and malrotated femurs following intramedullary nailing, Samuel[25] reported using an oblique derotational osteotomy to correct modest deformities. It is important to limit correction using this technique because large corrections create poor bony apposition at the osteotomy site. Direct surgical exposure is mandatory when performing a transverse osteotomy. Careful placement of Homan retractors is done to minimize stripping of soft tissue attachments. Threaded Kirschner wires are inserted at an angle mimicking the degree of malrotation, which had been determined preoperatively either by clinical exam or by CT scanning (**Figs. 5–8A,B; 5–9**). The osteotomy is performed with a saw with care to avoid thermal necrosis of the bone. Derotation is then performed using temporary external fixation or clamp fixation to stabilize the bone. Evaluation of the correction is then performed by comparing the positions of the implanted K-wires or by comparison with the contralateral limb.

Angular Deformities

Significant lower extremity single plane deformities are usually in the frontal plane. Often the goal is simple restoration of mechanical alignment. Although this is usually done by using an opening or closing wedge osteotomy,[20] superimposition of a tracing of the abnormal side over a tracing of the normal side will clarify what correction is needed (**Fig. 5–5A-D**).

Two-Plane Deformities

Paley[26] has pointed out that in a two-plane deformity, the degree of malalignment documented on standard anteroposterior (AP) and lateral radiographs underestimates the actual deformity. Therefore, a complete workup should include oblique films, which will often identify the true plane of deformity. It may be calculated from the AP and lateral views by plotting the degree of deformity in the coronal plane on the x-axis, and the degree of sagittal plane deformity on the y-axis. The resultant vector is the degree and direction of the maximal deformity. This can be done fluoroscopically as well as by rotating the image intensifier until the deformity demonstrates the greatest magnitude. The plane is then documented from the image intensifier.

A closing wedge or single oblique osteotomy is the best option for correction of a two-plane deformity. Treatment

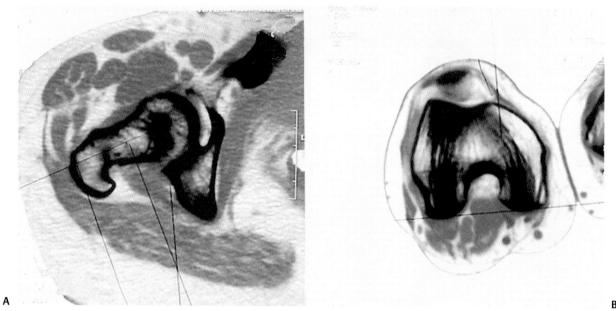

A   **B**

Figure 5–8 Computed tomographic scan cuts of the **(A)** proximal and **(B)** distal femur, demonstrating severe retroversion which clinically manifests as an external rotation deformity.

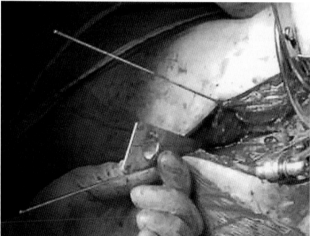

Figure 5–9 K-wire positioned on the proximal and distal fragments mimicking the deformity in preparation for surgical correction.

with the closing wedge technique requires determination of degree of correction in each plane and resection of a representative trapezoid (**Figs. 5–10A,B; 5–11A,B**). The disadvantage to this technique is the inability to place a lag screw following wedge resection because the resultant osteotomy is transverse. Another disadvantage is the osteotomy leads to additional leg length discrepancy.[27] In contrast, using a single oblique osteotomy[27] allows for lag screw placement and does not increase leg length discrepancy. The plane of the osteotomy cut is perpendicular to the malunion.[16,27]

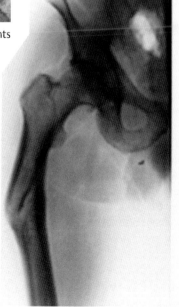

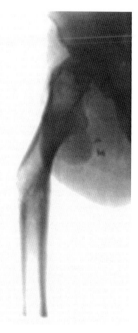

Figure 5–10 (A) AP and **(B)** lateral radiographs demonstrating proximal femoral malunion.   **A,B**

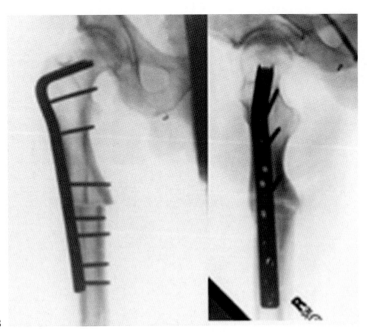

Figure 5–11 (A) Anteroposterior and **(B)** lateral radiographs after resection of a trapezoid to correct the deformity leaves a residual transverse osteotomy.

A,B

Three- and Four-Plane Deformities

Three- and four-plane deformities are best managed using a single oblique osteotomy.[17,28] If this method is chosen, trigonometric analysis[17] and the correct orientation of the cut will automatically correct rotation. Closing wedge osteotomy is another option. However, closing wedge osteotomy requires a resection of a trapezoid, and it is critical to correct rotation first. Failure to initially correct for rotation will impact the correction in the sagittal and coronal planes, especially in a curved bone such as the femur. In complex deformities preoperative planning can be aided by making a plastic model simulating the deformity. This will allow the opportunity to make the planned correction prior to surgery.

Osteotomies for Malunion Correction

The practice of malunion correction using an osteotomy requires knowledge of the advantages and disadvantages of the various osteotomy types. Anticipation of and preparation for the limitations of each osteotomy type will minimize complications. Whenever possible, choose an osteotomy that will help create inherent stability, thus protecting the hardware and construct from failure. Deformity correction should preferentially[7,28] take place at the deformity site to avoid creating a deformity to correct one. The exception would be in the case of poor local skin or bone quality where use of virgin skin or bone may be advantageous.[9,21]

Transverse Osteotomy

Transverse osteotomies in the diaphysis are useful for correcting malrotation. Transverse osteotomies are inher-

ently unstable in torsion and bending,[29] and therefore are best stabilized with a statically locked intramedullary nail. Care must be used in employing transverse osteotomies in the metaphysis due to the risk of invagination of the cortical step-off, which may lead to overcorrection[12] **(Fig. 5–12).**

Oblique Osteotomy

Oblique osteotomy provides an excellent tool in deformity correction because it can afford length and sagittal plane, in addition to coronal plane, correction. It also offers broader surface areas for healing, superior bending, and rotational stability, and can be compressed with a lag screw. Lag screws placed through the plate increase construct strength by 25%.[20]

Oblique osteotomies are useful in metaphyseal bone, especially when used with an incomplete cut to create a hinge for increased stability. The surgeon can add or remove wedges to adjust length, mechanical axis, and rotation. Oblique osteotomy also allows the hardware to be placed in a tension band fashion. It is important to make the cut without excessive obliquity to avoid shear unless resisted by an antiglide plate, as described by Brunner and Weber[30] **(Fig. 5–13A,B).**

Step-Cut Osteotomies

While seeming attractive during preoperative planning, step-cut osteotomies have significant disadvantages, such as requiring increased exposure, allowing only limited fixation, and limiting the potential for angular or rotational correction.

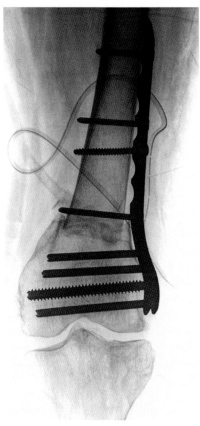

Figure 5–12 Radiograph demonstrating invagination of the osteotomy fragments with residual shortening.

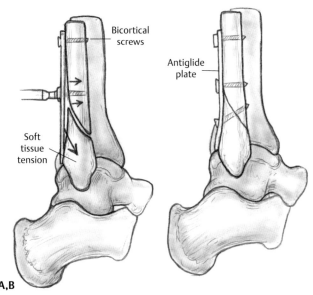

A,B

Figure 5–13 (A,B) Oblique osteotomy of the distal fibula stabilized with an antegrade plate.

Opening Wedge Osteotomy

In the diaphysis, opening wedge osteotomy allows for axial correction without sacrifice of length. However, opening wedge osteotomies are intrinsically unstable and should be managed with grafting of corticocancellous bone in the newly created defect. In the metaphysis the authors recommend grafting when the opening wedge correction is greater than 5 mm.

Surgical Techniques for Specific Malunions

The goal of malunion reconstruction in the proximal humerus is to reestablish the normal biomechanics of the shoulder. In terms of anatomy, this requires that the tuberosities be fixed to the metaphysis in their normal positions and orienting the articular surface to its normal 125 degrees. Normal alignment is established by taking a radiograph of the uninjured side and comparing tracings of the normal and abnormal side to determine the degree of malalignment. The osteotomy is planned and performed to leave residual obliquity, allowing for lag screw stabilization and also allowing correction of length. The osteotomy is finally stabilized with a plate applied at the end of the osteotomy, thus creating the additional structural benefit of an antiglide effect.

Proximal Humerus Malunion

Preoperatively, a radiographic evaluation is facilitated by placing the patient on a radiolucent table with a bump under the affected scapula elevating the patient to approximately a 45 degree angle. The image intensifier is then brought in on the contralateral side, and, by performing 45 degree oblique x-rays, one can see an AP view of the glenohumeral joint, as well as a scapular Y view by simply rotating the C-arm. A deltopectoral approach[31] is used for surgical exposure. Once exposure of the proximal humerus is achieved, retractors are placed to expose the malunion. Visualization is usually improved by passing a blunt Homan retractor around the superior and lateral aspects of the proximal humerus. Judicious retraction will prevent injury to the axillary nerve. More distally, exposure may be improved by sharply releasing a portion of the deltoid attachment off the humeral shaft. Threaded K-wires are then drilled in place so as to mimic the area of intended osteotomy **(Fig. 5–14)**. After resection of the wedge, the arm is adducted to close the osteotomy gap created. Fixation is performed with a fixed-angle construct such as a blade plate or locking plate and screws so as to ensure fixation in the metaphyseal bone. Compression is generated across the osteotomy site by loading the plate distally. Deep and superficial tissues are closed in the standard fashion.

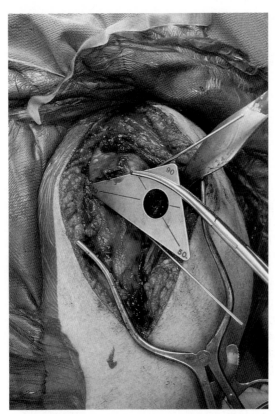

Figure 5–14 Kirschner wires mimicking the intended osteotomy of a proximal humerus malunion.

Distal Radius (see Video 5–1, Disk 1)

Distal radial malunions are common in the elderly and usually well tolerated due to the low functional demand in most of these patients. Patients with distal radial malunions experience a loss of strength due to loss of the normal volar tilt. Opening wedge or oblique osteotomy can reestablish the normal volar tilt, normalize the distal radial ulnar joint (DRUJ), and normalize length.

For an opening wedge osteotomy for the distal radius **(Fig. 5–15)**, a standard dorsal approach utilizing the fourth compartment is preferred. Radial and ulnar dissection will create access to the entire dorsal metaphysis. Once the dorsal radial surface is adequately exposed, threaded Kirschner wires are placed so as to mimic the proposed osteotomy. Proper wire placement is confirmed radiographically. Using a 1 in. microsagittal saw, the osteotomy is performed, leaving the volar cortex partially intact. An osteotome is inserted and gently used to lever the osteotomy site open. This will complete the osteotomy at the volar surface, but should be done so as to minimally disturb the soft tissues. Placement of the wrist on several towels will allow it to open on the dorsal surface.

Preoperatively, a tricortical wedge is planned to be taken from the iliac crest. The tricortical graft is planned so that the width of the wedge of crest taken is double the size needed to make the correction. This wedge is then split, and each piece is inserted to complete the correction. The depth of the graft harvest is the width of the radius on x-ray. One must recognize that measured lengths on nondigitalized plain radiographs have an approximate magnification of 20%. Once the graft is inserted, fixation is by a dorsally applied distal radial plate in compression **(Fig. 5–15)**. Closure is performed, with special attention to protecting the extensor pollicis longus from attritional rupture. This may be done by splitting the extensor retinaculum transversely and creating a slip to protect the extensor pollicis longus.

Distal Femur

Malunions of the distal femur are often multidimensional and can be in varus, valgus, flexion, or extension, and often have associated shortening **(Fig. 5–16A,B)**. Closing wedge osteotomies often exacerbate the shortening; therefore, planning should focus on oblique osteotomies, which allow the surgeon to regain length where necessary. Miranda and Mast have used a double oblique osteotomy to correct complex malunions of the distal femur (unpublished series). A case example of this technique is demonstrated in **Figs. 5–16A,B** and **5–17A,B**.

The authors prefer the standard lateral approach to the distal femur. Dissection remains extraperiosteal, save for the proposed osteotomy site. Homan retractors are placed to aid visualization and protect neurovascular structures. The leg is placed on a bump or triangle so as to take the tension of the gastrocnemius off the femoral condyles. A

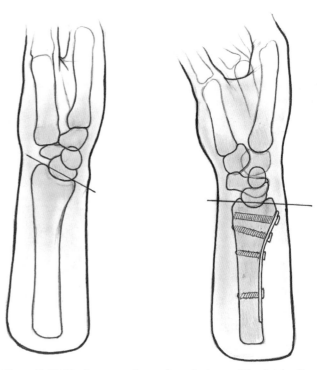

Figure 5–15 Plan for an opening wedge osteotomy of the distal radius with bone grafting.

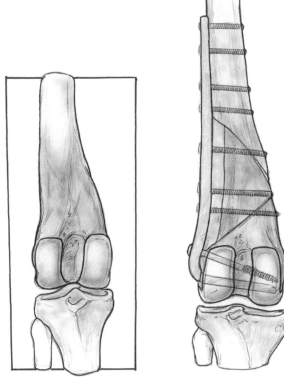

A,B

Figure 5–16 (A) A complex distal femoral malunion. **(B)** Blade plate fixation following double oblique osteotomies.

95 degree angle blade plate is the preferred implant because the placement of the angle blade plate parallel to the joint will re-create normal alignment if the osteotomy site is placed in compression.

Initially, Kirschner wires are placed mimicking the osteotomy cuts. The chisel is then used to create a channel for the blade plate **(Fig. 5–17A)**. It is notable that a 1.5 to 2.0 cm bridge is required between the chisel blade plate channel and the osteotomy site. Once seated, the blade must be loosened prior to the osteotomy cuts or the chisel

will be difficult to unseat. Once loosened, the cuts may be made. Next, seat the blade plate. At this point, using a Verbrugge clamp and the articulating tensioning device **(Fig. 5–17B)**, the distal fragment is distracted, and the intermediary segment is mobilized medially. Once in satisfactory position, the articulating tensioner is used to compress across the osteotomy sites. The Articulating Tensioning Device is employed to gain better than 100 kPa of compression. The intermediary segment will need to be stabilized or it will lateralize down the decline plane. Wherever possible, lag screws are placed across the osteotomy site to further enhance stability. Postoperatively, the patient ambulates with foot flat, touch down weight bearing. Active and passive ranges of motions are encouraged. No bracing or splinting is necessary.

Proximal Tibia

The goal of treatment of proximal tibial malunions is to minimize intra-articular step-off **(Fig. 5–2A,B)** and reestablish the normal mechanical alignment of the knee with a joint line that is parallel to the floor.

The surgical technique for an extra-articular proximal tibia malunion **(Fig. 5–18)** uses a medial approach, which allows adequate exposure for the osteotomy. The patient is positioned supine, a tourniquet is inflated to 250 mm Hg, and the knee is positioned in flexion by using a bump under the knee. A medial approach allows adequate exposure for the osteotomy. Using the image intensifier, the malunion is identified, and the intended line of osteotomy is noted and marked. Osteotomy is performed by using an osteotome. The surgeon should be sure that the meniscus is not trapped in the previous fracture site. A Kerrison rongeur is employed proximally and posteriorly so as to avoid injury to the posterior neurovascular structures. Fixation is with screws placed across the osteotomy in compression using lag technique, followed by buttress plate application **(Fig. 5–19A,B)**.

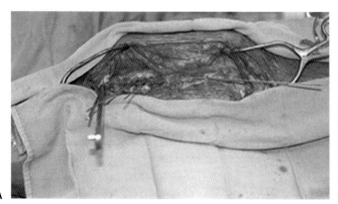

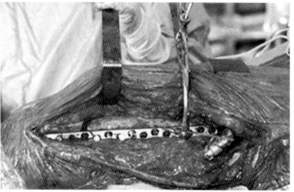

A **B**

Figure 5–17 (A) A clinical photograph demonstrating the channel for the blade plate. **(B)** A clinical photo demonstrating use of the articulating tensioning device.

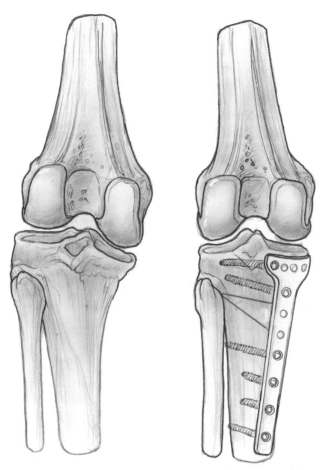

Figure 5–18 Illustration of a proximal tibial malunion treated by a medial opening wedge osteotomy.

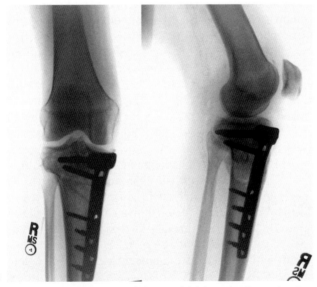

A,B

Figure 5–19 Postoperative **(A)** AP and **(B)** lateral radiographs after correction of the proximal tibial malunion.

New Techniques for Malunion Correction

Correction of complex malunions with a Taylor Spatial Frame (Smith & Nephew, Memphis, Tennessee), a relatively new development, allows correction in all three dimensions using a series of struts and a computer-controlled program that is downloaded from the manufacturer. The correction is automatically applied via the programmed system in a very gradual fashion. The early reports with this system are very encouraging, correcting complex deformities in all three planes with impressive accuracy.

Outcomes of Malunion Correction

Modern series of deformity correction show rates of success of 84 to 100% at correction of complex malunions.[17,19,21,29] Sanders et al[28] reviewed a series of 12 patients treated with oblique osteotomies of the tibia. In the patients who were compliant, all had excellent results. Sangeorzan et al[16] reported on four patients with tibial malunions. They described 100% union without complications after osteotomy. Chiodo et al[32] performed oblique osteotomies in six patients. They reported excellent results, with all deformities corrected to less than 10 degrees variance with the intact side. There were no major complications, and no patient required additional surgery.

Complications of Malunion

The most common complications associated with malunion surgery are under- or overcorrection (0 to 15%), nonunion (0 to 12%), nerve palsy (0 to 8%), infection (1 to 3%), delayed union (3 to 5%), and thromboembolism (2 to 4%).

- The most common (up to 15%) complication associated with surgical correction of malunions is failure to achieve correct anatomical alignment.
- You need to have good joint motion above and below a malunion to achieve a good functional result.
- Most malunions do not occur in strictly orthogonal planes. Make certain you have oblique radiographs to fully evaluate the deformity.

Epidemiology of Nonunions

Bhandari and Schemitsch[34] characterized the status of nonunions well. The published rates after long-bone fractures in the lower extremity range from 3 to 48%.[34] They pointed out that fracture healing is estimated to be delayed in 600,000 patients per year in the United States.[35] Approximately 100,000 of these fractures annually proceed to nonunion.[36] Risk factors associated with nonunion include fracture characteristics such as fracture displacement and segmental loss;[36–39] high-energy mechanism of injury;[38] severe soft tissue injuries;[40,41] and patient characteristics, for example, diabetes,[43,44] alcohol consumption,[44] smoking,[44,45] specific medications (steroids and nonsteroidal anti-inflammatories,[47–49] anticonvulsants,[50] antibiotics,[51] and anticoagulants);[52,53] and vasculopathy and vascular injuries.[54] Infection is an important and often catastrophic cause of nonunion.

Einhorn describes nonunion as the "cessation of all healing processes and union has not occurred."[55] Delayed union is defined as a continuation of healing processes, with union not occurring in the expected time and uncertainty regarding union.[55] In most instances a nonunion has been established when a fracture has not healed during the expected 3 to 9 months. Radiographically, this has been defined as a lack of bridging callus across the fracture site. Although bulky callus is reassuring on follow-up evaluation, cortical continuity has been found to be the single best predictor of fracture torsional strength, and callus size and area to be the least important indicator of union.[56]

Metaphyseal nonunions can be difficult to diagnose.[57] Exuberant callus is common with metaphyseal nonunions. This callus is a result of either motion or bone graft from previous surgery.[57] In actuality, metaphyseal healing takes place by the formation of new bone on existing trabecular bone at the fracture site. This mechanism means that there should be little callus formation seen on x-ray film. Again, cortical continuity is the most important radiographic indicator of healing.

Classification of Nonunions

Nonunions can be classified as either hypertrophic or avascular, each with additional subtypes[57] **(Fig. 5–20)**. Hypertrophic nonunions have an adequate blood supply but lack sufficient stability to generate union. The hypertrophic subtypes described by Weber and Cech[58] reflect the radiographic appearance of the nonunion. The elephant foot is rich in callus, usually caused by poor fracture stability in a milieu rich in blood supply. The next subtype is the horse's hoof nonunion. This subtype occurs as a result of moderately secure fixation with adequate blood supply. Radiographically, the horse's hoof nonunion has little callus and mild sclerosis. Last in this group is the oligotrophic nonunion, which has no callus and no hypertrophy. This subtype usually reflects fragment distraction or internal fixation without opposition.

Avascular nonunions lack blood supply but may also lack stability. Avascular nonunions are further divided into four subtypes. The first two subtypes identify nonunions with an intermediate fragment of decreased (torsion wedge) or absent blood supply (comminuted). The third subtype is nonunion where there is an absence of diaphyseal bone; these must be treated using a graft. The fourth subtype is the atrophic nonunion, which is the long-standing nonunion with osteoporotic ends lacking in osteogenic potential.

Evaluation of Nonunions

The initial evaluation of patients with a nonunion is detailed earlier in this chapter. Nonunion-specific laboratory workup should include complete blood count (CBC), erythrocyte sedimentation rate, and C-reactive protein. One should be careful, however, because in chronic conditions these laboratory studies can normalize. They are more useful when they are followed over time and a trend is established. Aspiration of a nonunion site suspected of infection can be helpful, but swabbing of open wounds and skin tracts is not usually accurate in identifying the infectious pathogens. The only accurate way to identify an infectious agent is by an open biopsy.

Radiographic evaluation specific for nonunions should include AP, lateral, and oblique views.[39] Stress radiographs are helpful to evaluate instability. MRI, especially when enhanced by intravenous gadolinium, is very accurate for evaluating pathological changes in bone and soft tissue. However, it is not as accurate for differentiating between edema, infection, and postoperative changes. MRI is also limited by any metallic implants in the region being evaluated. CT can be used in those patients with metallic implants and is helpful in evaluating the degree of union, subtle bone changes, sequestra, and devitalized bone.

Nuclear medicine scans are frequently used to evaluate for either acute or chronic infection. There are several

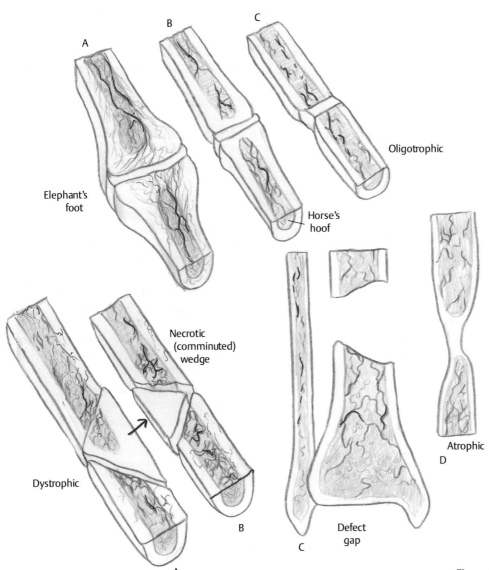

Figure 5–20 Classifications of nonunions.

radiopharmaceuticals available, each having different characteristics. Indium-labeled leukocyte scintigraphy, 99mTcABs immunoscintigraphy, and 99m-Tc-labeled nanocolloids are useful in the evaluation of infection, especially during the first year postoperatively, and when metallic implants are present. Suspected chronic, low-grade infections may be best evaluated by [111]Inleukocyte scintigraphy because it tracks cell migration over a 48 hour period.

Surgical Treatment of Nonunions (see Video 5–2, Disk 1)

The principle of nonunion treatment lies in reestablishing the environment required for healing a fracture. In other words, treatment requires ensuring the availability of the mesenchymal cells found in the periosteum of live bone,

the bone growth factors needed to evolve them, and an adequately vascularized environment with sufficient immobilization of the fracture fragments.[59-63] Preoperative evaluation should determine if each of these factors is available and also if there are factors that will negate their efficacy once the healing process has started. In the case of patients with an infection associated with a nonunion, adequate control of the infection is necessary to achieve union. Infection impacts on union by creating instability from bone as bone is reabsorbed by cytokines released during the acute inflammatory process.

With the exception of femoral and tibial nonunions, all other nonunions should be treated with a technique to generate compression across the nonunion site. Hypertrophic nonunions are typically the result of inadequate immobilization. Stable fixation without further disruption of the blood supply typically results in union in these cases. Tension band plating with interfragmentary screw fixation using indirect reduction[65] is an excellent approach to hypertrophic nonunions.

Atrophic nonunions are the result of an inadequate blood supply to the bone. Causes can include nonviable bone, bone stripped of its periosteum, yielding insufficient potential bone-forming cells, and inadequate immobilization of the fracture.[58] These conditions can be precipitated by severe displacement of fracture fragments where the bone ends are not in continuity, high-energy injuries, after internal fixation where the vascular supply is damaged, or with infection. In these situations, it is necessary to resect nonviable bone down to bleeding bone, place the fragments in compression, and then add bone graft to provide osteoinductive factors. In the case of nonunions where the surrounding soft tissue has little vascularity (e.g., the distal tibia), soft tissue transfer may be necessary.

Weber and Cech's defect nonunions require bone grafting or bone transport to achieve union. This type of nonunion can be found in patients having multiple prior procedures, prior infection, or extensive bony injury.[58] Failed internal fixation can also cause significant defects requiring grafting. Bone grafting should be supplemented by decortication, petaling, or shingling of the bone (**Fig. 5–21A,B**). Wave plate fixation[65,66] employs a plate contoured so that it stands away from the bone at the site of the nonunion (**Fig. 5–22**) so as to minimally interfere with vascular access or egress. Theoretically, this allows for more rapid and predictable incorporation of even large bone grafts in complex femoral[65] and humeral nonunions.[22]

Transfer of vascularized fibular autograph offers advantages because it creates immediate and lasting structural support.[67] This is in contrast to cancellous bone graft that is replaced by creeping substitution and weakens before union can be achieved. The disadvantage of vascularized fibular grafting is that it is time consuming and technically difficult. Distraction osteogenesis allows transportation of bone into the defect. The soft tissues are lengthened simultaneously, thereby limiting the necessity for soft tissue transfer. The drawbacks of this approach are that it is time and resource intensive and has a high complication rate.[68]

Electrical or ultrasound bone stimulators have been recommended for the treatment of well-vascularized nonunions.[69,70] The disadvantage of this approach is the inability to address deformity and the associated requirement of prolonged immobilization of the limb with the attendant complications of atrophy and contracture.

Femoral and tibial diaphyseal nonunions can be treated with an intramedullary rod. In such cases the medullary canal is accessed via the usual entry portals and reamed to a large size, permitting more secure fixation. The act of reaming causes a periosteal vascular reaction that stimulates bone formation.[71] Reaming also allows the deposi-

tion of bone at the nonunion site without stripping the nonunion site. In the instance where an intramedullary rod is fractured in situ, exposure of the nonunion site for extraction of the rod and debridement of devascularized tissues may be necessary. In this setting, plate fixation may be less traumatic than placement of another intramedullary rod.

Intertrochanteric Osteotomy for Femoral Neck Nonunion

Intertrochanteric osteotomy, as described by Pauwels, is a reliable and consistent method for treatment of nonunions of the femoral neck.[2] Preoperative plain radiographs of the hip in internal and external rotation, as well as a lateral view, are required for preoperative planning. The osteotomy planning described here is adapted from Müller.[71] The first step is to establish the inclination of the femoral neck nonunion. Using an AP film of the hip, the surgeon can draw a perpendicular line to the femoral shaft above the hip joint. A second line is drawn parallel to the femoral neck nonunion. The angle created by the intersection of these two lines is the angle of the femoral neck nonunion. The size or degree of closing wedge resected from the intertrochanteric area is the difference between the angle of nonunion and 25 degrees, which is the ideal angle for maximal joint reaction force across the nonunion.

The patient is placed in the supine position. The author's preferred approach is a direct lateral approach with the variation of taking down the vastus lateralis proximally off the trochanteric ridge in a horizontal T so that the vastus fascia may be closed over the implant. A 95 degree angled blade plate or the adult osteotomy plate (Synthes, Paoli, Pennsylvania) is the preferred implant in these cases. Initially, Kirschner wires are placed to mimic the osteotomy cut planned. Next, we prepare the proximal femur for the seating chisel by identifying the appropriate starting hole and then using the triple drill guide in the angled blade plate set to establish a channel for the blade. The authors find it helpful to insert three 4.5 mm drill bits in the guide and then check radiographs in both AP and lateral views with the three drill bits placed at 2 to 3 cm beyond the opening cortex. Radiographically, this will give an indication of the ultimate position of the blade. Once the seating chisel is placed across the nonunion and satisfactorily positioned on AP and lateral radiographs, the chisel is backed out and loosened prior to making the osteotomy cuts. When the osteotomy cuts are made and the wedge resected, the blade plate itself is seated. Please note that the blade should be seated with room to place the resected wedge between the blade and proximal fragment. This will lateralize the femur so as to avoid inadvertent valgus alignment at the knee. Once the blade is fixed to the proximal fragment, the shaft is ab-

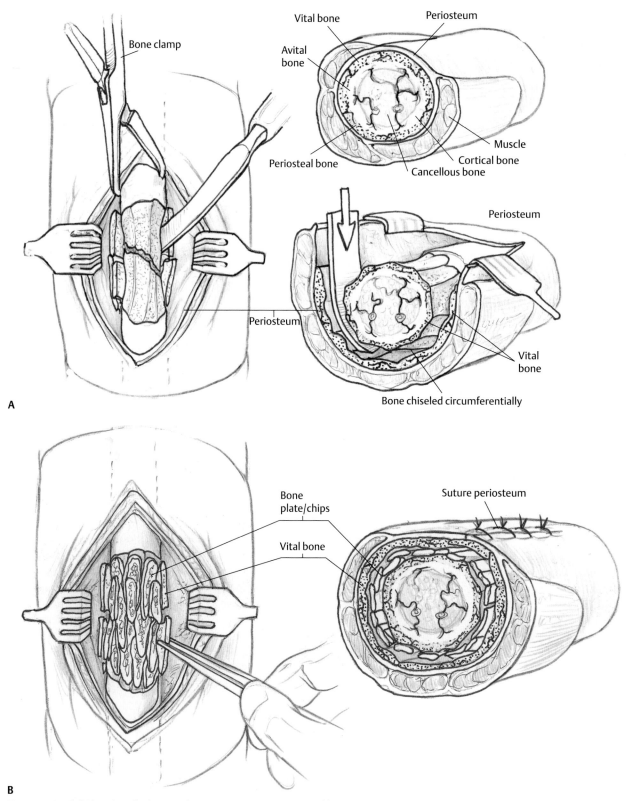

A

B

Figure 5–21 **(A)** Shingling the bone with an osteotome to expose vital bone. **(B)** Placing bone chips around the vital bone to obtain union.

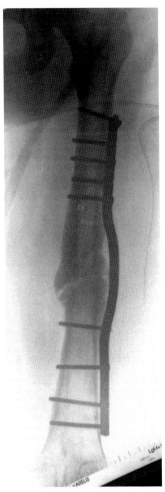

Figure 5–22 A "wave" plate applied to the diaphysis of the femur.

ducted until it meets the plate. One will note that the shaft has migrated proximally and that a mismatch has been created. Insertion of the distal screw of the plate fixes the shaft to the plate. Insertion of the most proximal screw will draw the shaft to the blade. As the screw is advanced, the oblique surface of the shaft contacts the proximal fragment with increasing compression. This increases the stability and stiffness of the construct. Due to the force generated by this technique, one must ensure that entrance for the osteotomy chisel is at least 1.5 to 2.0 cm away from the osteotomy site, or cut-out will occur (**Fig. 5–7**). **Fig. 5–23A–C** demonstrates a femoral neck nonunion and the 3 year follow-up results following an intertrochanteric osteotomy.

Hypertrophic Tibial Shaft Nonunion

Hypertrophic nonunion treatment has as its goal to increase the stiffness and stability of the nonunion, preferably in compression. An anterior approach is performed with careful dissection around the nonunion site. My initial approach relies on determining the true plane of the nonunion. This is done by evaluating the radiographs preoperatively or by using fluoroscopy intraoperatively. Once the plane is established, the approach is planned so as to place the plate on the tension side of the deformity. Dissection is performed in an extraperiosteal fashion. Homan retractors are placed around the nonunion. An osteotome is then driven across the nonunion to ensure mobility. Great effort is made to minimize disturbance to the blood supply. Once the alignment is corrected, a lag screw is placed across the nonunion site, and a plate is placed orthogonal to it. In serendipitous circumstances, the plate is applied, and the lag is placed through the plate. **Figs. 5–24A–D** and **5–25A–C** document the case of a 33-year-old woman with a hypertrophic nonunion of 13 years' duration.

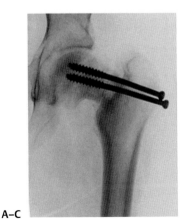
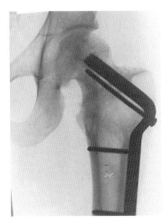
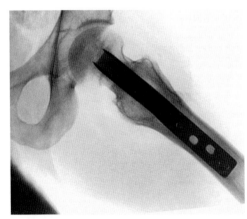

A–C

Figure 5–23 (A) Femoral neck nonunion following screw fixation. **(B)** AP and **(C)** lateral postoperative radiographs with 3 year follow-up using a blade plate to treat a femoral neck nonunion.

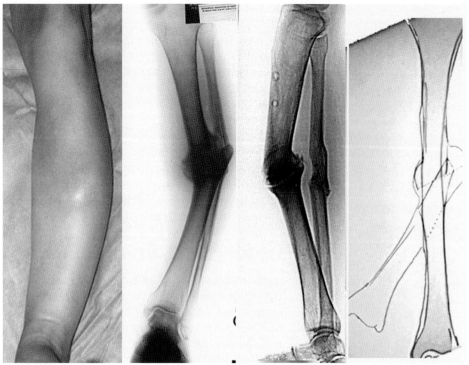

A–D

Figure 5–24 **(A)** A clinical photo showing deformity of the leg as a result of the nonunion. **(B)** Anteroposterior radiograph of the nonunion. **(C)** Lateral radiograph of the nonunion. **(D)** Preoperative plan with tracing of the deformity superimposed on a tracing of the contralateral leg.

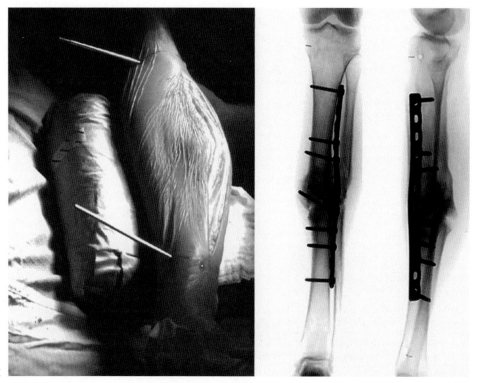

A–C

Figure 5–25 **(A)** Pin placement for using the large femoral distractor. **(B,C)** Postoperative radiographs following reduction and compression plating of the nonunion.

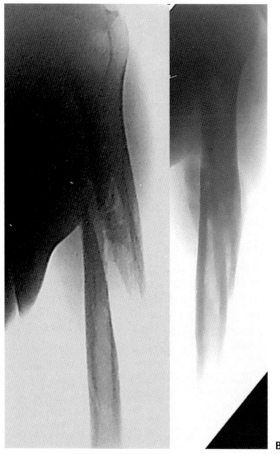

A   B

Figure 5–26 (A) Anteroposterior and **(B)** lateral radiographs demonstrating a nonunion of the diaphysis of the humerus.

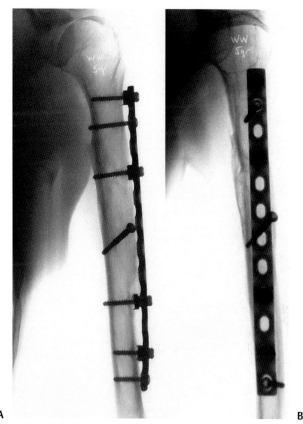

A   B

Figure 5–27 (A) Anteroposterior and **(B)** lateral radiographs following compression with a lag screw and placement of a neutralization plate with Schuli washers (Synthes, Paoli, Pennsylvania) to improve fixation and minimize plate disruption of blood flow.

Humeral Shaft Atrophic Nonunion

Plate fixation has a higher success rate than intramedullary nailing for nonunions of the humerus.[73] This likely reflects the bony anatomy of the distal humerus. The medullary canal of the distal humerus tapers distally and curves anteriorly, inviting reaming for larger nail placement. However, the cortical nature of the distal humerus causes it to undergo heat necrosis with reaming. **Figs. 5–26A,B** and **5–27A,B** demonstrate a nonunion treated by compression plate osteosynthesis.

The coracoid process and deltoid tubercle are palpated, and an anterolateral surgical approach is used for this nonunion. Distal extension is continued anterolaterally at the edge of the biceps brachii. Proximally, the interval is between the pectoralis major and the deltoid. In the distal portion of the wound, the biceps is mobilized medially, and the underlying brachii muscle is split. An extraperiosteal approach is used for deep tissue dissection. The dissection is carried proximally and distally enough to allow for plate placement. Once the nonunion is encountered, the periosteum is taken down around the nonunion with a sharp osteotome by flaking off pieces of cortex with it in a process called shingling. Often, the periosteum is absent, and the bone ends are covered with fibrous tissue.

The bone ends should be exposed and debrided until vascular bone is encountered, as indicated by the appearance of red specks that look like the spice paprika. If possible, shape the bone so it is stable when the bone ends are opposed. Insert bone graft at the nonunion site and around the surrounding tissues. A plate, usually 10 or 12 holes in length, is applied in compression across the nonunion site. Obtaining adequate compression often requires placing a screw outside the plate that is fixed on one side and use of a Verbrugge clamp **(Fig. 5–28A,B)**. Six to eight cortices of fixation are necessary on each side of the nonunion to resist the torsional forces created by the forearm.

Clavicle Nonunion

Clavicle nonunions treated by plate fixation require a transverse incision parallel to the clavicle. Sharp dissection is continued utilizing full-thickness flaps down to the level of the periosteum. An extraperiosteal approach is maintained except at the fracture site. The lateral end of the medial fragment is identified, and the bone end is exposed. The medial end of the lateral fragment is approached by carefully dissecting through the zone of nonunion. Once the medial end of the lateral fragment is

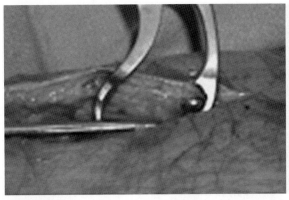
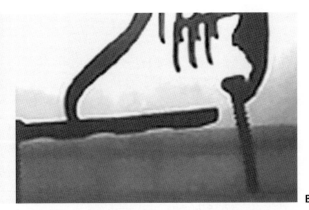

A   B

Figure 5–28 (A) Clinical photograph and **(B)** radiograph demonstrating the use of the Verbrugge clamp to obtain compression across nonunion site.

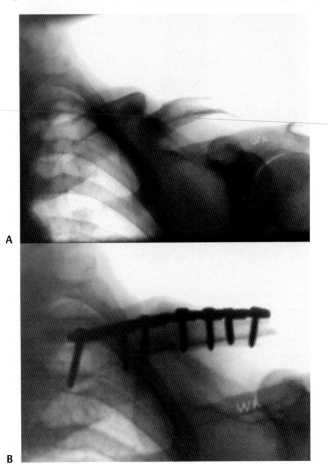

A

B

Figure 5–29 (A) Atrophic nonunion of the clavicle 10 months following fracture. **(B)** Healed nonunion 8 months following open reduction and internal fixation of the nonunion.

identified, a small, blunted Homan retractor is slipped over the edge of the fragment and levered against the lateral end of the medial fragment to bring them out to length and into opposition. On occasion, it may be necessary to square off the edges to create stability during this process or in the final reduction. Cancellous autograft is then placed below the nonunion in the defect of soft tissue created by the reduction of the clavicle. An eight- to 10-hole reconstruction plate is placed superiorly and applied in compression. The plate must be

twisted to accommodate the change in the anatomy as the superior border of the clavicle extends medial to lateral (**Fig. 5–29A,B**). Biplanar plate fixation is usually not necessary. Careful soft tissue closure is performed to maximize plate coverage with the full-thickness flaps. If the surgeon is suspicious that there is significant shortening of the clavicle, films of the contralateral clavicle should be taken for comparison and, if necessary, a tricortical iliac crest graft placed to reestablish the normal length.

Rehabilitation from Nonunion Surgery

The rehabilitation of a patient following surgical treatment of a nonunion varies depending on the location of the nonunion, as well as the treatment employed. In general, active range of motion is encouraged immediately postoperatively. Any strength training is deferred until cortical healing is seen on one view during clinical follow-up.

New Techniques for Malunions and Nonunions

Bone Grafts and Bone Graft Substitutes (see Video 5–3, Disk 1)

The use of bone graft and bone graft substitutes to augment stability and achieve union is integral to the treatment of nonunions and malunions. Although autologous bone grafting is the gold standard to which all other grafts are compared, there are circumstances where the appropriate use of allograft and bone graft substitutes can spare the patient the potential risks and complications of obtaining autograft. Any algorithm for bone graft use hinges on an understanding of when and what type of graft is necessary. A detailed description of all of the options currently available is beyond the scope of this chapter, but we will discuss the general principles and choices.

The biochemical and cellular environment of bone defects in fresh fractures differs greatly from nonacute scenarios. In the treatment of nonacute fractures, the surgeon must re-create the biochemical and cellular environment of the fresh fracture to generate union. Bone graft can provide the mesenchymal cells found in the periosteum of live bone and the bone growth factors needed to generate them. Bone graft can also be used to improve structural stability in large or diaphyseal defects. Both these circumstances necessitate that the mechanical environment has been optimized by creating sound bony fixation.[74] Assuming that stability has been created, then the size and location of the defect as well as the biological environment must be considered.

Diaphyseal defects less than 6 cm in a stable mechanical environment need both the scaffolding for osteoconduction and the cellular and chemical components to generate healing. Therefore, cancellous autograft is the best option. Cancellous allograft with bone marrow aspirate may yield similar rates of union, but this has not been clearly demonstrated in human prospective clinical studies.

For diaphyseal defects greater than 6 cm, a cortical autograft or allograft may be needed to provide structural stability. Vascularized cortical autografts are advantageous over nonvascularized autografts or allografts because of their more rapid and complete incorporation, as well as their ability to hypertrophy.[74] However, Finkemeier[74] points out that cortical allografts are best utilized in areas of excellent blood supply, such as the metaphyseal locations, or around the femur with its heavy muscular coat. In bony areas with poor or disrupted flow, the surgeon should strongly consider using vascularized autografts to achieve union.

Metaphyseal defects associated with nonunion are best treated with cancellous autograft for its osteoinductive properties. Those metaphyseal defects from impaction or cysts with a good vascular supply can be adequately treated with bone graft substitutes or corticocancellous allograft. Skeletal Repair System (SRS; Norian, Cupertino, California) stands out from other bone graft substitutes in that after 12 hours, this material hardens to form dahlite with a compressive strength of 55 mPa; because of its crystalline structure, it can eventually be resorbed and replaced by the host. This creates immediate stability as opposed to cancellous allograft, which will weaken with time as it is absorbed by creeping substitution.

Fracture healing is a complex process utilizing local and systemic regulatory factors. Bench and clinical research has begun to evaluate if the addition of some of these factors [e.g., bone morphogenetic proteins (BMPs), transforming growth factor-β (TGF-β), platelet-derived growth factor (PDGF), insulin-like growth factor (IGF), and fibroblast growth factor (FGF)] will improve union or can substitute for autograft. At present BMP 7 has been shown to yield results approaching autograft. The Food and Drug Administration (FDA) has concluded that, although the OP-1 implant (Howmedica, Rutherford, New Jersey) was an effective treatment for nonunions, BMP was not as effective as autograft. The FDA product labeling states that the commercially available BMP OP-1 is indicated "for use as an al-

ternative to autograft in recalcitrant long bone nonunions where use of autograft is unfeasible and alternative treatments have failed."

Tips and Tricks

- Successful nonunion treatment requires that compression be generated across the fragments.
- In addition to eccentric screw placement, there are three ways of generating compression for nonunions: a Verbrugge clamp, the Articulating Tensioning Device (Synthes), and the femoral distractor (Synthes). The latter two are useful for generating compression and distraction. The color guide in the Articulating Tensioning Device yields feedback about how much compression is being generated.
- We recommend the use of long plates to treat nonunions (80% of bone length).
- Whenever possible we use blade plate fixation or locked screws when working in the metaphyseal region.
- Lastly, we harvest bone graft using an acetabular reamer on the lateral cortex of the ilium. This is done through a vertical incision overlying the gluteal pillar just superior and posterior to the acetabulum. This will often generate 40 to 75 cc of graft easily **(Fig. 5–30).**

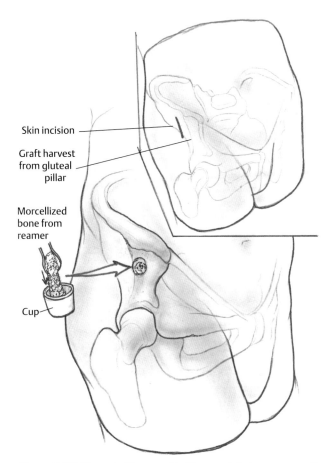

Skin incision

Graft harvest from gluteal pillar

Morcellized bone from reamer

Cup

Figure 5–30 Harvest of bone graft with an acetabular reamer on the lateral cortex of the ilium.

Outcomes of Nonunion Surgery

The outcomes for nonunions vary remarkably depending on patient comorbidities, available blood supply, index injury energy, and location of the nonunion. Ring et al[75] were able to unite a series of 14 recalcitrant nonunions (> 10 years) in an average of 4 months. These long bones included clavicle (two cases), humerus (five), femur (three), and tibial (four) nonunions. We believe that this demonstrates the excellent potential for long bones to heal with appropriate treatment.

Complications of Nonunion Surgery

Common complications[62,63,72,74] in nonunion surgery include persistent nonunion (0 to 20%), wound dehiscence (0 to 15%), and infection (0 to 3%). The harvesting of autologous bone is associated with a rate of major complications of 8.6% and a rate of minor complications of 20.6%.[75]

Pearls

- Delayed union occurs in 600,000 patients in the United States per year.
- Nonunion occurs in 100,000 fractures in the United States per year.
- Risk factors for nonunion include initial displacement, smoking, segmental bone loss, high-energy mechanism of injury, degree of soft tissue injury, diabetes, excessive alcohol consumption, vasculopathy, and certain medications.
- Elephant/horse's hoof nonunions are associated with unstable fixation.
- Oligotrophic nonunion is associated with distraction.
- Atrophic nonunions are associated with tissue interposition.
- Comminuted avascular nonunions are associated with sequestrum interposition.
- Two-part surgical neck fractures are the most common proximal humeral nonunion.
- Cortical continuity is the single best predictor of fracture torsional strength, and callus size and area are the least important indicators of union.
- The complication rate from the harvest of autologous bone is 8.6% major complications and 20.6% minor complications.

On the DVDs

Video 5–1   (Disk 1)   Correction of Varus Malunion of the Proximal Humerus by Osteotomy   The patient in this video has a varus malunion of the proximal humerus. He is treated with a closing wedge osteotomy and locked plating based on the preoperative surgical plan.

Video 5–2   (Disk 1)   Compression Plating of a Femur Nonunion   This video demonstrates compression plate fixation of a femur nonunion with a titanium broad LCDCP. The lateral approach to the femur, as well as the importance of debridement of the nonunion and compression of viable bone fragments are stressed.

Video 5–3   (Disk 1)   The Use of a Reamer-Irrigator-Aspirator   This video demonstrates a new technique for obtaining autologous bone graft and some bioactive substances using the Reamer-Irrigator-Aspirator (Synthes, Paoli, Pennsylvania).

References

1. Morscher E. Pathophysiology of posttraumatic deformities of the lower extremity. In: Hierholzer G, Muller KH, eds. Corrective Osteotomies of the Lower Extremity after Trauma. New York: Springer-Verlag; 1986:3–9
2. Pauwels F. Biomechanical principles of varus/valgus intertrochanteric osteotomy. In: The interotrochanteric osteotomy. J. Shatzker, ed. Springer Verlag 1984:3–24
3. Mast JW, Teitge RA, Gowda M. Preoperative planning for the treatment of nonunions and the correction of malunions of the long bones. Orthop Clin North Am 1990;21:693–714
4. Oest O. Special diagnosis and planning of corrective osteotomies. In: Hierholzer G, Muller KH, eds. Corrective Osteotomies of the Lower Extremity after Trauma. New York: Springer-Verlag; 1986:29–39
5. Dugdale TW, Degnan GG, Turen CH. The use of computerized tomographic scan to assess femoral malrotation after intramedullary nailing: a case report. Clin Orthop Relat Res 1992;279:258–263
6. Muller KH, Strosche H, Scheuer I. Plate osteosynthesis in posttraumatic deformities of the femoral shaft. Arch Orthop Trauma Surg 1984;103:303–319
7. Hierholzer G, Hax PM. Corrective osteotomies of the lower extremities after trauma. In: Hierholzer G, Muller KH, eds. Corrective Osteotomies of the Lower Extremity after Trauma. New York: Springer-Verlag; 1986:9–28
8. Liebrand B, MD de Ridder VA, De Lange, S, Ulrich C, Hermans F, Westeinde Hospital, Va Den Haag, Holland. The clinical relevance of the rotational deformity after femoral shaft fracture treated with intramedullary nailing. J Orthop Trauma 2000;14:133
9. Mast JW, Jakob R, Ganz R. Planning and Reduction Technique in Fracture Surgery. New York: Springer-Verlag; 1989
10. Oznur A, Cemalettin A, Mazhar TZ. Posteromedial approach and posterior plating of the tibia. J Trauma 2002;53:722–724
11. Hiem U, Muller-Gerbl M. The clinical consequences of the anatomy In: Hiem U. The Pilon Tibial Fracture; Classification, Surgical Techniques, and Results. Berlin: Springer-Verlag; 1991:31–32
12. Schatzker J. Intraarticular malunions and nonunions. Orthop Clin North Am 1990;21:743–759
13. Stahelin T, Hardegger F, Ward JC. Supracondylar osteotomy of the femur with the use of compression osteosynthesis with a malleable implant. J Bone Joint Surg Am 2000;82:712–722

14. Muller ME. Intertrochanteric osteotomy: indications, preoperative planning and technique. In: Schatzker J, ed. The Intertrochanteric Osteotomy. New York: Springer-Verlag; 1984:36–66

15. Perren S. Mechanical and technical principles of the internal fixation of corrective osteotomies. In: Hierholzer G, Muller KH, eds. Corrective Osteotomies of the Lower Extremity after Trauma. New York: Springer-Verlag; 1986:39–45

16. Sangeorzan BJ, Sangeorzan BP, Hansen ST Jr, Judd RP. Mathematically directed single-cut osteotomy for correction of tibial malunion. J Orthop Trauma 1989;3:267–275

17. Milch H. Osteotomy of the Long Bone. Springfield, IL: Thomas; 1947

18. Müller M, Allgöwer M, Willineger H. Manual of Internal Fixation. 2nd rev. ed. New York: Springer-Verlag; 1988

19. Klein MP, Rahn BA, Frigg R, et al. Reaming versus nonreaming in medullary nailing: interference with cortical circulation of the canine tibia. Arch Orthop Trauma Surg 1990;109:314–316

20. Stevens P. Principles of osteotomy. In: Chapman MW, ed. Operative Orthopedics. Philadelphia: Lippincott-Raven; 1993:489–509

21. Marti RK, Besselaar FP, Raaymakers ELFB. Malunion. In: AO Principles of Fracture Management. New York: Thieme; 2000:779–797

22. Ring D, Perey BH, Jupiter JB. The functional outcome of operative treatment of ununited fractures of the humeral diaphysis in older patients. J Bone Joint Surg Am 1999;81:177–190

23. Rozbruch SR, Muller U, Gautier E, Ganz R. The evolution of femoral shaft plating technique. Clin Orthop Relat Res 1998;354:195–208

24. Texshammar R, Colton C. AO/ASIF Instruments and Implants. New York: Springer-Verlag; 1984:67

25. Samuel AW. Malrotation of the femur after intramedullary nailing. Injury 1996;27:438–440

26. Paley D. Oblique plane deformity analysis. Bull Hosp Joint Dis; 52:35–36

27. Sanders R, Anglen JO, Mark JB. Oblique osteotomy for the correction of tibial malunion. J Bone Joint Surg Am 1995;77:240–246

28. Murray DW, Kambouroglou G, Kenwright J. One stage lengthening for femoral shortening with associated deformity. J Bone Joint Surg Br 1993;75:566–571

29. Evans EG, Dunn HK, Daniels HU. Comparison of transverse and oblique osteotomies. Trans Orthop Res Soc 1985;10:187

30. Brunner CF, Weber BG. Special techniques in internal fixation. New York: Springer-Verlag; 1982

31. Ruedi T, von Hochsteeer AHC, Schlumpf R. Surgical Approaches for Internal Fixation. New York: Springer-Verlag; 1984

32. Chiodo CP, Jupiter JB, Alvarez G, Chandler HP. Oblique osteotomy for multiplanar correction of malunions of the femoral shaft. Clin Orthop Relat Res 2003;406:185–194

33. Bhandari M, Schemitsch EH. Clinical advances in the treatment of fracture nonunion: the response to mechanical stimulation. Clin Orthop Relat Res 2000;11:372–377

34. Bhandari M, Guyatt GH, Adili A, et al. Reamed versus non-reamed IM nailing of lower extremity long bone fractures: a systematic overview and meta-analysis. J Orthop Trauma 2000;14:2–9

35. Caplan AI. Mesenchymal stem cells. J Orthop Res 1991;9:641–650

36. Sarmiento A, Sharpe FE, Ebramzadeh E, et al. Factors influencing the outcome of closed tibial fractures treated with functional bracing. Clin Orthop Relat Res 1995;315:8–24

37. Tytherleigh-Strong GM, Keating JF, Court-Brown CM. Extra-articular fractures of the proximal tibial diaphysis: their epidemiology, management and outcome. J R Coll Surg Edinb 1997;42:334–338

38. Oni OO, Dunning J, Mobbs RJ, et al. Clinical factors and size of the external callus in tibial shaft fractures. Clin Orthop Relat Res 1991;273:278–283

39. Sarmiento A. On the behaviour of closed tibial fractures: clinical/radiological correlations. J Orthop Trauma 2000;14:199–205

40. Gaston P, Will E, Elton RA, et al. Fractures of the tibia: can their outcome be predicted? J Bone Joint Surg Br 1999;81:71–76

41. Templeman DC, Gulli B, Tsukayama DT, et al. Update on the management of open fractures of the tibial shaft. Clin Orthop Relat Res 1998;350:18–25

42. Cozen L. Does diabetes delay fracture healing? Clin Orthop Relat Res 1972;82:134–140

43. Funk JR, Hale JE, Carmines D, et al. Biomechanical evaluation of early fracture healing in normal and diabetic rats. J Orthop Res 2000;18:126–132

44. Nyquist F, Berglund M, Nilsson BE, Obrant KJ. Nature and healing of tibial shaft fractures in alcohol abusers. Alcohol Alcohol 1997; 32:91–95

45. Schmitz MA, Finnegan M, Natarajan R, et al. Effect of smoking on tibial shaft fracture healing. Clin Orthop Relat Res 1999;365: 184–200

46. Kyro A, Usenius JP, Aarnio M, Kunnamo I, Avikainen V. Are smokers a risk group for delayed healing of tibial shaft fractures? Ann Chir Gynaecol 1993;82:254–262

47. Hogevold HE, Grogaard B, Reikeras O. Effects of short-term treatment with corticosteroids and indomethacin on bone healing: a mechanical study of osteotomies in rats. Acta Orthop Scand 1992;63:607–611

48. Altman RD, Latta LL, Keer R, et al. Effect of non-steroidal anti-inflammatory drugs on fracture healing: a laboratory study in rats. J Orthop Trauma 1995;9:392–400

49. Engesaeter LB, Sudmann B, Sudmann E. Fracture healing in rats inhibited by locally administered indomethacin. Acta Orthop Scand 1992;63:330–333

50. Frymoyer JW. Fracture healing in rats treated with diphenylhydantoin (Dilantin). J Trauma 1976;16:368–370

51. Huddleston PM, Steckelberg JM, Hanssen AD, et al. Ciprofloxacin inhibition of experimental fracture healing. J Bone Joint Surg Am 2000;82:161–173

52. Dodds RA, Catterall A, Bitensky L, et al. Effects on fracture healing of an antagonist of the vitamin K cycle. Calcif Tissue Int 1984;36:233–238

53. Stinchfield F, Sarkanan B, Samilson R. The effect of anticoagulant therapy on bone repair. J Bone Joint Surg Am 1956;38: 270–282

54. Dickson KF, Katzman S, Paiemont G. The importance of blood supply in the healing of tibial fractures. Contemp Orthop 1995;30: 489–493

55. Einhorn TA. Breakout session 1: definitions of fracture repair. Clin Orthop Relat Res 1998;355(Suppl):S353

56. Panjabi MM, Walter SD, Karuda M, et al. Correlations in radiographic analysis of healing fractures with strength: a statistical analysis of experimental osteotomies. J Orthop Res 1985;3:212–218

57. Ebraheim NA, Skie, MC, Heck BE, Jackson WT. Metaphyseal nonunion: a diagnostic dilemma. J Trauma 1995;38:261–268

58. Weber BG, Cech O. Pseudarthrosis. New York: Grune and Stratton; 1976

59. Bruder SP, Fink DJ, Caplan AI. Mesenchymal stem cells in bone development, bone repair and skeletal regeneration therapy. J Cell Biochem 1994;56:283–294

60. Lindholm TS, Nilsson OS, Lindholm TC. Extraskeletal and intraskeletal new bone formation induced by demineralized bone matrix combined with bone marrow cells. Clin Orthop Relat Res 1982;171:251–255

61. Takagi K, Urist MR. The role of bone marrow in bone morphogenetic protein-induced repair of femoral massive diaphyseal defects. Clin Orthop Relat Res 1982;171:224–231

62. Tiedman JJ, Connolly JF, Strates BS, Lippiello L. Treatment of nonunion by percutaneous injection of bone marrow and de-

mineralized bone matrix: an experimental study in dogs. Clin Orthop Relat Res 1991;268:294–302

63. Werntz JR, Lane JM, Burstein AH, et al. Qualitative and quantitative analysis of orthotopic bone regeneration by marrow. J Orthop Res 1996;14:85–93

64. Helfet DL, Jupiter JB, Gasser S. Indirect reduction and tension-band plating of tibial nonunion with deformity. J Bone Joint Surg Am 1992;74:1286–1297

65. Blatter G, Weber BG. Wave plate osteosynthesis as a salvage procedure. Arch Orthop Trauma Surg 1990;109:330–333

66. Weber BG, Brunner C. Special Techniques in Internal Fixation. Berlin: Springer-Verlag; 1982

67. Jupiter JB, Bour CJ, May JW Jr. The reconstruction of defects in the femoral shaft with vascularized transfers of fibular bone. J Bone Joint Surg Am 1987;69:365–374

68. Paley D. Problems, obstacles, and complications of limb lengthening by the Ilizarov technique. Clin Orthop Relat Res 1990;250:81–104

69. Brighton CT, Pollack SR. Treatment of recalcitrant non-union with a capacitively coupled electrical field: a preliminary report. J Bone Joint Surg Am 1985;67:577–585

70. Sharrard WJ. A double blind trial of pulsed electromagnetic fields for delayed union of tibial fractures. J Bone Joint Surg Br 1990;72:347–355

71. Müller M. Intertrochanteric osteotomies. In: Schatzker J, ed. The Intertrochanteric Osteotomy. New York: Springer-Verlag; 1984:25–35

72. Brav EA. The use of intramedullary nailing for nonunion of the femur. Clin Orthop Relat Res 1968;60:69–75

73. McKee MD, Miranda M, Riemer BL, et al. Management of humeral nonunion after failure of locking intramedullary nails. J Orthop Trauma 1996;10:492–499

74. Finkemeier CG. Bone-grafting and bone-graft substitutes J Bone Joint Surg Am 2002;84-A:454–464

75. Ring DB, Barrick WT, Jupiter JB. Recalcitrant nonunion. Clin Orthop Relat Res 1997;340:181–189

6 Injuries to the Cervicocranium

Carlo Bellabarba, Sohail K. Mirza, and Jens R. Chapman

The cervicocranium consists of the osseoligamentous and neurovascular structures that extend from the skull base to C2. It includes the craniocervical junction and the articulations between the first and second cervical vertebrae.

The cervicocranium's susceptibility to injury is related to (1) the large lever arm induced by the mass and immobility of the cranium combined with (2) the relative freedom of movement more caudally, with reliance on ligamentous structures rather than on intrinsic bony stability for the maintenance of craniocervical alignment. This tenuous functional unit is maintained by highly specialized C1 and C2 bony segments interconnected via a complex and incompletely understood ligamentous system whose vulnerability to injury may compromise the structural integrity of the entire craniocervical junction.

Due to the nearby neurovascular structures, injury to the upper cervical spine that results in loss of craniocervical integrity carries a high likelihood of death. However, improved trauma care has increased the likelihood of survival in patients with craniocervical injuries, raising the burden of responsibility to appropriately identify and treat these life-threatening injuries.

This chapter focuses primarily on the treatment of six injury types, many of which coexist: (1) occipital condyle fractures, (2) craniocervical dissociation, (3) fractures of the atlas, (4) C1–C2 instability patterns, (5) odontoid fractures, and (6) traumatic spondylolisthesis (hangman's fracture) of C2. In trying to achieve our main goal of describing the surgical treatment of craniocervical injuries, we also aim to impart a fundamental and prerequisite understanding of craniocervical instability patterns, the complexities involved in their diagnosis and classification, and the manner in which these principles apply to evolving treatment methods.

Nonoperative Treatment

General Concepts

The crucial first treatment step is timely injury recognition and determination of stability. Reduction maneuvers are typically performed with cranial skeletal traction in the emergency room using fluoroscopy. However, traction is contraindicated in distractive cervical spine injuries. Closed reduction of such distractive injuries may necessitate early application of a halo or postural reduction in a Rotorest

bed (Kinetic Concepts Inc., San Antonio, Texas) or with sandbags surrounding the head, both of which are usually temporizing measures pending operative stabilization.

Accompanying resuscitation efforts include vasopressor support for suspected neurogenic shock and emergent assessment for potential intracranial trauma. Patients with neurological injuries should be considered for intravenous methylprednisolone per the Third National Acute Spinal Cord Injury Study (NASCIS III) protocol, although the role of steroids in the treatment of acute spinal cord injuries has become increasingly unclear.

Emergent surgical intervention for patients with upper cervical spine injuries is rarely necessary. Open reduction and stable internal fixation are helpful intervention strategies for patients with dislocations and distractive upper cervical spine injuries. The presence of a spinal cord injury usually suggests the need for surgical stabilization and, possibly, decompression to maximize the chance for neurological recovery.

Nonoperative treatment options consist of recumbent skeletal traction, bracing, and halo immobilization. The reduction can be assessed by obtaining lateral recumbent and upright radiographs. The duration of external immobilization usually ranges from 2 to 4 months and depends on the type of injury and age of the patient. External immobilization is also commonly used for 6 to 12 weeks postoperatively after surgical stabilization. Recommendations vary widely with regard to the need for and duration of external support.

Bracing

In the presence of minimally or nondisplaced fractures of the upper cervical spine, external bracing alone can be considered. Sternal-occipital-mandibular immobilizer (SOMI)-type devices have been shown to allow the least upper cervical spine motion of nonhalo devices in cadaveric testing.[1]

Halo Orthosis

Halo-ring and vest orthotics offer the most stable form of external upper cervical spine immobilization.[1] The halo has been recommended for patients with isolated occipital condyle fractures, unstable atlas ring fractures, odontoid fractures, and displaced neural arch fractures of the axis.[2] Unlike bracing, the halo allows for some fracture manipulation and correction of malalignment. However, secondary loss of reduction has been noted in approximately half of patients.[3] A common mechanism of fracture displacement in a halo consists of a "snaking" of the cervical spine between supine and upright positions.[4] Although this phenomenon may not adversely affect the healing of inherently stable upper cervical spine fractures with large cancellous bone surfaces, unstable fractures with a small bony contact surface, such as type II odontoid fractures, may not be effectively immobilized.[5,6]

Skeletal Traction

Aside from its role in acute fracture reduction, traction can be used to maintain spinal alignment and stability for an extended period of time in an attempt to achieve initial consolidation of an unstable fracture prior to mobilizing the patient with a halo or rigid brace. Although there are no fixed guidelines for such a management strategy for cervical spine injuries, suggested time frames for traction have usually ranged from several days to weeks.[3,7] However, prolonged recumbency carries an increased morbidity and mortality risk, and consideration should be given to the use of a Rotorest bed and mechanical as well as pharmacological thromboembolism prophylaxis.[8]

Injury Classification and Indications for Surgical Treatment

Occipital Condyle Fractures

Classification

Although often inherently stable, occipital condyle fractures may be highly unstable if they represent bony avulsion of major craniocervical stabilizers. Anderson and Montesano described a classification system **(Fig. 6–1A–C)** consisting of three categories. Type I fractures are usually stable, comminuted axial loading injuries. Type II injuries are potentially unstable injuries caused by a shear mechanism that results in an oblique fracture extending from the condyle into the skull base. Type III injuries are unstable avulsion injuries that result in a transverse fracture line through the occipital condyle **(Fig. 6–2A,B).**[9] Any occipital condyle fracture should be considered a possible component of craniocervical dissociation.

Indications for Surgery

Operative treatment of occipital condyle fractures is generally reserved for the type III injuries that represent alar ligament avulsions and result in craniocervical instability **(Fig. 6–2A,B).** Surgical indications are therefore equivalent to those described following here for craniocervical dissociation.

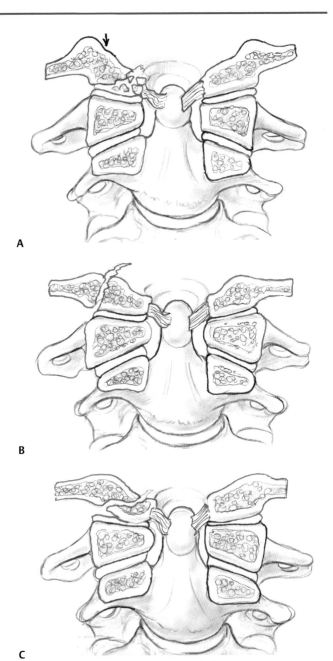

A

B

C

Figure 6–1 Anderson and Montesano classification of occipital condyle fractures. **(A)** Type I injuries are comminuted, stable impaction fractures caused by axial loading. **(B)** Type II injuries are impaction or shear fractures extending into the base of the skull and are usually stable. **(C)** Type III injuries are alar ligament avulsion fractures and represent unstable distraction injuries of the craniocervical junction.

Craniocervical Dissociation

Classification

Traynelis et al identified three craniocervical dissociation patterns according to the direction of displacement of the cranium relative to the cervical spine **(Fig. 6–3A–D).**[10] However, we have found that the extreme instability of these

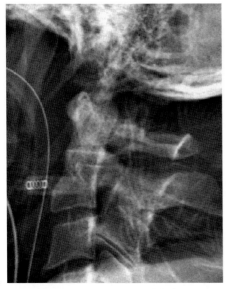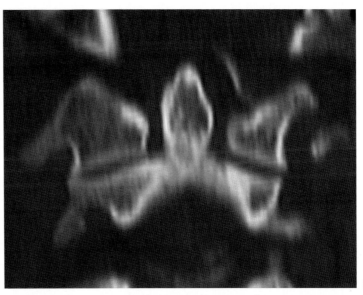

A   B

Figure 6–2 Type III occipital condyle fracture as a component of craniocervical dissociation. **(A)** Lateral cervical spine radiograph shows dislocation of the atlanto-occipital joints in a 48-year-old male involved in a high-speed motor vehicle collision. **(B)** Coronal computed tomographic image illustrates an associated avulsion fracture of the left occipital condyle, resulting in functional incompetence of the attached alar ligament.

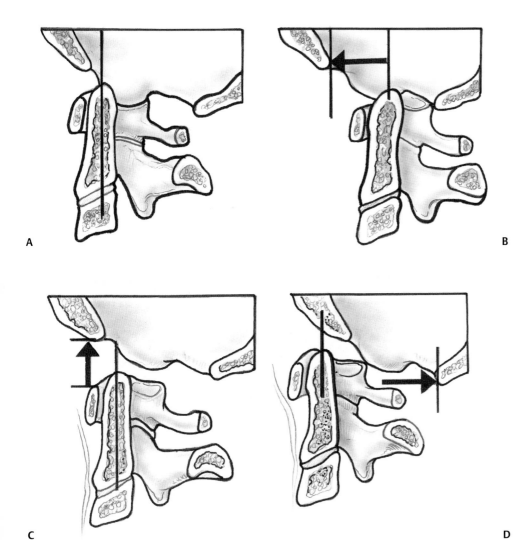

A   B

C   D

Figure 6–3 Traynelis classification of craniocervical dislocation. **(A)** Normal atlanto-occipital alignment. **(B)** Type I, anterior displacement. **(C)** Type II, distraction injury. **(D)** Type III, posterior displacement.

injuries renders the position of the head relative to the neck completely arbitrary and more dependent on external forces than on any intrinsic injury characteristic. In addition, this classification does not reflect injury severity or the potential for spontaneously reduced dislocations. These issues render directional classification systems less useful because the magnitude of displacement may underestimate the degree of instability, and the direction of displacement has little influence on prognosis or treatment method.

A useful classification system should quantify the stability of the craniocervical junction. Signs of instability are translation or distraction of more than 2 mm in any plane,[11] neurological injury, and concomitant cerebrovascular trauma.[12] The problem lies in segregating patients with minimally displaced ($\leq$ 2 mm) craniocervical injuries into those with relatively stable injuries that can be treated nonoperatively and those with highly unstable but partially reduced injuries that require operative stabilization in spite of a misleadingly low degree of displacement. We have found it useful to categorize these patients by using manual traction testing in minimally displaced injuries ($\leq$ 2 mm), reserving surgical stabilization for patients with type II and III injuries of the craniocervical junction, which we define as dissociations **(Table 6–1)**.

Indications for Surgery

Displacement of > 2 mm at the atlanto-occipital joint, either on static imaging studies or with provocative traction testing **(Table 6–1; Fig. 6–4A,B)**, or the presence of neurological injury is an indication for craniocervical stabilization. Particularly in the presence of neurological deficits, stabilization is performed as early as reasonably possible in the context of the frequently guarded condition of these polytraumatized patients.

Table 6—1 Harborview Classification of Craniocervical Injuries

Stage	Description of Injury
1	Magnetic resonance imaging evidence of injury to craniocervical osseoligamentous stabilizers Craniocervical alignment within 2 mm of normal Distraction of 2 mm or less on provocative traction radiograph
2	Magnetic resonance imaging evidence of injury to craniocervical osseoligamentous stabilizers Craniocervical alignment within 2 mm of normal Distraction of more than 2 mm on provocative traction radiograph
3	Craniocervical malalignment of more than 2 mm on static radiographic studies

Shaded areas represent injuries defined as craniocervical dissociation.

Fractures of the Atlas

Classification

It is useful to view atlas fractures as either stable or unstable injuries.[13] Instability invariably equates to the presence of transverse alar ligament (TAL) insufficiency, which can be diagnosed either by direct means, such as by identifying bony avulsion on computed tomographic (CT) scan or ligament rupture on magnetic resonance imaging (MRI), or indirectly by identifying widening of the lateral masses **(Fig. 6–5A–E)** with $\geq$ 7 mm lateral overhang relative to the lateral masses of C2,[14] appropriately corrected for radiographic magnification (see later discussion).[15]

Levine and Edwards[16] described a useful four-part classification system: (1) posterior arch fractures, (2) lateral

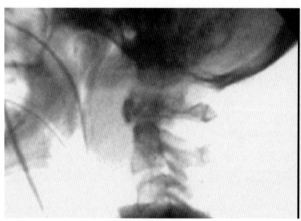

A

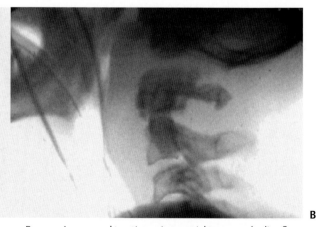

B

Figure 6–4 Provocative traction radiographs for staging of craniocervical instability. **(A)** Lateral cervical spine fluoroscopic view of a 22-year-old male involved in a high-speed motor vehicle collision who presented with neck pain and minimal (1 mm) subluxation with increased signal intensity at the atlantoaxial joints on computed tomography and magnetic resonance imaging, respectively (not shown). Progressive manual traction using cranial tongs under live fluoroscopic visualization demonstrates > 2 mm of widening across the atlantoaxial joints with no sensation of a solid end point. **(B)** This positive provocative traction test confirms a highly unstable craniocervical ligamentous injury that requires operative stabilization, defined as type II according to the Harborview classification system of craniocervical injuries.

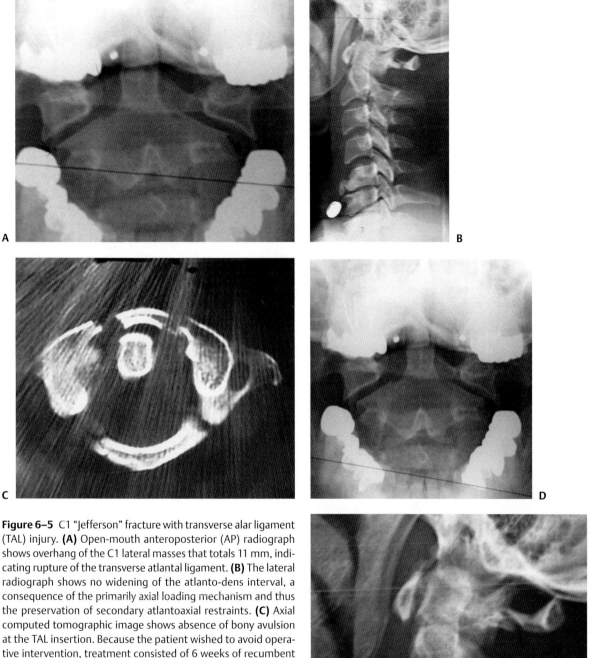

Figure 6–5 C1 "Jefferson" fracture with transverse alar ligament (TAL) injury. **(A)** Open-mouth anteroposterior (AP) radiograph shows overhang of the C1 lateral masses that totals 11 mm, indicating rupture of the transverse atlantal ligament. **(B)** The lateral radiograph shows no widening of the atlanto-dens interval, a consequence of the primarily axial loading mechanism and thus the preservation of secondary atlantoaxial restraints. **(C)** Axial computed tomographic image shows absence of bony avulsion at the TAL insertion. Because the patient wished to avoid operative intervention, treatment consisted of 6 weeks of recumbent cranial tong traction, followed by 6 weeks of ambulatory halo-vest immobilization. **(D)** Three months after injury, the open-mouth AP radiograph shows 9 mm of combined C1 lateral mass overhang. **(E)** The lateral radiograph, in conjunction with flexion-extension radiographs (not shown), shows no widening of the at-lanto-dens interval. The patient was asymptomatic at her last follow-up visit 1 year after her injury.

mass fractures, (3) isolated anterior arch fractures, and (4) bursting type fractures. As already mentioned, the extent of lateral mass separation is more relevant than the number of fracture fragments.

Indications for Surgery

Most C1 fractures are treated by nonoperative methods. Indications for operative management are related mainly to the loss of TAL integrity, as suggested by a combined lateral mass displacement of 7 mm or more (8.1 mm on x-ray with standard magnification), which introduces the potential for progressive lateral mass separation, C1–C2 instability, and pseudarthrosis.[14,15] Halo immobilization alone may be insufficient to maintain acceptable alignment in these patients. If upright radiographs in a halo show further lateral mass displacement or an anterior atlanto-dens interval (ADI) of > 3 mm, patients must be treated either with prolonged recumbency in cranial tong traction (**Fig. 6–5A–E**) or with operative stabilization, generally with posterior C1–C2 or occiput–C2 fixation.

Surgical stabilization options consist of C1–C2 transarticular screw fixation or segmental fixation with C1 lateral

mass and C2 pedicle screws connected by a plate or rod.[17] The latter method provides the opportunity to correct the C1 lateral mass widening by approximating the two rods with a cross-connector. Internal fixation of the C1 ring, by simply reapproximating the lateral masses to each other through lateral mass screws connected to a transversely oriented rod (**Fig. 6–6A–C**), is a potentially useful but not yet validated treatment option that theoretically preserves C1–C2 motion. A potential deficiency of directly repairing unstable C1 fractures is that the associated TAL deficiency may result in persistent C1–C2 instability. However, unlike with shear or distractive injuries, the axial loading mechanism that causes TAL rupture in displaced C1 ring fractures allows secondary restraints to remain intact, thus minimizing any remaining atlantoaxial instability once the atlas has been stabilized.[18]

Atlantoaxial Instability

Classification

Three atlantoaxial instability patterns present either as isolated or as combined injuries. Type A injuries are rotationally displaced in the transverse plane, type B injuries

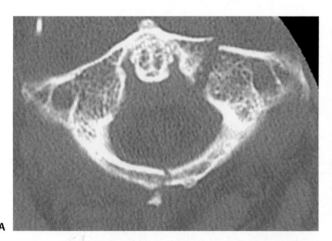

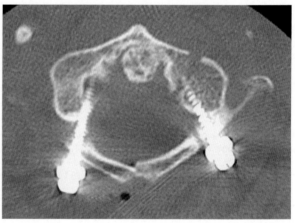

A

B

C

Figure 6–6 Direct repair of C1 lateral mass fracture. **(A)** Axial computed tomographic (CT) image shows a left C1 lateral mass fracture with associated posterior arch fracture in an elderly male who had difficulty tolerating rigid external immobilization. **(B)** Postoperative axial CT image shows direct repair of the C1 fracture with C1 lateral mass screws connected by a transverse bar, as illustrated **(C)** with an atlas model. The indications for this procedure have not been well established.

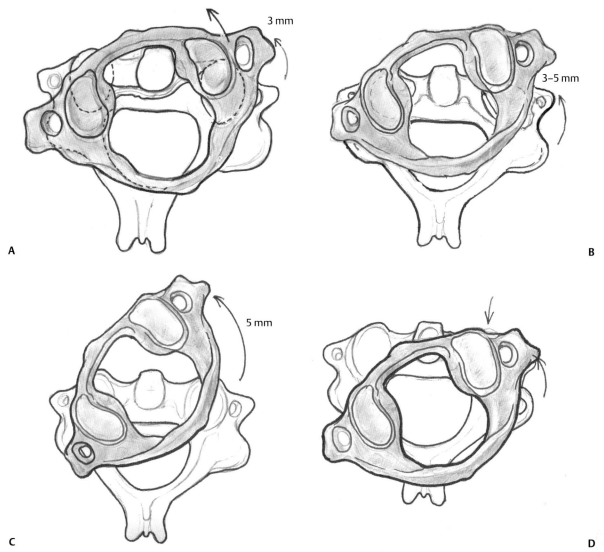

3 mm

3–5 mm

5 mm

A

B

C

D

Figure 6–7 Fielding and Hawkins classification of rotational (type A) atlantoaxial instability. **(A)** Type I. **(B)** Type II. **(C)** Type III. **(D)** Type IV.

are translationally unstable in the sagittal plane due to TAL insufficiency, and type C injuries are characterized by vertical atlantoaxial dissociation and represent a variant of craniocervical dissociation.

Type A injuries **(Fig. 6–7A–D)** Rotational displacement of the atlantoaxial motion segment is most commonly nontraumatic and will therefore not be described in detail. However, traumatic causes have been described and range in severity from mild rotational subluxation to complete dislocation of the atlantoaxial lateral masses.[19]

Type B injuries Translational atlantoaxial instability is the result of TAL insufficiency. Treatment of these highly unstable injuries depends on differentiating a ligamentous tear (type I) from a bony avulsion injury (type II) **(Fig. 6–8A–C)**.[13,20]

Type C injuries **(Fig. 6–9)** Distractive atlantoaxial injuries, or atlantoaxial dissociation, constitute a variant of craniocervical dissociation because the disrupted primary ligamentous stabilizers—the alar ligaments and tectorial membrane—extend from the C2 to the occiput. They frequently coexist with overt atlanto-occipital distraction injuries **(Fig. 6–10A–E)**.

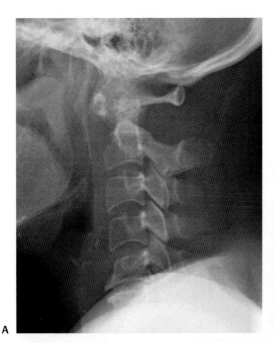

Figure 6–8 Translational (type B) atlantoaxial subluxation with bony transverse alar ligament (TAL) avulsion in a 65-year-old woman involved in a high-speed motor vehicle collision. **(A)** The lateral screening cervical spine radiograph shows widening of the atlanto-dens interval. **(B)** Axial computed tomographic (CT) image shows avulsion fracture at the left TAL insertion. An open reduction and posterior instrumented C1–C2 arthrodesis was performed. **(C)** Due to unfavorable vertebral artery anatomy for transarticular screw placement, fixation was achieved with a C1 lateral mass and C2 pars interarticularis screw construct.

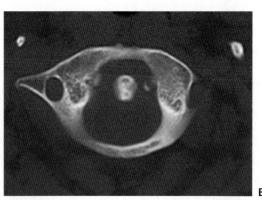

A

B

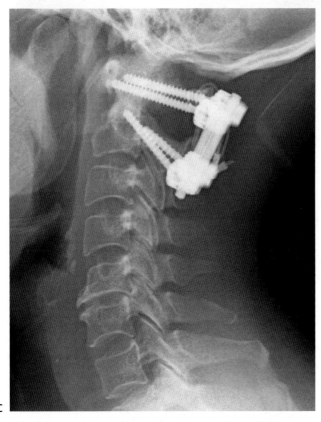

C

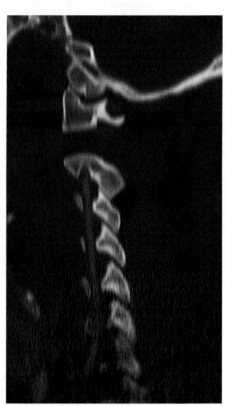

Figure 6–9 Distractive (type C) atlantoaxial instability. Sagittal computed tomographic image shows a craniocervical distractive injury, with wide displacement across the C1–C2 articulation. Note the subtle associated C0–C1 anterior subluxation. Because the major craniocervical ligamentous stabilizers extend from the foramen magnum to C2, distractive injuries at either of these two joints frequently result in instability at the adjacent articulation, which must be carefully evaluated to determine the extent of fixation required.

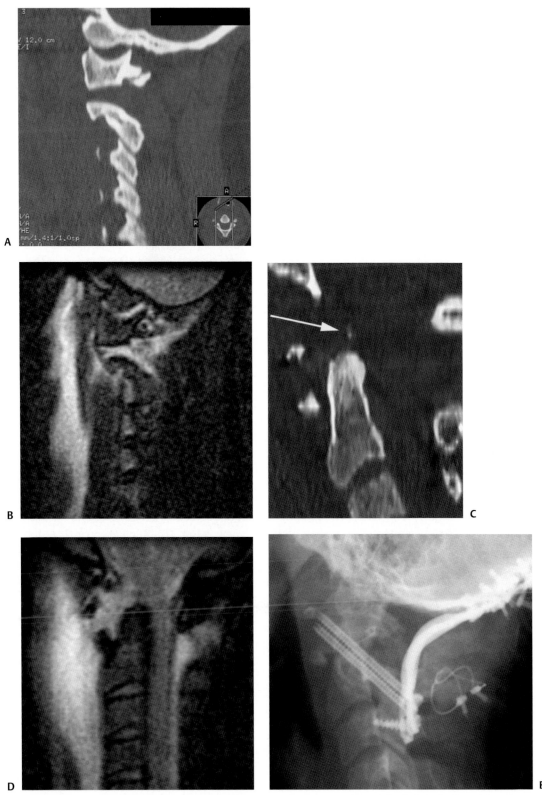

Figure 6–10 Craniocervical dissociation with subluxation at the atlanto-occipital and atlantoaxial joints. **(A)** Parasagittal computed tomographic (CT) and **(B)** magnetic resonance (MR) images and **(C)** midline sagittal CT and **(D)** MR image of the craniocervical junction in a 17-year-old woman involved in a high-speed motor vehicle collision show craniocervical dissociation with subluxation and distraction through both the C0–C1 and C1–C2 articulations and disruption of the tectorial ligament. The midline sagittal CT image **(C)** shows a type I odontoid fracture (arrow) as a component of the patient's craniocervical dissociation. **(E)** The patient had a progressive spinal cord injury and was taken emergently for occiput to C3 stabilization, after which her neurological status gradually normalized.

Indications for Surgery

Translational Instability

This highly unstable injury generally requires posterior atlantoaxial arthrodesis. However, in the presence of bony avulsion, successful healing may occur in approximately three fourths of patients with a period of recumbent traction followed by patient mobilization in a halo or SOMI.[13] An ADI of > 3 mm on flexion radiographs after 3 months of immobilization constitutes a failure of closed treatment and indicates the need for atlantoaxial arthrodesis.

Distraction Injuries

A distraction injury of C1–C2 with ≥ 2 mm of displacement requires surgical stabilization. This injury is analogous to craniocervical dissociation at the atlanto-occipital joint and should be treated under similar guidelines.

Odontoid Fractures

Classification

Fractures of the odontoid process are the most common of axis fractures (41%).[21] All odontoid fractures are considered unstable. Anderson and D'Alonzo's three-part system of odontoid fracture classification has become the basis for odontoid fracture management (**Fig. 6–11A–D**).[22] Type I injuries are considered bony avulsions of the alar ligament from the superolateral site of odontoid insertion and represent a component of a craniocervical dissociation. Type II injuries are located at the odontoid waist in the area covered by the TAL and have the highest propensity for pseudarthrosis, probably due to their small cross-sectional fracture surfaces and interruption in blood supply to the cephalad fragment. A type IIa subtype of odontoid fracture has been described by Hadley et al and consists of a highly unstable, segmentally comminuted injury extending from the waist of the odontoid into the body of the axis.[23] Type III fractures extend into the cancellous vertebral body and have wider, well-vascularized cancellous fracture surfaces.

Indications for Surgery

Type I

Because the treatment of type I odontoid fractures relates to how their associated alar ligament incompetence affects craniocervical stability,[22] indications for surgical management of these injuries are the same as those discussed for the treatment of craniocervical instability (**Fig. 6–10C**).

Type II

The management of type II odontoid fractures remains controversial. We advocate surgical stabilization for irreducible fractures, fractures with distractive patterns of displacement, or fractures with associated spinal cord injury (**Fig. 6–12A–D**). Relative indications include multiply injured patients, associated closed head injury, initial displacement of 4 mm or more, angulation > 10 degrees,[5,24] delayed presentation (> 2 weeks), multiple risk factors for nonunion,[23] the inability to treat with a halo due to advanced age,[8] associated cranial or thoracoabdominal injury or other medical factors, and the presence of associated upper cervical fractures.

Noncomminuted fractures in patients with favorable bone quality and appropriate body habitus are ideal for anterior odontoid screw fixation,[25] which allows preservation of some atlantoaxial motion. In patients with extensive fracture comminution or compromised bone quality or in whom achieving the requisite anterior odontoid screw trajectory is not feasible due to body habitus or the neck position required to maintain reduction, we favor a posterior atlantoaxial fusion using either transarticular screw fixation or segmental C1–C2 fixation.[17,26] Posterior atlantoaxial fusion is the recommended treatment for the two following subcategories of type II odontoid fractures that are not suitable for either nonoperative management or internal fixation with odontoid compression screws: type IIa dens fractures, which are inherently unstable due to a zone of segmental comminution at the odontoid base,[23] and "sagittally oblique" fractures,[27] in which the fracture line parallels the typical odontoid screw trajectory, leading to loss of reduction and inadequate fixation with attempts at interfragmentary compression.[28] Posterior C1–C2 arthrodesis with transarticular screws is ex-

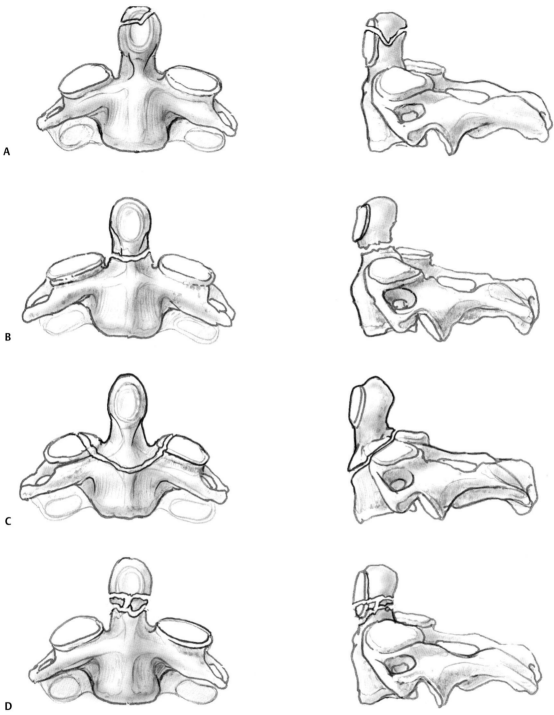

Figure 6–11 Anderson and D'Alonzo's odontoid fracture classification as appended by Hadley et al. **(A)** Type I fractures of the odontoid tip represent alar ligament avulsions. **(B)** Type II fractures occur at the odontoid waist, above the C2 lateral mass. **(C)** Type III fractures extend below the odontoid waist to involve the body and lateral masses of C2. **(D)** Hadley et al added the type IIa fracture with segmental comminution at the base of the odontoid.

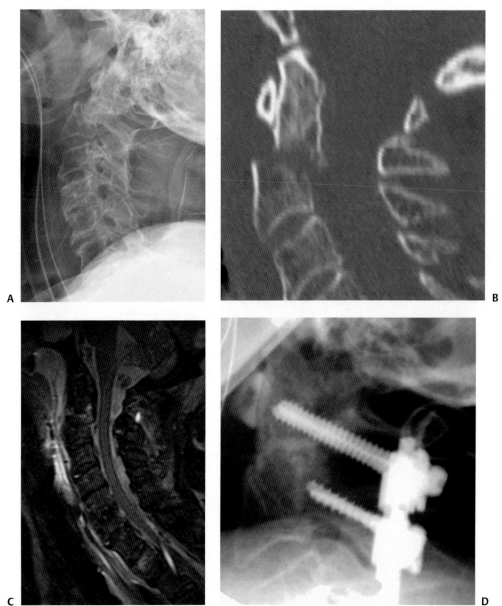

Figure 6–12 Type II odontoid fracture with incomplete spinal cord injury. **(A)** This 79-year-old woman sustained a displaced type II odontoid fracture, as shown on lateral radiograph and **(B)** sagittal computed tomographic image. **(C)** She sustained an American Spinal Injury Association (ASIA) D incomplete spinal cord injury with no evidence of spinal cord signal change on magnetic resonance imaging. **(D)** The patient was treated with posterior C1–C2 instrumented arthrodesis, as shown on postoperative lateral radiograph.

pected to have the most predictable healing results in the management of these two injury subtypes.[4,26,27]

Proper patient selection helps minimize the high complication rate of up to 28% that has been reported using anterior odontoid screw fixation.[25,27,29]

Type III

Type III odontoid fractures rarely require surgical stabilization. As with type II odontoid fractures, we advocate operative stabilization of fractures with associated spinal cord injury or distractive instability patterns (**Figs. 6–13A–C**). Posterior C1–C2 arthrodesis is the surgical treatment method of choice, since anterior odontoid screw fixation has a high failure rate with these injury types.[28] Relative indications include highly displaced irreducible fractures, patients with displaced injuries who cannot, for reasons cited above, be treated with a halo, and fractures with initial displacement of 5 mm or more, which have a high potential for nonunion, particularly in

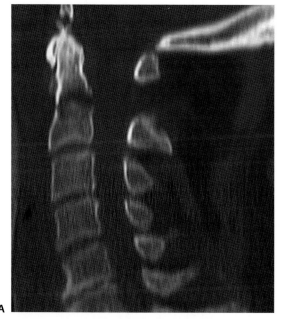
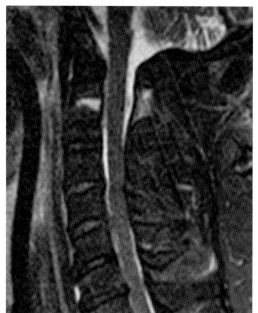

A

B

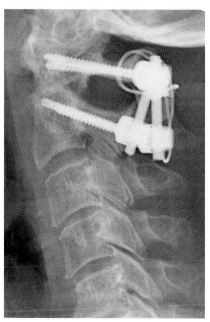

C

Figure 6–13 Type III odontoid fracture with distraction. **(A)** Sagittal computed tomography and **(B)** magnetic resonance imaging (MRI) show a distracted type III odontoid fracture. This atlantoaxial distractive injury is associated with extensive ligamentous disruption, as illustrated by the increased signal intensity between C1 and C2 posteriorly on MRI. **(C)** A lateral radiograph 3 months after posterior instrumented C1–C2 arthrodesis shows restoration of odontoid and atlantoaxial alignment.

the elderly population.[24] Results may be less predictable than is generally acknowledged, however, with delayed unions or pseudarthroses reported in up to 54% of nonoperatively treated patients,[24] which are also amenable to posterior C1–C2 fixation.

Traumatic Spondylolisthesis of the Axis (Hangman's Fractures)

Classification

Hangman's fractures are the second most common type of axis fracture (38%).[21] Effendi et al formulated the following simple classification, as subsequently modified by Levine and Starr and colleagues (**Fig. 6–14A–E**).[30–32]

Type I injuries consist of a minimally displaced, relatively stable fracture of the pars interarticularis that results from hyperextension and axial loading. Type Ia fractures are atypical unstable, lateral-bending fractures that are obliquely displaced and usually involve only one pars and extend anterior to the pars on the contralateral side.[32] The oblique plane of these fractures makes them less obvious on lateral radiographs, giving the appearance of an elongated pars (**Figs. 6–15A,B**). Type II fractures are displaced injuries that result when a flexion force follows the initial hyperextension and axial loading insult. Type II in-

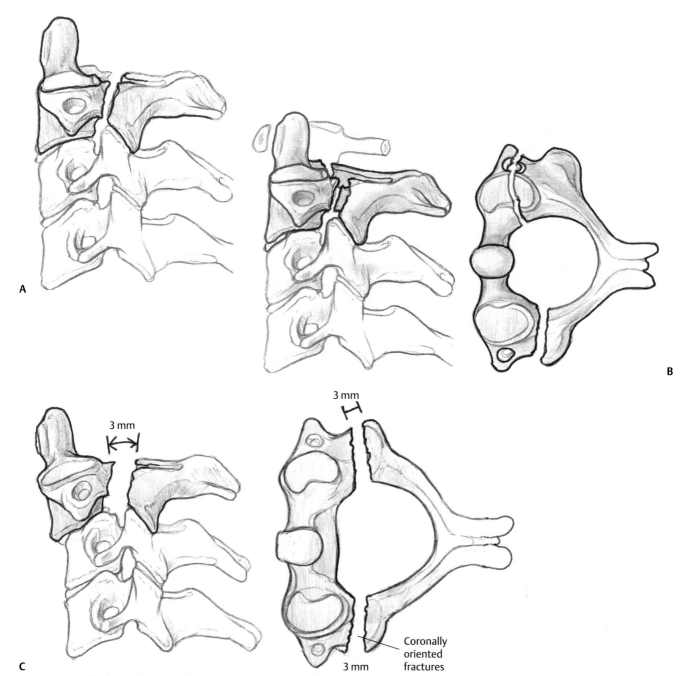

Figure 6–14 Effendi classification of hangman's fractures, as modified by Levine. **(A)** Type I. **(B)** Type Ia. **(C)** Type II.

juries are similar to type I injuries on supine radiographs but displace on upright radiographs. Physician-supervised flexion-extension radiographs of type I injuries have also been advocated to differentiate them from spontaneously reduced type II injuries.[7] Type IIa injuries are thought to occur from a flexion-distraction mechanism and are more unstable due to their associated C2–C3 disk disruption. Because they are flexion-distraction injuries, kyphosis is the prevailing deformity rather than translation **(Fig. 6–16A–C).** An inconsistent feature of type IIa injuries is that, because of the injury mechanism, the pars interartic-

ularis fractures tend to be more horizontal than in standard type II injuries. Levine has postulated that any injury where distraction of the C2–C3 disk space occurs with only 10 lb of traction should be considered type IIa. Type III injuries are unusual and highly unstable injuries in which the pars interarticularis fractures are associated with a complete unilateral or bilateral C2–C3 facet dislocation, which is not generally reducible by nonoperative means. On rare occasions, these injuries may also spontaneously reduce and have the more benign appearance of a type I injury on initial supine lateral radiographs

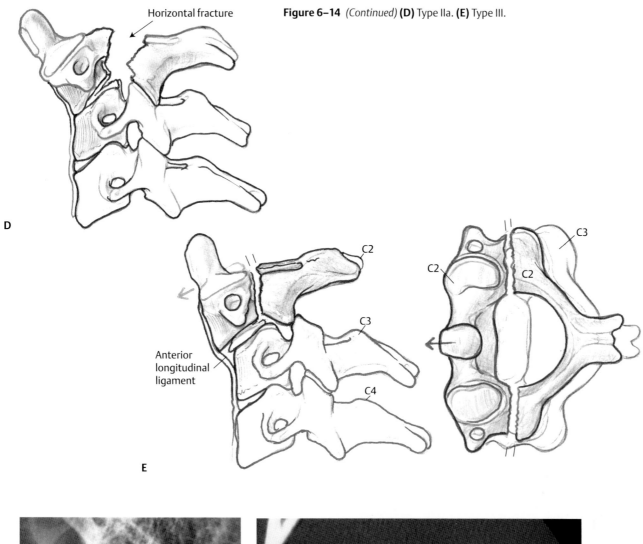

Horizontal fracture

Figure 6–14 *(Continued)* **(D)** Type IIa. **(E)** Type III.

D

C2

C3

C2

C2

Anterior
longitudinal
ligament

C3

C4

E

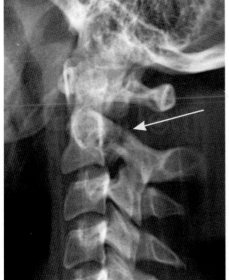

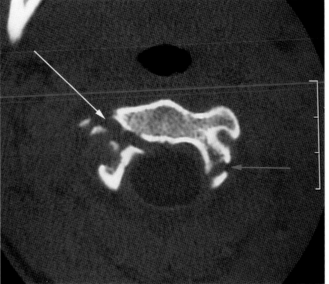

A

B

Figure 6–15 Type Ia traumatic spondylolisthesis of C2. **(A)** The fracture lines are "staggered" on the lateral view, giving the impression of an elongated pars (white arrow) on lateral radiograph. **(B)** Axial computed tomographic image shows typical position of pars interarticularis fracture (gray arrow) on one side, and atypical contralateral fracture extending into the vertebral body and foramen transversarium (white arrow). Displacement of the vertebral body fracture at the spinal canal results in a higher likelihood of spinal cord injury with type Ia injuries than with other type I or II injuries. This patient was neurologically intact and was treated successfully with a halo vest.

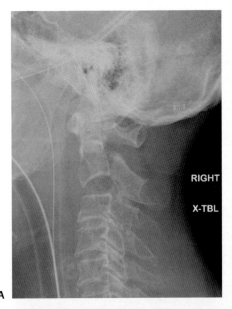

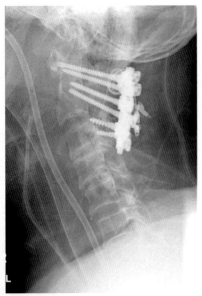

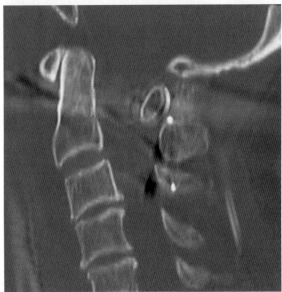

Figure 6–16 Type IIa traumatic spondylolisthesis of C2 due to motor vehicle collision in a 79-year-old male. **(A)** With type IIa injuries, a relative predominance of angulation over translation is seen on the lateral cervical spine radiograph. **(B)** Postoperative lateral radiograph and **(C)** postoperative sagittal CT image after open reduction and C1–C3 posterior instrumented arthrodesis. The C2–C3 segment must be stabilized due to the extensive disk disruption. Although interfragmentary screws were placed across the C2 pars interarticularis fractures bilaterally, the instrumentation was extended to C1 in this particular patient due to his advanced age and osteoporosis.

(Fig. 6–17A–C). Other classification systems have evaluated fracture stability based on the degree of translational and angulatory displacement as a measure of the integrity of C2–C3 diskoligamentous elements.[33]

Indications for Surgery

Operative stabilization is rarely indicated for traumatic spondylolisthesis of the axis.[33] Most injuries can be treated with early ambulatory immobilization with 12 weeks of

bracing for type I (and most Ia) fractures and of halo immobilization for most type II fractures.[30] Type IIa injuries may be treated with halo immobilization if their alignment can be successfully maintained, but traction is contraindicated in these injuries because it accentuates their kyphotic deformity.

If the kyphotic deformity in type IIa injuries cannot be controlled in a halo, surgery should be considered. A C2–C3 anterior cervical diskectomy and fusion (ACDF) with plating allows for fusion across the least number of levels and

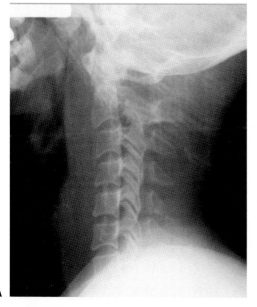

A

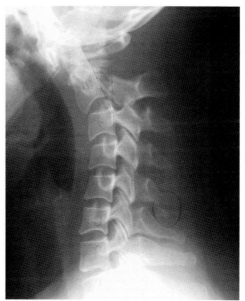

B

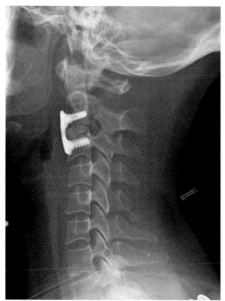

C

Figure 6–17 Type III traumatic spondylolisthesis of C2 treated with C2–C3 anterior diskectomy and fusion. **(A)** Lateral supine cervical spine radiograph showing what appears to be a type I traumatic spondylolisthesis of the axis sustained by a 37-year-old woman who was involved in a motor vehicle collision. The patient was discharged in a rigid cervical collar without upright radiographs. **(B)** The patient presented for evaluation with worsened neck pain and upper extremity paresthesias, at which time an upright lateral cervical radiograph in a rigid brace showed C2–C3 facet dislocation, consistent with a type III traumatic spondylolisthesis of C2. **(C)** After a gentle manipulative attempt at closed reduction of the facet dislocation was successful, a C2–C3 anterior cervical diskectomy and instrumented interbody arthrodesis was performed.

preserves atlantoaxial motion **(Fig. 6–17A–C)**.[34,35] However, because the anterior longitudinal ligament is often the only remaining intact C2–C3 stabilizing structure, posterior stabilization remains an appropriate option. A disadvantage of the posterior approach is that, absent the ability to gain acceptable purchase with C2 screws directly across the fracture, loss of atlantoaxial motion results from the need to extend the fixation to the C1 level **(Figs. 6–16A–C)**.

Type III injuries generally cannot be reduced by traction and require operative reduction and stabilization.

Stabilization options include (1) posterior C1–C3 fusion **(Fig. 6–18A,B)**; (2) posterior C2–C3 fusion using interfragmentary C2 screws across the fracture; (3) converting the fracture to a type I or II injury by posterior C2–C3 facet fusion using C2 screws, which stop short of the fracture, followed by collar or halo immobilization per the usual treatment for type I and II injuries; and (4) anterior C2–C3 ACDF **(Fig. 6–17A–C)**, in the unusual event that reduction occurs by closed methods. The advantage of the latter three options is their preservation of atlantoaxial motion.[7]

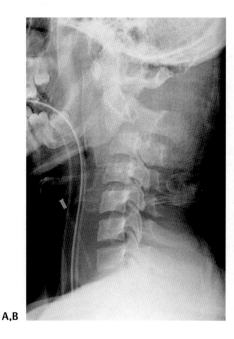 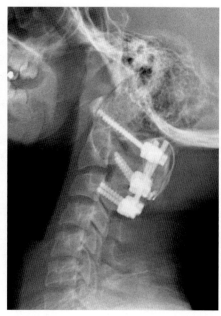

Figure 6–18 (A) Type III traumatic spondylolisthesis of C2 with American Spinal Injury Association (ASIA) C incomplete spinal cord injury sustained by a 19-year-old male unrestrained motor vehicle occupant involved in a collision. **(B)** As with most type III injuries, the facet dislocation could not be reduced by closed means and was treated with urgent open reduction and C1–C3 posterior instrumented arthrodesis.

A,B

Surgical Treatment

Surgical Options

Basic surgical options consist of decompressive procedures, fracture osteosynthesis, and fusion of vertebral motion segments.

Decompression

Because of the usually wide baseline spinal canal diameter, decompression of neural elements in upper cervical spine fractures is rarely necessary. In general, surgical decompression should only be performed if indirect decompression through fracture reduction maneuvers fails. Moreover, the posterior elements of the craniocervical junction provide important surfaces for bony healing of fusions and should therefore not be removed as a matter of routine. Case reports have described transoral dens resections for hypertrophic nonunion of dens fractures.[36] Occasionally, a depressed fracture of the atlas or the axis may have to be surgically elevated and removed. Posterior fossa decompression may be required in selected patients.

Osteosynthesis

The two indications for direct fracture repair in the upper cervical spine relate to the treatment of type II odontoid fractures[37] and surgical repair of a type II hangman's fracture with interfragmentary screw fixation. The validity of direct osteosynthesis for type II hangman's fractures has been questioned because this technique does not address the associated injury to the C2–C3 intervertebral disk.

Fusion

The mainstay of operative treatment of upper cervical fractures and dislocations remains fusion with instrumentation, most commonly performed from the posterior approach. In order of frequency, the most common upper cervical fusion procedures are atlantoaxial fusion, occipitocervical fusion, and, less commonly, C1–C3 fusion. Anterior upper cervical stabilization usually involves C2–C3 fusion for type IIa hangman's fractures. Anterior atlantoaxial fusion as a salvage procedure for previously failed posterior C1–C2 fusions and anterior occipitocervical techniques are rarely indicated and will not be discussed.

Patient Positioning

An unstable upper cervical spine fracture/dislocation requires atraumatic endotracheal airway access with minimal manipulation. Awake, fiberoptic intubation and positioning of a patient allows for clinical neurological monitoring. Electrophysiological neuromonitoring can be used as an alternative to awake positioning. For upper cervical spine injuries, the patient's head is generally secured with either Gardner-Wells or Mayfield three-pin tongs in patients without skull fractures. Operating tables should allow unobstructed image-intensifier access.

Supine positioning is used for odontoid screw placement and anterior C2–C3 diskectomy and fusion. Rarely, anterior occipitocervical approaches, including transoral and submandibular lateral approaches, are used. Prone positioning is used for atlantoaxial and occipitocervical fusions and most neural element decompressions. A slightly reversed Trendelenburg position reduces venous congestion in the upper cervical spine and may minimize blood loss. After patient positioning, fracture reduction is checked with an image intensifier, and neurological assessment is repeated with a clinical exam of an awakened patient, or electrophysiological testing.

Radiographic Imaging

Given the proximity of neural and vascular structures to the bony elements of the upper cervical spine, precise hardware placement requires intraoperative imaging. We favor fluoroscopic imaging, using concurrent biplanar fluoroscopy for selected procedures such as anterior odontoid screw placement, over more cumbersome three-dimensional systems. Visualization on the anteroposterior (AP) odontoid view can be enhanced with a radiolucent bite block.

Surgical Approaches

Posterior Upper Cervical Approach

Indications

Most upper cervical fractures are treated through the posterior approach. Indications range from purely decompressive procedures such as removal of the C1 posterior arch and posterior fossa decompression to procedures aimed at achieving a fusion between the C1–C2 segments alone or with the occiput (see **Video 6–1, Disk 1**). The posterior approach has the advantage of providing an anatomically familiar and extensile exposure. In addition, posterior spinal instrumentation techniques are generally biomechanically superior to anterior stabilization methods.

Technique

Posterior element integrity should be verified on imaging studies before performing a posterior dissection of the spine. Following a midline longitudinal incision, the midline intermuscular plane is developed, allowing subperiosteal exposure of the posterior elements. If the occiput is to be exposed, the incision is extended rostrally to the inion. The large, bifid spinous process of the axis is a helpful orientation aid during the early dissection. The C2–C3 interspinous ligament should be preserved if the intended fusion will not extend below C2. The atlas should be dissected in a strictly subperiosteal plane, keeping in mind the course of the vertebral artery on the superior aspect of its posterolateral arch. For the same reason sublaminar wire or cable passage around the atlas should be performed in an atraumatic, subperiosteal manner.

If screw fixation of the axis with pedicle or transarticular screws is desired, visualization of the superior and medial walls of the C2 pedicles as a reference point is recommended, which requires dissection of the atlantoaxial membrane off the superior lamina of the axis.[38] Exposure of the C1–C2 joints may be necessary for a formal arthrodesis of this motion segment, for instance, in the absence of an intact posterior arch of C1.[26] This dissection can result in considerable hemorrhage due to the overlying extensive epidural venous plexus. To facilitate exposure, the C2 nerve root is reflected cranially. When denuding or decorticating the atlantoaxial joint, the vertebral artery's course immediately lateral to the joint should be taken into account.

Anterior Upper Cervical Approach

Indications

There are three main indications for anterior upper cervical spine exposures in trauma. These are, in order of frequency: (1) screw fixation of a type II odontoid fracture (see **Video 6–2, Disk 1**), (2) anterior interbody fusion and plating of the C2–C3 interspace for a type IIa or III hangman's fracture, and (3) anterior arthrodesis of the atlantoaxial articulations as a rare salvage procedure for failed posterior atlantoaxial fusion attempts.[28,35,39]

Technique

The anterolateral approach to the cervical spine described by Smith and Robinson allows for anterior cervical spine exposure from the base of C2 to the cervicothoracic junction. McAfee et al described a submandibular retropharyngeal modification of this approach that provides exposure of the anterior atlantoaxial joints.[40] This procedure can be used if an anterior atlantoaxial arthrodesis is attempted.[41] For anterior transarticular screw placement, bilateral submandibular exposures have been reported to enable necessary screw trajectories. Fortunately, this procedure should rarely, if ever, be indicated because it is associated with increased morbidity.[41] Moreover, it has been shown that anterior transarticular screw fixation may be achieved through the standard and less morbid anterior cervical approach.[39]

Correct placement of the incision is important to minimize technical difficulties. For patients in whom odontoid screw or anterior transarticular screw placement is planned, a transverse Smith-Robinson–type approach is usually centered over C5. A transverse skin incision is made from the medial border of the sternocleidomastoid muscle to the midline. For C2–C3 anterior arthrodesis, a right-sided submandibular incision is used. The platysma is divided in line with its fibers for exposure of the interval between the sternohyoid muscles medially and the sternocleidomastoid muscle laterally. After the superficial layer of the deep cervical fascia has been incised longitudinally, the plane medial to the sternocleidomastoid muscle is developed to improve the exposure of the deeper layers. The carotid sheath is identified by palpation and is gently retracted laterally. After longitudinal incision of the middle layer of the deep cervical fascia medial to the carotid sheath, the trachea and esophagus are displaced medially as a unit using a blunt retractor. At the C2–C3 level the superior thyroid artery and vein may cross the operative field and require ligation. The remainder of the exposure is performed in the usual fashion. The prevertebral fascia is split longitudinally in the midline, and the longus colli muscle bellies are elevated off their vertebral attachments. Lateral dissection anterior to the longus colli muscle may lead to sympathetic chain injury and should be avoided. By limiting the extent of lateral vertebral body dissection to the lateral aspect of the uncovertebral joints, injury to the vertebral arteries can be avoided. Exposure of the C2–C3 interspace and odontoid process for odontoid screw fixation or of the anterior C2 lateral masses for anterior C1–C2 transarticular screw fixation is facilitated by the use of specialized retractor systems.

Transoral Approach

Indications

A transoral approach may be indicated for patients with spinal cord compression caused by a persistent mass effect from anterior elements of the upper cervical spine.[36] Rarely, the transoral approach is used for patients with mal- or hypertrophic nonunion of an odontoid fracture with neurological impairment. Although the transoral approach is effective for removal of the odontoid, it destabilizes the craniocervical junction and does not allow for anterior column reconstruction due to the limited exposure and an unduly high risk of infection.[42]

Technique

The transoral surgical exposure of the upper cervical spine can be deceptively straightforward. We recommend involving an otolaryngologist due to the inherent risk of infection or soft tissue dehiscence with potentially severe consequences. Also, one may need more complex osteotomy of the hard palate to gain sufficient exposure. An armored oral endotracheal tube and a self-retaining oral retractor are used. With the tube retracted laterally, sufficient access to the odontoid is usually gained by splitting and laterally retracting the overhanging soft palate with suture anchors. The anterior arch of the atlas, the odontoid process, and the vertebral body of the axis

are located directly beneath a thin layer of mucosal membrane and prevertebral fascia. If the goal is resection of the odontoid, the anterior arch of the atlas is resected between its junction with the left and right lateral masses, remaining within a maximum of 15 mm of the midline, as confirmed with anteroposterior fluoroscopy. The full length of the odontoid is then resected from apex to base. Predural soft tissues such as the tectorial membrane should be removed if they are a potential source of residual spinal cord impingement. The need for predural soft tissue resection should be carefully weighed against the severe potential morbidity of inadvertent dural tears in this area. A corrective osteotomy of an odontoid malunion can also be performed below the anterior arch of the atlas without resection of the entire odontoid and anterior arch.[6,43]

Surgical Techniques

Occipitocervical Fusion

Our preferred approach is to combine a rigid posterior segmental fixation construct with structural bone-grafting techniques.

Instrumentation Options

We prefer rigid fixation of the craniocervical junction with two separate parasagittal plates or cervical rods. Although plating constructs that gain purchase in the midline ridge of the occiput theoretically permit the use of longer screws into the occiput, this advantage is overshadowed by two distinct problems. First, the structural bone graft must be placed on top of the implant and may displace if the hardware pulls out or may need to be resected if hardware removal becomes necessary. Second, rotational stability provided by the implant is suboptimal, given the single midline plane of occipital fixation. We therefore do not recommend the use of such "Y-plates."

Bone Grafting

We prefer to secure a structural corticocancellous bone graft to the occiput and the upper cervical spine as an adjunct to the internal fixation. Typically, a pair of small bur holes is placed halfway between the inion and the foramen magnum on each side of the midline. On both sides, a cable with a locking device is passed in a superior to inferior direction, which is facilitated by using angled curets. Cervical fixation of the bone graft is achieved with a pair of sublaminar C2 cables. The bone graft is then attached to the craniocervical junction after decortication and placement of rigid internal fixation devices.

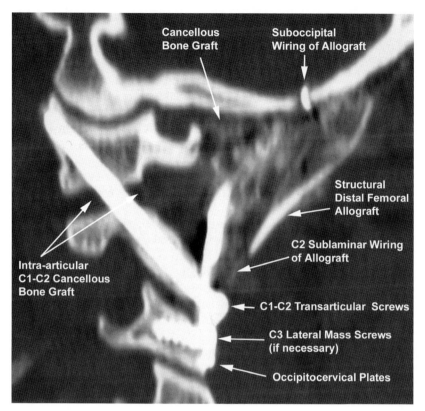

Cancellous
Bone Graft

Suboccipital
Wiring of Allograft

Structural
Distal Femoral
Allograft

C2 Sublaminar Wiring
of Allograft

Intra-articular
C1-C2 Cancellous
Bone Graft

C1-C2 Transarticular Screws

C3 Lateral Mass Screws
(if necessary)

Occipitocervical Plates

Figure 6–19 Technique of occipitocervical arthrodesis. Postoperative sagittal computed tomographic image of a 17-year-old male who sustained a craniocervical dissociation affecting the C0–C1 and C1–C2 articulations, with associated C2–C3 subluxation. The basic elements of our preferred technique for occipitocervical arthrodesis are outlined.

Technique

Prone positioning of the intubated patient is performed with Mayfield tongs or a halo on an operating table suitable for spine surgery, allowing full image-intensifier access. The craniocervical junction is reduced under image intensifier visualization with the goal of achieving neutral craniocervical alignment to avoid compensatory lower cervical malalignment. Midline exposure is performed from the inion to the C3 segment, or more caudally if necessary, and cables for bone graft attachment to the skull and the upper cervical spine are passed. A C1–C2 facet arthrodesis is then performed (see earlier description). A cervical rod or plate is contoured to fit the craniocervical junction. An improperly contoured plate can lead to a distraction or translation and should be avoided. With regard to the extent of caudal fixation, a pair of well-placed transarticular screws should be sufficient **(Fig. 6–19)** (see Transarticular Screw Technique).[44] Alternatively, individual C1 lateral mass screws may be added to this construct or may be used in conjunction with C2 pedicle screws rather than transarticular screws[17,45] (see C1 Lateral Mass and C2 Pedicle Screw Technique). Should rigid fixation to both C1 and C2 not be possible using one of these options, the instrumentation construct should include at least the C3 segment by means of lateral mass screws. Additional caudal fixation may be necessary in individual circumstances with associated cervical injuries or inadequate upper cervical fixa-

tion. The construct is then secured to the occiput with three to four bicortical 3.5 mm cortical screws. Drilling above the level of the inion should be avoided because of the risk of hardware prominence and possible injury to the transverse sinus, with potentially fatal consequences to the patient. A plate spacing of ~4 to 6 cm is desirable to accommodate a correspondingly sized structural graft. This graft is fashioned to cradle the occiput and straddle the C2 spinous process. The graft is then secured to the previously placed cervical and cranial wires or cables with drill holes placed through the graft. Prior to tightening these cables, the posterior bone elements of the craniocervical junction are decorticated, and morcellized iliac crest graft is placed between the host site and the structural allograft.

Atlantoaxial Fusion

Our preferred method for atlantoaxial fusion involves posterior transarticular screw fixation and direct decortication and bone grafting of the C1-C2 joints, augmented with a modified Gallie cabled structural bone graft. If transarticular screw placement is deemed either unsafe due to anomalous vertebral artery anatomy or technically implausible due to anatomical or positioning constraints, interconnected C1 lateral mass and C2 pedicle screw fixation is substituted for the transarticular screws, with other elements of the procedure remaining the same.

Cable Techniques and Sublaminar Hooks

Posterior cabling techniques are familiar, relatively easy, and have less risk of vertebral artery injury than screw fixation techniques.[46] The risk of neurological injury is also low, particularly if wire passage is avoided in the presence of persistent atlantoaxial subluxation when the space available for the spinal cord is decreased. The main disadvantages of these techniques when used alone are (1) relative lack of rotational stability requiring postoperative immobilization with cervicothoracic orthosis or halo; (2) incorrect force vectors for the treatment of posterior C1–C2 subluxation as with posteriorly displaced odontoid fractures, which are further displaced by this technique; and (3) the inability to use when the posterior C1 arch is absent or compromised. They serve as useful adjuncts to more rigid instrumentation methods.

Transarticular Screw Technique

Transarticular C1–C2 screws offer the stiffest form of atlantoaxial complex stabilization complex **(Fig. 6–20A–D)**.[47] Moreover, this stabilization technique does not require an intact neural arch of either C1 or C2. This procedure is technically challenging and requires congruous atlantoaxial joint reduction. Presence of anatomical variants, such as an excessively medial vertebral artery course across the C2 segment or skeletal dysplasia, can pose significant obstacles to safe completion of this procedure. Due to the presence of an aberrant vertebral artery course in up to 20% of the population,[48,49] careful evaluation of the preoperative CT scan is critical to determine the suitability of this technique. Furthermore, the possibility of achieving the necessary screw trajectory may be compromised by patient body habitus or by the head and neck position required for acceptable fracture alignment. If safe placement of transarticular screws appears doubtful, plate or rod fixation between screws in the C1 lateral mass and C2 pedicles should be considered. Alternative bail-out options, such as a Brooks-Jenkins wiring or extension of the fusion to the cranium, should be required in only a very few cases.

This procedure is performed with the patient in the prone position with the head secured by a halo ring or Mayfield tongs. An image intensifier is used in the lateral plane. Meticulous patient positioning is required. To achieve a sufficiently cranial transarticular drill trajectory, the patient's head and neck are gently flexed while maintaining fracture reduction under fluoroscopic control. Sufficient torso clearance to accommodate the intended transarticular drill trajectory must be verified externally with a metallic object held against the patient's side under fluoroscopy.

Surgical exposure from the occiput to the C3 is then performed as already described. The C1–C2 and the C2–C3 facet joints are identified bilaterally. If feasible without excessive hemorrhage, the atlantoaxial articulations are decorticated bilaterally. C1–C2 joint decortication should be considered if the posterior elements are not available for cabled bone grafting. When necessary, sublaminar wire passage is completed before drilling of the screws. To prevent spinal canal penetration, the medial wall of the isthmus of the axis is visualized with a neural elevator. Two small paramedian incisions are then placed at the cervicothoracic junction to allow the appropriate trajectory through percutaneous drilling and screw placement through a cannulated obturator and drill guide. The starting point for transarticular screws is located in the medial to central third of the inferior articular process of the axis. Drilling with a long Steinmann pin or guide wire for a cannulated screw system is then performed under lateral C-arm guidance, with a 45 to 60 degree vertical inclination trajectory aiming for the mid- to upper third of the anterior tubercle of the atlas. Intra-articular passage of the drill or guidewire can be ascertained by direct inspection of the joint. A medial angulation of 0 to 15 degrees is desirable to achieve optimal C1 lateral mass purchase while avoiding an excessively lateral course that may result in vertebral artery[38] and hypoglossal nerve injury.[26,50] Hypoglossal nerve injury can also be avoided by minimizing the extent to which the drill tip penetrates the anterior cortex of the C1 lateral mass or the placement of excessively long screws, the avoidance of which also prevents carotid artery injury.[26,51,52] Cadaveric and radiographic studies have shown that the anterior cortex of the lateral mass becomes engaged when the screw tip lies an average of ~7 mm posterior to the anterior tip of the arch of C1 on lateral radiographs.[51,52]

If cannulated screws are used, the guidewire should engage the anterior cortex of the C1 lateral mass without penetrating it. Drill length and tapping are then measured. If possible, cancellous bone graft is placed into the atlantoaxial joint. Then 3.5 or 4.0 mm diameter screws are placed, of sufficient length to just engage the anterior cortex of the lateral mass of the atlas. The optimal transarticular screw length ranges from 34 to 48 mm.[50,52,53] Due to the possibility of an unrecognized vertebral artery injury, screw placement on one side should be completed prior to starting the contralateral side. Doppler ultrasound evaluation of the vertebral artery above the arch of C1 is useful in assessing for potential injury in the case of uncertainty. Should a vertebral artery injury be suspected with the placement of the first screw, a contralateral transarticular screw should not be placed. Following placement of the transarticular screws, a formal midline fusion is performed using the Gallie technique.[46]

C1 Lateral Mass and C2 Pedicle Screw Technique

Posterior atlantoaxial fixation with individual C1 lateral mass and C2 pedicle screws[17,45] has evolved as a biomechanically[54] and clinically[45,55] equivalent method of restoring atlantoaxial stability while minimizing problems related

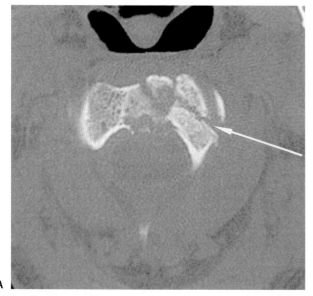
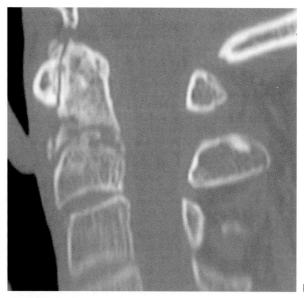

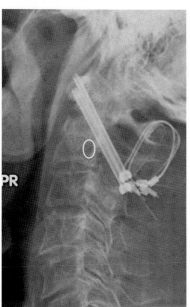
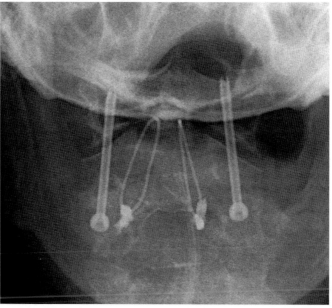

Figure 6–20 Transarticular screw technique for stabilization of un-stable odontoid fracture. **(A)** Axial and **(B)** sagittal computed tomo-graphic images showing a comminuted type III odontoid fracture with extension into the left C2 lateral mass (white arrow). The patient was treated with transarticular screw fixation. **(C)** The postoperative lateral radiograph illustrates the screw trajectory aimed toward the superior aspect of the C1 arch, which generally requires the use of percutaneous stab incisions parasagittally in the upper thoracic spine. A sufficiently cranial trajectory avoids the vertebral artery within the C2 foramen transversarium (white oval) and allows for

adequate purchase of the C1 lateral mass. **(D)** The postoperative open-mouth anteroposterior radiograph shows the orientation of the transarticular screws slightly medial to the sagittal plane. Later-ally directed screws should be avoided to prevent vertebral artery in-jury. The safety of this technique is greatly enhanced by direct visualization of the medial wall of the pars interarticularis, which al-lows the surgeon to (1) map a precise sagittal plane trajectory just lateral to this landmark and (2) select a starting point along this path just superior to the C2–C3 facet joint.

to transarticular screw trajectory and vertebral artery anatomy. Because this technique does not require drilling through the atlantoaxial joints, the possibility of restoring atlantoaxial motion by hardware removal after odontoid fracture healing has also been proposed.[45]

The technique of posterior atlantoaxial stabilization with C1 lateral mass and C2 pedicle screws **(Fig. 6–21A–H)**

(see **Video 6–1, Disk 1**) is a valuable alternative to C1–C2 transarticular screws, particularly in the elderly patient with exaggerated thoracic kyphosis, obese patients, and patients with vertebral artery anatomy that is unfavorable for transar-ticular screws.

Both the original description by Goel[55] and the modi-fication by Harms and Melcher[45] use a starting point on

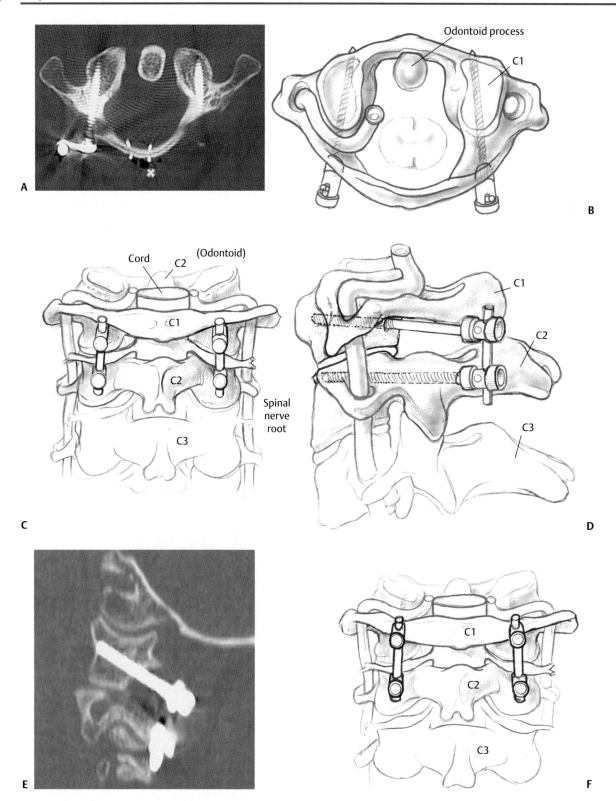

Figure 6–21 C1 lateral mass and C2 pedicle screw fixation. **(A)** Computed tomographic (CT) and **(B)** schematic axial images of C1 show the desired placement of C1 lateral mass screws. **(C)** Anteroposterior schematic image, **(D)** lateral schematic image and **(E)** sagittal CT image showing placement of C1 lateral mass screws with a starting point inferior to the C1 posterior arch on the posterior aspect of the lateral mass. This starting point requires manipulation of the C2 root and can result in problematic bleeding from the venous plexus that surrounds it. **(F,G)** An alternative starting point, along the posterior arch of C2 at its junction with the lateral mass, is illustrated schematically and **(H)** on sagittal CT image. This latter starting point may prevent the need for C2 manipulation and dissection through the surrounding venous plexus but is immediately adjacent to the vertebral artery, which must be protected as it courses along the posterior C1 arch.

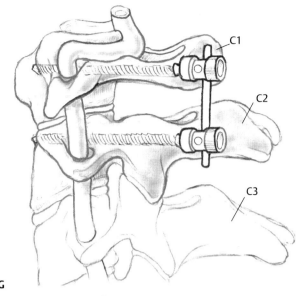

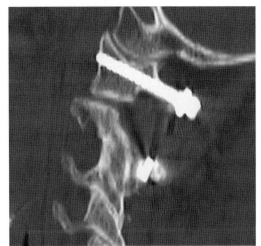

Figure 6–21 (Continued)

the posterior aspect of the C1 lateral mass proper, caudal to the prominence where the posterior arch meets the lateral mass. Access to this starting point requires dissection through the extensive overlying venous plexus, which may lead to problematic bleeding[55] and requires retraction[45] or transection of the C2 root,[17] either of which may result in occipital numbness and dysesthesias. We prefer a C1 screw starting point at the more readily accessible junction of the posterior arch and lateral mass, which minimizes the need for dissection through the previously mentioned venous plexus and the likelihood of injury to the C2 root. An additional potential benefit may be that screw purchase is enhanced by exploiting the thick cortical bone at the confluence of the posterior arch and lateral mass.

The technique is performed with the patient positioned prone and the head secured with a halo or Mayfield tongs. Head and neck manipulation is performed as required to achieve an acceptable reduction. The limitations in head and neck position required for feasibility of this technique are much less than with transarticular screw fixation.

A midline dorsal exposure is performed as described for transarticular screw fixation. Blunt dissection of the C1 posterior arch is carried laterally to the junction of the arch with the lateral mass. Circumferential subperiosteal dissection of the C1 posterior arch is performed with narrow angled curets to allow for visualization or palpation of the medial wall of the C1 lateral mass. This dissection is performed in a strictly subperiosteal manner over the superior aspect of the arch to avoid injury to the vertebral artery, which is identified. The medial wall of the C2 neural arch is also identified in a fashion similar to that described for transarticular screw and C2 pedicle screw placement. If direct bone grafting is planned, the C1–C2 joint is visualized by incising the posterior joint capsule after dissecting along the pars interarticularis of C2, generally requiring

extensive bipolar coagulation of the abundant overlying venous plexus.

A true lateral fluoroscopic view of C1 is then obtained and used to guide a bicortical channel with a 2.0 mm smooth drill bit starting ~2 mm lateral to the junction of the lateral mass with the posterior arch of C1, generally just medial to where the posterior arch narrows at the vertebral artery sulcus. A curved instrument is placed over the superior margin of the posterior arch, between the starting point and the vertebral artery. Creating a bony concavity with a bur is advisable to prevent the drill bit from migrating along this relatively narrow and convex bony ridge. The drill is directed bicortically in the true sagittal plane toward the middle of the anterior margin of C1 on lateral fluoroscopy. This starting point and trajectory helps avoid the vertebral artery foramen, the spinal canal, and the atlanto-occipital joint. A bicortical 3.5 or 4.0 mm screw is then placed. Issues regarding radiographic identification of appropriate screw length and the dangers to the carotid artery and hypoglossal nerve with excessive anterior drill or screw penetration are similar to those already described for transarticular screws.[26,50–52]

Anterior Odontoid Screw Fixation

This procedure is advocated for the treatment of noncomminuted odontoid fractures with intact vertebral body of the axis (**Fig. 6–22A–F**) (see **Video 6–2, Disk 1**).[25,28,29] Prudent patient selection and meticulous technical execution are necessary to avoid perioperative complications and high failure rates. Vertebral body fracture of the axis, comminution of the odontoid, and patients with osteoporosis offer a poor prognosis for successful instrumentation. Treatment of odontoid nonunions with anterior fixation alone is generally not recommended, although success has been reported in delayed unions up to 6 months

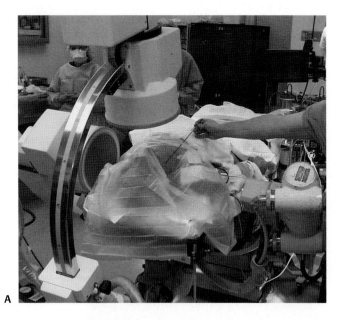

A

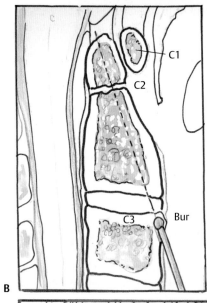

B

C1
C2
C3
Bur

C1
C2
C3

Midline positioning

C

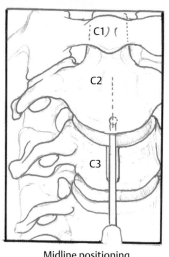

C2

C2
Tap penetrates
cortical tip
of odontoid

C2

C3
Screw in place

F

D,E

C3

C3

Drill bit penetrates
tip of odontoid

postinjury.[28] Because this procedure is entirely dependent upon radiographic visualization, the most critical part of this procedure is the ability to obtain adequate lateral and open-mouth odontoid views with preferably two image intensifiers, while maintaining an anatomical, closed reduction of the odontoid fracture with a head and neck position that is amenable to the required screw trajectory. Should any of these prerequisites not be attainable, the surgical plan should be adjusted, and a posterior atlantoaxial stabilization procedure should be considered. Another potential obstacle is the patient's chest size, which may interfere with the horizontal inclination angle required for this instrumentation technique. Large, barrel-chested patients or patients with excessive fixed cervical or cervicothoracic kyphosis may therefore be unsuitable for this technique. Fine adjustment of the patient's head position under fluoroscopy by extending the neck gently can aid in attaining the desired trajectory. The presence of sufficient torso clearance to allow for the intended odontoid screw trajectory is then verified externally with a metallic object held against the patient's chest under fluoroscopy. Because of the possibility that odontoid screw fixation cannot be performed, alternative plans should always be made.

The procedure is performed with the patient supine and the head secured by a fixed cranial holding device, such as Mayfield tongs. A conventional right- or left-sided Smith-Robinson approach is usually centered over C5. Upon reaching the prevertebral fascia, the dissection is carried rostrally to the C2–C3 disk space, which is exposed by reflecting the longus colli muscles laterally. A curved, radiolucent submandibular retractor is placed on the anterior vertebral body of C2. The anterior anulus of the C2–C3 disk is excised along with a small wedge of the anterosuperior C3 end plate to expose the anteroinferior lip of C2. This cortical lip is removed with a high-speed bur to prepare a smooth bony surface for instrumentation that minimizes the risk of anterior cortical breakout at the base of the axis. An odontoid screw should allow for fracture compression either with the use of terminal threads or by overdrilling the caudal fragment. Fixation can be performed with either one or two screws. Single small fragment screws have been reported to provide adequate stability in clinical and biomechanical testing.[37] Well-placed dual screws have the advantage of minimizing ro-

tational displacement but are considered to be technically more challenging. Our preference has been the placement of two 3.5 versus 4.0 mm screws, if possible, and to resort to dual 2.7 mm screws if the two larger screws cannot be accommodated. The goals of screw placement are to be collinear to the longitudinal axis of the odontoid, to have screw thread purchase rostral to the fracture only, and to engage the posterior cortex of the odontoid tip with the terminal screw threads. The specific technique (single or dual, cannulated or solid screws) remains a matter of surgeon preference and should take individual patient factors into consideration. If conventional solid screws are used, we prefer the use of a Steinmann pin over a drill bit, due to a lower risk of breakage and the absence of bone removal with drilling.

Anterior C2–C3 Diskectomy and Fusion

This procedure is primarily considered for treatment of displaced type II or IIa hangman's fractures. It should be emphasized that the majority of patients with type II injuries can be treated nonoperatively. The surgical approach, diskectomy and fusion with bone grafting, and plating are similar to that employed in the lower cervical spine and will therefore not be reiterated (see earlier discussion). Due to intricacies of fracture reduction and hardware placement, we recommend performing an anterior C2–C3 fusion with an image intensifier in a lateral projection plane. The Smith-Robinson approach centered over the C3–C4 disk space usually allows for exposure of the C2–C3 disk space. A long, angled, radiolucent retractor such as that described for odontoid screw fixation is helpful in gaining adequate exposure of the upper cervical spine. Alternatively, a right-sided retropharyngeal modification of the exposure, as described by McAfee et al, can be useful in large patients.[40]

Technical challenges associated with an anterior C2–C3 fusion consist mainly of obtaining adequate exposure, avoiding anterior translation of the axis relative to the C3 vertebral body, and placing the anterior plate flush with the ventral vertebral bodies. If placed for a hangman's type fracture, the anterior plate serves as a buttress plate. To avoid secondary loss of reduction, this anterior cervical plate should feature a low-profile locking screw mechanism.

Figure 6–22 Technique of anterior odontoid screw fixation. **(A)** The use of biplanar fluoroscopy greatly facilitates this procedure. Prior to draping the operative field, it is useful to use a metallic marker and lateral fluoroscopy to confirm that the patient's neck position and chest morphology will allow the desired screw trajectory. A radiolucent bite block is useful to enhance anterior fluoroscopic visualization. **(B)** An essential initial step is the excision of the anterior anulus of C2–C3 and removal of the anterosuperior C3 vertebral body and end plate to allow for a sufficiently posterior starting point and sufficiently cranial screw trajectory. **(C)** Appropriate positioning of the screw starting point in the coronal plane must be confirmed with an anteroposterior fluoroscopic view. Midline positioning for single

screw placement is demonstrated for simplicity. The authors prefer using two screws, which requires a slightly paramedian starting point for each screw. **(D)** The drill trajectory tends to parallel the anterior odontoid cortex. It is essential to penetrate the cortex of the proximal odontoid, preferably at or just posterior to the odontoid tip. **(E)** Tapping of the entire trajectory, including the far cortex at the odontoid tip, is recommended. **(F)** The use of partially threaded screws simplifies interfragmentary compression. To achieve optimal fixation and fracture compression, the screw threads should engage the cortex at the tip of the odontoid as the screw head contacts the base of the odontoid, and all screw threads must be within the proximal fragment.

Tips and Tricks

- A slightly reversed Trendelenburg position reduces venous congestion in the upper cervical spine during surgery and may minimize blood loss.
- Postoperative airway management is very important for patients who have undergone surgical stabilization of the upper cervical spine. Premature extubation can lead to airway obstruction and a need for emergent reintubation. Assessment of airway swelling prior to routine postoperative extubation and a low threshold for delaying extubation until swelling has diminished minimize complications. Temporary loss of a patient's gag reflex should also be taken into consideration in the initial postoperative phase as a means of minimizing the risk of aspiration.
- Intraoperative imaging of the upper cervical spine on the AP odontoid view can be enhanced with a radiolucent bite block.
- Type IIa hangman's fractures are potentially unstable, but may spontaneously reduce and have the more benign appearance of a type I injury on initial supine lateral radiographs. Traction is contraindicated in type IIA hangman's injuries because it accentuates associated kyphotic deformity.
- We prefer rigid fixation of the craniocervical junction with two separate parasagittal plates or cervical rods. Dual-plate fixation provides improved rotational stability compared with a single midline or Y-plate, and facilitates bone grafting.
- Due to the possibility of an unrecognized vertebral artery injury during transarticular C1–C2 fixation, screw placement on one side should be completed prior to starting the contralateral side. Intraoperative Doppler ultrasound evaluation of the vertebral artery above the arch of C1 is useful in assessing for potential injury in the case of uncertainty.

Postoperative Care

Postoperative airway management is crucial for patients who have undergone surgical stabilization of the upper cervical spine. Premature extubation can lead to airway obstruction and a need for emergent reintubation.[56] Assessment of airway swelling prior to postoperative extubation and a low threshold for delaying extubation until swelling has diminished are important early postoperative management issues. Temporary loss of a patient's gag reflex should also be taken into consideration in the initial postoperative phase as a means of minimizing the risk of aspiration.

The type and duration of external postoperative immobilization vary and should consider many factors. Patients should generally be mobilized in an upright position following surgical stabilization. A rigid brace such as a Miami-

J or Philadelphia collar usually provides adequate postoperative external support, assuming that the patient was treated with stable internal fixation. In unusual circumstances a halo remains a desirable form of supplemental immobilization, particularly in patients with facial fractures, multilevel injuries, osteopenic bone, and uncertain implant fixation. External immobilization should rarely be required beyond 2 to 3 months postoperatively. When discontinuing external immobilization, regardless of treatment form, stability of the injury should be reassessed with flexion-extension and open-mouth odontoid radiographs. Traction films are obtained if necessary to confirm a stable craniocervical junction.

New Technology

The major advance in instrumentation has consisted of the development of polyaxial screw systems that have allowed for new atlantoaxial fixation techniques.[17,45,57] These techniques have provided increased versatility in treating atlantoaxial instability and have practically eliminated technical and anatomical barriers to achieving rigid C1–C2 fixation. C1–C2 stabilization by means of C1 lateral mass screws and C2 screws placed either in the pedicle, pars interarticularis, or lamina have proven, for the most part, to be biomechanically equivalent to the extremely rigid yet less accommodating transarticular screw technique.

The evolution of various intraoperative image guidance systems also presents the potential for safer placement of hardware in the anatomically complex craniocervical region, which often provides little room for error due to its proximity to vital neurovascular and visceral structures. The three main categories of systems currently available include the following:

1. *Three-dimensional CT- or fluoroscopy-based virtual imaging systems that require specialized equipment and the integration of imaging studies with some type of marker attached to the area being instrumented.* These systems allow for virtual, real-time intraoperative images that demonstrate the intended trajectory during screw placement and allow for measurement of appropriate screw length and diameter. Disadvantages of these systems include expense, increased operative time, and the potential that recording errors may cause a discrepancy between the true anatomy and the virtual images being relied upon intraoperatively.

2. *Three-dimensional fluoroscopy that provides axial, coronal, and sagittal reformations created by integrating multiple fluoroscopy images obtained at various angles.* The main disadvantage of this technique is that, given that the quality of the three-dimensional (3-D) images is entirely dependent on the quality of the fluoroscopic images from which they are being reconstructed, recon-

struction of the regions that are most difficult to visualize fluoroscopically, and would therefore benefit most from 3-D visualization, tend to have the lowest resolution and are therefore the least useful. Also, this 3-D visualization can only be used to verify screw position rather than to correctly guide the initial screw trajectory, as with the imaging systems previously described.

3. *Intraoperative CT scanners.* These are somewhat more cumbersome, yet may also provide suboptimal resolution. Because of their relative lack of versatility and their awkwardness, these devices may soon become supplanted by the three-dimensional fluoroscopy imaging systems already described. Although the various imaging techniques described earlier continue to improve, at this juncture they are all fraught with various impracticalities that hinder their widespread use. Moreover, there is little clinical validation regarding the increased safety of these systems as compared with the use of standard fluoroscopy and sound anatomical principles. The evolution of intraoperative imaging systems, however, may eventually serve not only to improve the safety of current techniques but also to permit the development of new fixation methods.

Outcomes and Complications

The outcome of patients who sustain upper cervical injuries is often more dependent on associated intracranial injury than on the injury to the spine. Patient comorbidities, subtle differences among similar injuries, and a wide range of treatment options add confusion regarding realistically attainable clinical results. Knowledge of problem areas surrounding certain injury types is, however, a necessary first step in minimizing their occurrence.

Injury-Specific Outcomes and Complications

Occipital Condyle Fractures

Little is known about the morbidity associated with occipital condyle fractures.[58] Outcome likely depends on the presence of various comorbidities, such as associated head injury. The outcome of type III fractures is better represented in the subsequent discussion of craniocervical dissociation outcomes. Although the incidence of posttraumatic arthritis is unknown, outcome is contingent on the presence or absence of symptoms of posttraumatic arthritis such as neck pain, occipital headaches, and restricted craniocervical motion. Torticollis may result from chronic atlanto-occipital subluxation. An association between occipital condyle fractures and palsy of their most closely associated cranial nerves (IX, X, XI, XII) in up to a third of cases has also been described.[59,60]

Craniocervical Dissociation

Most craniocervical dissociations are fatal. The outcome of survivors is dependent on (1) the type and severity of associated injuries, particularly the closed head injuries; (2) the severity of neurological injury; and (3) the timeliness with which the diagnosis of craniocervical dissociation is recognized and can be operatively stabilized. Logic dictates that survivors have less displaced or even spontaneously reduced injuries, and neurological deficits in survivors are likely to be less severe. Partly because of these reasons and despite substantial advances in neuroimaging, craniocervical dissociations continue to be frequently missed. Early recognition and timely fixation of these injuries improve outcome by protecting against neurological deterioration. Delayed diagnosis in these highly unstable injuries has been associated with secondary neurological deterioration and possibly death in up to 75% of patients.[61] These unacceptably high numbers underscore the importance of improving our current cervical spine trauma screening measures.

Fractures of the Atlas

Severe complications associated with an isolated fracture of the atlas are rare. With the exception of pain or loss of sensation in the greater occipital nerve distribution, neurological sequelae are uncommon, and, if present, likely to be related to associated injuries. Patients with posterior arch fractures are expected to heal with few or no symptoms. Osteoarthritis of the upper cervical spine may occur as a result of a displaced lateral mass fracture. Minimally displaced lateral mass or Jefferson (burst) fractures treated nonoperatively are associated with an 80% incidence of some residual neck pain and a 17% nonunion rate.[20] The amount of displacement tolerated by the upper cervical spine articulations without developing posttraumatic arthritis is unknown. Severe malunion of an unstable atlas fracture resulting in a painful torticollis, such as with a highly displaced lateral mass fracture, may require realignment and occiput to C2 fusion (**Fig. 6–23A–D**).

Atlantoaxial Instability

Traumatic Transverse Ligament Insufficiency: Acute traumatic rupture of the TAL, excluding that which occurs due to axial loading with associated displaced fracture of the atlas, is usually fatal.[62] In the occasional survivor, profound neurological deficits may be present, although patients may be neurologically intact on presentation.[63] Because of the common mechanism of forced forward flexion or translation of C1 on C2 due to a blow to the occiput, head injuries are a common associated finding and may be the predominant influence on outcome in survivors.[18,62] Syncope and vertigo may result from injury to the vertebrobasilar arterial system.

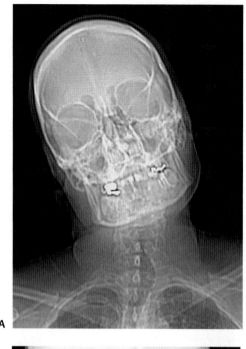

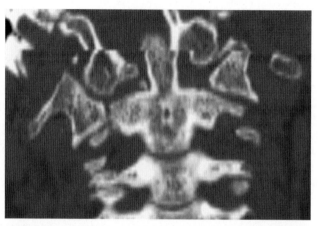

Figure 6–23 Malunion of lateral mass fracture of the atlas with craniocervical malalignment. **(A)** Anteroposterior radiograph of a 47-year-old woman who sustained a right C1 lateral mass fracture that was treated nonoperatively. She developed progressive tilt and rotation at the craniocervical junction. **(B)** Coronal computed tomographic image illustrates malunion with lateral displacement of the right C1 lateral mass, resulting in articulation of the right occipital condyle directly with the C2 lateral mass. **(C)** Anterioposterior and **(D)** lateral radiographs taken after the patient had undergone corrective osteotomy with instrumented posterior craniocervical arthrodesis.

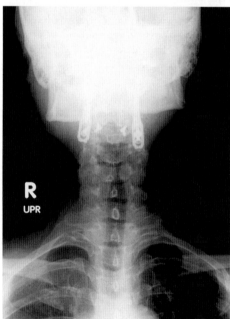

A

C

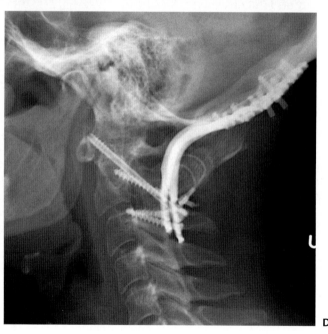

B

D

Patients with type II bony avulsion injuries of the TAL have a 26% reported likelihood of instability after nonoperative treatment.[13] Patients with late atlantoaxial instability as demonstrated on flexion-extension radiographs, or painful atlantoaxial arthritis as shown on CT scan and bone scan, can be considered for C1–C2 fusion. In the case of long-standing and irreducible deformities, treatment may require adjunctive decompression and cranial extension of the fusion to the occiput.

TAL rupture that may occur in a minority of odontoid fractures has been described as an indication for early C1–C2 stabilization due to the high likelihood of persistent C1–C2 instability, even in the presence of a successfully healed odontoid process.[64]

Atlantoaxial Distraction: The prognosis for outcome and complications with this injury pattern are best represented by the previous section on craniocervical dissociation outcomes.

Odontoid Fractures

Odontoid fractures are associated with significant morbidity and even mortality. Fracture nonunion and missed injuries are the most common causes of complications.

Primary neurological injury or secondary deterioration associated with odontoid fractures is rarely encountered.[43] Pseudarthrosis of a type II odontoid fracture is a leading cause of secondary neurological deterioration.[43] A pseudarthrosis of the odontoid has been defined as the absence of fracture site bridging after 4 months of treatment.[65] Most cases of os odontoideum may in fact represent a nonunion of a type I or II odontoid fracture.[22]

Type I injuries are rarely encountered. Based on the limited number of cases described[5,66] in the absence of associated craniocervical instability, few complications or residual symptoms result from treatment of an isolated type I fracture with external immobilization.

Type II odontoid fractures have been associated with a high nonunion rate regardless of the type of nonoperative treatment. Without immobilization, type II fractures have been found to have a 100% risk of nonunion.[5,66] Nonoperative treatment with either bracing or halo has been reported to result in nonunion rates ranging from 15 to 85%.[5,22,65] Prerequisites for a successful nonoperative treatment are maintenance of a nearly anatomical fracture reduction without distraction.[5,67] More than 20% translation of a type II odontoid fracture, as seen on open-mouth or lateral radiograph, implies a fracture surface area insufficient for meaningful bony union.[68] Of many potential predisposing risk factors for fracture nonunion, fracture displacement of 4 to 5 mm has been the most consistently identified factor.[5,65,66] Other risk factors for nonunion include age above 60 years, fracture angulation > 9 degrees, and delay in the institution of treatment.[4,27,67,68]

Nonunion with odontoid screws has been described in 10% of patients, with an overall perioperative complication rate of up to 28%.[27,29] C1–C2 fusions have reported nonunion rates of $\leq$ 4% using transarticular screw and wired structural bone-graft constructs.[5,26,69]

Nonoperative treatment of type III odontoid fractures in a halo is associated with pseudarthrosis rates from 9 to 13%.[5,22] Fracture displacement $\geq$ 4 mm or angulation $\geq$ 10 degrees have been associated with nonunion rates of 22 to 54%.[5,24,65] If surgical stabilization of a type III odontoid fracture is undertaken, it should be in the form of atlantoaxial fixation because excessively high failure rates (55%) have been reported for odontoid screw fixation.[28]

Although spinal cord injury as a result of fractures in the upper cervical spine is less common than in the lower cervical or thoracic spine, type II odontoid fractures are the most common nondistractive fracture of the upper cervical spine to present with primary neurological injury. The frequency of neurological injury with type II odontoid fractures ranges from 18 to 25%,[5,22] and the severity of neurologic injury ranges from isolated cranial nerve injury to pentaplegia.

A considerable mortality rate is associated with upper cervical spine fractures. Although, fractures in healthy individuals have a high mortality because they generally result from high-energy trauma, the overall high mortality rates appear to be primarily related to the high proportion of elderly patients in whom these fractures occur as a marker for progressively frail health. The in-hospital mortality rate for elderly patients with type II odontoid fractures has been reported to be 27 to 42%.[8,67,70] In one series, this high mortality rate was reduced to 0 after institution of an early surgical stabilization protocol.[8] Early surgical stabilization and immobilization with a neck collar is considered the generally preferred treatment strategy for upper cervical spine injuries in this age group.[8,70]

Traumatic Spondylolisthesis of the Axis (Hangman's Fracture)

Although fractures of the axis account for 25 to 71% of deaths at the scene of injury,[66] acute postadmission mortality after hangman's fractures is as low as 2 to 3%.[66] Neurological injury resulting from this fracture type has been identified in 3 to 10% of patients.[31,33] Type III injuries are at highest risk for neurological injury due to the facet dislocation component, with a reported incidence of up to 60%.[7] Type Ia fractures have a 33% incidence of associated spinal cord injury, probably due to the canal compromise, which occurs with fracture displacement in this atypical oblique fracture pattern (**Fig. 6–15A,B).** Type Ia injuries also have a greater potential for vertebral artery injury because of common foramen transversarium involvement.[32] Successful healing of C2 traumatic spondylolisthesis is reported to approach 95%.[31] This is most commonly achieved with nonoperative measures, even in the presence of displacement of the pars interarticularis. Associated upper cervical (15%), subaxial (23%), or head injuries are usually greater contributors to prognosis than the C2 fracture itself. Fractures of type Ia, IIa, and III subcategories constitute a greater treatment challenge due to either their atypical fracture orientation or their inherent ligamentous injury component.

Symptomatic degeneration of the C2–C3 articulations, potentially requiring arthrodesis, is thought to occur in 10% of patients and is more likely to occur in type I injuries because most patients with type II injuries progress to spontaneous anterior ankylosis.[23] This may explain why patients with displaced injuries rarely develop long-term symptoms despite the frequent absence of bony healing across the pars fracture. Patients who heal in severe kyphosis may have difficulty with neck extension.

Symptomatic pseudarthrosis is unusual. In the case of type I injuries, treatment involves either direct osteosynthesis with interfragmentary compression across the pars interarticularis fracture through a posterior approach, or C2–C3 arthrodesis through an anterior approach.[33] In type II injuries, because of the greater deformity and displacement, anterior fusion is usually more appropriate than attempts at direct osteosynthesis.

Vascular Injuries

Vascular injuries are not infrequent with upper cervical spine trauma, although the incidence remains unclear and depends on the diagnostic modalities used.[12,71] Vertebral artery disruption should be considered in any distractive upper cervical spine injury, such as atlantoaxial dissociation or in patients with type III or IV atlantoaxial rotary subluxation. In addition, vertebral artery injuries should be considered in any displaced fracture involving the transverse foramen. Despite the vertebral artery running in close proximity to the rostral lamina of the posterior ring of the atlas, fractures to the atlas ring have not been commonly associated with local vertebral artery trauma. Forced hyperflexion injuries, such as with anteriorly displaced type III odontoid fractures, may leave the vertebral arteries spared but can lead to thrombosis of the carotid arteries.

Treatment-Specific Outcomes and Complications

Skeletal Traction and Halo Vest

Complications of skeletal traction include local complications or systemic ailments resulting from prolonged recumbency. Local complications include pin tract infection, loss of fixation, occipital decubitus formation, dural pin penetration, and propagation of a skull fracture. Systemic complications associated with prolonged skeletal traction may include respiratory compromise, thromboembolism, decubitus ulcers, and sepsis.[72] Pharmacological thromboembolism prophylaxis in patients with acute spine fracture is associated with an increased risk of epidural hematoma formation. In general, prolonged traction for upper cervical spine fractures has become increasingly unpopular, despite the absence of specific data delineating the incidence of medical complications. Judicious use of cervical traction therefore remains a valid treatment option under certain circumstances. For elderly patients prolonged traction is associated with a significant morbidity and usually less desirable.[8]

Halovests have relatively high associated complications. These include loss of reduction in 46% of patients, pressure sores in 11%, and dural pin penetration in 1% of patients. Pin complications are commonly encountered: loosening was found in 36% of patients, infections in 20%, pain at the pin site in 18%, and disfiguring scars in 9%. Increased incidence of pulmonary complications and aspiration are associated with use of halovest devices for elderly patients.[8] Despite these complication rates, halos remain a popular treatment choice for a variety of upper cervical spine fractures in North America.

Craniocervical Fusion

Craniocervical dissociation is fatal in the majority of cases, allowing for few meaningful descriptions of treatment results. Pseudarthrosis rates of up to 23% have been reported with onlay grafting and nonrigid fixation (wiring) methods.[73–76] An 89% fusion rate has been reported using onlay grafting alone, which eliminates hardware-associated complications but requires the use of aggressive postoperative immobilization techniques, including recumbency and skull tong traction, Minerva jacket, and halo.[77] Onlay structural autograft with cerclage wire alone resulted in comparatively improved fusion rates[75] but had the disadvantage of requiring more comprehensive postoperative external immobilization and was complicated by wire breakage in 78% of patients[78] and late fracture of the graft in up to 15% of patients.[79] These problems were initially addressed by substituting a contoured loop for onlay bone graft.[80,81]

The use of rigid fixation with plates or rods and screws has improved nonunion rates to < 6%.[74,76] Rigid craniocervical fusion techniques using screw and plate constructs with suboccipital- and sublaminar-cabled structural graft has resulted in fusion rates approaching 100% with no incidence of hardware failure or need for revision surgery due to reasons of instability despite, in general, the inclusion of fewer motion segments.[82] Potential technical problems include malreduction, which may result in neurological worsening and possible penetration of the inner cortex of the skull, which can lead to injury to neural or vascular structures. The bigger challenge in treating survivors of craniocervical dissociation lies in recognizing their often radiographically subtle yet highly unstable injuries and maintaining sufficient stability to protect neurological function during the initial preoperative treatment phase, which includes the requisite resuscitation and multisystem evaluation in these universally polytraumatized patients. Posterior craniocervical stabilization has recently been shown to be largely neuroprotective after craniocervical dissociation versus an ~40% incidence of neurological worsening in patients who had a delay in diagnosis.[82a]

Posterior Atlantoaxial Fusion

Structural Bone Graft and Wiring

Although wiring techniques are a safe and straightforward method of atlantoaxial stabilization, pseudarthrosis occurs in up to 25% of cases despite the use of more rigid adjunctive external immobilization methods.[46,83] This problem is related to the relative inability of posterior wiring alone to neutralize mainly rotational, and to some extent translational, forces.[65,84] Another described complication is extension of the fusion mass to the occiput.[85] With the advent of modern internal fixation techniques, wiring techniques remain useful as adjunctive methods for stabilization and securing structural bone graft.[86]

Posterior wiring techniques are not effective for injuries where the atlas is displaced posteriorly relative to the axis. In such injuries, posterior wiring tends to accentuate rather than correct the deformity.

Because posterior wiring does not provide rigid fixation, and because wiring is not ideal for posteriorly displaced odontoid fractures, loss of reduction has been reported to occur with the use of posterior bone-graft and wiring techniques alone. Although uncommon, spinal cord injury may occur, presumably during wire passage, and may be avoided by not passing wires before complete reduction has been achieved.[5]

Transarticular Screws

The advent of transarticular screw fixation has allowed a greater degree of atlantoaxial stability than was previously achievable and has become practically indispensable in the treatment of upper cervical injuries.[44,53,84] Fusion rates approaching 100% have been reported following transarticular screw fixation, usually with adjunctive posterior bone grafting and wiring techniques.[26,69] The main concerns pertain to the potential for screw malposition resulting in injury to the vertebral artery, spinal cord, hypoglossal nerve, and carotid artery.

The proximity of the vertebral artery to the transarticular screw pathway has led to a reported clinical incidence of vertebral artery injury that ranges from 0 to 6%, with an associated 0.2% risk of immediate neurological deficit and 0.1% mortality.[38,86,87] Should a vertebral artery injury be suspected, local hemostasis can be achieved with bone wax or placement of the transarticular screw on the affected side. There should, however, be no attempt to place the contralateral transarticular screw. Postoperatively, selective angiographic embolization can ensure satisfactory hemostasis and prevent occurrence of an arteriovenous fistula and embolic stroke.

Excessive drill penetration of the anterior cortex of the atlas can lead to injury of the internal carotid artery or the hypoglossal nerve.[26] Carotid artery injury is not likely to be recognized intraoperatively. Excessive retropharyngeal soft tissue swelling as seen on a lateral cervical radiograph can lead to the diagnosis. Angiographically aided embolization following trial occlusion with an intra-arterial balloon can be used to control local hemorrhage. These complications can be avoided by appreciating that the anterior cortex of the C1 lateral mass lies posterior to the anteriormost projection of the C1 anterior arch on a lateral radiograph by an average of 7 mm, and can be estimated by evaluating preoperative axial images of the atlas.[51]

Fusion rates with transarticular screw fixation are reported to be above 95%. Early hardware failure is an unusual occurrence that usually consists of screw cutout either in the atlas or of the screw shaft within the pars

of the axis. Anatomical patient variations such as a very shallow and arcuate isthmus can predispose to limited screw purchase within the axis. Similarly, an insufficiently cephalad drill trajectory can lead to limited screw purchase at the anteroinferior edge of the C1 lateral mass. Late hardware failure can result from a pseudarthrosis, the salvage of which may consist of revision posterior atlantoaxial fusion, occipitocervical fusion, or anterior atlantoaxial arthrodesis.[39,41,88] Removal of a broken distal transarticular screw is usually unnecessary and impractical.

Proximity of the C2 nerve root to the posterior isthmus of the atlas exposes it to potential injury during posterior C1–C2 facet arthrodesis. The resulting symptoms of occipital numbness or dysesthesias, however, have only rarely been reported.[26,69]

One can anticipate ~50% loss of head rotation following successful C1–C2 arthrodesis.[89] Although this may lead to a certain degree of functional impairment, the functional consequences have not been well documented in the posttraumatic patient population.

C1 Lateral Mass and C2 Pedicle Screws

Fixation that connects individual screws in the C1 lateral masses to C2 pedicle or pars interarticularis screws has become more popular over the last decade, presumably because of the greater versatility this technique affords as compared with transarticular screw fixation.[45] This construct alone has been noted to be biomechanically similar to transarticular screws with adjunctive posterior bone graft and wiring.[54] The main advantages of this technique relate to the use of a pedicle screw at C2, which has a more easily achievable trajectory and carries a lower theoretical risk of vertebral artery injury than the transarticular screw. This stabilization method is particularly valuable as an alternative to transarticular screw fixation when the latter procedure is deemed unsafe or technically implausible due to anomalous vertebral artery anatomy or when issues related to patient anatomy or positioning interfere with acceptable transarticular screw trajectory. Only small, uncontrolled case series have been published to date using this technique, with equivalently high fusion and low loss of fixation rates to transarticular screw techniques.[17,45,55]

Anterior Approach

Risks of the anterior surgical approach to the neck include neurological injury and injury to the esophagus, trachea, or vascular structures. All of these are relatively infrequent events and should occur in < 5% of patients. Dysphagia as a result of anterior surgical exposure is relatively common and may be more prevalent in the upper than in the lower cervical spine.[40,41,56,90] There does not seem to be any difference in the frequency of recurrent laryngeal nerve injury between right- versus left-sided upper cervical spine approaches.

Anterior Odontoid Screw Fixation

Results of anterior odontoid screw fixation have varied in the literature. Although some large series have shown excellent success rates, with healing rates approaching 90% in patients treated within 6 months of injury regardless of patient age and bone quality,[28,91,92] other series have shown higher complication rates, particularly loss of fixation, in patients with osteoporosis.[93] In addition to bone quality, sagittal plane fracture obliquity in the anterior direction similar to that of intended screw placement appears to be associated with lower (75%) healing rates.[28] In general, patients with anteriorly displaced odontoid fractures pose a greater challenge to odontoid screw fixation, compared with those with posteriorly displaced fractures. Lack of an anatomical reduction or inability to achieve interfragmentary compression across the fracture can greatly impair the efficacy of odontoid screw fixation.

Major complication rates of up to 28% have been reported with odontoid screw fixation[25,27–29,37] and consisted mainly of hardware-related complications (10%) and superficial wound infections (2%) in the largest published series.[28] Of the hardware-related complications, half consisted of screw disengagement from the C2 body in patients with type III odontoid fractures, putting into question whether this technique is appropriate for odontoid fractures that extend into the C2 body. A second commonly seen hardware-related complication is backing out of the odontoid screw, which occurs primarily when the screw tip has not acceptably engaged the apical cortex of the odontoid. Failure of screw fixation may have catastrophic consequences, as demonstrated by a report of quadriplegia and death from respiratory failure that resulted from fracture displacement after loss of fixation.[28] Similar sequelae of odontoid screw fixation have been reported on other occasions.[91] A third hardware-related complication pertains to screw malposition. The failure rate of odontoid screw fixation does not appear to be influenced by the use of one versus two screws.[28,37,94] Other technical mistakes include an excessively anterior starting point, which can leave a thin anterior bony shell in the axis that is unable to contain the screw shaft. If a cannulated screw system is used, care should be taken to avoid advancement of a guide wire rostral to the tip of the odontoid. Although rare, intraoperative spinal cord and cranial nerve injury has been described.[27,29] It is apparent from the literature that a considerable learning curve exists with this complex procedure.[5,27]

Although fracture union does not appear to be affected by delay in surgery of up to 6 months, long-standing odontoid pseudarthrosis responds poorly to anterior screw fixation, as demonstrated by a mere 25% healing rate in a series of 18 patients who were operated for pseudarthrosis between 18 and 48 months postinjury.[28] The 25% hardware-related complication rate in this group of patients, consisting mainly of screw fracture, was consistent with previously reported experiences with odontoid screw fixation of pseudarthroses.[27]

Complications already described for the Smith-Robinson approach, such as esophageal or neurovascular injury, dysphagia, and pharyngeal edema, have been reported to occur when placing anterior odontoid screws.[27,28,91,95]

Technical considerations that may preclude the use of odontoid screw fixation pertain primarily to physical characteristics that do not allow for acceptable screw trajectory, such as prominent thoracic kyphosis, barrel chest, and fracture characteristics that require a flexed position to maintain an acceptable reduction.

C2–C3 Anterior Diskectomy and Fusion

Because surgery is not commonly necessary for the treatment of traumatic spondylolisthesis of the axis, there are few reports on the results of anterior C2–C3 diskectomy and fusion for the treatment of traumatic conditions. One series of five patients[35] describes the successful use of this technique without complications, using autologous tricortical iliac crest graft and anterior plating with subsequent external immobilization in a halo, for the treatment of type II traumatic spondylolisthesis of the axis with associated upper cervical injuries. Patients presenting with neurological deficits had profound postoperative recovery.

Complications related to this procedure pertain to the anterior approach to the upper cervical spine, which are well described,[56] and to the potential for pseudarthrosis or loss of fixation, the frequency of which is not well documented. Upper cervical approaches appear to have a higher risk of airway-related problems.[56] Due to small patient numbers, there is also no comparison to posterior instrumentation approaches for the same conditions. The mandible commonly obstructs the surgical exposure of the anterior upper neck, adding to the complexity of the procedure. Reported problems with anterior C2–C3 fusion are primarily technical, such as achieving an adequate anterior decompression, proper bone graft positioning, and placement of stable low-profile instrumentation. Prominent hardware could potentially lead to swallowing difficulties and even esophageal erosion and should therefore be avoided. Horner's syndrome and suboccipital pain with associated C2–C3 degenerative changes have been reported as frequent complications of this procedure for the treatment of traumatic spondylolisthesis of the axis.[34]

Due to the presence of an aberrant vertebral artery course in up to 20% of the population, careful evaluation of the preoperative CT scan is critical before performing transarticular screw fixation of C1–C2.

Pearls

- Vertebral artery disruption should be considered in any distractive upper cervical spine injury, or in patients with type III or IV atlantoaxial rotary subluxation, as well as in any displaced fracture involving the transverse foramen.
- Any occipital condyle fracture should be considered a possible component of craniocervical dissociation and potentially unstable.
- The integrity of the TAL is the primary determinant of instability associated with injuries of the atlas. Signs of TAL insufficiency include bony avulsion, widening of the lateral masses on radiographs or CT scan, and ligament rupture on MRI.
- Type II odontoid fractures are the most common nondistractive fracture of the upper cervical spine to present with primary neurological injury. The frequency of neurological injury with type II odontoid fractures ranges from 18 to 25%, and the severity ranges from isolated cranial nerve injury to pentaplegia.

- Type II odontoid fractures have a 100% risk of nonunion when treated without immobilization. Initial nonoperative treatment consisting of either bracing or halo result in nonunion rates ranging from 15 to 85%. Of many potential risk factors for odontoid nonunion, fracture displacement of 4 to 5 mm has been the most consistently identified factor.
- In contrast to item 5, nonoperative treatment of type III odontoid fractures in a halo is associated with pseudarthrosis rates from 9 to 13%.
- For type III odontoid fractures, posterior C1–C2 arthrodesis is the surgical treatment method of choice because anterior odontoid screw fixation has a high failure rate with these injury types.[28]
- Direct osteosynthesis of type II hangman's fractures does not address the associated injury to the C2–C3 intervertebral disk.

On the DVDs

Video 6–1 (Disk 1) Posterior Instrumentation and Fusion C1–C3 This patient sustained an irreducible fracture subluxation of C1–C2. Treatment consisted of posterior instrumentation and fusion of C1 to C3 with lateral mass screw fixation in C1.

Video 6–2 (Disk 1) ORIF of an Odontoid Fracture This patient sustained a type 2 odontoid fracture and was treated with open reduction and internal fixation with placement.

References

1. Johnson RM, Hart DL, Simmons EF, Ramsby GR, Southwick WO. Cervical orthoses: a study comparing their effectiveness in restricting cervical motion in normal subjects. J Bone Joint Surg Am 1977;59:332–339
2. Govender S, Grootboom M. Fractures of the dens: the results of non-rigid immobilization. Injury 1988;19:165–167
3. Whitehill R, Richman JA, Glaser JA. Failure of immobilization of the cervical spine by the halo vest: a report of five cases. J Bone Joint Surg Am 1986;68:326–332
4. Lind B, Nordwall A, Sihlbom H. Odontoid fractures treated with halo-vest. Spine 1987;12:173–177
5. Clark CR, White AA III. Fractures of the dens: a multicenter study. J Bone Joint Surg Am 1985;67:1340–1348
6. Guiot B, Fessler RG. Complex atlantoaxial fractures. J Neurosurg 1999;91(Suppl 2):139–143
7. Levine AM, Edwards CC. The management of traumatic spondylolisthesis of the axis. J Bone Joint Surg Am 1985;67:217–226
8. Bednar DA, Parikh J, Hummel J. Management of type II odontoid process fractures in geriatric patients: a prospective study of sequential cohorts with attention to survivorship. J Spinal Disord 1995;8:166–169
9. Anderson PA, Montesano PX. Morphology and treatment of occipital condyle fractures. Spine 1988;13:731–736
10. Traynelis VC, Marano GD, Dunker RO, Kaufman HH. Traumatic atlanto-occipital dislocation: case report. J Neurosurg 1986;65:863–870
11. Dvorak J, Schneider E, Saldinger P, Rahn B. Biomechanics of the craniocervical region: the alar and transverse ligaments. J Orthop Res 1988;6:452–461

12. Song WS, Chiang YH, Chen CY, Lin SZ, Liu MY. A simple method for diagnosing traumatic occlusion of the vertebral artery at the craniovertebral junction. Spine 1994;19:837–839
13. Dickman CA, Greene KA, Sonntag VK. Injuries involving the transverse atlantal ligament: classification and treatment guidelines based upon experience with 39 injuries. Neurosurgery 1996;38: 44–50
14. Spence KF Jr, Decker S, Sell KW. Bursting atlantal fracture associated with rupture of the transverse ligament. J Bone Joint Surg Am 1970;52:543–549
15. Heller JG, Viroslav S, Hudson T. Jefferson fractures: the role of magnification artifact in assessing transverse ligament integrity. J Spinal Disord 1993;6:392–396
16. Levine AM, Edwards CC. Fractures of the atlas. J Bone Joint Surg Am 1991;73:680–691
17. Goel A, Laheri V. Plate and screw fixation for atlanto-axial subluxation. Acta Neurochir (Wien) 1994;129:47–53
18. Fielding JW, Cochran GB, Lawsing JF, Hohl M. Tears of the transverse ligament of the atlas: a clinical and biomechanical study. J Bone Joint Surg Am 1974;56:1683–1691
19. Fielding JW, Hawkins RJ. Atlanto-axial rotatory fixation: fixed rotatory subluxation of the atlanto-axial joint. J Bone Joint Surg Am 1977;59:37–44
20. Levine AM. Avulsion of the transverse ligament associated with a fracture of the atlas: a case report. Orthopedics 1983;6:1467–1471
21. Ryan MD, Henderson JJ. The epidemiology of fractures and fracture-dislocations of the cervical spine. Injury 1992;23:38–40
22. Anderson LD, D'Alonzo RT. Fractures of the odontoid process of the axis. J Bone Joint Surg Am 1974;56:1663–1674

23. Hadley MN, Browner CM, Liu SS, Sonntag VK. New subtype of acute odontoid fractures (type IIa). Neurosurgery 1988;22(1 Pt 1): 67–71

24. Apuzzo ML, Heiden JS, Weiss MH, Ackerson TT, Harvey JP, Kurze T. Acute fractures of the odontoid process: an analysis of 45 cases. J Neurosurg 1978;48:85–91

25. Bohler J. Anterior stabilization for acute fractures and non-unions of the dens. J Bone Joint Surg Am 1982;64:18–27

26. Jeanneret B, Magerl F. Primary posterior fusion C1/2 in odontoid fractures: indications, technique, and results of transarticular screw fixation. J Spinal Disord 1992;5:464–475

27. Aebi M, Etter C, Coscia M. Fractures of the odontoid process: treatment with anterior screw fixation. Spine 1989;14:1065–1070

28. Apfelbaum RI, Lonser RR, Veres R, Casey A. Direct anterior screw fixation for recent and remote odontoid fractures. J Neurosurg 2000;93(Suppl 2):227–236

29. Etter C, Coscia M, Jaberg H, Aebi M. Direct anterior fixation of dens fractures with a cannulated screw system. Spine 1991;16(Suppl 3): S25–S32

30. Effendi B, Roy D, Cornish B, Dussault RG, Laurin CA. Fractures of the ring of the axis: a classification based on the analysis of 131 cases. J Bone Joint Surg Br 1981;63:319–327

31. Levine AM, Edwards CC. Traumatic lesions of the occipitoatlantoaxial complex. Clin Orthop Relat Res 1989;239:53–68

32. Starr JK, Eismont FJ. Atypical hangman's fractures. Spine 1993; 18:1954–1957

33. Francis WR, Fielding JW, Hawkins RJ, Pepin J, Hensinger R. Traumatic spondylolisthesis of the axis. J Bone Joint Surg Br 1981;63: 313–318

34. Cornish BL. Traumatic spondylolisthesis of the axis. J Bone Joint Surg Br 1968;50:31–43

35. Tuite GF, Papadopoulos SM, Sonntag VK. Caspar plate fixation for the treatment of complex hangman's fractures. Neurosurgery 1992;30:761–764

36. Goto S, Tanno T, Moriya H. Cervical myelopathy caused by pseudoarthrosis between the atlas and axis associated with diffuse idiopathic skeletal hyperostosis. Spine 1995;20:2572–2575

37. Sasso R, Doherty BJ, Crawford MJ, Heggeness MH. Biomechanics of odontoid fracture fixation. Comparison of the one- and two-screw technique. Spine 1993;18:1950–1953

38. Solanki GA, Crockard HA. Peroperative determination of safe superior transarticular screw trajectory through the lateral mass. Spine 1999;24:1477–1482

39. Reindl R, Sen M, Aebi M. Anterior instrumentation for traumatic C1–C2 instability. Spine 2003;28:E329–E333

40. McAfee PC, Bohlman HH, Riley LH, Robinson RA, Southwick WO, Nachlas NE. The anterior retropharyngeal approach to the upper part of the cervical spine. J Bone Joint Surg Am 1987;69:1371–1383

41. Vaccaro AR, Ring D, Lee RS, Scuderi G, Garfin SR. Salvage anterior C1–C2 screw fixation and arthrodesis through the lateral approach in a patient with a symptomatic pseudoarthrosis. Am J Orthop 1997;26:349–353

42. Zavanone M, Guerra P, Rampini P, Crotti F, Vaccari U. Traumatic fractures of the craniovertebral junction: management of 23 cases. J Neurosurg Sci 1991;35:17–22

43. Fairholm D, Lee ST, Lui TN. Fractured odontoid: the management of delayed neurological symptoms. Neurosurgery 1996;38:38–43

44. Magerl FSCS. Stable posterior fusion of the atlas and axis by transarticular screw fixation. In: Kehr PWA, ed. Cervical Spine. Berlin: Springer-Verlag; 1986:322–327

45. Harms J, Melcher RP. Posterior C1–C2 fusion with polyaxial screw and rod fixation. Spine 2001;26:2467–2471

46. Gallie WE. Fractures and dislocations of the cervical spine. Am J Surg 1939;46:494–499

47. Grob D, Magerl F. Surgical stabilization of C1 and C2 fractures [in German]. Orthopade 1987;16:46–54

48. Madawi AA, Casey AT, Solanki GA, Tuite G, Veres R, Crockard HA. Radiological and anatomical evaluation of the atlantoaxial transarticular screw fixation technique. J Neurosurg 1997;86:961–968

49. Tokuda K, Miyasaka K, Abe H, et al. Anomalous atlantoaxial portions of vertebral and posterior inferior cerebellar arteries. Neuroradiology 1985;27:410–413

50. Ebraheim NA, Misson JR, Xu R, Yeasting RA. The optimal transarticular C1–2 screw length and the location of the hypoglossal nerve. Surg Neurol 2000;53:208–210

51. Nadim Y, Sabry F, Xu R, Ebraheim N. Computed tomography in the determination of transarticular C1–C2 screw length. Orthopedics 2000;23:373–375

52. Gebhard JS, Schimmer RC, Jeanneret B. Safety and accuracy of transarticular screw fixation C1–C2 using an aiming device: an anatomic study. Spine 1998;23:2185–2189

53. Hanson PB, Montesano PX, Sharkey NA, Rauschning W. Anatomic and biomechanical assessment of transarticular screw fixation for atlantoaxial instability. Spine 1991;16:1141–1145

54. Melcher RP, Puttlitz CM, Kleinstueck FS, Lotz JC, Harms J, Bradford DS. Biomechanical testing of posterior atlantoaxial fixation techniques. Spine 2002;27:2435–2440

55. Goel A. C1–C2 pedicle screw fixation with rigid cantilever beam construct: case report and technical note. Neurosurgery 2002;51: 853–854

56. Sagi HC, Beutler W, Carroll E, Connolly PJ. Airway complications associated with surgery on the anterior cervical spine. Spine 2002;27:949–953

57. Wright NM. Posterior C2 fixation using bilateral, crossing C2 laminar screws: case series and technical note. J Spinal Disord Tech 2004;17:158–162

58. Noble ER, Smoker WR. The forgotten condyle: the appearance, morphology, and classification of occipital condyle fractures. AJNR Am J Neuroradiol 1996;17:507–513

59. Urculo E, Arrazola M, Arrazola M, Riu I, Moyua A. Delayed glossopharyngeal and vagus nerve paralysis following occipital condyle fracture: case report. J Neurosurg 1996;84:522–525

60. Crisco JJ III, Panjabi MM, Dvorak J. A model of the alar ligaments of the upper cervical spine in axial rotation. J Biomech 1991;24: 607–614

61. Montane I, Eismont FJ, Green BA. Traumatic occipitoatlantal dislocation. Spine 1991;16:112–116

62. Krantz P. Isolated disruption of the transverse ligament of the atlas: an injury easily overlooked at post-mortem examination. Injury 1980;12:168–170

63. Wigren A, Sweden U, Amici F Jr. Traumatic atlanto-axial dislocation without neurological disorder: a case report. J Bone Joint Surg Am 1973;55:642–644

64. Greene KA, Dickman CA, Marciano FF, Drabier J, Drayer BP, Sonntag VK. Transverse atlantal ligament disruption associated with odontoid fractures. Spine 1994;19:2307–2314

65. Schatzker J, Rorabeck CH, Waddell JP. Fractures of the dens (odontoid process): an analysis of thirty-seven cases. J Bone Joint Surg Br 1971;53:392–405

66. Greene KA, Dickman CA, Marciano FF, Drabier JB, Hadley MN, Sonntag VK. Acute axis fractures: analysis of management and outcome in 340 consecutive cases. Spine 1997;22:1843–1852

67. Alander DH, Andreychik DA, Stauffer ES. Early outcome in cervical spinal cord injured patients older than 50 years of age. Spine 1994;19:2299–2301

68. Southwick WO. Management of fractures of the dens (odontoid process). J Bone Joint Surg Am 1980;62:482–486

69. Haid RW, Subach BR, McLaughlin MR, Rodts GE, Wahlig JB. C1–C2 transarticular screw fixation for atlantoaxial instability: a 6-year experience. Neurosurgery 2001;49:65–68

70. Lieberman IH, Webb JK. Cervical spine injuries in the elderly. J Bone Joint Surg Br 1994;76:877–881

71. Friedman D, Flanders A, Thomas C, Millar W. Vertebral artery injury after acute cervical spine trauma: rate of occurrence as detected by MR angiography and assessment of clinical consequences. AJR Am J Roentgenol 1995;164:443–447

72. Garfin SR, Botte MJ, Waters RL, Nickel VL. Complications in the use of the halo fixation device. J Bone Joint Surg Am 1986;68: 320–325

73. Sherk HH, Snyder B. Posterior fusions of the upper cervical spine: indications, techniques, and prognosis. Orthop Clin North Am 1978;9:1091–1099

74. Abumi K, Takada T, Shono Y, Kaneda K, Fujiya M. Posterior occipitocervical reconstruction using cervical pedicle screws and plate-rod systems. Spine 1999;24:1425–1434

75. Wertheim SB, Bohlman HH. Occipitocervical fusion: indications, technique, and long-term results in thirteen patients. J Bone Joint Surg Am 1987;69:833–836

76. Smith DC. Atlanto-occipital dislocation. J Emerg Med 1992;10: 699–703

77. Elia M, Mazzara JT, Fielding JW. Onlay technique for occipitocervical fusion. Clin Orthop Relat Res 1992;280:170–174

78. Haher TR, Yeung AW, Caruso SA, et al. Occipital screw pullout strength: a biomechanical investigation of occipital morphology. Spine 1999;24:5–9

79. Hamblen DL. Occipito-cervical fusion: indications, technique and results. J Bone Joint Surg Br 1967;49:33–45

80. Ransford AO, Crockard HA, Pozo JL, Thomas NP, Nelson IW. Craniocervical instability treated by contoured loop fixation. J Bone Joint Surg Br 1986;68:173–177

81. Itoh T, Tsuji H, Katoh Y, Yonezawa T, Kitagawa H. Occipito-cervical fusion reinforced by Luque's segmental spinal instrumentation for rheumatoid diseases. Spine 1988;13:1234–1238

82. Sasso RC, Jeanneret B, Fischer K, Magerl F. Occipitocervical fusion with posterior plate and screw instrumentation: a long-term follow-up study. Spine 1994;19:2364–2368

82a. Bellabarba C, Mirza SK, West GA, Mann FA, Dailey AT, Newell DW, Chapman JR. Diagnosis and treatment of craniocervical dislocation in a series of 17 consecutive survivors during an 8-year period. J Neurosurg Spine 2006 4:429–440

83. Hajek PD, Lipka J, Hartline P, Saha S, Albright JA. Biomechanical study of C1–C2 posterior arthrodesis techniques. Spine 1993;1 8:173–177

84. Grob D, Crisco JJ, Panjabi MM, Wang P, Dvorak J. Biomechanical evaluation of four different posterior atlantoaxial fixation techniques. Spine 1992;17:480–490

85. Fielding JW, Hawkins RJ, Ratzan SA. Spine fusion for atlanto-axial instability. J Bone Joint Surg Am 1976;58:400–407

86. Grob D, Jeanneret B, Aebi M, Markwalder TM. Atlanto-axial fusion with transarticular screw fixation. J Bone Joint Surg Br 1991;73: 972–976

87. Wright NM, Lauryssen C. Vertebral artery injury in C1–2 transarticular screw fixation: results of a survey of the AANS/CNS section on disorders of the spine and peripheral nerves. American Association of Neurological Surgeons/Congress of Neurological Surgeons. J Neurosurg 1998;88:634–640

88. Vaccaro AR, Lehman AP, Ahlgren BD, Garfin SR. Anterior C1–C2 screw fixation and bony fusion through an anterior retropharyngeal approach. Orthopedics 1999;22:1165–1170

89. Panjabi M, Dvorak J, Duranceau J, et al. Three-dimensional movements of the upper cervical spine. Spine 1988;13:726–730

90. Bazaz R, Lee MJ, Yoo JU. Incidence of dysphagia after anterior cervical spine surgery: a prospective study. Spine 2002;27:2453–2458

91. Henry AD, Bohly J, Grosse A. Fixation of odontoid fractures by an anterior screw. J Bone Joint Surg Br 1999;81:472–477

92. Borm W, Kast E, Richter HP, Mohr K. Anterior screw fixation in type II odontoid fractures: is there a difference in outcome between age groups? Neurosurgery 2003;52:1089–1092

93. Andersson S, Rodrigues M, Olerud C. Odontoid fractures: high complication rate associated with anterior screw fixation in the elderly. Eur Spine J 2000;9:56–59

94. Graziano G, Jaggers C, Lee M, Lynch W. A comparative study of fixation techniques for type II fractures of the odontoid process. Spine 1993;18:2383–2387

95. Daentzer D, Deinsberger W, Boker DK. Vertebral artery complications in anterior approaches to the cervical spine: report of two cases and review of literature. Surg Neurol 2003;59:300–309

7 Lower Cervical Spine Injuries

John Charles France

Injury to the lower cervical spine can be devastating to the trauma patient, and it remains the responsibility of all those involved in trauma care to ensure that all such injuries are properly detected and treated. Because the anatomy of the lower cervical vertebrae (C3–C7) is essentially identical, the injury patterns are similar across each segment and can be discussed together. This differs from the upper cervical spine (occiput–C2), where each segment is unique, creating distinctly different injuries. Much of the existing literature on subaxial spine injuries is of poor methodological quality. Therefore, practice standards cannot be established, only guidelines.[1] This must be kept in mind in the course of reading any chapter on the topic.

Injury Evaluation and Classification

Lower cervical spine injuries can be classified by bony morphology, anatomy, mechanism, nature of neurological injury, or combinations of these. Each of these systems has value, and they can be used together to give an accurate representation of a particular injury and to guide development of a treatment plan for that injury. One of the primary factors is the neurological status of the patient. If a patient is determined to have a neurological deficit, it is further characterized as complete or incomplete. This distinction affects treatment decisions as well as timing of treatment. For a deficit to be considered complete, there can be no motor or sensory function below the level of injury. Any discernible motor or sensory function below the level of injury makes it incomplete. Because the zone of neurological injury can vary relative to the bony injury, it is not uncommon to see function at the levels immediately caudal to the bony injury and still be considered complete. Additionally, there can be a "veil" of intact sensation about the shoulders because roots exiting from within more cephalad levels of the cervical spine supply this area. A patient's injury cannot reliably be considered complete during the period of spinal shock (the first 24 to 48 hours), but the likelihood of neurological recovery is less than 3% if there is no evidence of distal function or sacral sparing within the first 24 hours.[2,3] An incomplete neurological deficit may be manifested as only sacral sparing, with intact perianal sensation or toe flexion, meaning that there is potential for neurological recovery. Incomplete deficits are further subdivided into several distinct patterns. Central cord syndrome is the most common and typically occurs from an impact to the spinal cord, compressing it peripherally toward the central core. The applied forces are greatest in the center of the cord, resulting in a distribution of injury that is explained by the anatomical organization of the spinal tracts. Because the cervical portion is more centrally located and the sacral tracts are at the periphery, the upper extremities are more affected than the lower extremities. The prognosis to regain ambulatory function is relatively good. Anterior cord syndrome involves the anteriorly based tracts of the spinal cord, sparing the posterior columns, which preserves vibration sense, proprioception, and deep pressure. Motor functions, along with pain/temperature sensation, are the most severely affected. The prognosis for recovery is poor because this syndrome often has a vascular basis. Posterior cord syndrome is essentially the opposite of anterior cord syndrome but is rarely seen as a result of trauma. Only the posterior columns are involved, perhaps secondary to impact from a lamina fracture. Brown-Séquard syndrome is interesting due to the anatomical explanation for the resultant neurological pattern of injury. Motor function is impaired ipsilateral to the injury, whereas pain and temperature sensation is impaired contralateral to the injury. This is due to the fact that the decussation of the nerve fibers for the motor tracts occurs proximally within the brainstem and the pain/temperature fibers cross immediately upon arrival to the cord. This injury is most often the result of penetrating trauma but can also be seen after a blunt impact applied laterally to the cord. Lastly, root injury differs from the above incomplete syndromes in that it involves lower motor neuron function with improved potential for recovery.

A further application of the neurologically based classification is to apply it to the functional status of the patient, as in the Frankel classification.[4] Functional level A is complete loss of sensory and motor function below the level of injury, level B is preservation of sensory but no motor function below the level of injury, level C is useless motor function below the level of injury, level D is useful sensory and motor function below the level of injury, and level E is normal motor and sensory function below the level of injury.

A mechanistic classification was developed by Allen et al based on a retrospective review of 165 injuries of the cervical spine (**Fig. 7–1**).[5] They described six patterns according to the presumed attitude of the cervical spine at the time of injury (e.g., flexion or extension) and the predominant mode of failure (e.g., compression or distraction). This classification is relatively complex and infers a mechanism based on interpretation of the static x-ray image. Treatment can be deduced based on reversal of the mechanism and stabilization in such a way that prevents reproduction of the destabilizing force. For example, a

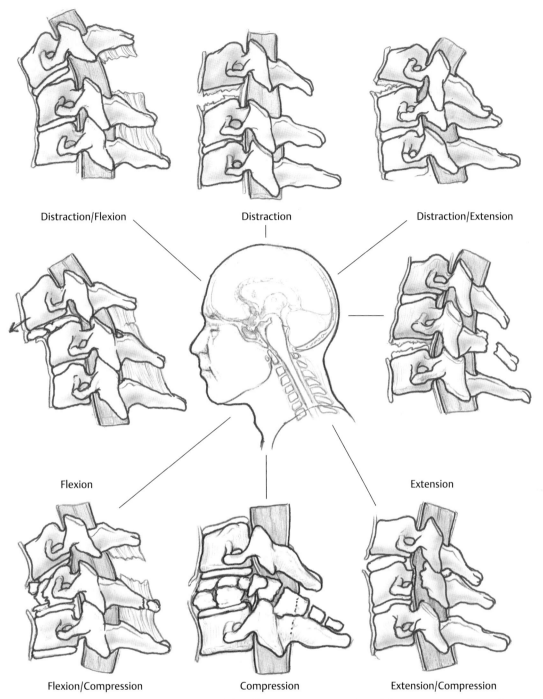

Figure 7–1 A diagrammatic representation of the Allen-Ferguson mechanistic classification on subaxial cervical spine fractures. (From Chapman JR, Anderson PA. Cervical spine trauma. In: Frymoyer J, ed. The Adult Spine: Principles and Practice. 2nd ed. Philadelphia: Lippincott-Raven; 1997:1270, with permission.)

flexion-distraction injury results in disruption of the posterior ligaments and facet capsules and can extend into the posterior anulus if the force is severe enough. Thus the posterior tension band is disrupted, making the logical choice for treatment one that restores that tension band via a posterior approach. However, the mechanism of injury does not always correlate with the resultant fracture pattern. Torg et al[6] looked at the National Football Head and Neck Injury Registry and found that the same mecha-

nism of injury can result in different fracture patterns depending on the level at which the injury occurs. For example, an axial loading mechanism to the middle cervical spine (i.e., C3–C4) is more likely to result in a facet dislocation or disk herniation than the expected burst or teardrop fracture that occurs in the lower cervical spine.[7] Additionally, rotational forces are not well accounted for and can play an important role in the fracture pattern.[8] Many different forces can come into play within the same patient. For example, a fall that involves landing on the head can force the neck into flexion and at the same time rotate as the body twists to the side.

The most popular classification used in the literature is a simple descriptive one based on the pathoanatomy. Typical injury patterns include facet fracture dislocations (unilateral or bilateral), axial injuries (compression, teardrop, burst fractures), and extension fractures (teardrop avulsion, spinous process, lateral mass). With this system, however, the nuances of any particular group of fractures are difficult to distinguish, and these factors can have important implications in determining treatment. For example, facet dislocation associated with fracture of either the inferior or the superior facet can be more unstable than those without fracture; therefore, reduction is more easily achieved but also more easily lost. This can have implications for choosing an anterior or posterior approach, as will be discussed later. Efforts have been made to correlate neurological and morphological classifications but are of limited value for the individual patient.[9]

Imaging

To classify an injury, the proper radiographs are necessary.[10] Anteroposterior (AP), lateral, and odontoid views are generally accepted for initial screening. To better visualize the cervicothoracic junction, a swimmer's view or trauma obliques (obtained by rotating the x-ray beam rather than the patient) can be utilized.[11] A variety of radiographic signs, such as the "naked facet" and "reverse hamburger bun" signs, have been described to aid in the diagnosis and characterization of an injury.[12,13] More than 90% of injuries can be detected on the plain radiographs.[14] However, the low cervical vertebrae and cervicothoracic junction can be difficult to visualize, making computed tomography (CT) necessary for full evaluation.[15] Lateral mass fractures[16–19] and fractures in severely degenerative necks[20] are also notoriously difficult to visualize on plain radiographs, and CT scanning may be necessary to detect subtle fractures in those trauma patients with neck pain despite normal-appearing plain radiographs.[21] Helical CT scanning affords excellent resolution for sagittal and coronal reconstructions and may become the imaging modality of choice. Helical CT scanning has been suggested as a means of dividing fractures into major or minor injuries.[22] Greater caution must be exercised in the elderly patient with spondylotic changes creating a rigid spine. Although their fractures may be atypical and more subtle radiographically, they may be unstable, putting them at risk for late neurological compromise **(Fig. 7–2A,B)**.[23] If a fracture is identified on plain films, then a CT scan is also warranted to further define the nature of that fracture.[24,25] Once a cervical fracture is identified, AP and lateral radiographs of the thoracic and lumbar spine are indicated to rule out noncontiguous fractures that are present in 6.4% of patients.[26] Myelography may be necessary to assess the canal for disk herniation or epidural hematoma in those patients unable to have a magnetic resonance imaging (MRI) scan.[27,28]

The role of MRI in the assessment of cervical spine injuries is evolving. It is ideal for evaluation of ligament, disk, and neurological structures.[29] A small group of patients exist with ligamentous injuries that have normal initial radiographs **(Fig. 7–3A–C)**.[30,31] The extent of instability or in-

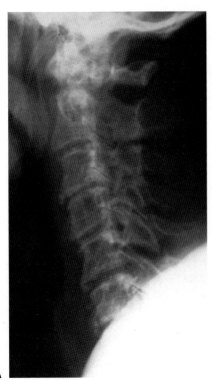

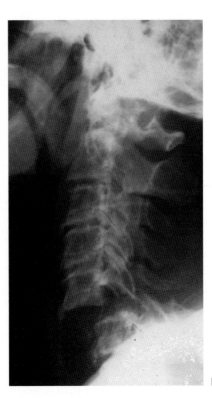

Figure 7–2 (A) An elderly patient whose initial x-ray was misinterpreted as negative **(B)** suffered a bilateral facet dislocation upon removal of the collar. The degenerative process made the radiographs more difficult to interpret, and the loss of elasticity made the spine more rigid, allowing it to fracture more easily.

A

B

jury in these patients can only be determined with risky flexion/extension radiographs, clinical follow-up allowing the injury to manifest itself with late displacement (an unfortunate means of diagnosis), or MRI scanning. These patients may be young with an otherwise normal-appearing spine or elderly with advanced degenerative changes that mask the underlying ligamentous injury. In the latter group the ligaments are stiff and act more like a fracture than a ligamentous tear. At this time, the role of MRI in the assessment of facet dislocations is well established, but

the timing of the study and how to utilize the information remain controversial.[32] Vaccaro et al used MRI to demonstrate the extent of ligamentous damage associated with unilateral and bilateral facet dislocations.[33] MRI was also used to assess the likelihood of a disk herniation associated with facet dislocation pre- and postreduction in 11 patients.[34] Two of the 11 patients were found to have a herniation prior to reduction. Nine of the 11 were successfully reduced using closed serial traction with the patient awake, and five of those nine were found to have a hernia-

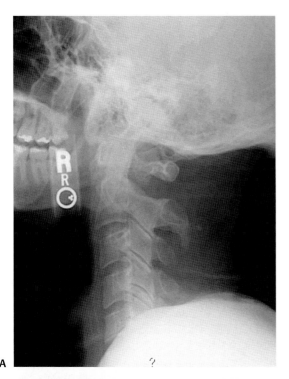

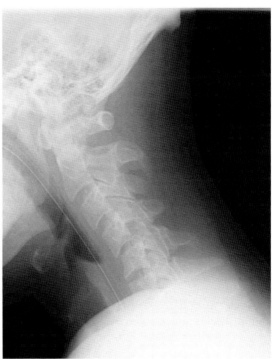

A

B

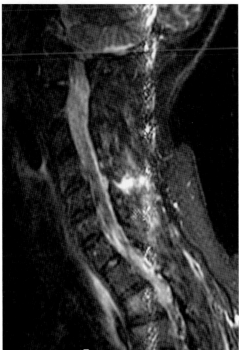

C

Figure 7–3 **(A)** Pure ligamentous injury can be missed on the initial lateral x-ray if the image is taken while the spine is properly aligned. **(B)** The instability can be revealed on a flexion lateral film or **(C)** predicted with a sagittal inversion recovery magnetic resonance imaging.

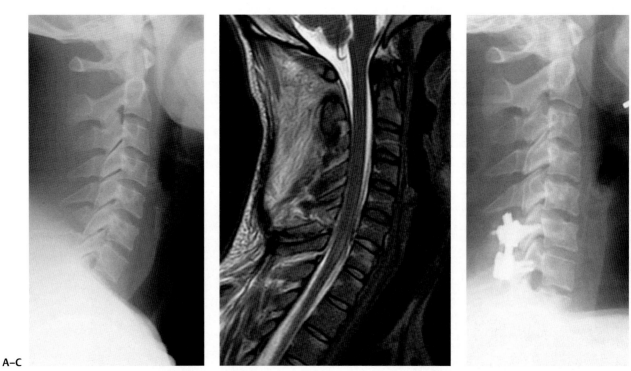

A–C

Figure 7–4 An atypical spinous process fracture occurring at the base of the spinous process and associated with posterior ligamentous injury as well as disruption of the posterior annulus. **(A)** Lateral radiograph of the cervical spine showing a C6 fracture at the base of the spinous process. **(B)** Sagittal T2 MRI image showing disruption of the posterior annulus of the disk and increased signal on the disk space signifying a significant flexion injury. **(C)** These findings imply a flexion component and may warrant surgical stabilization.

tion postreduction. No patient suffered neurological deterioration. Lastly, MRI may be useful in evaluating the cervical spine in the obtunded patient. Under these circumstances a screening MRI should include inversion recovery or fat-saturated T2-weighted sequences and be done in a timely fashion to make edema and ligamentous disruption more obvious.[35] Other means of clearance in the obtunded patient include dynamic fluoroscopy for distraction and flexion/extension testing.[36]

Nonoperative Treatment

Many injuries of the lower cervical spine are treated nonoperatively. Nonoperative management can range from benign neglect to halo vest immobilization. For example, spinous process fractures and transverse process fractures are stable and amenable to simple hard collar immobilization for 6 weeks, or even comfort care only with soft collars or benign neglect. However, one must be aware that spinous process fractures can, at times, occur from a flexion mechanism[37] rather than from the usual extension, muscle pull (classic clay shoveler's),[38,39] or direct blow[38] mechanisms. When flexion is the mechanism of injury, a more substantial posterior ligamentous injury may coexist, creating a potentially unstable pattern warranting more aggressive management and possibly even surgical stabilization **(Fig. 7–4A–C).** Either dynamic flexion/extension radiographs or MRI can be used to distinguish a flexion injury from a more benign extension

injury. Isolated fractures through the transverse foramen are usually benign and treated with collar immobilization until it is clear that there is no other subtle instability, at which time treatment is symptomatic. One must beware of the possibility of vertebral artery injury when the vertebral foramen is involved.[40]

Teardrop avulsion fractures are typically minor extension injuries involving a small fleck of bone pulled off the anteroinferior aspect of the vertebral body by the anulus. They are treated with collar immobilization for 6 weeks. On occasion the hyperextension may be more severe, resulting in a hyperextension dislocation.[41] These are often associated with other facial trauma. The teardrop avulsion injury is not to be confused with the more ominous teardrop fracture that is the result of a compression-flexion mechanism **(Fig. 7–5A–C).** The latter is also referred to as a quadrangular fragment fracture. It signifies a much more unstable injury that is only rarely treated nonoperatively. Distinguishing radiographic criteria of a teardrop fracture include a larger anteroinferior fragment (a chunk rather than a chip), posterior retropulsion of the cephalad vertebrae, widening of the facets, and a characteristic sagittal split in the vertebral body.[42,43]

Lateral mass fractures vary in severity, and many can be treated successfully in a nonoperative mode. The first factor to consider in making the determination for treatment is the neurological status of the patient. If a spinal cord injury exists, it is assumed that the skeletal injury is unstable, and the patient is treated with operative stabilization.

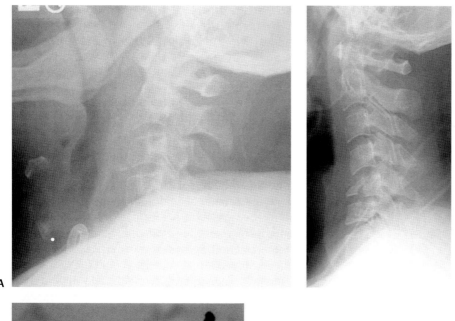

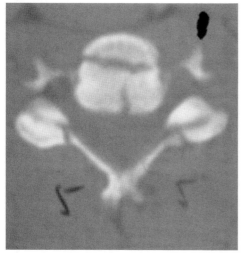

Figure 7–5 (A) A teardrop avulsion fracture is a relatively benign injury represented by the small "chip" of bone off the anteroinferior aspect of the vertebral body. **(B)** This is in contrast to the much more ominous teardrop fracture **(C)** with a larger "chunk" from the anteroinferior body, retropulsion of the cephalad body, and sagittal split on computed tomographic scanning.

If only an isolated root injury exists, nonoperative treatment is possible, with anticipated recovery of the root deficit. If the fracture is minimally or nondisplaced, the root injury occurred at impact, and external immobilization in a rigid collar or more substantial brace such as a sternal-occipital-mandibular immobilizer (SOMI) or Minerva should be utilized, followed by close radiographic observation for displacement. If enough fracture displacement exists to compromise the neural foramen, creating residual root compression, then operative treatment should be considered. Such displacement is often a rotational problem that can be reduced with traction but tends to redisplace even with rigid halo immobilization.[44]

In the case of facet dislocations, there is little role for nonoperative management, particularly with bilateral facet dislocations. This is due to the fact that the posterior ligamentous injury does not tend to heal well enough to restore structural stability to the spinal column, and recurrent dislocation despite rigid external immobilization in a halo vest is well documented.[45,46] In one study,[44] only 44% of the facet dislocations (unilateral similar to bilateral) treated with halo vest achieved clinical stability, and many of those that were stable had poor anatomical results. Interestingly, a poor anatomical result did not correlate with a poor clinical outcome.[44] The exception to this generalization may be the case of unilateral facet dislocations. Occasionally, a patient who has a history of an untreated neck injury is found to have an old unilateral facet dislocation **(Fig. 7–6)**. Because the opposite facet capsule is intact, the dislocated facet tends to "lock" into its new position, making it relatively stable. As long as bony integrity remains, the patient may be asymptomatic and have suffered a new injury or request evaluation for chronic neck pain. Spontaneous fusion of the injured facet can occur. In fact, in the past, viable treatment options have included simply allowing the facet dislocation to persist or reducing the dislocation followed by a period of external immobilization, but these approaches tend to have a higher incidence of late pain.

Fractures that result from axial loads such as compression, burst, and teardrop fractures also have potential for nonoperative management **(Fig. 7–7A–C)**. Surgical treatment is more appropriate when a spinal cord injury ex-

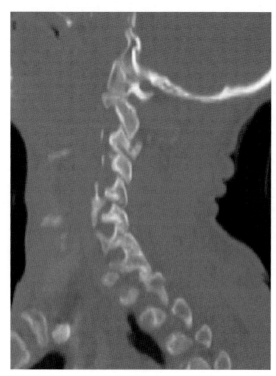

Figure 7–6 A healed unilateral facet dislocation in an asymptomatic patient who presented with an independent second spinal fracture.

ists. When no spinal cord injury exists, the degree of bony and ligamentous injury dictates how aggressive one should be with treatment. Defining stability can be difficult under these circumstances. White and Panjabi attempted to define cervical spine stability with a numerical grading system that attached points to various factors associated with the injury.[47] If a definite posterior ligamentous injury exists along with the anterior bony injury, then operative treatment is appropriate. Sometimes, such an injury is apparent from plain radiographs or CT scan, but an MRI may be helpful if some question remains. Nonoperative treatment should only be undertaken if the amount of deformity on the initial films is acceptable because external immobilization is unlikely to maintain any correction in alignment achieved with longitudinal traction. Because these injuries tend to result in kyphosis, any external support should apply a good extension moment and be fairly rigid. Cadaver studies have shown canal compromise to increase with compression and extension positioning, putting the neural elements at greater risk.[48] Thus the use of a SOMI, Minerva, or halo is the best option. In a direct comparison of halo vest management versus anterior corpectomy with stabilization, Fisher et al[49] noted greater residual kyphosis in the halo vest group (11.4 vs 3.5 degrees) but were unable to correlate the greater residual deformity with poorer outcomes. However, four of 24 patients required conversion to surgical treatment due to either loss of alignment or neurological deterioration.

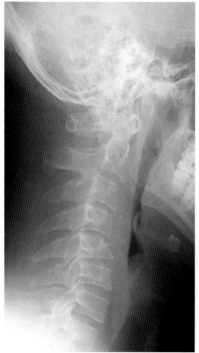
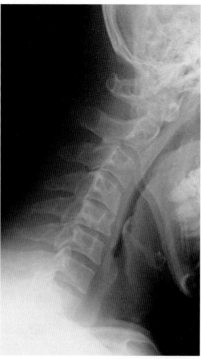
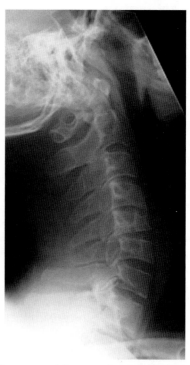

A–C

Figure 7–7 **(A)** A patient who presented 4 days postinjury with neck pain and a lateral x-ray demonstrated a teardrop axial compression-flexion fracture. Because he had already been fully mobile for 4 days without displacement or neurological sequelae, he was treated successfully with Minerva brace immobilization, shown by stability on flexion extension radiographs at 6 months. **(B)** Flexion radiograph at 6 months post injury. **(C)** Extension radiograph at 6 months post injury.

Indications for Surgical Treatment

General Indications

The goals of surgical treatment are essentially the same as nonoperative treatment: to achieve stability, restore and maintain spinal alignment, decompress and protect neurological elements, and minimize late pain. Surgical management should be considered when it is unlikely that these goals can be achieved by nonoperative means. Although indications for surgical treatment focus on the fracture pattern and neurological status of the patient, one must also take into account factors such as age, preexisting medical problems, body habitus, additional injuries, patient compliance, and patient expectations or desires.

Neurological Deficit

Neurological deficit is the most common indication for surgery. When considering neurological injury, one should assess whether it is a spinal cord deficit or nerve root deficit. Spinal cord injuries are further divided into incomplete or complete lesions. When the neurological deficit is isolated to a nerve root, then the surgical indication is less strong. Because the root is a lower motor nerve, the potential for recovery is greater, even with nonoperative treatment. When root deficits are present in a spine fracture that is nondisplaced or minimally displaced, nonoperative management should be considered. An exception to this occurs when the associated bony injury is unstable, and repetitive damage could result from continued motion at the fracture site. When the neurological injury involves the spinal cord, it is generally presumed that the associated bony injury is unstable. Although a significant component of the neurological injury occurred at the time of impact, there is often residual cord compression, and the risk of repetitive trauma from the bony instability is high. Thus surgical intervention is indicated to relieve the residual pressure on the cord and prevent further damage. These principles hold true across the array of lower cervical injury patterns, but the means of achieving the desired effect varies with the injury pattern. For example, neurological decompression in a facet dislocation can be achieved nonoperatively with traction to realign the bony elements, at which point surgical stabilization is performed to prevent redislocation and further neurological injury. This is different from a burst fracture with retropulsion of bone onto the spinal cord. Under these circumstances traction has a limited ability to decompress the cord, and complete decompression can only be achieved surgically by direct removal of bone from the canal.

Stability

Another reason for surgery is to achieve stability in a position of anatomical alignment. Defining the degree of instability that warrants surgical stabilization is controversial. An important distinction is made between bony and ligamentous injury because stability can eventually be achieved with healing in a bony injury, whereas instability often persists in a predominantly ligamentous injury.

Facet Joint Dislocation

It is accepted that surgical stabilization is warranted in bilateral facet dislocation due to the degree of ligamentous injury.[50] With unilateral facet dislocation there is more controversy regarding treatment. Once reduced, a unilateral facet dislocation is more stable than a reduced bilateral dislocation. One factor determining stability after reduction is an associated fracture of either the superior or the inferior facet. If a facet fracture exists, then redislocation will occur more easily. If reduction by traction occurs easily with low weights, then redislocation will also occur more easily. Rather than dislocating at the extreme of flexion, the dislocation can occur earlier with less flexion by anterior translation of the inferior facet on the superior facet. Without a fracture the reduced facet is often reasonably stable; in fact, spontaneous fusion will occur in ~50%.[51] This can also be true of the unreduced unilateral facet dislocation. Once a unilateral dislocated facet undergoes closed reduction, it can actually be more unstable than prior to reduction,[52] perhaps further justifying surgical management. Beyer et al compared patients treated with nonoperative halo vest immobilization with patients treated with posterior fusion.[51,53] They found that anatomical reduction was achieved and maintained in only 25% of halo patients as compared with 60% of surgical patients; as a result, late pain was more frequent in the nonoperative group. Surgical fusion in these patients is indicated as a means of minimizing late pain.[53–55] The author's preferred treatment for unilateral facet dislocations is surgical stabilization, assuming no extraneous circumstances.

Burst and Teardrop Fractures

Because burst fractures and teardrop fractures are the result of compression, the ligaments can be preserved, resulting in a predominantly bony injury. When a component of flexion is added to the mechanism of injury, there will be a greater degree of ligamentous disruption that increases the likelihood of late instability.[56] When the patient is neurologically intact, the amount of deformity and the degree of ligamentous injury are the primary determinants of treatment. Unfortunately, many patients suffer neurological injury with the fracture, which is an indication for surgery because it allows the canal to be decompressed. The presence of neurological injury indicates that more energy was imparted on the spine, increasing the likelihood of instability.[57] In a review of surgical versus conservative treatment of burst and teardrop fractures, a statistically significant neurological recovery (as measured by Frankel grade), canal restoration, and overall sagittal alignment was noted in the surgical group.[58,59] Even if the neurological injury is deemed complete, aggressive decompression is warranted to improve the possibility of regaining root function caudal to the level of injury.[60,61]

Lateral Mass Fractures

Lateral mass fractures seldom present with spinal cord injury; the majority of neurological deficits associated with this fracture pattern are single-root injuries. Thus the neurological deficit itself is usually not the indication for surgery. These injuries are often difficult to detect on plain radiographs and are typically identified on CT scans. However, the degree of instability is based on the degree of associated ligamentous and disk disruption, which is best seen on MRI scans. Instability in these injuries is generally rotational, which is difficult to control nonoperatively, even in a halo vest.[62] If greater than 15% subluxation or greater than 10 degrees of angulation exists on the plain radiographs or CT, enough instability can be implied to warrant surgical stabilization.[44] Such small amounts of displacement may not be noted on the original films, so Halliday et al postulated that the degree of instability could be predicted by the amount of ligamentous involvement noted on an MRI.[63] They concluded that if at least three of the following ligaments were involved—the facet capsule, the interspinous ligament, the anterior longitudinal ligament (ALL), and the posterior longitudinal ligament (PLL)—then operative stabilization should be considered.

Surgical Treatment

General Considerations

Surgery of the cervical spine for fracture can only accomplish three goals: alter/restore alignment, achieve stability via fusion, and decompress the neurological elements. When undertaking surgical treatment, the most appropriate procedure depends on the fracture pattern, spinal alignment and stability, and the need for neurological decompression. These goals can be accomplished through anterior, posterior, or combined approaches. The most important factor determining treatment is the neurological status of the patient, and this should be considered first.

If neurological impairment exists, relieving pressure on the spinal cord is the first factor to consider for surgical planning. The urgency of decompression is a matter of debate. Indirect decompression of the spinal cord may be accomplished with traction. For example, reduction of a facet dislocation realigns the bony rings of the spinal canal. In other cases, such as a burst fracture, decompression may require direct surgical removal of retropulsed bone fragments from the spinal canal. Ideally, the surgical approach used for spinal decompression can also be used to stabilize the spine. If this is not possible, two approaches may be necessary. These issues are discussed in the sections that follow with regard to particular fracture patterns.

Facet Joint Fracture-Dislocations

Facet joint fracture-dislocation is the result of a flexion-distraction mechanism causing disruption of the posterior ligamentous tension band. An additional rotational component must be present when the dislocation is unilateral. Thus a posterior approach is most appropriate to restore the posterior tension band (see **Video 7–1, Disk 1**). As a general rule, reduction of the dislocation is accomplished with cervical traction prior to proceeding to the operating room. Usually the reduction is performed in the emergency department immediately after the injury is clarified radiographically using plain radiographs and CT scanning. This can be accomplished safely in the awake patient who is capable of cooperating with serial neurological exams during the course of the reduction process.[64] This step has the most urgency if the patient is neurologically impaired, particularly in those patients with incomplete neural deficits.[65,66] Some surgeons suggest obtaining an MRI prior to closed reduction with plans for an open anterior cervical diskectomy if a herniation is identified.[67] However, current literature does not appear to indicate that the finding of a herniated disk is clinically significant prior to awake, closed reduction.[68,69] For reduction of facet dislocations, Gardner-Wells tongs are positioned with the points in line with the external auditory meatus. They can be positioned slightly anterior or slightly posterior depending on whether extension or flexion, respectively, is desired. Patient positioning can also be used to maintain a flexion or extension moment during traction.[70] Care is taken to ensure that the points of the tongs are below the maximum circumference of the skull to avoid cephalad migration of the tongs, resulting in loss of fixation. In addition, one should ensure that no skull fracture exists that would compromise pin position in those patients with concomitant closed head injuries.

Initially, 10 to 15 lb of weight is applied to accommodate the weight of the head. After traction is applied, a cross-table lateral x-ray should be obtained to ensure that excessive distraction does not occur at the facet dislocation or that an occult concomitant injury such as occipital cervical dissociation is present. Weight is then added in 5 to 10 lb increments, followed by serial neurological exams and repeated cross-table lateral x-rays. Mild sedation is useful to relax the patient, and adequate time should be allowed between radiographs to allow the patient to relax the neck muscles. It is critical that the patient remains alert and cooperative throughout the procedure to facilitate an effective neurological exam. One continues to add weight until either reduction is achieved, two thirds body weight has been applied,[71] overdistraction of the injured or adjacent segments occurs, or the patient develops neurological complaints or excessive pain. Clinical and cadaveric studies both support traction weights up to 140 lb.[72,73] If heavy weight is to be utilized, then standard steel Gardner-Wells tongs should be used because carbon fiber MRI-compatible tongs typically are limited to 60 lb. Applying traction with some flexion aids in unlocking bilateral facet dislocations; once reduction is achieved, then the neck can be extended to maintain anatomical alignment.

Most bilateral facet dislocations can be reduced prior to surgery with this technique. Unilateral facet dislocations may be more difficult to reduce because of their tendency to "lock," as noted earlier. Sometimes, gentle manipulation into flexion with rotation away from the dislocated side can aid in final reduction once traction has been applied to distract the facet into a perched position.[70] When a neurological deficit develops during the course of reduction with traction, it should not be assumed that the etiology is a herniated nucleus pulposus. In this situation, an MRI is warranted to accurately diagnosis the cause and plan the surgical approach before proceeding to the operating room. Ludwig et al describe a case of epidural hematoma that developed during reduction resulting in a progressive neurological deficit.[74] However, in this case the neural compression was found to be posterior to the cord, warranting a posterior laminectomy rather than an anterior diskectomy.

In the unusual circumstance that closed reduction fails, one must proceed to an open reduction.[75] Prior to performing open reduction, an MRI is warranted to rule out an associated herniated nucleus pulposus, which can cause an increase in neurological deficit during open reduction.[76] In a study of 55 patients with cervical trauma evaluated with an MRI, a 42% incidence of acute disk herniation was identified.[77] In patients with an anterior cord syndrome, the incidence was 100%. If a significant disk herniation exists, then an anterior procedure to evacuate the disk material prior to open reduction is indicated. There are a variety of techniques to gain reduction of the facets after the diskectomy.[78] During anterior surgery, direct visualization of the anterior alignment of the vertebral bodies is possible. However, a lateral radiograph should still be used intraoperatively to verify that the reduction is adequate. Radiographic visualization to confirm reduction can prove to be difficult at the more caudal levels, such as C6–C7 **(Fig. 7–8)**. Stabilization with an anterior intervertebral bony strut and plate seems to be clinically adequate although not as biomechanically sound as a posterior stabilization.[79–81] If an anterior approach alone is to be utilized, then care must be taken to verify that the bone graft does not overdistract the facet joints. One must be especially careful in cases with a substantial facet fracture, which makes the fracture pattern more unstable with translation alone, rather than flexion and distraction **(Fig. 7–9A,B)**. Under these circumstances, consideration should be given to performing a posterior stabilization as well. In the absence of a documented disk herniation, a posterior stabilization can be performed. If the reduction remains difficult, some gentle intralaminar distraction can be used to unlock the facet prior to translating it posteriorly.[82] Alternatively, a partial facetectomy can be performed to allow more direct translation, decreasing the need for excessive distraction. The downside to the latter technique is that there is less remaining facet bone available to abut the opposite facet, which decreases the

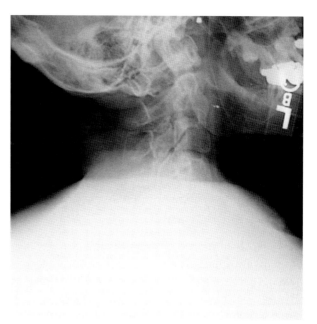

Figure 7–8 A lateral image in an obese patient with poor visualization of the subaxial spine. This would make intraoperative radiographic verification of facet reduction via an anterior approach extremely difficult.

postreduction stability. Partial facet resection is typically reserved for patients presenting in a delayed manner, which is usually associated with a more difficult reduction.[83–85]

Successful closed reduction decompresses the spinal canal, and spinal stabilization can proceed at a more convenient time. An MRI should be performed at this juncture to assess for disk herniation that may continue to compromise the canal or could be retropulsed when the facets are compressed during restoration of the posterior tension band. If a significant disk herniation exists, one should proceed with an anterior approach, as already discussed. If no disk herniation is identified, posterior stabilization is preferred and performed with the patient in the prone position. Turning the patient prone is one of the most dangerous parts of the procedure. Some form of neurological monitoring should be considered; options include awake intubation and positioning of the awake patient to allow a neurological exam after positioning, or evoked potential monitoring prior to and after positioning. In addition, a lateral fluoroscopic image should be obtained immediately upon turning to the prone position to verify the alignment of the neck.

The posterior surgical approach is a standard midline exposure, taking care not to disrupt adjacent soft tissue stabilizers. Many techniques of interspinous wiring with or without bone grafting have been described.[86–91] Hadra is given credit for the first interspinous wiring as a means of internal fixation in 1891,[86] and Rogers' technique of interspinous process wiring was popularized in 1942.[87] Davey et al[88] and Segal et al[89] described the Dewar technique in which K-wires are passed percutaneously through adjacent spinous processes and a structural iliac graft followed by a figure-of-eight wire wrapped around the construct to hold everything in place. Others have offered modifications of

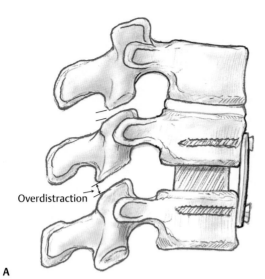

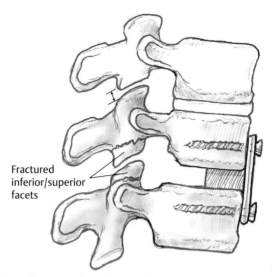

A

B

Figure 7–9 (A) Overdistraction of the facets by the intervertebral graft can unlock the facets, decreasing mechanical stability of stand-alone anterior plate fixation. **(B)** The same effect can occur if there is a significant fracture of the facets allowing posterior to anterior translation to occur without the need for flexion to unlock the facets.

the Dewar technique.[90] The Bohlman triple-wire technique minimizes wire cut out by looping over the spinous process in addition to passing through it, and included a wire to directly secure a structural graft to the spinous process.[91] Although somewhat historic, these techniques remain viable options for stabilization as isolated techniques or in conjunction with more modern means of instrumentation. Feldborg et al described posterior wiring without the use of bone grafting or other fusion techniques in 34 fracture patients.[92] With a mean follow-up of 38 months (12 to 78 months), mean loss of lordosis was 7.5 degrees, eight of 34 had wire breakage, 10 had pin migrations, but 26 had some evidence of either anterior or posterior fusion. Twenty-four of the 34 complained of late pain, most of which was considered minor. These poor results confirm the need for concomitant fusion at the time of instrumentation. Biomechanical studies demonstrate that polymethyl methacrylate in conjunction with inter-spinous wiring improves the initial angular stiffness over wiring with bone graft,[93] but concerns about long-term stability exist, and the failure rate when used clinically in the traumatic patient is excessive.[94]

Because wiring constructs are located posterior and directly in the midline, they are at a biomechanical disadvantage in controlling rotational forces such as those that exist in unilateral facet dislocation. To counter this, an oblique facet wiring can be included that involves passing a wire through the cephalad-dislocated facet, then through the caudal spinous process. Oblique wiring is also useful whenever the posterior neural arch is disrupted, precluding use of one spinous process for wiring.[95] Hook plates have been specifically developed for use in posterior cervical stabilization and allow compression across an inter-spinous process graft while locking the facets in place **(Fig. 7–10A,B).**[96] This device offers increased biomechanical resistance to flexion strain over posterior wiring tech-

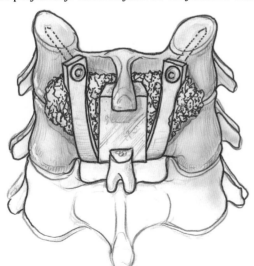

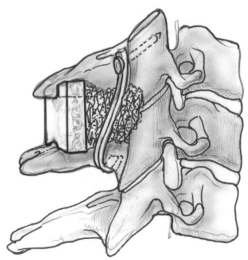

A

B

Figure 7–10 The hook plate construct. **(A)** Posterior view. **(B)** Lateral view. (From Jeanneret B, Magerl F, Ward EH, Ward JC. Posterior stabilization of the cervical spine with hook plates. Spine 1991;16(Suppl 3):S56–S63, with permission.)

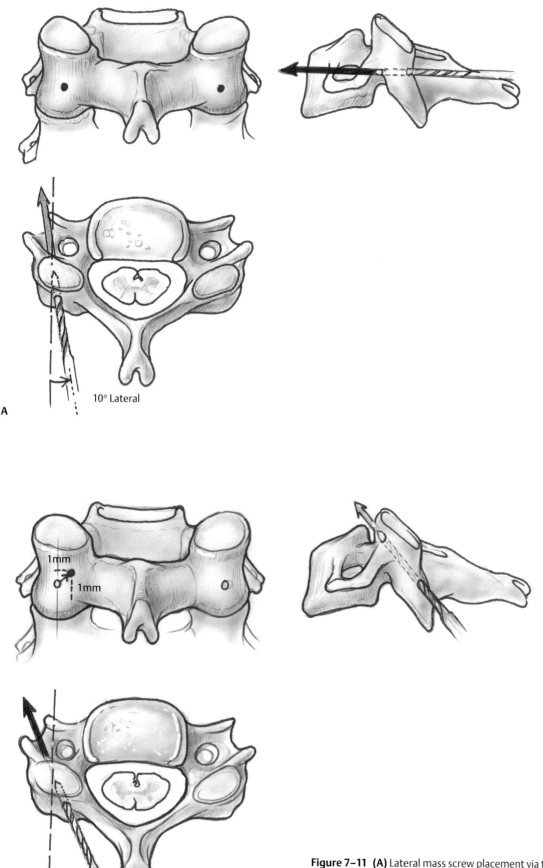

Figure 7–11 (A) Lateral mass screw placement via the Roy-Camille and **(B)** Magerl techniques. (From Choueka J, Spivak JM, Kummer FJ, Steger T. Flexion failure of posterior cervical lateral mass screws: influence of insertion technique and position. Spine 1996;21:462– 468, with permission.)

A

B

niques.[81] There is no role for laminectomy in the management of facet dislocation unless there is direct pressure on the posterior cord from a lamina fracture.[97] This is because laminectomy tends to further decrease spinal stability and the surface area available for fusion.

Roy-Camille et al first described plates and screws applied posterior to the lateral masses to improve posterior surgical fixation.[98] Plate fixation offers better rotational stability because the plates are applied away from the midline, making plates applicable for unilateral facet dislocations as well as bilateral dislocations. Grob and Magerl[99] noted that a biomechanically superior[100] method of lateral mass screw fixation is achieved by directing the screw 30 degrees cranially and 10 degrees laterally, rather than aiming straight forward (**Fig. 7–11A,B**). Numerous variations on the techniques that utilize lateral mass fixation have been reported,

and it has become a preferred method of posterior stabilization.[101,102] At C7 the lateral mass can be inadequate for screw fixation, but the screw can be directed into the pedicle under those circumstances (**Fig. 7–12A–C**). Transfacet screws have been described as a means of salvaging the stabilization if lateral mass screws strip or under circumstances of atypical anatomy. The biomechanical pullout in a cadaver study is comparable to lateral mass screws, but that model did not simulate the situation where a lateral mass screw has already failed.[103] Recently, the technique of percutaneous lateral mass screw placement has been published,[104] and the future of this type of minimally invasive procedure in the trauma setting is in its infancy.

The author's (JCF) preferred technique of posterior stabilization include an interspinous process cable to lock in the facets followed by lateral mass plating (**Fig. 7–13A,B**).

Figure 7–12 (A) An axial diagram of C7 pedicle screw placement. **(B)** A posterior view demonstrating the difference in starting position for a lateral mass screw at C5 (upper level) as compared to a pedicle screw at C7 (lower level). **(C)** A lateral view showing the cephalad-caudal trajectory.

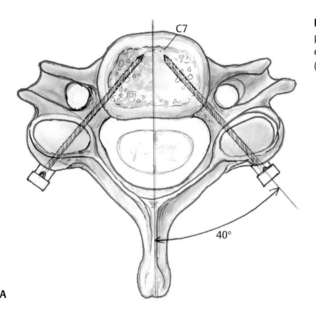

A

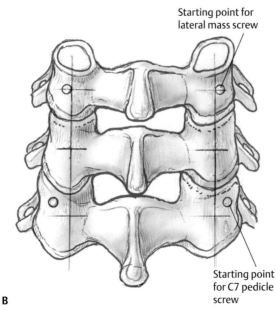

Starting point for lateral mass screw

Starting point for C7 pedicle screw

B

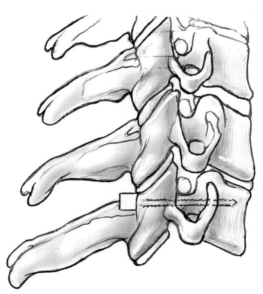

C

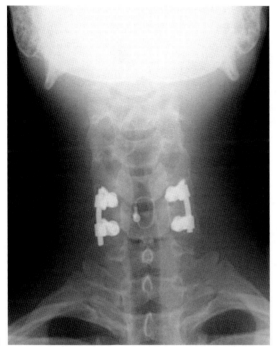
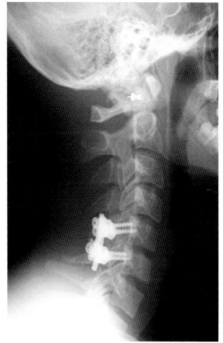

A

B

Figure 7–13 Authors' (JCF) preferred method of stabilization of facet dislocation when the posterior approach is utilized. An interspinous process cable is first used to lock in the facets, followed by lateral mass plating. The hole through the base of the spinous process is cheated toward the upper end of the cephalad spinous process and toward the lower side of the caudal one to minimize the risk of cutout as the cable is tightened. **(A)** Anteroposterior postoperative fixation view. **(B)** Lateral postoperative view.

The posterior dissection is performed in standard subperiosteal fashion, but great care should be exerted to maintain all soft tissue attachments at the adjacent uninjured segments. The lateral border of the dissection should be the lateral edge of the lateral mass but not beyond nor anterior to that edge to avoid venous bleeding. The first step toward stabilization is a simple spinous process wiring. A drill hole is placed at the base of the spinous processes on either side of the injury, cheating to the superior end of the cephalad spinous process and the lower end of the caudal spinous process to avoid cable cutout. After the cable is locked, attention is directed to placement of the lateral mass screws. The borders of the lateral mass are defined, the centerpoint identified, then an awl is used to perforate the anticipated starting point 1 mm medial to the centerpoint. This perforation minimizes the risk of the drill walking laterally during drilling. The author prefers to use a K-wire to drill, which packs the bone about the drill hole to aid in screw purchase. Prior to placing the connecting rods to the lateral mass, the facets are decorticated, and iliac bone graft is packed directly into the facet. After the rods are connected, the remainder of the bone graft is packed over the exposed lamina and spinous processes. Postoperative immobilization is a rigid collar for 6 to 12 weeks, depending on intraoperative assessment of the stability obtained.

There has been increasing interest in the anterior approach for the stabilization of facet dislocations.[105,106] Aebi et al reported on 64 patients treated by anterior plating, with only one loss of fixation.[107] Razack et al also report favorable stabilization outcomes utilizing unicortical anterior plates.[108] The anterior approach can easily be used in all facet dislocations following closed reduction. If a closed reduction cannot be obtained, then use of the anterior approach presents some challenges. First, if one intends to use an anterior approach for an irreducible dislocation, then the reduction will need to be obtained intraoperatively. Several techniques have been described to accomplish this task **(Fig. 7–14A–C)**.[78,109] Second, it is necessary to verify that a reduction has been obtained and that no overdistraction exists, prior to proceeding with internal fixation. Intraoperative imaging of the cervical spine can be a daunting task in the obese, in patients with heavy shoulder musculature, and in patients with a short neck, particularly if the dislocation is at a lower level, such as C6–C7. At times, the patient may have to be turned prone for an additional posterior reduction prior to returning to the anterior approach for internal fixation; this has been called "the 720 degree approach." Finally, if a larger facet fracture exists, then the stability of the spine is further dimin-

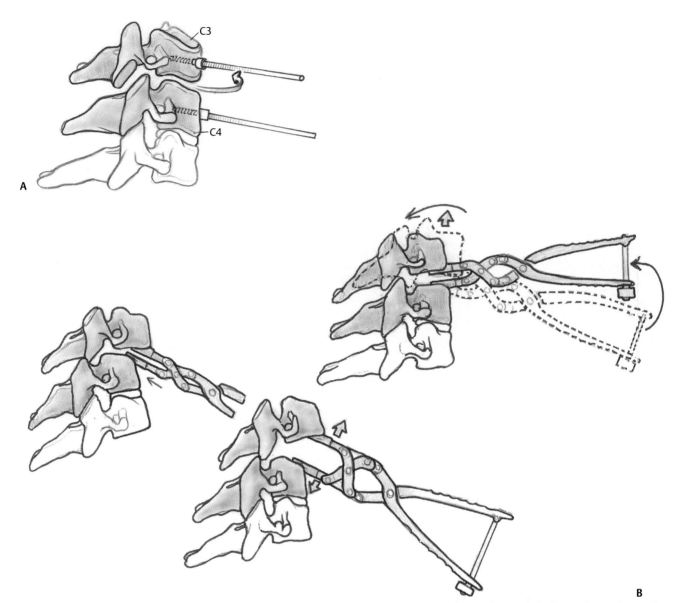

Figure 7–14 (A–C) A variety of techniques can be employed to achieve reduction of the facets from the anterior approach. **(A)** The retractor pins from the Caspar set can be placed at the trajectory shown to allow rotation and flexion-distraction of the facet to facili- tate reduction. **(B)** Alternately, a vertebral spreader can be used to distract and translate the upper body posteriorly as a means of re- duction. (*Continued on page 153.*)

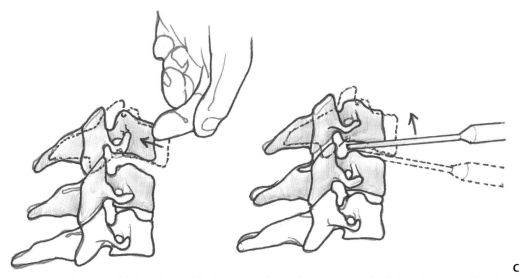

C

Figure 7–14 *(Continued)* **(C)** Lastly, a Cobb elevator can be used posteriorly in the disk to distract and flex the neck so that the upper vertebrae can be pushed posteriorly. (From Ordonez BJ, Benzel EC, Naderi S, Weller SJ. Cervical facet dislocation: techniques for ventral reduction and stabilization. J Neurosurg 2000;92(Suppl 1):18–23, with permission.)

ished,[110] and greater surgical stability must be achieved. Under these circumstances, an additional posterior procedure should be considered. One should be familiar with and adept at all of these techniques to effectively manage the array of injury combinations.

Pearls

- The posterior approach is the most biomechanically sound method of stabilization and is preferred in those patients without disk herniation.
- The anterior approach can be clinically adequate for stabilization if a disk herniation exists, dictating that approach to achieve decompression.
- If the anterior approach is used, care must be taken to ensure that reduction is verified, the facets are not overdistracted, and any associated fractures of the facets are minimal so that the facets can be locked in place to achieve translational stability.

Compression, Burst, and Teardrop Fractures

Fractures that involve a component of axial loading causing loss of anterior column height that are deemed appropriate for surgical management are best treated via an anterior approach to directly address the pathology.[105] A classic example of such an injury is a burst fracture. Historically, a posterior fusion alone was performed if the fracture was considered unstable. However, Favero and Van Peteghem[111] looked at their series of patients treated

with posterior wiring and found the rate of loss of fixation, kyphosis, and pain to be unacceptable. Their treatment protocol was changed to utilize anterior procedures, and a second group of patients was studied, demonstrating a significant improvement in those same factors. Interestingly, the degree of residual kyphosis did correlate with pain in their study. Advantages of the anterior approach are that the anterior column can be directly supported biomechanically, and any retropulsed bone can be visualized and reliably removed from the canal.[107,112] The anterior approach for corpectomy is suitable for most compression, burst, and teardrop fracture patterns. The corpectomy is completed at least the width of the cord and from the inferior end plate of the vertebrae above to the superior end plate of the vertebrae below. This decompression defect is reconstructed with allograft or autologous structural bone, then plated. An additional posterior stabilization is indicated in those patients that also have either significant posterior fracture or ligamentous injury (**Fig. 7–15A–D**).[113] The teardrop fracture is often associated with posterior injury because the mechanism includes flexion combined with

Pearls

- The primary procedure should be anterior to reconstruct the anterior column support and accomplish any necessary decompression.
- The addition of a posterior procedure should be based on the degree of posterior injury to the facets and ligamentous structures.

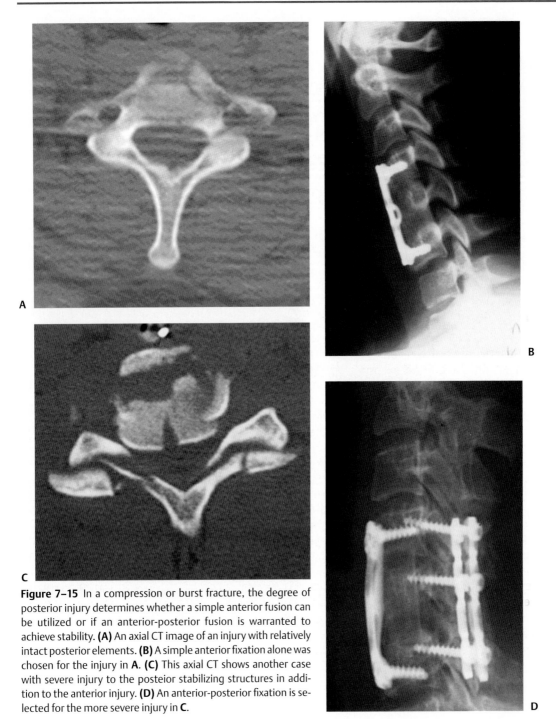

Figure 7–15 In a compression or burst fracture, the degree of posterior injury determines whether a simple anterior fusion can be utilized or if an anterior-posterior fusion is warranted to achieve stability. **(A)** An axial CT image of an injury with relatively intact posterior elements. **(B)** A simple anterior fixation alone was chosen for the injury in **A**. **(C)** This axial CT shows another case with severe injury to the posteior stabilizing structures in addition to the anterior injury. **(D)** An anterior-posterior fixation is selected for the more severe injury in **C**.

an axial load. Lateral mass fixation is preferred when additional posterior instrumentation is warranted.

Lateral Mass Fractures

Lateral mass fractures are thought to occur as a result of an extension-compression mechanism. Because the lateral mass contains both the superior and inferior facets of the fractured vertebrae, they typically affect two adjacent motion segments. In some fractures there is a rotational component to the injury, which generally occurs through only one disk level and can make the fracture more unstable, perhaps warranting surgical stabilization. The affected disk level can sometimes be determined on plain radiographs but is more clearly delineated with an MRI scan. Because the injury primarily involves the posterior ele-

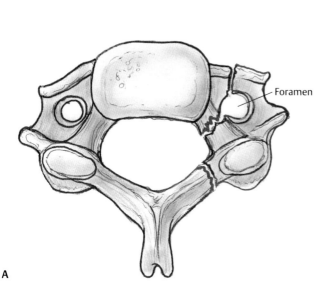

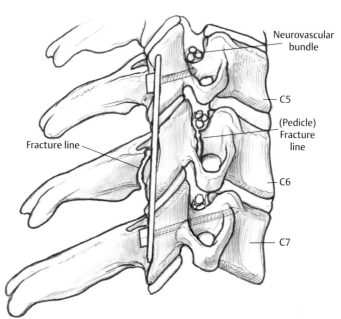

A

B

Figure 7–16 **(A)** If posterior stabilization is chosen for a lateral mass fracture, the construct must span two segments to effectively immobilize the fracture. **(B)** This is because when the lateral mass is frac-tured free from the remainder of the vertebral body, the inferior and superior facets are rendered unstable.

ments, the preferred method of surgical stabilization has traditionally been posterior. The posterior fixation should span two motion segments to adequately control the instability due to the fact that the fractured lateral mass is no longer attached to the remainder of the vertebral body.[114] From a biomechanical standpoint, straight midline fixation, such as spinous process wiring, is inadequate for controlling rotation (similar to unilateral facet dislocations). Thus a C5 lateral mass fracture would undergo a posterior C4–C6 fusion, spanning the fractured segment. Lateral mass screws could be placed at all three levels opposite the fractured side, and at C4 and C6 on the side of the fracture.

In an attempt to avoid a two-level fusion, an anterior diskectomy and fusion at the level of the rotational injury has been postulated as a better way to stabilize this

fracture pattern **(Fig. 7–16A,B).**[115] The level above or below the anterior fusion is still affected by the fracture and must be protected in a rigid collar immobilization. Lifeso and Colucci[115] compared cohorts of posterior and anteriorly stabilized lateral mass fractures and found that anteriorly stabilized patients had less collapse and a lower incidence of late kyphosis. The anterior approach is the author's preferred method of stabilization to limit the fusion to a single motion segment. The disk level to be fused is based on the level of subluxation or injury identified on MRI. It is understood that the adjacent level has sustained an injury, but this can usually be treated nonoperatively with a postoperative collar. Another possible but rarely employed technique is direct screw fixation of the lateral mass via the pedicle, which offers the advantage of direct osteosynthesis of the fracture while avoiding fusion across motion segments. The technique was described by Magerl, but there is little clinical data on the results of this procedure[116] **(Fig. 7–17A–C)**, and it is technically demanding.

Outcomes

In patients with subaxial (C3–C7) trauma, the neurological status is the primary determinant of the patient's function. Residual pain also affects outcome. Unfortunately, pain is a very subjective outcome measure with many influences, including spinal alignment, overall mobility, residual root compression, nonunion, and a host of psychosocial issues.

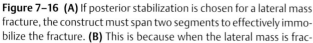

Pearls

- The posterior elements are affected across two motion segments, but anterior disruption is generally localized to one motion segment.
- Anterior fixation can usually fuse only one level, whereas posterior fixation must include two levels.
- MRI can be useful in delineating the anterior level or levels of injury.

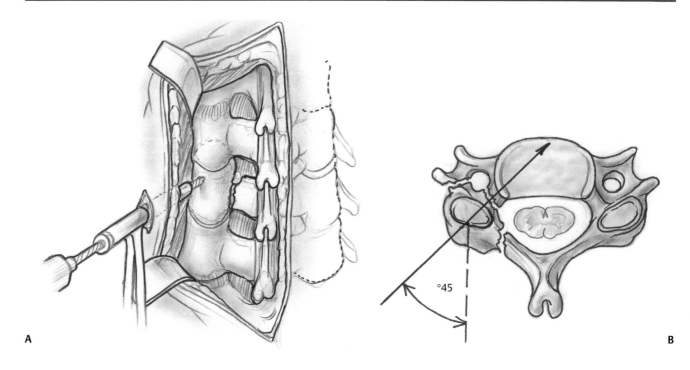

A

B

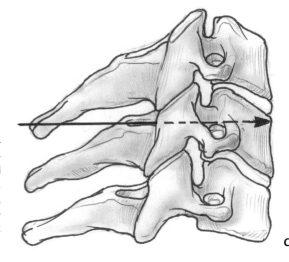

C

Figure 7–17 Direct osteosynthesis of the fractured pedicle in a lateral mass fracture. **(A)** A diagrammatic illustration of screw placement for direct osteosynthesis of the pedicle. One can see that the drill trajectory requires a separate stab incision outside the surgical incision. **(B)** The proper trajectory in the axial plane. **(C)** The proper trajectory in the sagittal plane. (From Jeanneret B, Gebhard JS, Magerl F. Transpedicular screw fixation of articular mass fracture-separation: results of an anatomical study and operative technique. J Spinal Disord 1994; 7:222–229, with permission.)

Factors That Influence Outcome

Spinal Canal Dimension

Although the preinjury spinal canal dimensions influence the severity of spinal cord injury that results from a cervical fracture or dislocation,[117,118] it does not appear to impact the potential for recovery in general.[119] However, the amount of canal compromise noted on the posttraumatic CT scan can offer some predictability about the resultant neurological deficit and the potential for recovery in patients with burst fractures.[120]

Interval to Decompression

The interval between injury and spinal cord decompression may affect the likelihood of neurological recovery and therefore outcome. Hadley et al reviewed 68 patients with spinal cord injury from cervical facet fracture-dislocations treated with either closed or open reduction.[66] In those patients with significant neurological recovery, the timing of decompression was a greater influence than the means of treatment. More recently, Papadopoulos et al developed an early decompression protocol at their institution based on persistent, MRI-documented canal compromise.[121]

They prospectively studied 91 consecutive patients, 66 treated according to protocol and 25 cases that deviated from the protocol because the decompression of their spinal cord was delayed for various reasons. Fifty percent of the patients in the protocol made significant improvement in Frankel grade as compared with only 24% in the delayed treatment group. Animal models have similarly demonstrated the benefit of early decompression on neurological recovery,[122–125] but the times to decompression shown to be beneficial in those studies are very short and may not be feasible in a clinical setting. From accident videos we know that the degree of deformity that results at the time of impact is substantially greater than the residual deformity seen in the emergency department. Thus much of the injury to the spinal cord is the result of that initial impact and cannot be altered surgically. However, any remaining compression on the spinal cord can potentially continue to cause primary injury to the cord as the patient is moved about and may contribute to the secondary cord injury as a result of ongoing ischemia or other mediators. Early decompression may help minimize secondary damage, similar to giving methylprednisolone.

Jarmundowicz et al used a rabbit model to demonstrate the improvement in spinal cord microcirculation that results from decompression, further supporting this theory.[126] Intuitively, early decompression makes sense to most spine surgeons but must be weighed against the difficulty of performing very technical operative procedures, at odd hours, with unfamiliar teams. This issue has received a great deal of attention recently,[127] and Fehlings et al[128] and others[129] have attempted to set forth some guidelines based on the current literature. Fehlings et al, in a very thorough review of the literature, point out that, although level II and III evidence exists to support early decompression, there are no level I data. Fehlings et al conclude by emphasizing the need for well-controlled, prospective studies to better define the role of timing of decompression on neurological outcomes.

Cost Effectiveness

If the economic impact of treatment of cervical fractures is analyzed, it is clear that the potential for rehabilitation is enhanced by surgical stabilization, and the length of stay in rehabilitation facilities is diminished.[130] Cotler et al looked at the financial impact of surgical stabilization versus nonoperative treatment on acute hospital costs and found an average savings of $18,407.00 in the operative group.[131]

Pain

The role of pain as it influences outcome is a topic in itself and is clearly influenced by psychosocial factors such as litigation, workmen's compensation, depression, and narcotic dependence. These are complicated issues worthy of mention but cannot be fully explored in the scope of this chapter. Restoration of anatomical alignment is one of the goals of any treatment, whether it is nonoperative or operative, and was commonly examined in the papers referenced throughout this chapter. In those papers comparing nonoperative to operative treatment (using modern stabilization techniques) of similar fracture patterns, the consensus is clearly in favor of surgical stabilization as a way to restore and maintain spinal alignment. However, the correlation between the final alignment and pain is less consistent.[44,49,51,53] Perhaps this would change with long-term follow-up as the adjacent motion segments develop degenerative changes because of residual imbalance. In the case of unilateral facet dislocations that were allowed to remain in the displaced position, there appears to be a higher incidence of late pain.[132]

Choice of Surgical Technique

As noted in the section on surgical stabilization, there are a variety of studies looking at the different fusion techniques but very few directly comparing the efficacy of one technique versus another. Shapiro et al compared two types of posterior stabilization and fusion for unilateral locked facets.[133] They looked at interspinous braided cable with lateral mass plate fixation (the author's preferred technique) compared with interspinous wiring with facet wiring using iliac struts. They concluded that the group that underwent lateral mass plating had significantly less kyphosis and tended to have better clinical outcomes. This result is likely a reflection on the greater rigidity of lateral mass plating as compared with wiring, which may be even more pronounced with current locked plating constructs.

Complications

Many of the potential complications of treatment of subaxial cervical injuries have been addressed in the preceding text. Complications specific to the techniques of internal fixation should be considered, particularly with respect to posterior cervical plating, which has become commonplace. Heller et al[134] reviewed 654 lateral mass screws inserted in 78 patients for a variety of indications. Complications per screw inserted included nerve root injury in 0.6%, facet violations in 0.2%, no vertebral artery injuries, broken screw in 0.3%, and screw loosening in 1.1%. To minimize the risk of nerve root injury, one must understand the anatomy of the lateral mass and the relationship to the surrounding structures. Xu et al analyzed this in a cadaver study to determine that the midpoint of the lateral mass is a safe place to initiate screw insertion.[135] Fixation failure has been evaluated as it relates to the technique of screw insertion. Choueka et al compared the Roy-Camille technique to the Magerl and found the Magerl technique to be advantageous for placement of the end screws.[136]

It is important to remember that vertebral artery injury can be associated with a variety of cervical fractures and not just those fractures involving the vertebral foramen.[137–139] The incidence has been reported to be as high as 46% in those cervical fractures severe enough to warrant surgical stabilization.[140] Flexion-distraction injuries may be the most common cause of vertebral artery injuries,[141] and the more severe the flexion-distraction type injury, the more likely it is that an occult vertebral artery injury exists.[142] Magnetic resonance angiography (MRA) has proven useful in detecting these injuries,[143] but no consensus exists as to whether or how vertebral artery injuries should be treated in asymptomatic patients. At this time, MRA is reserved for patients with symptoms consistent with an arterial injury or in those patients with recognized injury to one artery and whose opposite artery could be endangered during treatment. Bilateral vertebral artery injury has been described and has devastating consequences, including death.[144] Once detected, treatment involves reduction and stabilization of any malalignment and possible anticoagulation, assuming that no other contraindications to anticoagulation exist as a result of the overall trauma. In addition to vertebral artery injury, carotid artery and esophageal injuries have been described.[145]

New Technology and Future Treatments

As in many other areas of fracture treatment, the current push is to develop less invasive techniques that better preserve uninjured tissue and hopefully enhance return to function. Currently, iliac crest bone graft remains the most common means of creating a fusion but carries with it a measurable morbidity. As bone morphogenetic protein (BMP) technology becomes more readily available, the need for harvesting bone from the iliac crest should be diminished. At the time this chapter was written, recombinant BMP was only available for use in anterior spinal fusion and only specifically approved by the Food and Drug Administration in the United States for use with lumbar anterior interbody fusion cages. In addition, the current costs are prohibitive to its routine use in fusion procedures. As these issues improve, the morbidity associated with iliac crest bone graft can be eliminated, and the door to percutaneous fusion technology can be opened.

Percutaneous instrumentation of the spine is in its infancy, with most of the current data involving thoracoscopically applied scoliosis instrumentation, anterior cage devices, and posterolateral fusion techniques. Very little has been written regarding percutaneous cervical instrumentation. As image-guided technology advances, the risk of such procedures in the cervical spine should decrease, and the accuracy of application should improve. Any such procedures for use with subaxial cervical trauma would still be considered experimental.

On the DVDs

Video 7–1 (Disk 1) Posterior Open Reduction C6–C7 with Posterior Fusion C6 to T1 with Instrumentation This patient sustained a bilateral facet fracture dislocation at C6, C7 with a spinal cord injury. Operative treatment consisted of open reduction of a persistent subluxation, followed by posterior instrumentation and fusion of C6 to T1. Pedicle screw instrumentation was placed in T1.

References

1. Hadley MN. Treatment of subaxial cervical spinal injuries. Neurosurgery 2002;50(3 Suppl):S156–S165
2. Stauffer ES. Neurologic recovery following injuries to the cervical spinal cord and nerve roots. Spine 1984;9:532–534
3. Bohlman HH. Acute fractures and dislocations of the cervical spine. J Bone Joint Surg Am 1979;61:1119–1142
4. Frankel HL, Hancock DO, Hyslop G, et al. The value of postural reduction in the initial management of closed injuries of the spine with paraplegia and tetraplegia, I. Paraplegia 1969;7:179–192
5. Allen BL Jr, Ferguson RL, Lehmann TR, O'Brien RP. A mechanistic classification of closed, indirect fractures and dislocations of the lower cervical spine. Spine 1982;7:1–27
6. Torg JS, Sennett B, Vegso JJ, Pavlov H. Axial loading injuries to the middle cervical spine segment: an analysis and classification of twenty-five cases. Am J Sports Med 1991;19:6–20

7. Torg JS, Pavlov H, O'Neill MJ, Nichols CE Jr, Sennett B. The axial load teardrop fracture: a biomechanical, clinical and roentgenographic analysis. Am J Sports Med 1991;19:355–364
8. Argenson C, de Peretti F, Ghabris A, Eude P, Hovorka I. Traumatic rotatory displacement of the lower cervical spine. Bull Hosp Jt Dis 2000;59:52–60
9. Dall DM. Injuries of the cervical spine, I: Does the type of bony injury affect spinal cord recovery? S Afr Med J 1972;46:1048–1056
10. Babcock JL. Cervical spine injuries: diagnosis and classification. Arch Surg 1976;111:646–651
11. Ireland AJ, Britton I, Forrester AW. Do supine oblique views provide better imaging of the cervicothoracic junction than swimmer's views? J Accid Emerg Med 1998;15:151–154
12. Lingawi SS. The naked facet sign. Radiology 2001;219:366–367

13. Daffner SD, Daffner RH. Computed tomography diagnosis of facet dislocations: the "hamburger bun" and "reverse hamburger bun" signs. J Emerg Med 2002;23:387–394

14. Diliberti T, Lindsey RW. Evaluation of the cervical spine in the emergency setting: who does not need an x-ray? Orthopedics 1992;15:179–183

15. Matz SR, Reeder JD. Spinous process fractures in a jockey: a case report. Am J Orthop 1999;28:365–366

16. Smith GR, Beckly DE, Abel MS. Articular mass fracture: a neglected cause of post-traumatic neck pain? Clin Radiol 1976; 27:335–340

17. Pech P, Kilgore DP, Pojunas KW, Haughton VM. Cervical spinal fractures: CT detection. Radiology 1985;157:117–120

18. Lee C, Woodring JH. Sagittally oriented fractures of the lateral masses of the cervical vertebrae. J Trauma 1991;31:1638–1643

19. Nyunt BA. Unrecognized fracture through the base of superior articular facet of cervical spine presenting with transient tetraparesis. Injury 1995;26:563–564

20. King SW, Hosler BK, King MA, Eiselt EW. Missed cervical spine fracture-dislocations: the importance of clinical and radiographic assessment. J Manipulative Physiol Ther 2002;25:263–269

21. Yetkin Z, Osborn AG, Giles DS, Haughton VM. Uncovertebral and facet joint dislocations in cervical articular pillar fractures: CT evaluation. AJNR Am J Neuroradiol 1985;6:633–637

22. Daffner RH, Brown RR, Goldberg AL. A new classification for cervical vertebral injuries: influence of CT. Skeletal Radiol 2000; 29:125–132

23. Mahale YJ, Silver JR. Progressive paralysis after bilateral facet dislocation of the cervical spine. J Bone Joint Surg Br 1992;74:219–223

24. Clark CR, Igram CM, el-Khoury GY, Ehara S. Radiographic evaluation of cervical spine injuries. Spine 1988;13:742–747

25. Shanmuganathan K, Mirvis SE, Levine AM. Rotational injury of cervical facets: CT analysis of fracture patterns with implications for management and neurologic outcome. AJR Am J Roentgenol 1994;163:1165–1169

26. Keenen TL, Antony J, Benson DR. Noncontiguous spinal fractures. J Trauma 1990;30:489–491

27. Apple DF Jr, McDonald AP, Smith RA. Identification of herniated nucleus pulposis in spinal cord injury. Paraplegia 1987;25: 78–85

28. Harrington JF, Likavec MJ, Smith AS. Disc herniation in cervical fracture subluxation. Neurosurgery 1991;29:374–379

29. Leite CC, Escobar BE, Bazan C III, Jinkins JR. MRI of cervical facet dislocation. Neuroradiology 1997;39:583–588

30. Herkowitz HN, Rothman RH. Subacute instability of the cervical spine. Spine 1984;9:348–357

31. Rifkinson-Mann S, Mormino J, Sachdev VP. Subacute cervical spine instability. Surg Neurol 1986;26:413–416

32. Hart RA. Cervical facet dislocation: when is magnetic resonance imaging indicated? Spine 2002;27:116–117

33. Vaccaro AR, Madigan L, Schweitzer ME, Flanders AE, Hilibrand AS, Albert TJ. Magnetic resonance imaging analysis of soft tissue disruption after flexion-distraction injuries of the subaxial cervical spine. Spine 2001;26:1866–1872

34. Vaccaro AR, Falatyn SP, Flanders AE, Balderston RA, Northrup BE, Cotler JM. Magnetic resonance evaluation of the intervertebral disc, spinal ligaments, and spinal cord before and after closed traction reduction of cervical spine dislocations. Spine 1999; 24:1210–1217

35. Stabler A, Eck J, Penning R, et al. Cervical spine: postmortem assessment of accident injuries–comparison of radiographic, MR imaging, anatomic, and pathologic findings. Radiology 2001; 221:340–346

36. Davis JW, Parks SN, Detlefs CL, Williams GG, Williams JL, Smith RW. Clearing the cervical spine in obtunded patients: the use of dynamic fluoroscopy. J Trauma 1995;39:435–438

37. Matar LD, Helms CA, Richardson WJ. "Spinolaminar breach": an important sign in cervical spinous process fractures. Skeletal Radiol 2000;29:75–80

38. Dellestable F, Gaucher A. Clay-shoveler's fracture. Stress fracture of the lower cervical and upper thoracic spinous processes. Rev Rhum Engl Ed 1998;65:575–582

39. Meyer PG, Hartman JT, Leo JS. Sentinel spinous process fractures. Surg Neurol 1982;18:174–178

40. Rodriguez M, Tyberghien A, Matge G. Asymptomatic vertebral artery injury after acute cervical spine trauma. Acta Neurochir (Wien) 2001;143:939–945

41. Edeiken-Monroe B, Wagner LK, Harris JH Jr. Hyperextension dislocation of the cervical spine. AJR Am J Roentgenol 1986;146: 803–808

42. Kim KS, Chen HH, Russell EJ, Rogers LF. Flexion teardrop fracture of the cervical spine: radiographic characteristics. AJR Am J Roentgenol 1989;152:319–326

43. Lee C, Kim KS, Rogers LF. Sagittal fracture of the cervical vertebral body. AJR Am J Roentgenol 1982;139:55–60

44. Sears W, Fazl M. Prediction of stability of cervical spine fracture managed in the halo vest and indications for surgical intervention. J Neurosurg 1990;72:426–432

45. Whitehill R, Richman JA, Glaser JA. Failure of immobilization of the cervical spine by the halo vest: a report of five cases. J Bone Joint Surg Am 1986;68:326–332

46. Stauffer ES. Subaxial injuries. Clin Orthop Relat Res 1989;239: 30–39

47. White AA 3rd, Southwick WO, Panjabi MM. Clinical instability of the lower cervical spine: a review of past and current concepts. Spine 1976;1:15–27

48. Ching RP, Watson NA, Carter JW, Tencer AF. The effect of post-injury spinal position on canal occlusion in a cervical spine burst fracture model. Spine 1997;22:1710–1715

49. Fisher CG, Dvorak MF, Leith J, Wing PC. Comparison of outcomes for unstable lower cervical flexion teardrop fractures managed with halo thoracic vest versus anterior corpectomy and plating. Spine 2002;27:160–166

50. Wolf A, Levi L, Mirvis S, et al. Operative management of bilateral facet dislocation. J Neurosurg 1991;75:883–890

51. Beyer CA, Cabanela ME, Berquist TH. Unilateral facet dislocations and fracture-dislocations of the cervical spine. J Bone Joint Surg Br 1991;73:977–981

52. Crawford NR, Duggal N, Chamberlain RH, Park SC, Sonntag VK, Dickman CA. Unilateral cervical facet dislocation: injury mechanism and biomechanical consequences. Spine 2002;27:1858–1864

53. Beyer CA, Cabanela ME. Unilateral facet dislocations and fracture-dislocations of the cervical spine: a review. Orthopedics 1992; 15:311–315

54. Andreshak JL, Dekutoski MB. Management of unilateral facet dislocations: a review of the literature. Orthopedics 1997;20: 917–926

55. Shapiro SA. Management of unilateral locked facet of the cervical spine. Neurosurgery 1993;33:832–837

56. Romanelli DA, Dickman CA, Porter RW, Haynes RJ. Comparison of initial injury features in cervical spine trauma of C3–C7:

predictive outcome with halo-vest management. J Spinal Disord 1996;9:146–149

57. Carter JW, Mirza SK, Tencer AF, Ching RP. Canal geometry changes associated with axial compressive cervical spine fracture. Spine 2000;25:46–54

58. Koivikko MP, Myllynen P, Karjalainen M, Vornanen M, Santavirta S. Conservative and operative treatment in cervical burst fractures. Arch Orthop Trauma Surg 2000;120:448–451

59. Bohlman HH, Anderson PA. Anterior decompression and arthrodesis of the cervical spine: long-term motor improvement, I: Improvement in incomplete traumatic quadriparesis. J Bone Joint Surg Am 1992;74:671–682

60. Yablon IG, Palumbo M, Spatz E, Mortara R, Reed J, Ordia J. Nerve root recovery in complete injuries of the cervical spine. Spine 1991;16(Suppl 10):S518–S521

61. Anderson PA, Bohlman HH. Anterior decompression and arthrodesis of the cervical spine: long-term motor improvement, II: Improvement in complete traumatic quadriplegia. J Bone Joint Surg Am 1992;74:683–692

62. Bucholz R, Cheung KC. Halo vest versus spinal fusion for cervical injury: evidence from an outcome study. J Neurosurg 1989;70: 884–892

63. Halliday AL, Henderson BR, Hart BL, Benzel EC. The management of unilateral lateral mass/facet fractures of the subaxial cervical spine: the use of magnetic resonance imaging to predict instability. Spine 1997;22:2614–2621

64. Grant GA, Mirza SK, Chapman JR, et al. Risk of early closed reduction in cervical spine subluxation injuries. J Neurosurg 1999;90 (Suppl 1):13–18

65. Lee AS, MacLean JC, Newton DA. Rapid traction for reduction of cervical spine dislocations. J Bone Joint Surg Br 1994;76:352–356

66. Hadley MN, Fitzpatrick BC, Sonntag VK, Browner CM. Facet fracture-dislocation injuries of the cervical spine. Neurosurgery 1992;30:661–666

67. Doran SE, Papadopoulos SM, Ducker TB, Lillehei KO. Magnetic resonance imaging documentation of coexistent traumatic locked facets of the cervical spine and disc herniation. J Neurosurg 1993;79:341–345

68. Hadley MN. Initial closed reduction of cervical spine fracture-dislocation injuries. Neurosurgery 2002;50(Suppl 3):S44–S50

69. Vaccaro AR, Nachwalter RS. Is magnetic resonance imaging indicated before reduction of a unilateral cervical facet dislocation? Spine 2002;27:117–118

70. Cotler HB, Miller LS, DeLucia FA, Cotler JM, Davne SH. Closed reduction of cervical spine dislocations. Clin Orthop Relat Res 1987; 214:185–199

71. Sabiston CP, Wing PC, Schweigel JF, Van Peteghem PK, Yu W. Closed reduction of dislocations of the lower cervical spine. J Trauma 1988;28:832–835

72. Star AM, Jones AA, Cotler JM, Balderston RA, Sinha R. Immediate closed reduction of cervical spine dislocations using traction. Spine 1990;15:1068–1072

73. Cotler JM, Herbison GJ, Nasuti JF, Ditunno JF Jr, An H, Wolff BE. Closed reduction of traumatic cervical spine dislocation using traction weights up to 140 pounds. Spine 1993;18:386–390

74. Ludwig SC, Vaccaro AR, Balderston RA, Cotler JM. Immediate quadriparesis after manipulation for bilateral cervical facet subluxation: a case report. J Bone Joint Surg Am 1997;79:587–590

75. Lu K, Lee TC, Chen HJ. Closed reduction of bilateral locked facets of the cervical spine under general anaesthesia. Acta Neurochir (Wien) 1998;140:1055–1061

76. Eismont FJ, Arena MJ, Green BA. Extrusion of an intervertebral disc associated with traumatic subluxation and dislocation of cervical facets. J Bone Joint Surg Am 1991;73:1555–1560

77. Rizzolo SJ, Piazza MR, Cotler JM, Balderston RA, Schaefer D, Flanders A. Intervertebral disc injury complicating cervical spine trauma. Spine 1991;16 Suppl 6):S187–S189

78. Allred CD, Sledge JB. Irreducible dislocations of the cervical spine with a prolapsed disc: preliminary results from a treatment technique. Spine 2001;26:1927–1930

79. Do Koh Y, Lim TH, Won You J, Eck J, An HS. A biomechanical comparison of modern anterior and posterior plate fixation of the cervical spine. Spine 2001;26:15–21

80. Coe JD, Warden KE, Sutterlin CE, McAfee PC. Biomechanical evaluation of cervical spinal stabilization methods in a human cadaveric model. Spine 1989;14:1122–1131

81. Sutterlin CE III, McAfee PC, Warden KE, Rey RM Jr, Farey ID. A biomechanical evaluation of cervical spinal stabilization methods in a bovine model: static and cyclical loading. Spine 1988;13:795–802

82. Fazl M, Pirouzmand F. Intraoperative reduction of locked facets in the cervical spine by use of a modified interlaminar spreader: technical note. Neurosurgery 2001;48:444–445

83. Kahn A, Leggon R, Lindsey RW. Cervical facet dislocation: management following delayed diagnosis. Orthopedics 1998;21:1089–1091

84. Bartels RH, Donk R. Delayed management of traumatic bilateral cervical facet dislocation: surgical strategy: report of three cases. J Neurosurg 2002;97(Suppl 3):362–365

85. Thompson GH, Hohl M. Healed untreated anterior cervical spine dislocation: a case report. Spine 1978;3:113–115

86. Hadra BE. Wiring the spinous process in injury and Pott's disease. Trans Am Orthop Assoc 1891;4:206–210

87. Rogers W. Treatment of fracture-dislocation of the cervical spine. J Bone Joint Surg Am 1942;24A:245–258

88. Davey JR, Rorabeck CH, Bailey SI, Bourne RB, Dewar FP. A technique for posterior cervical fusion for instability of the cervical spine. Spine 1985;10:722–728

89. Segal D, Whitelaw GP, Gumbs V, Pick RY. Tension band fixation of acute cervical spine fractures. Clin Orthop Relat Res 1981;159: 211–222

90. al Baz MO, Mathur N. Modified technique of tension band wiring in flexion injuries of the middle and lower cervical spine. Spine 1995;20:1241–1244

91. Bohlman HH. Acute fractures and dislocations of the cervical spine: an analysis of three hundred hospitalized patients and review of the literature. J Bone Joint Surg Am 1979;61:1119–1142

92. Feldborg Nielsen C, Annertz M, Persson L, Wingstrand H, Saveland H, Brandt L. Posterior wiring without bony fusion in traumatic distractive flexion injuries of the mid to lower cervical spine. Long-term follow-up in 30 patients. Spine 1991;16:467–472

93. Whitehill R, Reger S, Weatherup N, et al. A biomechanical analysis of posterior cervical fusions using polymethylmethacrylate as an instantaneous fusion mass. Spine 1983;8:368–372

94. Whitehill R, Cicoria AD, Hooper WE, Maggio WW, Jane JA. Posterior cervical reconstruction with methyl methacrylate cement and wire: a clinical review. J Neurosurg 1988;68:576–584

95. Cahill DW, Bellegarrigue R, Ducker TB. Bilateral facet to spinous process fusion: a new technique for posterior spinal fusion after trauma. Neurosurgery 1983;13:1–4

96. Jeanneret B, Magerl F, Ward EH, Ward JC. Posterior stabilization of the cervical spine with hook plates. Spine 1991;16(Suppl 3): S56–S63

97. Jacobs B. Cervical fractures and dislocations (C3–7). Clin Orthop Relat Res 1975;109:18–32

98. Roy-Camille R, Saillant G, Berteaux D, Marie-Anne S. Early management of spinal injuries. In: McKibbin B, ed. Recent Advances in Orthopaedics. Edinburgh: Churchill-Livingstone; 1979:57–87

99. Grob D, Magerl F. Dorsal spondylodesis of the cervical spine using a hooked plate. Orthopade 1987;16:55–61

100. Montesano PX, Juach EC. Anatomic and biomechanical study of posterior cervical plate arthrodesis. Orthop Trans 1989;13: 205–206

101. Anderson PA, Henley MB, Grady MS, Montesano PX, Winn HR. Posterior cervical arthrodesis with AO reconstruction plates and bone graft. Spine 1991;16(Suppl 3):S72–S79

102. Ebraheim NA, Rupp RE, Savolaine ER, Brown JA. Posterior plating of the cervical spine. J Spinal Disord 1995;8:111–115

103. Klekamp JW, Ugbo JL, Heller JG, Hutton WC. Cervical transfacet versus lateral mass screws: a biomechanical comparison. J Spinal Disord 2000;13:515–518

104. Wang MY, Prusmack CJ, Green BA, Gruen JP, Levi AD. Minimally invasive lateral mass screws in the treatment of cervical facet dislocations: technical note. Neurosurgery 2003;52:444–447

105. Goffin J, Plets C, Van den Bergh R. Anterior cervical fusion and osteosynthetic stabilization according to Caspar: a prospective study of 41 patients with fractures and/or dislocations of the cervical spine. Neurosurgery 1989;25:865–871

106. Jonsson H Jr, Cesarini K, Petren-Mallmin M, Rauschning W. Locking screw-plate fixation of cervical spine fractures with and without ancillary posterior plating. Arch Orthop Trauma Surg 1991 ;111:1–12

107. Aebi M, Zuber K, Marchesi D. Treatment of cervical spine injuries with anterior plating: indications, techniques, and results. Spine 1991;16(Suppl 3):S38–S45

108. Razack N, Green BA, Levi AD. The management of traumatic cervical bilateral facet fracture-dislocations with unicortical anterior plates. J Spinal Disord 2000;13:374–381

109. Ordonez BJ, Benzel EC, Naderi S, Weller SJ. Cervical facet dislocation: techniques for ventral reduction and stabilization. J Neurosurg 2000;92(Suppl 1):18–23

110. Raynor RB, Pugh J, Shapiro I. Cervical facetectomy and its effect on spine strength. J Neurosurg 1985;63:278–282

111. Favero KJ, Van Peteghem PK. The quadrangular fragment fracture: roentgenographic features and treatment protocol. Clin Orthop Relat Res 1989;239:40–46

112. Cabanela ME, Ebersold MJ. Anterior plate stabilization for bursting teardrop fractures of the cervical spine. Spine 1988;13: 888–891

113. Richman JD, Daniel TE, Anderson DD, Miller PL, Douglas RA. Biomechanical evaluation of cervical spine stabilization methods using a porcine model. Spine 1995;20:2192–2197

114. Levine AM, Mazel C, Roy-Camille R. Management of fracture separations of the articular mass using posterior cervical plating. Spine 1992;17(Suppl 10):S447–S454

115. Lifeso RM, Colucci MA. Anterior fusion for rotationally unstable cervical spine fractures. Spine 2000;25:2028–2034

116. Jeanneret B, Gebhard JS, Magerl F. Transpedicular screw fixation of articular mass fracture-separation: results of an anatomical study and operative technique. J Spinal Disord 1994;7:222–229

117. Kang JD, Figgie MP, Bohlman HH. Sagittal measurements of the cervical spine in subaxial fractures and dislocations: an analysis of two hundred and eighty-eight patients with and without neurological deficits. J Bone Joint Surg Am 1994;76:1617–1628

118. Ersmark H, Lowenhielm P. Factors influencing the outcome of cervical spine injuries. J Trauma 1988;28:407–410

119. Lintner DM, Knight RQ, Cullen JP. The neurologic sequelae of cervical spine facet injuries: the role of canal diameter. Spine 1993;18:725–729

120. Sapkas G, Korres D, Babis GC, et al. Correlation of spinal canal posttraumatic encroachment and neurological deficit in burst fractures of the lower cervical spine (C3–7). Eur Spine J 1995;4:39–44

121. Papadopoulos SM, Selden NR, Quint DJ, Patel N, Gillespie B, Grube S. Immediate spinal cord decompression for cervical spinal cord injury: feasibility and outcome. J Trauma 2002;52:323–332

122. Delamarter RB, Sherman J, Carr JB. Pathophysiology of spinal cord injury: recovery after immediate and delayed decompression. J Bone Joint Surg Am 1995;77:1042–1049

123. Dolan EJ, Tator CH, Endrenyi L. The value of decompression for acute experimental spinal cord compression injury. J Neurosurg 1980;53:749–755

124. Carlson GD, Minato Y, Okada A, et al. Early time-dependent decompression for spinal cord injury: vascular mechanisms of recovery. J Neurotrauma 1997;14:951–962

125. Guha A, Tator CH, Endrenyi L, Piper I. Decompression of the spinal cord improves recovery after acute experimental spinal cord compression injury. Paraplegia 1987;25:324–339

126. Jarmundowicz W, Tosik D, Chlebinski J, Gorkiewicz Z. The effect of early decompression on the extent of changes in spinal cord microcirculation in experimental traumatic injury to the cord in rabbits [in Polish]. Neurol Neurochir Pol 1997;31:1167–1175

127. Rosenfeld JF, Vaccaro AR, Albert TJ, Klein GR, Cotler JM. The benefits of early decompression in cervical spinal cord injury. Am J Orthop 1998;27:23–28

128. Fehlings MG, Sekhon LH, Tator C. The role and timing of decompression in acute spinal cord injury: what do we know? What should we do? Spine 2001;26(Suppl 24):S101–S110

129. Silber JS, Vaccaro AR. Summary statement: the role and timing of decompression in acute spinal cord injury: evidence-based guidelines. Spine 2001;26(Suppl 24):S110

130. Murphy KP, Opitz JL, Cabanela ME, Ebersold MJ. Cervical fractures and spinal cord injury: outcome of surgical and nonsurgical management. Mayo Clin Proc 1990;65:949–959

131. Cotler HB, Cotler JM, Alden ME, Sparks G, Biggs CA. The medical and economic impact of closed cervical spine dislocations. Spine 1990;15:448–452

132. Rorabeck CH, Rock MG, Hawkins RJ, Bourne RB. Unilateral facet dislocation of the cervical spine: an analysis of the results of treatment in 26 patients. Spine 1987;12:23–27

133. Shapiro S, Snyder W, Kaufman K, Abel T. Outcome of 51 cases of unilateral locked cervical facets: interspinous braided cable for lateral mass plate fusion compared with interspinous wire and facet wiring with iliac crest. J Neurosurg 1999;91(Suppl 1):19–24

134. Heller JG, Silcox DH, Sutterlin CE. Complications of posterior cervical plating. Spine 1995;20:2442–2448

135. Xu R, Ebraheim NA, Nadaud MC, Yeasting RA, Stanescu S. The location of the cervical nerve roots on the posterior aspect of the cervical spine. Spine 1995;20:2267–2271

136. Choueka J, Spivak JM, Kummer FJ, Steger T. Flexion failure of posterior cervical lateral mass screws: influence of insertion technique and position. Spine 1996;21:462–468

137. Handa Y, Hayashi M, Kawano H, Kobayashi H, Hirose S. Vertebral artery thrombosis accompanied by burst fracture of the lower cervical spine: case report. Neurosurgery 1985;17:955–957

138. Vaccaro AR, Urban WC, Aiken RD. Delayed cortical blindness and recurrent quadriplegia after cervical trauma. J Spinal Disord 1998;11:535–539

139. Schwarz N, Buchinger W, Gaudernak T, Russe F, Zechner W. Injuries to the cervical spine causing vertebral artery trauma: case reports. J Trauma 1991;31:127–133

140. Willis BK, Greiner F, Orrison WW, Benzel EC. The incidence of vertebral artery injury after midcervical spine fracture or subluxation. Neurosurgery 1994;34:435–441

141. Louw JA, Mafoyane NA, Small B, Neser CP. Occlusion of the vertebral artery in cervical spine dislocations. J Bone Joint Surg Br 1990;72:679–681

142. Sim E, Vaccaro AR, Berzlanovich A, Pienaar S. The effects of staged static cervical flexion-distraction deformities on the patency of the vertebral arterial vasculature. Spine 2000;25: 2180–2186

143. Veras LM, Pedraza-Gutierrez S, Castellanos J, Capellades J, Casamitjana J, Rovira-Canellas A. Vertebral artery occlusion after acute cervical spine trauma. Spine 2000;25:1171–1177

144. Vishteh AG, Coscarella E, Nguyen B, Sonntag VK, McDougall CG. Fatal basilar artery thrombosis after traumatic cervical facet dislocation. Case report. J Neurosurg Sci 1999;43:195–199

145. Tomaszek DE, Rosner MJ. Occult esophageal perforation associated with cervical spine fracture. Neurosurgery 1984;14:492–494

8 Thoracic Spine Fractures

Rajiv K. Sethi, Kirkham B. Wood, and Mitchel B. Harris

Fractures of the thoracic spine are generally considered to include the first through tenth vertebrae; fractures involving the eleventh and twelfth vertebrae are considered to be those involving the thoracolumbar junction. Fractures in this region account for only 10 to 20% of all spine fractures.[1-3] Thoracic spine injuries are often overlooked in the emergency department due to other concomitant injuries and difficulties with emergent radiographic imaging; they nonetheless can be a significant source of morbidity. Because of the anatomy of this region and the forces necessary for bony injury, thoracic spine fractures are often associated with polytrauma and are often complicated by spinal cord injury.[4-8] Meyer[1] reported that 63% of the fractures of the upper thoracic spine seen during a 15-year period resulted in complete neurological injury to the spinal cord. Thus practitioners involved with trauma should be well versed in the fracture patterns, biomechanics, and treatment of thoracic spine fractures.

Biomechanics

The biomechanics of the thoracic spine differ from those of the cervical or lumbar spine. The thoracic spine is connected to the rib cage by the costovertebral joints, consisting of the costotransverse articulations and the heads of the ribs, which impart a great deal of stability to this region, especially in extension, lateral bending, and axial rotation.[9] Most bony injuries of the thoracic spine therefore occur in flexion with varying degrees of axial loading because the rib cage is less able to resist these forces. The stability of thoracic motion segments is significantly diminished when the costovertebral joints have been disrupted. When evaluating patients who have injuries to the costovertebral joints, the clinical stability of the spine must be carefully determined. Although the rib cage provides a great deal of rigidity, lateral rib fractures, by themselves, have not been shown to correlate with late deformity in patients treated nonoperatively.[7]

The sternum is another vital component of overall stability of the thoracic spine. In patients with high-energy trauma to the thorax, the sternum may be buckled or even fractured. This injury pattern is more commonly seen in those who have struck the steering wheel or dashboard in deceleration motor vehicle accidents.[10] This buckling or fracturing of the sternum is important because the rib cage and intact sternum serve as the "fourth column" (anteriorly), helping to stabilize the thoracic spine against deforming flexion and extension forces.[11,12] Andriacchi and associates calculated that the compression tolerance of the spinal column in the presence of the rib cage and sternum is increased by a factor of 4.[13] Removal of one or two ribs, as is commonly done for exposure during spinal surgery, did not significantly affect the stiffness of the thoracic spine unless a portion of the sternum was removed as well.[13] Thus, when even a trivial thoracic wedge compression fracture is associated with a displaced or overriding sternal fracture, the spine should be considered potentially unstable and aggressively evaluated to avoid further kyphosis and the potential for chronic pain, deformity, and neurological injury.[14]

Fracture Classification

A commonly used classification of thoracic and lumbar fractures is based on a system first offered by Magerl and associates.[15,16] The proposal is an open-ended, mechanistic classification that includes nearly every fracture pattern (**Fig. 8–1A–C).** Fractures are listed in increasing severity of bone and soft tissue disruption leading to increasing instability. Three main fracture types exist. Type A fractures are compression injuries primarily involving the anterior vertebral body. Type B are distraction injuries through either primarily ligamentous structures (B1) or osseous elements (B2) posteriorly. Type C injuries are multidirectional, typically with translation or rotation, and involve both the anterior and posterior columns of the spine. Type C fractures often represent fracture-dislocations and are the most unstable of all spinal injuries and the most prone to neurological deterioration while the patient is hospitalized.[17]

Minor Injuries

Minor injuries to the thoracic spine include fractures of the spinous or transverse processes and the pars interarticularis, or of an isolated vertebral facet or lamina. Such injuries rarely cause neurological sequelae and are inherently stable. Almost exclusively, they are managed non-surgically with either careful observation or an orthosis. Pain control and activity restrictions are based on the degree of symptoms present.

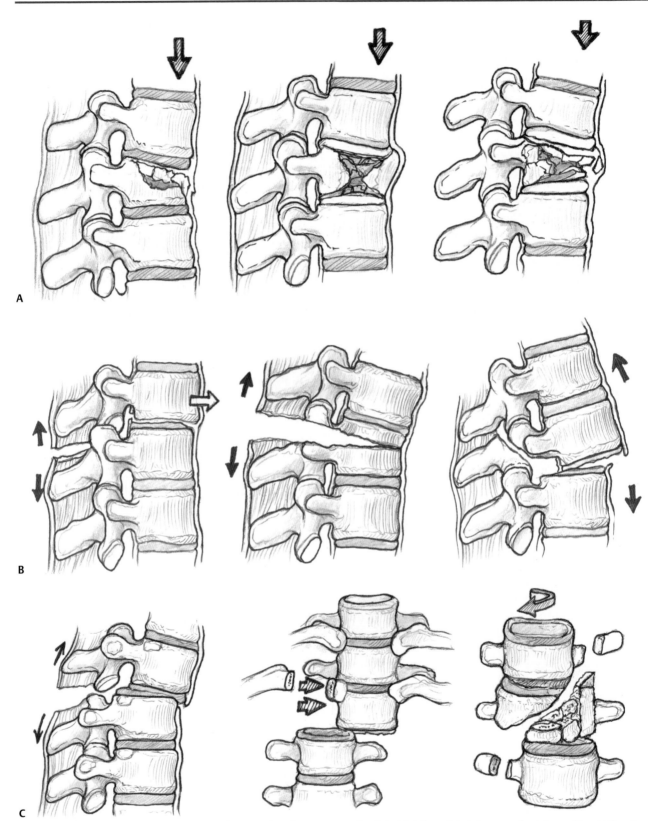

Figure 8–1 Schematic view of the thoracic fracture classification system proposed by Gertzbein. **(A,** left to right**)** Impaction compression fracture; sagittal split compression fracture; burst fracture. **(B,** left to right**)** Posterior disruption primarily ligamentous; posterior disruption primarily bony; anterior disruption through the disk. **(C,** left to right**)** Compression injury with rotation; type B injury with rotation; rotational shear injury. (Adapted from Gertzbein SD. Spine update: classification of thoracic and lumber fractures. Spine 1994;19:626–628.)

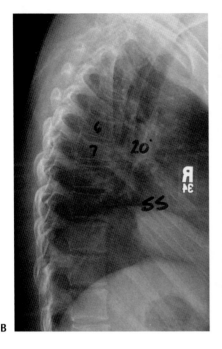
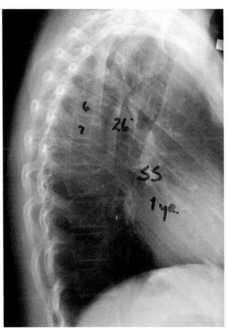

A,B

Figure 8–2 (A) Lateral radiograph of a T7 compression fracture in a 23-year-old woman involved in a motor vehicle accident. Treatment consisted of 2 months of a thoracolumboscacral orthosis. **(B)** Lateral radiograph 12 months later shows minimal residual wedging. The patient did not complain of pain.

Major Injuries

Compression Fractures

Compression fractures of the thoracic spine (types A1 and A2) represent anterior failure of the vertebral body due to a compressive force **(Fig. 8–2A,B)**. The posterior vertebral body cortex remains undisturbed in a true compression fracture, and thus no retropulsion of bone into the spinal canal occurs. Compression fractures are the most common injury to the thoracic spine and represent more than 50% of all major spinal trauma.[13] Although these fractures can occur throughout the thoracic spine, they most commonly occur at the level of T6–T8 because of the high degree of axial loading of the anterior column that takes place at the apex of the spine's natural kyphosis.

Burst Fractures

Compared with simple compression fractures, burst fractures of the thoracic spine (type A3) represent a more substantial degree of axial loading of the vertebral body, such that fracture of the posterior cortex occurs with retropulsion of bone into the spinal canal. This can result in compromised neurological function. Within the thoracic spine, burst fractures are not nearly as common as they are in the lower thoracolumbar region (T10–L2). This is thought to be due to several factors, principally the more kyphotic nature of this region of the spine that directs loads to the anterior aspect of the vertebral body, as well as the support provided by the surrounding rib cage.[3,18]

When performed, lateral radiographs show that the posterior vertebral body line is disrupted, with visible loss of overall vertebral height **(Fig. 8–3A,B)**. Because of the proximity of the spinal cord and the relatively small area of the spinal canal compared with the lower thoracolumbar and lumbar regions, burst fractures of the upper thoracic spine more commonly result in some degree of neurological impairment.

Flexion-Distraction Injuries

Flexion-distraction (seat-belt) injuries of the thoracic spine (types B1 and B2) represent primary failure of the posterior ligamentous (B1) or bony (B2) complex under flexion and tension **(Fig. 8–4)**. Flexion-distraction fractures are actually somewhat rare in the thoracic spine and are more commonly seen in the thoracolumbar or lumbar spine regions, areas not supported by the rib cage and sternum. Many subtypes have been described based on the degree of bony or ligamentous involvement.[19] Anteriorly, the vertebral body wedging is typically mild, and the anterior longitudinal ligament (ALL) remains intact.

Fracture-Dislocations

Fracture-dislocations of the thoracic spine (type C) are the most unstable of all thoracic spine injuries and represent failure of both anterior and posterior aspects of the spine under combinations of compression, tension, rotation, and shear forces.[18] Fracture-dislocations result from

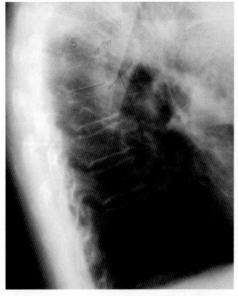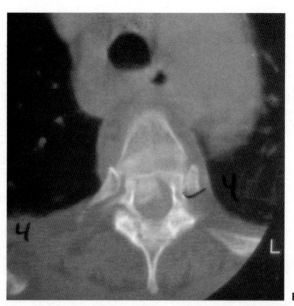

A   B

Figure 8–3 (A) Lateral radiograph of a T4 burst fracture in a 39-year-old man caused when a large metal beam struck him in the upper back. Note the collapse of both the anterior and the posterior verte-bral body heights. **(B)** Axial computed tomographic image through the fracture gives excellent detail of the fracture morphology. Note that the costovertebral articulations remain intact.

the highest levels of force and are the thoracic spine injuries most commonly associated with neurological deficits.[1,3]

The radiographic hallmark of fracture-dislocations is translation or rotation of a vertebral body on coronal or sagittal images **(Fig. 8–5A,B)**. Computed tomography (CT) aids strongly in fracture identification; however, subtle vertebral translation may be difficult to appreciate on axial images, and sagittal reformatting may be necessary.

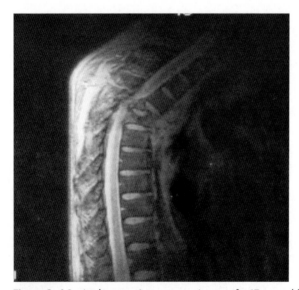

Figure 8–4 Sagittal magnetic resonance image of a 17-year-old boy who fell from a second-story balcony, suffering a flexion-distraction injury to the midthoracic spine.

Hyperextension Injuries

Hyperextension injuries of the thoracic spine (B3) represent primary failure of the anterior column in extension and are rare, again reflecting the protective role of the sternum, rib cage, and ALL. Apparent damage to the anterior column may be minimal in some hyperextension injuries, the most common of these fractures being seen when the posterior column fails in compression. Anterior disk-space widening, sagittal translation, and a small avulsion fracture of the inferior vertebral end plate are the radiographic features of these injuries **(Fig. 8–6)**. The anterior ligamentous disruptions are best seen on magnetic resonance imaging (MRI).

Because of the disruption of the ALL and the compression injuries to the posterior column, these fractures are inherently unstable. Surgical stabilization must avoid overdistraction and cannot serve simply as a posterior tension band. Pedicle screw systems that provide segmental three-dimensional fixation of the spine work especially well in these unstable injuries.

Ankylosing Spondylitis/Diffuse Idiopathic Skeletal Hyperostosis

Pathological bone disorders such as ankylosing spondylitis (AS) and diffuse idiopathic skeletal hyperostosis (DISH) produce a brittle spine that puts patients with these disorders at increased risk for fracture after even minor trauma.[20] Fractures associated with DISH most commonly occur through the vertebral body, whereas the pattern in ankylosing spondylitis is typically fractured through the disk. Overall, the prognosis is determined by the mechanism of injury, the degree of osteoligamentous damage,

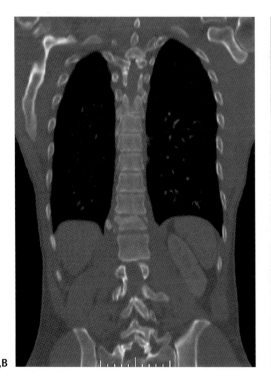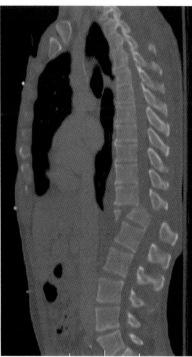

A,B

Figure 8–5 A 35-year-old male who fell 20 feet from a roof, landing on his back with complete paralysis of the lower extremities. **(A)** Anteroposterior computed tomographic (CT) reconstruction. **(B)** Sagittal CT reconstruction.

and whether a neurological deficit is present.[21] In the AS patient, most of the ligaments have become ossified and therefore provide minimal resistance under tension strains. Patients with AS are more prone than patients without the disease to develop posttraumatic spinal

epidural hematomas, even after relatively minor trauma. Best demonstrated on MRI, a spinal epidural hemorrhage appears as a tapered epidural mass compressing the cord. Urgent decompression is the usual method of treatment depending on the degree and status of potential neurological compromise. Noteworthy is the high incidence of increased morbidity and mortality in these patients.

Radiological Assessment

The diagnosis of upper thoracic fractures in polytrauma patients remains a challenge. The clinical findings are often difficult to detect, especially in the presence of associated extremity fractures, head injuries, or chest injury requiring ventilatory support.[21] When neurological impairment is absent, a potentially unstable fracture may initially go undetected. In 5 to 27% of cases, multiple, often noncontiguous spinal fractures can be found, typically in the low lumbar spine or cervicothoracic junction.[4,5,8,22,23] The discovery of a significant fracture involving the thoracic spine should prompt a detailed radiographic evaluation of the remainder of the spinal column. Conversely, any fracture identified in the cervical or lumbar region should lead to a full axial skeletal evaluation. This is currently addressed by high-speed CT scans with advanced reformatting programs.

Radiographic examination of the presumed isolated thoracic spine injury begins with adequate supine anteroposterior (AP) and cross-table lateral radiographs. Often the trauma patient has already been through the

Figure 8–6 Extension-type fracture-dislocation in a 63-year-old woman struck by an automobile. Lateral radiograph shows the anterior opening of the disk space and posterior vertebral translation.

CT scanner, and reformatted images of the spine have been done. Imaging of the cervicothoracic junction may be difficult; the lateral x-ray of the neck does not usually show the sixth and seventh cervical vertebrae. Frequently, a swimmer's view with the arms extended will image the lower cervical and upper thoracic spine. Alternatively, a CT scan may be necessary to view this region. Historically, it has been the lateral view that demanded our keen attention. However, the AP view also warrants close inspection. The AP radiograph, with proper settings, can be very helpful in identifying end plate injuries as well as subtle malalignment.

CT has long been considered the examination of choice in detailing the nature of bony injuries to the spine. Because of advances in imaging technology, CT is often available in the emergency or trauma room setting and is often performed in lieu of plain radiographs. CT should always be obtained in obtunded or sedated polytrauma patients or patients whose mechanism of injury has a recognized association with thoracic fractures. Albrecht et al have recently done a large comparison between plain films and CT in polytrauma patients and have shown that plain films can miss up to 50% of unstable spine fractures, all of which were readily identified by CT.[24] In this study, all spinal injuries relevant to acute management were seen on CT but not on conventional radiography.

MRI is increasingly used in trauma settings, especially for the assessment of soft tissue injuries and spinal cord pathology. MRI provides several different views of the traumatized area relatively quickly, including the spinal cord, intervertebral disks, cerebrospinal fluid, epidural space, posterior ligamentous structures (e.g., seat-belt injuries), and the bone marrow. MRI is capable of identifying edema, hemorrhage, and spinal cord disruption. MRI findings have been shown to correlate reasonably well with potential neurological recovery.[25,26] MRI also provides information regarding the ALL and PLL, structures often difficult to evaluate on CT.[27] A disadvantage of MRI in the acute trauma setting is the fact that monitoring of the injured patient within the enclosed magnetic resonance scanner can be difficult, and many life-support systems are incompatible with MRI equipment.[28]

An important aspect of the radiological workup of thoracic spine trauma is the evaluation of aortic injury, which may have similar clinical and radiographic findings to a thoracic spine injury. Because aortic rupture can compromise the collateral circulation from the spinal arteries and cause ischemic necrosis of the cord, aortic rupture can cause paraparesis or paraplegia. Mediastinal widening, pleural fluid, hemothorax, pneumomediastinum, obliteration of the paraspinous stripe, and an apical cap are all radiographic characteristics of potential aortic transection.[29,30] However, similar findings on plain radiographs can be seen in many patients with otherwise uncomplicated upper thoracic bony injuries.[5,29]

Initial clues to the presence of an aortic injury can be seen on plain AP radiographs of the chest. With a vertebral fracture, the left main-stem bronchus remains in its normal position, whereas with injuries to the aorta, the bronchus is depressed somewhat. If a nasogastric tube is in place, it will be displaced to the right in cases of aortic transection.[4] Because of the high level of mortality associated with aortic injury (historically, 80% of these patients would die before they could be transported to the hospital), Bolesta and Bohlman recommend ruling out an aortic injury with a vascular study before stabilizing the thoracic spine in any situation of high-energy trauma.[29]

Treatment Planning

Determining the stability of the injured thoracic spine is the most important and often the most difficult step in deciding the treatment plan. According to White and Panjabi, clinical instability is defined as "the loss of the ability of the spine to maintain its pattern of displacement under physiologic loads, so that there is no initial or additional neurological deficit, no major deformity, and no incapacitating pain."[31] Several factors need to be assessed to ultimately define the stability of a given thoracic injury, including the mechanism of injury, the amount of force involved, the quality of the bone, the radiographic appearance of the particular structures involved, and the neurological status of the victim. Spinal instability exists as a continuum and is not an all-or-nothing phenomenon. As suggested previously, any thoracic injury associated with a concomitant fracture of the sternum should be considered potentially unstable. The presence of any posterior element injury (spinous process fractures, facet subluxations, or dislocations) can reduce spinal stability, especially with concomitant injury to the anterior ligamentous structures. Rotational forces in association with flexion are also capable of injuring the ALL and rendering the spine unstable. Clinical instability, however, cannot consistently be predicted from simple static radiographs because similar biomechanical forces often produce dissimilar injuries. A thorough understanding of the biomechanical and biological aspects of an injury becomes crucial in adequately planning treatment.

The goals of treatment are well defined: (1) to stabilize the spine to prevent further deformity, (2) to allow early mobilization, (3) to avoid (further) neurological injury, (4) to relieve pain, and (5) to reduce health care cost as much as possible.

Nonoperative Treatment

The majority of thoracic spine injuries are relatively stable and can be treated nonsurgically. Compression and most burst fractures in patients with intact costovertebral connections, intact rib cages, and stable neurological findings can be treated with a variety of orthoses for 6 to 12 weeks. Increasingly, minor compression fractures are being treated with early ambulation and no orthosis, with similar results.[7,32] Most patients will benefit from a program of back strengthening exercises. When a flexion-distraction injury (seat-belt) fracture presents with a purely osseous fracture component (B2), these injuries may heal with bony union in an orthosis. Injuries of the uppermost thoracic spine (above T6), however, are often difficult to immobilize in an orthosis without incorporating the head and neck, and these cervical-thoracic orthoses typically are poorly tolerated.

Surgical Treatment

The indications for surgical intervention are based primarily on the stability of the injured spine and its neurological status. Fracture-dislocations (type C) are the injuries that are most commonly treated with surgical reduction, stabilization, and fusion. However, compression fractures with loss of more than 50% of anterior vertebral body height may develop progressive painful kyphosis, and surgical

stabilization may be considered.[3,7,33,34] Hanley and Eskay found that six of eight compression fractures treated non-operatively complained of long-standing pain related to bony collapse and kyphosis.[3] On occasion, compression fractures, especially in the elderly, may be associated with some element of neurological deficit—usually from a herniated disk or from progressive kyphosis and angular deformity.[33] Early decompression in conjunction with stabilization in this age group may be of some benefit. On the other hand, if there is no radiographic evidence of spinal cord compression, and CT or MR imaging has not demonstrated ligamentous injury, the risks of surgical intervention for compression fractures must be carefully considered.

The specific approach (anterior vs posterior) to the thoracic fracture pattern is dictated not only by the need to decompress in the setting of neurological injury, but also by the specifics of the fractured vertebra. The various approaches and their utility are illustrated in **Fig. 8–7A–D.** Anterior reconstruction may be needed for reconstitution

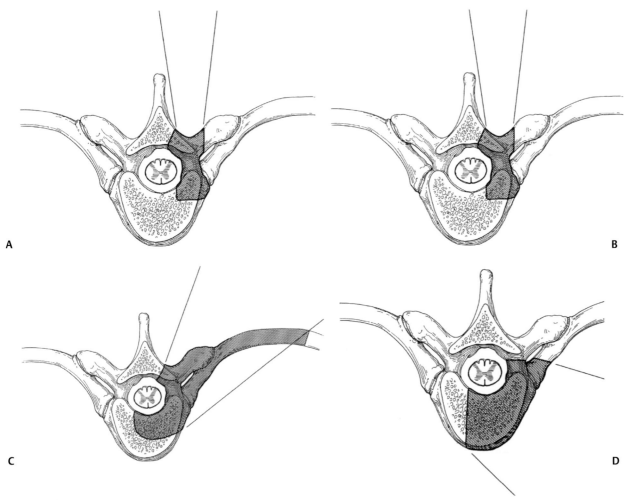

Figure 8–7 The various approaches for decompressing the thoracic spinal canal. **(A)** Laminectomy for posterior compression. **(B)** Transpedicular approach allows decompression of the lateral aspect of the spinal canal. **(C)** Costotransversectomy allows similar exposure of the lateral spinal canal plus access to the anterior vertebral body.

(D) Transthoracic exposure requires a thoracotomy but affords the best exposure of the anterior canal. (From Lemole GM, Henn JS, Sonntag VKS. Thoracic fractures. In: Vaccaro AR, ed. Fractures of the Cervical, Thoracic and Lumbar Spine. New York: Marcel Dekker; 2003:407–439, with permission.)

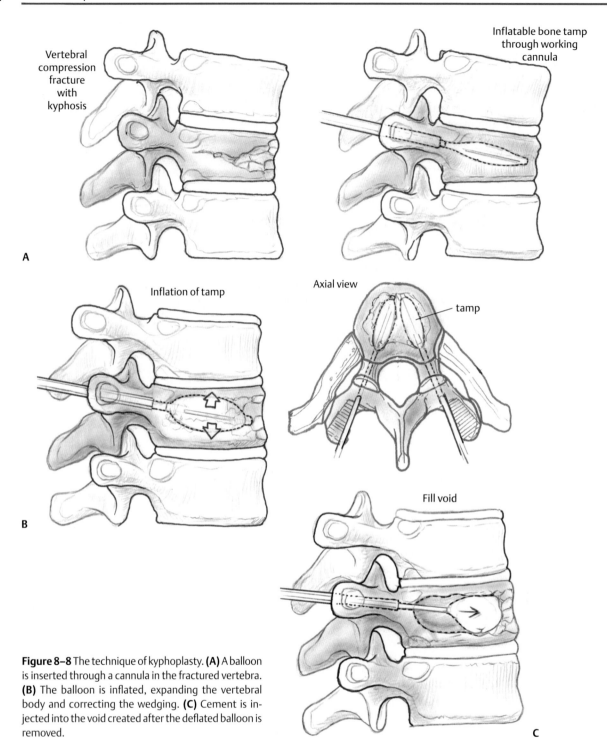

Figure 8–8 The technique of kyphoplasty. **(A)** A balloon is inserted through a cannula in the fractured vertebra. **(B)** The balloon is inflated, expanding the vertebral body and correcting the wedging. **(C)** Cement is injected into the void created after the deflated balloon is removed.

of a capable load-bearing anterior column. If the load-bearing anterior column is not dramatically comminuted, then a posterior procedure might be indicated, especially for the polytrauma patient.

Vertebroplasty and Kyphoplasty

In recent years, there has been a significant increase in the number of patients with compression fractures, particularly in osteoporotic bone, that have been treated with either vertebroplasty or kyphoplasty.[35–37] Vertebroplasty is a procedure whereby, under fluoroscopic guidance, polymethyl methacrylate (bone cement) is percutaneously injected into the fractured vertebral body from a posterior transpedicular approach. It is often performed in an outpatient setting by musculoskeletal or neuroradiologists as well as spine surgeons. The procedure was first developed for use in isolated vertebral body metastases such as occur in multiple myeloma, but quickly became useful for nonpathological compression fractures. Kyphoplasty is a similar procedure; however, before instilling the bone cement, a small balloon is inflated within the fractured vertebra to elevate the collapsed vertebral end plates and restore some of the normal sagittal profile of the injured segment. After reduction of the fracture, the balloon is decompressed and the cement is instilled, filling the defect and maintaining the correction of the deformity (**Fig. 8–8A–C**). This provides both the benefit of increasing the strength of the vertebra and improving the sagittal balance of the kyphotic thoracic spine.

Both vertebroplasty and kyphoplasty have been shown to reduce pain and expedite discharge from the hospital as well as improve physical and mental function. Coumans et al have shown from their experience at the Massachusetts General Hospital that there is a significant improvement in short form (SF)-36 scores after kyphoplasty and that the results of kyphoplasty persisted at 1 year post-treatment.[38] McKiernan et al prospectively followed 46 patients to 6 months postvertebroplasty. They found immediate and statistically significant reduction in pain and improvement in all domains of the osteoporosis quality of life questionnaire that remained improved at each evaluation point throughout the 6-month period ($p < .007$).[39] However, long-term comparison of these procedures with more conservative treatment such as bracing, bed rest, and medication has not yet been provided. Because both involve the instillation of cement into a relatively controlled space, the procedure is generally contraindicated when the posterior vertebral body is compromised. When posterior vertebral fractures are present, such as in a burst fracture, the injection of cement risks compromise of the spinal canal from extravasation of the liquefied cement. In addition, extrusion of polymethyl methacrylate into the surrounding tissues, or even embolization to distant organs such as the heart or the lungs, can occur.[35,37]

Posterior Instrumentation

In most cases of unstable traumatic deformity (burst fractures, flexion-distraction injuries, and fracture-dislocations), multisegmental posterior instrumentation is applicable. Typically, because of the strong bending forces existing in the normally kyphotic spine, many levels above and below the injury need to be included in the fusion (see **Video 8–1, Disk 1**), and postoperative orthotic containment may also be beneficial (**Fig. 8–9**).[40–42] Modern multisegmental instrumentation systems may allow more rigid fixation, sometimes over a slightly shorter area, especially if pedicle screws can be employed (**Fig. 8–10A–E**).[8,43,44] These intrapedicular screws are particularly indicated when strong three-dimensional control of the displaced spine is necessary, such as in a fracture-dislocation or hyperextension injury.

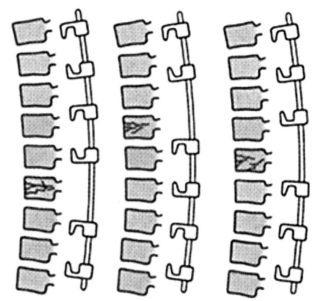

Figure 8–9 Illustration of various segmental posterior constructs for a thoracic-level fracture. Note the multiple points of fixation above and below the fracture. (From Lewandroski KU, McLain RG. Thoracolumbar fractures: evaluation, classification, and treatment. In: Frymoyer JW, Weisel SW, eds. The Adult and Pediatric Spine. 3rd ed. Philadelphia: Lippincott, Williams and Wilkins; 2004:817–843, with permission.)

Another relatively recent addition to the array of surgical options for thoracic fractures is endoscopic osteosynthesis and instrumentation.[45,46] The learning curve of thoracoscopic surgery is admittedly somewhat steep, but in practiced hands, the major complication rate is fairly low ($< 2\%$), and when compared with patients treated with open thoracotomy, less postoperative pain medication seems to be required.

Spinal Decompression

General guidelines for decompressive surgery of the spine include neurological deterioration or an incomplete neurological deficit, including sacral sparing, with confirming radiographic evidence of an offending soft tissue or osseous lesion. The extent of neurological injury at presentation helps guide the surgeon's decision to perform the decompression. The presence of a complete spinal cord deficit may indicate severe anatomical compromise or functional transection of the spinal cord. Historically, such patients have shown a low incidence of improvement with surgery.[5,7,34,47] Age is another factor; patients older than 50 years of age with a spinal cord injury have been shown to have a poorer prognosis for neurological recovery than younger patients.[48]

When indicated, most fractures are best decompressed by an anterior approach for removal of the retropulsed bone.[34,47] Posterior decompression with ma-

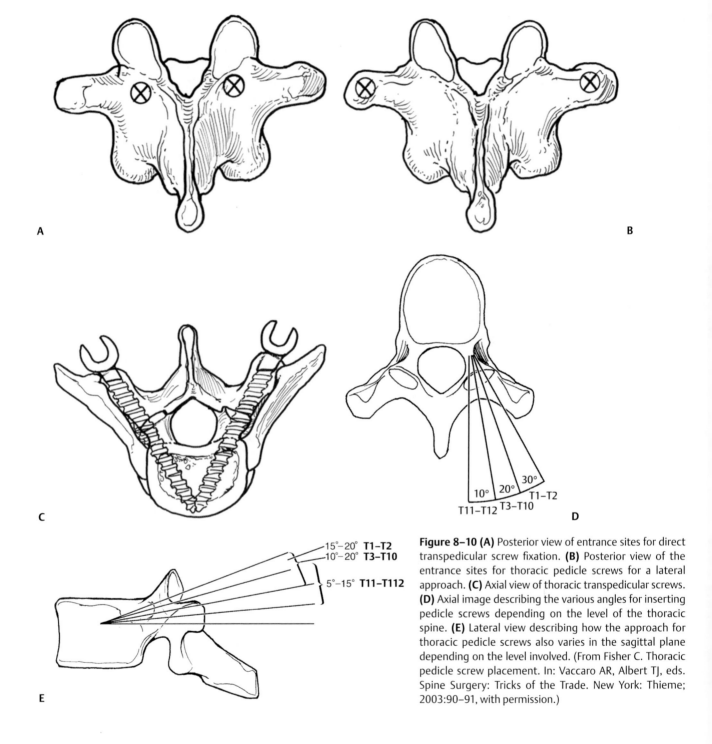

Figure 8–10 (A) Posterior view of entrance sites for direct transpedicular screw fixation. **(B)** Posterior view of the entrance sites for thoracic pedicle screws for a lateral approach. **(C)** Axial view of thoracic transpedicular screws. **(D)** Axial image describing the various angles for inserting pedicle screws depending on the level of the thoracic spine. **(E)** Lateral view describing how the approach for thoracic pedicle screws also varies in the sagittal plane depending on the level involved. (From Fisher C. Thoracic pedicle screw placement. In: Vaccaro AR, Albert TJ, eds. Spine Surgery: Tricks of the Trade. New York: Thieme; 2003:90–91, with permission.)

nipulation of the spinal cord has been associated with a higher degree of worsening neurological injury compared with the more preferred anterior approach.[5,47,49] Incomplete spinal cord injuries may improve with reduction of the fracture and restoration of spinal alignment and definitive stabilization.

The timing of surgical decompression remains controversial. There remains no strong correlation between the degree of initial neurological impairment and the amount of narrowing of the spinal canal diameter; hence the mere presence of an offending lesion in the canal is not by itself an indication for decompression.[5,50] On the other hand, several experimental studies in animals have shown that neurological recovery can be directly related to the duration of spinal cord compression.[51,52] In humans, evidence of favorable outcomes after acute decompression does exist but remains anecdotal.[12,53–56] Krengel and associates[57] and others[3,5,22,58] have shown dramatic improvement and varying degrees of neurological recovery in individuals with incomplete spinal cord injuries from thoracic trauma treated with early decompression, spinal realignment, and surgical stabilization. These studies compare favorably to the historical controls that were treated with either postural reduction or late surgical intervention. The lack of comparative studies makes it difficult to show a true cause-and-effect relationship between the timing of decompression and the degree of neurological recovery that is appreciably different from the natural history of limited neurological recovery in nonoperative cases. It is accepted that early surgery in the polytrauma victim does decrease the medical complications associated with spinal cord injury such as pneumonia, deep vein thrombosis, pulmonary embolism, and skin breakdown. The number of hospital and intensive care unit (ICU) days and the overall cost of care are lower as well.[59]

One area of controversy is whether to surgically stabilize thoracic fractures in the setting of complete neurological injury.[5,47] Proponents point out the advantages of shortened hospital stays, less total cost, more rapid mobilization, earlier rehabilitation, and avoidance of progressive and possibly painful kyphosis.[60] On the other hand, many authors have reported complications that can accompany lengthy thoracic fusions, including ascending paraplegia, wound infections, pneumonia, cerebrospinal fluid leaks, and pseudarthosis.[5,7,34,41,60,61]

Surgical Technique of Anterior Decompression and Fusion

As stated previously, the main accepted indications for anterior surgical procedures in thoracic spine trauma include acute decompression and stabilization of unstable burst fractures with neurological injury, correction of posttraumatic kyphosis, and reconstruction of the load-bearing anterior column to further prevent progression of kyphotic deformity.

The anterior approach to the spine is transthoracic when working from T4–T9, thoracoabdominal from T10–L1, and retroperitoneal from T12–L5. In transthoracic surgery, a right-sided approach is often used for levels above T10 to avoid vital structures. The rib at the level of the vertebra one to two segments above the desired level is resected. Subsequently, the parietal pleura is exposed and incised halfway between the neuroforamen and the anterior vertebral level. A radiograph should be obtained to document the correct spinal level. The segmental vessels overlying the injured vertebral body are identified and ligated. The pleura and periosteum are subsequently elevated. This allows placement of a blunt retractor between the anterior spine and the vessels. Another blunt narrow retractor is placed within the neuroforamen at the lateral border of the spinal canal to facilitate tissue retraction laterally. Next, adjacent disks are sharply incised and removed. The pedicle is identified once the rib head is resected. It is subsequently removed with a Kerrison punch or high-speed bur. Once the pedicle has been removed, the posterior

boundary of the vertebral body is identified to facilitate removal of the vertebral body. Decompression is continued until the medial border of the contralateral pedicle is identified.[62] Once the decompression is completed, a suitable anterior column reconstruction is performed, followed by either anterior or posterior stabilization. Subsequent pleural closure is achieved, and a chest tube is left in place. Standard wound closure techniques with superficial drains can then be utilized.

In the absence of significant posterior osseous or ligamentous disruption, anterior fusion, with a dual rod or plating fixation device, can suffice. Structural allograft, autograft, or cage devices can be used to reconstruct the anterior load-bearing column.

Surgical Technique and Instrumentation of Posterior Decompression and Fusion (see Video 8–1, Disk 1)

Standard posterior decompression techniques will be described as utilized by the authors. A midline skin incision is made extending from the most cephalad spinous process to the most caudal one. Localization of the incision is done with careful radiographic correlation. After the skin incision, subsequent electrocautery is used to dissect down to the level of the spinous process. Once the dissection is carried lateral to the spinous processes, an intraoperative radiograph is used to document level. A towel clamp on the spinous process of interest is used.

Once the correct level has been confirmed, electrocautery is used to cut muscle attachments to the spinous processes and laminae. Care should be taken to protect the capsules of the facet joints if fusion is not planned at the level of the decompression. The interspinous ligament is subsequently removed with a Leksell rongeur, and a bone cutter is used to remove the spinous processes en bloc. Decompression of the spinal canal is subsequently undertaken. Central canal decompression should be undertaken first. A high-speed bur is used to thin the laminae down, leaving the ligamentum flavum intact to protect the dura. The surgeon must exercise caution to spare the pars interarticularis. Subsequently, a Kerrison rongeur is used to remove the laminae in a caudad to cephalad fashion. In the case of a burst fracture, debris within the central canal can be removed once the laminectomy is completed. If needed, the surgeon can proceed with decompression of the lateral recesses and individual foramina, which would involve a partial medial facetectomy. The need for decompression of the lateral recesses and individual foramina will be determined by the specifics of the fracture pattern as seen on preoperative studies. Laminectomy over one or more levels affords direct exposure of the posterior canal. Costotransversectomy and a transpedicular approach can further allow removal of lateral and in some cases anterior impingement.

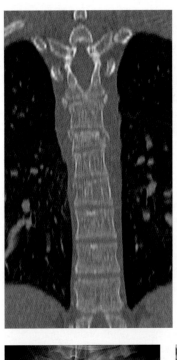
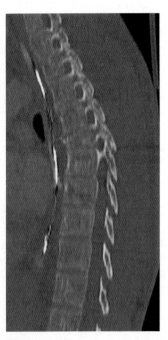

A,B

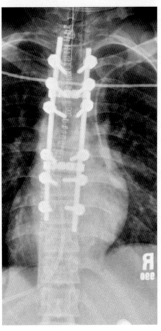
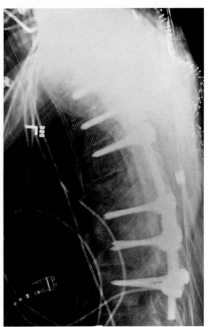

C,D

Figure 8–11 (A) Anteroposterior (AP) and **(B)** sagittal computed tomographic (CT) reconstructions of a T4 burst fracture. **(C)** AP and **(D)** sagittal CT reconstructions showing stabilization over multiple levels using pedicle screws.

Techniques of instrumentation have been evolving over the past several decades from fusion without instrumentation, to the use of hooks, rods, and wires, and in recent years increasing use of pedicle screws **(Fig. 8–11A–D Video 8–1, Disk 1)**. Pedicle screws stabilize both columns of the vertebral axis, effecting application of corrective forces in three planes. Ideally, this technique is preferred for the treatment of fracture-dislocations where fixation can usually be extended over multiple levels without sacrificing important motion segments as in the lumbar spine. All posterior instrumented constructs need to be supplemented with careful decortication and some form of bone graft, preferably autograft. Newer instrumentation does not obviate the need for careful fusion techniques.

Inserting screws into thoracic pedicles can be difficult. Careful radiological examination is needed preoperatively to assess the feasibility of screw placement. The overlying costotransverse and articular facets may obscure the anatomy of the thoracic pedicles. In addition, the thecal sac cannot be retracted to visualize the medial wall of the pedicle, as is commonly done in the lumbar spine. Image-guided surgery might provide some assistance in determining both the feasibility and a safe trajectory.[63] In a recent cadaveric study, Fayyazi et al found CT to be relatively insensitive when compared with open dissection in assessing thoracic pedicle screw position. This type of data may lead to further acceptance of the need for image-guided surgery.[64]

Rehabilitation

Rigid fixation with newer instrumentation systems has allowed for quicker postoperative rehabilitation. Before the development of instrumentation systems, the spine surgeon would use an external orthosis to obtain and maintain the desired spinal alignment while the fusion would take place. With the use of pedicle screws and newer, stronger instrumentation, the period of postoperative immobilization is now decreasing. The decision to use an orthosis is one that should take into account the patient's biology, the biomechanics of the instrumentation, and psychosocial considerations. In the setting of thoracolumbar trauma, the surgeon should take into account the extent of the fusion performed in addition to patient biology. For example, a smoker will require more time for the fusion to mature and therefore may need a brace to reduce some of the forces on the hardware that might otherwise result in fatigue failure before fusion maturation.

In designing a specific rehabilitation program, one must take into account patient factors such as age, health, and anticipated activity level. Many surgeons recommend active rehabilitation as early as 4 to 6 weeks after surgery. This may include back strengthening exercises and a cardiovascular fitness program. The end goal is to enable the patient to return to work and have an acceptable level of function.

Outcomes

Compression Fractures

Most compression fractures have been shown to do well with brace or cast immobilization. Poor outcomes have been shown with compression fractures with more than 30 degrees of kyphosis and more than 50% destruction of the anterior weight-bearing column.[22]

Burst Fractures

Most burst fractures without neurological deficit will do well if treated nonsurgically. It is important to verify that neither posterior ligamentous incompetence nor anterior sternal fractures exist that would threaten the overall sagittal plane stability of the spine. As discussed earlier in this chapter, these associated injuries have been shown to lead to increasing kyphosis and poor clinical outcomes.

General Outcomes after Thoracic Spine Fracture

McLain et al prospectively followed 70 consecutive patients treated with posterior instrumentation for unstable thoracic and thoracolumbar fractures, half of whom had neurological injuries, to assess return to work and functional recovery over the 5 year postoperative period. They found that 70% of the patients returned to work, 54% of which were at their previous level of employment with no functional limitations. Neurological injury had a much greater impact on functional outcome than did any other variable.[65] The ability of modern multisegmental instrumentation to distribute the corrective forces over many levels seems to reduce the risk of hook or rod failure, something seen in up to 15% of patients treated with first-generation Harrington rods.

Outcome studies of patients treated with surgery for flexion-distraction injuries as well as fracture-dislocations tend to be case series with little comparative data or functional outcome information. Such studies would be helpful in determining not only treatment options, surgical versus nonsurgical, but approach, surgical technique, time to surgery, methods of rehabilitation, and long-term outcome.

Complications

Anterior surgical treatment provides predictable decompression of the spinal cord with predictable fusion rates. Nonetheless, complications do exist.[66–69] Oskouian and Johnson retrospectively reviewed 207 patients who underwent anterior decompression and reconstruction. Vascular complications developed in 12 patients (5.8%), and two patients (1%) died. Deep venous thrombosis developed in five patients (2.4%), with one patient dying from a pulmonary embolism.[70]

Vascular injury is best treated by immediate direct repair. Occasionally, nonthreatening venous bleeding can be allowed to tamponade. Careful closure of the parietal pleura helps to contain postoperative bleeding. Drains placed percutaneously into the retroperitoneal space or chest tubes in the thoracic cavity can be used to remove hematomas, but a sudden increase in output can signal new injury. Injury to the lymphatic system is also possible during anterior exposure and may go undetected at the time of surgery. In the event such an injury is suspected, the chest tube output can be analyzed for fat content to confirm the diagnosis. Chest tube drainage is then typically extended until the lipid-laden output decreases. A diet low in fat content can aid in the reduction of lymphatic output. Injury to the pulmonary system can range from postoperative atelectasis to parenchymal injury at the time of exposure. The former is treated with aggressive pulmonary toilet, antibiotics if necessary, and drainage when indicated. Parenchymal injury, including pneumothorax, is managed with negative pressure chest tube decompression until stabilized. Occasionally significant and obvious damage to the lungs may require thoracic surgical consultation and repair. Postoperative pain from thoracotomy can be treated with subcostal anesthesia with long-acting agents. Postoperative infections, although less common than with posterior surgery, are treated with the same principles of debridement, irrigation, drainage, and appropriate antibiotics. Injury to the spinal cord is possible, especially during decompressions. The use of postoperative steroids in such an event remains controversial. Careful intraoperative neurophysiological monitoring, including somatosensory and motor evoked potentials, can be used, especially in the setting of a procedure requiring decompression. Blood pressure should be maintained by the anesthesia team to avoid hypotension, especially in the face of suspected potential cord injury.

On the other hand, the posterior approach offers an extensile and more familiar means for stabilizing thoracolumbar spine injuries while still giving sufficient access to decompress the spinal canal posteriorly if necessary. Danisa et al have shown through a retrospective analysis of surgical treatment of unstable thoracolumbar burst fractures that there was equal neurological improvement in the groups treated with anterior or posterior surgery and decreased operative time and blood loss in the posterior treated group.[71]

Potential complications during the posterior approach may be less life threatening, but may well be more common than following anterior surgery. Early postoperative infections are typically treated with aggressive irrigation and debridement and appropriate antibiotics. In the case of an early postoperative infection, if the instrumentation is stable, it need not be removed because the stability it affords aids in infection resolution. If the infection occurs or is diagnosed after solid fusion has occurred, then the instrumentation can be removed. Newer devices employing vacuum suction not only aid in the resolution of an acute infection but also facilitate wound closure. Injury to the spinal cord, especially during decompression, is possible during posterior approaches just as it is during anterior surgery, and is similarly managed. Postoperative hematomas can be a potential source of pain as well as wound dehiscence and potential infection. Drains should be placed following meticulous closure, and suction is employed until the daily output is minimal. Instrumentation failure is another potential complication. If indicated, prompt repair, removal, or reinstrumentation should be performed.

New Techniques

New techniques have had moderate influence on the treatment of thoracic fractures. Cervical, thoracolumbar, and low lumbar fractures have benefited more substantially from newer technologies due to their increased incidence and the importance of maximizing residual mobile spinal segments. Modern posterior instrumentation systems have led to an increase in the use of pedicle screws in the thoracic spine. Their use has increased the strength of fixation and the versatility of posterior instrumentation while virtually eliminating the iatrogenic loss of normal thoracic kyphosis commonly seen after the use of pure distraction devices (such as Harrington rods). Pedicle insertion techniques and the understanding of pedicle morphometry are essential tools for the experienced spinal surgeon. Of particular importance is the appreciation of the "watershed area" found between T3 and T7, where the thoracic pedicles are often too small for intrapedicular insertion.[72]

Vertebroplasty and kyphoplasty procedures have been used with increasing popularity in the thoracic spine.[73–75] The original use of this technique was in myeloma and other osteolytic spinal tumor lesions.[76,77] However, as the tumor experience increased and the degree of pain relief was appreciated, vertebroplasty and kyphoplasty procedures were initiated for the osteoporotic compression fractures commonly seen in the thoracic spine.[78] The general impression gleaned from the current literature is favorable for the use of both vertebroplasty and kyphoplasty in the treatment of compression fractures of the thoracic spine; however, there is still insufficient "hard scientific data" to state with certainty that this form of intervention improves the functional outcome without significant risk.[79]

The movement toward endoscopic, minimally invasive techniques applicable to spinal surgery continues. Currently, endoscopic thoracic diskectomies have proven effective, albeit with a large learning curve.[80] This technique can be used for the rare thoracic herniated disk with myelopathy, but is far more popular in the setting of an anterior release in combination with correction of deformity. More importantly, with the improvement in techniques and endoscopic instruments, this technique has obvious implications for endoscopic thoracic spine fracture management. In a similar fashion, metastatic disease of the thoracic spine similarly can be addressed through endoscopic techniques.[81] As our experience with endoscopic technique matures, and our equipment develops to address minimal access surgery, thoracic spine fracture management will be added to the list of pathologies safely and effectively managed via endoscopic techniques.

On the DVDs

Video 8–1 (Disk 1) Posterior Open Reduction T4–T5, Posterior Fusion T2–T7 with Instrumentation This patient sustained a fracture dislocation of T4–T5 with a spinal cord injury. It was treated with open reduction and posterior pedicle screw instrumentation and fusion from T2–T7. Instrumentation spanned two full levels above and below the injured motion segments to ensure adequate fixation.

References

1. Meyer PRJ. Fractures of the thoracic spine: T1 to T10. In: Meyer PRJ, ed. Surgery of Spine Trauma. New York: Churchill Livingstone; 1989:525–571

2. Miyasaka Y, Satomi K, Sugihara S, Tahara Y, Hayashi T, Ishii Y. Posterior fracture dislocation of the thoracic spine without neurologic deficit: a case report and short literature review. Spine 1993;18:2351–2354

3. Hanley EN, Eskay ML. Thoracic spine fractures. Orthopedics 1989;12:689–696

4. Brandser EA, el-Khoury GY. Thoracic and lumbar spine trauma. Radiol Clin North Am 1997;35:533–557

5. Petitjean ME, Mousselard H, Pointillart V, Lassie P, Senegas J, Dabadie P. Thoracic spinal trauma and associated injuries: should early spinal decompression be considered? J Trauma 1995;39:368–372

6. Saboe L, Reid DC, Davis LA. Spine trauma and associated injuries. J Trauma 1991;31:43–48

7. Capen DA, Gordon ML, Zigler JE, Garland DE, Nelson RW, Nagelberg S. Nonoperative management of upper thoracic spine fractures. Orthop Rev 1994;23:818–821

8. Argenson C, Boileau P, de Peretti F, Lovet J, Dalzotto H. Fractures of the thoracic spine (T1–T10): Apropos of 105 cases [in French]. Rev Chir Orthop Reparatrice Appar Mot 1989;75:370–386

9. Oda I, Abumi K, Lu D, Shono Y, Kaneda K. Biomechanical role of the posterior elements, costovertebral joints, and rib cage in the stability of the thoracic spine. Spine 1996;21:1423–1429

10. Hills MW, Delprado AM, Deane SA. Sternal fractures: associated injuries and management. J Trauma 1993;35:55–60

11. Berg EE. The sternal-rib complex: a possible fourth column in thoracic spine fractures. Spine 1993;18:1916–1919

12. Grootboom MJ, Govender S. Acute injuries of the upper dorsal spine. Injury 1993;24:389–392

13. Andriacchi T, Schultz A, Belytschko T, Galante J. A model for studies of mechanical interactions between the human spine and rib cage. J Biomech 1974;7:497–507

14. Lund JM, Chojnowski A, Crawford R. Multiple thoracic spine wedge fractures with associated sternal fracture: an unstable combination. Injury 2001;32:254–255

15. Gertzbein SD. Spine update: classification of thoracic and lumbar fractures. Spine 1994;19:626–628

16. Magerl F, Aebi M, Gertzbein SD, Harms J, Nazarian S. A comprehensive classification of thoracic and lumbar injuries. Eur Spine J 1994;3:184–201

17. Gertzbein SD. Neurologic deterioration in patients with thoracic and lumbar fractures after admission to the hospital. Spine 1994;19:1723–1725

18. Denis F. The three column spine and its significance in the classification of acute thoracolumbar spinal injuries. Spine 1983;8:817–831

19. Gertzbein SD, Court-Brown CM. Rationale for the management of flexion-distraction injuries of the thoracolumbar spine based on a new classification. J Spinal Disord 1989;2:176–183

20. Israel Z, Mosheiff R, Gross E, Muggia-Sullam M, Floman Y. Hyperextension fracture-dislocation of the thoracic spine with paraplegia in a patient with diffuse idiopathic skeletal hyperostosis. J Spinal Disord 1994;7:455–457

21. van Beek EJ, Been HD, Ponsen KK, Maas M. Upper thoracic spinal fractures in trauma patients: a diagnostic pitfall. Injury 2000;31:219–223

22. Bohlman HH. Treatment of fractures and dislocations of the thoracic and lumbar spine. J Bone Joint Surg Am 1985;67:165–169

23. Marczynski W, Kroczak S, Baranski M. Fractures of thoracic and lumbar spine; treatment and follow-up. Ann Transplant 1999;4:46–48

24. Albrecht T, von Schlippenbach J, Stahel PF, Ertel W, Wolf KJ. The role of whole body spiral CT in the primary workup of polytrauma patients: comparison with conventional radiography and abdominal sonography. Rofo 2004;176:1142–1150. German

25. Bondurant FJ, Colter HB, Kulkarni MV, McArdle CB, Harris JHJ. Acute spinal cord injury: a study using physical examination and magnetic resonance imaging. Spine 1990;15:161–168

26. Kulkarni MV, McArdle CB, Kopanicky D. Acute spinal cord injury: MR imaging at 1.5T. Radiology 1987;164:837–843

27. Brightman RP, Miller CA, Rea GL, Chakeres DW, Hunt WE. Magnetic resonance imaging of trauma to the thoracic and lumbar spine: the importance of the posterior longitudinal ligament. Spine 1992;17:541–550

28. Meyer S. Thoracic spine trauma. Semin Roentgenol. 1992;27:254–261

29. Bolesta MJ, Bohlman HH. Mediastinal widening associated with fractures of the upper thoracic spine. J Bone Joint Surg Am 1991;73:447–450

30. Groskin SA. Selected topics in chest trauma. Radiology 1992;183:605–617

31. White AA, Panjabi MM. Clinical Biomechanics of the Spine. 2nd ed. Philadelphia: Lippincott; 1990

32. Ohana N, Sheinis D, Rath E, Sasson A, Atar D. Is there a need for lumbar orthosis in mild compression fracture of the thoracolumbar spine? A retrospective study comparing the radiographic results between early ambulation with and without lumbar orthosis. J Spinal Disord 2000;13:305–308

33. Nash CLJ, Schatzinger LH, Brown RH, Brodkey J. The unstable thoracic compression fracture: its problems and the use of spinal cord monitoring in the evaluation of treatment. Spine 1977;2:261–265

34. Schweighofer F, Hofer HP, Wildburger R, Stockenhuber N, Bratschitsch G. Unstable fractures of the upper thoracic spine. Langenbecks Arch Chir 1997;382:25–28

35. Lee BJ, Lee SR, Yoo TY. Paraplegia as a complication of percutaneous vertebroplasty with polymethylmethacrylate: a case report. Spine 2002;27:E419–E422

36. Kallmes DF, Schweickert PA, Marx WF, Jensen ME. Vertebroplasty in the mid- and upper thoracic spine. AJNR Am J Neuroradiol 2002;23:1117–1120

37. Zoarski GH, Snow P, Olan WJ, et al. Percutaneous vertebroplasty for osteoporotic compression fractures: quantitative prospective evaluation of long-term outcomes. J Vasc Interv Radiol 2002;13:139–148

38. Coumans JV, Reinhardt MK, Lieberman IH. Kyphoplasty for vertebral compression fractures: 1 year clinical outcomes from a prospective study. J Neurosurg 2003;99(Suppl 1):44–50

39. McKiernan F, Faciszewski T, Jensen R. Quality of life following vertebroplasty. J Bone Joint Surg Am 2004;86-A:2600–2606

40. Nasca R, Lemons JE, Walker J, Batson S. Multiaxis cyclic biomechanical testing of Harrington, Luque, and Drummond implants. Spine 1990;15:15–20

41. Sasso RC, Colter HB, Reuben JD. Posterior fixation of thoracic and lumbar spine fractures using DC plates and pedicle screws. Spine 1991;16(Suppl 3):S134–S139

42. Sasso RC, Colter HB. Posterior instrumentation and fusion for unstable fractures and fracture-dislocations of the thoracic and lumbar spine: a comparative study of three fixation devices in 70 patients. Spine 1993;18:450–460

43. Yue JJ, Sossan A, Selgrath C, et al. The treatment of unstable thoracic spine fractures with transpedicular screw instrumentation: a three-year consecutive series. Spine 2002;27:2782–2787

44. Suk SI, Kim WJ, Lee SM, Kim JH, Chung ER. Thoracic pedicle screw fixation in spinal deformities: are they really safe. Spine 2001;26:2049–2057

45. Khoo LT, Beisse R, Potulski M. Thoracoscopic-assisted treatment of thoracic and lumbar fractures: a series of 371 consecutive cases. Neurosurgery 2002;51(Suppl):S104–S117

46. Hertlein H, Hartl WH, Piltz S, Schurmann M, Andress HJ. Endoscopic osteosynthesis after thoracic spine trauma: a report of two cases. Injury 2000;31:333–336

47. Bohlman HH, Freehafer A, DeJak J. The results of treatment of acute injuries of the upper thoracic spine with paralysis. J Bone Joint Surg Am 1985;67:360–369

48. Bracken MB, Shepard MJ, Collins WF. A randomized, controlled trial of methylprednisolone or naloxone in the treatment of acute spinal-cord injury: results of the Second National Acute Spinal Cord Injury Study. N Engl J Med 1990;322:1405–1411

49. Morgan TH, Wharton GW, Austin GN. The results of laminectomy in patients with incomplete spinal cord injuries. Paraplegia 1971;9:14–23

50. Braakman R, Fontijne WP, Zeegers R, Steenbeek JR, Tanghe HL. Neurological deficit in injuries of the thoracic and lumbar spine: a consecutive series of 70 patients. Acta Neurochir (Wien) 1991;111:11–17

51. Carlson GD, Minato Y, Okada A. Early time-dependent decompression for spinal cord injury: vascular mechanisms of recovery. J Neurotrauma 1997;14:951–962

52. Guha A, Tator CH, Endrenyi L, Piper I. Decompression of the spinal cord improves recovery after acute experimental spinal cord compression injury. Paraplegia 1987;25:324–339

53. Aebi M, Mohler J, Zach G, Morscher E. Indication, surgical technique, and results of 100 surgically-treated fractures and fracture-dislocations of the cervical spine. Clin Orthop Relat Res 1986;203:244–257

54. Wilberger JE. Diagnosis and management of spinal cord trauma. J Neurotrauma 1991;8(Suppl 1):S21–S30

55. Tator CH, Duncan EG, Edmonds VE, Lapczak LI, Andrews DF. Comparison of surgical and conservative management in 208 patients with acute spinal cord injury. Can J Neurol Sci 1987;14:60–69

56. Benzel EC, Larson SJ. Functional recovery after decompressive operation for thoracic and lumbar spine fractures. Neurosurgery 1986;19:772–778

57. Krengel WFI, Walter F, Anderson PA, Henley MB. Early stabilization and decompression for incomplete paraplegia due to a thoracic-level spinal cord injury. Spine 1993;18:2080–2087

58. Sapkas GS, Papagelopoulos PJ, Papadakis SA, Themistocleous GS, Stathakopoulos DP, Efstathiou P. Thoracic spinal injuries: operative treatment and neurologic outcomes. Am J Orthop 2003;32:85–88

59. McKinley W, Meade MA, Kirschblum S, Barnard B. Outcomes of early surgical management versus late or no surgical intervention after acute spinal cord injury. Arch Phys Med Rehabil 2004;85:1818–1825

60. Place HM, Donaldson DH, Brown CW, Stringer EA. Stabilization of thoracic spine fractures resulting in complete paraplegia: a long-term retrospective analysis. Spine 1994;19:1726–1730

61. Rechtine GR, Bono PL, Cahill D, Bolesta MJ, Chrin AM. Postoperative wound infection after instrumentation of thoracic and lumbar fractures. J Orthop Trauma 2001;15:566–569

62. Singh K, Eichenbaum M, Fitzhenry L, et al. Evaluation and management of thoracolumbar fractures: anterior approach. In: Reitman CA, ed. Management of Thoracolumbar Fractures. Rosemont, IL: American Academy of Orthopaedic Surgeons; 2004:79–84

63. Lemole GM, Bartolomei J, Henn JS, Sonntag VKH. Thoracic fractures. In: Vaccaro A, ed. Fractures of the Thoracic, Cervical and Lumbar Spine. Manhattan: Marcel Dekker. 2002:407–441

64. Fayyazi AH, Hugate RR, Pennypacker J, Gelb DE, Ludwig SC. Accuracy of computed tomography in assessing thoracic pedicle screw malposition. J Spinal Disord Tech 2004;17:367–371

65. McLain RF, Burkus JK, Benson DR. Segmental instrumentation for thoracic and thoracolumbar fractures: prospective analysis of construct survival and five-year follow-up. Spine J 2001;1:310–323

66. Hamilton A, Webb JK. The role of anterior surgery for vertebral fractures with and without cord compression. Clin Orthop Relat Res 1994;300:79–89

67. Bradford DS, McBride GG. Surgical management of thoracolumbar spine fractures with incomplete neurologic deficits. Clin Orthop Relat Res 1987;218:201–216

68. Knop C, Fabian HF, Bastian L, et al. Fate of transpedicular intervertebral bone graft after posterior stabilization of thoracolumbar burst fractures. Eur Spine J 2002;11:251–257

69. Knop C, Bastian L, Lange U, Oeser M, Zdichavsky M, Blauth M. Complications in the surgical treatment of thoracolumbar burst injuries. Eur Spine J 2002;11:214–226

70. Oskouian RJ, Johnson JP. Vascular complications in anterior thoracolumbar spinal reconstruction. J Neurosurg 2002;96:1–5

71. Danisa OA, Shaffrey CI, Jane JA, et al. Surgical approaches for the correction of unstable thoracolumbar burst fractures: a retrospective analysis of treatment outcomes. J Neurosurg 1995;83: 977–983

72. McLain RF, Ferrara L, Kabins M. Pedicle morphometry in the upper thoracic spine: limits to safe screw placement in older patients. Spine 2002;27:2467–2471

73. Chiras J, Depriester C, Weill A, Sola-Martinez MT, Deramond H. Percutaneous vertebral surgery: technics and indications. J Neuroradiol 1997;24:45–59

74. Heini PF, Walchli B, Berlemann U. Percutaneous transpedicular vertebroplasty with PMMA: operative technique and early results: a prospective study for the treatment of osteoporotic compression fractures. Eur Spine J 2000;9:445–450

75. Cortet B, Cotten A, Boutry N, et al. Percutaneous vertebroplasty in the treatment of osteoporotic vertebral compression fractures: an open prospective study. J Rheumatol 1999;26:2222–2228

76. Galibert P, Deramond H, Rosat P, Le Gars D. Preliminary note on the treatment of vertebral angioma by percutaneous acrylic vertebroplasty. Neurochirurgie 1987;33:166–168

77. Cotten A, Dewatre F, Cortet B, et al. Percutaneous vertebroplasty for osteolytic metastases and myeloma: effects of the percentage of lesion filling and the leakage of methylmethacrylate at clinical follow-up. Radiology 1996;200:525–530

78. Lieberman IH, Dudeney S, Reinhardt MK, Bell G. Initial outcome and efficacy of "kyphoplasty" in the treatment of painful osteoporotic vertebral compression fractures. Spine 2001;26:1631–1637

79. Jarvik JG, Kallmes DF, Mirza SK. Vertebroplasty: learning more, but not enough. Spine 2003;28:1487–1489

80. Huntington CF, Murrell WD, Betz BR, Cole BA, Clements DH, Balsara RK. Comparison of thoracoscopic and open thoracic discectomy in a live bovine model for anterior spinal fusion. Spine 1998;23:1699–1702

81. McLain RF, Lieberman IH. Endoscopic approaches to metastatic thoracic disease. Spine 2000;25:1855–1857

9 Thoracolumbar and Lumbar Spine Trauma

Steven M. Theiss

Though the most common spine fracture, thoracolumbar and lumbar spine fractures are relatively rare, occurring at a rate estimated at 64 injuries per 100,000 persons per year. These fractures are commonly associated with concomitant injuries and prolonged hospitalization.[1] In evaluating a series of blunt trauma patients presenting to a level 1 trauma center, just over 6% of the patients who underwent thoracolumbar radiography had vertebral injuries. The most common level injured is L1, followed by L2, L3, and then T12.[2] The most common injury at the thoracolumbar junction was a compression fracture, whereas the most common injury to the lumbar spine was a spinous process fracture.

The high prevalence of injuries at the thoracolumbar junction, as well as the specific vertebral injuries seen, has been attributed to several factors. First are the anatomical differences in the thoracic and lumbar regions. These include the transition from thoracic kyphosis to lumbar lordosis, the change in the orientation of the facet joints from a coronal to a sagittal orientation, and a change in the relative flexibility of the spine as one transitions from the thoracic to the lumbar region.[2] Specific anatomical features of the vertebral bodies themselves also influence the pattern of fractures seen in this region. Stress concentrations in the vertebral bodies tend to be greatest at the base of the pedicles where there is thinning of the posterior vertebral body cortex. This is also the area of greatest tensile and compressive strain, therefore causing this to be a common area of fracture initiation.[3,4]

Classification

There are several purposes and requirements for any classification system. It should provide understandable terminology to allow communication and research, supply information concerning the severity of injury, and guide choice of treatment.[5] Numerous classification systems have been proposed for fractures of the lumbar spine and thoracolumbar junction.[5–13] These classifications have been based on various aspects of the injury, including the anatomy of the injury, the mechanism of the injury, or the resultant stability of the injury. Yet, despite the variety of classifications available, there is no single classification that is universally accepted. In fact, there really is no classification that the clinician can use to unequivocally plan

appropriate treatment for the majority of thoracolumbar injuries.

Perhaps the simplest and most widely utilized modern classification is that of Denis.[8,9] Denis was the first to introduce the concept of the three-column spine and describe its relationship to spinal stability. In defining three columns of the spine, he simply expanded upon the two-column concepts that had previously existed. According to Denis, the posterior column consists of the posterior bony arch (specifically the pedicles, lamina, spinous process, and transverse process) as well as the alternating ligamentous structures, namely, the supraspinous ligament, interspinous ligament, facet capsule, and ligamentum flavum. The middle column is the posterior longitudinal ligament, the posterior anulus, and the posterior wall of the vertebral body, whereas the anterior column consists of the anterior longitudinal ligament, the anterior anulus, and the anterior part of the vertebral body. Using these definitions, Denis then described four anatomical types of thoracolumbar injuries, along with subclassifications. The mechanism of each type of fracture was also described, but this classification was an anatomical classification. The first type of fracture described was a compression fracture, which consisted of failure of the anterior column under compression, with tensile failure of the posterior column associated with severe anterior collapse **(Fig. 9–1)**. The defining feature of this injury is that the middle column is intact, and there is no subluxation or retropulsion of bone toward the neural elements. Compression fractures are subdivided into anterior and lateral compression subtypes. The second type of fracture, the so-called burst fracture, results from an axial loading force. In this type of fracture, there is failure of both the anterior and middle columns with retropulsion of the posterior cortex of the vertebral body back toward the neural elements. The posterior column is often involved as well, usually with a vertical split of the lamina and widening of the interpedicular distance **(Fig. 9–2)**. These fractures are further subclassified into types A through E. Types A, B, and C represent retropulsion and fracture of both end plates, the superior end plate and the inferior end plate, respectively. Type D burst fractures represent a combined burst rotation fracture that can radiographically mimic a fracture dislocation, but with primary pathognomonic features of a burst fracture, whereas type E describes a lateral burst fracture with preferential involvement of the lateral cortex of the vertebral body. The third anatomical type of

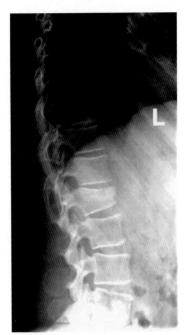

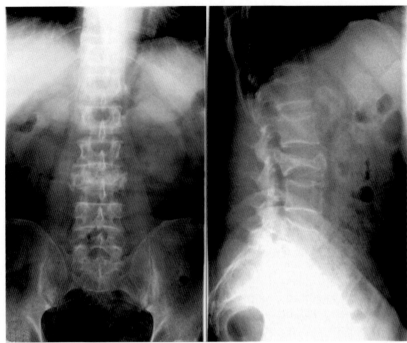

Figure 9–1 This patient sustained a compression fracture of L1 with compression of the anterior column but intact posterior cortex of the vertebral body. Tensile failure of the posterior column is associated with anterior collapse of 50% or greater.

A,B

Figure 9–2 **(A)** Anteroposterior (AP) and **(B)** lateral lumbar radiographs show an L3 burst fracture with loss of height and retropulsion of the posterior vertebral cortex. Note the widening of the interpedicular distance on the AP radiograph.

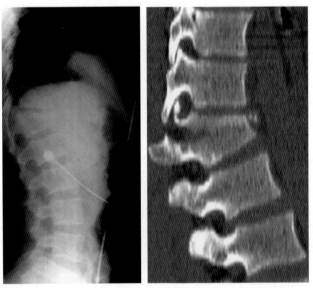

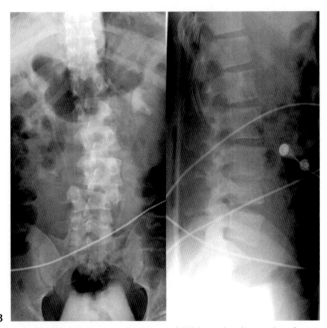

A,B

Figure 9–3 **(A)** Lateral radiograph and **(B)** sagittal computed tomographic reconstruction of a seat-belt-type injury with tensile failure of the posterior and middle column. This particular fracture shows compression of the anterior column.

A,B

Figure 9–4 **(A)** Anteroposterior and **(B)** lateral radiographs of a patient with an L3– L4 fracture dislocation. This injury results in failure of all three columns of the spine.

fracture described by Denis is the seat-belt-type injury. This describes failure of the posterior and middle columns under tension, with the axis of rotation about the anterior column, which acts as a hinge (**Fig. 9–3**). Finally, Denis described the fracture dislocation, which involves failure of all three columns (**Fig. 9–4**).[9] Instability was then defined as mechanical, neurological, or both, and depends upon the integrity of the middle column. Denis hypothesized that loss of the integrity of the middle column, in conjunction with injury to either the anterior or posterior column, resulted in instability. Yet, despite the popularity of this classification, it does not give any specific treatment recommendations.

In an effort to help the surgeon plan specific treatment, others have developed more detailed and comprehensive classification systems that take into account other factors associated with the injury, including comminution, deformity, and displacement.[6,7,11,14] The most comprehensive of these is the classification of Magerl et al.[5] This classification is outlined in **Table 9–1** and is based on the pathomorphological characteristics of the injury; it is comprehensive and can also help guide treatment. The first category is based on one of three types of spinal injury, which can be discerned on routine radiographs. These three types of injury are vertebral body compression, resulting from a compressive force; anterior and posterior element injury with distraction, resulting from a tensile force; and anterior and posterior element injury with rotation, resulting from axial torques. Each type of injury is then divided into three groups and then subgroups according to more detailed morphological criteria. This classification, though more complicated than that postulated by Denis, is comprehensive and can be used to help formulate both operative and nonoperative treatment options.[5]

Clinically, perhaps the most useful classification system is the load-sharing classification of McCormack et al.[11] This is the only classification that is used exclusively to plan surgical intervention. This classification applies specifically to three-column fractures that require operative treatment, and attempts to define which fractures are most amenable to short-segment stabilization and which require more significant intervention consisting of either anterior structural bone grafting or multilevel fixation. This classification considers the comminution, displacement, and deformity of the fractured segment and assigns 1 to 3 points for each category, with 3 being more

severe (**Fig. 9–5**). A score of 9 indicates the most instability possible. The authors recommend that fractures with scores less than 7 are amenable to short-segment posterior instrumentation, whereas those with scores of 7 or greater require anterior structural grafting or multilevel fixation.[11]

Nonoperative Treatment

The goals of treatment of thoracolumbar fractures are clear: to ensure spinal stability, ensure spinal alignment, and potentiate neurological recovery. As with any fracture, nonoperative treatment of thoracolumbar injuries is desirable if the treatment leads to clinical success without increased morbidity. Although the role of nonoperative treatment for thoracolumbar fractures is clearly established for some fracture types, its utility in others is highly debatable. In fact, the clinician really has very little level 1 evidence to support decision making. Unfortunately, even the ultimate anatomical parameters that need to be achieved to ensure a good result are debatable.[15–17] Clearly, spinal stability must be achieved to avoid a new or progressive neurological injury either during or following treatment. Spinal stability, though, is difficult to define. Whitesides defined a stable spine as a spine that can withstand forces in multiple directions without progressive deformity or progressive neurological deficit.[18] The most important aspect of spinal stability to achieve is protection of the neural elements. In injuries with complete bony and diskoligamentous disruption, the spine is unstable to all and any forces, and the need for operative stabilization is clear. Although some authors have advocated prolonged recumbency as treatment in some patients, it should be used only if operative stabilization is not possible.[19–21] In instances where spinal stability to only isolated forces is compromised, the relative merits of operative repair are less clear and are dependent on the nature of the injury. We therefore will discuss nonoperative treatment for each specific Denis fracture type.

Compression Fractures

Nonoperative treatment is appropriate for the vast majority of Denis compression fractures. These fractures correspond with Magerl type A1 and A2 injuries. By definition,

Table 9—1   The AO Thoracolumbar Fracture Classification

Type A. Vertebral Body Compression
A1 Impaction Fractures
    A1.1 End plate impaction
    A1.2 Wedge impaction features
        1. Superior wedge impaction fracture
        2. Lateral wedge impaction fracture
        3. Inferior wedge impaction fracture
A2 Split Fractures
    A2.1 Sagittal split fracture
    A2.2 Coronal split fracture
    A2.3 Pincer fracture
A3 Burst Fractures
    A3.1 Incomplete burst fracture
        1. Superior incomplete burst fracture
        2. Lateral incomplete burst fracture
        3. Inferior incomplete burst fracture
    A3.2 Burst-split fracture
        1. Superior burst-split fracture
        2. Lateral burst-split fracture
        3. Inferior burst-split fracture
    A3.3 Complete split fracture
        1. Pincer burst fracture
        2. Complete flexion burst fracture
        3. Complete axial burst fracture

Type B. Anterior and Posterior Element Injury with Distraction
B1 Posterior Disruption Predominantly Ligamentous (Flexion-Distraction)
    B1.1 With transverse disruption of the disk
        1. Flexion-subluxation
        2. Anterior dislocation
        3. Flexion-subluxation/anterior dislocation with fracture of the articular process
    B1.2 With type A fracture of the vertebral body
        1. Flexion-subluxation + type A fracture
        2. Anterior dislocation + type A fracture
        3. Flexion-subluxation/anterior dislocation with fracture of the articular process + type A fracture
B2 Posterior disruption predominantly osseous (flexion-distraction injury)
    B2.1 Transverse bicolumn fracture
    B2.2 With disruption of the disk
        1. Disruption through the pedicle and disk
        2. Disruption through the pars interarticularis and disk (flexion-spondylolysis)
    B2.3 With type A fracture of the vertebral body
        1. Fracture through the pedicle + type A fracture

        2. Fracture through the pars interarticularis (flexion-spondylolysis) + type A fracture
B3 Anterior disruption through the disk (hypertension-shear injury)
    B3.1 Hyperextension-subluxation
        1. Without injury of the posterior column
        2. With injury of the posterior column
    B3.2 Hyperextension-spondylolysis
    B3.3 Posterior dislocation

Type C. Anterior and Posterior Element Injury with Rotation
C1 Type A injuries with rotation (compression injuries with rotation)
    C1.1 Rotational wedge fracture
    C1.2 Rotational split fractures
        1. Rotational sagittal split fracture
        2. Rotational coronal split fracture
        3. Rotational pincer split fracture
        4. Vertebral body separation
C2 Type B injuries with rotation
    C1.1-B.1 Injuries with rotation (flexion-distraction injuries with rotation)
        1. Rotational flexional subluxation
        2. Rotational flexional subluxation with unilateral articular process fracture
        3. Unilateral dislocation
        4. Rotational anterior dislocation without/with fracture of the articular processes
        5. Rotational flexional subluxation without/with unilateral articular process fracture + type A fracture
        6. Unilateral dislocation + type A fracture
        7. Rotational anterior dislocation without/with fracture of articular processes + type A fracture
    C2.2-B.2 Injuries with rotation (flexion-distraction injuries with rotation)
        1. Rotational transverse bicolumn fracture
        2. Unilateral flexion-spondylolysis with disruption of the disk
        3. Unilateral flexion-spondylolysis + type A fracture
    C2.3-B.3 Injuries wih rotation (hyperextension-shear injuries with rotation)
        1. Rotational hyperextension-subluxation without/with fracture of posterior vertebral elements
        2. Unilateral hyperextension-spondylolysis
        3. Posterior dislocation with rotation
C3 Rotational-shear injuries
    C3.1 Slice fracture
    C3.2 Oblique fracture

Source: Adapted with permission from Data from Magerl F, Aebi M, Gertzbein SD, Harms J, Nazarian S. A comprehensive classification of thoracic and lumbar injuries. Eur Spine J 1994;3:184–201.

Comminution/Involvement

1. Little: < 30% comminution on sagittal plane section CT

2. More: 30%–60% comminution

3. Gross: > 60% comminution

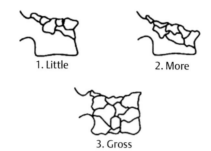

1. Little 2. More

3. Gross

Figure 9–5 The load-sharing classification is used to determine which three-column fractures are amenable to short-segment posterior instrumentation. Fractures with scores less than 7 are amenable to short-segment posterior stabilization. (With permission from Parker JW, Lane JR, Karaikovic EE, Gaines RW. Successful short-segment instrumentation and fusion for thoracolumbar spine fractures: a consecutive 4-year series. Spine 2000;25:1157–1170.)

Apposition of Fragments

1. Minimal: Minimal displacement on axial CT cut

2. Spread: At least 2 mm displacement of < 50% cross-section of body

3. Wide: At least 2 mm displacement of > 50% cross-section of body

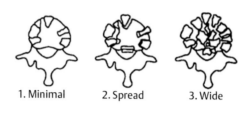

1. Minimal 2. Spread 3. Wide

Deformity Correction

1. Little: Kyphotic corrections ≤ 3° on lateral plain films

2. More: Kyphotic correction 4°–9°

3. Most: Kyphotic correction ≥ 10°

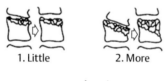

1. Little 2. More

3. Most

compression fractures are not associated with a neurological deficit; however, they are potentially unstable to flexion and compression forces.[5] Thus nonoperative treatment has focused on resisting these forces. Classically, the need for operative stabilization has depended on the degree of vertebral body collapse and resultant kyphosis, although the thresholds for operative intervention are variable.[15,22–24] Acceptable amounts of local kyphosis at the fracture site have varied by author to between 15 and 50 degrees.[15] To further complicate the issue, some studies have not been able to identify a strong correlation between final kyphosis and residual pain or disability.[15,23,25] The ability to significantly change the degree of collapse and kyphosis nonoperatively is questionable. Hyperextension bracing or casting can initially improve kyphosis and collapse, but the deformities tend to recur over time.[15,26,27]

Currently, the vast majority of compression fractures are treated nonoperatively. Surgery should be considered for patients with greater than 20 degrees of local kyphosis or progressive deformities indicating possible disruption of the posterior ligamentous tension band. This has been associated with anterior collapse of the vertebral body greater than 50%.[28] Recently, magnetic resonance imaging (MRI) has been used to evaluate the integrity of the posterior ligamentous complex in an effort to predict those fractures that will progressively collapse if treated non-operatively. However, an absolute threshold for surgical intervention does not exist. Other factors that must be considered are the overall sagittal alignment of the spine, pain, and the level of injury. Patients should be aggressively mobilized, and prolonged recumbency should be avoided.[15,26,29] A hyperextension brace can be used, but with the knowledge that this should not be counted on to significantly change the degree of collapse or kyphosis. Although braces are not structurally necessary in patients with 30% collapse or less, use of a brace may lessen pain.[15] Upright, weight-bearing radiographs are obtained prior to discharge and during follow-up. Bracing, if used, is recommended for 3 months, and fractures are followed for 6 months. With careful follow-up, fractures with progressive collapse or unacceptable kyphosis can be identified and stabilized.

Burst Fractures

The fracture type that generates the most controversy when discussing the role of nonoperative treatment is the Denis burst fracture, or Magerl type A3 fracture. Nonoperative treatment of burst fractures may be appropriate for patients without a neurological deficit or with an isolated root deficit only. Though there is no level 1 evidence that patients with a significant neurological deficit improve more reliably following decompression and stabilization,[30] accepted treatment of patients with significant neurological deficit is clearly surgical intervention. Traditionally, there have been three factors that have been relative indications for operative intervention in lumbar burst fractures: canal compromise, vertebral collapse, and kyphosis.[31] Each of these parameters has been studied in patients that are treated nonoperatively for thoracolumbar burst fractures. Several authors have found that retropulsed bone is resorbed from the spinal canal in patients that are treated nonoperatively.[26,32–36] Neurological deterioration has been observed, but the incidence is quite low.[37,38] Therefore, given that the degree of canal compromise reliably improves and that the incidence of neurological deterioration is low, the decision to treat a burst fracture surgically in a neurologically normal patient based on canal compromise alone is unfounded.

Although canal compromise reliably improves nonoperatively, the same cannot be said for kyphosis and vertebral body collapse. Vertebral collapse in and of itself is not a strong indication for operative intervention. The main issue pertaining to vertebral collapse is the resulting spine deformity, chiefly kyphosis. Numerous authors have observed that kyphosis cannot be improved with nonoperative treatment.[16,36,39–42] Initial improvement in kyphosis is often lost, even when the reduction is held with a rigid cast.[16,43] In fact, patients treated with no ex-

ternal mobilization, even in the presence of posterior element fractures, don't seem to develop any more deformity than patients that are braced.[44] Therefore, if the degree of kyphosis postinjury needs to be reduced, it must be done operatively. However, the degree of acceptable kyphosis is debatable. Long-term follow-up studies indicate that the degree of kyphosis does not correlate with pain and disability in a group of patients with deformities averaging 20 to 25 degrees.[23,41] Therefore, given the limitations of nonoperative management to correct deformity, local kyphosis of greater than 30 degrees resulting from a Denis burst or Magerl type A3 fracture should be treated with operative reduction and stabilization. Local kyphosis of 20 to 30 degrees should be considered for operative intervention. Other factors relating to the injury need to be considered, including overall spine sagittal alignment, concomitant injuries, medical comorbidities, and rate of progression. Patients without other operative indicators should be treated in a thoracolumbosacral orthosis (TLSO) to be worn whenever they are upright.

Patients with less than 20 degrees of kyphosis can be treated nonoperatively. This has been clearly shown by a prospective randomized study comparing operative and nonoperative treatment of thoracolumbar burst fractures without neurological deficit. In this study, patients without neurological deficit, with an average kyphosis of just over 10 degrees, had a superior outcome when treated nonoperatively compared with operative treatment.[36] Given this evidence, the vast majority of thoracolumbar burst fractures without neurological deficit should be treated nonoperatively. Operative intervention should be reserved for fractures with deformity at least greater than 20 degrees or progressive collapse. Low lumbar burst fractures, defined as fractures at L3 or below, are more amenable to nonoperative treatment than are fractures at the thoracolumbar junction. Some reports have indicated that patients with isolated root injuries can improve nonoperatively, although the results of surgery in this setting are superior.[45,46] Low lumbar burst fractures, due to the strong ligamentous attachments to the pelvis, have less propensity for kyphosis and deformity than those at the thoracolumbar junction.[47]

Flexion-Distraction Injuries

The indications for nonoperative management of Magerl type B fractures, which include Denis seat-belt-type injuries, are limited. By definition, these injuries involve at least two columns, and, therefore, they are all unstable to some, if not all, forces. In those injuries that consist primarily of soft tissue disruption, nonoperative treatment is not appropriate due to poor healing potential. These patients require operative stabilization. However, patients with transverse bony disruption of the posterior elements and middle vertebral column can be treated nonoperatively. These injuries are classified as Magerl Type B2.1, or the single-level Chance fracture, according to Denis.[9] These patients can be treated by extension reduction and immobilization in either a TLSO or a cast. If a TLSO is used, it must be worn at all times. Because the injury is entirely bony, there is excellent healing potential. Upright, weight-bearing radiographs should be closely followed to recognize loss of reduction or progressive deformity. Brace or cast immobilization should continue for a total of 12 weeks. Flexion and extension radiographs should be obtained at the completion of immobilization to ensure full union.

Fracture-Dislocations

Nonoperative treatment of Magerl type C fractures or Denis fracture-dislocations is mentioned only to discourage it. Because of the global instability resulting from the multicolumn injury, there is no way to mobilize the patient and still maintain spinal alignment nonoperatively. When used, nonoperative treatment must consist of prolonged recumbency. In turn, prolonged recumbency results in prolonged hospitalization and a high rate of complications associated with prolonged bed rest, such as venous thromboembolism, stasis ulcers, and pulmonary complications. Although some retrospective data exist that suggest prolonged bed rest on a kinetic bed does not result in any greater incidence of complications compared with a group treated operatively, it does result in significantly prolonged hospitalization.[21] The standard of care for fracture-dislocations is operative treatment and early mobilization.

Surgical Treatment

Indications for Surgical Treatment

Operative indications differ among the various types of fractures and will be discussed relative to each separate fracture type.

Compression Fractures

As mentioned, Denis compression fractures, corresponding to Magerl type A1 and type A2 fractures, rarely require surgical intervention. By definition, these fractures do not result in neurological injury. Surgical intervention is indicated in cases of thoracolumbar kyphosis greater than 30 degrees, or occasionally more minimal kyphosis resulting in overall sagittal decompensation. This most commonly occurs with multiple-level fractures. The final surgical indication is a Magerl split fracture (A2) with a resultant nonunion, or wide displacement of the split fragment indicating a potential nonunion.

Burst Fractures

The operative indications in Denis burst fractures, or Magerl type A3 injuries, are still controversial. The only absolute operative indication is a neurological deficit due to the injury. As discussed, there may be a role for nonoperative treatment of an isolated root injury due to a lower lumbar burst fracture, specifically in L3, L4, or L5. However, the literature justifying this is scant.[48] As a general rule, all patients with thoracolumbar burst fractures and neurological deficit should undergo operative treatment. Operative indications based upon degrees of canal compromise, percent of vertebral body collapse, and resultant deformity are relative indications, and the decision to operate should be made on a case-by-case basis. This is particularly true in light of the available data that fail to correlate patient outcome with ultimate degrees of deformity or vertebral collapse.[36,49,50] There are occasions, however, when operative intervention is indicated for deformity or collapse. Established parameters for surgery in the absence of neurological deficit are kyphosis of greater than 20 degrees, greater than 50% collapse, and greater than 50% canal compromise.[51] Of these parameters, the most important factor in deciding upon operative treatment is the degree of deformity, or kyphosis. Canal compromise reliably improves in patients treated nonoperatively, and neurological deterioration is very rare.[33,34,52] Therefore, the decision for surgery in neurologically normal patients should be made on the basis of kyphosis and vertebral body collapse. These indicators must be considered in the context of the overall clinical picture.

There is no absolute value that mandates surgery for any one of these parameters. Surgical intervention should be strongly considered in patients with greater than 30 degrees of kyphosis, or in patients with either progressive kyphosis or overall sagittal decompensation. In patients with stable kyphosis of less than 20 degrees, operative intervention is rarely indicated. As with patients with compression fractures, an MRI scan can be used to evaluate the posterior ligamentous complex. Injury to the posterior ligaments may help predict which patients will progressively collapse when treated nonoperatively. Finally, burst fractures with a split fragment may require surgical intervention when there is wide displacement of the split fragment or a nonunion develops (**Fig. 9–6**).

Flexion-Distraction Injuries

Operative treatment of flexion-distraction injuries, or Magerl type B injuries, is the rule. Nonoperative treatment is appropriate in the rare instance when the injury involves predominantly the osseous structures and the facet joints are intact in a patient without neurological injury. If the fracture can be posturally reduced and the reduction maintained with either a custom-molded hyperextension TLSO or cast, it will reliably heal because these injuries are stable in extension. However, full-time brace wear is

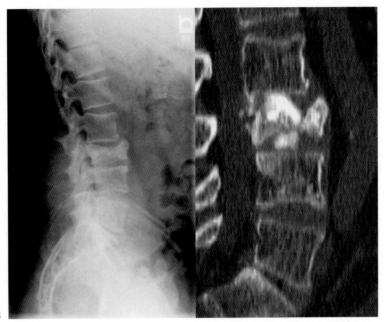

Figure 9–6 (A) This lateral radiograph shows a burst fracture in a patient with persistent pain. **(B)** The postdiskogram computed tomographic reconstruction shows contrast dye that has entered the nonunion site of a split fragment.

A,B

cumbersome, and the patient must be carefully followed for loss of reduction. Admittedly, the patient with a flexion-distraction injury amenable to nonoperative treatment is rare. Most commonly, these injuries require surgery. This is particularly true in injuries that disrupt the ligamentous structures or disk, which have no ability to heal nonoperatively even if anatomically reduced. Therefore, flexion-distraction injuries through the disk by definition require surgery. Surgery is also indicated when predominantly bony injuries cannot be anatomically reduced or concomitant vertebral body injuries result in significant deformity.

Fracture-Dislocations

Denis fracture-dislocations or Magerl type C injuries (rotational) are universally unstable and, of all the injuries, are most commonly associated with neurological injury.[5] Due to the inherent instability of these injuries, they are very difficult to treat nonoperatively and maintain stability and alignment. Therefore, they all require surgery. Nonoperative treatment is only appropriate in a patient who is unable to undergo operative intervention for medical reasons.

Surgical Anatomy and Approaches

Once the decision has been made to treat a fracture surgically, there are usually three options as to the surgical approach that can be used. These options are an anterior approach, a posterior approach, or a circumferential approach (both). The decision as to which approach is the most appropriate is based on several factors. The goals of the surgery are decompression of the neurological structures, restoration of spinal alignment, rigid stabilization of

the unstable spinal segments, and ultimate bony healing of the affected motion segments. If arthrodesis is involved, it is also desirous to fuse as few motion segments as possible.

Neurological Decompression

The first goal of surgery, in the face of a neurological injury, is decompression of the affected neural elements. The approach that best accomplishes this depends upon the region of the spine affected, the degree of compression, and the location of the compression in the spinal canal. For thoracolumbar junction and lumbar injuries, the compressed neurological structures consist of the spinal cord, the conus medullaris, and the cauda equina. The conus medullaris has a variable location in the thoracolumbar spine but is typically located at the level of the L1 vertebral body, or the L1–L2 disk. Caudad to the conus lies the cauda equina, with a corresponding nerve root exiting beneath each pedicle in the lumbar spine. Determining the location of the conus medullaris is paramount because this structure should not be directly manipulated during the surgical decompression. Decompression of this region should consist of a technique that spares traction or manipulation of the subarachnoid space. Both anterior and posterior approaches can be used to reduce anterior compression, whereas a posterior approach is necessary to address posterior neural compression due to soft tissue or bony impingement. The cauda equina can be carefully retracted during surgical decompression to assist in removal of bony or soft tissue fragments. This allows more flexibility in this anatomical region of the various surgical approaches. Anterior compression of the cauda equina can be addressed either anteriorly or posteriorly, whereas posterior compression is best corrected posteriorly. A further consideration in the lumbar spine is compromise of the intervertebral neuroforamen. This can also be decompressed through either approach, but only if recognized in the diagnostic evaluation. A circumferential (combined anterior-posterior) approach is almost never necessary to fully decompress the neural elements.

Reduction of Spinal Deformity

The next factor that must be considered in choosing the most suitable surgical approach is the ability to reduce the injury from the selected approach. This is most relevant in injuries that result in dislocation of the facet joints. It is often difficult to indirectly reduce facet dislocations from an anterior approach alone, and plans should be made to reduce facet dislocations posteriorly, with the facet joint under direct vision and manipulation. Aside from this consideration, good surgical outcomes can be expected with either anterior or posterior approaches for the vast majority of thoracolumbar injuries.[53–82] For a given injury, a logical assessment of the injury pattern and associated instability can guide the choice of surgical approach. Whenever possible, stabilization of a thoracolumbar fracture should directly reconstruct the bony and ligamentous structures that have been injured and have caused the resulting deformity or instability. The surgeon should avoid disrupting any remaining intact stabilizers. Forces can then be placed on the instrumentation to restore alignment, as well as sagittal and coronal balance. The ultimate stability of the construct depends on the number of motion segments instrumented, the forces that must be resisted by the construct following reduction, and the initial degree of instability. In general, the technique that ultimately results in the fewest motion segments being fused is preferable. Finally, the chosen approach must give a reasonable chance of a solid arthrodesis to maintain ultimate correction and alignment. Bone grafting techniques of the posterior elements alone, especially in the setting of high-energy fractures, results in less predictable arthrodesis compared with intervertebral bone grafting techniques that take advantage of the richly vascular vertebral bodies for bone grafting.[66,83]

Besides the considerations already discussed, there are some anatomical considerations that could influence the approach used for a specific injury. We have already mentioned the pertinent neuroanatomy and its influence on the decompression portion of the procedure. The main factor in determining the suitability of the anterior approach for a specific injury is the vascular anatomy. In the thoracolumbar region, the anterior approach is preferably retroperitoneal from the left side. This is desirable because the aorta on the left is easier to manipulate and retract than the vena cava on the right. The diaphragm often has to be taken down for exposure and reconstruction of injuries above L2. However, this consideration alone should not preclude treatment of upper lumbar injuries from an anterior approach if other aspects of the injury are better dealt with anteriorly. The biggest deterrent to anterior treatment for thoracolumbar injuries is the vascular anatomy in the lower lumbar region. The aortic bifurcation occurs in the region of the L4, L5 disk space, with the common iliac artery and vein usually crossing the L5 vertebral body. This makes anterior instrumentation of L5 or S1 difficult, if not impossible, due to the proximity of the vascular structures. The posterior approach to this region has no such anatomical constraints. Unfortunately, significant reconstruction of the anterior column is difficult from a posterior approach. This is particularly true when the injury has resulted in significant comminution of the anterior vertebral bodies necessitating placement of a large structural strut.

Posterior Surgical Approach

The surgical technique for the basic posterior approach and anterior approach is similar throughout the different regions of the thoracolumbar spine. The posterior approach is performed through a longitudinal incision over the spinous processes of the vertebrae to be exposed (see **Video 9–1, Disk 1**). During elective procedures, incisional blood loss can be reduced by injecting the dermis with 1:500,000 epinephrine. This is not done in the face of acute trauma because the epinephrine could injure exposed neural elements. Following dissection down to the thoracolumbar fascia, the fascia is split with electrocautery over the spinous processes. Using a Cobb elevator, the erector spinae musculature is then stripped subperiosteally from the spinous processes, lamina, and facet capsules of the posterior elements, working in a caudad to cephalad direction. This direction is necessary to effectively elevate the multifidi muscle, which attaches obliquely on the posterior elements in a caudad to cephalad direction. Dissection can then be carried laterally to expose the transverse processes, which are lateral to the superior facet at each level. Hemostasis is achieved by ensuring subperiosteal elevation of the erector spinae as well as local packing of previously exposed areas, while exposing other areas.

Anterior Surgical Approach

The preferred anterior approach to the thoracolumbar junction and distally is the retroperitoneal approach **(Fig. 9–7)** (see **Video 9–2, Disk 1**). This can either be done through an oblique incision in the flank, centered at the level of interest, or through a longitudinal paramedian incision parallel with the lateral border of the rectus sheath. The paramedian incision is best for lower lumbar exposure from L4 to S1. The oblique incision allows exposure of multiple levels, including the lumbosacral junction, but also allows takedown of the diaphragm, rib resection, and exposure of the lower thoracic spine. With either incision, the deep dissection is retroperitoneal. The transperitoneal approach can be used for exposure of the lumbosacral junction, but retroperitoneal exposure is generally quite comparable, with less potential risk of complications related to intra-abdominal

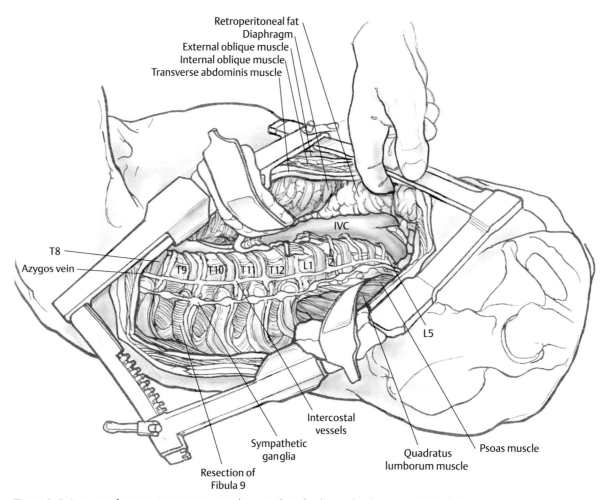

Retroperitoneal fat
Diaphragm
External oblique muscle
Internal oblique muscle
Transverse abdominis muscle

IVC

T8
Azygos vein

T9 T10 T11 T12 L1 2

L5

Intercostal
vessels

Sympathetic
ganglia

Quadratus
lumborum muscle

Psoas muscle

Resection of
Fibula 9

Figure 9–7 Drawing of an anterior retroperitoneal approach to the thoracolumbar spine. IVC, inferior vena cava.

exposure. Superficially, after dissection through the skin and subcutaneous fat, the three layers of the oblique musculature are split parallel with the skin incision. After the internal and external oblique are divided with electrocautery, the transversalis muscle is bluntly split until the retroperitoneal cavity is identified and entered. The peritoneum is stripped from the undersurface of the transversalis fascia, and the retroperitoneal cavity is entered, protecting the peritoneum. Once the retroperitoneal space is entered, the segmental artery and vein at each level are isolated and ligated. This allows exposure of the anterolateral aspect of the vertebral bodies and disks. The lumbosacral junction can be identified by palpating the sacral promontory, though a radiograph should be obtained intraoperatively to identify the proper level. Exposure of the lumbosacral junction is easiest between the two common iliac vessels, carefully retracting the ipsilateral iliac vein laterally. Exposure of the L4–L5 disk and above is best performed lateral to the aorta.

Timing of Surgery

There is no consensus regarding the optimal timing of surgery in patients with thoracolumbar injuries. The ideal time for surgical intervention to maximize neurological recovery is unknown. Animal studies have suggested that earlier decompression results in improved neurological recovery, but decompression had to be completed within 6 hours of the neurological insult.[84] These results have not been replicated in human trials. Early surgery in the setting of acute spinal cord injury does not seemingly lead to an increased chance of neurological deterioration, as was once thought.[85] There are retrospective cohort studies that suggest improved neurological recovery for patients undergoing earlier surgery, although a specific optimal time is not evident.[86,87] Prospective analysis is necessary before any definitive conclusions can be reached.[88] One setting where urgent surgery seems to be warranted is in the patient with a progressive neurological deficit.[85] The other factor influencing timing of surgical intervention in patients with acute thoracolumbar injuries is the overall medical condition of the patient. As previously mentioned, patients with thoracolumbar injuries often have other significant injuries.[1] With the lack of clear evidence regarding the benefit of urgent surgery, it is important to ensure that the patient is medically optimized prior to surgical intervention.

Surgical Techniques

Compression Fractures

Denis compression fractures, or Magerl type A1 fractures, that require operative stabilization are best treated with posterior instrumentation and arthrodesis. By definition, a compression fracture that results in severe deformity or unacceptable kyphosis is associated with disruption of the posterior ligamentous tension band. Therefore, surgical reconstruction should focus on reconstruction of this tension band.

As already discussed, the instrumentation and arthrodesis should span as few segments as possible. For injuries at the thoracolumbar junction, instrumentation can include two segments proximal to the injury and one segment distally.[64] Lumbar injuries should be instrumented one level above and below the level of the injury. The exception to these recommendations is an injury with significant comminution of the vertebral body. Although the classification by McCormack et al applies to three-column thoracolumbar fractures, the concept of avoiding short-segment constructs in fractures with significant comminution applies to compression fractures as well. Appropriate options in this circumstance include a longer posterior construct or anterior reconstruction.[11] For the more common posterior approach, patients are positioned prone on a radiolucent table. Prone positioning alone often helps to reduce the fracture. Thoracolumbar kyphosis can be reduced by fully extending the hips and placing padding under the anterior thighs on the table **(Fig. 9–8)**. A posterior approach as described earlier is performed to expose the posterior elements of the relevant levels. A radiograph or fluoroscopic image is always taken to verify the level. The exposure includes the transverse processes of all levels to be instrumented. By definition, with this specific type of injury there is no neurocompression, obviating the need for a decompressive procedure. Pedicle screw instrumen-

tation should be used whenever possible because it is biomechanically superior to a hook construct.[89] Following exposure, the landmarks for the placement of the pedicle screws are identified. The start position of the screws in the lumbar spine is the point where the transverse process, the superior facet, and the pars interarticularis intersect. The start hole is made with a pneumatic bur or handheld awl, and the pedicle is sounded with a blunt probe. Orientation of the pedicle in the sagittal plane can be judged on the localizing image taken during exposure. Orientation of the pedicle in the coronal plane varies according to the level being instrumented. The lateral to medial orientation of the pedicle decreases as the vertebral level moves from caudad to cephalad. At S1, the medial angulation of the pedicle is 35 degrees, and the medial angulation progressively decreases until T11 or T12, where the medial orientation of the pedicle is less than 10 degrees. Fluorography can be used as an aid during screw insertion but is not necessary in cases where landmarks are clear.

After placement of the screws, their position should be verified radiographically. The start position for placement of the thoracic pedicle screws is along the superior ridge of the transverse process in the cephalad/caudad direction, where it intersects with the lateral third of the superior facet **(Figs. 9–9A,B)**. After all screws are placed, the fracture can be reduced and stabilized. The rods are slightly undercontoured in the sagittal plane and seated initially in the screws superior to the fracture. The rods can then be carefully seated in the inferior screws, though care should be taken not to excessively torque the superior screws, particularly in patients with osteopenia, resulting in relatively poor screw purchase. The superior screws are then provisionally tightened, and compression is placed across the construct. This compression is the main reduction maneuver for this type of injury, rather than cantilever bending. Cantilever bending, or in situ bending during reduction, has been associated with increased screw pullout in short-segment constructs.[90] Following placement of the

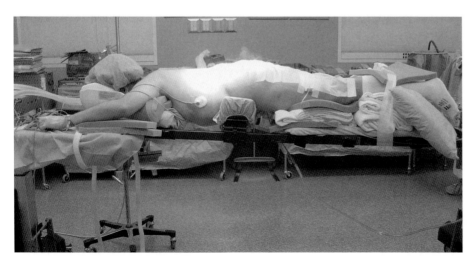

Figure 9–8 Prone positioning of a patient on a radiolucent Jackson table. The hips are fully extended in this patient with a kyphotic deformity to allow optimal correction of the deformity.

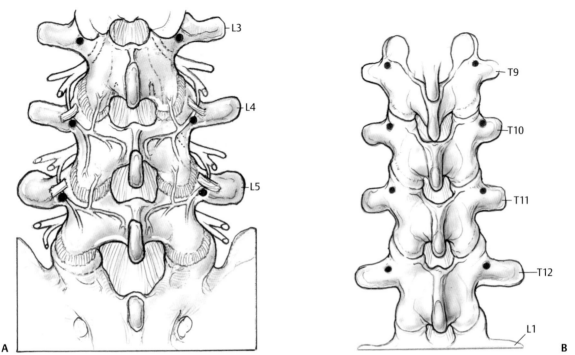

Figure 9–9 The anatomical landmarks for the start positions of the **(A)** lumbar and **(B)** lower thoracic pedicle screws are shown.

rods, autogenous iliac crest is harvested from the posterior superior iliac spine region either through a separate skin or through a fascial incision. Bone graft is placed between the transverse processes after decortication of the processes. Although autogenous bone graft is still preferred, other grafting options incorporating bone morphogenetic proteins and autogenous stem cells have shown promise in early clinical studies.[91] Finally, two-cross links are placed to increase the rigidity of the construct.

Burst Fractures

Just as there is considerable controversy in determining which burst fractures require operative intervention, there is also debate as to the best operative approach in those that require surgery. Numerous approaches have been advocated, including anterior alone, posterior alone, combined anterior-posterior through two incisions, and anterior and posterior constructs through a single posterior incision.[54,63,83,91–94]

Perhaps the most challenging aspect of treating these fractures is choosing which approach to use because there is scant scientific evidence to help decide which approach is best for a particular fracture. Good results have been shown with all of the approaches.[53,87,93,95] In general, studies directly comparing anterior and posterior approaches have shown comparable results, but with significantly reduced operative time and blood loss when addressing the fracture posteriorly.[91,92,96] However, posterior short-segment fixation alone for burst fractures with significant

vertebral body comminution has been shown to have a high rate of failure with residual kyphosis (**Fig. 9–10**).[11]

Ideal candidates for anterior surgery are patients with canal compromise greater than 80% with incomplete neurological deficit, severe vertebral body comminution, or kyphosis greater than 30 degrees (**Fig. 9–11A–E**) (see **Video 9–2,**

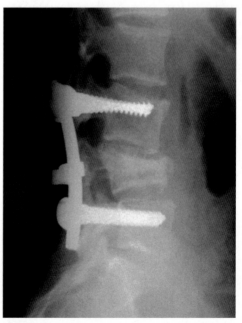

Figure 9–10 This patient underwent short-segment posterior instrumentation for an L4 burst fracture. This radiograph is 6 weeks postoperative and demonstrates loss of correction with increased kyphosis.

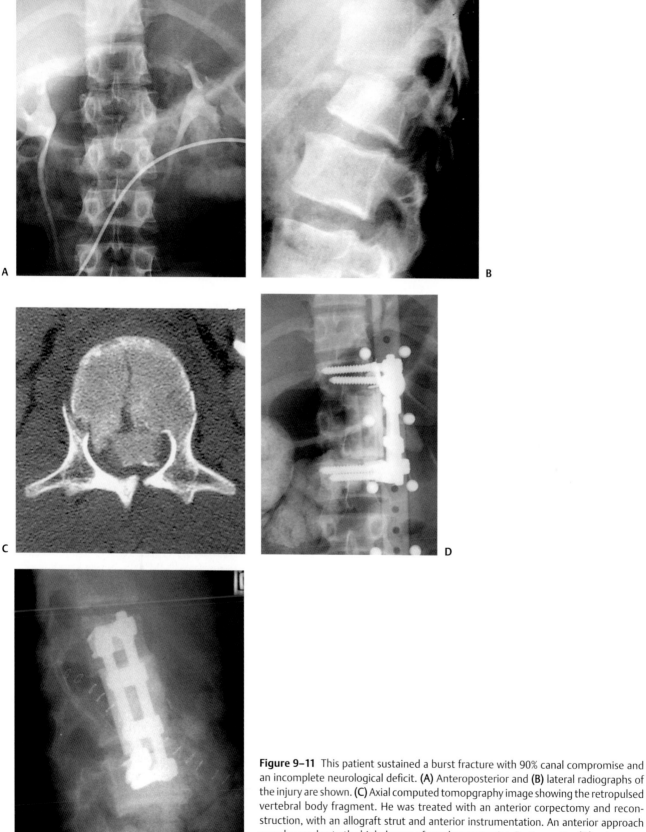

Figure 9–11 This patient sustained a burst fracture with 90% canal compromise and an incomplete neurological deficit. **(A)** Anteroposterior and **(B)** lateral radiographs of the injury are shown. **(C)** Axial computed tomopgraphy image showing the retropulsed vertebral body fragment. He was treated with an anterior corpectomy and reconstruction, with an allograft strut and anterior instrumentation. An anterior approach was chosen due to the high degree of canal compromise. Postoperative **(D)** anteroposterior and **(E)** lateral radiographs of the reconstruction.

Disk 1).[97] To perform an anterior decompression, reduction, and stabilization, the patient is positioned in the right lateral decubitus position on the operating table with the use of a beanbag. A kidney rest is elevated, and the table is flexed to stretch the oblique musculature and create more room between the inferior costal margin and the iliac crest. The bottom knee is flexed to help stabilize the patient in this position, but the peroneal nerve of this leg must be padded and protected. Thigh-high antiembolism stockings hose and pneumatic compression stockings are placed on both legs for deep vein thrombosis (DVT) prophylaxis. Anterior retroperitoneal exposure should extend from the superior end plate of the vertebral body cephalad to the fracture, to the inferior end plate of the body caudad to the fracture. A radiograph should verify the level. Care should be taken not to surgically violate the disk spaces, which are not to be included in the fusion or reconstruction. The fractured body, as well as the bodies above and below the injured level, is then exposed by subperiosteally elevating the psoas muscle, with the aid of electrocautery. The psoas should be elevated laterally until the base of the pedicle is exposed. Again, this should include the ipsilateral pedicles of the levels above and below the fracture to aid in accurate placement of the instrumentation.

After exposure is completed, the disks above and below the fractured body should first be removed. A Cobb elevator and curet can be used to separate the cartilaginous end plate from the subchondral bone, greatly aiding the diskectomy. The diskectomy then defines the extent of the vertebral body and can aid in identification of the spinal canal. The corpectomy can then be performed. Every effort should be made to first identify the spinal canal prior to removing significant portions of the vertebral body to reduce blood loss from the richly vascular cancellous vertebrae. The canal can be identified along the end plates of the vertebral bodies above or below the fracture or by resecting the ipsilateral pedicle at the level of the fracture. After the canal is identified, the anterior two thirds of the vertebral body can be removed quickly with an osteotome and rongeur. Blood loss can be reduced with bone wax and packing. Preoperatively, it should be determined what portion of the vertebral body has been retropulsed into the spinal canal and the maneuver required to remove this fragment. For instance, if this fragment comes from the superior end plate, it is best removed by rotating the fragment out of the canal inferiorly **(Fig. 9–12)**. Oftentimes, significant epidural bleeding accompanies the decompression. If such bleeding cannot be controlled with bipolar electrocautery, it is best to complete the entire decompression prior to gaining hemostasis by gently packing the epidural space with Gelfoam. A disadvantage to an anterior procedure is that traumatic posterior dural tears cannot be directly repaired. In this instance, cerebrospinal fluid (CSF) leakage should be treated with strict supine bed rest postoperatively.

After the corpectomy and hemostasis, attention is turned to the reconstruction and fusion. Bone grafting options for the fusion include tricortical iliac crest autograft, structural

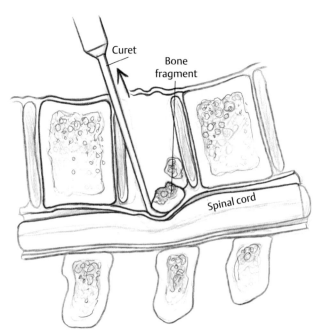

Figure 9–12 When a fragment from the superior end plate is retropulsed into the spinal canal, it is best removed by rotating the fragment with a curet in an inferior and anterior direction to avoid iatrogenic neurological injury.

allograft, or a fusion cage. Each grafting method has specific advantages and disadvantages. Autograft harvest risks donor site morbidity, whereas structural allograft is associated with a higher pseudarthrosis rate.[98] Perhaps the best solution is a fusion cage. This can provide not only structural anterior column support but also the benefits of autograft fusion rates because the cage can be packed with autograft harvested from the removed vertebral body.[99] Anatomical reduction must be achieved prior to grafting. In anterior burst fracture surgery, this is accomplished by distraction across the corpectomy site. Several different anterior instrumentation systems are available, including screw–rod systems, conventional plates, and locking plates. All have been documented to have similar results.[63,66,96,100,101] Distraction is best placed across the corpectomy site after screws are placed in the vertebrae above and below the fracture site. To place the instrumentation correctly, it is imperative to identify the base of the pedicle of the vertebrae in which the screws will be placed. This allows proper identification of the starting point for the posterior screw in the posterior half of the vertebral body. The screw can then be safely oriented away from the spinal canal while still achieving maximum length and purchase. Errors particularly occur when the instrumentation is placed too far anteriorly. This actually causes the screws to be angled toward the spinal canal. After distraction is placed across the corpectomy site, the graft of choice can be placed **(Fig. 9–13A,B)**. The end plates should be decorticated to aid in fusion. The remainder of the instrumentation can then be placed. Postoperatively, the patient is mobilized as quickly as possible and fitted with a TLSO that is worn for 3 months.

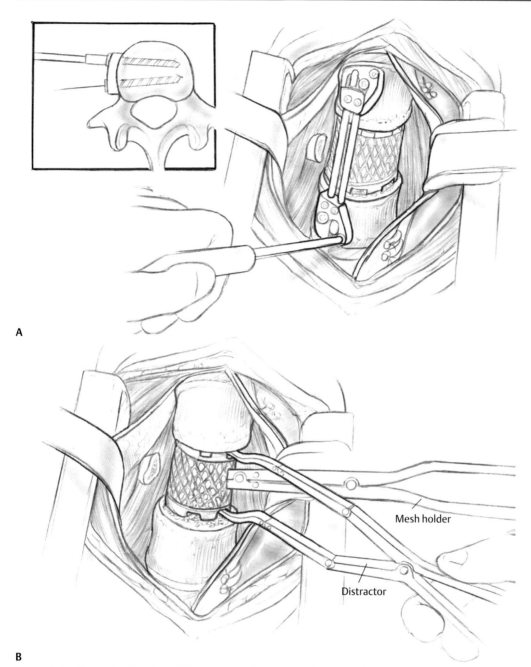

A

B

Mesh holder

Distractor

Figure 9–13 Illustration showing **(A)** the insertion of screws into the vertebral body, followed by **(B)** distraction of the corpectomy site and placement of the graft. The vertebral screws can easily be used to distract the corpectomy site.

Alternatively, a posterior approach can be used. This is best for fractures that are amenable to a short-segment posterior construct according to the load-sharing classification.[11] In fractures that are not amenable to a short-segment posterior construct, the posterior approach can still be used, but it may need to include more motion segments. The procedure is performed with the patient positioned prone on a radiopaque table. The patient's hips are fully extended in an effort to reduce the kyphotic deformity at the fracture site. Antiembolism stockings and pneumatic compression boots are applied for DVT prophy-

laxis. A posterior approach is performed, exposing the posterior elements and transverse processes of the fractured level, as well as the levels to be instrumented.

First, the instrumentation is placed. For a short-segment construct, this consists of pedicle screws in the levels above and below the fractured vertebrae. The screws are placed using the routine anatomical landmarks previously described with the aid of fluorography. Next, a single rod is placed unilaterally, and distraction is placed across the fracture site. This indirectly begins to decompress the neural elements through ligamentotaxis. Attention is now

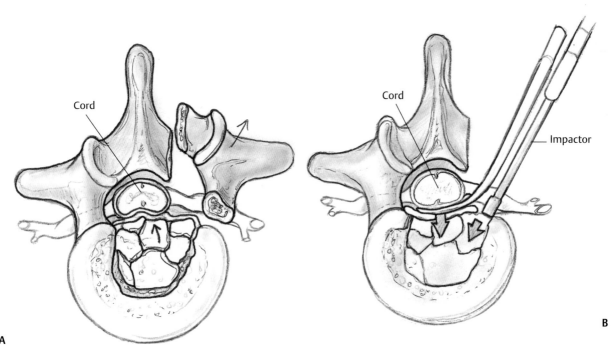

Figure 9–14 **(A)** A posterolateral decompression is done by first removing the ipsilateral facet and pedicle. **(B)** Next, a cavity is created in the vertebral body, and the retropulsed fragments are reduced into the cavity.

turned to direct decompression of the neural elements. In the region of the conus medullaris and above, this should be done by a posterolateral approach, whereas in the region of the cauda equina, it can be done posteriorly. A posterolateral technique begins by removing the lateral portion of the ipsilateral lamina, including the adjacent facet joint **(Fig. 9–14A,B)**. The pedicle is identified, as well as the root exiting caudad to the pedicle. While protecting the root and dura, a pneumatic bur is used to drill out the middle of the pedicle, and a curet is then used to remove the medial wall. This allows visualization of the posterior cortex of the fractured vertebral body. A void can then be created in the body with tamps and curets, and the retropulsed fragments can be pushed anteriorly into the void, directly decompressing the subarachnoid space. If a dorsal dural tear is encountered, it should be primarily repaired. Routinely, the posterolateral decompression need only be performed from one side to fully decompress the entire spinal canal. In the cauda equina region, a routine laminectomy can be performed, and the retropulsed fragment can be manipulated after carefully retracting the ipsilateral neural elements. Following decompression, the contralateral rod is placed, and distraction is placed across this segment as well. Because distraction results in relative kyphosis, the rods should be contoured in a lordotic posture prior to placing the rod to avoid a flatback deformity after distraction **(Fig. 9–15)**. The reduction of the posttraumatic kyphosis is therefore gained by patient positioning and rod contouring. In situ bending should never be used because this has been associated with loss of reduction postoperatively in short-segment constructs.[102] Two cross-

links are placed, and autogenous iliac crest is harvested and placed posterolaterally between the decorticated remaining posterior elements. The patient is quickly mobilized and fitted with a TLSO postoperatively.

Circumferential surgery is also appropriate treatment for thoracolumbar burst fractures. Good results have been documented, though the precise indications are somewhat unclear.[59,91,93] This approach is best used when the indications for anterior surgery are present, along with suspected posterior column instability. When performing the procedure, the anterior decompression and fusion are first completed. Distraction is placed across the corpectomy site, and the anterior strut graft is placed without instrumentation. Posteriorly, compression is applied to the pedicle screw construct to both secure the interbody graft and increase lordosis.

Flexion-Distraction Injuries

By definition, flexion-distraction injuries produce distraction of the posterior column through either the ligaments of the posterior column or the posterior bony elements. The seat-belt injury described by Denis and the classic Chance fracture are only a subset of the injuries that can be produced by a flexion-distraction force.[8] The classifications by Magerl and Gertzbein comprehensively describe the injuries that are caused by a flexion-distraction force.[5,103] When planning surgical intervention, it is important to identify the stabilizing structures that are disrupted. In virtually all these injuries the posterior column fails under tension. The middle column almost always fails under tension as well, with either

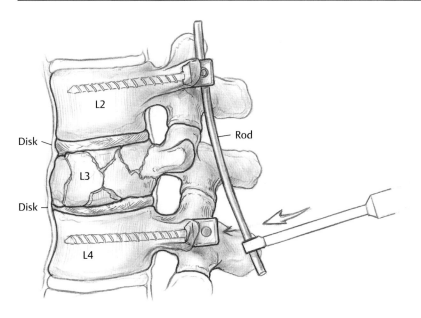

L2

Disk

Rod

L3

Disk

L4

Figure 9–15 As distraction across the lumbar spine restores vertebral body height, it causes relative kyphosis and a flatback deformity. Therefore, lordosis should be achieved by rod contouring.

a ligamentous and disk injury or tensile failure of the posterior vertebral body cortex. The type of injury to the anterior column depends on the location of the axis of rotation within the spinal column. If the axis of rotation is anterior to the anterior longitudinal ligament, the anterior column will also fail under tension. Conversely, if the axis of rotation is located in the vertebral body itself, the anterior column may fail under compression. It is important to distinguish this type of anterior compression injury from a compression fracture because the flexion-distraction injury has a significantly higher rate of progressive deformity and subluxation **(Fig. 9–16A–E).** Because the main instability associated with flexion-distraction injuries is in flexion, reconstruction of these injuries is typically best accomplished by posterior compression instrumentation (see **Video 9–1, Disk 1**). This allows reduction of the deformity using the middle column as a fulcrum, reestablishing the height lost from any anterior column compression. To accomplish this, the patient is positioned prone on a radiopaque table. The hips are fully extended to posturally reduce the deformity as much as possible. A standard posterior approach is performed, exposing the posterior elements above and below the injured motion segment. A fracture through the lamina and spinous process needs to be recognized preoperatively to avoid iatrogenic neurological injury during exposure. Pedicle screws are then placed using routine anatomical landmarks in the pedicles above and below the injured motion segment. A short-segment construct is appropriate in cases of both ligamentous and bony posterior column injury.[104] For a ligamentous injury, this means that the instrumentation need only include a single motion segment. The number of segments instrumented in posterior bony injuries depends on the integrity of the involved pedicles.

Oftentimes the fracture involves only the inferior aspect of the pedicles, and screws can still be placed in the injured vertebrae. In this instance, occasionally, a fracture can be treated with compression instrumentation across a single vertebra with no fusion. The fracture is thus reduced and stabilized by placing compression across pedicle screws and infralaminar hooks at the same level. In instances when the injured pedicle cannot be instrumented, the instrumentation needs to be extended to the next most cephalad level.[105] Following placement of the pedicle screws and verification of screw position with fluorography, the rods are contoured and placed. Compression is placed across the construct to reduce the deformity and restore the posterior tension band. Prior to compression, any infolded and/or torn ligamentum flavum is removed to avoid any chance of iatrogenic neurological injury with reduction. In cases of disk disruption, the surgeon must be cognizant of the possibility of injury to the posterior anulus and disk herniation occurring at the time of construct compression. Thus any change in neurological status postoperatively needs to be emergently investigated with neuroimaging followed by diskectomy if appropriate.[106] Finally, the posterior elements are decorticated across the fused segments and bone graft, and two cross-links are placed.

One unique injury pattern in flexion-distraction injuries is the rare case when the fracture results in a compression injury to the posterior vertebral body cortex, with retropulsion of bone into the spinal canal. This injury pattern therefore results in distraction of the posterior column but compression of the middle and anterior columns. Posterior compression instrumentation using the posterior vertebral cortex as a fulcrum is no longer appropriate because the posterior cortex has been disrupted. Therefore, posterior instrumentation of this injury is similar to that of a burst fracture where distraction is necessary to restore middle column height and indirectly decompress the spinal canal. However, because the posterior elements have experienced tensile failure—unlike a burst fracture—distraction must be done carefully because

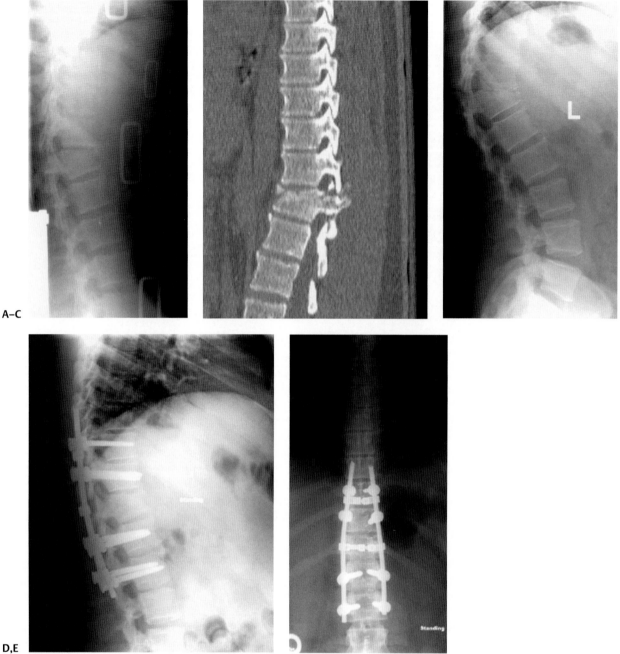

A–C

D,E

Figure 9–16 **(A)** The injury radiograph of a patient incorrectly diagnosed with a compression fracture. **(B)** The sagittal computed tomographic reconstruction shows this to be a flexion-distraction injury. **(C)** At 8 weeks the patient presented with a progressive deformity. He required surgical intervention. Due to the subacute nature of his injury, he required instrumentation two levels above and below the fracture to correct and maintain correction of his deformity. The postoperative **(D)** anteroposterior and **(E)** lateral radiographs show reduction and stabilization of the deformity.

in this particular injury overdistraction is possible. Distraction also predictably increases the kyphosis across the fracture site, so the kyphotic deformity must be reduced through rod contouring and patient positioning. Once the posterior tension band is restored, if further decompression is required, this can be accomplished posterolaterally. Short-segment instrumentation may still be appropriate, but this needs to be decided based on the amount of anterior comminution, similar to the criteria

that need to be met to treat a burst fracture with short-segment instrumentation **(Fig. 9–17A,B)**.

In the patient with a flexion-distraction injury, anterior surgery alone is not indicated. An anterior strut graft is not able to adequately stabilize the flexion instability that is associated with a flexion-distraction injury. The anterior strut inevitably is at or very close to the axis of the instability, placing the graft at a distinct mechanical disadvantage. Anterior distraction alone cannot adequately restore lordosis

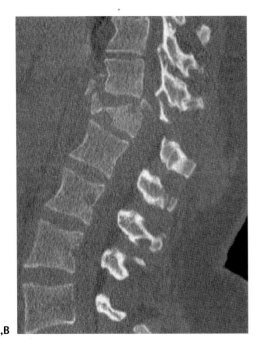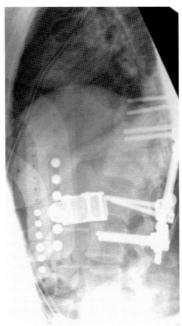

A,B

Figure 9–17 (A) This sagittal computed tomographic reconstruction shows a flexion-distraction injury with posterior vertebral body cortex retropulsion and paraparesis. This is distinctly different from a burst fracture due to the tensile failure of the posterior column. **(B)** This patient underwent posterior decompression and reduction/fusion.

in the absence of an intact posterior tension band. Therefore, if vertebral body comminution or canal compromise requires anterior reconstruction, it should be done following posterior stabilization and reduction.

Fracture-Dislocations

Fracture-dislocations can result from numerous forces on the spine, including distraction, rotation, and shear.[5,8] In every instance, these injuries involve all three columns and are highly unstable and are often associated with neurological injury. Consequently, except in extraordinary circumstances, operative treatment is indicated. As a result of the dislocation, displacement of the affected motion segments can be significant and in multiple planes. Reduction and stabilization from an anterior approach is difficult, and, therefore, posterior surgery is the mainstay of operative treatment. The posterior approach allows for wide exposure of multiple motion segments, accurate reduction of the fracture, and rigid stabilization.[105] Any decompression required can also be safely performed from the posterior approach **(Fig. 9–18A,B).**

The patient is positioned prone on a radiopaque table, as previously described. A standard posterior approach to the thoracolumbar spine is performed, exposing at least two motion segments cephalad and caudad to the injured level. During the exposure, care must be taken to avoid iatrogenic neurological injury. This is most likely in areas of fractured or deficient posterior elements that are not anticipated preoperatively. Following exposure, instrumentation is placed. Due to the markedly unstable nature of fracture-dislocations, short-segment instrumentation in general is not indicated, with a documented high failure rate.[107] Instrumentation should consist of pedicle screws if at all possible.[108] The

three-column fixation achieved by pedicle screws is especially helpful in fracture dislocations where wide displacement can require multiplanar forces to achieve reduction. Pedicle screws can be placed safely throughout the thoracic and lumbar spine, even after fracture dislocations, but the surgeon must be aware of any posttraumatic spine deformity that could alter the orientation of the nearby pedicles.[108] Instrumentation should include at least two vertebrae above and below the level of the injury. One exception to this would be the rare case of a pure dislocation. In this instance, short-segment instrumentation can adequately stabilize the area of injury, where the intact posterior elements can also add stability to the final construct. After placement of the pedicle screws, any fracture fragments directly impinging on the neuroelements are removed, and any dural tear is directly repaired. Finally, the fracture is reduced. The specific reduction maneuver required varies, depending on the type of displacement caused by the injury. In general, though, correction can be obtained by first fixing a physiologically contoured rod to the caudad screws and then sequentially translating the cephalad segments to the rod. Distraction or compression can then be applied to the construct to get the final reduction. Two cross-links are placed, and the remaining posterior elements are decorticated prior to placing bone graft.

Predictably good outcomes have been documented for numerous instrumentation systems following posterior reduction and stabilization of thoracolumbar fracture dislocations.[58,60,69,80,108–112] Yet some authors acknowledge the occasional need for anterior surgery following the posterior procedure.[59,105] A subsequent anterior procedure should be reserved for cases with persistent anterior neurocompression following posterior surgery, or when anterior vertebral body comminution is sufficient to necessitate an

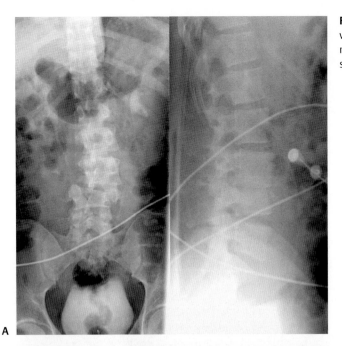

Figure 9–18 **(A)** Pre- and postoperative radiographs of a patient who sustained an L3–L4 fracture dislocation. He underwent posterior reduction/decompression and instrumented fusion. **(B)** His construct included fusion two levels above and below the level of injury.

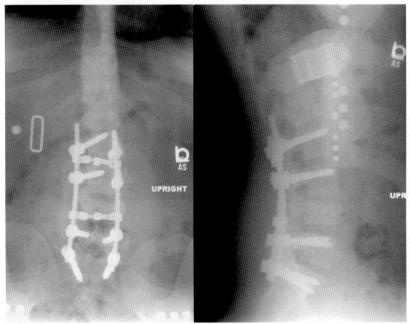

anterior structural graft. However, there are no specific data that can help the surgeon predict failure of a long-segment posterior construct in the face of anterior comminution. Therefore, the decision to perform an anterior corpectomy or add a structural anterior graft is often based on the individual preferences of each treating surgeon.

Complications

As with any significant injury requiring extensive reconstruction, the surgical treatment of thoracolumbar fractures can

be associated with a variety of complications. These complications can be similar to complications seen with any major surgical procedure, or specifically related to reduction and stabilization of thoracolumbar fractures. In fact, the complication rate can be significant. A review by Knop et al shows the perioperative complication rate to be as high as 15%, with almost half of those patients ultimately requiring revision surgery.[113] Therefore, the surgeon must always be aware of emerging complications and treat them appropriately.

Perhaps the most lethal complication in patients with thoracolumbar fractures is DVT and pulmonary embolus

Tips and Tricks

- In the lumbar spine, the lateral to medial orientation of the pedicles decreases as the vertebral level moves from caudad to cephalad. At S1, the medial angulation of the pedicle is 35 degrees, but at T11 or T12 the medial orientation of the pedicle is less than 10 degrees.
- When they exist as part of the injury pattern, facet dislocations should be reduced under direct vision posteriorly.
- The biggest deterrent to anterior treatment for thoracolumbar injuries is the vascular anatomy in the lower lumbar region. The aortic bifurcation occurs in the region of the L4–L5 disk space, with the common iliac artery and vein usually crossing the L5 vertebral body. This makes anterior instrumentation of L5 or S1 difficult, if not impossible, due to the proximity of the vascular structures.
- For compression fractures occurring at the thoracolumbar junction, instrumentation should include two segments proximal to the injury and one segment distally.[64] Lumbar compression injuries only require instrumentation one level above and below the level of the injury.
- For lumbar burst fractures with significant vertebral body comminution, posterior short-segment fixation alone has a high rate of failure with residual kyphosis.[11]
- During treatment of burst fractures, posterolateral decompression need only be performed from one side to fully decompress the entire spinal canal.
- When using posterior distraction instrumentation to reduce and stabilize a lumbar burst fracture, one should remember that distraction results in relative kyphosis. To avoid a flatback deformity after distraction, the rods should be contoured in a slightly lordotic posture prior to insertion.
- For lumbar burst fractures, ideal candidates for anterior surgery are patients with canal compromise greater than 80% with incomplete neurological deficit, severe vertebral body comminution, or kyphosis greater than 30 degrees.[97]
- When treating burst fractures from an anterior approach, a common error is to insert the instrumentation too far anteriorly. This actually causes the screws to be angled toward the spinal canal.
- When combined anterior and posterior approaches are used to treat a thoracolumbar burst fracture, the anterior decompression and fusion should be completed first.
- When evaluating flexion-distraction injuries, one must carefully analyze the fracture pattern and understand three possible variations, depending on the location of the axis of rotation (fulcrum) within the spinal column:

- If the fulcrum is anterior to the anterior longitudinal ligament, the anterior column will also fail under tension.
- Conversely, if the axis of rotation is located in or behind the vertebral body, the anterior column will fail under compression. It is important to distinguish this type of anterior compression injury from a compression fracture because the flexion distraction injury has a significantly higher rate of progressive deformity and subluxation.
- Rarely, there is a compression injury to the posterior vertebral body cortex, with retropulsion of bone into the spinal canal. This injury pattern occurs when the fulcrum is at the spinal canal, resulting in distraction of the posterior column and compression of the middle and anterior columns. In this case, posterior compression instrumentation using the posterior vertebral cortex as a fulcrum is not appropriate because the posterior cortex has been disrupted. Posterior instrumentation of this injury must produce distraction to restore middle column height and indirectly decompress the spinal canal. However, because the posterior elements have experienced tensile failure—unlike a burst fracture—distraction must be done carefully because in this particular injury overdistraction is possible.
- Disruption of the posterior elements should be recognized on preoperative imaging studies to avoid incarcerating the neural elements in the lamina fracture during fracture reduction.
- In cases of disk disruption associated with flexion-distraction injuries, the surgeon must be cognizant of the possibility of injury to the posterior anulus and disk herniation occurring at the time of construct compression.
- Because reduction and stabilization of thoracolumbar fracture-dislocations from an anterior approach is difficult, posterior surgery is the mainstay of operative treatment.
- Due to the unstable nature of fracture-dislocations, short-segment instrumentation is not usually indicated, with a documented high failure rate.[107]
- After posterior reduction and fixation of a thoracolumbar fracture-dislocation, a subsequent anterior procedure is needed for cases with persistent anterior neurocompression or when anterior vertebral body comminution is sufficient to necessitate an anterior structural graft.
- When a wound infection is identified, it should be aggressively treated with surgical drainage, debridement, and intraoperative cultures.

(PE). It is known that the overall risk of DVT in patients following major spine reconstructive procedures for a variety of diagnoses is low.[114] However, these data cannot be extrapolated to the patient with acute thoracolumbar spine trauma because the incidence of DVT and PE increases significantly in this population. The incidence of thromboembolism has been shown to be highest in patients who have sustained a spinal cord injury or a long bone fracture, or in patients with advanced age.[115,116] Yet, even in those populations at particularly high risk for thromboembolism, recommended prophylaxis regimens are often based on opinion and cohort studies, rather than class 1 data. In fact, a recent meta-analysis suggested that the incidence of DVT and PE may be similar in trauma patients whether or not they receive any prophylaxis.[117] Nevertheless, DVT prophylaxis is essential in all thoracolumbar fracture patients. The simplest form of prophylaxis is sequential pneumatic mechanical compression, which has been shown to decrease thromboembolic complications when exclusively used in a cohort of patients undergoing spine reconstructive procedures and in a cohort of patients with spinal cord injuries (SCIs).[114,115] In patients with SCI, the presence of a long bone fracture increased the risk of DVT significantly. Therefore, in high-risk patients, particularly those with traumatic spinal cord injury and concomitant long bone fracture, prophylaxis should consist of both mechanical as well as pharmacological prophylaxis. The placement of a prophylactic inferior vena cava filter (VCF) does not appear to be warranted.[118] However, in patients with a documented PE in the acute postoperative period, therapeutic anticoagulation is associated with a high complication rate, and placement of a VCF should be considered instead.[119]

More commonly, complications related to surgical intervention for thoracolumbar fractures are associated with the surgical procedure or injury itself. These include infection, pseudomeningocele, posttraumatic deformity, pseudarthrosis, and progressive neurological deficit. Postoperative wound infection following surgical treatment of thoracolumbar fractures must be diagnosed promptly and treated aggressively. Infection is most common following posterior stabilization procedures.[120] However, there is no indication that the infection rate following fracture stabilization is any different from the infection rate following other spine reconstructive procedures. The infection rate varies by report but is most likely between 5 and 10%.[21,59,121,122] The most important aspect of treating a postoperative wound infection is prompt diagnosis. Any patient with a draining wound should be suspected of having a postoperative wound infection until proven otherwise. Treating a draining wound following posterior instrumentation and fusion with local wound care and oral antibiotics should be avoided at all costs because this form of treatment is doomed to failure. When a wound infection is identified, it should be aggressively treated with surgical drainage, debridement, and intraoperative cultures.[120] The superficial layer is exposed and thoroughly debrided. If the fascia is completely intact, the deep portions

of the wound should be aspirated through a remote site to ensure that the infection has not entered the subfascial space. If a defect in the fascia is seen, the wound should be opened in its entirety and meticulously debrided. The instrumentation is left in place, though any obviously necrotic bone graft should be removed. Superficial infections where little necrotic tissue is present may be closed after initial debridement over a drain. If significant necrotic tissue is present, or in the case of a deep infection, repeat debridement is indicated. I prefer to pack the wound with a vacuum-assisted closure (VAC) sponge to facilitate drainage of persistent infection and promote formation of granulation tissue. The sponge should be placed into the depths of the wound and may lie directly on exposed bone or instrumentation.[123] The patient then returns to the operating room in 48 to 72 hours for repeat debridement. If healthy granulation tissue is present throughout, the wound may then be closed over deep and superficial drains. Should significant necrosis still be present, packing is repeated until the wound is clean. Local wound care is combined with long-term IV antibiotic treatment, with agents chosen based on culture data.

Dural tears commonly occur in conjunction with thoracolumbar fractures and have been documented in association with flexion-distraction injuries, fracture-dislocations, and burst fractures.[124–126] Yet, most commonly, the literature discusses the association between burst fractures and dural lacerations. Whether or not specific fracture characteristics predict an increased chance of a dural tear is debatable, but tears have been associated with neurological injuries and lamina fractures.[124,127–129] The lacerations may be on the anterior or the posterior portions of the dura.[130] Elements of the cauda equina can even become entrapped in the lamina fracture in a small percentage of cases. It is important to recognize this on preoperative imaging studies to avoid incarcerating the neural elements in the lamina fracture during fracture reduction.[127,131] When dural tears are encountered, they should be treated by direct repair. Persistent pseudomeningoceles may be treated by either reexploration and repair or closed subarachnoid drainage.[132]

Following treatment for a thoracolumbar fracture, patients can develop a posttraumatic deformity. This complication has been associated with all types of thoracolumbar injuries. There are numerous causes, including inadequate initial stabilization, implant failure, pseudarthrosis, and subsequent laminectomy.[133] The most common posttraumatic deformity is increased thoracolumbar kyphosis, and pain is the predominant symptom (**Fig. 9–19**). Gertzbein, in a multicenter retrospective study of patients with thoracolumbar injuries, found that patients with residual kyphosis of greater than 30 degrees following treatment have an increased incidence of pain.[134] Progressive kyphosis following thoracolumbar fracture treatment has also been associated with increased pain.[135] Clearly, the most effective treatment of posttraumatic deformity is prevention. Progressive deformities result from inadequate immobilization of unstable three-column injuries. Most often this is

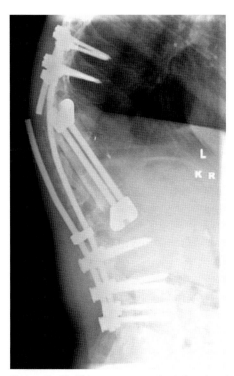

Figure 9–19 This posttraumatic deformity developed following multilevel corpectomy and posterior stabilization for contiguous level fractures. The deformity developed due to a pseudarthrosis.

due to an unrecognized posterior column injury combined with anterior column compression. Careful clinical and radiological evaluation is critical to avoid posttreatment deformity. MRI may be helpful in this regard, particularly when looking for a posterior ligamentous injury.[135] When a deformity does develop, treatment can be difficult. Surgical treatment is reserved for patients with progressive deformity or worsening neurological deficit. Pain alone is not a surgical indication because pain relief following deformity correction is unreliable, though Vaccaro and Silber, and Bohlman et al did report consistent pain relief following surgery for patients with residual posttraumatic canal compromise.[133,136] When planning surgical intervention for patients with posttraumatic deformity, a variety of surgical approaches have been described, including anterior surgery alone, posterior osteotomies, and stabilization, as well as combined anterior and posterior procedures.[133]

Virtually every published series of surgical treatment of thoracolumbar fractures describes pseudarthrosis as a complication, regardless of the surgical approach.[55–57,64,66,71,74,80,93,98,100,137,138] The true pseudarthrosis rate is unknown, though some authors feel that the pseudarthrosis rate following thoracolumbar fracture stabilization is lower than that for elective fusions.[139] However, there are several factors that have been shown to increase the rate of pseudarthrosis. These factors are the use of allograft, smoking, anti-inflammatory drug use, and poor nutrition.[98,140] For this reason, autograft should be used when possible, and aggressive nutritional support should be instituted. The diagnosis of a pseudarthrosis is usually

best made with a combination of dynamic radiographs and thin-cut computed tomography (CT) with sagittal and coronal reconstructions. Surgical indications for the treatment of a pseudarthrosis are a progressive deformity or progressive neurological deficit. Because pseudarthroses can be asymptomatic, surgical treatment of a pseudarthrosis for pain relief only gives unpredictable results.[140]

Neurological deterioration following surgical treatment of a thoracolumbar fracture needs to first be promptly diagnosed and then urgently evaluated. Diagnosis, though, can be difficult, particularly in an obtunded patient. In this instance, the surgeon should consider intraoperative neurological monitoring with somatosensory evoked potentials (SSEPs) to help recognize a potentially undetectable neurological injury. Although the experience with SSEPs in fracture surgery is not as great as the experience with deformity surgery, consistently diminished amplitudes have been associated with postoperative neurological deficit in the fracture patient.[141] If a change in the neurological status of the patient is detected postoperatively, urgent evaluation is necessary. Potentially reversible causes include misplaced hardware, a disk herniation resulting from reduction, increased bone retropulsion, and an epidural hematoma. Nonreversible causes are neurological injury from manipulation during the procedure or cord ischemia. Regardless, prompt neuroimaging should be obtained. If a reversible lesion is diagnosed, particularly at the level of the spinal cord or conus medullaris, the patient should emergently return to the operating room.

Outcomes

Given the wide range of thoracolumbar injuries, as well as the diverse surgical approaches, techniques, and instrumentation systems used for treatment, it is difficult to generalize about the outcomes of treatment. One reason for this is that most all outcome studies involve small cohorts only and are largely retrospective.[72,134,142–146] In analyzing the outcomes, though, there are really two factors that need to be examined. One is the rate of neurological recovery, and the other is the overall functional recovery of the patient. Following surgical treatment for thoracolumbar fractures, neurological deficits reliably improve. This is particularly true for patients with incomplete neurological injuries, regardless of the specific procedure performed.[72,142,143,145] As mentioned previously, the effect of the timing of surgical intervention on neurological recovery is unknown.[88] The final neurological status of the patient most closely predicts the patient's ultimate functional outcome.[144] When looking specifically at functional outcomes, cohort studies have indicated that between 70 and 80% of patients return to work, though a significant percentage return with restrictions.[70,143–145] Patients with advanced academic achievement were more likely to return to work.[145] In patients with residual pain, neurological pain is usually more debilitating than axial back pain. A large percentage of patients with significant back pain have a potentially identifiable cause, including pseudarthrosis, deformity, and instability.[144] Prospective studies are needed to determine which of the many treatment options offer the patient the best chance of returning to preinjury activities.

New Techniques

Surgical procedures to treat thoracolumbar fractures are often extensive procedures associated with significant morbidity. Some new techniques, therefore, focus on achieving the goals of surgery in a minimally invasive fashion. One such goal of surgery is reduction of spinal deformity or kyphosis, particularly in patients with compression or burst fractures. Kyphoplasty has been successfully used in patients with osteoporotic compression fractures to reduce kyphotic deformities as well as to stabilize painful vertebral segments.[147] This technique has been applied to patients with acute traumatic burst fractures. A kyphoplasty is done on the fractured vertebrae to help reduce kyphosis and reinforce the anterior column. This construct is then supplemented with short-segment posterior instrumentation and fusion. Initial results have suggested that patients in which the fractured segment is augmented with a kyphoplasty have better maintenance of kyphosis correction.[148]

Minimally invasive instrumentation systems also have applications for patients with thoracolumbar fractures. These techniques have been applied to both anterior and posterior stabilization and fusion procedures. The goal is to stabilize and reduce fractures through smaller incisions with less morbidity. To date, most experience in thoracolumbar fractures has been with minimally invasive anterior instrumentation systems.[79,149–151] Posterior systems are commonly used to treat other thoracolumbar pathologies and undoubtedly can be adapted for trauma applications.[152] Image-guided surgery may also aid the surgeon in treating thoracolumbar injuries. For instance, pedicle screws can be accurately placed using image guidance throughout the thoracolumbar spine.[153] This technology may also be helpful in decompressive procedures, decreasing both operative time and potential for iatrogenic neurological injury.

Finally, the ever-expanding role of growth factors and bone morphogens in spine surgery will surely have applications in the treatment of thoracolumbar fractures. Thus far, bone morphogenic proteins (BMPs) have achieved clinical success in elective interbody and posterolateral lumbar fusions.[154] One potential trauma application is using these growth factors locally to stimulate bone formation in fractured vertebral bodies, resulting in decreased healing time. Although a single limited trial with BMP-7 failed to demonstrate increased bone formation with transpedicular transplantation, the cohort was very small.[155] Perhaps further research can identify a role for these biological agents in reconstruction of patients following thoracolumbar trauma.

Pearls

- Six percent of the blunt trauma patients presenting to a level 1 trauma center have vertebral injuries.
- The conus medullaris has a variable location in the thoracolumbar spine but is typically located at the level of the L1 vertebral body, or the L1–L2 disk.
- Established parameters for surgery in patients with burst fractures and no neurological deficit are kyphosis of greater than 20 degrees, greater than 50% collapse, and greater than 50% canal compromise.[156] Of these, the degree of canal compromise in a neurologically normal patient is probably least important, whereas the degree of kyphotic deformity is the most important criterion.

- In contrast, all patients with thoracolumbar burst fractures and neurological deficit should undergo operative treatment.
- Nonoperative treatment of thoracolumbar fracture-dislocations is inappropriate except in rare cases where that patient cannot undergo surgery. Because reduction and stabilization of these injuries from an anterior approach is difficult, posterior surgery is the mainstay of operative treatment.
- Potentially reversible causes of intraoperative neurological injury include misplaced hardware, a disk herniation resulting from reduction, increased bone retropulsion, and an epidural hematoma.
- Patients with residual kyphosis of greater than 30 degrees following treatment have an increased incidence of pain.

On the DVDs

Video 9–1 (Disk 1) Open Reduction, Posterior Lateral Decompression T12, Posterior Fusion T10–L2 with Instrumentation This patient sustained a flexion distraction injury at T12 with a spinal cord injury. Operative treatment consisted of open reduction of the fracture followed by instrumentation and fusion from T10–L2 with posterolateral decompression at T12.

Video 9–2 (Disk 1) Anterior L1 Corpectomy, Anterior Fusion T12–L2 with an Expandable Cage and Instrumentation This patient sustained an L1 burst fracture with a neurologic injury. An anterior corpectomy was performed, with reconstruction and fusion using an expandable cage and anterior instrumentation from T12 to L2.

References

1. Hu R, Mustard CA, Burns C. Epidemiology of incident spinal fracture in a complete population. Spine 1996;21:492–499
2. Holmes JF, Miller PQ, Panacek EA, Lin S, Horne NS, Mower WR. Epidemiology of thoracolumbar spine injury in blunt trauma. Acad Emerg Med 2001;8:866–872
3. Heggeness MH, Doherty BJ. The trabecular anatomy of thoracolumbar vertebrae: implications for burst fractures. J Anat 1997;191(Pt 2):309–312
4. Hongo M, Abe E, Shimada Y, Murai H, Ishikawa N, Sato K. Surface strain distribution on thoracic and lumbar vertebrae under axial compression: the role in burst fractures. Spine 1999;24:1197–1202
5. Magerl F, Aebi M, Gertzbein SD, Harms J, Nazarian S. A comprehensive classification of thoracic and lumbar injuries. Eur Spine J 1994;3:184–201
6. Aligizakis AC, Katonis PG, Sapkas G, Papagelopoulos PJ, Galanakis I, Hadjipavlou A. Gertzbein and load sharing classifications for unstable thoracolumbar fractures. Clin Orthop Relat Res 2003;411:77–85
7. Capen DA. Classification of thoracolumbar fractures and posterior instrumentation for treatment of thoracolumbar fractures. Instr Course Lect 1999;48:437–441
8. Denis F. The three column spine and its significance in the classification of acute thoracolumbar spinal injuries. Spine 1983;8:817–831
9. Denis F. Spinal instability as defined by the three-column spine concept in acute spinal trauma. Clin Orthop Relat Res 1984;189:65–76
10. Ferguson RL, Allen BL Jr. A mechanistic classification of thoracolumbar spine fractures. Clin Orthop Relat Res 1984;189:77–88
11. McCormack T, Karaikovic E, Gaines RW. The load sharing classification of spine fractures. Spine 1994;19:1741–1744
12. Vollmer DG, Gegg C. Classification and acute management of thoracolumbar fractures. Neurosurg Clin N Am 1997;8:499–507
13. Magerl F, Aebi M, Gertzbein SD, Harms J, Nazarian S. A comprehensive classification of thoracic and lumbar injuries. Eur Spine J 1994;3:184–201
14. Gertzbein SD. Spine update: classification of thoracic and lumbar fractures. Spine 1994;19:626–628
15. Folman Y, Gepstein R. Late outcome of nonoperative management of thoracolumbar vertebral wedge fractures. J Orthop Trauma 2003;17:190–192
16. Tropiano P, Huang RC, Louis CA, Poitout DG, Louis RP. Functional and radiographic outcome of thoracolumbar and lumbar burst fractures managed by closed orthopaedic reduction and casting. Spine 2003;28:2459–2465
17. Weinstein JN, Collalto P, Lehmann TR. Thoracolumbar "burst" fractures treated conservatively: a long-term follow-up. Spine 1988;13:33–38
18. Whitesides TE Jr. Traumatic kyphosis of the thoracolumbar spine. Clin Orthop Relat Res 1977;128:78–92
19. Hartman MB, Chrin AM, Rechtine GR. Non-operative treatment of thoracolumbar fractures. Paraplegia 1995;33:73–76
20. Ramieri A, Domenicucci M, Passacantilli E, Nocente M, Ciappetta P. The results of the surgical and conservative treatment of non-neurologic comminuted thoracolumbar fractures. Chir Organi Mov 2000;85:129–135
21. Rechtine GR, Cahill D, Chrin AM. Treatment of thoracolumbar trauma: comparison of complications of operative versus nonoperative treatment. J Spinal Disord 1999;12:406–409
22. Denis F, Armstrong GW, Searls K, Matta L. Acute thoracolumbar burst fractures in the absence of neurologic deficit: a comparison between operative and nonoperative treatment. Clin Orthop Relat Res 1984;189:142–149
23. Weinstein JN, Collalto P, Lehmann TR. Long-term follow-up of nonoperatively treated thoracolumbar spine fractures. J Orthop Trauma 1987;1:152–159
24. Whitesides TE Jr. Traumatic kyphosis of the thoracolumbar spine. Clin Orthop Relat Res 1977;128:78–92
25. Chow GH, Nelson BJ, Gebhard JS, Brugman JL, Brown CW, Donaldson DH. Functional outcome of thoracolumbar burst fractures managed with hyperextension casting or bracing and early mobilization. Spine 1996;21:2170–2175
26. Aligizakis A, Katonis P, Stergiopoulos K, Galanakis I, Karabekios S, Hadjipavlou A. Functional outcome of burst fractures of the thoracolumbar spine managed non-operatively, with early ambulation, evaluated using the load sharing classification. Acta Orthop Belg 2002;68:279–287
27. Chow GH, Nelson BJ, Gebhard JS, Brugman JL, Brown CW, Donaldson DH. Functional outcome of thoracolumbar burst fractures managed with hyperextension casting or bracing and early mobilization. Spine 1996;21:2170–2175
28. Denis F, Armstrong GW, Searls K, Matta L. Acute thoracolumbar burst fractures in the absence of neurologic deficit: a comparison between operative and nonoperative treatment. Clin Orthop Relat Res 1984;189:142–149
29. Chow GH, Nelson BJ, Gebhard JS, Brugman JL, Brown CW, Donaldson DH. Functional outcome of thoracolumbar burst fractures managed with hyperextension casting or bracing and early mobilization. Spine 1996;21:2170–2175
30. Boerger TO, Limb D, Dickson RA. Does "canal clearance" affect neurological outcome after thoracolumbar burst fractures? J Bone Joint Surg Br 2000;82:629–635
31. McAfee PC, Yuan HA, Lasda NA. The unstable burst fracture. Spine 1982;7:365–373
32. Cantor JB, Lebwohl NH, Garvey T, Eismont FJ. Nonoperative management of stable thoracolumbar burst fractures with early ambulation and bracing. Spine 1993;18:971–976
33. Dai LY. Remodeling of the spinal canal after thoracolumbar burst fractures. Clin Orthop Relat Res 2001;382:119–123
34. de Klerk LW, Fontijne WP, Stijnen T, Braakman R, Tanghe HL, van Linge B. Spontaneous remodeling of the spinal canal after conservative management of thoracolumbar burst fractures. Spine 1998;23:1057–1060
35. Mumford J, Weinstein JN, Spratt KF, Goel VK. Thoracolumbar burst fractures: the clinical efficacy and outcome of nonoperative management. Spine 1993;18:955–970
36. Wood K, Butterman G, Mehbod A, Garvey T, Jhanjee R, Sechriest V. Operative compared with nonoperative treatment of a thoracolumbar burst fracture without neurological deficit: a prospective, randomized study. J Bone Joint Surg Am 2003;85-A:773–781
37. Denis F, Armstrong GW, Searls K, Matta L. Acute thoracolumbar burst fractures in the absence of neurologic deficit: a comparison between operative and nonoperative treatment. Clin Orthop Relat Res 1984;189:142–149
38. Mumford J, Weinstein JN, Spratt KF, Goel VK. Thoracolumbar burst fractures: the clinical efficacy and outcome of nonoperative management. Spine 1993;18:955–970
39. Cantor JB, Lebwohl NH, Garvey T, Eismont FJ. Nonoperative management of stable thoracolumbar burst fractures with early ambulation and bracing. Spine 1993;18:971–976
40. Chow GH, Nelson BJ, Gebhard JS, Brugman JL, Brown CW, Donaldson DH. Functional outcome of thoracolumbar burst fractures

managed with hyperextension casting or bracing and early mobilization. Spine 1996;21:2170–2175

41. Domenicucci M, Preite R, Ramieri A, Ciappetta P, Delfini R, Romanini L. Thoracolumbar fractures without neurosurgical involvement: surgical or conservative treatment? J Neurosurg Sci 1996;40:1–10

42. Shen WJ, Liu TJ, Shen YS. Nonoperative treatment versus posterior fixation for thoracolumbar junction burst fractures without neurologic deficit. Spine 2001;26:1038–1045

43. Cantor JB, Lebwohl NH, Garvey T, Eismont FJ. Nonoperative management of stable thoracolumbar burst fractures with early ambulation and bracing. Spine 1993;18:971–976

44. Shen WJ, Shen YS. Nonsurgical treatment of three-column thoracolumbar junction burst fractures without neurologic deficit. Spine 1999;24:412–415

45. Mick CA, Carl A, Sachs B, Hresko MT, Pfeifer BA. Burst fractures of the fifth lumbar vertebra. Spine 1993;18:1878–1884

46. Seybold EA, Sweeney CA, Fredrickson BE, Warhold LG, Bernini PM. Functional outcome of low lumbar burst fractures: a multicenter review of operative and nonoperative treatment of L3–L5. Spine 1999;24:2154–2161

47. An HS, Simpson JM, Ebraheim NA, Jackson WT, Moore J, O'Malley NP. Low lumbar burst fractures: comparison between conservative and surgical treatments. Orthopedics 1992;15:367–373

48. Mick CA, Carl A, Sachs B, Hresko MT, Pfeifer BA. Burst fractures of the fifth lumbar vertebra. Spine 1993;18:1878–1884

49. Shen WJ, Liu TJ, Shen YS. Nonoperative treatment versus posterior fixation for thoracolumbar junction burst fractures without neurologic deficit. Spine 2001;26:1038–1045

50. Weinstein JN, Collalto P, Lehmann TR. Thoracolumbar "burst" fractures treated conservatively: a long-term follow-up. Spine 1988;13:33–38

51. McAfee PC, Yuan HA, Lasda NA. The unstable burst fracture. Spine 1982;7:365–373

52. Mumford J, Weinstein JN, Spratt KF, Goel VK. Thoracolumbar burst fractures: the clinical efficacy and outcome of nonoperative management. Spine 1993;18:955–970

53. Akalm S, Kis M, Benli IT, Citak M, Mumcu EF, Tuzuner M. Results of the AO spinal internal fixator in the surgical treatment of thoracolumbar burst fractures. Eur Spine J 1994;3:102–106

54. Akbarnia BA, Crandall DG, Burkus K, Matthews T. Use of long rods and a short arthrodesis for burst fractures of the thoracolumbar spine: a long-term follow-up study. J Bone Joint Surg Am 1994; 76:1629–1635

55. Aydin E, Solak AS, Tuzuner MM, Benli IT, Kis M. Z-plate instrumentation in thoracolumbar spinal fractures. Bull Hosp Jt Dis 1999;58:92–97

56. Bailey SI, Bartolozzi P, Bertagnoli R, et al. The BWM spinal fixator system: a preliminary report of a 2-year prospective, international multicenter study in a range of indications requiring surgical intervention for bone grafting and pedicle screw fixation. Spine 1996;21:2006–2015

57. Carl AL, Tranmer BI, Sachs BL. Anterolateral dynamized instrumentation and fusion for unstable thoracolumbar and lumbar burst fractures. Spine 1997;22:686–690

58. Chavda DV, Brantigan JW. Technique of reduction and internal fixation of thoracolumbar fracture-dislocation using pedicle screws and variable screw placement plates. Orthop Rev 1994; Suppl:25–31

59. Defino HL, Rodriguez-Fuentes AE. Treatment of fractures of the thoracolumbar spine by combined anteroposterior fixation using the Harms method. Eur Spine J 1998;7:187–194

60. Devilee R, Sanders R, de Lange S. Treatment of fractures and dislocations of the thoracic and lumbar spine by fusion and Harrington instrumentation. Arch Orthop Trauma Surg 1995; 114:100–102

61. Fabris D, Costantini S, Nena U, Gentilucci G, Ricciardi A. Cotrel-dubousset instrumentation in thoracolumbar seat belt-type and flexion-distraction injuries. J Spinal Disord 1994;7:146–152

62. Gardner VO, Thalgott JS, White JI, Lowery GL. The contoured anterior spinal plate system (CASP): indications, techniques, and results. Spine 1994;19:550–555

63. Ghanayem AJ, Zdeblick TA. Anterior instrumentation in the management of thoracolumbar burst fractures. Clin Orthop Relat Res 1997;335:89–100

64. Glaser JA, Estes WJ. Distal short segment fixation of thoracolumbar and lumbar injuries. Iowa Orthop J 1998;18:87–90

65. Hamilton A, Webb JK. The role of anterior surgery for vertebral fractures with and without cord compression. Clin Orthop Relat Res 1994;300:79–89

66. Kaneda K, Taneichi H, Abumi K, Hashimoto T, Satoh S, Fujiya M. Anterior decompression and stabilization with the Kaneda device for thoracolumbar burst fractures associated with neurological deficits. J Bone Joint Surg Am 1997;79:69–83

67. Khoo LT, Beisse R, Potulski M. Thoracoscopic-assisted treatment of thoracic and lumbar fractures: a series of 371 consecutive cases. Neurosurgery 2002;51(Suppl 5):S104–117

68. Korovessis P, Piperos G, Sidiropoulos P, Karagiannis A, Dimas T. Spinal canal restoration by posterior distraction or anterior decompression in thoracolumbar spinal fractures and its influence on neurological outcome. Eur Spine J 1994;3:318–324

69. Korovessis PG, Baikousis A, Stamatakis M. Use of the Texas Scottish Rite Hospital instrumentation in the treatment of thoracolumbar injuries. Spine 1997;22:882–888

70. Leferink VJ, Keizer HJ, Oosterhuis JK, van der Sluis CK, ten Duis HJ. Functional outcome in patients with thoracolumbar burst fractures treated with dorsal instrumentation and transpedicular cancellous bone grafting. Eur Spine J 2003;12:261–267

71. Liu CL, Wang ST, Lin HJ, Kao HC, Yu WK, Lo WH. AO fixateur interne in treating burst fractures of the thoracolumbar spine. Zhonghua Yi Xue Za Zhi (Taipei) 1999;62:619–625

72. Louis CA, Gauthier VY, Louis RP. Posterior approach with Louis plates for fractures of the thoracolumbar and lumbar spine with and without neurologic deficits. Spine 1998;23:2030–2039

73. Macchiarola A, Di Carlo FP, Di Pietro FP, Scisco A. USS internal fixator in lumbar and thoracolumbar vertebral fractures. Chir Organi Mov 2000;85:177–184

74. Markel DC, Graziano GP. A comparison study of treatment of thoracolumbar fractures using the ACE Posterior Segmental Fixator and Cotrel-Dubousset instrumentation. Orthopedics 1995;18:679–686

75. Matsuzaki H, Tokuhashi Y, Wakabayashi K, Ishihara K, Shirasaki Y, Tateishi T. Rigix plate system for anterior fixation of thoracolumbar vertebrae. J Spinal Disord 1997;10:339–347

76. Okuyama K, Abe E, Chiba M, Ishikawa N, Sato K. Outcome of anterior decompression and stabilization for thoracolumbar unstable burst fractures in the absence of neurologic deficits. Spine 1996; 21:620–625

77. Parker JW, Lane JR, Karaikovic EE, Gaines RW. Successful short-segment instrumentation and fusion for thoracolumbar spine fractures: a consecutive 41/2-year series. Spine 2000;25:1157–1170

78. Ruan DK, Shen GB, Chui HX. Shen instrumentation for the management of unstable thoracolumbar fractures. Spine 1998;23: 1324–1332

79. Schultheiss M, Kinzl L, Claes L, Wilke HJ, Hartwig E. Minimally invasive ventral spondylodesis for thoracolumbar fracture treatment: surgical technique and first clinical outcome. Eur Spine J 2003;12: 618–624

80. Shiba K, Katsuki M, Ueta T, et al. Transpedicular fixation with Zielke instrumentation in the treatment of thoracolumbar and lumbar injuries. Spine 1994;19:1940–1949

81. Thalgott JS, Kabins MB, Timlin M, Fritts K, Giuffre JM. Four year experience with the AO Anterior Thoracolumbar Locking Plate. Spinal Cord 1997;35:286–291

82. Zheng ZG, Cheng MH, Dong TH. Unstable fracture of thoracolumbar spine treated with pedicle screw plating: a report of 90 cases. Chin Med J (Engl) 1994;107:281–285

83. Schnee CL, Ansell LV. Selection criteria and outcome of operative approaches for thoracolumbar burst fractures with and without neurological deficit. J Neurosurg 1997;86:48–55

84. Delamarter RB, Sherman J, Carr JB. Pathophysiology of spinal cord injury: recovery after immediate and delayed decompression. J Bone Joint Surg Am 1995;77:1042–1049

85. Fehlings MG, Sekhon LH, Tator C. The role and timing of decompression in acute spinal cord injury: what do we know? What should we do? Spine 2001;26(Suppl 24):S101–S110

86. Clohisy JC, Akbarnia BA, Bucholz RD, Burkus JK, Backer RJ. Neurologic recovery associated with anterior decompression of spine fractures at the thoracolumbar junction (T12–L1). Spine 1992;17(Suppl 8):S325–S330

87. Gaebler C, Maier R, Kutscha-Lissberg F, Mrkonjic L, Vecsei V. Results of spinal cord decompression and thoracolumbar pedicle stabilisation in relation to the time of operation. Spinal Cord 1999;37:33–39

88. Fehlings MG, Tator CH. An evidence-based review of decompressive surgery in acute spinal cord injury: rationale, indications, and timing based on experimental and clinical studies. J Neurosurg 1999;91(Suppl 1):1–11

89. An HS, Singh K, Vaccaro AR, et al. Biomechanical evaluation of contemporary posterior spinal internal fixation configurations in an unstable burst-fracture calf spine model: special references of hook configurations and pedicle screws. Spine 2004;29:257–262

90. Yerby SA, Ehteshami JR, McLain RF. Offset laminar hooks decrease bending moments of pedicle screws during in situ contouring. Spine 1997;22:376–381

91. Been HD, Bouma GJ. Comparison of two types of surgery for thoraco-lumbar burst fractures: combined anterior and posterior stabilisation vs. posterior instrumentation only. Acta Neurochir (Wien) 1999;141:349–357

92. Danisa OA, Shaffrey CI, Jane JA, et al. Surgical approaches for the correction of unstable thoracolumbar burst fractures: a retrospective analysis of treatment outcomes. J Neurosurg 1995;83:977–983

93. Dimar JR, Wilde PH, Glassman SD, Puno RM, Johnson JR. Thoracolumbar burst fractures treated with combined anterior and posterior surgery. Am J Orthop 1996;25:159–165

94. Muller U, Berlemann U, Sledge J, Schwarzenbach O. Treatment of thoracolumbar burst fractures without neurologic deficit by indirect reduction and posterior instrumentation: bisegmental stabilization with monosegmental fusion. Eur Spine J 1999;8:284–289

95. Arino VL. Our experience in 33 cases of thoracolumbar fracture treated by transpedicle instrument. Chir Organi Mov 2000;85:161–165

96. Stancic MF, Gregorovic E, Nozica E, Penezic L. Anterior decompression and fixation versus posterior reposition and semirigid fixation in the treatment of unstable burst thoracolumbar fracture: prospective clinical trial. Croat Med J 2001;42:49–53

97. Kirkpatrick JS. Thoracolumbar fracture management: anterior approach. J Am Acad Orthop Surg 2003;11:355–363

98. Finkelstein JA, Chapman JR, Mirza S. Anterior cortical allograft in thoracolumbar fractures. J Spinal Disord 1999;12:424–429

99. Lange U, Knop C, Bastian L, Blauth M. Prospective multicenter study with a new implant for thoracolumbar vertebral body replacement. Arch Orthop Trauma Surg 2003;123:203–208

100. Kirkpatrick JS, Wilber RG, Likavec M, Emery SE, Ghanayem A. Anterior stabilization of thoracolumbar burst fractures using the Kaneda device: a preliminary report. Orthopedics 1995;18:673–678

101. Mariotti AJ, Diwan AD. Current concepts in anterior surgery for thoracolumbar trauma. Orthop Clin North Am 2002;33:403–412 vii.

102. McLain RF, Sparling E, Benson DR. Early failure of short-segment pedicle instrumentation for thoracolumbar fractures: a preliminary report. J Bone Joint Surg Am 1993;75:162–167

103. Gertzbein SD, Court-Brown CM. Rationale for the management of flexion-distraction injuries of the thoracolumbar spine based on a new classification. J Spinal Disord 1989;2:176–183

104. Finkelstein JA, Wai EK, Jackson SS, Ahn H, Brighton-Knight M. Single-level fixation of flexion distraction injuries. J Spinal Disord Tech 2003;16:236–242

105. Bellabarba C, Mirza SK, Chapman JR. Surgical treatment of thoracolumbar fractures-posterior approach. In: Reitman CA, ed. Management of Thoracolumbar Fractures. Rosemont, IL: American Academy of Orthopaedic Surgeons; 2004:65–78

106. Heller JG, Garfin SR, Abitbol JJ. Disk herniations associated with compression instrumentation of lumbar flexion-distraction injuries. Clin Orthop Relat Res 1992; 284:91–98

107. Yu SW, Fang KF, Tseng IC, Chiu YL, Chen YJ, Chen WJ. Surgical outcomes of short-segment fixation for thoracolumbar fracture dislocation. Chang Gung Med J 2002;25:253–259

108. Yue JJ, Sossan A, Selgrath C, et al. The treatment of unstable thoracic spine fractures with transpedicular screw instrumentation: a 3-year consecutive series. Spine 2002;27:2782–2787

109. Katonis PG, Kontakis GM, Loupasis GA, Aligizakis AC, Christoforakis JI, Velivassakis EG. Treatment of unstable thoracolumbar and lumbar spine injuries using Cotrel-Dubousset instrumentation. Spine 1999;24:2352–2357

110. Razak M, Mahmud M, Mokhtar SA, Omar A. Thoracolumbar fracture-dislocation results of surgical treatment. Med J Malaysia 2000;55(Suppl C):14–17

111. Stambough JL. Posterior instrumentation for thoracolumbar trauma. Clin Orthop Relat Res 1997;335:73–88

112. Stavrev P. Thoracolumbar spine stabilization in fracture-dislocations. Folia Med (Plovdiv) 1994;36:59–65

113. Knop C, Bastian L, Lange U, Oeser M, Zdichavsky M, Blauth M. Complications in surgical treatment of thoracolumbar injuries. Eur Spine J 2002;11:214–226

114. Smith MD, Bressler EL, Lonstein JE, Winter R, Pinto MR, Denis F. Deep venous thrombosis and pulmonary embolism after major reconstructive operations on the spine: a prospective analysis of three hundred and seventeen patients. J Bone Joint Surg Am 1994;76:980–985

115. Maxwell RA, Chavarria-Aguilar M, Cockerham WT, et al. Routine prophylactic vena cava filtration is not indicated after acute spinal cord injury. J Trauma 2002;52:902–906

116. Velmahos GC, Kern J, Chan LS, Oder D, Murray JA, Shekelle P. Prevention of venous thromboembolism after injury: an evidence-based report, II: Analysis of risk factors and evaluation of the role of vena caval filters. J Trauma 2000;49:140–144

117. Velmahos GC, Kern J, Chan LS, Oder D, Murray JA, Shekelle P. Prevention of venous thromboembolism after injury: an evidence-based report, I: Analysis of risk factors and evaluation of the role of vena caval filters. J Trauma 2000;49:132–138

118. Deep K, Jigajinni MV, McLean AN, Fraser MH. Prophylaxis of thromboembolism in spinal injuries: results of enoxaparin used in 276 patients. Spinal Cord 2001;39:88–91

119. Cain JE Jr, Major MR, Lauerman WC, West JL, Wood KB, Fueredi GA. The morbidity of heparin therapy after development of pulmonary embolus in patients undergoing thoracolumbar or lumbar spinal fusion. Spine 1995;20:1600–1603

120. Theiss SM, Lonstein JE, Winter RB. Wound infections in reconstructive spine surgery. Orthop Clin North Am 1996;27:105–110

121. Boriani S, Palmisani M, Donati U, et al. The treatment of thoracic and lumbar spine fractures: a study of 123 cases treated surgically in 101 patients. Chir Organi Mov 2000;85:137–149

122. Shen WJ, Liu TJ, Shen YS. Nonoperative treatment versus posterior fixation for thoracolumbar junction burst fractures without neurologic deficit. Spine 2001;26:1038–1045

123. Yuan-Innes MJ, Temple CL, Lacey MS. Vacuum-assisted wound closure: a new approach to spinal wounds with exposed hardware. Spine 2001;26:E30–E33

124. Cammisa FP Jr, Eismont FJ, Green BA. Dural laceration occurring with burst fractures and associated laminar fractures. J Bone Joint Surg Am 1989;71:1044–1052

125. Denis F, Burkus JK. Shear fracture-dislocations of the thoracic and lumbar spine associated with forceful hyperextension (lumberjack paraplegia). Spine 1992;17:156–161

126. Sar C, Bilen FE. Thoracolumbar flexion-distraction injuries combined with vertebral body fractures. Am J Orthop 2002;31:147–151

127. Aydinli U, Karaeminogullari O, Tiskaya K, Ozturk C. Dural tears in lumbar burst fractures with greenstick lamina fractures. Spine 2001;26:E410–E415

128. Pau A, Silvestro C, Carta F. Can lacerations of the thoraco-lumbar dura be predicted on the basis of radiological patterns of the spinal fractures? Acta Neurochir (Wien) 1994;129:186–187

129. Silvestro C, Francaviglia N, Bragazzi R, Piatelli G, Viale GL. On the predictive value of radiological signs for the presence of dural lacerations related to fractures of the lower thoracic or lumbar spine. J Spinal Disord 1991;4:49–53

130. Carl AL, Matsumoto M, Whalen JT. Anterior dural laceration caused by thoracolumbar and lumbar burst fractures. J Spinal Disord 2000;13:399–403

131. Denis F, Burkus JK. Diagnosis and treatment of cauda equina entrapment in the vertical lamina fracture of lumbar burst fractures. Spine 1991;16(Suppl 8):S433–S439

132. Nairus JG, Richman JD, Douglas RA. Retroperitoneal pseudomeningocele complicated by meningitis following a lumbar burst fracture: a case report. Spine 1996;21:1090–1093

133. Vaccaro AR, Silber JS. Post-traumatic spinal deformity. Spine 2001;26(Suppl 24):S111–S118

134. Gertzbein SD. Scoliosis Research Society: multicenter spine fracture study. Spine 1992;17:528–540

135. Oner FC, van Gils AP, Faber JA, Dhert WJ, Verbout AJ. Some complications of common treatment schemes of thoracolumbar spine fractures can be predicted with magnetic resonance imaging: prospective study of 53 patients with 71 fractures. Spine 2002;27:629–636

136. Bohlman HH, Kirkpatrick JS, Delamarter RB, Leventhal M. Anterior decompression for late pain and paralysis after fractures of the thoracolumbar spine. Clin Orthop Relat Res 1994;300:24–29

137. Razak M, Mahmud MM, Hyzan MY, Omar A. Short segment posterior instrumentation, reduction and fusion of unstable thoracolumbar burst fractures: a review of 26 cases. Med J Malaysia 2000;55(Suppl C):9–13

138. Stambough JL. Cotrel-Dubousset instrumentation and thoracolumbar spine trauma: a review of 55 cases. J Spinal Disord 1994;7:461–469

139. Edward CCLAM. Complications associated with posterior instrumentation in the treatment of thoracic and lumbar injuries. In: Garfin S, ed. Complications of Spine Surgery. Baltimore: Williams and Wilkins; 2004:164–199

140. Reitman CA. Complications. In: Reitman CA, ed. Management of Thoracolumbar Fractures. Rosemont, IL: American Academy of Orthopaedic Surgeons; 2004:119–128

141. Tsirikos AI, Aderinto J, Tucker SK, Noordeen HH. Spinal cord monitoring using intraoperative somatosensory evoked potentials for spinal trauma. J Spinal Disord Tech 2004;17:385–394

142. Gaebler C, Maier R, Kukla C, Vecsei V. Long-term results of pedicle stabilized thoracolumbar fractures in relation to the neurological deficit. Injury 1997;28:661–666

143. McLain RF, Burkus JK, Benson DR. Segmental instrumentation for thoracic and thoracolumbar fractures: prospective analysis of construct survival and five-year follow-up. Spine J 2001;1:310–323

144. McLain RF. Functional outcomes after surgery for spinal fractures: return to work and activity. Spine 2004;29:470–477

145. Tasdemiroglu E, Tibbs PA. Long-term follow-up results of thoracolumbar fractures after posterior instrumentation. Spine 1995;20:1704–1708

146. Weyns F, Rommens PM, Van Calenbergh F, Goffin J, Broos P, Plets C. Neurological outcome after surgery for thoracolumbar fractures: a retrospective study of 93 consecutive cases, treated with dorsal instrumentation. Eur Spine J 1994;3:276–281

147. Berlemann U, Franz T, Orler R, Heini PF. Kyphoplasty for treatment of osteoporotic vertebral fractures: a prospective non-randomized study. Eur Spine J 2004;13:496–501

148. Cho DY, Lee WY, Sheu PC. Treatment of thoracolumbar burst fractures with polymethyl methacrylate vertebroplasty and short-segment pedicle screw fixation. Neurosurgery 2003;53:1354–1360

149. Horn EM, Henn JS, Lemole GM Jr, Hott JS, Dickman CA. Thoracoscopic placement of dual-rod instrumentation in thoracic spinal trauma. Neurosurgery 2004;54:1150–1153

150. Olinger A, Hildebrandt U, Mutschler W, Menger MD. First clinical experience with an endoscopic retroperitoneal approach for anterior fusion of lumbar spine fractures from levels T12 to L5. Surg Endosc 1999;13:1215–1219

151. Schultheiss M, Hartwig E, Kinzl L, Claes L, Wilke HJ. Thoracolumbar fracture stabilization: comparative biomechanical evaluation of a new video-assisted implantable system. Eur Spine J 2004;13:93–100

152. Khoo LT, Palmer S, Laich DT, Fessler RG. Minimally invasive percutaneous posterior lumbar interbody fusion. Neurosurgery 2002;51(Suppl 5):S166–1

153. Gebhard F, Weidner A, Liener UC, Stockle U, Arand M. Navigation at the spine. Injury 2004;35(Suppl 1):S-A35–45

154. Boden SD, Kang J, Sandhu H, Heller JG. Use of recombinant human bone morphogenetic protein-2 to achieve posterolateral lumbar spine fusion in humans: a prospective, randomized clinical pilot trial: 2002 Volvo Award in clinical studies. Spine 2002;27:2662–2673

155. Laursen M, Hoy K, Hansen ES, Gelineck J, Christensen FB, Bunger CE. Recombinant bone morphogenetic protein-7 as an intracorporal bone growth stimulator in unstable thoracolumbar burst fractures in humans: preliminary results. Eur Spine J 1999;8:485–490

156. McAfee PC, Yuan HA, Lasda NA. The unstable burst fracture. Spine 1982;7:365–373

10 Shoulder Girdle Injuries

Peter Alexander Cole and Daniel Joseph Marek

Acromioclavicular Joint Dislocation

Acromioclavicular (AC) dislocation is a common injury due to the prominence of the AC joint on the superolateral aspect of the shoulder. The bony anatomy of the shoulder girdle makes the AC joint vulnerable to direct force with any blow to the shoulder, such as during a fall onto the shoulder.

The AC joint is a synovial joint that contains a round meniscus composed of fibrocartilage. The lateral clavicle is connected to the upper extremity by the coracoclavicular (CC) and coracoacromial (CA) ligaments and AC joint capsule. AC joint dislocation occurs when there is at least partial disruption of these structures. Proper diagnosis of "AC separations" and careful selection of patients for surgical intervention following AC joint injury are required to minimize arthrosis, instability, and dysfunction.

The AC joint plays an important role in suspension of the upper extremity to the axial skeleton. This articulation may allow for up to 20 degrees of rotation[1] and is further affected by the weight of the upper extremity as well as large muscular forces that act across a small surface area. These factors help to explain why internal fixation failures are common, and why there are so many described techniques to repair fractures and dislocations of this joint.

Distal clavicle fractures will be handled separately at the end of this chapter; however, much of the same discussion regarding the diagnosis and treatment of AC dislocations is relevant to the displaced or intra-articular distal clavicle fracture as well.

Classification

Both Tossy et al[2] and Allman[3] developed classification systems for AC dislocations based on the degree of ligament injury and radiographic evidence of displacement **(Table 10–1)**. Rockwood et al[4] later described three additional types of more severe injury (types IV through VI)

based on the direction as well as the amount of dislocation. Rockwood's type IV AC dislocation is complete, and the clavicle is displaced posteriorly. The type V injury is an extreme variation of type III, where the clavicle buttonholes through the trapezius into the subcutaneous tissue, whereas the type VI dislocation is an inferiorly displaced clavicle below the coracoid process.

Clinical Assessment

The injured AC joint is swollen and tender. If a visual or palpable step-off exists, or the distal clavicle feels unstable, then there is at least a type II injury. It is not uncommon for type I and II injuries to hurt for a longer period of time than type III injuries due to residual articular contact and tethering of partially torn ligamentous structures. Abrasions over the superolateral area of the shoulder must be noted if surgery is considered because surgery should be delayed until skin care and reepithelialization have occurred.

An anteroposterior (AP) x-ray of the shoulder reveals the injury; however, visualization of the joint is improved with a 10 degree cephalic tilt view centered over the AC joint, also known as a Zanca x-ray view. Imaging of both AC joints on the same large x-ray cassette helps to demonstrate relative displacement, as well as anatomical variations of the AC facets.

Nonoperative Treatment

Indications for Nonoperative Treatment

Rockwood type I and II AC injuries should be treated nonoperatively with the expectation of excellent short- to midterm results. In the event that late, symptomatic AC arthrosis occurs, elective distal clavicle excision can predictably relieve pain and restore function.[5] Comparing operative versus nonoperative treatment of type III AC

Table 10—1   Combined Tossy and Allman Classification for Acromioclavicular Joint Separation

Type I	Partial tear of ligaments, minimal pain, point tenderness over the acromioclavicular (AC) joint, and no laxity of the AC joint; normal plain films
Type II	Rupture of the capsule and AC ligament. Intact coracoclavicular (CC) ligaments; pain and point tenderness over the AC joint; deformity may be present; plain films reveal an elevated clavicle extending less than the diameter of the clavicle
Type III	Rupture of both AC and CC ligaments; pain and point tenderness are noted over the AC joint and distal third of the clavicle; marked deformity is present; plain films reveal a wide separation between the clavicle and coracoid process

dislocations, the collective weight of evidence reveals no benefit from surgical treatment,[6,7] though some authors believe that the overhead throwing athlete and manual laborer should undergo reconstruction.[8,9]

Reductions, Casting Techniques, Orthoses

Ice should be provided in the acute setting to relieve pain and swelling, and a sling is useful for support of the upper extremity against gravity. There is no benefit to closed reduction because a located joint cannot be maintained with any orthosis, including a figure-of-eight sling.

Rehabilitation

A sling may be used for 2 to 3 weeks to support the extremity during the acute phase of pain. Function is advanced as discomfort allows. Shorter or longer periods with relative rest are required according to the severity of the sprain or dislocation. Patient reassurance is necessary during months of resolving symptoms.

Indications for Surgical Treatment

Surgical reconstruction is indicated in patients with Rockwood type IV to VI AC injuries to prevent chronic dysfunction and pain. The management of type III injuries remains controversial. Most experts recommend nonoperative management, whereas others believe that overhead throwing athletes and manual laborers should undergo operative treatment for Rockwood type III AC injuries.[10–12]

Surgical Treatment

Surgical Anatomy

Fusion of the secondary ossification centers about the AC joint occurs at ~17 years of age for the acromial portion and 24 years of age for the distal clavicle.[10] The average size of the joint is 9 × 19 mm.[11,12] Branches of the axillary, suprascapular, and lateral pectoral nerve innervate the AC joint.[4] Urist found that the clavicle slightly overrides the acromion process in about half of people, and that 21% of AC joints are incongruent.[7] The lateral clavicular facet actually underrides the acromion 3% of the time[8,12] Knowledge of individual variation is helpful during diagnostic and surgical interpretation of anatomy. Furthermore, Moseley stated that the vertical and underriding variations are more likely to have chronic problems after dislocation.[12] The AC joint capsule is strongest at its superior and posterior margin. The scapula is suspended from the clavicle via the CC ligaments, consisting of the well-defined trapezoid and conoid ligaments. These structures run from the base of the coracoid to the undersurface of the clavicle. The trapezoid ligament spans from the coracoid base just lateral to the conoid ligament.

These strong ligaments provide restraint against clavicular elevation.

Surgical Techniques

Many surgical procedures have been described to repair an AC dislocation. The strategies have included fixing the distal clavicle directly to the acromion, augmenting the CC ligaments, or both. Though each strategy can be employed in the acute or delayed setting, if a late reconstruction is done, it is usually combined with a distal clavicle resection.

The most widely known procedure is that described by Weaver and Dunn, in which the CA ligament is transferred through the end of a resected distal clavicle.[13] Many surgeons augment some variation of this repair with fixation across the AC joint, or into or around the coracoid neck.[12]

The same procedures have been employed for distal clavicle fractures, particularly those in which the shaft displaces superiorly due to ruptured CC ligaments (**Fig. 10–1**). The fixation and repair challenges of distal clavicle fractures, regarding maintaining reduction, are similar to the surgical challenges of AC dislocations.

Positioning

The beach-chair position is utilized, and the entire forequarter and extremity are prepped and draped well up onto the neck. An intrascapular or ipsilateral towel is not used for positioning of this surgery because this maneuver will tend to accentuate the deforming force of the clavicle. It is helpful to place an x-ray cassette optimally before draping so that the shoulder is accurately centered, facilitating a good intraoperative radiographic opportunity. Prep the entire extremity to facilitate evaluation of rotational nuances at the time of AC reduction.

Incisions

A 6 cm incision centered over the anterior edge of the distal clavicle is made to expose the dislocated AC joint. The incision is made in Langer's lines, and thus is vertically oriented, as in the shape of a saber, allowing for direct exposure of the torn ligaments, and an adequate exposure of the coracoid. Carefully develop the flaps between the deltoid and trapezius for later accurate closure of this deltotrapezial tissue plane. After the distal clavicle and AC joint are exposed, the typically shredded AC joint capsule is debrided. An evaluation of the articular integrity is made, removing pieces of detached articular cartilage if present. In the acute setting, the clavicle should be noted to reduce rather readily. The CC ligaments are then inspected for integrity, with the intention of repairing these if possible.

If the surgeon elects to save the distal clavicle, as in the acute AC disruption, a drill hole is made in the clavicle adjacent to where the native CC ligament attaches. Mersilene

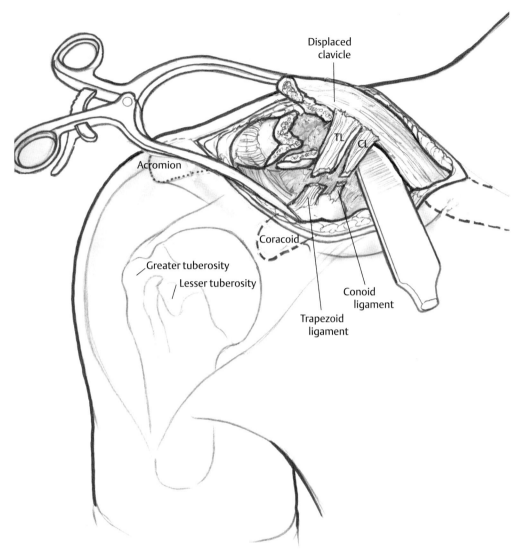

Figure 10–1 An extra-articular distal clavicle fracture. Note that the coracoclavicular ligaments are torn, allowing the clavicle to be displaced superiorly by the sternocleidomastoid. Whether there is intra-articular extension of the clavicle fracture or not, direct and primary reduction of these fragments is unnecessary and perhaps deleterious. Co, coracoid; LT, lesser tuberosity; GT, greater tuberosity; TL, trapezoid ligament; CL, conoid ligament.

tape is then passed along the base of the coracoid under the conjoint tendon and anterior to the hook-shaped coracoid, then up through the drill hole in the clavicle, and sutured secure after reduction. The nonabsorbable synthetic tape is preferable to heavy suture due to the increased likelihood of "cutting out" the drill hole with suture, though certainly, given the strong deforming forces, the tape has been described to cut through as well. The CC ligaments are then sutured primarily. Enhancement of fixation is then executed with the addition of a screw from the superior clavicle down into the coracoid base. A 6.5 mm partially threaded screw is used for this purpose, so that with the lag effect, the Mersilene tape is offloaded. As mentioned before it is the authors' preference to plan for elective removal of the screw approximately 3 months postoperatively, after CC ligament healing.

In the case of a symptomatic chronic dislocation, arthritic joint, or comminuted distal clavicle, the surgeon should perform a distal clavicle resection and subsequent reconstruction of the CC ligaments. The clavicle is simply burred back from its distal end to the area of insertion of the CC ligaments, ~1.5 cm proximal on the bone. The distal clavicle is prepared by opening and smoothing the exit point of the medullary canal, and a slightly more proximal hole is drilled in the cephalad surface of the clavicle. The CA ligament is then detached from its insertion on the acromion, and a no. 2 braided suture is passed in a Krackow or modified Bunnell technique fashion through the end of the clavicle up through the drill hole, where it is then sutured as a loop around the distal resected clavicle. This is the Weaver-Dunn procedure described[13] and popularized for this clinical problem.

Tips and Tricks

- Augmentation of a ligament reconstruction with some type of fixation to offload the repair is wise. It is likely that a screw, such as a modified Bosworth screw[4,14] or a partially threaded 6.5 mm screw, from the superior clavicle down into the coracoid, is superior to Kirschner wires that cross the AC joint or a plate that traverses (bridges) the AC joint because the fixation is perpendicular to the deforming force. Due to the rotational motion of the AC joint, however, the surgeon should expect loosening of this screw over time, and therefore should plan elective removal. Due to the curved and slender shape of the distal coracoid, the surgeon should dissect along the proximal and posterior edge to appreciate the broader base into which fixation should be purchased. Otherwise, it is not uncommon to either fracture the coracoid or simply obtain poor purchase.

- Supplemental forms of anesthesia are useful for shoulder surgery. Begin with the infusion of a subdermal and subcutaneous local anesthetic mixed with epinephrine to decrease bleeding and intercept local pain pathways. Furthermore, it is useful to perform an interscalene block to supplement anesthesia. An indwelling interscalene catheter is used for 1 to 2 days to facilitate early therapy.

Rehabilitation

Patients undergoing surgical reconstruction of AC injuries should be protected in a sling for 4 to 6 weeks. Passive range of motion (PROM) exercises should be encouraged over this time period, but pushing, pulling, or reaching activities should not be allowed. Active range of motion (AROM) may commence at 6 weeks postoperatively, and strengthening exercises at 8 weeks. Contact sports may be initiated at 16 to 20 weeks postop.[14]

New Techniques

A new device called the hook plate (Synthes USA, Paoli, Pennsylvania) is gaining popularity[15,16] and may lessen the risk of loss of fixation. The plate is fixed to the cephalad border of the distal clavicle, and a terminal hook sweeps under the posterior acromion so that the clavicle is restrained from springing superiorly **(Fig. 10–2)** (see **Video 10–1, Disk 2**). It can also be used in combination glenoid neck and distal clavicle injuries **(Fig. 10–3A–D)**, where the surgeon can effectively operate on both locations during the same prep and drape.

Though it provides tremendous leverage against the deforming forces of the distal clavicle, it is associated with a risk of "erosion" of the undersurface of the acromion, and possible fracture.[17,18] It is also prominent, and for these two reasons the surgeon should plan for elective removal of the implant after fracture (or ligamentous) healing.

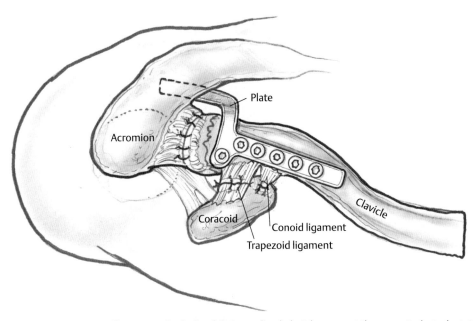

Figure 10–2 A very effective method of stabilizing a distal clavicle fracture or acromioclavicular dislocation is the Hook Plate (Synthes USA, Paoli, Pennsylvania). This implant provides a powerful indirect reduction of the fracture, taking advantage of screw fixation in the clavicular diaphysis, and the stable lever of the acromion, under which the hook is placed, as shown. The Hook Plate should be removed 4 to 6 months after surgery because motion normally occurs at the acromioclavicular joint and may cause loosening or fracture of the implant and osteolysis of the acromion. Accordingly, it is imperative to perform a soft tissue repair to promote healing of either or both the ligaments or joint capsule as shown. If the distal clavicle is comminuted, one may perform a resection of the distal 1 cm of the clavicle and repair the coracoacromial ligament into the distal clavicle through a drill hole. Co, coracoid.

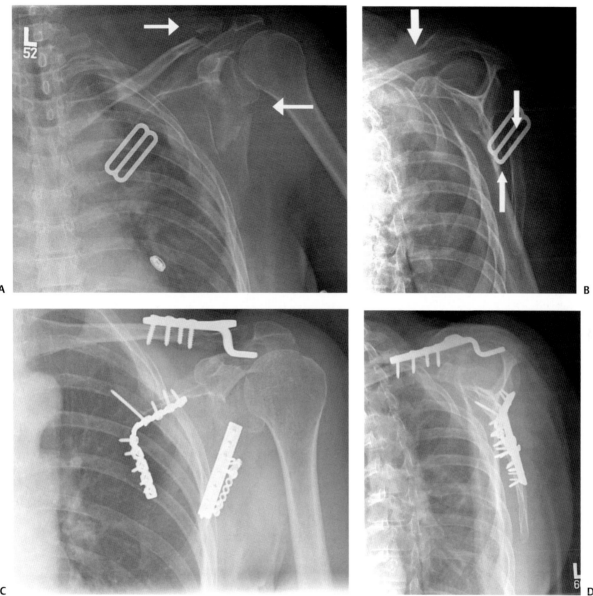

Figure 10–3 (A) Anteroposterior shoulder x-ray demonstrating multiple injuries, including a distal clavicle fracture (rightward arrow), a glenoid neck fracture (leftward arrow), and multiple rib fractures. **(B)** The scapula Y view highlights the clavicular displacement (wide arrow). Furthermore, translation of the lateral border fragments is depicted (narrow arrows), along with mild angular deformity between these fragments and bayonet apposition of the lateral border, though the sling clip in this x-ray unfortunately obscures this. **(C)** Anteroposterior x-ray taken 3 months after fixation of the distal clavicle and glenoid neck fracture. The distal clavicle was effectively fixed with a hook plate. **(D)** Scapula Y x-ray postoperatively showing the restored relationship of the lateral border and acromioclavicular joint.

Outcomes

The prognosis for type I injuries managed nonoperatively is excellent, whereas type II injuries have a good to excellent long-term prognosis.[4] A small percentage of patients, mostly with type II injuries, will develop symptomatic AC joint arthritis, requiring a distal clavicle resection.[4,19] If conservative management of this fails, arthroscopic or open resection of the distal clavicle can be done by removing the distal 1.5 to 2.0 cm of bone, and results have generally been favorable.[4]

Complications

Most of the complications related to surgery involve failure of fixation, causing instability, recurrent prominence of the distal clavicle, and pain. Hardware failure occurs with any technique and may include slippage of Kirschner wires, cutout of CC screws, failure of grafts, or suture cutting through the distal clavicle or coracoid. These various modes of failure underscore the technically demanding nature of the reconstruction.

Scapula Fractures

Fractures of the scapula account for 3 to 5% of all fractures about the shoulder girdle[20-26] and make up less than 1% of all broken bones, according to a review of 4390 cases by Wilson in 1938.[21] Scapula fractures are evidence that significant trauma has occurred. The forces required to cause a scapula fracture are large because of the well-endowed muscular envelope in which it lies, the mobility of the scapula on the thoracic cage, and surrounding musculoskeletal structures (proximal humerus, AC joint, and clavicle), which usually yield first.[22]

Similarly, fractures involving the glenoid neck and body usually occur after high-energy trauma, in patients who sustain a direct impact to the posterosuperior and lateral forequarter. Based on this mechanism, it is not surprising that associated injuries occur in ~90% of these patients.[23,24]

Classification

Because of the rarity of this injury, only a few classifications are commonly recognized for fractures of the scapula. The classifications of Ada and Miller,[25] as well as that of Hardegger et al,[26] are comprehensive and anatomically defined.

Two classifications were developed specifically for intra-articular glenoid fractures: those of Ideberg[27] and Mayo et al.[28] The Ideberg classification is based on 100 glenoid fractures. The scheme of Mayo et al is actually a reorganized version of the Ideberg classification but takes into account the imaging and operative findings of 27 intra-articular glenoid fractures (**Table 10–2**). The intent of Mayo et al was to create a classification scheme that would direct surgical decision making. In so doing, there is emphasis on the associated scapula body and process fractures with which glenoid fractures commonly occur. This application may be the most useful for glenoid surgery.

The Orthopaedic Trauma Association (OTA) classification system is an alphanumeric system that classifies both intra- and extra-articular variants. Its main weakness is that it was not developed by correlating identified patterns of injury with treatment or outcome.

Clinical Evaluation

First and foremost, the physical examination should reflect an understanding of the commonly associated injuries,

Table 10–2   Ideberg Classification Modified by Mayo et al [28]

Type I	Transverse, anterior glenoid
Type II	Transverse, superior glenoid
Type III	Transverse, inferior glenoid
Type IV	Transverse, through body
Type V	Transverse through body and glenoid with associated coracoid, acromion, or neck fractures

particularly those that are life threatening. It is important to disrobe the patient and appreciate whether or not the affected forequarter is medialized or depressed. Frequently, this displacement is obvious and disfiguring. This deformity is also a clue as to the amount of medialization, and thus whether the patient should undergo surgery.

Shoulder girdle injuries are frequently associated with neurovascular lesions and demand an appropriate assessment of the brachial plexus and distal perfusion because 13% of patients with scapula fractures sustain a brachial plexus injury.[28] The suprascapular and axillary nerves are at particular risk (**Fig. 10–4A,B**), yet it is usually impossible to assess their motor function because of fracture displacement and pain; however, axillary nerve sensation should be documented. Abrasions over the scapula spine and acromion are common; therefore, skin integrity should be assessed for appropriate timing of surgery.

Regarding the radiographic examination, it is important to follow the displaced neck or body fracture closely. In the authors' experience, it is not uncommon to see worsening angulation and medialization over the initial 2 to 3 weeks when the lateral border is "unhitched" or comminuted (**Fig. 10–5A,B**).

Nonoperative Treatment

Indications for Nonoperative Treatment

The management of scapula fractures has historically been nonoperative, perhaps in part because of the paucity of information regarding outcomes, combined with a relative unfamiliarity in treating these injuries.[28] Certainly, isolated and minimally displaced scapula fractures should be treated expectantly. Treatment has emphasized symptom relief and early motion. In fact, because the shoulder is such a mobile joint, it can tolerate some degree of displacement, although the limits of tolerable displacement are not well identified by clinical studies. After motion is restored in the first 4 to 6 weeks, therapy is directed at rehabilitating the rotator cuff and strengthening parascapular musculature. Because more than 90% of scapula fractures are minimally displaced,[29] this noninvasive approach is effective for most.[24,25,30-40]

Reduction and Casting Techniques and Functional Bracing

There is no known or identified role for closed reduction or casting. No brace has proven to be efficacious for scapula fractures.

Rehabilitation

If the scapula fracture is treated nonoperatively, a 2-week period of immobility while the arm is supported with a sling is appropriate. Active mobility of the elbow and

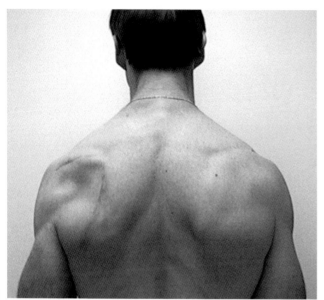

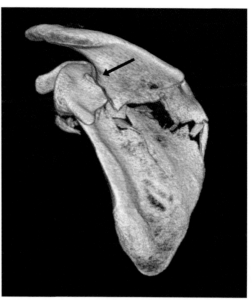

A

Figure 10–4 (A) Clinical photograph of a patient 3 years after he underwent open reduction and internal fixation of a modified Ideberg type VI fracture. Note the atrophy of the infraspinatus muscle. He was diagnosed postoperatively with a suprascapular nerve injury by a electromyographic and nerve conduction study. **(B)** Suprascapular nerve injury is more likely with displaced fracture variants of the modified Ideberg type V variety like the one shown. In this pattern,

B

the fracture extends into the supraglenoid notch, as shown in this three-dimensional computed tomographic image. The arrow depicts the critical location where the neurovascular bundle exits from under the acromion. If a patient has this type of fracture and is more than 2 weeks from the time of injury, it is wise to obtain a study to assess neurological integrity.

wrist are encouraged in the immediate phase to reduce swelling and deconditioning. After this, the patient should begin passive motion, advancing to a full range as symptoms allow. It is helpful to begin with pendulum exercises and increase the PROM under the guidance of a therapist.

The patient should be taught to use the uninvolved extremity to assist with exercises. Scapula fractures will heal rapidly due to a well-endowed blood supply. Therefore, AROM can be started at 4 weeks and maximized quickly. Resistive exercises are begun by 8 weeks, and

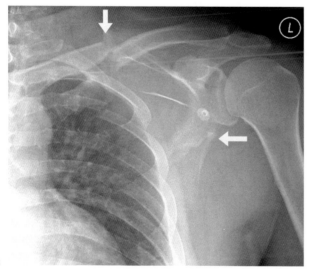

A

Figure 10–5 (A) Anteroposterior view of a shoulder that reveals a scapula neck and ipsilateral clavicle fracture (arrows) shortly after injury. The clavicle is not shortened, and it does not appear as though the glenoid is medialized significantly. For these reasons, nonoperative management was initially chosen. **(B)** Anteroposterior x-ray taken 1 week later shows a significant change in alignment, despite

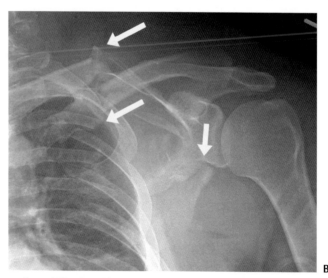

B

immobilization. The patient was concerned that his shoulder appeared more droopy and was more painful. Note the increased shortening of the clavicle, and the increased downward angulation and medial displacement of the glenoid (top and bottom arrows). The ribs were also far more displaced (middle arrow). The patient chose surgical intervention.

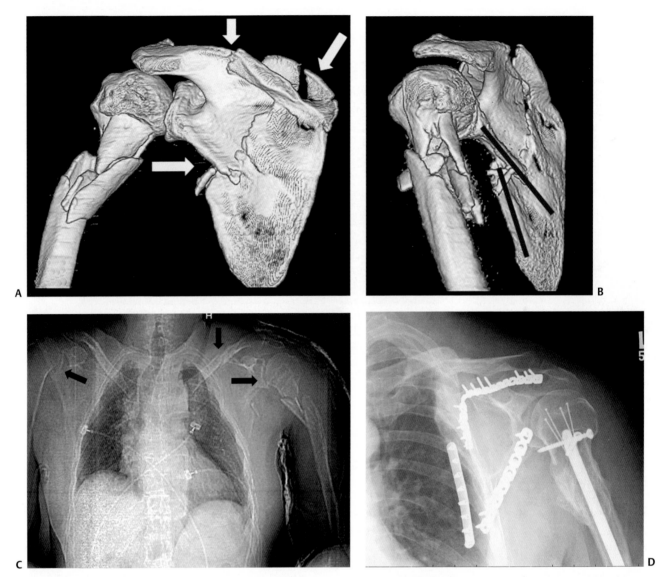

Figure 10–6 (A) A three-dimensional (3-D) computed tomographic (CT) reconstruction of the scapula of a 52-year-old patient who was injured in a motor vehicle collision. He had displaced rib fractures and fractures of the left clavicle, proximal humerus, and scapular neck. His glenoid was displaced approximately 15 mm medially. The arrows depict the fractured superior scapula. **(B)** Lateral 3-D CT of the same patient reveals angular deformity in the semicoronal plane of 15 degrees at the lateral border, as depicted by the corresponding lines on the image. **(C)** A "scout" film of the chest capturing both shoulders is helpful to evaluate any asymmetry of the shoulders. Notice the apparent medialization of the left shoulder girdle over multiple rib fractures. Also notice that the left glenoid faces more inferiorly than the right (depicted by respective left and right arrows), a typical deformity in floating shoulder injuries. The injury is a floating shoulder because of the ipsilateral clavicle fracture (downward arrow). **(D)** Operative repair of all fractures was performed. This is a 6-month postoperative anteroposterior x-ray showing fixation and healing of the scapula and humerus.

restrictions lifted (including weight bearing) as symptoms allow by 3 months.

Indications for Surgical Treatment

Displaced (> 4 mm) articular fractures of the glenoid are the clearest indication for surgery. If humeral head subluxation, early arthrosis, and a poor outcome are to be prevented, open reduction and internal fixation (ORIF) should be performed.[23,29,31,32]

Fractures of the scapula neck should be treated operatively if displacement or angulation causes functional imbalance of the parascapular musculature. Miller and Ada have recommended ORIF if the glenoid is medially displaced more than 9 mm or there is more than 40 degrees of angular displacement.[33] We recommend consideration for operative intervention if glenoid medialization exceeds 15 mm, or lateral border angular deformity exceeds 25 degrees.

Double disruption of the superior shoulder suspensory complex (SSSC) is another indication for surgical treatment

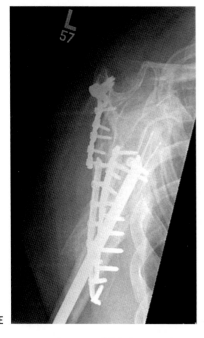
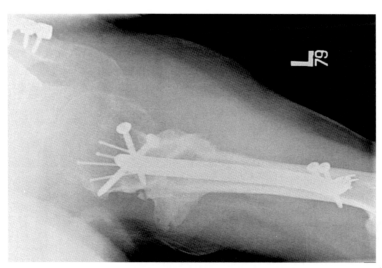

E   F

Figure 10–6 *(Continued)* **(E)** The scapular Y view 6 months postoperatively. A retrograde humeral nail was done to stabilize the proximal humerus fracture so that both fixation procedures could be done from the floppy lateral position. **(F)** The axillary view of the shoulder shows accurate reduction of the humeral head in the joint and confirms that the hardware is extra-articular. At 2 year follow-up, his shoulder motion revealed 165 degrees of forward flexion, 40 degrees of external rotation, and symmetric internal rotation and abduction. Maximal strength and endurance exams were nearly identical, though his DASH score at 6 months was 43.

of scapula fractures. The SSSC is a bony–soft tissue ring made up by the glenoid, coracoid, and acromion processes, as well as the distal clavicle, the AC joint, and the CC ligaments.[34] The superior strut is the middle clavicle, and the inferior strut is the lateral scapula. Lesions to two or more of these structures theoretically destabilize the shoulder and create the "floating shoulder" lesion. Therefore, stabilization of one or both lesions has been recommended to restore integrity to the SSSC, thereby preserving its function of maintaining a stable relationship between the upper extremity and axial skeleton and providing a firm attachment for the many soft tissues that enable shoulder function.[41]

The presence of a scapula neck fracture with an ipsilateral clavicle fracture is a controversial indication for surgical management. In general, the authors' approach to these double lesions is to restore integrity of the SSSC with open reduction and internal fixation of the clavicle or AC joint if it would be otherwise surgically indicated (i.e., type IV AC dislocation or medial clavicular displacement > 2 cm). Subsequent to fixation of the clavicle or AC joint, fixation of the scapula should be executed if it meets the surgical indications already discussed, 15 mm of medialization, or 25 degrees of angular deformity to restore appropriate biomechanical function of the glenohumeral joint **(Fig. 10–6A,B).** I use an opposite shoulder AP radiograph and a computed tomographic (CT) scan to make such a determination. A chest x-ray may be used as well **(Fig. 10–6C).** One can be misled by a single AP x-ray of the injured shoulder because the glenoid may be significantly displaced and angulated, making it impossible to get a "true" AP view of the glenohumeral joint perpendicular to the normal plane of the scapula, because a clear view through the glenohumeral joint is often used as the criteria for determining whether a true AP view has been obtained.

In summary, in our opinion, operative indications for performing open reduction and fixation of extra-articular scapula fracturesare : 100% translation of the lateral border of the scapula, 25 degrees of angular deformity of the glenoid in the semicoronal plane (as determined on a scapula Y view), or 1.5 cm of medialization of the glenoid. These criteria are not absolute and must be placed in the context of the patient's age, activity demands, and extremity dominance **(Fig. 10–6D–F).** Other extra-articular fractures that require open reduction and internal fixation include displaced fractures of the scapular spine, coracoid, and acromion processes. These fractures carry a poor prognosis when treated nonoperatively.[30,31,33,35–37]

Indications for operative treatment of intra-articular fractures include articular step-off or gap of 4 mm or more, if more than 20% of the articular surface is involved or if the defect causes instability of the humeral head **(Fig. 10–7A,B).**

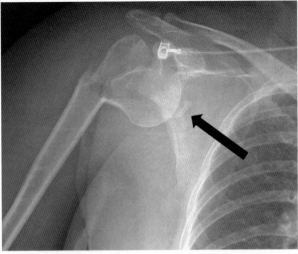

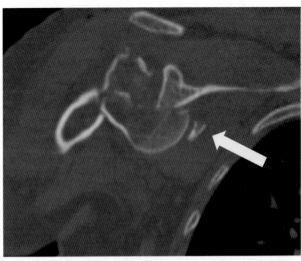

A

B

Figure 10–7 (A) Anteroposterior view of the shoulder of a 72-year-old female, showing a three-part fracture dislocation of the proximal humerus with an associated anterior glenoid fracture depicted by the arrow. The scapula Y and axillary views did not reveal the fragment clearly. **(B)** A computed tomographic scan helped to determine that the fragment was 3 cm in length. The arrow depicts the glenoid fragment seen on this coronal reconstruction image. Because the patient required a deltopectoral approach for the humerus reduction and fixation, the glenoid fracture was fixed as well (see also **Fig. 10–22**).

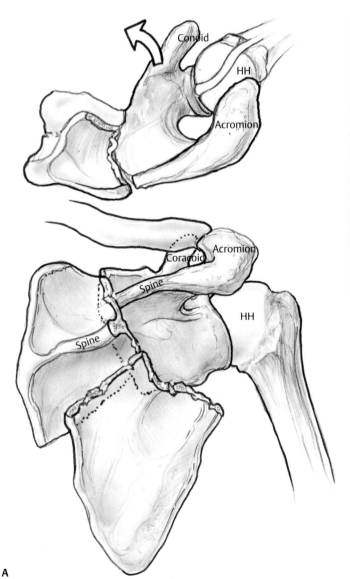

A

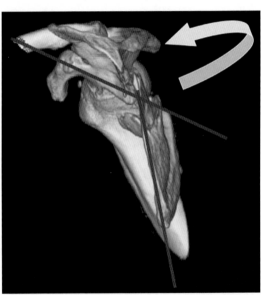

B

Figure 10–8 (A) A common pattern of extra-articular scapula fracture is illustrated. The primary fracture line extends from the lateral border to the vertebral border and/or acromial spine as shown. Less commonly, the primary fracture line goes from the lateral border right up through the glenoid notch. In the lower illustration, note the medial displacement of the glenoid relative to the body fragment. The surgeon will typically encounter a large step-off at the lateral border of the scapula as shown. The typical anteversion deformity of the glenoid neck is reflected in the upper illustration by the rotating arrow in this top-down view (looking down at the superior surface). **(B)** An example of a three-dimensional computed tomographic reconstruction of the scapula as seen from the vertebral border. This patient's fracture demonstrates the typical pattern illustrated in **Fig. 10–8A**. Note this common anteversion of the glenohumeral joint relative to the rest of the scapula body. Therefore, there is not just angular deformity of the lateral border as in this case, but rotational deformity of the glenoid neck as well (curved arrow). HH, humeral head; Spine, acromial spine.

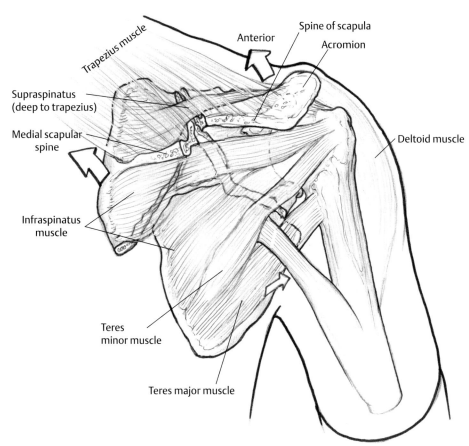

Figure 10–9 Though a dynamic balance of muscular forces comes to bear on the deformity of individual fragments, it is not exactly known how each contributes to displacement. This illustration shows the overlying musculature of the broken scapula and makes it easier to appreciate how such muscles may act to deform the fragments. Other important muscles that are not shown include the levator scapula inserting at the superomedial angle, as well as the major and minor rhomboid muscles inserting at the vertebral border. The latissimus dorsi (not shown) would exacerbate medialization and depression of the glenoid indirectly through the proximal humerus. Appreciate how such muscles may act to deform the fragments (see arrows).

Surgical Treatment

Surgical Anatomy

The scapula is approximately flat and triangular, with a thin translucent body, surrounded by borders that are well developed because of their positions as muscular origins and insertions. When fractured, landmarks are a bit harder to appreciate because predictable deforming vectors are at work based on muscular forces (**Fig. 10–8A,B**). The scapular spine divides the superior and inferior angles of the scapula, thus forming the supraspinatus and infraspinatus fossae, which are origins for their respectively named muscles (**Fig. 10–9**). Its concave anterior surface serves as a broad origin for the subscapularis muscle.

The spine of the scapula ends laterally as the acromion, which arches over the humeral head from which it is separated by the rotator cuff and subacromial bursa. Along with the clavicle, it serves as the origin of the deltoid muscle. The trapezius also originates on the acromion and scapular spine anteriorly. The medial border of the scapula is the site of attachment of the serratus anterior, which functions during scapula protraction, and the rhomboid

muscles, which assist with scapular retraction. The levator scapulae muscle inserts on the superior medial border and is specifically named for its function. The lateral border of the scapula sweeps up from the inferior angle, forming a thick condensation of bone that ends in the neck of the scapula. The lateral border is the site of origin of the teres major and minor muscles, as well as the insertion for the long head of the triceps on the neck and part of the latissimus dorsi at the inferior angle. The coracoid process is a curved osseous projection medial to the anterior neck of the scapula, which serves as the origin for the CC and CA ligaments as well as for the coracobrachialis, short head of the biceps, and pectoralis minor muscles. Just above the coracoid process on the superior margin of the scapula is the scapular incisura, traversed by the transverse scapular ligament, above which lies the suprascapular artery and below which runs the same nerve.

The pear-shaped glenoid fossa lies at the lateral angle of the scapula, its peripheral margin covered by a fibrocartilaginous labrum that is confluent above with the long head of the biceps tendon at the supraglenoid tubercle. The labrum increases the depth of the glenoid by 50%.[38] The glenoid fossa is ~39 mm in a superior-inferior direction and 29 mm in an anterior-posterior direction in its lower half, which is 20% wider than the top half.[39]

The scapula is part of the superior shoulder suspensory mechanism, which attaches the upper extremity to the axial skeleton by the clavicle. Eighteen muscular origins and insertions on the scapula[33] aid in its function to provide a stable base from which glenohumeral mobility can occur.[40]

Surgical Techniques

Logical operative approaches should provide adequate exposure of the fracture, add as little structural damage as possible, and consider the restorative capacity of the biological repair process.[42] Most scapula fractures are best operated by the posterior approach of Judet or the anterior deltopectoral approach.

Posterior Approach

Positioning First, the patient is placed in the lateral decubitus position, "flopping" slightly forward for better access to the posterior shoulder. An axillary roll must be appropriately positioned. Arm rests, towels, or specially designed positioning bumps should support the extremity in 90 degrees of forward flexion and slight abduction (**Fig. 10–10**) (see **Video 10–2, Disk 2**). The entire upper ex-

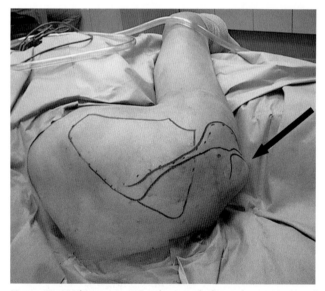

Figure 10–10 This preoperative photograph shows the positioning of the patient for the posterior shoulder approach. The patient is in the lateral decubitus position (floppy forward) with the arm draped free. A wide surgical field is favored. The injured arm is draped free to assess range of motion intraoperatively, to manipulate the extremity if needed to assist with fracture reduction, and to allow for manipulation of the shoulder after fixation to release extrinsic adhesions. The acromioclavicular dislocation in this case is appreciated (arrow), and the glenohumeral joint is very depressed by virtue of the fracture pattern. It is a good habit to palpate and draw bony landmarks for incision planning.

tremity and forequarter should be prepped and draped to allow for manipulation of the shoulder. From a posterior view, the prep should include the inferior neck superiorly, the vertebral column medially, and the latissimus fold caudally.

Incisions The posterior shoulder joint is enveloped by muscular tissue, including the rotator cuff muscles and deltoid. The key to a successful surgical incision is accurate palpation of the bony landmarks of the acromial spine and vertebral border of the scapula. The prominent posterolateral acromion is palpated and followed medially to the superomedial angle of the scapula, and then caudad along the vertebral (medial) border. It is very helpful to manually protract and retract the scapula by grabbing the arm and "shucking" it medially and laterally to create scapulothoracic excursion. This allows the surgeon to feel the vertebral border as it is indirectly manipulated. Note that the incision makes an acute angle at the superomedial corner of the scapula.

A Judet posterior incision is planned using these landmarks, with the horizontal limb 1 cm caudad/distal to the acromial spine and the vertical limb 1 cm lateral to the medial vertebral border. This adjustment places the scar off the prominent bony border for better plate coverage and allows for lateral retraction of a slightly less voluminous flap.

The incision is made through subcutaneous tissue and then directly down onto the bony ridge of the acromial spine all the way around to the superior medial angle and down the medial vertebral border. For access to the lateral border of the scapula, the incision must be generous to allow for easy flap retraction. Properly executed, the fascial incision along the acromial spine and medial border should yield a cuff of tissue to suture back to its bony origin at the end of the procedure.

Exposure Options At this juncture, the operative approach depends upon whether the surgeon desires limited or complete exposure to the posterior scapula (see Tips and Tricks). Limited operative "windows" can be used to access specific portions of the fractures involving the lateral border, acromial spine, and vertebral border (see **Video 10–2, Disk 2**); or an extensive approach can be executed to expose the entire posterior scapula. Keep in mind that the open, extensile approach, though seemingly devitalizing, still preserves the entire subscapularis muscular sleeve on the anterior surface of the scapula, and the elevated flap respects an intravascular plane, raising the flap on the neurovascular pedicle of the suprascapular artery. In this context, this extensile approach is biologically respectful, and nonunion of the scapula body or neck has not occurred in the authors' experience of over 100 posterior approaches for scapular fixation, more than half utilizing the extensile method.

Limited windows are created around the posterior scapular perimeter as needed to address certain fracture

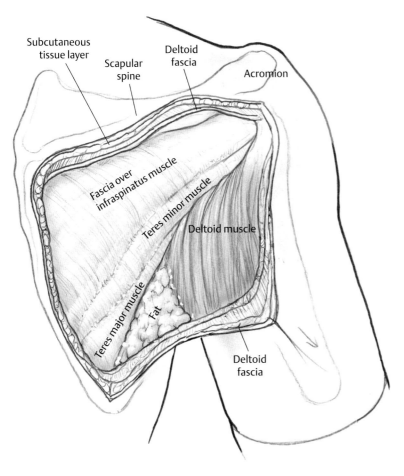

Subcutaneous
tissue layer

Scapular
spine

Deltoid
fascia

Acromion

Fascia over
infraspinatus muscle

Teres minor muscle

Deltoid muscle

Teres major muscle

Fat

Deltoid
fascia

Figure 10–11 A view of the posterior shoulder muscula-ture after skin incision and dissection of the subcuta-neous tissue and deltoid from the acromial spine and vertebral border. This approach is used when the surgeon intends to enter the interval between the infraspinatus and teres minor to access the lateral border, as shown in **Fig. 10–13A.** If the surgeon prefers to elevate the entire muscular envelope off the infraspinatus fossa, then the deltoid and subcutaneous dissection should be deferred to a single musculocutaneous flap, as shown in **Figs. 10–14** and **10–15A–E.** If a single musculocutaneous flap is elevated, the surgeon will not be able to perform a pos-terior capsulotomy and assess intra-articular displace-ment because the large flap will prevent the surgeon from getting enough lateral retraction and exposure.

locations. The muscle plane entered at the acromial border is between the trapezius, originating at the superior mar-gin (left undisturbed), and the deltoid at the inferior mar-gin, which is elevated. The deltoid should then be dis-sected off the muscular origin of the infraspinatus and tagged for reattachment later **(Fig. 10–11).** An elevator is used to elevate the infraspinatus from its origin in the in-fraspinatus fossa, either near the acromial superior border or at the medial vertebral border **(Fig. 10–12).**

At the vertebral border of the scapula, the intermuscular plane is between the infraspinatus and the rhomboids (left undisturbed), which function in scapular retraction. The most important window is between the infraspinatus and teres minor, which must be developed to access the lateral border of the scapula and the glenohumeral joint if neces-sary (see **Video 10–2, Disk 2**). The fascia of these muscles must be clearly exposed to appreciate the interval between these two muscles. The course of the muscle fibers varies slightly, and their character is subtly different. If the surgeon enters too superior, denervation of a part of the infraspina-tus will be inevitable; if too inferior, then the axillary nerve and posterior humeral circumflex artery are at risk in the quadrangular space. Once this important interval is devel-oped, the lateral border of the scapula can be accessed,

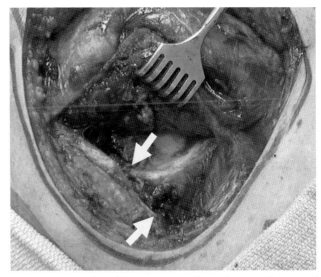

Figure 10–12 A clinical intraoperative photo showing elevation of the infraspinatus muscle from the superior medial angle of the scapula at the vertebral (medial border). The posterior Judet incision has already been made and the deltoid dissected off the rotator cuff musculature, allowing for creation of the two medial and lateral win-dows for reduction and fixation. Appreciate the displacement of the fracture, approximately 4 cm at the superomedial angle, as depicted by the arrows.

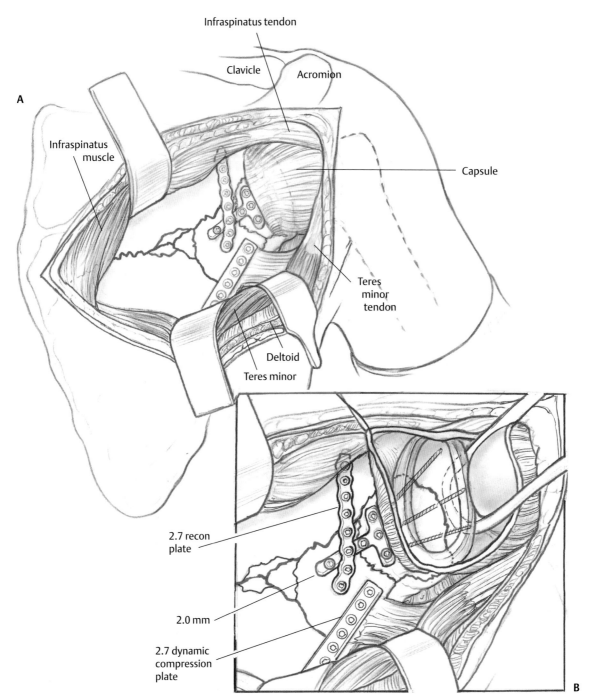

Figure 10–13 (A) Shown is the approach between the muscular interval of the teres minor and infraspinatus, after a straight skin incision, yielding access to the lateral border, glenoid neck, and acromial base. This approach is quite adequate within days of a fracture when reduction of the fragments is easier. Minifragment (2.0 mm) plates are used for smaller articular fragments, and 2.7 mm reconstruction plates are used to contour along the acromial base. **(B)** The inset shows the introduction of a Fukuda retractor through a posterior capsulotomy into the glenohumeral joint to retract the humeral head and allow improved visualization of the glenoid fossa.

which is a critical location to correct glenoid version and medialization, and apply fixation. Note that these two intervals at the vertebral border and lateral border can also be accessed through a straight incision, as shown in **Fig. 10–13A.** The straight incision can be used when there is a simple medial to lateral body fracture pattern, or when there is an isolated posterior glenoid fracture. If the glenoid articular surface must be assessed, then a vertical capsulotomy can be made in such a way as to leave a repairable cuff of tissue on the glenoid side of the glenohumeral joint **(Fig. 10–13B).**

A more extensile approach can be done by elevating the infraspinatus and teres minor, with the deltoid, off their origins as one musculocutaneous flap, but this may be more devitalizing and limits the ability to see within the

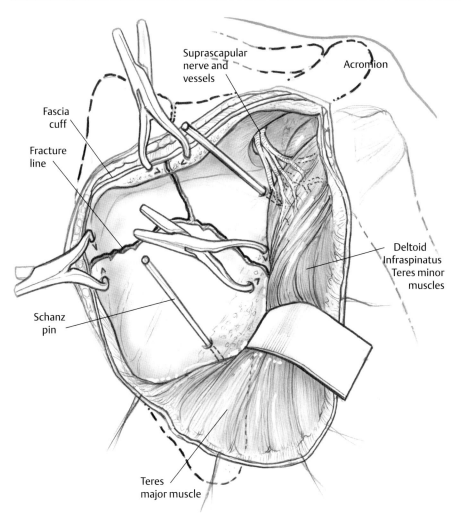

Suprascapular
nerve and
vessels

Acromion

Fascia
cuff

Fracture
line

Deltoid
Infraspinatus
Teres minor
muscles

Schanz
pin

Teres
major muscle

Figure 10–14 For an extensile approach, one may elevate the infraspinatus and teres minor along with the deltoid off their origins as one musculocutaneous flap, but this may be more devitalizing and limits exposure of the intra-articular glenoid fossa.

joint **(Fig. 10–14)**. It is important to repair the muscular origin back through drill holes at the end of such an exposure.

Reduction Technique The lateral border of the scapula and glenoid neck is where the best bone stock is found, so manual reduction maneuvers and fixation are best performed in this region **(Fig. 10–15A,B)**. Schanz pins (4 mm) and T-handled chucks can be used to manipulate main fragments but should be set out of the way of preferred plate placement **(Fig. 10–15C)** (see **Video 10–2, Disk 2**). Generally, at least one straight 2.7 mm plate is placed along the lateral border to stabilize fractures in this region **(Fig. 10–15D)**.

Once reduction is obtained, either it is stable or it must be held for plate and screw application. If the reduction is not stable when the Schanz pins are released, then small, pointed bone reduction clamps can be used to hold the reduction **(Fig. 10–15E)**. If the reduction is still not stable, then an assistant can place a provisional 2.0 mm plate and screws slightly more medial to hold the lateral border in proper relation but remaining out of the

way of desired definitive (2.7 mm dynamic compression (DC) plate) plate fixation **(Figs. 10–3C; 10–15D)**.

If the fracture is significantly displaced and deforming forces are difficult to overcome, a small-fragment external fixator can be used at this juncture to maintain the reduction of the lateral border.

Occasionally, reduction of the lateral border is hindered by displacement of other fracture lines elsewhere in the scapula. If this is the case, one should obtain anatomical reduction of these other areas by accessing the acromial spine and/or medial vertebral border as the pattern dictates. These regions present other opportunities to gain fixation. Often a combination of clamps on the lateral and medial border and acromion is what it takes to perfect the reduction before plate application **(Fig. 10–14)**.

Implant Choice In general, 2.7 mm low-profile plates are the best suited for placement on the scapula borders and have sufficient strength. Larger 3.5 mm plates do not provide as many points of fixation, are difficult to contour, and are too prominent along the acromial and vertebral borders.

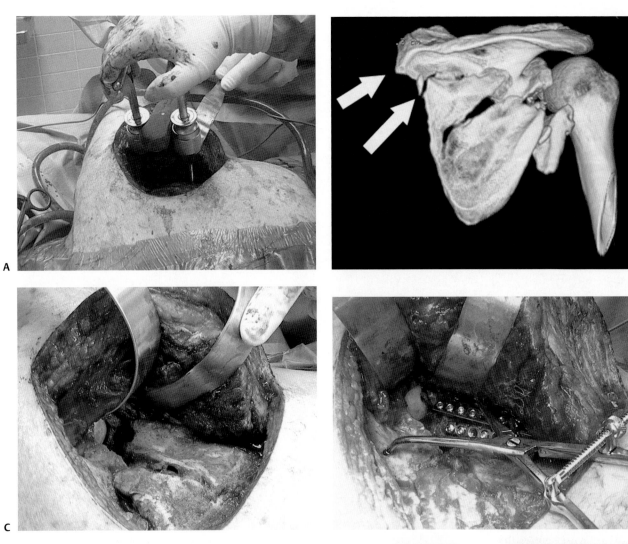

Figure 10–15 (A) An intraoperative image of the posterior approach is shown after the placement of two 5 mm Schanz pins. One Schanz pin is in the proximal glenoid neck fragment, and one is in the distal lateral border fragment. Four millimeter Schanz pins are more optimally sized for these fragments but are not strong enough when great reduction forces are needed. A T-handled chuck is placed on each so that the surgeon can manipulate the fragments into place. Also shown is a mallet handle placed between the two Shanz pins that can be used as a fulcrum to "stretch out" contractures and to get the fragments loosened to mobilize. This is a helpful maneuver in cases where surgery is delayed for more than 3 weeks. **(B)** A three-dimensional computed tomographic reconstruction of a 34-year-old patient who sustained an intra-articular modified Ideberg type IV fracture from a snowmobile accident. It is viewed from the posterior surface of the scapula, showing an intra-articular step-off of about 2 cm, and displacement of both the glenoid neck and superomedial angle (arrows). This image corresponds to the intraoperative images of **Fig. 10–15A,C,E. (C)** This open extensile posterior exposure reveals the displaced fracture fragments. The infraspinatus and teres minor are behind the retractors, and the reader is viewing from medial to lateral into the wound. Note the humeral head "falling" through the displaced fragments as the inferior glenoid is completely displaced, as in **Fig. 10–15B. (D)** The inferior glenoid and its corresponding neck component are now fixed to the distal lateral border with a 2.7 mm reconstruction plate. The 2.0 mm plate was used to provisionally hold the glenoid neck reduced while the Schanz pins were

removed, after which the larger 2.7 mm plate could be secured. The Weber clamp is placed on the inferior neck (tong out of site), while the other tong is placed through a strategic drill hole to set up for the reduction of the two main articular fragments shown in **Fig. 10–15B. (E)** The final reduction maneuver to bring the articular and corresponding body fragments together, done by squeezing the clamp. The next steps will include creating a plate montage to connect the main superior and inferior fragments at the medial and lateral borders.

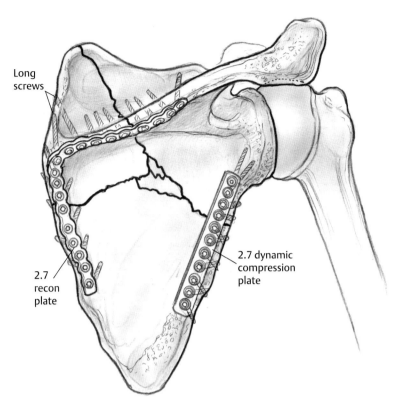

Long screws

2.7 recon plate

2.7 dynamic compression plate

Figure 10–16 A successful formula for stabilizing most of the commonly encountered scapula neck and body fracture variants. The use of a single 2.7 mm dynamic compression plate on the lateral border, placed without need for contouring, allows for balanced fixation. Longer plates must be used for a comminuted border, but in simple patterns an eight-hole plate is sufficient. A 2.7 mm reconstruction plate is used to span fractures exiting the acromial spine and vertebral border. Contouring a plate to fit the superomedial angle is difficult but is an effective strategy to offload the stresses on the lateral border fixation. Note the variably angled screws that are used through the plates to enhance fixation, which is important, given the thin borders of the scapula that are only 8 to 10 mm thick medially. Generally, comminution within the central scapular body can be ignored.

Because the lateral border withstands the most stresses, a 2.7 mm dynamic compression plate should be used **(Fig. 10–16)**. These can generally be applied straight without contouring. Optimally, there should be at least four screws distal to the fracture and three in the glenoid neck to obtain balanced fixation for a simple fracture pattern.

On the other hand, for the acromial and vertebral borders of the scapula, 2.7 mm reconstruction plates are sufficiently strong and are more conducive to contouring along the superomedial border where the plate often spans two fracture lines **(Fig. 10–16)**. Contouring a plate to fit the superomedial angle is difficult because it requires bending the implant in three planes **(Fig. 10–17)**. Two small Kocher clamps are useful to create this contour. One should strive to place six screws on either side of the fracture in this region because each screw is typically 8 to 10 mm long, and fixation may be poor. It is also helpful to angle these screws in different directions to enhance screw purchase.

Closure Once fixation has been accomplished, perform a manipulation of the free extremity and visualize scapular motion for stability. Ensure that all extrinsic adhesions and stiffness be eliminated prior to awaking the patient, especially if the patient's surgery was delayed for an extended period due to referral or other injuries.

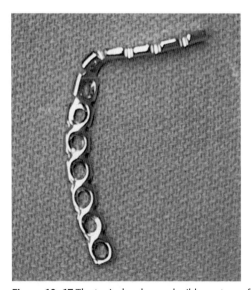

Figure 10–17 The typical and reproducible contour of the superomedial angle of the scapula, reflected in a 2.7 mm reconstruction plate. The superior limb wraps around the medial acromial spine, and the inferior limb stems down the vertebral border. This plate fixes the vertebral border, which helps to offload the lateral border fixation and allows the scapula to move as a unit.

Debride any devitalized muscle prior to closure. A drain should be placed under the myocutaneous flap and exit proximal and anterior to the wound through a long subcutaneous tunnel to lessen persistent drainage due to dependency in the supine position.

For repair of the myocutaneous flap, make three 2.5 mm drill holes in the acromial spine and three more in the vertebral border to repair the fascia back to its bony origin. It is imperative that this myofascial closure be secure to prevent an avulsion of the deltoid, infraspinatus, or teres minor origin during rehabilitation.

With a heavy, braided, nonabsorbable, no. 2 suture, reduce the myofascial flap back to its bony origin (through the drill holes). Supplement the fascial closure with no. 1 absorbable braided suture. The authors prefer an absorbable subcuticular stitch for the skin if the injury is more than a week old because scar formation in this region can be excessive.

Anterior Approach

Positioning   The patient is placed in a beach chair position with an arm board attached to support the extremity. An x-ray plate is positioned behind the shoulder during the setup so that an intraoperative film can be taken. Place a small towel roll under the ipsilateral shoulder to help thrust it forward. Because the anterior approach is used for the fixation of anterior glenoid fractures, a direct intra-articular view of the joint obviates the need for intraoperative fluoroscopy.

Incisions   An incision is made from the palpable coracoid to a point just lateral to the axillary fold, commonly named the deltopectoral groove **(Fig. 10–18).** This incision is taken down to the deltopectoral interval where the cephalic vein is identified. The incision can be extended distally to the deltoid insertion and proximally to the clavicle for greater exposure.

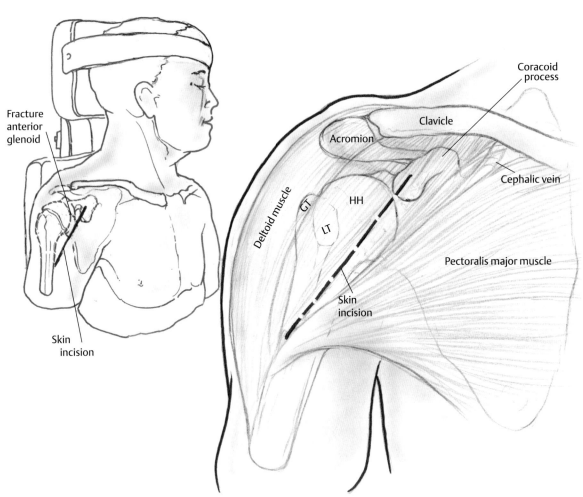

Figure 10–18 The deltopectoral incision is made from the palpable coracoid process along the deltopectoral interval toward the deltoid insertion. The cephalic vein marks the interval between the muscles. The inset shows the patient properly positioned in the beach chair position, with the head angled toward the opposite side and secured. The anterior approach is used for Ideberg type II fractures and anterior glenoid fractures. GT, greater tuberosity; LT, lesser tuberosity; HH, humeral head.

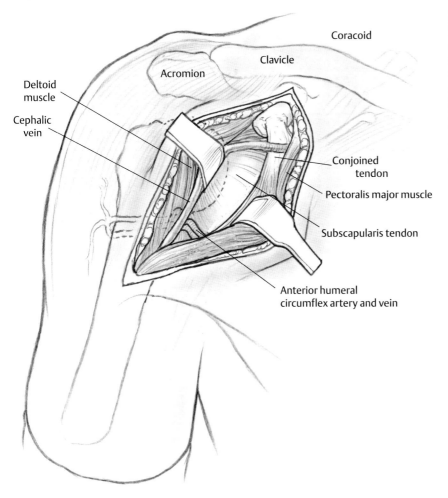

Coracoid

Clavicle

Acromion

Deltoid
muscle

Cephalic
vein

Conjoined
tendon

Pectoralis major muscle

Subscapularis tendon

Anterior humeral
circumflex artery and vein

Figure 10–19 The interval between the pectoralis major and deltoid has been developed, and the cephalic vein retracted laterally (or medially). After incising the clavipectoral fascia (not shown), the coracobrachialis is exposed and retracted medially, thus exposing the broad, flat subscapularis tendon, under which lies the capsule of the shoulder joint. Dissection is preferably limited to the anatomy above the leash of blood vessels of the anterior humeral circumflex artery.

Exposure   Once the cephalic vein is identified in the deltopectoral interval, it should be retracted laterally with the deltoid and preserved through the duration of the procedure. The interval between the deltoid and pectoralis major is dissected down to the clavipectoral fascia that covers the coracobrachialis and subscapularis tendons (**Fig. 10–19**).

Superior and inferior retractors are first placed, and the humerus is rotated to appreciate the tension on the subscapularis tendon and its insertion onto the lesser tuberosity. At the inferior margin of the tendon lie the transversely running anterior humeral circumflex vessels, which should be ligated or cauterized. Below this leash of vessels, the axillary nerve is at risk, and there is no need to extend the incision inferiorly. With the humerus in neutral position, the subscapularis tendon should be incised 1 cm medial to its insertion to maintain a cuff of tissue for later repair. Often the subscapularis is difficult to separate from the joint capsule. Although it is helpful to discriminate these two layers for an accurate closure, occasionally it is necessary to repair the two jointly due to inadvertent dissection into the capsule.

Stay sutures should be placed on each side of the subscapularis muscle to identify for closure, as well as to prevent medial displacement of the muscle.

The joint capsule is now appreciated. An arthrotomy can be performed by dividing the capsule vertically just medial to the palpable glenoid rim to allow intra-articular inspection (**Fig. 10–20**). Alternatively, the surgeon can work through the fracture to wash out the joint and then obtain an indirect articular reduction by reducing the extra-articular component of the fragment. If there is articular comminution, then capsulotomy is mandatory, and the surgeon needs to work on either side of the capsule. For optimal joint inspection, the surgeon should place a retractor in the joint, on the posterior edge of the glenoid, to lever the humeral head laterally away from the scapular articular surface (**Fig. 10–21**).

Reduction can be effected with a dental pick or shoulder hook, and provisional fixation obtained with Kirschner wires. Fluoroscopy is not needed because direct inspection of the joint is performed. Depending on the size of the fragment or the degree of comminution, implant (screw) choices may range in size from 2.0 to 3.5 mm

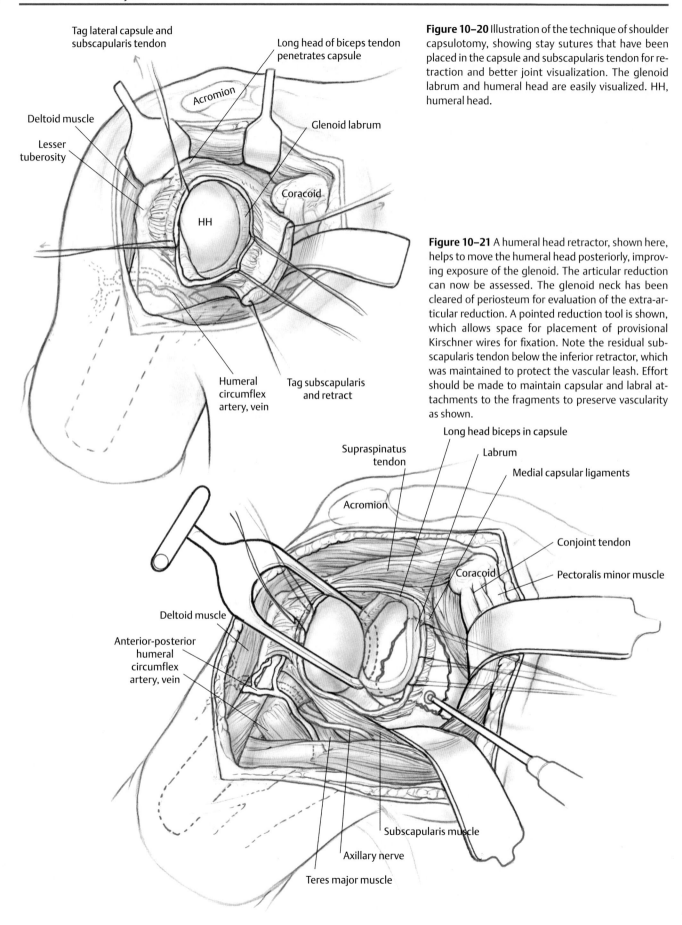

Tag lateral capsule and
subscapularis tendon

Long head of biceps tendon
penetrates capsule

Acromion

Deltoid muscle

Glenoid labrum

Lesser
tuberosity

Coracoid

HH

Humeral
circumflex
artery, vein

Tag subscapularis
and retract

Figure 10–20 Illustration of the technique of shoulder capsulotomy, showing stay sutures that have been placed in the capsule and subscapularis tendon for retraction and better joint visualization. The glenoid labrum and humeral head are easily visualized. HH, humeral head.

Figure 10–21 A humeral head retractor, shown here, helps to move the humeral head posteriorly, improving exposure of the glenoid. The articular reduction can now be assessed. The glenoid neck has been cleared of periosteum for evaluation of the extra-articular reduction. A pointed reduction tool is shown, which allows space for placement of provisional Kirschner wires for fixation. Note the residual subscapularis tendon below the inferior retractor, which was maintained to protect the vascular leash. Effort should be made to maintain capsular and labral attachments to the fragments to preserve vascularity as shown.

Long head biceps in capsule

Labrum

Supraspinatus
tendon

Medial capsular ligaments

Acromion

Conjoint tendon

Coracoid

Pectoralis minor muscle

Deltoid muscle

Anterior-posterior
humeral
circumflex
artery, vein

Subscapularis muscle

Axillary nerve

Teres major muscle

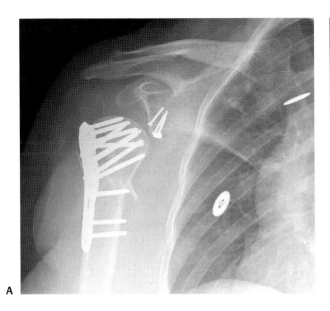

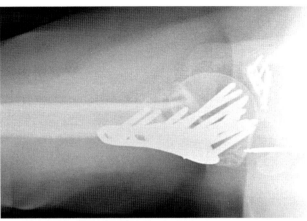

A

B

Figure 10–22 (A) This is an anteroposterior shoulder x-ray taken 6 weeks after open reduction and internal fixation of the proximal humerus and anterior glenoid of the same patient depicted in **Fig. 10–7.** The inferior subluxation of the humeral head is caused by deltoid atony that commonly occurs after such injuries. **(B)** Axillary view demonstrating articular restoration and congruity of both the humeral and glenoid side of the joint.

(Fig. 10–22A,B). Frequently, a mini buttress plate can be applied on the anteroinferior edge of the glenoid, particularly if there is any comminution **(Fig. 10–23).**

Closure of the capsule and subscapularis may be performed with no. 2 braided suture. The subcutaneous tissue is approximated with 2–0 suture, and the skin is closed with a monofilament, subcuticular, absorbable suture.

Rehabilitation

Rehabilitation for the anterior and posterior approaches is similar. The goal of surgery is to obtain stable fixation, defined as a construct that withstands physiological passive motion. The adult shoulder has a propensity to stiffen quickly. Every effort must be directed at maintaining full range of motion, which is verified during surgery

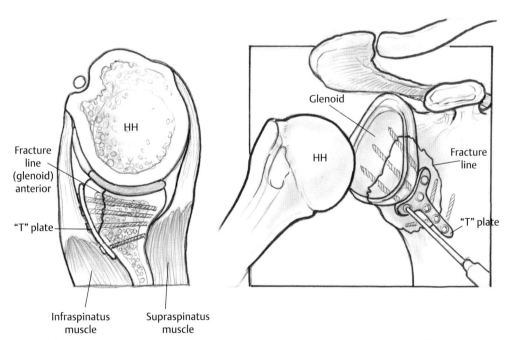

Figure 10–23 The technique of buttress plating of the anterior-inferior glenoid is shown in two views. Minifragment 2.0 mm screws and plates tend to work well, particularly when the fracture is impacted or multiple fragments are present. The inset (left panel) shows a cross section of the glenoid and highlights the buttress effect of the plate, with subchondral screws compressing the glenoid fragment. HH, humeral head.

Tips and Tricks

Posterior Approach

- *Delay in Treatment*   Because patients with scapular fractures often have other serious injuries that require immediate attention, it is not uncommon for a patient with a complex scapula fracture to be referred relatively late to an orthopaedic specialist. Nevertheless, it is feasible to operate on scapular fractures within 6 weeks of injury, although the operation is more difficult, requires patience to take down callus, and depends on a thorough understanding of characteristic fracture patterns and deforming forces. Even with delayed reconstruction, patient satisfaction is high because of improved cosmesis, decreased pain, and improved mobility.

- *Associated Spine Injury*   Cervical and thoracic spine injury is associated with scapula fractures in over one fifth of cases.[26] In such cases, care must be coordinated with a neurological or orthopaedic spine surgeon prior to positioning and induction of anesthesia. If possible, spinal internal stabilization should be performed first; if nonoperative spine management is chosen, care must be taken to establish intraoperative in-line halo traction. Traction is preferable to working around a cervical collar, with regard to both safety and draping.

- *Abrasions*   Because scapula fractures are commonly caused by blunt trauma, abrasions and road rash are common findings. These skin lesions must resolve or be excluded from the surgical field prior to incisions. These lesions usually reepithelialize within 2 weeks using simple wound care—a very reasonable period of time to wait for optimal soft tissue circumstances.

- *Positioning for a Posterior Approach*   Positioning may vary depending on the goal of surgery. For repair of extra-articular fractures, the patient should be allowed to tilt slightly forward from the lateral decubitus position, whereas if posterior access to the glenohumeral joint is desired, then the patient's torso should remain vertical to properly accommodate the anteverted position of the scapula on the thorax. This prevents the surgeon from having to fight gravity, as well as from having to work "upside down" while performing articular reconstruction of the glenoid.

Selection of Posterior Approach

- *Extensile Exposure*   The choice of exposure depends on the fracture pattern and the time to surgery. When the fracture is more than a week old, or the fracture is complex with more than three exit points around the "ring" of the scapula, it is helpful to utilize a completely open approach, with elevation of the entire deltoid, infraspinatus, and teres minor. The extensile exposure allows the surgeon to visualize and manipulate the fracture at multiple points to effect the reduction, as well as the ability to mobilize the fractures by breaking up intervening callus in cases operated late. Care must be taken in such cases not to overretract the flap, which threatens the suprascapular neurovascular bundle. It is also important to understand that direct access to the joint (intra-articular inspection) is not possible when retracting the whole rotator cuff flap.

- *Straight Incision*   A posterior glenoid fracture or an intra-articular glenoid fracture with involvement of the glenoid neck, with minimal involvement or displacement of the acromial spine and vertebral border, can be approached with a simple straight posterior incision. For these simpler fractures, all of the pathology, reduction maneuvers, and fixation can be accessed through the interval between the teres minor and infraspinatus.

- *Infraspinatus Tenotomy*   If greater exposure to the glenoid fossa or superior glenoid is desired, an infraspinatus tenotomy can be performed, leaving 1 cm of cuff insertion at the greater tuberosity for repair **(Fig. 10–24)**. This allows the slender musculotendinous portion of the infraspinatus to be retracted off the superior glenoid region for easy access to the glenohumeral joint. This maneuver is particularly helpful in large muscular patients with Ideberg type II fractures.

Reduction and Fixation

- *Lateral Border Reduction*   In the common scapula neck variants, it is essential to have a joystick in the distal aspect of the lateral border and medial aspect of the neck. Low-profile devices such as 4 mm Schanz pins or a small fragment external fixator are useful to maintain the reduction of the lateral neck. These devices provide enough additional space for correct drill direction, clamp application, and screw placement. In contrast, standard bone reduction clamps do not suit these fracture patterns well due to interference with the flap.

- *Vertebral Border Reduction*   Because the vertebral border of the scapula is quite thin, it is helpful to place vertically oriented, pointed bone reduction forceps into small drill holes through the posteromedial aspect of the body, rather than clamping the medial border itself, which makes plate application nearly impossible without clamp removal.

- *Enhancing Implant Contour and Purchase*
  - To enhance screw purchase at the medial border of the scapula, direct each screw ~30 degrees in a different direction to minimize pullout. This strategy also adds another 1 to 2 mm of length to each screw, which further improves purchase. In the authors' experience, applying six 8 mm long screws at different angles has proven sufficient to avoid failure of fixation.
  - To enhance fixation at the superior medial angle of the scapula is to utilize the excellent bone stock at the base of the supraspinatus fossa (anterosuperior). Screws in excess of 20 mm long can be obtained with the correct drill vector in this area. Palpate this region under the levator scapulae origin to appreciate the proper vector for placement of screws.

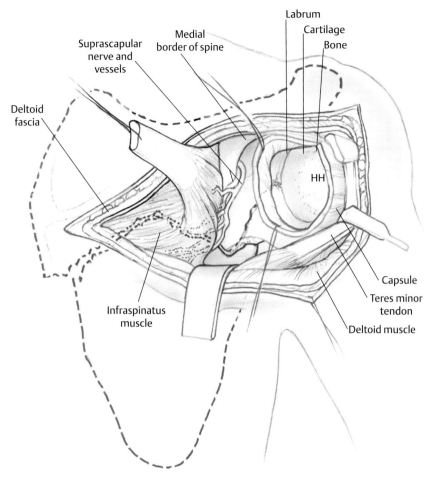

Suprascapular
nerve and
vessels

Medial
border of spine

Labrum
Cartilage
Bone

Deltoid
fascia

HH

Infraspinatus
muscle

Capsule

Teres minor
tendon

Deltoid muscle

Figure 10–24 The surgical exposure possible when utilizing the interval between the infraspinatus and teres minor, with the addition of an infraspinatus tenotomy to enhance exposure to the glenoid. This approach is shown with a posterior capsulotomy over the glenoid rim, with care not to cut the labrum. The suprascapular neurovascular bundle must be protected from excessive retraction. Note the modification in the skin incision, which is straight. This incision would still allow for access to the superomedial angle of the scapula if necessary for plating through a different window. HH, humeral head.

while the stability of the fracture can be directly visualized. If the fracture is not stable, then every attempt should be made to gain such stability, lest the surgeon accept either stiffness from immobilization, or failure of fixation. Following surgery, full PROM should be instituted immediately.

The goal of rehabilitation during the first 4 weeks postoperatively is to regain and maintain motion. The goal should not be strength acquisition, and the patient must be reminded of this. A stably fixed fracture can feel quite comfortable quickly, and the patient will be inclined to use it. The surgeon should stress to the patient that no active motion, no lifting, and no weight bearing are done for 4 weeks.

A continuous passive motion (CPM) machine can be used selectively by patients demonstrating problems with standard physiotherapy. CPM should be considered in all patients with brachial plexopathy. Pulleys and push-pull sticks powered by the opposite extremity, and supine assisted motion are necessary modalities. Appropriate pain control is necessary for the patient to obtain maximum movement. A regional anesthetic block with an indwelling interscalene catheter for the first 48 to 72 hours postoper-

atively is an excellent adjunctive method to promote early gains in confidence. Ipsilateral elbow, wrist, and hand exercises using 3 to 5 lb weights (on a supported elbow) are encouraged. These exercises will lessen upper extremity muscular atrophy and promote edema reduction.

Postoperative Care

Postoperative Orders

- Sling for comfort
- Full shoulder PROM
- No shoulder AROM, lifting, or weight bearing
- Hand, wrist, and elbow exercises (3 to 5 lb) with full PROM + AROM
- D/C drain when less than 15 mL/8 hour shift

Follow-Up

The patient should generally be seen at 2, 6, and 12 weeks postoperatively. At each of these visits, AP, scapular Y, and axillary radiographs should be obtained. Thereafter, follow-up at 6-month intervals for 1 year is appropriate to document maximum function in most cases. A simple AP radiograph at these intervals is all that is necessary. Patients with associated injuries may warrant longer follow-up, especially those with a brachial plexopathy.

At 2 weeks the wound should be checked, and patients should be encouraged and reassured to push PROM, until 4 weeks, at which time they may begin lifting their shoulder and use their own shoulder muscles, though not against resistance (except gravity).

At the 6-week follow-up visit, the patient begins a program of weight lifting that begins with 3 to 5 lb and accelerates as the patient's symptoms allow. At the 6-week interval, the physician must intercept the occasional patient that is not progressing with motion. This is more common in patients who have a brachial plexus injury, a head injury, a halo vest for spine injury, or complex associated fractures of the ipsilateral extremity. This is an excellent time for a manipulation under anesthesia to jumpstart the motion for the patient. If range of motion is not regained during this period, the patient may have permanent loss of function.

At the 3-month follow-up, the patient is reassured of progress. Slow improvements in strength, endurance, and conditioning continue to be noted for up to 18 months; it is important to educate patients on the expected length of convalescence.

Caveats

For anterior approaches to the shoulder, external rotation should be protected against forced passive external rotation past neutral, or internal rotation against resistance for a full 6 weeks. This is needed to protect the repair of the subscapularis tenotomy during exposure of the glenohumeral joint. After 6 weeks, these restrictions may be removed.

For posterior approaches in which the infraspinatus and teres minor have been mobilized from their origins (see extensile posterior approach), and in which the deltoid is taken off the acromial spine, these muscles must be protected for 6 weeks as well. The postoperative regimen as already described generally achieves this automatically. The active external rotation and shoulder extension allowed at 4 weeks do not stress these muscular repairs excessively.

It is important to emphasize that the patient who is slow to progress at the 6-week interval should undergo shoulder manipulation under anesthesia because it will be too late after 3 months of scarring. Patients at increased risk for stiffness include those with head or brachial plexus injury (who may be totally dependent upon others for their therapy), as well as those with complex associated ipsilateral injuries and patients with a halo vest for spine fractures. After manipulation, intra-articular injection of 10 mL of local anesthetic and steroid may lessen reformation of intra-articular adhesions.

Outcomes

Operative management of displaced intra-articular glenoid fractures is clearly indicated. Mayo et al[28] have reported the largest operative series of intra-articular glenoid fractures and documented 82% good or excellent results among 27 patients evaluated clinically and radiographically at 43 months postoperatively.

Studies support the notion that scapular neck fractures should be treated operatively if displacement or angulation renders functional imbalance to the parascapular musculature. Miller and Ada recommend ORIF if the glenoid is medially displaced more than 9 mm or there is more than 40 degrees of angular displacement.[33] This recommendation is based on a follow-up of 16 such patients treated nonoperatively, of whom 50% had pain, 40% had exertional weakness, and 20% had decreased motion at a minimum of 15 months' follow-up. A group of eight patients in this same study were treated operatively, and all achieved a painless range of motion. Hardegger et al[26] achieved 79% good or excellent results in a series of 37 patients treated operatively, although only five cases were "severely displaced or unstable" scapula neck fractures, and these were not analyzed separately. Nordqvist and Petersson[43] analyzed 68 patients with a mean 14-year follow-up and found that 50% of patients with residual deformity have shoulder symptoms. Armstrong and Van Der Spuy[30] noted that six of 11 patients with displaced scapula neck fractures had residual stiffness at 6 months.

Several papers discuss the management of double disruptions of the superior shoulder suspensory complex. Herscovici et al[35] reported on ORIF of seven clavicle fractures in patients with ipsilateral scapula neck fractures. In this series, all patients achieved excellent functional results with no deformity at 48.5-month follow-up. Two other patients in this series treated nonoperatively had significant shoulder drooping and decreased range of motion. Others have also advocated internal fixation of just the clavicle for restoration of length and sufficient stability of the shoulder.[26,44] Leung and Lam[45] treated 15 such patients with internal fixation of both the fractures and discovered good or excellent results in 14 patients 25 months after surgery. On the other hand, Ramos et al[46] reviewed 16 patients with ipsilateral clavicle and scapula neck fractures treated conservatively. Ninety-two percent had good or excellent results at 7.5-year follow-up. A significant shortcoming of these three studies is that none documented the degree of displacement of the scapula neck fracture, and in the latter, the radiological outcome was noted to be good in all but one, suggesting minimal original displacement. In a recent retrospective study by Edwards et al,[47] the outcome of noninvasive treatment of ipsilateral clavicle and scapula fractures was assessed at a mean 28-months follow-up. Nineteen of 20 healed uneventfully, with excellent range of motion and function. This study did document the degree of displacement of the clavicle and scapula fracture. Interestingly, this is a study of mostly minimally displaced injuries; only two of 20 scapulas and eight of 20 clavicles were displaced more than 1 cm.

Complications

The most serious complications associated with scapular fractures do not actually involve the scapula itself, but rather pertain to accompanying injuries of adjacent and distant structures that occurred at the time of injury. Because scapula fractures are seen in high-energy trauma, the most common injuries are the ipsilateral shoulder, upper extremity, lung, and chest wall. In fact, the mortality rate of patients with a scapula fracture is 2%. Ten to 40% of cases are associated with a cerebral contusion and 15 to 55% of patients have a pulmonary lesion such as pneumothorax or contusion.

Complications from a fracture of the scapula itself are extremely rare. Such reported complications include nonunion, malunion, glenohumeral degenerative joint disease, and instability. Also, shoulder instability can arise from angulation of the glenoid neck. If a glenoid neck fracture is angulated, glenohumeral pain, and dysfunction may arise. Finally, an improper rehabilitation program may lead to increased shoulder stiffness.[48]

Fractures of the Clavicle

The clavicle is the bony linkage between the axial and appendicular skeleton. Any force absorbed by the upper extremity is transmitted to the thorax through the clavicle via the AC and sternoclavicular joints. Clavicle fractures are the most common fracture, constituting 5 to 10% of all fractures[49,50] and accounting for ~35% of all shoulder girdle fractures.[51] Though most commonly seen in children and young adults,[52] they are diagnosed with increasing frequency in later decades, particularly in the context of the epidemic of osteoporosis.

Classification

Though there are several classifications proposed, Allman simply divided the clavicle fracture into anatomical thirds, with the middle third being group I, the distal third group II, and the proximal third group III **(Table 10–3)**.[3] Neer[53] further classified distal third clavicular fractures, which he defined as being lateral to the medial edge of the trapezoid ligament **(Table 10–4)**.

Table 10—3   Allman's Classification for Fractures of the Clavicle

Group I	Middle third
Group II	Distal third
Group III	Proximal third

Table 10—4   Neer's Classification for Fractures of the Distal Third of the Clavicle

Type I	Involves the distal end of clavicle with intact coracoclavicular ligaments
Type II	Involves the distal end of clavicle with tearing of coracoclavicular ligaments and wide displacement of fragments—higher risk for nonunion

Pearl

Pain and deformity localized to the clavicle are the most typical presentation. Ecchymosis and tenting of the skin may be recognized. Physical exam will frequently detect bony crepitus and should include inspection of the skin for punctures or lacerations consistent with an open fracture. Because the clavicle is directly anterior to the brachial plexus and the subclavian artery, physical examination should also include neurovascular assessment, particularly in injuries associated with high-energy mechanisms.

Nonoperative Treatment

Indications for Nonoperative Treatment

The mainstay of treatment for proximal, middle, and minimally displaced distal clavicular fractures is nonoperative. With distal-third clavicle fractures, there will not be much displacement of the proximal clavicle if the CC ligaments are intact. Extra-articular fractures, displaced less than 1 cm, are treated with a simple sling or a sling-and-swath immobilizer for comfort.

Intra-articular distal clavicle fractures most often also warrant nonoperative treatment. In the case of intra-articular clavicle fractures, the patient should be warned of the possibility of arthritic symptoms if there is step-off or comminution at the AC joint. This outcome can be treated on a delayed basis with distal clavicle resection. In children 2 weeks of relative immobilization are required before callus begins to provide the splinting necessary for healing of the bone ends. In adults, a month of such immobilization will provide the same relief. The patient must be followed on a weekly basis; however, until consolidation, because these injuries can displace substantially **(Fig. 10–25A,B,C)**. If they do, it is possible that operative intervention may become warranted.

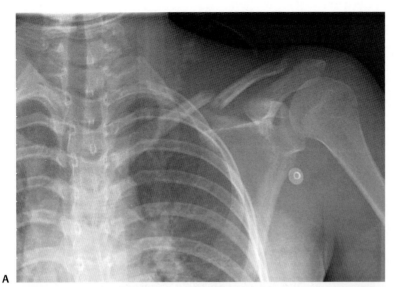

A

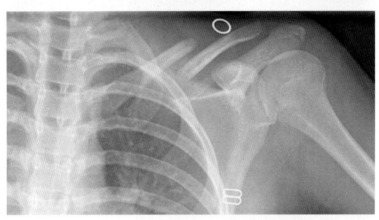

B

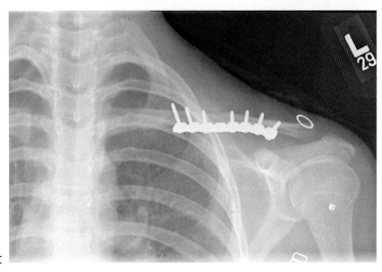

C

Figure 10–25 (A) Anteroposterior shoulder image of a 16-year-old female figure skater whose left middle third clavicle fracture was treated nonoperatively. **(B)** Follow-up anteroposterior radiograph taken 2 weeks later, demonstrating marked shortening of the clavicle with overlap more than 2 cm. At this juncture, surgery was recommended because of the potential functional embarrassment associated with malunions of the clavicle, as well as the cosmetic deformity of the shoulder. **(C)** Postoperative anteroposterior x-ray of the patient. She regained normal shoulder function by week 6 after surgery.

Reduction and Casting Techniques

The typical deformity seen after clavicle fracture is caused by the proximal (medial) fragment being pulled superiorly by the sternocleidomastoid muscle that inserts on the proximal clavicle. The deformity is accentuated by the weight of gravity acting on the upper extremity pulling downward on the distal (lateral) fragment **(Fig. 10–26)**. Closed reductions of displaced clavicle fractures, much like AC dislocations, are not routinely done due in large part to instability and the difficultly of providing an external support once reduced.

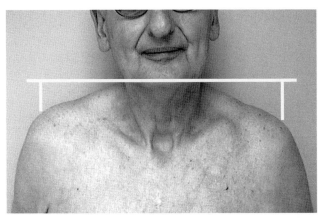

Figure 10–26 This patient had a markedly displaced clavicle fracture with approximately 3 cm of overlap on an anteroposterior x-ray view. This picture shows the patient 3 months after the injury, after being asked to retract his shoulders. The lines help to define the amount of shoulder depression. The patient had poor function and substantial symptoms with yardwork and particularly overhead activities. He claimed it felt like he was slugging around a great weight on the left side. He opted for surgical reconstruction.

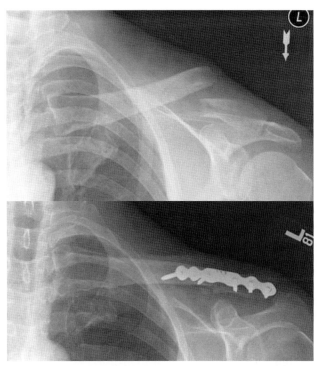

Figure 10–27 Anteroposterior x-ray of the shoulder of a 42-year-old 3 months after he fell off his bicycle and sustained a displaced distal one-third clavicle fracture (upper panel). He complained of shoulder pain and weakness and was disappointed in his deformity. He opted for surgical reconstruction at this juncture. Also shown is an antero-posterior radiograph of the shoulder taken after repair (lower panel). His distal clavicle was fixed with a special plate designed for the pubic symphysis, which has a central buildup that makes the plate more rigid in this area and allows aggressive rehabilitation.

Functional Bracing

Patients are managed symptomatically by immobilizing the shoulder using a sling. Though some orthopedists favor a figure-of-eight sling,[54-56] it is generally well accepted that this modality offers no advantage over simple support with a sling. Comparative studies have demonstrated no difference in shoulder function, residual deformity, or time to return to full range of motion and activity when a sling is used.[55] The figure-of-eight bandage or sling may be discontinued at 3 to 4 weeks for young children, 4 to 6 weeks for teenagers and young adults, or 6 to 8 weeks for adults.[57]

Rehabilitation

Exercises to increase range of motion such as passive shoulder pendulum and active forward flexion/abduction can be initiated once the sling is removed. After healing has been demonstrated, patients may begin to progressively strengthen the muscles of their affected shoulder.

Indications for Surgical Treatment

There are several indications for operative management of clavicle fractures. The clearest indication is the case of an open fracture, which requires irrigation, debridement, and stabilization. The most common form of internal fixation is with plate and screws. Fractures lateral to the coracoid may be associated with torn CC ligaments, in which case the shaft of the clavicle tends to displace proximally while the distal fragment remains anchored to the acromion (**Fig. 10–27**). This injury variant is associated with a higher rate of nonunion. Conservative management should be

discussed with the patient and placed in the context of the patient's activity level, hand dominance, age, and comorbidities. If this lateral fracture variant is displaced more than 1 cm, strong consideration should be given to open reduction and stabilization (**Fig. 10–27**).

Another relative indication for surgery is medialization of the shoulder by more than 2 cm, as indicated by the amount of overriding of the clavicle shaft fragments (**Fig. 10–25A–C**). McKee et al documented poorer performance on endurance testing, as well as on a validated outcome test, in patients with more than 2 cm of shortening,[58] and showed that operative correction of malunions of this type can improve function and strength (see **Video 10–3, Disk 2**).[59]

If the neck of the scapula (glenoid) is fractured along with the clavicle, surgery to repair the clavicle may be considered[41] to stabilize the "floating shoulder" (**Figs. 10–3A-D; 10–5A,B**). This injury complex has been described as a "double disruption of the superior shoulder suspensory complex" and implies that the glenohumeral joint has no support.[34] Other authors have suggested the alternative of scapula fixation in this setting instead,[25] and yet others have advocated fixation of both injuries.[45]

Surgical Treatment

Surgical Anatomy

The surgical anatomy of the clavicle has been extensively described by Abbott and Lucas[60] and reviewed by Craig.[61] The sternocleidomastoid muscle inserts on the medial third of the clavicle; just superior to the clavicle, a space containing only loose adipose tissue exists. The superficial fascia further extends laterally to make up the undersurface of the trapezius muscle. The superior aspect of the deep fascial layer extends laterally to form an inverted sling for the omohyoid muscle, and the inferior portion blends with a fascia encompassing the subclavius muscle.[54,62]

The anterior wall of the axilla is made up of two layers. The superficial layer contains the pectoralis major muscle and the pectoral fascia, whereas the deep layer contains the pectoralis minor muscle and clavipectoral fascia. The pectoral fascia inserts onto the inferior aspect of the clavicle. The infraclavicular triangle is formed by the borders of the clavicle superiorly, pectoralis major inferomedially, and the anterior deltoid inferolaterally. The clavipectoral fascia encompasses the subclavius muscle, attaches to the clavicle, and extends inferiorly to make up the axillary fascia. The subclavius muscle originates from the first rib and the manubrium and inserts on the inferior surface of the clavicle.[60,61]

Behind the clavicle and in front of the large vessels and nerves that extend from the neck to the axilla lies a myofascial layer that is made up of the omohyoid fascia and the clavipectoral fascia. This myofascial layer protects the junction of the subclavian and axillary veins, which lies in close proximity to the clavicle near its medial-middle border. The myofascial layer also protects the internal jugular and subclavian veins that unite to form the innominate vein near the sternoclavicular joint.[54,62]

Surgical Technique

Make a straight horizontal incision approximately 1 cm inferior to the palpable clavicle and centered over the fracture (see **Video 10–3, Disk 2**). In the subcutaneous tissue are supraclavicular nerves, which are difficult to identify. Usually two or three may be seen. Injury to these nerves may result in numbness or, less commonly, painful dysesthesias over the anterior chest. When there is a comminuted zone of injury so that greater exposure of the clavicle is necessary, these nerves are more difficult to preserve. Nevertheless, the authors recommend a dissection that accounts for their identification and protection when possible (**Fig. 10–28**).

After the superficial dissection, the platysma is divided sharply with a scalpel along the anterior border of the clavicle. A supraperiosteal dissection of the anterior margin of the clavicle is done to appreciate the fracture. Extending the dissection inferior or caudad on the bone mobilizes some of the pectoralis origin, which is well tolerated due to its broad origin. In simple oblique patterns, fracture reduction is easily obtained with a pointed bone tenaculum, followed by a 2.7

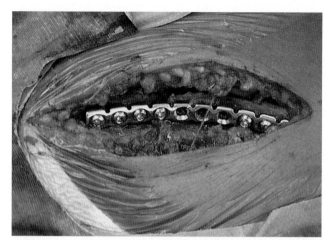

Figure 10–28 Intraoperative photograph of the anterior exposure for a clavicle fracture. In this case, anteroinferior plating was done; with this technique the plate is less prominent and less likely to bother the patient. A branch of the supraclavicular nerve is visible crossing the plate. When possible the authors try to preserve these nerves to avoid sensory changes that sometimes occur following surgery. Although this case shows the use of reconstruction plates, they may be more prone to failure than standard plates, and we do not advocate their routine use except in young patients, who will likely heal quickly.

or 3.5 mm lag screw placed perpendicular to the fracture. If necessary, a provisional Kirschner wire may be used to help maintain the reduction while the clamp is removed and the plate is contoured. A neutralization plate is then applied with at least six cortices of purchase on either side of the fracture (**Fig. 10–28**). Anteroinferior placement of the hardware is preferred to lessen prominence of the hardware under the skin, particularly in slender patients or those who don a backpack (**Fig. 10–29**). This position also allows the surgeon to drill away from the critical neurovascular structures beneath the clavicle. Furthermore, a 3.5 mm dynamic compression plate is preferred for its strength in most, though in smaller individuals, a 2.7 mm dynamic compression plate

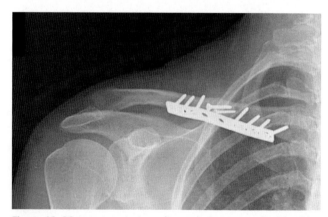

Figure 10–29 Anteroposterior radiograph showing preferable placement of a plate on the anteroinferior border of the clavicle, where it will not be palpable postoperatively. In this case, healing by primary intention occurred using a 3.5 mm dynamic compression plate in a neutralization fashion after placing lag screws. Currently, precontoured implants must be applied to the superior surface of the clavicle, which is one disadvantage to using them.

may be warranted, and in younger patients, a 3.5 mm reconstruction plate is sufficient due to faster healing times.

One of the main difficulties during clavicle fracture surgery is to counteract the deforming forces acting on the superiorly displaced proximal (medial) fragment, accentuated by the distal fragment falling inferiorly due to gravity. Fracture reduction is particularly difficult when there is significant intercalary comminution, so that a pointed bone tenaculum can't be easily used. Rather than attempting to put together a comminuted segment, which invariably will devitalize blood supply and slow healing (or promote nonunion), a bridge plate should be used. First, a plate of adequate length is applied to the medial fragment with no less than six cortices of purchase. Then, with manipulation of the shoulder through the arm, the lateral fragment may be reduced to the medial fragment. If the arm is not draped free, this maneuver can be done through the drapes. Using a pointed bone reduction clamp lateral to the fracture, the length of the distal fragment can be restored to match the contour of the plate. Fixation can be achieved without "touching" the fracture. Distal fixation is then performed with no less than six cortices of purchase.

Skin closure is accomplished with a 2-0 braided, absorbable suture for the platysma and subcutaneous tissue. The epidermis is approximated with a running subcuticular, monofilament, absorbable 4–0 suture.

Tips and Tricks

- Occasionally, it is very helpful to precontour a plate to the anterior surface of a bone model prior to entering the operation because this contour is very difficult to judge intraoperatively, particularly when the bone is malreduced or the fracture severely comminuted. This is an area where the precontoured superior plates are helpful.
- Although six cortices of fixation are considered to be adequate for a simple fracture pattern, more screws should be used on each side of the fracture in comminuted injuries or patients with osteoporosis. In both these circumstances, a locking plate may provide better fixation. The locking plate is also helpful when there is not enough distance on the bone to gain more than six cortices of purchase.
- It is helpful to place a single x-ray cassette behind the shoulder under the drapes while positioning the patient, so that at the end of the procedure, a radiograph can be taken with accurate placement of the cassette. Fluoroscopy is not necessary for this operation.

Rehabilitation

Patients should be seen in the office a week after surgery, during which time their extremity has been supported by a sling. During the first week they are encouraged to perform pendulum activities, but after this juncture, passive and gentle active-assisted range of motion should be encouraged up to the sixth week. The patient can then begin more aggressive AROM and light lifting, starting with 3 to 5 lb repetitions. Good function is usually restored by 3 months postinjury, at which time restrictions can usually be lifted. Radiographic healing should be nearly complete by this juncture, but the shoulder can take months to strengthen, particularly in the elderly.

New Techniques

Clavicular hook plate fixation is a relatively new surgical technique for managing distal clavicle fractures, as well as AC dislocations as previously discussed (see AC section, New Techniques) (see **Video 10–1, Disk 2**). A study comparing K-wires to clavicular hook plate fixation demonstrated an adequate reduction in symptoms as well as restoration of function by both methods, but clavicular hook plates had fewer complications.[63]

Precontoured clavicle implants have been recently introduced to fit the cephalad border of the clavicle. These are helpful in that they obviate the need for contouring plates in the curvaceous zone of the middle and distal one third of the clavicle. This fact allows one to use indirect reduction with greater ease, particularly in comminuted fractures. They do not accommodate the "lower contour" geography of the anterior clavicle but are placed on the biomechanically advantageous "tension" side of the fracture (**Fig. 10–30**).

Outcomes

Many authors believe that the routine surgical management of clavicular fractures is not indicated.[49,57] With conservative management, the nonunion rate is stated to be small, between 0.1 and 0.8%.[49,57] However, these data can be misleading because a majority of patients with clavicular fractures are children and young adults, and undisplaced midclavicular fractures occur more readily in children, whereas displaced proximal clavicular fractures occur more often in the elderly.[51,63] Therefore, elderly patients may have

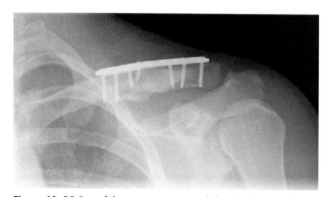

Figure 10–30 One of the new precontoured clavicle plates, preferred by some surgeons for its better biomechanical position on the tension side of the bone, and its ease of application without need for contouring. The authors use this implant in cases of ipsilateral scapula neck and clavicle surgery, where the superior clavicle is accessed at the same prep and drape as the posterior glenoid process.

a higher nonunion rate because of the higher frequency of displaced fractures. Stanley and Norris[56] reported that the patient's age at the time of the injury affected recovery, with 33% of those over the age of 20 years still having symptoms 3 months after they had sustained their fracture.

Complications

Patients should be counseled from the start that they should anticipate a lump in the region of the fracture if treated nonoperatively. Previous reports of nonunion rates were in the range of 0.1 and 0.8%.[49,57] However, studies have shown higher nonunion rates for the distal clavicle in the range of 30%.[45,64,65] Identified risk factors for nonunion include displacement and age.[66] It is possible that the higher nonunion rates of more recent studies reflect different fracture patterns from higher-energy mechanisms.

Complications associated with nonunion include limited function of the shoulder, neurological symptoms, thoracic outlet syndrome, and arterial ischemia.[67–70]

Pearls

- Fusion of the secondary ossification centers about the AC joint occurs at ~17 years of age for the acromial portion and 24 years of age for the distal clavicle.
- The AC joint capsule is strongest at its superior and posterior margins.
- Associated injuries occur in ~90% of patients with scapula fractures.
- Thirteen percent of patients with scapula fractures sustain a brachial plexus injury. Cervical and thoracic spine injury is associated with scapula fractures in over one fifth of cases.

On the DVDs

Video 10–1 (Disk 2) ORIF of Distal Clavicle Fracture Using a Hook Plate This video shows the application of a clavicular hook plate to reduce and stabilize the distal clavicle and AC joint in a patient who also underwent open reduction and internal fixation of his associated scapula fracture.

Video 10–2 (Disk 2) ORIF Scapula Using a Posterior Approach and Intermuscular Windows This video demonstrates repair of a comminuted scapular fracture utilizing the Judet approach com-

bined with an intermuscular window to approach and repair the lateral border of the scapula.

Video 10–3 (Disk 2) Reconstruction of Clavicular Malunion This video demonstrates the open reduction and internal fixation of a malunited clavicle fracture that was 6 to 8 weeks old had displaced significantly, and was causing pain in this overhead laborer. Lag screw fixation through the plate was employed after callus was debrided and an anatomic reduction was obtained.

References

1. Inman VT, Savujon JB, Abbot LC. Observation in the function of the shoulder joint. J Bone Joint Surg Am 1944;26A:1–70
2. Tossy JD, Mead NC, Sigmond HM. Acromioclavicular separations: useful and practical classification for treatment. Clin Orthop Relat Res 1963;28:111–119
3. Allman FL Jr. Fractures and ligamentous injuries of the clavicle and its articulation. J Bone Joint Surg Am 1967;49:774–784
4. Rockwood CA Jr, Williams GR Jr, Young DC. Disorders of the acromioclavicular joint. In: Rockwood CA Jr, Matsen FA III, eds. The Shoulder. Vol 1. 2nd ed. Philadelphia: WB Saunders; 1998: 483–553
5. Shaffer BS. Painful conditions of the acromioclavicular joint. J Am Acad Orthop Surg 1999;7:176–188
6. Bannister GC, Wallace WA, Stableforth PG, Hutson MA. The management of acute acromioclavicular dislocation: a randomized prospective controlled trial. J Bone Joint Surg Br 1989;71:848–850
7. Urist MR. Complete dislocation of the acromioclavicular joint: the nature of the traumatic lesion and effective methods of treatment with an analysis of 41 cases. J Bone Joint Surg Am 1946;28A:813–837
8. Powers JA, Bach PJ. Acromioclavicular separations: closed or open treatment? Clin Orthop Relat Res 1974;104:213–233
9. Buss DD, Watts JD. Acromioclavicular injuries in the throwing athlete. Clin Sports Med 2003;22:327–341
10. Tiurina TV. Age-related characteristics of the human acromioclavicular joint [in ???] Arkh Anat Gistol Embriol 1985;89:75–81
11. Bosworth BM. Complete acromioclavicular dislocation. N Engl J Med 1949;241:221–225
12. Moseley HF. Athletic injuries to the shoulder region. Am J Surg 1959;98:401–422

13. Weaver JK, Dunn HK. Treatment of acromioclavicular injuries, especially complete acromioclavicular separation. J Bone Joint Surg Am 1972;54:1187–1194
14. Kwon YW, Iannotti JP. Operative treatment of acromioclavicular joint injuries and results. Clin Sports Med 2003;22: 291–300
15. Faraj AA, Ketzer B. The use of a hook-plate in the management of acromioclavicular injuries: report of ten cases. Acta Orthop Belg 2001;67:448–451
16. Ryhanen J, Niemela E, Kaarela O, Raatikainen T. Stabilization of acute, complete acromioclavicular joint dislocations with a new C hook implant. J Shoulder Elbow Surg 2003;12:442–445
17. Sim E, Schwarz N, Hocker K, Berzlanovich A. Repair of complete acromioclavicular separations using the acromioclavicular hook plate. Clin Orthop Relat Res 1995;314:134–142
18. Flinkkila T, Ristiniemi J, Hyvonen P, Hamalainen M. Surgical treatment of unstable fractures of the distal clavicle: a comparative study of Kirschner wire and clavicular hook plate fixation. Acta Orthop Scand 2002;73:50–53
19. Mumford EB. Acromioclavicular dislocation. J Bone Joint Surg 1941;23:799–802
20. Butters KP. The Scapula. Philadelphia: WB Saunders; 1990
21. Wilson PD. Experience of the Management of Fractures and Dislocations (based on analysis of 4,390 cases) by Staff of the Fracture Service MGH Boston. Philadelphia: JB Lippincott; 1938
22. Cole PA. Scapula fractures. Orthop Clin North Am 2002;33:1–18
23. Ideberg R, Grevsten S, Larsson S. Epidemiology of scapular fractures: incidence and classification of 338 fractures. Acta Orthop Scand 1995;66:395–397

24. McGahan JP, Rab GT, Dublin A. Fractures of the scapula. J Trauma 1980;20:880–883

25. Ada JR, Miller MD. Scapular fractures: analysis of 113 cases. Clin Orthop Relat Res 1991;269:174–180

26. Hardegger FH, Simpson LA, Weber BG. The operative treatment of scapular fractures. J Bone Joint Surg Br 1984;66:725–731

27. Ideberg R. Fractures of the scapula involving the glenoid fossa. In: Bateman JE, Welsh RP, eds. Surgery of the Shoulder. Philadelphia: Decker; 1984:63–66

28. Mayo KA, Benirschke SK, Mast JW. Displaced fractures of the glenoid fossa: results of open reduction and internal fixation. Clin Orthop Relat Res 1998;347:122–130

29. Goss TP. Scapular fractures and dislocations: diagnosis and treatment. J Am Acad Orthop Surg 1995;3:22–33

30. Armstrong CP, Van Der Spuy J. The fractures scapula: importance and management based on a series of 62 patients. Injury 1984; 15:324–329

31. Goss TP. Fractures of the glenoid cavity. J Bone Joint Surg Am 1992;74:299–305

32. Guttentag IJ, Rechtine GR. Fractures of the scapula: a review of the literature. Orthop Rev 1988;17:147–158

33. Miller MR, Ada JR. Injuries to the shoulder girdle. In: Browner BD, Jupiter JB, Levine AM, eds. Skeletal Trauma. Philadelphia: WB Saunders; 1998:1657–1670

34. Goss TP. Double disruptions of the superior shoulder suspensory complex. J Orthop Trauma 1993;7:99–106

35. Goss TP. The scapula, coracoid, acromial and avulsion fractures. Am J Orthop 1996;25:106–115

36. Ogawa K, Naniwa T. Fractures of the acromion and the lateral scapular spine. J Shoulder Elbow Surg 1997;6:544–548

37. Ogawa K, Yoshida A. Fracture of the superior border of the scapula. Int Orthop 1997;21:371–373

38. Howell SM, Galinat BJ. The glenoid-labral socket: a constrained articular surface. Clin Orthop Relat Res 1989;243:122–125

39. Iannotti JP, Gabriel JP, Schneck SL, et al. The normal glenohumeral relationships. an anatomical study of one hundred and forty shoulders. J Bone Joint Surg Am 1992;74:491–500

40. Van der Helm FC, Pronk GM. Three dimensional recording and description of motions of the shoulder mechanism. J Biomech Eng 1995;117:27–40

41. Herscovici D Jr, Fiennes AGW, Allgöwer M, et al. The floating shoulder: ipsilateral clavicle and scapular neck fractures. J Bone Joint Surg Br 1992;74B:362–364

42. Bateman JE. Surgical approaches to the shoulder. Orthop Clin North Am 1980;11:349–366

43. Nordqvist A, Petersson C. Fracture of the body, neck or spine of the scapula: a long-term follow-up study. Clin Orthop Relat Res 1992;283:139–144

44. Reüdi T, Chapman MW. Fractures of the scapula and clavicle. In: Chapman MW, ed. Operative Orthopaedics. Philadelphia: JB Lippincott; 1998:197–202

45. Leung KS, Lam TP. Open reduction and internal fixation of ipsilateral fractures of the scapular neck and clavicle. J Bone Joint Surg Am 1993;75:1015–1018

46. Ramos Mencia R, Alonso A, Ferrandez L. Conservative treatment of ipsilateral fractures of the scapula and clavicle. J Trauma-Injury Infection & Critical Care 1997;42:239–242

47. Edwards SG, Whittle AP, Wood GW. Nonoperative treatment of ipsilateral fractures of the scapula and clavicle. J Bone Joint Surg Am 2000;82A:774–780

48. Goss TP, Cantu RV. Scapula Fracture. eMedicine. 2002; http://www.emedicine.com/orthoped/topic554.htm

49. Neer CS II. Nonunion of the clavicle. JAMA 1960;172:1006–1011

50. Moore TO. Internal pin fixation for fracture of the clavicle. Am Surg 1951;17:580–583

51. Nordqvist A, Petersson C. The incidence of fractures of the clavicle. Clin Orthop Relat Res 1994;300:127–132

52. Robinson CM, Cairns DA. Primary nonoperative treatment of displaced lateral fractures of the clavicle. J Bone Joint Surg Am 2004;86-A:778–782

53. Neer CS. Fractures of the distal third of the clavicle. Clin Orthop Relat Res 1968;58:43–50

54. McCandless DN, Mowbray MAS. Treatment of displaced fractures of the clavicle: Sling versus figure-of-eight bandage. Practitioner 1979;223:266–267

55. Andersen K, Jensen PO, Lauritzen J. Treatment of clavicular fractures: figure-of-eight bandage versus a simple sling. Acta Orthop Scand 1987;58:71–75

56. Stanley D, Norris SH. Recovery following fractures of the clavicle treated conservatively. Injury 1988;19:162–164

57. Rowe CR. An atlas of anatomy and treatment of midclavicular fractures. Clin Orthop Relat Res 1968;58:29–42

58. McKee MD, Pederson EM, Wild LM, et al. Previously unrecognized deficits after nonoperative treatment of displaced midshaft fracture of the clavicle detected by patient based outcome measures and objective muscle strength testing. Conference Proceedings, Defining Indications for New Techniques in Fracture Fixation, OTA Specialty Day, 2003, San Francisco, CA

59. McKee MD, Wild LM, Schemitsch EH. Midshaft malunions of the clavicle. J Bone Joint Surg Am 2003;85-A:790–797

60. Abbott LC, Lucas DB. The function of the clavicle: its surgical significance. Ann Surg 1954;140:583–599

61. Craig EV. Fractures of the clavicle. In: Rockwood CA Jr, Matsen FA III, eds. The Shoulder. Vol 1. 2nd ed. Philadelphia, PA: WB Saunders; 1998:428–482

62. Flinkkila T, Ristiniemi J, Hyvonen P, Hamalainen M. Surgical treatment of unstable fractures of the distal clavicle. Acta Orthop Scand 2002;73:50–53

63. Taylor AR. Some observations on fractures of the clavicle. Proc R Soc Med 1969;62:1037–1038

64. Edwards DJ, Davanagh TG, Flannery MC. Fractures of the distal clavicle: a case for fixation. Injury 1992;23:44–46

65. Anderson K. Evaluation and treatment of distal clavicle fractures. Clin Sports Med 2003;22:319–326

66. Robinson CM, Court-Brown CM, McQueen MM. Estimation of the risk of nonunion after a fracture of the clavicle. Paper presented at: Defining Indications for New Techniques in Fracture Fixation, OTA Specialty Day, 2003, San Francisco, CA

67. Jupiter JB, Leffert RD. Non-union of the clavicle: associated complications and surgical management. J Bone Joint Surg Am 1987;69:753–760

68. Der Tavitian J, Davison JN, Dias JJ. Clavicular fracture non-union surgical outcome and complications. Injury 2002;33: 135–143

69. Toledo LC, MacEwen GD. Severe complication of surgical treatment of congenital pseudarthrosis of the clavicle. Clin Orthop Relat Res 1979;139:64–67

70. Guilfoil PH, Christiansen T. An unusual vascular complication of fractured clavicle. JAMA 1967;200:72–73

11 Proximal Humeral Fractures and Shoulder Dislocations

Andrew H. Schmidt

Proximal humeral fractures represent up to 5% of all fractures and most often occur in the elderly patient with osteoporosis as the result of a fall. Their incidence is increasing with the aging of the population. The proximal humerus may also be fractured in younger patients, usually as the result of high-energy trauma. In this circumstance, there is a high incidence of associated injuries, including neurovascular lesions of the injured arm and injuries of the cervical spine and chest. Over the past decade, there has been ongoing controversy about the relative merits of operative versus nonoperative treatment for proximal humeral fractures, as well as uncertainty about whether better results are achieved with internal fixation or hemiarthroplasty.[1–4] Improved techniques and implants for both reduction and fixation of proximal humeral fractures and for shoulder hemiarthroplasty after fracture have been developed,[5–7] and outcome studies are now being performed that will help dictate treatment of these diverse injuries.[8]

Dislocations of the glenohumeral joint are also common and affect persons of all ages. The goal of treatment is expedient reduction with recovery of full function. The natural history of shoulder dislocation with respect to the risk of recurrent dislocation continues to be defined.[9,10] Young patients with traumatic dislocation are those most likely to develop recurrent instability. Although early surgery is traditionally not considered, arthroscopic evaluation of the recently dislocated shoulder may play a role in defining lesions associated with late instability and may allow for early repair, with decreased morbidity from chronic instability.[11,12] Elderly patients often have an associated injury to the rotator cuff; if present, surgical repair should be considered.[11,13]

Proximal Humeral Fractures

The overriding principle in the treatment of proximal humeral fractures is the need to restore functional range of motion. Shoulder movement depends on the relative gliding of the humeral head, rotator cuff, and deltoid muscle. Capsular restriction or loss of these gliding surfaces will render the shoulder stiff and painful and lead to a poor outcome. The importance of early mobilization following even nondisplaced fracture of the proximal humerus has been demonstrated.[14] Improved results are seen when active mobilization is allowed before 14 days after injury, compared with delayed mobilization.[14] If a fracture of the proximal humerus is either unacceptably displaced or too unstable to allow early motion, then operative intervention should be considered in any patient that needs or desires to regain useful function of the shoulder. Whether this is best done by reduction and fixation of the fracture or by prosthetic replacement of the shoulder depends on the patient's needs and expectations, fracture pattern, bone quality, implants available, and experience of the surgeon. Stabilization of the proximal humerus in polytrauma patients by methods that allow early motion and weight bearing on the injured limb continue to be advocated, and new devices such as intramedullary nails and locking plates have been developed that may allow this to be done with less invasive techniques.[15] Only a few studies of these procedures have been reported, however, and these techniques should be considered unproven.

Classification

The management of proximal humeral fractures begins with a thorough assessment of the functional needs and abilities of the patient, the presence of cognitive or physical impairments, the fracture pattern, bone density, the patient's expectations, and the ability of the patient to comply with a rehabilitation program. The goal of treatment is to obtain fracture union and maintain function of the shoulder while avoiding complications. The skills of the surgeon and the resources available must also be considered.

The complex anatomy of the shoulder girdle must be understood to successfully treat proximal humerus fractures and shoulder dislocations. Fractures of the proximal humerus occur in typical patterns that are influenced by muscular insertions that cause predictable displacement of each fragment (**Fig. 11–1**). The muscular and neurovascular anatomy of the proximal humerus also influence treatment and complications.

The classification proposed by Neer remains the worldwide standard for the evaluation and discussion of these injuries.[16] The Neer classification considers the presence of displacement or angulation of each of the four major segments of the proximal humerus: the humeral head, greater tuberosity, lesser tuberosity, and shaft. The AO/OTA (Arbeitsge-meinschaft für Osteosynthesefragen/Orthopaedic

Figure 11–1 The pathoanatomy of proximal humeral fractures. Notice the predictable displacement caused by deforming muscle insertions.

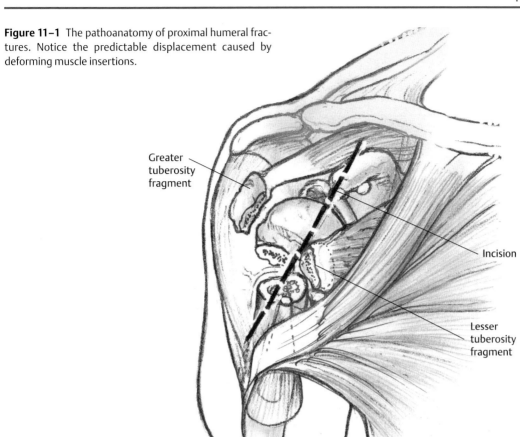

Greater tuberosity fragment

Incision

Lesser tuberosity fragment

Trauma Association) classification system emphasizes the blood supply to the humeral head and has 27 subdivisions that allow very specific identification of fractures. However, the nomenclature of this fracture is alphanumeric rather than descriptive and is difficult to apply and understand.

Proximal humerus fractures have proven to be very difficult to classify in a reproducible manner, with several studies documenting poor inter- and intraobserver reliability. The reliability is not improved with simplified classification schemes or the additional use of computed tomography.[17-20] Four-part fractures are commonly subclassified because the valgus-impacted type appears to have a better prognosis than other types of four-part fractures.[7]

The diagnosis of a fracture of the proximal humerus is straightforward. The patient presents with pain and swelling about the shoulder after an injury. The diagnosis is confirmed with imaging. Initially, plain radiographs are obtained, consisting of the well-known shoulder trauma series: true anteroposterior (AP) and lateral x-rays in the plane of the scapula and the axillary lateral view **(Fig. 11–2).** Although the importance of the axillary view in classifying the fracture has been highlighted,[21] one should be aware of the limitations of this view. Patients and technologists are often reluctant to obtain the axillary view because of pain and the need to move the injured arm, and it has been shown that the axillary radiograph does not accurately

represent the amount of angulation of the surgical neck that is present.[22] An alternative to the axillary view is to take a similar image in the opposite direction, with the arm kept immobilized in a sling, or to utilize the transverse cuts of a computed tomographic (CT) scan. In either case, the axillary view or axial CT image confirms that the shoulder is reduced, details whether any defects are debris within the joint, diagnoses glenoid fractures, and reveals the amount and direction of displacement of the tuberosities.

Even though advanced imaging may not improve classification reliability, CT is a useful and sometimes necessary adjunct to the assessment of the proximal humerus for the treatment of a specific fracture.[23] CT provides valuable information about the degree of comminution, the presence of intra-articular fracture lines, the presence of glenohumeral subluxation or articular impaction, and whether the lesser tuberosity is fractured **(Fig. 11–3).** With respect to clinical decision making, a key distinction is that between the so-called three- and four-part fractures.[23] This question is answered by determining the status of the lesser tuberosity. When the lesser tuberosity is not fractured and remains attached to the humeral head, the vascular supply of the humeral head can be assumed to be intact, and the fracture may be treated by restoring normal alignment of the head and shaft and ensuring that tuberosity displacement is corrected. If the lesser tuberosity is

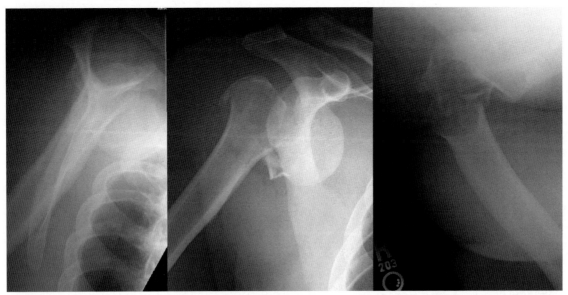

Figure 11–2 The shoulder trauma series, consisting of anteroposterior (middle panel), scapular lateral (left panel), and axillary lateral (right panel) views.

displaced in addition to the greater tuberosity, the fracture is classified as a four-part fracture, and the prognosis and treatment are instead determined by the high likelihood of avascular necrosis that follows this injury.[23]

One particular fracture pattern has been recognized that is worthy of special consideration. In 1991, Jakob et al

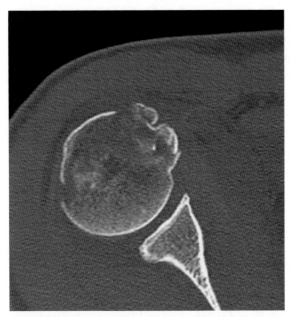

Figure 11–3 An axial computed tomographic cut of a proximal humeral fracture, showing several nondisplaced fracture lines in the vicinity of the lesser tuberosity. These fracture lines may have implications for the vascularity of the articular segment. A normal glenohumeral relationship is noted. If the shoulder were dislocated, it would be apparent in this view, which would also reveal any impaction of the humeral head.

described the four-part valgus-impacted fracture of the proximal humerus.[24] This fracture is easily recognized by the "popsicle" appearance of the articular segment that has fallen into the void left by displacement of the greater tuberosity so that the articular surface faces superiorly **(Fig. 11–4)**. In this circumstance, despite comminution, soft tissue attachments to the articular segment remain intact that both facilitate fracture reduction and maintain the viability of the articular segment. In their initial description of this fracture, Jakob et al noted that the rate of osteonecrosis was just 26% in their series of 19 such fractures, lower than typically expected in a series of four-part fractures.[24]

Nonoperative Treatment

The majority of proximal humeral fractures are minimally displaced. These stable fractures may be managed with only brief immobilization in a sling **(Fig. 11–5A,B)**. Functional exercises are begun when pain permits. Koval and coworkers have shown that institution of therapy within 14 days leads to improved functional outcomes.[14]

For proximal humeral fractures in particular, the lack of consistently successful surgical techniques and the frequent complications associated with operative management have led to a large number of these cases being treated nonoperatively. In general, the literature does not provide much high-quality evidence comparing the results of nonoperative treatment to specific surgical techniques. A recently published meta-analysis of the treatment of three- and four-part fractures found that conservatively managed patients had more pain and worse range of motion than those managed by either fixation or arthroplasty.[2] Court-Brown reported a series of 125 valgus-impacted fractures treated nonoperatively. One year after injury, 80%

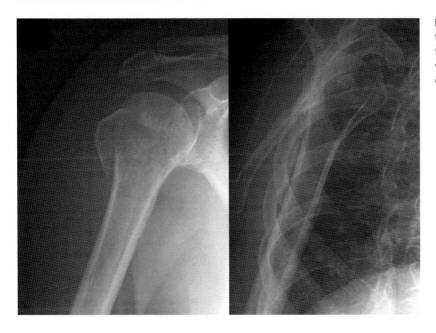

Figure 11–4 X-rays of a stable valgus-impacted fracture. The hallmark of this fracture pattern is that the humeral head is pointing upward rather than toward the glenoid. The greater tuberosity is usually displaced.

of the primarily elderly patients had a good to excellent outcome, despite residual deficits in strength and range of motion.[25]

Indications for Nonoperative Treatment

Fractures that are treated nonoperatively should be stable enough to allow early functional use and be minimally dis-

placed **(Fig. 11–5A,B)**. At the time of the initial evaluation, the arm should be examined to ensure that the proximal part of the humerus could be moved, with motion occurring at the shoulder joint and not at the fracture site. There should not be significant posterior or superior displacement of the greater tuberosity; uncorrected displacement of the tuberosities has adverse effects upon rotator cuff function, whereas surgical neck malunion may affect range

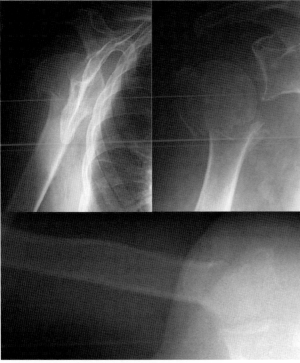

A

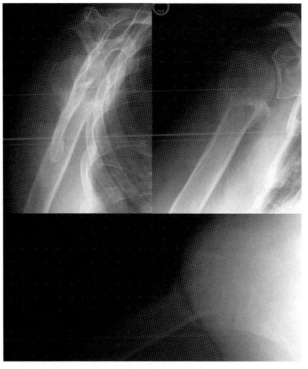

B

Figure 11–5 (A) A three-part (surgical neck and greater tuberosity) fracture in an elderly female patient. The patient was treated in a sling with early range of motion exercises. **(B)** Follow-up films after

12 weeks show healing and acceptable alignment. The patient had no pain and was able to reach the top of her head easily.

of motion. A patient with reasonably high functional demands and a displaced proximal humeral fracture will be better treated with surgery so that early range of motion can be instituted.

Reduction and Splinting Techniques

Tuberosity displacement is difficult to reduce nonoperatively. The exception is a tuberosity fracture associated with shoulder dislocation; in this case, reduction of the shoulder dislocation may effect reduction of the tuberosity as well.

Displaced surgical neck fractures can sometimes be reduced by applying longitudinal traction to the arm with the arm in an adducted position. Adduction of the humerus neutralizes the deforming force of the pectoralis muscle insertion on the distal fragment. If the fracture can be impacted and remains in a stable position, nonoperative management would be appropriate.

Functional Bracing

Functional bracing per se is not very feasible in proximal humeral fractures because of the significant deforming forces of the many muscular insertions on the various fracture fragments. In rare instances, it might be feasible to immobilize the arm in a so-called airplane splint with the shoulder abducted or in a forward-elevated position. Because such a position is poorly tolerated, there is little indication for this manner of treatment.

Rehabilitation

Early institution of functional range of motion is important to achieve the best outcomes. Koval et al showed improved outcomes when such exercises were begun within 14 days of injury.[14] Their protocol consisted of using a sling for initial pain relief. All patients were seen again within 1 week after the injury, were given instructions for range of motion exercises for the arm, and were referred to a physical therapist. The physical therapist supervised active range of motion exercises for the elbow, wrist, and hand combined with passive range of motion exercises for the shoulder twice a week. The shoulder exercises were begun with the patient in the supine position for forward elevation, external rotation, and internal rotation to the chest. In addition, patients were asked to perform the exercises up to four times daily at home. The sling was continued for 4 to 6 weeks until the fracture had united clinically. Once the sling was discontinued, active range of motion exercises were initiated, starting with the patient in the supine position and gradually progressing to a sitting position. Finally, isometric deltoid and rotator cuff–strengthening exercises were added. Once reasonable active motion of the shoulder was achieved, resistive exercises for the deltoid and rotator cuff muscles were

added. Approximately 12 weeks after the fracture, a more vigorous stretching program was begun.

Indications for Surgical Treatment

Although the Neer classification is often used for surgical decision making, a more descriptive approach is followed here, based upon an understanding of the fracture lines and displacements. Fractures of the proximal humerus can be thought of as involving either or both the surgical neck and the tuberosities. In turn, fracture displacement affects the biomechanical function of the shoulder and the vascularity of the fracture fragments. Both aspects must be considered for each fracture fragment identified. Another key aspect of decision making is the stability of the fracture; stable fractures are considered to be those that will tolerate early functional motion. In general, surgery is indicated when fracture instability would prevent early functional use or when the fracture pattern has sinister features, as discussed in later sections.

Surgical neck fractures can be nondisplaced or displaced, and simple or comminuted. Displaced surgical neck fractures should be treated with correction of translational displacement and angulation. A variety of useful fixation techniques exist, including plate fixation, percutaneous pins, or tension-band wires, and intramedullary nailing with either flexible or interlocking devices **(Fig. 11–6A,B)**. Occasionally, hemiarthroplasty is the preferred option. The ideal choice of fixation for a given patient depends on many factors, including the degree of comminution, bone quality, and experience of the surgeon. Isolated anatomical neck fractures are exceedingly rare and may be treated with pin or screw fixation in young patients or hemiarthroplasty in the elderly. More often, so-called anatomical neck fractures are described in association with more complex injuries that also involve the tuberosities and the metaphyseal region **(Fig. 11–7A,B)**. In these injuries, the metaphysis is comminuted, and the articular segment remains as a well-defined fragment. Surgical indications in these more complex fractures are more controversial and are discussed later in this section.

Isolated greater tuberosity fractures are often associated with anterior shoulder dislocation. After fracture, the greater tuberosity fragment typically displaces superiorly or posteriorly or both. Posterior displacement is more difficult to assess on radiographs, and CT scanning may be necessary. Both patterns of displacement are associated with potential impingement against the acromion. Displaced tuberosity fragments should be reduced and fixed **(Fig. 11–8)**. The degree of acceptable displacement is controversial. One study suggested that displacement of as little as 3 mm is associated with impingement symptoms in athletic individuals.[26] It is well accepted that more than 5 mm of displacement is an indication for surgery in patients that require overhead function of the arm. Tension-band techniques using wire or heavy suture have excellent

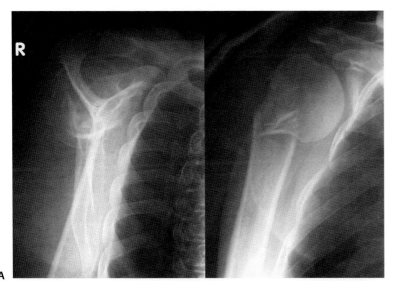

A

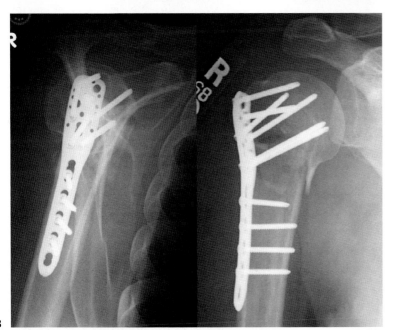

B

Figure 11–6 (A) Example of a displaced surgical neck fracture in a young patient. In this case, the humeral head is angulated in varus. Some comminution is evident. Notice that the profile of the bicipital groove is visible on the scapular lateral view (left panel). **(B)** Postoperative views after fixation with a locking proximal humeral plate. Note that one of the anterior screws is slightly long and appears to extend beyond the subchondral bone.

Figure 11–7 (A) Example of a comminuted fracture. Careful inspection of these views demonstrates that the greater and lesser tuberosities as well as the humeral head have been fractured, making this a four-part fracture. **(B)** X-rays 6 months after limited internal fixation using a semitubular plate and nonabsorbable suture. There is slight residual displacement and some collapse of the metaphysis. The patient returned to work as a plumber.

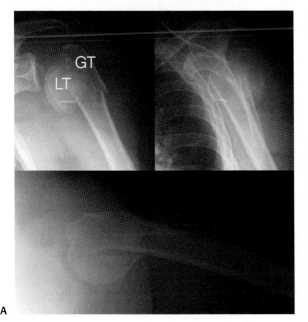

A

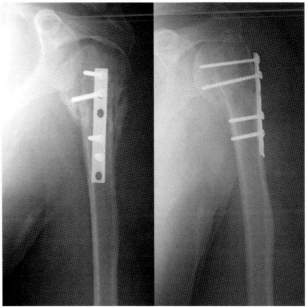

B

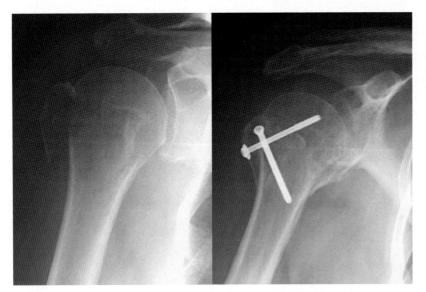

Figure 11–8 Displaced greater tuberosity fracture. In this case, there is a stable, valgus-impacted fracture of the humeral head. The greater tuberosity was reduced by elevating the humeral head and fixed with two screws as well as a tension-band suture (not visible).

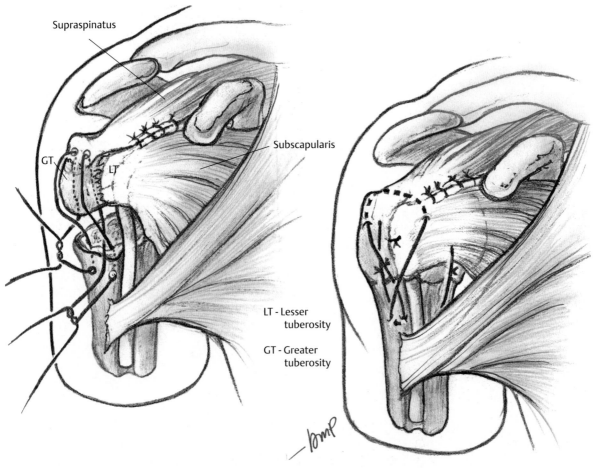

Figure 11–9 A tension band in a displaced three-part fracture treated by open reduction and suture fixation. There are sutures capturing the displaced greater tuberosity fragment and the lesser tuberosity/humeral head fragment.

results **(Fig. 11–9);** screw fixation may be considered when comminution is minimal and the bone quality good. One should remember that rotator cuff tears are associated with displaced tuberosity fractures, and rotator cuff repair should be performed when such fractures require surgery.

Isolated lesser tuberosity fractures are rare and may occur with posterior dislocations. Large fragments of the lesser tuberosity may require open reduction and fixation if they are displaced.

Many proximal humeral fractures consist of various combinations of these more elementary fracture patterns. So-called three-part fractures generally represent the combination of a surgical neck fracture and greater tuberosity fracture **(Figs. 11–4; 11–5A,B).** For these injuries, treatment results are related primarily to the degree of residual tuberosity displacement or head and neck angulation.[23] Avascular necrosis may occur in up to 27% of three-part fractures but is often asymptomatic because only a portion of the humeral head is involved **(Fig. 11–10).**[23] Therefore, treatment of three-part fractures of the proximal humerus should be based on the biomechanical consequences of the fracture rather than on concern about the vascularity of the humeral head.[23] In a patient that requires functional restoration of the injured arm, reduction of displaced tuberosity fragments and correction of malalignment of the humeral head are necessary **(Fig. 11–7A,B).** Any technique can be utilized

for the repair of the surgical neck fracture, combined with pinning or tension-band fixation of the greater tuberosity.[27]

In contrast, avascular necrosis is a more common sequela of four-part fractures and typically results in complete involvement of the humeral head and severe pain and stiffness.[23,28] In addition, the poor bone quality and degree of comminution usually associated with these fractures make open reduction and internal fixation of these injuries prone to failure. Therefore, for displaced four-part fractures, treatment is based on biological principles rather than mechanical principles and many experts recommend hemiarthroplasty. However, several authors report successful results with open reduction and limited internal fixation for four-part fractures, and this treatment should be considered in more active patients.[27] Interestingly, complications after operative repair of valgus-impacted four-part fractures seem to be much less frequent than in other types of four-part fractures, and these fractures are a good indication for internal fixation.[7] When a valgus-impacted fracture is identified, one must carefully look for evidence of lateral displacement of the humeral head fragment **(Fig. 11–11).**[7] If this occurs, the medial periosteal vessels that perfuse the articular segment may in fact be ruptured, and avascular necrosis is more likely to result. In the absence of lateral displacement of the humeral head fragment, the humeral head is likely to remain viable.

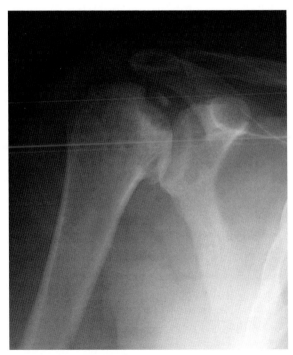

Figure 11–10 Example of osteonecrosis of the humeral head occurring after a minimally displaced fracture. The patient was minimally symptomatic.

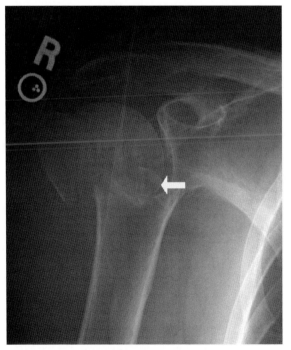

Figure 11–11 A valgus-impacted fracture with more than 1 cm of lateral displacement of the humeral head compared with the humeral shaft (arrow). This may signify disruption of the blood vessels supplying the humeral head.

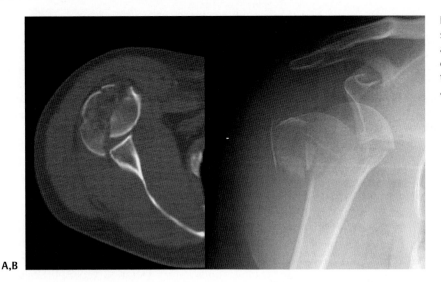

Figure 11–12 (A) Anteroposterior x-ray showing a head-splitting fracture. Note the appearance of the "double-bubble." **(B)** Axial computed tomographic cut demonstrating the fracture of the humeral head splitting the articular surface.

A,B

However, recent work has shown that the results of nonoperative treatment of valgus-impacted fractures are also satisfactory.[25] Randomized clinical trials are necessary to completely define the indications for surgical treatment of valgus-impacted fractures; until such data are available, surgeons must rely on their own judgment and the wishes of the patient. It has been shown that the severity of symptoms associated with avascular necrosis correlates the best with the residual displacement of the fracture fragments. If the humeral head anatomy has been restored following fracture, the clinical results for patients that develop avascular necrosis are comparable with those for patients without avascular necrosis.[28]

Indications for shoulder hemiarthroplasty are classically the displaced four-part fracture in an elderly patient, four-part fracture dislocations, "head-splitting fractures," and fractures with significant articular impaction **(Fig. 11–12A,B).** Certain displaced three-part fractures in patients with severe osteoporosis have also been considered for arthroplasty, but newer techniques of fixation are changing the indications for these fractures for which osteonecrosis is uncommon.

Surgical Treatment

Surgical Anatomy

There are two main approaches to the surgical reconstruction of proximal humeral fractures: open or percutaneous surgery. Open procedures are mostly done through the utility deltopectoral approach **(Fig. 11–13),** whereas a deltoid-splitting approach is occasionally used for isolated greater tuberosity fractures **(Fig. 11–14).**

Percutaneous approaches are used for pinning the proximal humerus and for interlocking screw insertion when intramedullary nails are used. The main concern with percutaneous approaches is the risk of iatrogenic injury to branches of the axillary nerve **(Fig. 11–15).**[29,30] The axillary nerve exits the quadrilateral space and arborizes on the undersurface of the deltoid. In a cadaveric study assessing the risk of percutaneous pinning, the proximal lateral pin was found to be a mean of 3 mm from the axillary nerve.[30] Additional anatomical structures at risk of injury from anterior pins include the long head of the biceps tendon (mean 2 mm from the anterior pin; in three of 10 specimens the tendon was impaled) and the cephalic vein (mean distance 11 mm; perforated in one instance). Finally, tuberosity pins were 6 to 7 mm from the axillary nerve and posterior humeral circumflex artery, respectively.[30] Similar concerns apply to antegrade nails; blunt dissection and the use of drill sleeves will make interlocking screw insertion safer. Despite these theoretical risks, clinically significant neurovascular complications are very rare.

There are few significant risks with the deltopectoral approach **(Fig. 11–13).** The cephalic vein defines the deltopectoral interval and should be identified and retracted laterally with the deltoid muscle. During deep dissection, an important landmark for the deltopectoral approach is the coracoid process and its associated strap muscles. The long head of the biceps tendon serves as a reference to identify the lesser (medial to the tendon) and greater tuberosity (lateral to the tendon). During the initial exposure and mobilization of the fracture, one should keep in mind that important vascular contributions to the articular segment are made by the arcuate branch of the anterior humeral circumflex artery that ascends along the bicipital groove, as well as the rotator cuff insertions **(Fig. 11–13).**

Although fracture patterns are quite variable, the proximal humerus fractures into fairly consistent fragments **(Fig. 11–1).** Most often, there are fracture lines in the region of the surgical neck and comminution of the greater

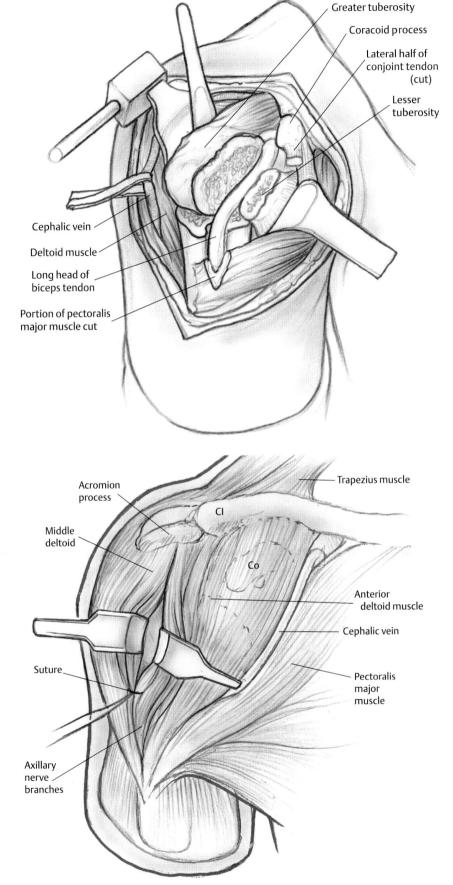

Greater tuberosity

Coracoid process

Lateral half of
conjoint tendon
(cut)

Lesser
tuberosity

Cephalic vein

Deltoid muscle

Long head of
biceps tendon

Portion of pectoralis
major muscle cut

Figure 11–13 The anatomy of the deltopectoral approach.

Acromion
process

Middle
deltoid

Trapezius muscle

Cl

Co

Anterior
deltoid muscle

Cephalic vein

Suture

Pectoralis
major
muscle

Axillary
nerve
branches

Figure 11–14 The deltoid-splitting approach.
Note the axillary nerve branches that are at
least 5 cm distal to the acromion. The suture in
the muscle avoids inadvertent injury.

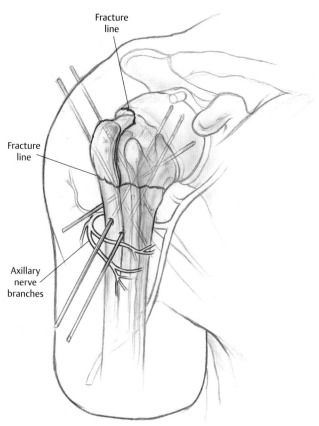

Figure 11–15 The desired placement of percutaneous pins and their relationship to the axillary nerve.

tuberosity. The articular segment will be displaced in a manner that is dictated by the remaining soft tissue attachments to the humeral head and the type of injury. Careful assessment of the fracture anatomy and the displacement of the humeral head will often lead to a logical plan for the steps needed to reduce the fracture. For example, in a valgus-impacted fracture, the greater tuberosity is displaced and the humeral head "falls" into the resultant void. There is often an intact medial soft tissue attachment between the humeral head and shaft. Reduction of this fracture requires restoration of the normal position of the humeral head by pushing proximally and medially on the lateral aspect of the humeral head, thereby rotating the humeral head on the intact soft tissue hinge. Once the humeral head is reduced, the greater tuberosity may be reduced into its bed, after which it serves to maintain reduction of the humeral head.

Surgical Techniques

General Considerations

Patients undergoing surgery for repair of proximal humeral fractures should receive prophylactic antibiotics within an

hour of surgery. Multiply injured patients should have their cervical spine cleared because of issues with positioning the head during surgery.

The fixation of all devices in the proximal humerus is limited by the frequent osteopenia of the humeral head associated with these injuries. In a recent biomechanical study, the strength of screw fixation was related to screw position within the humeral head.[31] Using paired cadaveric specimens, it was found that the pull-out strength was greatest when the screws had subchondral fixation in the center of the humeral head.[31]

Recent biomechanical studies have evaluated the relative strength of various methods of fixation of the proximal humerus.[5] When plate fixation is performed, the use of a fixed-angle plate appears to be better than a standard buttress plate.[5] Koval et al compared 10 fixation techniques for fractures of the proximal humerus, using both fresh-frozen and embalmed cadaver specimens.[6] In the frozen specimens (representing patients with good bone quality), the T-plate provided the strongest fixation. In the embalmed specimens (representing patients with osteoporosis), the Enders nail/tension-band technique provided the strongest fixation. In both types of bone, tension-band fixation alone provided the least effective fixation.[6] In an osteotomy model, the addition of calcium phosphate cement improved the strength of fixation after pinning or use of either a cloverleaf or blade plate, even in osteoporotic bone.[32]

Percutaneous Pinning

Percutaneous pinning is a versatile technique that is potentially applicable to many proximal humeral fractures; the only prerequisite is the ability to reduce the fracture by closed or percutaneous methods (see **Video 11–1, Disk 2**). Therefore, a thorough understanding of the anatomy of a given fracture is mandatory to enable the surgeon to recognize and correct deforming forces. Besides getting the fracture reduced, one of the most important steps when using multiple pins to stabilize fractures of the proximal humerus is to ensure that the pins are divergent in multiple planes (**Fig. 11–15**). Biomechanical studies demonstrate that fixation rigidity is greatest when bicortical tuberosity pins and AP pins are added to at least two lateral pins.[33]

The procedure is performed with the patient in the supine or beach chair position. The image intensifier is placed on the same side, parallel to the operating table, next to the patient's head. This allows for imaging in the AP and axillary projections.

The steps necessary to reduce the fracture should be practiced before proceeding with the surgical preparation. Nearly always, there is an apex-anterior angulation that is corrected by pushing toward the floor at the fracture site while lifting up on the arm (**Fig. 11–16**). Reduction of the tuberosities and final reduction of the humeral head may require percutaneous joysticks.

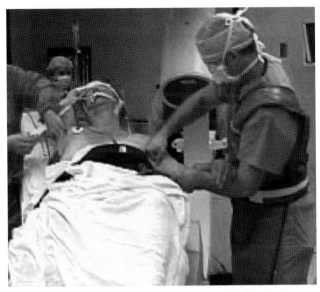

Figure 11–16 Intraoperative photograph demonstrating how a posteriorly directed force applied to the proximal humerus will reduce the common apex-anterior angulation of the surgical neck.

With this technique, the fracture is stabilized with multiple terminally threaded 2.5 mm pins (**Figs. 11–15; 11–17A–D**). The pins are drilled through the near cortex but should be impacted by hand into the humeral head. First, reduction of the humeral head and the shaft is accomplished with the maneuver already described. When needed, a separate pin is inserted into the humeral head to use as a joystick and reduce the head onto the shaft. The first pin is drilled retrograde into the anterolateral humeral shaft and into the proximal segment. A second pin can be inserted at a slightly different angle and should diverge in the head of the humerus. The pins are carefully advanced. Additional pins are inserted as necessary from the tip of the greater tuberosity to the medial humeral neck, and anteriorly into the lesser tuberosity to posterior humerus. Often, as many as seven or eight pins may be necessary. Following insertion, the pins are cut as far as possible beneath the skin.

Aftercare requires careful follow-up. Unfortunately, the pins limit shoulder range of motion, but patients are

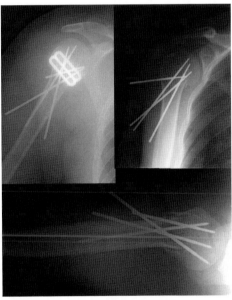

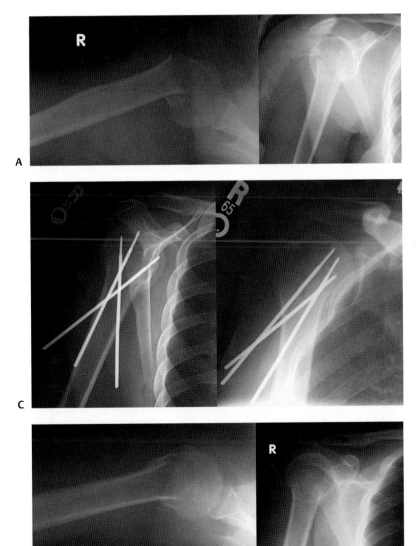

Figure 11–17 (A) Example of an angulated surgical neck fracture. **(B)** Postoperative views after closed reduction and pinning with four terminally threaded pins. **(C)** X-rays at 6 weeks. Note that one pin was removed because of loosening. **(D)** Healed x-rays taken at 3 months.

encouraged to perform pendulum exercises. Weekly follow-up may be necessary to monitor progress; occasionally pins become prominent as soft tissue swelling decreases and may need to be shortened. The greater tuberosity pins are removed at 4 weeks, and the remaining pins at 6 to 8 weeks. Following pin removal, the patient is started on a more aggressive physiotherapy program.

Plate Fixation

Osteosynthesis of the proximal humerus with plates is another versatile procedure applicable to many fracture patterns, from simple displaced surgical neck fractures to complex multifragment injuries **(Figs. 11–6A,B; 11–7A,B)** (see **Videos 11–2** and **11–3, Disk 2**). Although limited deltoid-splitting approaches have been described, such fixation is best done through the deltopectoral approach.

With the patient in a beach chair position, an image intensifier is placed parallel to the table at the patient's head. Intraoperative imaging in the AP and axillary planes is used. The deltopectoral interval is developed. Abduction of the shoulder during the approach relaxes the deltoid and facilitates exposure. A blunt retractor may be placed around the lateral aspect of the proximal shaft, and the anterior portion of the deltoid insertion may be released from the humerus if necessary. The conjoined tendon is identified, and another blunt retractor can be used to retract this structure medially, being cognizant of the musculocutaneous nerve and axillary nerve. The upper portion of the pectoralis major insertion on the humerus may also be released if needed **(Fig. 11–13)**.

The fracture fragments are atraumatically identified and exposed. The long head of the biceps tendon is a useful landmark for identifying the tuberosities. Sutures are placed in the rotator cuff insertions. The greater tuberosity is often displaced posteriorly and can be retrieved with the arm abducted. Traction sutures in the tendinous insertions hold the fragments more securely than bone clamps. Soft tissue attachments should be maintained, but when needed the rotator interval may be opened. In the case of a dislocated humeral head, a K-wire may be used to help reduce the articular segment.

A low-profile, precontoured plate is utilized. The humeral head is reduced with manipulation by blunt elevators or joysticks using image intensification. The author prefers a plate with locking, angular stable screws, especially in osteoporotic bone **(Fig. 11–6A,B)**. The plate is applied along the humeral shaft with one or two screws. The height of the plate must be evaluated with the image intensifier to ensure that the plate is not prominent. A second screw is placed in the distal plate to be sure that the plate is well aligned with the humeral shaft. With a locking plate, a triple drill guide is threaded into a specific hole. A guide pin is advanced into the reduced humeral head using image intensification in two planes. A second guide pin can be inserted in a different hole. When using a nonlocking plate, the surgeon must be sure that the screws

appropriately diverge within the humeral head. The screws are measured and inserted. Remaining screws are placed into the humeral head and shaft.

The tuberosities are reduced to the humeral shaft. The traction sutures that were previously placed can be replaced with nonabsorbable suture, and the sutures can be tied to the plate or to a hole in the bone. It is preferable to have sutures placed between the tuberosity and the humeral shaft as well as in a horizontal cerclage fashion, even incorporating the plate. The tuberosities must be repaired to their anatomical position and must be stable so that the musculotendinous unit of the rotator cuff is restored and can tolerate early motion. While directly observing the repair, the surgeon moves the shoulder through a range of motion so that limits of motion are determined for postoperative exercises.

After final repair of the tuberosities and confirmation of the reduction and fixation with imaging, the deltopectoral interval is closed. Drains are not typically used.

Intramedullary Nailing

Intramedullary nailing of the proximal humerus is of potential advantage in patients with osteoporotic bone or metastatic lesions and in fractures with diaphyseal extension **(Fig. 11–18A–C)** (see **Videos 11–4** and **11–5, Disk 2**). The procedure may be done percutaneously with surgical neck fractures but requires some further splitting of the anterolateral deltoid when three- or four-part fractures are treated. Image intensification is necessary; a reasonable experience with nailing humeral shaft fractures is beneficial.

There are two approaches to positioning the patient and the C-arm. My preferred approach is to place the patient supine with the torso tilted ~30 degrees toward the uninjured side. The C-arm is brought in from the opposite side, and by simply arcing the image intensifier over the patient, AP and lateral views of the shoulder can be obtained. The alternative approach is to position the patient in the beach chair position and place the C-arm on the injured side, next to the patient's head (see description in the section on percutaneous pinning). Regardless of the approach, "practice" images with the C-arm should be done before the patient is prepped and draped to confirm adequate visualization and reduction maneuvers.

The patient's arm is prepped and draped free. The initial incision is made obliquely off of the anterolateral acromion for 2 cm. For more complex fracture patterns, an incision up to 5 cm may be made. Lateral deltoid-splitting approaches should be discouraged because of the increased risk of shoulder pain and more difficulty with nail insertion.[34]

Image intensification should be used to assist with identifying the starting point. At this point, if the tuberosities are fractured, sutures should be placed in the rotator cuff insertions and the tuberosities mobilized. A K-wire is inserted into the humeral head and used to derotate the humeral head so that is has the normal relationship to the

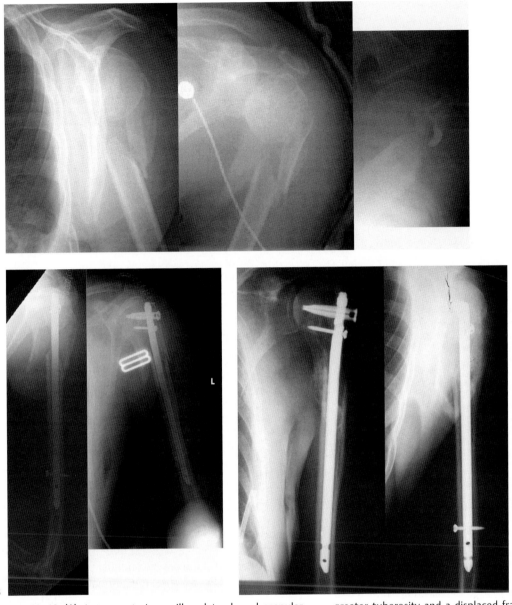

Figure 11–18 (A) Anteroposterior, axillary lateral, and scapular lateral x-rays of a proximal humeral fracture associated with extension and comminution of the upper third of the humeral shaft. The humeral head component includes a nondisplaced fracture of the greater tuberosity and a displaced fracture of the surgical neck. **(B)** Postoperative views after intramedullary nailing with a proximal humeral nail. **(C)** Final x-rays after fracture union.

glenoid. The specific maneuver that is needed will depend on the fracture pattern. One should be able to visualize the normal sulcus between the lateral edge of the articular surface of the humeral head and the greater tuberosity. If needed, the humeral head can be pinned to the glenoid to temporarily maintain it in the reduced position.

A guide pin is then inserted into the proximal humerus and directed down the humeral shaft. The precise entry point will depend on the shape of the chosen nail; one should consult with the recommendations of the manufacturer of the device that is used. The pin should be well centered on the lateral view. The surgical neck component of the fracture is typically reduced by manipulation of the arm.

After the guide pin is inserted into the humeral shaft, the starting point is opened with a cannulated drill. The humeral shaft is reamed at the surgeon's discretion; it is often not necessary in older patients with wide medullary canals. The length of the nail is confirmed. The nail is inserted gently.

The proximal interlocking screws are inserted using a jig. Usually, a combination of screws in multiple planes is used. The tuberosities are reduced with a combination of traction applied to the previously placed sutures, K-wires, or pointed clamps. Using the attached jigs, the interlocking screws are inserted into the reduced tuberosities. Finally, more sutures are used to further reinforce the repair of the tuberosities.

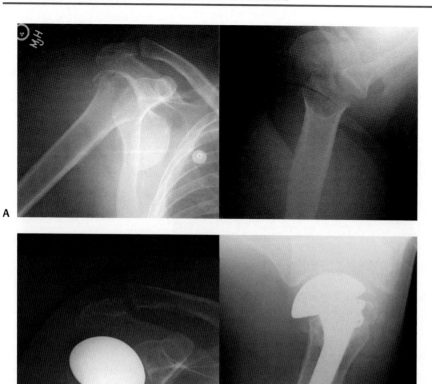

Figure 11–19 A comminuted four-part fracture-dislocation treated by hemiarthroplasty. **(A)** Anteroposterior (AP) and axillary lateral views of the injury. **(B)** AP and axillary views 1 year after hemiarthroplasty with a low-profile fracture stem and tuberosity reconstruction.

Distal interlocking is performed at the discretion of the surgeon, but probably recommended in most cases.

Hemiarthroplasty

The role of prosthetic replacement for proximal humeral fractures continues to be controversial (**Figs. 11–19A,B**).[4] Recent reports suggest that the outcome after hemiarthroplasty is not as good as what has generally been considered.[1,4,35] Furthermore, the results of early arthroplasty are better than when it is performed after failed internal fixation or malunion following nonoperative treatment.[1] Secure tuberosity repair, restoration of normal retroversion of the humeral head, and restoration of proper length of the humerus are the keys to obtaining good results with hemiarthroplasty after proximal humerus fracture (**Fig. 11–20**).

The technique of shoulder hemiarthroplasty following proximal humeral fracture differs in several important aspects from the more familiar technique of shoulder arthroplasty for arthrosis (see **Video 11–6, Disk 2**). These differences arise primarily from the disruption of anatomy and loss of bone stock, both of which render prosthetic positioning more difficult. Because the ultimate function of the shoulder depends so greatly on the rotator cuff, one of the most important steps in shoulder hemiarthroplasty following fracture is the secure reconstruction of the rotator cuff and tuberosities around the implant.

Even when arthroplasty is planned, careful preoperative assessment of plain radiographs is an important step in preoperative planning. When possible, an AP x-ray of the uninjured limb should be obtained. With this comparison x-ray, one can often begin to assess the height of the humeral head and the offset and angulation of the neck.

The deltopectoral approach is utilized as previously described. Often, the upper 1 to 2 cm of the pectoralis major tendon is released off of its humeral insertion. Blunt, curved retractors can be placed beneath the deltoid and conjoined tendon. The coracoacromial ligament is preserved.

The first step is to identify the biceps tendon, which in turn serves as a key to the identification of the tuberosity fragments. A vessel-loop can be secured around the biceps tendon. Multiple heavy nonabsorbable horizontal sutures

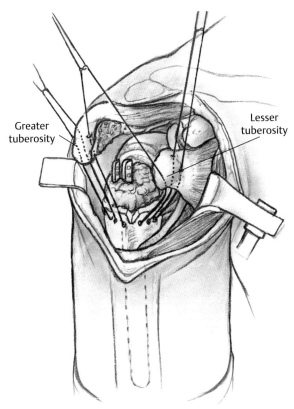

Figure 11–20 The tuberosity reconstruction after hemiarthroplasty. Vertical sutures are placed into both tuberosities, and a horizontal cerclage suture is placed between the tuberosities.

are placed within the rotator cuff insertions on the lesser and greater tuberosities. The rotator interval is opened to increase access to the joint, and the tuberosity fragments mobilized. The humeral head fragments are removed; if possible the removed head is measured with calipers or a template to determine the appropriate prosthetic size.

The humeral stem is identified and the medullary canal debrided. Gentle reaming is done, primarily to size the stem. An appropriately sized trial stem is inserted. If available, the stem is attached to the arm with a stabilizing jig. The stem should be placed in 20 degrees of retroversion compared with the transepicondylar axis. A trial head of similar size to the removed specimen is attached, and trial reduction is performed. Finally, the tuberosities are reduced into position using their attached sutures.

The trial reduction is assessed in multiple steps. First, the height of the stem is checked by assessing the tension on the biceps and noting any overlap of the greater tuberosity and the stem. The tip of the greater tuberosity should be slightly lower than the top of the humeral head. Rotation is assessed by noting that the prosthetic humeral head faces the glenoid with the arm in neutral rotation, and the greater tuberosity should overlap the lateral fin. Once the correct position is obtained, reference marks for height and rotation should be made. After the trial stem is removed, at least two drill holes are made in the anterolateral part of the shaft, and two large, nonabsorbable sutures are placed in them.

The definitive humeral stem is cemented in place; a cement plug is not necessary. After the cement has cured, the definitive humeral head can be placed after repeated trials if needed. Stepwise, secure repair of the tuberosities is the final and most important step. First of all, two of the horizontal sutures in the greater tuberosity are passed around the medial humeral neck and tied. The remaining two horizontal sutures are also passed medially around the neck, but in addition are passed around the lesser tuberosity, which is also secured. The two sutures placed in the humeral shaft are then used to create a vertical tension band. Additional sutures in the rotator interval and between the tuberosities complete the repair. Cancellous bone graft from the resected fragments can be placed around the proximal shaft to promote bony healing of the tuberosities to the shaft. Following repair, the shoulder should be brought through a range of motion. The soft tissue reconstruction should be stable and watertight.

Tips and Tricks

- Nearly always, there is an apex-anterior angulation of the surgical neck of the humerus that is corrected by pushing toward the floor at the fracture site while lifting up on the distal arm.
- Regardless of the approach used for fracture fixation, "practice" images with the C-arm should be done before the patient is prepped and draped to confirm adequate visualization and reduction maneuvers.
- When multiple percutaneous pins are used, the pins are drilled through the near cortex but should be impacted by hand into the humeral head.
- During plate fixation, abduction of the shoulder during the approach relaxes the deltoid and facilitates exposure.

Rehabilitation

Rehabilitation after surgical repair of proximal humeral fractures is similar to that already described for nonoperative treatment. Hodgson et al found that patients who started immediate physiotherapy had less pain and better motion compared with patients that were immobilized for 3 weeks.[36] Pendulum exercises are generally begun immediately. Once the wound is benign, gentle active-assisted range of motion exercised are begun. After percutaneous pinning, range of motion exercises must be limited to some degree because of pain and the relatively weak fixation. After plate fixation and nailing, passive exercises are usually appropriate, with the considerations that follow. When greater tuberosity fractures have been repaired, active abduction and external rotation should be delayed for soft tissue healing. After hemiarthroplasty or in fractures with lesser tuberosity repair, the subscapularis must be protected from active internal rotation or passive external rotation. In general, active motion is begun within 6 to 8 weeks, and resisted exercises in 10 to 12 weeks after the fracture has united.

New Techniques

There are several new options and implants available for the fixation of proximal humerus fractures. Many of these have not been validated by comparative trials. There has been an explosion of bone-graft substitutes on the market. Kwon et al studied the use of calcium phosphate cement on the fixation of proximal humeral osteotomies in a cadaveric model. Regardless of the type of fixation (multiple pins, cloverleaf plate, blade plate), the biomechanical properties of fixation were significantly improved by the addition of calcium phosphate cement.[32] Furthermore, the addition of cement improved the stiffness of the most osteoporotic specimens to levels above those of the most osteodense specimens treated with internal fixation alone.[32]

Outcomes

Many studies have reported on the outcomes of treatment following proximal humeral fracture, utilizing various methods of assessment.[3,37] Retrospective studies seem to indicate that the functional outcome of elderly patients with three-part fractures or valgus-impacted fractures is favorable irrespective of whether they are treated conservatively or surgically.[3,25] In one study, 96% of elderly patients were satisfied with their shoulder function 3 years after they had sustained a three-part fracture.[3] In contrast, 67% of patients that had a four-part fracture could not accept their shoulder function, and most of the unhappy patients had radiographic evidence of osteoarthritis or avascular necrosis. The Constant score seems to correlate well with the patients' own opinions, whereas the Neer score was less predictive.[3] In one of the only prospective, randomized studies that have been performed to date, Zyto et al could find no functional differences between patients with three- and four-part fractures treated conservatively or with tension-band osteosynthesis.[8]

One potential determinant of outcome is rotator cuff function. In one study, outcomes according to the Constant score were correlated with the integrity of the rotator cuff as assessed by ultrasonography.[37] It was found that rotator cuff pathology was indeed related to fracture displacement, as expected, and that the integrity of the cuff was associated with outcome.[37] This finding may argue for more aggressive diagnosis and treatment of rotator cuff lesions in patients with fractures of the proximal humerus.

The outcome following hemiarthroplasty is difficult to assess when compared with the results of internal fixation.[4] After hemiarthroplasty, pain relief appears to be satisfactory, but restoration of functional range of motion is less predictable.[35] There seems to be quite a difference in results depending on the specific method of assessment.[1] Clearly, more randomized, prospective comparative studies are needed before these questions can be definitively answered.

Locking Plates

So-called locking plates are popular new devices with very little published data so far about their efficacy in proximal humeral fractures (**Fig. 11–6A,B**). In theory, locking plates have better fixation in osteoporotic bone, making them ideal for proximal humeral fractures. Case series have been presented at national meetings, indicating results that are equally good in elderly patients as in younger patients with few complications, but we must await the publication of comparative, peer-reviewed studies to define the indications and expected results with these devices. Despite the lack of published results, many surgeons are very enthusiastic about their use.

Hemiarthroplasty

In 1970, Neer reported satisfactory results in 90% of patients undergoing shoulder hemiarthroplasty for the treatment of proximal humeral fractures.[16] Ever since, it has been considered that hemiarthroplasty is a predictably successful way to manage these complex fractures in elderly patients. However, more thorough analyses using contemporary outcomes assessment methodologies indicate that the results of hemiarthroplasty may not be quite so good. Although outcomes after hemiarthroplasty may be satisfactory with regard to pain relief, they are inconsistent regarding functional measures.[35] Movin et al evaluated 29 patients between 2 and 12 years after undergoing humeral hemiarthroplasty for fracture, and found disappointing results.[38] All patients had compromised function, with a mean Constant score of just 38 (range 16 to 69). Pain, as measured by a visual analog score, was a mean of 21 at rest and 47 with movement of the shoulder.[38] Differences in outcome were not related to the timing of surgery or the type of prosthesis used.[38]

Complications

General Considerations

The best results after repair of proximal humeral fractures occur with anatomical reduction, stable fixation without impingement, no vascular embarrassment of the humeral head, normal neurological function, and early functional rehabilitation. Achieving all of these goals has proven elusive, and complications are frequent with these injuries. Poor bone density is a nearly universal constant in these injuries, making rigid fixation difficult. Numerous muscles insert on the proximal humerus and exert deforming forces that must be neutralized; these forces commonly lead to loss of fixation or inadequate initial reduction (**Fig. 11–1**). The subdeltoid and subacromial gliding mechanism must be restored to restore motion; adhesions in these regions as a result of the initial trauma, surgical intervention, or immobilization contribute to poor function.

Clinically evident neurovascular complications occur in ~5 to 6% of proximal humeral fractures. Subclinical neurological findings documented on electromyography may be seen in the majority of patients.[39] The axillary artery is the most common vascular structure injured, whereas the axillary nerve is the most common neurological injury.

The vascular supply to the humeral head is limited and is at risk following fracture. Avascular necrosis is a well-known sequela of complex fractures of the proximal humerus, but its significance is unclear.[28] The risk of osteonecrosis is related to the fracture pattern, degree of displacement, and method of treatment. The risk is highest among four-part fractures (up to 40%), less in three-part fractures (up to 15%), and very rare in surgical neck fractures. It has been pointed out that the risk of osteonecrosis is much less with four-part valgus-impacted fractures compared with other four-part fractures.[24] Recent studies have clarified this issue, showing that avascular necrosis is rare after three-part fractures, and when it does occur, it involves only a portion of the humeral head and causes little discomfort.[23] In contrast, complete avascular necrosis is common after most displaced four-part fractures and often leads to more disabling symptoms.[23,28] Gerber et al pointed out that the clinical outcome in patients with osteonecrosis is dependent on the anatomical alignment of the fracture; patients with osteonecrosis but no malalignment had much better results than those with both osteonecrosis and malalignment.[28]

Nonunions are rare and most often associated with surgical neck fractures. They are usually obvious on plain radiographs, but tomography may be necessary. Salvage is usually possible with open reduction and stable fixation; we have found the use of intramedullary fibular strut allografts to be of benefit (**Fig. 11–21A–D**). Rarely, prosthetic replacement may be a better option.

Malunion is a much more frequent problem that can be very difficult to manage. Tuberosity malunion can impair rotator cuff function as well as cause subacromial impingement (**Fig. 11–22**). In a biomechanical study, 5 mm of superior displacement of the greater tuberosity increased the deltoid force required for abduction by 16%. Combined posterior/superior displacement of 1 cm increased the deltoid force by 29%.[40] Humeral head or surgical neck malunion can impair range of motion and overall shoulder function (**Fig. 11–23A,B**) (see **Video 11–7, Disk 2**).

Open Reduction and Internal Fixation

The potential complications of attempted open reduction and internal fixation of the proximal humerus fall into several broad categories. Those complications include osteonecrosis, loss of fixation, and malunion or nonunion.

Because of the association of proximal humeral fractures and osteoporosis, loss of fixation and implant migration is a common problem with these injuries. The risk varies with the technique chosen. Malunion had been reported in 19% of patients undergoing closed reduction and percutaneous pinning.[41] Loss of fixation may be less common with newer plates that incorporate fixed-angle screws.

Osteonecrosis of the humeral head following fracture may be partial or complete; the significance of this complication continues to be debated. Wijgman et al examined 60 patients with three- or four-part proximal humerus fractures that were managed with either plate or cerclage wire fixation at an average of 10 years after injury.[42] Although 22 of the 60 patients (37%) had osteonecrosis, 17 of them (77% of those with osteonecrosis) had good or excellent functional outcomes. There did not appear to be any correlation between the type of fixation and the development of osteonecrosis.[42]

Complications of closed reduction and percutaneous pinning include malreduction and malunion, pin track infection, and pin loosening. The risk of osteonecrosis appears to be related to the fracture pattern and is probably unaffected by the technique. Similarly, loss of fixation is more common among three- and four-part fractures.

Open reduction and internal fixation with plates requires a more invasive approach and may be associated with an increased risk of osteonecrosis, depending on one's particular technique. On the other hand, more rigid fixation may promote better revascularization of the humeral head by creeping substitution and may lessen the risk of articular collapse when osteonecrosis occurs. Complications that are unique to internal fixation of proximal humeral fractures include technical errors (inadequate reduction, oversize or incorrectly positioned implants), loss of fixation, and iatrogenic rotator cuff disruption. In the past, late loss of reduction has occurred in up to 14% of patients treated with traditional T-plates.[43] The use of plates with angular stability such as blade plates or plates with locking screws and/or augmentation of the fracture with polymethyl methacrylate (PMMA) or calcium phosphate cement lessen this risk.

Intramedullary nailing of the proximal humerus is appealing because the implant does not rely so much on screw purchase in the humerus and may therefore have less risk of fixation failure. However, screw purchase in the humeral head has been problematic in some series.[44] Furthermore, reduction is not facilitated by the implant, and the approach requires violation of the rotator cuff with potential chronic shoulder pain.

Hemiarthroplasty

Potential complications of shoulder arthroplasty following proximal humeral fracture are numerous and include shoulder instability (dislocation of the prosthetic humeral

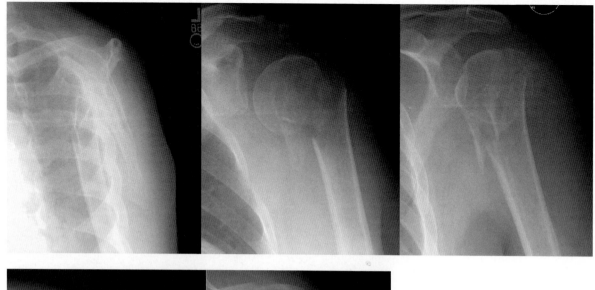

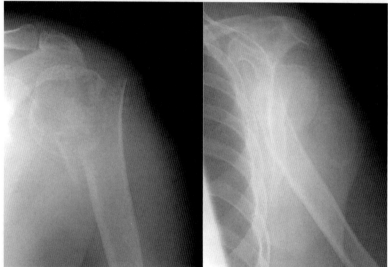

Figure 11–21 **(A)** X-rays of a comminuted surgical neck fracture. **(B)** Follow-up x-rays taken 8 weeks later suggest a nonunion. **(C)** An axial computed tomographic cut confirming a nonunion. **(D)** The fracture united 6 months after fixation with a locking blade plate made from a standard 3.5 mm reconstruction plate.

head from the glenoid), tuberosity malunion, and component malposition (errors in reestablishing height or rotation or both).

Component malposition is common and occurs in part as a result of the problems with instability of the trial humeral stem. Most often, the residual humeral shaft is a "pipe," and it is very difficult to ascertain and maintain the correct height and rotation of the stem during trial reduction and during stem insertion. Errors in restoring the correct height of the humeral head can lead to pain and poor motion if the prosthesis is too proud, or instability and weakness if it is too distal. Errors in rotation of the humeral stem affect the degree of retroversion of the shoulder, and hence its biomechanics. Because there is such a wide variation in normal humeral retroversion, restoring this anatomical feature is that much more difficult. The proximal bicipital groove is often used as a reference to rotation, but this anatomical feature is most often absent in these cases. Variations in elbow carrying angle make the forearm axis unreliable. These

problems can be obviated by use of the fracture stem with a mounting sleeve for trial reduction, as well as markings on the stem for the assessment of height.

Shoulder Dislocations

Shoulder stability is a complex phenomenon that is still the subject of intensive research. The mechanisms that contribute to shoulder stability continue to be defined. With the absence of intrinsic osseous support, shoulder stability is provided primarily by soft tissues, with capsuloligamentous structures providing static restraint while muscles provide dynamic stability.

Classification

Shoulder dislocations are classified by their etiology, direction, and time to diagnosis. Only traumatic dislocations are

Figure 11–21 *(Continued)*

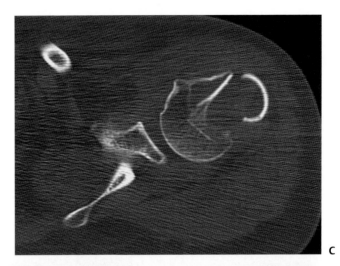

C

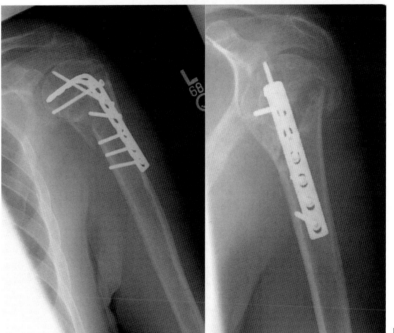

D

considered in this chapter. Most dislocations are anterior-inferior, but posterior dislocation and the unusual inferior dislocation (luxatio erecta) are also described. Posterior dislocations of the glenohumeral joint must always be considered in anyone with a shoulder injury. The diagnosis of posterior shoulder dislocation is often delayed and may be missed on AP radiographs.

Early magnetic resonance imaging appears to be better than delayed imaging at defining the presence of intra-articular pathology.[45] In general, the factors associated with an increased risk of recurrent dislocation are the age of the patient, the degree of violence producing the injury, and the nature of the damage to the anterior labrum and capsular attachments. Arthroscopic examination soon after acute dislocation may help identify those patients with high-risk lesions, allowing early repair and less long-

term disability.[12] Rotator cuff tear is more likely to be associated with dislocation in patients older than 40 years and may be a source of continued disability if not identified and repaired.[9]

Nonoperative Treatment

Acute anterior shoulder dislocations are treated by immediate, gentle, closed reduction. Neurological injury may accompany shoulder dislocation.[39] The axillary nerve is most commonly injured, although any part of the brachial plexus may be affected. A thorough neurological examination must be documented both before and after reduction. Prereduction x-rays are taken to document the dislocation and to identify any associated fractures. Although postreduction radiographs are routinely ordered, one study found that the

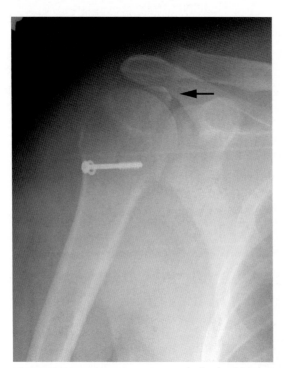

Figure 11–22 An anteroposterior x-ray of a shoulder showing residual displacement of the greater tuberosity (arrow) after an attempt at open reduction and fixation with a screw.

yield of this practice is so low that the time and expense of obtaining routine radiographs is not justified.[46] The need for postreduction immobilization remains controversial.

Indications for Nonoperative Treatment

Essentially all acute shoulder dislocations are managed nonoperatively. Closed reduction under general anesthesia is rarely indicated for irreducible dislocations, dislocations associated with nondisplaced surgical neck fractures that

might displace during manipulative reduction, and those with displaced greater tuberosity fractures.[47]

Reduction Techniques

There are a multitude of techniques described to reduce the dislocated shoulder; most rely on either or both longitudinal traction and leverage of the injured arm with the patient appropriately relaxed. The classic "Hippocratic" method involves the use of vigorous force with the heel of the person's foot effecting the reduction placed in the axilla of the patient. Another traditional method involves the application of traction to the arm by one person and the use of countertraction applied to the patient's torso by another, usually with a sheet wrapped around the patient's chest. These methods are painful, occasionally unsuccessful, and may be associated with complications, including humeral fracture and neurovascular injury.

Numerous "atraumatic" methods have been described. One of the most widely known methods is the so-called Kocher method, which is performed by first flexing the elbow, fully externally rotating the arm, adducting the externally rotated arm, lifting the point of the olecranon, and finally internally rotating the shoulder to effect reduction. As reported by Zahiri et al, this method was first described by Kocher in 1869 and has been repeatedly criticized ever since.[48] Nevertheless, Thakur and Narayan report the successful use of this technique in 16 dislocations, without any anesthesia or sedation and without any complications.[49]

In 1938, Milch described another simple method.[50] The clinician stands to the injured side of the patient and places the near hand in front of the shoulder with the thumb against the dislocated humeral head and the opposite hand gripping the forearm of the patient. The clinician then abducts and externally rotates the shoulder, with the elbow partly flexed, until the arm is above the patient's head. The humeral head should rotate into a reduced position, assisted by gentle pressure of the thumb.

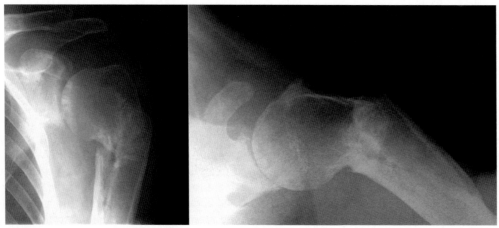

A   B

Figure 11–23 **(A)** Anteroposterior and **(B)** axillary lateral views of a surgical neck malunion. This case demonstrates the nearly universal tendency for such fractures to develop varus and apex-anterior deformities.

A more recently described technique, known as the external rotation method, is also safe, reliable, and comfortable for the patient.[51] The patient is in the supine position, with the clinician standing on the injured side. The elbow is flexed to 90 degrees with the arm against the side of the chest. The arm is gently lifted until the shoulder is in 20 degrees of forward elevation. With the patient's wrist and elbow supported by the clinician, the shoulder is gently externally rotated until reduction occurs, and then internally rotated to lie across the patient's chest. In a recent report, the external rotation method was successful in 36 of 40 acute anterior dislocations; in 29 cases no premedication was needed.[47] However, the method was not successful in four cases, including both patients in the series that also had displaced greater tuberosity fractures. The authors suggest that patients with displaced greater tuberosity fractures should be reduced under general anesthesia.[47]

Another useful technique is the method of Stimson, in which the patient is placed prone and a weight is attached to the injured arm that dangles off of the side of the table. With time, the shoulder may reduce without manipulation, although scapular manipulation may assist the reduction.

Regardless of the technique that is used, adequate muscular relaxation and analgesia are very helpful. Newer rapid-acting anesthetic agents such as propofol and methohexital (both dosed at 1 mg/kg bolus, with follow-up doses of 0.5 mg/kg every 2 minutes) may be safely administered in an emergency department setting.[52] Intra-articular injection of local anesthetic is another valuable method of analgesia, especially if intravenous sedation is not available or is contraindicated. Miller et al compared the ability of intravenous sedation or intra-articular lidocaine to facilitate reduction of a simple anterior shoulder dislocation using a modified Stimson method in 30 patients.[53] The group receiving local anesthesia spent less time in the emergency department (75 minutes vs 185 minutes in the sedation group, $p < .01$). There were no significant differences between the two groups regarding pain, success of the Stimson technique, or the time required to reduce the shoulder. Intravenous sedation was much more expensive than the use of lidocaine ($97.64 per patient compared with $0.52 for lidocaine).[53]

Rehabilitation

It remains very controversial whether to immobilize the shoulder following a traumatic shoulder dislocation. Although it has been suggested that immobilization will allow for better healing of injured soft tissues, some studies have not shown a clear benefit to prolonged immobilization.[10] Maeda et al found that the recurrence rate in young male rugby players during the first 2 years was lower in patients immobilized 4 to 7 weeks than in those with less than 3 weeks of immobilization.[54]

More recently, the position of immobilization has been of interest. Itoi et al performed a cadaveric study in which they noted that there was better apposition of the anterior shoulder capsule with the arm in external rotation.[55] In a clinical follow-up study, 40 patients with acute shoulder dislocations were assigned to conventional immobilization in internal rotation or immobilization in external rotation.[56] The recurrence rate was 30% in the internal rotation group and zero in the external rotation group at a mean follow-up of 15.5 months. The difference in recurrence rate was even greater among those who were aged less than 30 years (45% in the internal rotation group vs 0% in the external rotation group). The authors conclude that immobilization with the arm in external rotation is more effective in reducing the rate of recurrence after initial dislocation of the shoulder.[56]

Indications for Surgical Treatment

There are two aspects to consider in the management of shoulder dislocation: management of the acute injury and definitive repair of injured structures. Traumatic shoulder dislocation is associated with stretching and tearing of the capsuloligamentous structures of the shoulder and is associated with hematoma formation. Some investigators have suggested that early arthroscopic lavage of the shoulder may decompress the shoulder, provide better coaptation of the torn anterior capsule, and improve proprioception.[57] Although controversial, definitive early operative stabilization for anterior shoulder dislocation may be considered for young, high-demand patients who are unwilling to modify their lifestyle and have no prior dislocation, subluxation, or impingement history, no neurological injury, and no greater tuberosity fracture.[58] Noting that 21% of all patients presenting to their unit with shoulder dislocation had already suffered recurrence at 1 year (43% among those 15 to 22 years old), Davy and Drew suggest that young patients presenting with first-time traumatic anterior dislocations receive arthroscopic lavage within 10 days of injury.[59]

Patients who experience early redislocation should be carefully evaluated. Robinson et al showed that patients that sustain redislocation within 1 week may have either a large rotator cuff tear, fracture of the glenoid rim, or fractures of both the glenoid rim and the greater tuberosity.[60] Early operative repair is justified for patients in whom the dislocation is associated with one of these other injuries and who have evidence of gross instability.

Locked posterior dislocations are an especially difficult situation. Open reduction may be required if the dislocation is subacute or chronic. If there is a small reverse Hill-Sachs lesion, transfer of the lesser tuberosity into the defect is appropriate. If there is extensive damage to the articular cartilage, a reverse Hill-Sachs lesion of more than 45% of the humeral head, or duration of dislocation greater than 6 months, total shoulder arthroplasty is indicated.[61]

During total shoulder replacement for locked posterior dislocation, a secondary posterior incision may be necessary to extract the dislocated humeral head.[61]

Surgical Treatment

Surgical Anatomy

Traumatic shoulder dislocation is associated with much possible pathology. The classic Bankart (also referred to as the Perthes) lesion is avulsion of the anterior-inferior labrum from the glenoid. Although this lesion is commonly seen, it has been emphasized that some degree of capsular stretching always occurs as well. Less commonly, there is tearing of the glenohumeral ligaments off the humerus—the so-called humeral avulsion of glenohumeral ligament (HAGL) lesion.

Hintermann and Gachter performed shoulder arthroscopy on 212 patients with at least one shoulder dislocation and found a wide variety of pathology.[11] Anterior labral tears were the most common finding, occurring in 87% of cases. Other pathologies (in decreasing order of frequency) were anterior capsular insufficiency (79%), Hill-Sachs lesions of the humeral head (68%), glenohumeral ligament insufficiency (55%), complete rotator cuff tear (14%), posterior labral tears (12%), and superior labrum anterior and posterior SLAP lesions (7%). A similar spectrum of findings was identified by Taylor and Arciero.[12]

Surgical Techniques

A detailed description of the many methods and controversies associated with late repair of patients with recurrent shoulder instability is beyond the scope of this chapter, and readers are directed to other texts for a discussion of this topic. In the following paragraphs, the role of early arthroscopic lavage and arthroscopically assisted capsulorrhaphy are briefly discussed because these methods have some utility in the immediate postinjury period and may be of interest to the clinician initially responsible for treating patients with shoulder dislocation.

Arthroscopy

Early arthroscopy following traumatic shoulder dislocation has been advocated by many authors and may be of both diagnostic and therapeutic benefit.[12,57,59] Arthroscopic lavage may decompress the shoulder and allow better coaptation of the injured tissues or improve proprioceptive function. However, one recent study refuted the concept that early arthroscopy was of benefit. In a series of 31 patients aged 16 to 39, te Slaa et al found that the intra-articular pathology discovered during arthroscopy was not predictive of shoulder instability. In addition, there was no correlation between sporting activities and shoulder instability, and the authors found it unlikely that arthroscopic lavage reduces redislocation rates after acute dislocation in the young patient.[62]

Arthroscopic-Assisted Capsulorrhaphy

Bottoni et al performed a randomized comparison of arthroscopic stabilization of the shoulder within 10 days of injury to nonoperative management.[63] Ten patients were treated surgically with an arthroscopic Bankart repair using the Suretac device (Acufex Microsurgical, Inc., Mansfield, Massachusetts). Only one of these patients developed recurrent instability, compared with 75% of those treated nonoperatively. Larrain et al, in a nonrandomized study, found a redislocation rate of 95% compared with 4% after acute arthroscopic repair with either transglenoid sutures or a bone anchor.[64] The reader is referred to texts on shoulder surgery for a detailed description of the techniques of arthroscopic shoulder surgery.

Outcomes

Surprisingly, the natural history of traumatic shoulder dislocation is not well known. Recently, the results of a 3 year observational study of 538 consecutive patients with a first-time anterior dislocation of the shoulder was reported.[60] Seventeen (3.2%) of the patients sustained an early redislocation within 1 week of the original dislocation. Risk factors associated with early redislocation included high-energy trauma (relative risk = 13.7), associated neurological deficit (relative risk = 2.0), large rotator cuff tear (relative risk = 29.8), fracture of the glenoid rim (relative risk = 7.0), and fracture of both the glenoid rim and greater tuberosity (relative risk = 33.5).[60]

Complications

Neurological injury accompanies shoulder dislocation, and assessment of neurological function is difficult because the pain associated with the injury itself can cause varying degrees of apparent weakness. Visser et al performed electromyographic (EMG) studies in a cohort of 215 patients with shoulder trauma and documented abnormal findings in 62%. Motor and sensibility testing was not predictive of EMG-documented neurological injury; therefore, a large number of these lesions are not detected.[39]

Pearls

- Subclinical neurological abnormalities are detectable in 60% of patients with shoulder trauma.
- Rotator cuff tear is more likely to be associated with dislocation in patients older than 40 years.

On the DVDs

Video 11–1 (Disk 2) Closed Reduction and Percutaneous Pinning This video demonstrates the technique of closed reduction and pinning of an unstable surgical neck fracture.

Video 11–2 (Disk 2) ORIF of an Anterior Shoulder Fracture—Dislocation with a Non-locking Periarticular Plate This patient had both an anterior dislocation of the humeral head and an oblique fracture of the proximal humeral shaft. This video demonstrates repair of this injury using a periarticular plate.

Video 11–3 (Disk 2) Open Reduction of a Comminuted Proximal Humeral Fracture with a Locking Plate This video demonstrates the repair of a valgus-impacted fracture associated with displacement and comminution of both tuberosities, using a locking proximal humerus plate.

Video 11–4 (Disk 2) Intramedullary Nailing of the Proximal Humerus with a Locking Nail This video demonstrates repair of an unstable surgical neck fracture with an intramedullary nail that incorporates locking screws for humeral head fixation.

Video 11–5 (Disk 2) Intramedullary Nailing of the Proximal Humerus with a Spiral Blade Nail This video demonstrates repair of an unstable surgical neck fracture with an intramedullary nail that uses a spiral blade for fixation of the humeral head.

Video 11–6 (Same as Video 5–1, Disk 1) Shoulder Hemiarthroplasty for Proximal Humerus Fracture This video demonstrates the technique of shoulder hemiarthroplasty for management of a proximal humeral fracture, specifically highlighting the technique of tuberosity reconstruction.

Video 11–7 (Same as Video 5, Disk 2) Correction of Varus Malunion of the Proximal Humerus by Osteotomy This video shows correction of a varus malunion of the proximal humerus that was treated with a closing wedge osteotomy and locked plating.

References

1. Bosch U, Skutek M, Fremerey R, Tscherne H. Outcome after primary and secondary hemiarthroplasty in elderly patients with fractures of the proximal humerus. J Shoulder Elbow Surg 1998;7:479–484

2. Misra A, Kapur R, Mafulli N. Complex proximal humeral fractures in adults: a systematic review of management. Injury 2001;32:363–372

3. Zyto K, Kronberg M, Broström L-Å. Shoulder function after displaced fractures of the proximal humerus. J Shoulder Elbow Surg 1995;4:331–336

4. Zyto K, Wallace WA, Frostick SP, Preston BJ. Outcome after hemiarthroplasty for three- and four-part fractures of the proximal humerus. J Shoulder Elbow Surg 1998;7:85–89

5. Chudik SC, Weinhold P, Dahners LE. Fixed-angle plate fixation in simulated fractures of the proximal humerus: a biomechanical study of a new device. J Shoulder Elbow Surg 2003;12:578–588

6. Koval KJ, Blair B, Takei R, Kummer FJ, Zuckerman JD. Surgical neck fractures of the proximal humerus: a laboratory evaluation of ten fixation techniques. J Trauma 1996;40:778–783

7. Resch H, Povacz P, Frohlich R, Wambacher M. Percutaneous fixation of three- and four-part fractures of the proximal humerus. J Bone Joint Surg Br 1997;79:295–300

8. Zyto K, Ahrengart L, Sperber A, Törnkvist H. Treatment of displaced proximal humeral fractures in elderly patients. J Bone Joint Surg Br 1997;79:412–417

9. Pevny T, Hunter RE, Freeman JR. Primary traumatic anterior shoulder dislocation in patients 40 years of age and older. Arthroscopy 1998;14:289–294

10. Hovelius L, Augustini BG, Fredin H, Johansson O, Norlin R, Thorling J. Primary anterior dislocation of the shoulder in young patients: a ten-year prospective study. J Bone Joint Surg Am 1996;78:1677–1684

11. Hintermann B, Gachter A. Arthroscopic findings after shoulder dislocation. Am J Sports Med 1995;23:545–551

12. Taylor DC, Arciero RA. Pathologic changes associated with shoulder dislocations: arthroscopic and physical examination findings in first-time, traumatic anterior dislocations. Am J Sports Med 1997;25:306–311

13. Gumina S, Postacchini F. Anterior dislocation of the shoulder in elderly patients. J Bone Joint Surg Br 1997;79:540–543

14. Koval KJ, Gallagher MA, Marsicano JG, Cuomo F, McShinawy A, Zuckerman JD. Functional outcome after minimally displaced fractures of the proximal part of the humerus. J Bone Joint Surg Am 1997;79:203–207

15. Lin J, Hou S-M, Hang Y-S. Locked nailing for displaced surgical neck fractures of the humerus. J Trauma 1998;45:1051–1057

16. Neer CS II. Displaced proximal humerus fractures: part I. Classification and evaluation. J Bone Joint Surg Am 1970;52:1077–1089

17. Bernstein J, Adler LM, Blank JE, et al. Evaluation of the Neer system of classification of proximal humerus fractures with computerized tomographic scans and plain radiographs. J Bone Joint Surg Am 1996;78:1371–1375

18. Brien H, Noftall F, MacMaster S, Cummings T, Landells C, Rockwood P. Neer's classification system: a critical appraisal. J Trauma 1995;38:257–260

19. Sallay PI, Pedowitz RA, Mallon WJ, Vandemark RM, Dalton JD, Speer KP. Reliability and reproducibility of radiographic interpretation of proximal humeral fracture pathoanatomy. J Shoulder Elbow Surg 1997;6:60–69

20. Sjödén GO, Movin T, Güntner P, et al. Poor reproducibility of classification of proximal humeral fractures: additional CT of minor value. Acta Orthop Scand 1997;68:239–242

21. Sidor ML, Zuckerman JD, Lyon T, Koval K, Cuomo F, Schoenberg N. Classification of proximal humerus fractures: the contribution of the scapular lateral and axillary radiographs. J Shoulder Elbow Surg 1994;3:24–27

22. Simon JA, Puopolo SM, Capla EL, Egol KA, Zuckerman JD, Koval KJ. Accuracy of the axillary projection to determine fracture angulation of the proximal humerus. Orthopedics 2004;27:205–207

23. Schai P, Imhoff A, Preiss S. Comminuted humeral head fractures: a multicenter analysis. J Shoulder Elbow Surg 1995;4:319–330

24. Jakob RP, Miniaci A, Anson PS, Jaberg H, Osterwalder A, Ganz R. Four-part valgus impacted fractures of the proximal humerus. J Bone Joint Surg Br 1991;73:295–298

25. Court-Brown CM, Cattermole H, McQueen MM. Impacted valgus fractures (B1.1) of the proximal humerus: the results of nonoperative treatment. J Bone Joint Surg Br 2002;84:504–508

26. Park TS, Choi IY, Kim YH, Park MR, Shon JH, Kim SI. A new suggestion for the treatment of minimally displaced fractures of the

greater tuberosity of the proximal humerus. Bull Hosp Jt Dis 1997; 56:171–176

27. Ko J-Y, Yamamoto R. Surgical treatment of complex fractures of the proximal humerus. Clin Orthop Relat Res 1996;327:225–237

28. Gerber C, Hersche O, Berberat C. The clinical significance of post-traumatic avascular necrosis of the humeral head. J Shoulder Elbow Surg 1998;7:586–590

29. Kamineni S, Ankem H, Sanghavi S. Anatomical considerations for percutaneous proximal humeral fracture fixation. Injury 2004;35: 1133–1136

30. Rowles DJ, McGrory JE. Percutaneous pinning of the proximal part of the humerus: an anatomic study. J Bone Joint Surg Am 2001;83:1695–1699

31. Liew AS, Johnson JA, Patterson SD, et al. Effect of screw placement on fixation in the humeral head. J Shoulder Elbow Surg 2000;9: 423–426

32. Kwon BK, Goertzen DJ, O'Brien PJ, Broekhuyse HM, Oxland TR. Biomechanical evaluation of proximal humeral fracture fixation supplemented with calcium phosphate cement. J Bone Joint Surg Am 2002;84:951–961

33. Naidu SH, Bixler B, Capo JT, Moulton MJR, Radin A. Percutaneous pinning of proximal humerus fractures: a biomechanical study. Orthopedics 1997;20:1073–1076

34. Riemer BL, Butterfield SL, D'Ambrosia R, Kellam J. Seidel intramedullary nailing of humeral diaphyseal fractures: a preliminary report. Orthopedics 1991;14:239–246

35. Wretenberg P, Ekelund A. Acute hemiarthroplasty after proximal humerus fracture in old patients: a retrospective evaluation of 18 patients followed for 2–7 years. Acta Orthop Scand 1997;68:121–123

36. Hodgson SA, Mawson SJ, Stanley D. Rehabilitation after two-part fractures of the neck of the humerus. J Bone Joint Surg Br 2003;85:419–422

37. Wilmanns C, Bonnaire F. Rotator cuff alterations resulting from humeral head fractures. Injury 2002;33:781–789

38. Movin T, Sjödén GOJ, Ahrengart L. Poor function after shoulder replacement in fracture patients: a retrospective evaluation of 29 patients followed for 2–12 years. Acta Orthop Scand 1998;69: 392–396

39. Visser CP, Tavy DL, Coene LN, Brand R. Electromyographic findings in shoulder dislocations and fractures of the proximal humerus: comparison with clinical neurologic examination. Clin Neurol Neurosurg 1999;101:86–91

40. Bono CM, Renard R, Levine RG, Levy AS. Effect of displacement of fractures of the greater tuberosity on the mechanics of the shoulder. J Bone Joint Surg Br 2001;83:1056–1062

41. Jaberg H, Warner JJ, Jakob RP. Percutaneous stabilization of unstable fractures of the humerus. J Bone Joint Surg Am 1992;74: 508–515

42. Wijgman AJ, Roolker W, Patt TW, et al. Open reduction and internal fixation of three and four-part fractures of the proximal part of the humerus. J Bone Joint Surg Am 2002;84-A:1919–1925

43. Hessmann MH, Blum J, Hofmann A, Küchle R, Rommens PM. Internal fixation of proximal humeral fractures: current concepts. Eur J Trauma 2003;5:253–261

44. Bernard J, Charalambides C, Aderinto J, Mok D. Early failure of intramedullary nailing for proximal humeral fractures. Injury 2000; 31:789–792

45. Wintzell G, Haglund-Akerlind Y, Tengvar M, Johansson L, Eriksson E. MRI examination of the glenohumeral joint after traumatic primary anterior dislocation: a descriptive evaluation of the acute lesion and at 6-month follow-up. Knee Surg Sports Traumatol Arthrosc 1996;4:232–236

46. Hendey GW, Kinlaw K. Clinically significant abnormalities in postreduction radiographs after anterior shoulder dislocation. Ann Emerg Med 1996;28:399–402

47. Eachempati KK, Dua A, Malhotra R, Bhan S, Bera JR. The external rotation method for reduction of acute anterior dislocations and fracture-dislocations of the shoulder. J Bone Joint Surg Am 2004; 86-A:2431–2434

48. Zahiri CA, Zahiri H, Tehrany F. Anterior shoulder dislocation reduction technique – revisited. Orthopedics 1997;20:515–521

49. Thakur AJ, Narayan R. Painless reduction of shoulder dislocation by Kocher's method. J Bone Joint Surg Br 1990;72:524

50. Milch J. Treatment of dislocation of the shoulder. Surgery 1938;3:732–740

51. Plummer D, Clinton J. The external rotation method for reduction of acute anterior shoulder dislocation. Emerg Med Clin North Am. 1989;7:165–175

52. Miner JR, Biros M, Krieg S, Johnson C, Heegaard W, Plummer D. Randomized clinical trial of propofol versus methohexital for procedural sedation during fracture and dislocation reduction in the emergency department. Acad Emerg Med 2003;10:931–937

53. Miller SL, Cleeman E, Auerbach J, Flatow EL. Comparison of intra-articular lidocaine and intravenous sedation for reduction of shoulder dislocations: a randomized, prospective study. J Bone Joint Surg Am 2002;84-A:2135–2139

54. Maeda A, Yoneda M, Horibe S, Hirooka A, Wakitani S, Narita Y. Longer immobilization extends the "symptom-free" period following primary shoulder dislocation in young rugby players. J Orthop Sci 2002;7:43–47

55. Itoi E, Hatakeyama Y, Urayama M, Pradhan RL, Kido T, Sato K. Position of immobilization after dislocation of the shoulder: a cadaveric study. J Bone Joint Surg Am 1999;81:385–390

56. Itoi E, Hatakeyama Y, Kido T, et al. A new method of immobilization after traumatic anterior dislocation of the shoulder: a preliminary study. J Shoulder Elbow Surg 2003;12:413–415

57. Wintzell G, Hovelius L, Wikblad L, Saebo M, Larsson S. Arthroscopic lavage speeds reduction in effusion in the glenohumeral joint after primary anterior shoulder dislocation: a controlled randomized ultrasound study. Knee Surg Sports Traumatol Arthrosc 2000;8:56–60

58. Arciero RA, St. Pierre P. Acute shoulder dislocation: indications and techniques for operative management. Clin Sports Med 1995;14: 937–953

59. Davy AR, Drew SJ. Management of shoulder dislocation: are we doing enough to reduce the risk of recurrence? Injury 2002;33:775–779

60. Robinson CM, Kelly M, Wakefield AE. Redislocation of the shoulder during the first six weeks after a primary anterior dislocation: risk factors and results of treatment. J Bone Joint Surg Am 2002;84-A:1552–1559

61. Cheng SL, Mackay MB, Richards RR. Treatment of locked posterior fracture-dislocations of the shoulder by total shoulder arthroplasty. J Shoulder Elbow Surg 1997;6:11–17

62. te Slaa RL, Brand R, Marti RK. A prospective arthroscopic study of acute first-time anterior shoulder dislocation in the young: a five-year follow-up study. J Shoulder Elbow Surg 2003;12: 529–534

63. Bottoni CR, Wilckens JH, DeBerardino TM, et al. A prospective, randomized evaluation of arthroscopic stabilization versus nonoperative treatment in patients with acute, traumatic, first-time shoulder dislocations. Am J Sports Med 2002;30:576–580

64. Larrain MV, Botto GJ, Montenegro HJ, Mauas DM. Arthroscopic repair of acute anterior shoulder dislocation in young athletes. Arthroscopy 2001;17:373–377

12 Humeral Shaft Fractures

David C. Templeman and Stephen Andrew Sems

Humeral shaft fractures account for ~1% of acute fractures in trauma registries. Despite the nearly universal acceptance of intramedullary nailing for fractures of the long bones of the lower extremity, nonoperative management remains the treatment of choice for many humeral shaft factures. For those fractures that require stabilization, both plating and nailing have similar results, although with slightly different complications. Each method has its advantages and disadvantages, which are discussed at length in this chapter.

Associated injuries to the radial nerve occur in 6 to 17% of humeral shaft fractures; these are most commonly seen in displaced transverse fractures in the mid-diaphysis. This fact mandates that a motor examination specifically testing wrist extension be documented for every humeral fracture at the time of initial presentation. It should be noted that a common mistake, often made after splinting the arm and wrist, is to observe extension of the fingers, which is a test of the intrinsic muscles of the hand and their innervation by the ulnar nerve. Evaluation of the radial nerve is performed by testing wrist extension with grading of the motor function.

Nonoperative Treatment

General Concepts

Presently, nonsurgical management is considered the treatment of choice for most isolated humeral shaft fractures. The predictably good results achieved with functional bracing in particular have been noted by Sarmiento, who reported union rates near 99% when treating closed and low-energy open fractures.[1–3] Other methods of nonoperative management include coaptation splints, hanging arm casts, and varieties of slings and swaths. Each of these methods is discussed in the following paragraphs.

Nonoperative management is not ideal for certain fractures and in certain situations. For example, problems with the nonoperative management of isolated humeral shaft fractures are more common when treating displaced transverse fractures, which are prone to nonunion, and in fractures with persistent angulation greater than 20 degrees. This amount of angulation may contribute to decreased range of motion of the shoulder; in particular, varus angulation is associated with loss of functional shoulder abduction. In contrast, shortening of the humerus does not appear to cause a functional problem. Castellá et al recently reported on a series of 30 humeral nonunions occurring after nonoperative management; nine were in elderly women with the same fracture pattern: a long lateral butterfly fragment at the junction of the middle and distal thirds of the humerus.[4]

Coaptation Splinting

Coaptation splints are often the first choice for the initial stabilization of humeral shaft fractures in the emergency department. The splint is U-shaped and should be advanced as far up into the axilla as possible on the medial side of the arm and extend around the elbow to end above the deltoid on the lateral side (**Fig. 12–1A–D**). For more proximal fractures, extending the lateral segment of the splint above the shoulder to the side of the neck will increase the amount of shoulder immobilization, which may result in improved pain control during the first week after injury. Tubular stockinette can be placed around the splint and tied loosely around the neck to prevent the splint from slipping when above-the-shoulder immobilization is desired. Fractures treated in coaptation splints may develop varus angulation due to the positioning of the arm against the body, especially if the axillary segment of the cast ends at or distal to the fracture (**Fig. 12–2**). To prevent varus deformity, the splint must often be molded into valgus (banana shaped). The axillary end of the splint should be well padded, and dessicating powder can be applied to avoid skin complications in this area. Weekly radiographs should be monitored to ensure appropriate fracture positioning with this technique. Like the hanging arm cast, coaptation splinting may be used for the initial postinjury period before conversion to functional bracing for definitive treatment.

Functional Bracing

Functional bracing is an effective method of obtaining union in humeral shaft fractures that allows shoulder and elbow motion while promoting fracture union. Functional bracing works by providing circumferential compression to the soft tissue, resulting in an increase in the hydrostatic pressure around the fracture. Functional bracing allows motion of the adjacent joints while immobilizing the fracture. Active muscle use assists in reducing fracture angulation and rotation.[3]

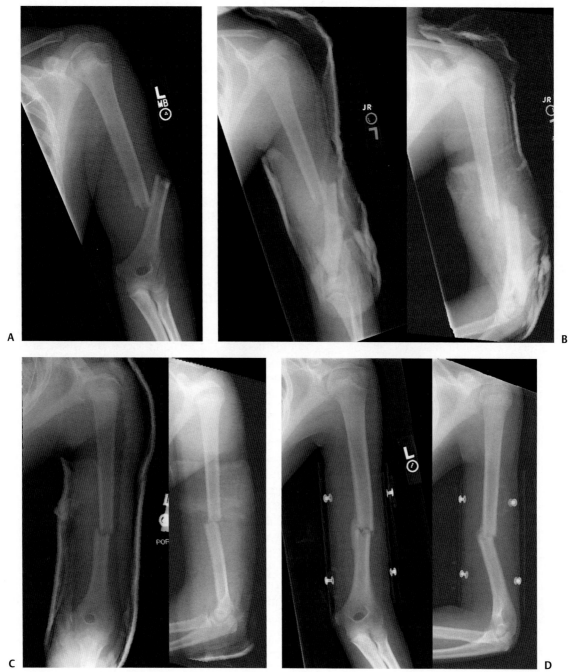

Figure 12–1 Example of a humeral coaptation splint. **(A)** Anteroposterior (AP) radiograph of a midshaft humerus fracture. **(B)** AP and lateral radiographs in a poorly applied plaster coaptation splint, with little change in fracture position. **(C)** After resplinting with a tighter splint, showing improved reduction. **(D)** Final radiographs in a functional brace.

Humeral fracture braces consist of two shells, one fitting inside the other **(Fig. 12–3).** One shell is formed to fit the bicep muscle belly, and the other fits the triceps. The shells should not impinge on the elbow area or impede elbow motion. Two or three Velcro straps allow tightening of the brace to a snug fit. The adjustability of the braces allow them to be placed as early as 5 to 7 days after injury, regard-

less of the amount of swelling, and subsequent tightening of the brace is done as swelling subsides. Functional braces are poorly tolerated immediately following injury. Therefore, initial immobilization for 1 to 2 weeks with a coaptation splint, hanging arm cast, or Velpeau sling is recommended. Patients are allowed to perform activities as tolerated with the extremity; however, shoulder abduction should be lim-

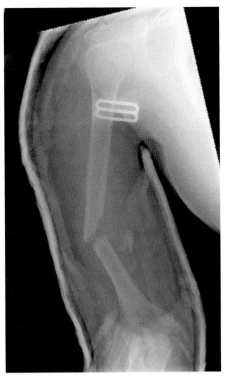

Figure 12–2 X-ray of varus deformity of a fracture immobilized with a coaptation splint. This deformity is difficult to prevent in a patient who is not able to be upright; this patient was in an intensive care unit. Gravity helps align the fracture in an upright patient.

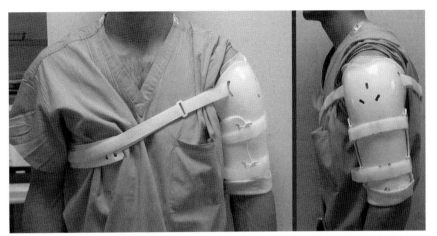

Figure 12–3 Humeral fracture brace. Tubular stockinette is applied followed by the clamshell orthosis. The patient must tighten the straps daily to keep the brace snug.

ited until the fracture unites to decrease the tendency for varus angulation to occur. Brace treatment will be necessary for approximately 8 weeks or until the patient has pain-free motion with radiographic evidence of union. There are several large series documenting that nonunions are uncommon with the use of functional orthosis.[1–3]

Hanging Arm Casts

So-called hanging arm casts have been traditionally used for the management of displaced humeral shaft fractures. Their use was based on the rationale that gravity, acting upon the weight of the cast, would align the arm. Humeral fractures amenable to treatment with hanging arm casts include fractures with shortening and those having a long oblique or spiral pattern. These fractures can withstand the potential lengthening that occurs with this method of treatment. In contrast, transverse fracture patterns are not ideally treated with this method, due to the potential for overdistraction and resultant nonunion that may occur. A hanging cast may be applied in the first week following injury to obtain reduction. After this time, transition to functional bracing is preferred due to the risk of shoulder and elbow stiffness following the prolonged immobilization that is required with a hanging arm cast. This technique is gravity dependent and requires the patient to stay in an upright position at all times to keep the fracture reduced. Otherwise, the weight of the cast could actually contribute to fracture displacement. Patients may dislike this technique due to the need to sleep upright in a chair or recliner. The hanging cast should be lightweight to minimize the potential for overdistraction and should extend from a point proximal to the fracture, holding the elbow at 90 degrees of flexion with the forearm in neutral rotation. The cast should leave the hand free to allow wrist and finger motion. The cast is suspended from a loop around the patient's neck and connected to the cast near the wrist. Adjustments in the position of the loop can be made depending on the type of deformity that is present. Varus deformities require moving the loop more laterally (away from the body), and fractures in valgus can be corrected by connecting the loop more medially (toward the abdomen). Apex anterior angulation can be corrected by moving the attachment more distally, whereas apex posterior angulation requires moving the loop to a more proximal attachment.

Other Nonoperative Treatment Methods

There are several other nonoperative methods that have been described to treat humeral shaft fractures. Velpeau dressings completely immobilize the upper extremity and should be used only as a temporizing method until other methods are appropriate. Shoulder spica casting has been used for fractures requiring significant abduction to reduce. These casts are difficult to apply and awkward to wear. Surgical treatment is preferred for fractures that would otherwise require shoulder spica casting to treat. Skeletal traction utilizing a transolecranon pin has been previously used for treatment. External fixation is much simpler to use and has replaced any indication for skeletal traction in the treatment of humeral shaft fractures.

Injury Classification

Classification of humeral shaft fractures is done on a descriptive basis, with multiple features of the fracture taken into account. Diaphyseal fractures can be classified by location: proximal third, middle third, and distal third. However, a more useful description of location depends on the location of the fracture with respect to the muscular insertions on the humerus. In the proximal aspect of the diaphysis, the deforming forces on fractures include the pectoralis major and deltoid. Thus fractures occurring above the pectoralis major insertion will be deformed, with the distal segment being displaced medially by the pull of the pectoralis major muscle. In this case, the proximal fragment will be abducted and externally rotated by the forces applied by the rotator cuff. In a humeral shaft fracture occurring between the insertions of the pectoralis major and the deltoid, the proximal shaft will displace medially due to the pull of the pectoralis major, whereas the distal shaft will be displaced proximally and laterally by the pull of the deltoid (**Fig. 12–4A–C**). In fractures occurring below the insertion of the deltoid, the stronger deltoid will cause the proximal fragment to displace into abduction, overpowering the pectoralis major.

In addition to localization of the fracture, the classification should include a description of the fracture pattern, using terms such as *transverse, spiral, oblique, comminuted,*

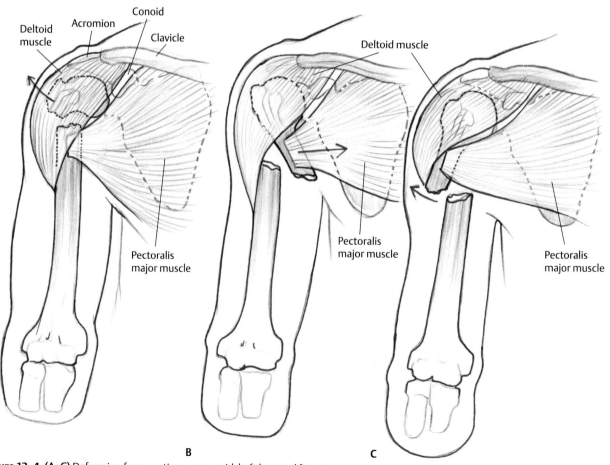

Figure 12–4 (A–C) Deforming forces acting upon a midshaft humeral fracture.

and *segmental.* Finally, the classification should include a description of the soft tissue status of the limb, utilizing the classifications of Tscherne and Gotzen for closed fractures[5] and Gustilo and Anderson for open fractures.[6]

Indications for Surgical Treatment

Failure to Maintain Appropriate Alignment

Closed treatment can be expected to result in union in over 90% of cases. However, surgical treatment of these fractures is indicated in specific instances. Nonoperative treatment that fails to maintain reduction within accepted parameters should result in a change to surgical treatment. Klenerman showed that humeral angulation of up to 20 degrees in the anteroposterior (AP) plane and 30 degree in varus or valgus and up to 3 cm of shortening are well tolerated.[7]

Open Fractures

Fractures with communication to the environment through a traumatic skin lesion should be managed operatively, with thorough debridement of all devitalized soft tissue and bone, and stabilization of the fracture. The importance of skeletal stability in the setting of open fractures should be appreciated for the role the stability plays in protecting the soft tissue from further injury and allowing better, faster recovery of the injured extremity.

Associated Articular Injuries

Diaphyseal humerus fractures associated with intra-articular fractures of the shoulder or elbow that require internal fixation should be stabilized at the same time (**Fig. 12–5A–E**). These fractures could either be a diaphyseal fracture that extends into the adjacent joint, or a segmentally fractured humerus that includes a diaphyseal fracture and a separate intra-articular shoulder or elbow fracture. Following fixation of the articular component of the fracture, postoperative care should include early mobilization of the joint, and a stable humeral diaphysis is necessary for this. Failure to stabilize the humeral shaft will prevent this mobilization and result in increased incidence of joint stiffness.

Neurovascular Injuries

Radial nerve injuries are the most common nerve injury associated with humeral shaft fractures, with a reported incidence ranging from 1.8 to 34%.[8-11] Most primary and secondary radial nerve palsies associated with a humeral shaft fracture are due to neurapraxia and resolve spontaneously. Therefore, there is no consensus about which lesions might demand open exploration. Radial nerve lesions associated with fractures of the distal third of the diaphysis with a longitudinal or spiral component (the Holstein-Lewis fracture) are an example of an instance where operative intervention might be considered. In this fracture pattern, the nerve may be lacerated or impaled by a sharp spike of bone, or trapped between the fracture fragments.[8] In contrast, most fractures of the middle third of the humerus are more likely to result in a bruised or contused nerve when there is nerve dysfunction.[12] In general, excellent results following conservative treatment of radial nerve lesions associated with humeral shaft fractures have been reported.[10,11]

One of the most controversial indications for operative intervention is the iatrogenic radial nerve palsy following closed manipulation, especially in the fractures of the distal third of the shaft with a long, spike-type configuration. Although these lesions are commonly said to require operative intervention, it has been shown that the vast majority of secondary radial nerve palsies also recover spontaneously.[13] Finally, it has been shown that radial nerve deficits in open humeral shaft fractures are often due to nerve laceration.[14] A final, but very subjective, finding is the presence of a gap in an otherwise benign fracture pattern with a nerve lesion; in such a case the gap may be evidence of nerve interposition (**Fig. 12–6A–E**).

Vascular injuries in the setting of humeral shaft fractures are more commonly associated with penetrating trauma.[15] Surgical stabilization of the extremity is necessary to provide a stable setting for the vascular repair to function without kinking or being stretched because of lack of skeletal stability. Whenever possible, skeletal stabilization should be completed prior to vascular repair or grafting for this reason. Cooperative multidisciplinary management of these cases is necessary.

Floating Elbow Injuries

Forearm fractures associated with humeral shaft fractures are optimally treated with surgical stabilization of all fractures to allow early mobilization of the extremity (**Fig. 12–5A–E**).[16,17] Failure to stabilize one or both fractures would require prolonged immobilization and potentially result in elbow and shoulder stiffness.

Impending Pathological Fractures

Pathological fractures of the humerus are a significant source of pain and disability for patients with metastatic disease or metabolic bone disease. Impending fractures of the humerus can be stabilized by multiple operative techniques. Stabilization should be considered when 50 to 75% of the bone is destroyed by the lesion as evaluated on biplanar radiographs.[18] Combined internal fixation and external beam radiation is effective in providing pain relief, as well as a stable limb, which will allow function. Internal fixation can be combined with cement augmentation to provide improved stability and subsequent pain relief.

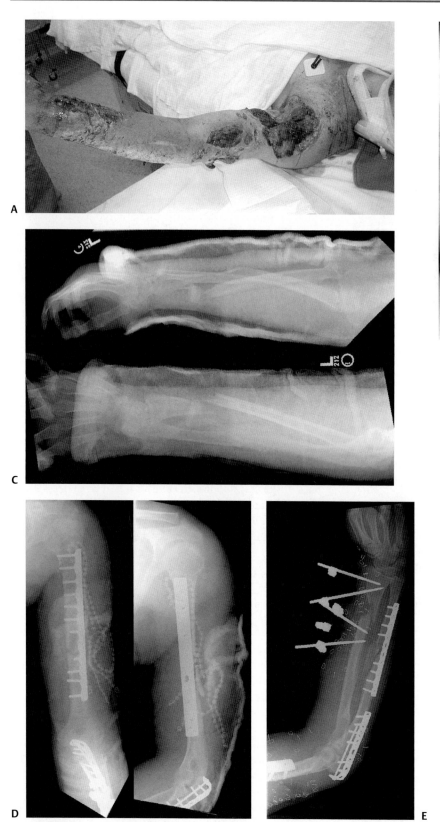

Figure 12–5 Ipsilateral open humeral shaft fracture and forearm fractures. **(A)** Clinical photos of the patient's arm, which was rolled over by his car. **(B)** Anteroposterior (AP) radiograph of the humerus; also visible is a dislocation of the radial head and proximal ulna fracture. **(C)** AP and lateral radiographs of the forearm, showing comminuted midshaft radius and ulna fractures in addition to the elbow fracture-dislocation. **(D)** AP and lateral radiographs of the humerus after open reduction and plate fixation. Note the antibiotic beads in the soft tissues. **(E)** Radiograph of the forearm after initial fixation.

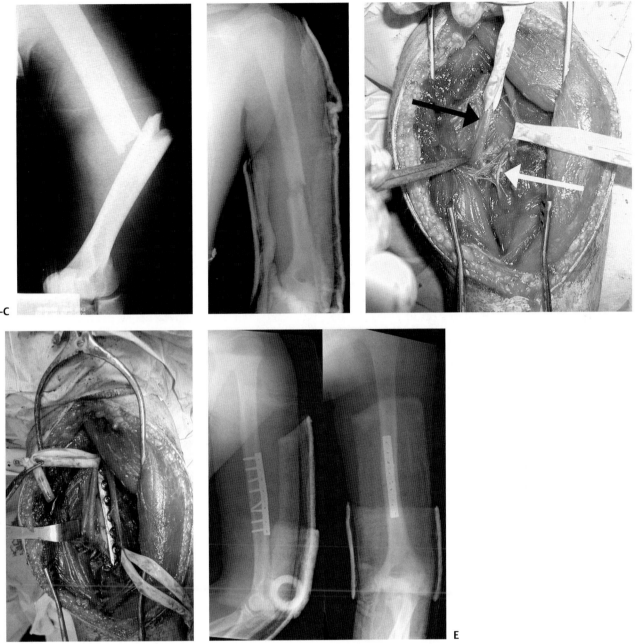

A–C

D

E

Figure 12–6 (A) Anteroposterior radiograph showing a displaced, angulated midhumeral fracture. The patient's radial nerve was functioning. (B) Postreduction radiograph showing good alignment but a residual gap at the fracture. Transverse humeral fracture with a gap and a radial nerve palsy. (C) Intraoperative exploration demonstrated the radial nerve (black arrow) entrapped within the fracture site (white arrow). (D) Intraoperative photo after repositioning of the nerve and plate fixation. (E) Postoperative radiograph after open reduction and internal fixation.

Polytrauma Patients

Patients with multiple extremity fractures, including diaphyseal humerus fractures, are candidates for surgical stabilization of the humerus. In patients with head injuries and expected prolonged intensive care unit stays, rigid fixation aids in nursing care, transport, and limited mobilization of these patients. Patients with multiply injured extremities should be given consideration for fixation of their humerus when they will require the fractured arm for assistance with weight bearing on crutches or a walker, or for transfers. Internal fixation of humeral shaft fractures with a plate has allowed full weight bearing on the extremity with no increased risk of complication.[19] In patients with bilateral upper extremity fractures, consideration of operative stabilization should be given to hasten the ability to allow self-care and activities of daily living.

Surgical Treatment

General Concepts

There are several indications for surgical stabilization of humerus fractures as reviewed previously; generally accepted indications include open humeral fractures, bilateral humeral fractures, pathological fractures, ipsilateral humerus and forearm fractures (the floating elbow), and multiply injured patients where fixation assists patient care and mobilization. An important element of nonoperative care is the ability of the patient to sit, and often sleep, in a semiupright position that allows for gravity to help reduce the fracture through the weight of the arm.

For patients with a fracture of the humerus and an associated lower extremity that requires restricted weight bearing, fixation of the humerus can provide such a patient with the ability to use crutches or other assistive devices. Tingstad et al note that others have estimated that the use of bilateral axillary crutches places up to 80% of body weight on the upper extremity, and documented that plate fixation is secure enough to provide these patients with the ability to use crutches when the principles of internal fixation are achieved.[19] In addition, many orthopaedic trauma surgeons believe that it is possible to allow weight bearing after intramedullary nailing of the humerus when the fracture patterns are stable. An example would be intramedullary fixation of a transverse midshaft humerus fracture. Currently, evidence is lacking to recommend weight bearing after intramedullary fixation of comminuted fractures or other unstable fracture patterns.

Plate fixation and intramedullary nailing are the most common methods for the stabilization of humeral shaft fractures. External fixation is rarely used because of the risk of damaging neurovascular structures with pin placement and the subsequent problems of pin track infections with motion of the shoulder and elbow.

The choice of plate fixation or use of an intramedullary nail is controversial and dependent upon many factors, including the fracture pattern and location, associated soft tissue injuries and neurovascular injury, the presence of osteoporosis, associated ipsilateral injuries, and the method preferred by the operating surgeon.

Intramedullary nailing of humeral shaft fractures was not widely practiced until the advent of interlocking nails, which expanded the indications for nailing humeral shaft fractures and made the procedure more predictably successful. Currently, union rates seem to be comparable for plates and nails; the controversy exists because of the apparently increased risk of shoulder pain after antegrade nailing versus the benefits of using a closed technique. Proponents of plating also point out the risk of radial nerve injury from blind nail placement, whereas nailing advocates claim that the risk to the nerve is greater during open procedures. There have been several attempts to compare the relative advantages and problems experienced with the use of plate fixation as opposed to intramedullary nailing.[20–23] Small, prospective, randomized trials and meta-analyses conclude that both plate fixation and intramedullary nailing achieve high and comparable rates of union. The major difference between the two methods has been in the complications that are specific to the two techniques.

Surgical Techniques: Open Reduction and Internal Fixation with Plates

Patient Positioning

The choice of patient position depends on the approach chosen to expose the humeral fracture. Generally, the anterolateral approach will necessitate supine positioning with a radiolucent armboard attached to the table. In the setting of polytrauma, the supine position is preferred, especially when there is a spinal injury or if spine clearance is not complete. The patient can be positioned with the head turned away from the operative side slightly to allow easier draping as well as protection from misplaced instruments on the facial area during the procedure. The endotracheal tube is preferably placed so that it exits on the far side of the mouth from the operative side. The patient should be positioned with the torso as close to the armboard as possible. A small bump placed under the scapula will slightly elevate the shoulder and allow easier access for draping the arm to the shoulder. Shoulder abduction of approximately 60 degrees allows exposure of the humeral shaft. Use of a nonsterile tourniquet will result in the inability to adequately approach humeral fractures in the middle or proximal third, so a sterile tourniquet is helpful in these circumstances if a tourniquet is desired.

Lateral decubitus positioning is useful when a lateral or posterior approach is used. The patient can be supported with a beanbag, and a large bump of linen can be taped to the patient's chest to act as an operative surface. Alternatively, a popliteal roll leg holder may be positioned in the antecubital area and fastened to the table to provide a similar working surface. When positioning the patient in the lateral position, the torso should be brought toward the edge of the table as far as safely possible. The shoulder is abducted 90 degrees for maximal exposure.

The posterior approach is easily accomplished in the prone position (see **Video 12–1, Disk 2**). The shoulder is abducted 90 degrees and in neutral extension. Chest rolls appropriately positioned will allow a small amount of forward flexion of the shoulder to prevent excessive stretch of the brachial plexus. A radiolucent armboard attached to the operative table will provide an adequate working surface and still allow intraoperative fluoroscopy use.

Radiographic Imaging

Preoperative radiographic evaluation should include two views of the entire humerus in orthogonal planes. This is

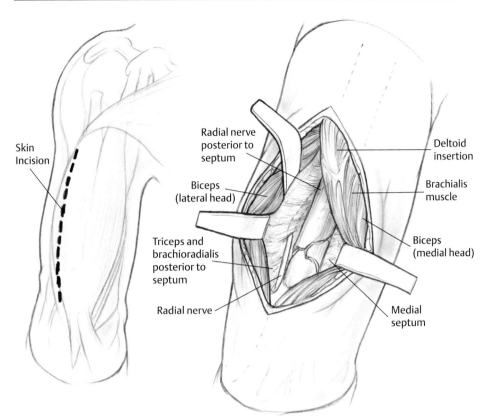

Figure 12–7 Anterolateral approach to the humerus.

Labels in figure:

Skin Incision

Radial nerve posterior to septum

Biceps (lateral head)

Triceps and brachioradialis posterior to septum

Radial nerve

Deltoid insertion

Brachialis muscle

Biceps (medial head)

Medial septum

typically accomplished by an AP and lateral x-ray of the humerus. Many special views exist for proximal and distal humeral imaging, but the humeral diaphysis is best viewed with these two simple views.

Whereas much of the humerus can be reduced and secured under direct visualization, intraoperative fluoroscopy is a useful tool for almost every humerus fracture. Imaging can aid in judging reduction as well as hardware position and screw placement and length. In the lateral decubitus position, the C-arm is brought in from the front side of the patient in the vertical direction. This arrangement will produce an AP view of the humerus, and a lateral view can be obtained by externally rotating the shoulder 90 degrees. Imaging in the supine or prone position is performed by keeping the C-arm in a vertical position and rotating the shoulder to obtain AP and lateral images through the radiolucent arm table.

Surgical Approaches

Anterior Approach

The anterolateral approach **(Fig. 12–7)** is commonly used for open reduction and internal fixation (ORIF) of the humeral shaft. This approach provides access to the entire diaphysis of the humerus and can be extended both proximally and distally. The approach is made lateral to the palpable mass of the biceps and brachialis muscles. The brachialis is dissected to the bone at a point just anterior to the lateral intermuscular septum. Dissection and mobilization of the radial nerve

are not mandatory with this approach, although some care should be taken to avoid injury to the lateral antebrachial cutaneous nerve in the distal portion of the incision.

Posterior Approach

The posterior approach provides exposure of the lower three fourths of the humerus and is most often used for fractures of the distal third of the humerus. For these injuries, the posterior surface of the humerus is relatively flat and is therefore ideal for placing a plate **(Fig. 12–8)**. The radial nerve is at risk during posterior exposures and it must be identified and protected.[24] The posterior approach is easier to perform when the patient is prone, although the lateral decubitus position may be used. The skin incision is made in the posterior midline of the arm. Superficially, the interval between the long and lateral heads of the triceps is separated **(Fig. 12–9A,B)**. The deep dissection requires splitting the medial head, with identification of the radial nerve and profunda brachii artery in the spiral groove

Other Approaches

Rarely, direct medial or lateral approaches to the humerus may be considered. Medial approaches are usually performed for exposure of open fractures with a medial wound or when vascular exposure is necessary. The lateral approach is an extensile approach that allows supine positioning and requires no muscle splitting.[25]

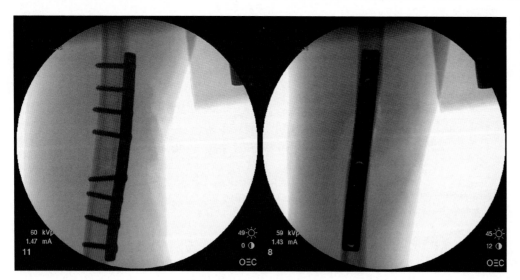

Figure 12–8 Posterior plating of the humerus. Note how the plate is bent slightly at its midpoint to apply compression uniformly across the fracture.

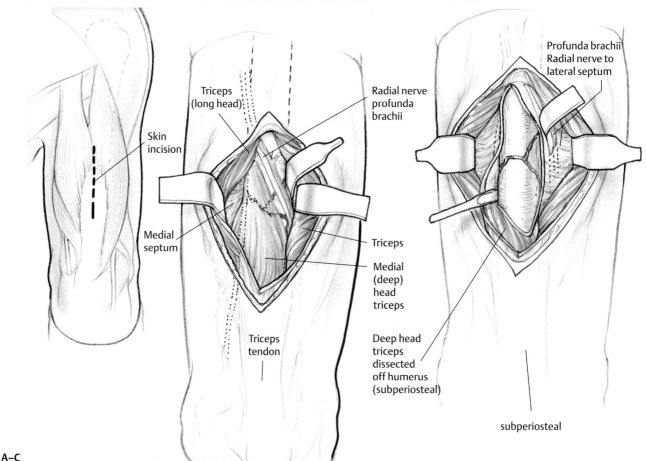

A–C

Figure 12–9 Posterior approach to the humerus. **(A)** The skin incision is shown on the dotted line. **(B)** superficial dissection. Deep dissection.

Reduction and Fixation

Typically, standard techniques of open reduction and plate fixation as advocated by the Arbeitsgemeinschaft für Osteosynthesefragen/Association for the Study of Internal Fixation (AO/ASIF) are employed.[26] This involves selecting a plate of appropriate size for the patient and fracture pattern (see later discussion). Simple fractures, including transverse, short oblique, and bending-wedge patterns, are treated with direct open reduction. Soft tissue attachments to bone are respected, and circumferential clamps are avoided. The plate is often used as a reduction aid. Comminuted fractures are best treated by bridge plating—in essence, spanning the fracture with fixation of the plate to the intact proximal and distal segments so that length, rotation, and alignment are restored. This limits dissection and soft tissue stripping around the zone of comminution but may place the radial nerve at greater risk of injury.[27] Percutaneous plating has recently been described, utilizing two small incisions proximal and distal to the fracture and sliding the plate across the fracture.[28]

Instrumentation Options

Typically, a 4.5 mm dynamic compression plate (DCP) of appropriate length (long enough to apply at least four bicortical screws in each fragment) is used. Although the so-called broad DCP was initially recommended for the humerus and the femur, in many smaller patients, a narrow 4.5 mm DCP is appropriate. In very small patients, a 3.5 mm DCP may even be used. A current trend is to utilize longer plates, with fewer screw holes utilized

When plating a transverse fracture, the plate should be prebent to apply compression uniformly across the fracture surface (**Fig. 12–8**). For oblique and spiral fractures, lag screws may be placed as needed, ideally through the plate. When treating fractures of the distal humeral shaft, it may not be possible to obtain eight cortices of fixation without the plate impinging upon the olecranon fossa. In this circumstance, a second plate may be placed at 90 degrees to the first and advanced down either the medial or lateral columns of the distal humerus (**Fig. 12–10A–C**).

Bone Grafting

It is not possible to provide definitive recommendations about the need for bone grafting during plating of humeral shaft fractures. Most of the existing literature that addresses the topic consists of retrospective cohort studies or case-control studies that were performed before the current emphasis on indirect reduction techniques, and bone grafting was done according to the preference of the surgeon. There is one published randomized trial comparing dynamic compression plating with or without bone grafting to Enders nailing.[29] In this study, Chiu et al found that the use of bone grafting during plating accelerated union by 3 weeks compared with plating without bone grafting.[29] However, no data exist regarding the need for bone grafting with contemporary plating techniques, and the authors do not perform prophylactic bone grafting, choosing instead to use indirect reduction and bridge plating techniques to manage comminuted fractures.

Postoperative Care of Humeral Plating

After adequate plating of humeral shaft fractures, no further external form of immobilization is necessary unless it is deemed necessary to protect the wound with a posterior splint for a short period of time. Otherwise, a soft dressing is applied postoperatively. Range of motion exercises of the shoulder and elbow are begun immediately, and active motion of the elbow and shoulder is encouraged. Patients are allowed to use the extremity for crutch walking and

transfers if necessary. Patients are encouraged to progress as tolerated with respect to activity, but they are restricted from heavy lifting and higher-stress activities until healing is radiographically documented.

Intramedullary Nailing of Humeral Shaft Fractures

Intramedullary nailing of humeral shaft fractures is considered by some to be a sound and even preferred approach for the stabilization of humeral shaft fractures.[30,31] However, the relative merits of nailing versus plating are less clear for the humerus as compared with other long bones, and the relative role of these two techniques remains very controversial.

The initial techniques described for intramedullary nailing of humeral fractures involved the use of small, flexible nails; Enders nails and Rush rods were frequent choices. The advantage of flexible nails was their ability to be inserted through portals that were eccentric to the intramedullary canal and did not require insertion through the rotator cuff. Retrograde insertion through the humeral epicondyles was also possible. The primary disadvantage of these flexible nailing systems was that the fixation was less rigid, and nail migration was common. When used correctly union rates as high as 90% were reported with the use of both Enders nails, Hackethal nails, and Rush rods.[29,32–35]

The introduction of locked nails overcame the stability problems associated with flexible nails and maintained the ability to use a closed technique of fracture fixation. Locked nails also allow surgeons to use this technique for more comminuted fracture patterns that would not have been easily treated with flexible nails. Unfortunately, the expanded indications for interlocking nailing come at a higher price in terms of potential complications.[36,37] The insertion of interlocking screws presents the potential for additional neurovascular injury.[38,39] In addition, rigid interlocking nails require a starting point that is more or less coaxial with the medullary canal, so that different entry points are necessary than those used for flexible nailing. For antegrade nailing, the starting portal requires an incision of the rotator cuff, whereas for retrograde nailing, a large portal in or just above the olecranon fossa is necessary. These approaches, and the unique complications associated with each, are described following here.

Interlocking nails may be reamed or unreamed; as in other long bones there is controversy about which method is better. Unlike the femur and tibia, reaming the intramedullary canal has not been shown to increase the union rates reported for humeral nailing.[40] However, because of the small diameter of the humerus and the lack of a wide distal metaphysis, some traumatologists believe that reaming helps to avoid nail incarceration and distraction at the fracture site, which is considered to increase the risk of nonunion. Others argue that reaming produces thermal necrosis that can lead to nonunion. Nevertheless, due to the small diameter of the intramedullary canal, reaming allows larger-diameter (and stronger) nails to be

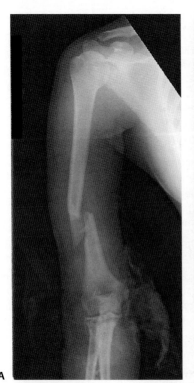

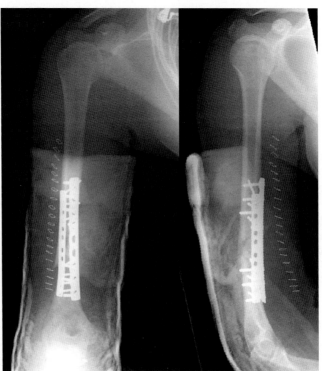

A

B

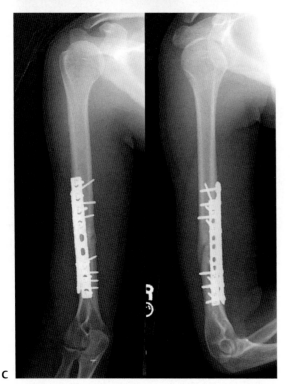

C

Figure 12–10 **(A)** Anteroposterior radiograph of the humerus showing a comminuted fracture of the distal third. The patient had a traumatic elbow arthrotomy with complete avulsion of the medial collateral ligament. **(B)** After internal fixation utilizing two plates at right angles. Use of a single plate would not provide enough fixation. **(C)** Final radiographs.

inserted. So-called limited reaming, in which no attempt is made to perform aggressive reaming of the endosteal surface, provides a way to determine appropriate nail diameter. To avoid injuring the radial nerve, one should push the unmoving reamer across a comminuted segment rather than ream with power. One study that compared nailing with and without reaming was unable to document differences in union rates or complications.[40] Because of the small diameter of the distal humerus, some degree of reaming is required for the retrograde insertion of humeral nails.

Preoperative Preparation and Intraoperative Imaging

Antegrade Intermedullary Nailing

Antegrade humeral nailing is performed with the patient in one of two positions; for either position, the patient's injured extremity is moved to the edge of the table. The first approach is to place the patient in a slight beach chair position, with the C-arm placed above the head of the table and extending distally over the shoulder (**Fig. 12–11**). In this manner, one can easily obtain an AP view of the humerus. Additionally, by moving the C-arm to a horizontal position, a standard axillary lateral view can be obtained. The second method is to keep the patient supine, rolled 30 to 45 degrees toward the uninjured side, propped on towels. The C-arm is then brought in from across the table. By arcing the C-arm over and back, true AP and transscapular Y views are easy to obtain without moving the arm (**Fig. 12–12A–C**) (see **Videos 12–2, 12–3, Disk 2**).

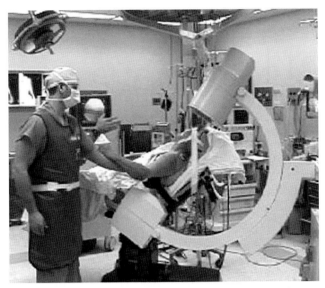

Figure 12–11 Beach chair position for antegrade humeral nailing.

Once adequate imaging is assured, the shoulder and arm are prepped and draped. Open wounds are extended, irrigated, and debrided. With open fractures, it is useful to manually reduce the fracture and to visually ensure that the radial nerve is not trapped within the fracture.

Anterior Acromial Approach for Antegrade Nailing

- *Indications* Humeral nailing is usually described using a lateral deltoid-splitting approach, identical to that used for repair of a greater tuberosity fracture. However, this approach has been shown to lead to much higher rates of shoulder pain and dysfunction than the anterior acromial approach first reported by Riemer et al.[41] A review of anatomical specimens demonstrates that the lateral deltoid insertion leads to an incision in the rotator cuff that cuts transversely across the insertion of the infraspinatus, whereas the anterior incision is oriented directly in line with the fibers of the supraspinatus.

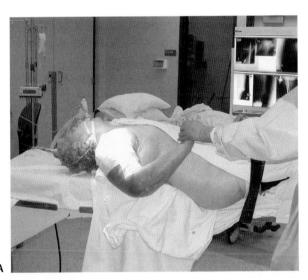

A

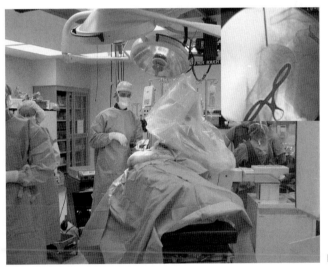

B

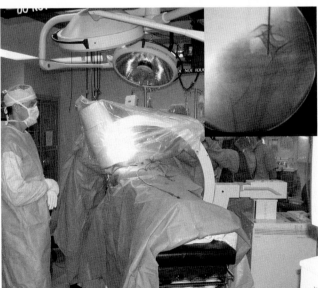

C

Figure 12–12 Alternative positioning of the patient and the C-arm, providing anteroposterior and scapular Y views. **(A)** The patient is supine, "log-rolled" toward the uninjured side with a large towel. **(B)** The C-arm is positioned for an anteroposterior (AP) view of the shoulder, with the corresponding image shown in the upper right panel. Because the patient's torso is tilted away from the operative side, the C-arm must be rotated over the top to obtain a true AP view. **(C)** Without moving the patient, the C-arm is arced backward, and a lateral scapular view can be obtained as seen in the upper right panel.

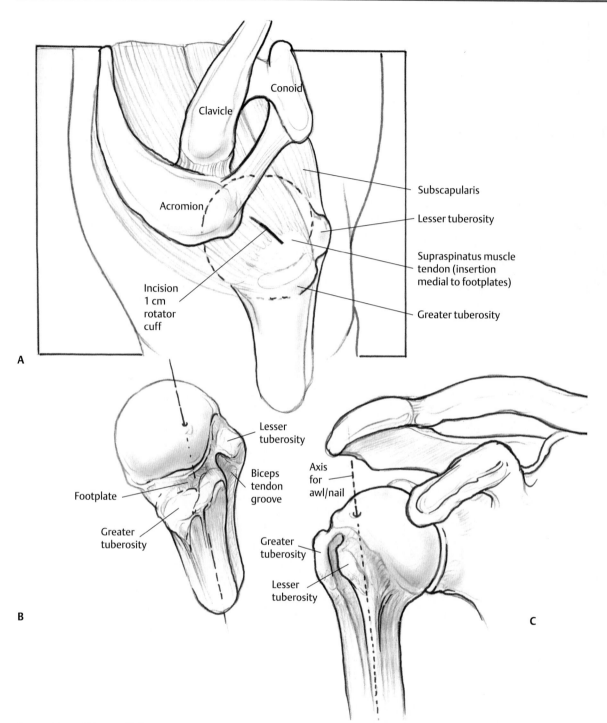

Figure 12–13 **(A)** A small skin incision is made at the anterolateral corner of the acromion, extending obliquely forward and laterally. This incision is in line with the supraspinatus tendon. **(B)** Access to the medullary canal is achieved by making an entry hole 1 cm medial to the greater tuberosity, at the edge of the articular cartilage. **(C)** This drawing shows the relationship of the starting point to the surrounding bones. By extending and adducting the shoulder, the nail can be safely inserted past the acromion.

Furthermore, the anterior approach allows nail insertion in front of the acromion so as to remove this structure as an impediment to nail insertion. For these reasons, the anterior acromial approach is preferred for all cases and is described as follows.

Technique   An incision 2 to 3 cm long is made extending off the anterolateral corner of the acromion **(Fig. 12–13A–C)**. The deltoid and its deep fascia are split

and gently retracted. The underlying supraspinatus tendon is exposed and divided sharply, and retraction sutures are placed. A guide pin is placed in the sulcus between the greater tuberosity and the articular surface, and its position is confirmed on both AP and lateral C-arm images **(Fig. 12–12A–C)**. The guide pin should be centered on the medullary canal in both views. The pin is advanced several centimeters into the humerus, and a cannulated awl or drill is used to enlarge the portal manually **(Fig. 12–14)**. A reaming guidewire can then be advanced across the fracture and into the distal segment. Minimal reaming should be done to ensure that the nail does not get "jammed" into the distal fragment.

Next, the nail is inserted over a guidewire. Care should be taken to ensure that the fracture is not distracted during nail insertion; axial compression on the proximal ulna helps to prevent distraction of the fracture site. Proximal interlocking is done with the attached jig. Lateral to medial screws are preferred, although, regardless of the direction of insertion, care should be taken to avoid penetrating the opposite cortex by more than a few millimeters because of the risk of neurovascular injury.[39] Distal interlocking should be performed from an anterior to posterior direction using a 3 to 4 cm incision placed two to four fingerbreadths proximal to the crease of the antecubital fossa. The biceps and brachialis are split bluntly. The median nerve and brachial artery are retracted medially, and the bone is visualized with retractors before drilling is begun **(Fig. 12–15A–C)**.

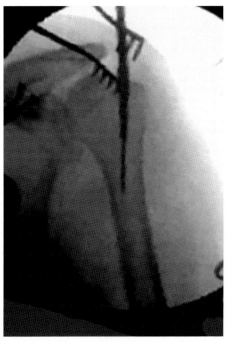

Figure 12–14 Intraoperative fluoroscopic view of a cannulated drill being used over a guidewire to open up the intramedullary canal of the proximal part of the humerus.

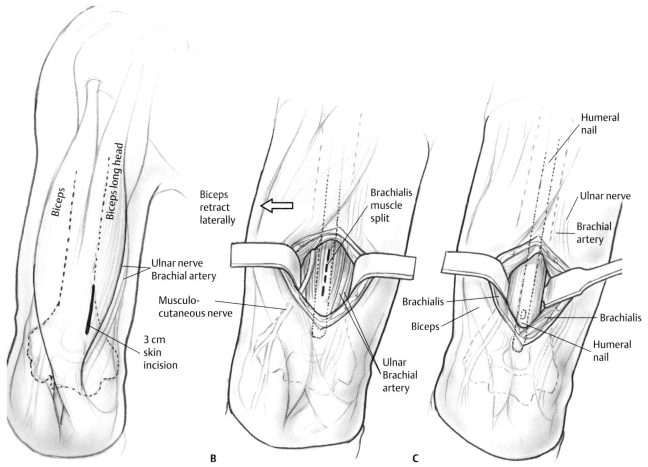

A   B   C

Figure 12–15 **(A)** A 3 cm skin incision is made over the interlocking hole (using fluoroscopy). **(B)** The biceps is retracted laterally, exposing the fibers of the brachialis. **(C)** The brachialis muscle fibers are split longitudinally, exposing the bone. Blunt retractors are shown maintaining the exposure.

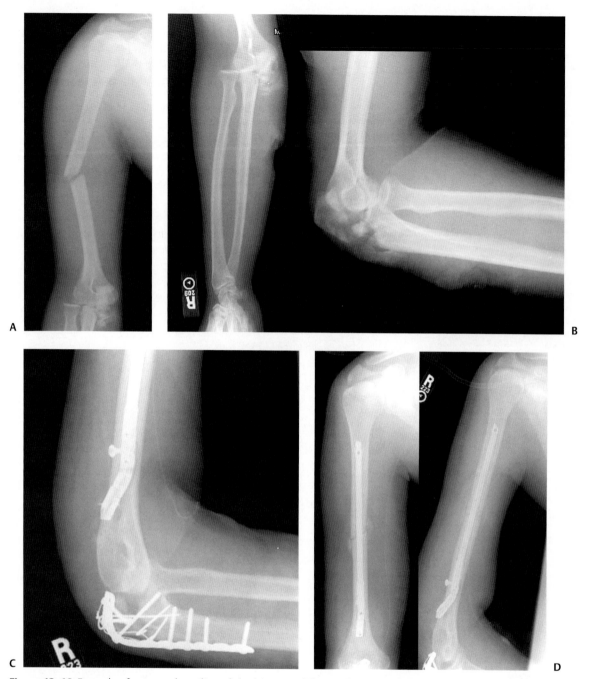

Figure 12–16 Example of retrograde nailing of the humerus. **(A)** Radiographs of a humerus fracture above a comminuted fracture of the proximal ulna. **(B)** Lateral radiograph **(C)** of the elbow after plate fixation of the ulna and retrograde nailing of the humerus, performed through the same incision. **(D)** Follow-up anteroposterior and lateral radiographs of the humerus.

Retrograde Intramedullary Nailing

To avoid the complication of shoulder pain associated with antegrade nailing, retrograde insertion of humeral nails has been advocated by some.[42] An especially good indication would be the patient with ipsilateral olecranon and humeral fractures; with retrograde nailing both injuries could be treated with one incision over the posterior elbow **(Fig. 12–16A–D).**

Triceps Splitting Approach for Retrograde Nailing

- *Indications* Fractures in the diaphysis and proximal third of the humerus are amenable to retrograde nailing.

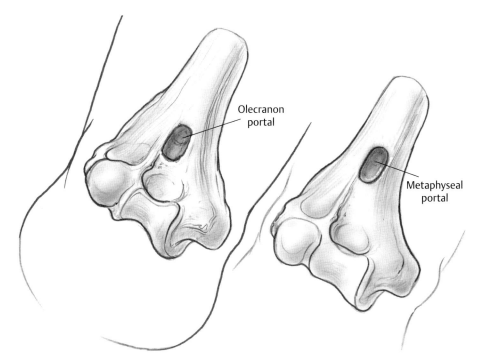

Figure 12–17 Two possible portals for retrograde nailing. The left drawing shows a portal on the cephalad portion of the olecranon fossa, whereas the right shows the portal more proximally located on the dorsal cortex.

Olecranon portal

Metaphyseal portal

Distal third fractures are better suited to antegrade nailing or plate fixation because retrograde nailing provides poor fixation of more distal fractures.

Technique   Retrograde nailing of the humerus is easiest to perform when the patient is in the prone position, using an armboard or other radiolucent device to support the arm. The entire arm should be prepped within the surgical field; in most cases a tourniquet is not needed. The elbow is flexed to gain access to the olecranon fossa, and the incision is made in the midline of the distal humerus. The triceps muscle is split in line with its fibers, and the posterior surface of the humerus is exposed. Two entry portals have been described. Ingman and Waters[31] created an entry site on the posterior aspect of the humerus on the slope of the olecranon fossa (**Fig. 12–17,** left), whereas Rommens et al[42] created an entry site proximal to the olecranon fossa in the metaphysis of the distal humerus (**Fig. 12–17,** right). Because these entry sites are eccentric to the intramedullary canal, an oblique portal in the longitudinal axis of the humerus must be made to insert the relatively rigid interlocking nails. In general, a combination of drills is used to create the insertion site, which must be oval and ~1 cm wide and 2 to 3 cm long. It is critical to avoid reaming of the anterior cortex, which weakens the bone (**Fig. 12–18**). Nail insertion is done according to the recommended technique for the specific nail being used; however, if any resistance is encountered, the entry site should be enlarged to avoid fractures of the distal humerus. Fluoroscopic imaging is used to verify reduction of the fracture, passing of the nail across the fracture, and insertion of the locking bolts.

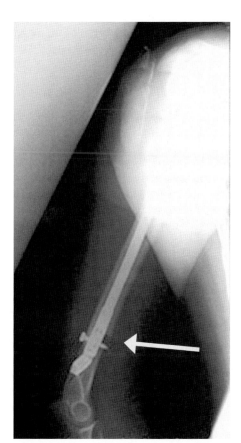

Figure 12–18 Example of eccentric reaming of the anterior humeral cortex (arrow) during retrograde nailing.

Reporting on a series of 84 humeral nailings performed at four different centers, Blum et al[43] observed that retrograde nailing is a more technically demanding procedure than antegrade nailing, due to the unique shape of the distal humerus and the high stresses caused by the insertion of stiff nails. In addition, fractures and fissures of the distal humerus were observed during nail insertion. To avoid this complication, an insertion portal of 10 mm in width and 20 mm in length was recommended for insertion of an unreamed humeral nail.[43]

Postoperative Care Following retrograde nailing of humerus fractures, a soft postoperative dressing is applied because the rigid internal fixation obviates the need for external immobilization. The patient is encouraged to begin early range of motion of the elbow and shoulder. Weight-bearing status of the extremity is determined on a case by case basis. Fractures with significant comminution and little direct contact of the fracture ends may be kept from weight bearing until some sign of fracture healing is appreciated. However, in fractures with some cortical contact, the patient may be allowed to bear weight on the arm immediately.

External Fixation

External fixation as a method of treatment of diaphyseal humerus fractures is reserved for fractures that cannot be treated by any other method. This group includes fractures with extensive soft tissue injury that requires access to the extremity, such as fractures associated with severe burns, combat wounds, and those caused by projectiles.[44–46] Patients who are not candidates for internal fixation due to soft tissue injury or extensive, segmental bone loss that also require stability for mobilization may be treated with external fixation. External fixation can be used to treat fractures until union, but it is more commonly used as a temporary method of achieving stabilization until soft tissue concerns are corrected and another method of fixation can be used.

Technique

The patient is positioned supine with a radiolucent armboard attached to the table. The patient is positioned so that the entire humerus can be visualized with the C-arm. Two bicortical Schanz pins are placed in the proximal-most segment and two are placed distal to the fracture. Direct visualization of pin placement is recommended to avoid neurovascular injury. The fracture is aligned and the fixator secured under live fluoroscopy. External fixation allows the late application of compression to fractures that do not show acceptable levels of healing in the initial postoperative period.

Complications

Pin track infection following external fixation of humeral shaft fractures has been reported in up to 53% of patients.[47]

This complication can be attributed to the robust amount of muscle covering the humerus that the pins must traverse. The continuous motion of the soft tissues around the pins may contribute to the high rate of complications involving the pin tracks. Radial nerve injury following placement of external fixation in the treatment of diaphyseal humerus fractures has also been reported.[48] Should this occur, immediate exploration of the nerve is indicated.

Postoperative Care

Following placement of external fixation for treatment of humeral shaft fractures, the patient is mobilized as tolerated. Weight-bearing use of the arm for lifting is progressed when radiographic evidence of healing is appreciated. Immediate weight bearing is not allowed as it is in fractures treated with plates or intramedullary rods. Immediate range of motion of the shoulder and elbow is encouraged.

Outcomes and Complications

Malunion

Malunion following diaphyseal humerus fractures is generally well tolerated, with acceptable angulation of up to 30 degrees and shortening of 2 or 3 cm rarely causing any functional problems. Treatment of a symptomatic humeral malunion is done in the same manner as the original fracture would have been approached. A corrective osteotomy followed by rigid internal fixation generally provides acceptable outcomes.

Nonunion

Nonunion following nonoperatively treated humeral shaft fractures has been found to occur in up to 5% of cases.[3] The incidence of nonunion is marginally greater following operative management; 7% of cases were associated with nonunion or loss of fixation in one of the larger series of patients treated by open reduction and plate fixation.[49] Hypertrophic nonunions result from inadequate stability of a fracture with adequate osteogenic stimulus, whereas atrophic nonunions occur when the fracture-healing cascade fails to begin in the fracture region. The successful treatment of a nonunion depends on addressing the underlying reason for failure of the fracture to unite initially. First, the patient's nutritional status should be evaluated with measurement of the white blood cell count, total protein and albumin, and transferrin levels. Any malnutrition should be aggressively treated. Fractures exhibiting a hypertrophic pattern of nonunion without significant bone loss are considered to need more stability and may be initially treated with external immobilization. Ultimately, rigid stabilization of the nonunion is typically followed by bony union. Fixation may be accomplished with intramedullary nailing or plating.

Internal fixation with compression plates is the standard treatment of both hypertrophic and atrophic nonunions. Following exposure of an atrophic nonunion, aggressive debridement of the fibrous tissue is performed, and the bone edges are scalloped. It is important to remove any interposed fibrous tissue that may hinder bony union. Bone grafting in the form of autologous cancellous bone from the iliac crest can supplement plate fixation in cases of minimal amount of bone loss, whereas nonunions in the setting of segmental bone loss may require more complex bone grafting methods such as corticocancellous struts or vascularized fibular autografts. Hypertrophic nonunions may simply be plated and compressed. Debridement and bone grafting of these nonunions are not required.

Intramedullary rodding of established nonunions is an alternative to plating in patients without segmental bone loss or a significant amount of fibrous tissue interposed between the fracture ends. Nailing is particularly helpful in patients with nonunion following pathological fractures or in patients with poor bone quality that would not be amenable to plating. Nails should be locked at both ends to provide rotational stability as well as maintaining length in cases of segmental bone loss. Closed nailing can be augmented with directed bone grafting placed through a chest tube to deliver bone to the nonunion site.

Neurovascular

In closed fractures, radial nerve palsies are usually due to neuropraxia from displacement of the fracture at the time of the injury. Spontaneous recovery occurs within 3 to 4 months after injury in nearly 90% of patients. Patients should be placed in forearm-based wrist splints to support the wrist and fingers until motor function returns. When recovery does not occur within this time period, an electromyogram (EMG) should be obtained to determine if exploration is indicated. Early exploration of the radial nerve in patients with closed fractures has not been shown to improve the rate of recovery.[50] In contrast, early exploration of open fractures is recommended because in this setting many radial nerve palsies are due to lacerations.[14] A recent review of early repair of lacerated radial nerves found a poor rate of recovery, which was thought to be due to the large zone of injury associated with the radial nerve laceration.[51]

The management of radial nerve palsies that occur at the time of closed reduction and splinting of the humerus fractures is controversial. Only a small number of these cases have been reported, so a general consensus to management has not been established. However, one review of 20 years of experience reported on 16 secondary palsies; early surgical exploration did not favorably influence the rate of recovery.[13]

Treatment-Specific Outcomes and Complications

Plating

Plate fixation is associated with the complications of radial nerve palsy, infection, and failure of fixation. Radial nerve palsy is uncommon; it occurs in no more than 1 to 2% of cases after open reduction and internal fixation and is likely due to intraoperative traction upon the radial nerve. The choice of surgical approach does not appear to affect the incidence of nerve palsy. When observed after plate fixation, the common opinion is to observe for functional recovery. The rates of infection with the plating of closed fractures are 1 to 2% and are consistent with the infection rates observed after plate fixation of other upper extremity fractures. Fixation failure after plate fixation is also uncommon and is rarely noted as being higher than 5%. Failures of plate fixation are commonly associated with poor surgical technique or patient-specific factors such as alcohol use. Inadequate surgical technique is usually due to the use of a plate that is too short or an inadequate number of screws placed proximal and distal to the fracture site. The inappropriate use of small fragment plates for fixation of the humeral shaft in large individuals is occasionally responsible. Patient-related factors include smoking, which delays fracture healing, and alcoholism. This second factor should be carefully studied in determining whether a given patient should be treated with fixation. In our experience, alcoholic patients sustain their fractures from falls while intoxicated, a situation that is likely to be repeated after they are discharged from the hospital and are coping with postoperative pain and restrictions for their injuries.

Antegrade Nailing

The major complications associated with antegrade intramedullary nailing of the humerus include nonunion and shoulder pain. Nonunion is more common after nailing than plating and is reported to range from 5 to 10%. Distraction of the fracture site during insertion of the nail is strongly implicated in the development of nonunion and must be avoided. Shoulder pain seems to be related to the specifics of the entry portal used for insertion of the nail. Initial reports of shoulder pain in early series were as high as 20 to 40%. Later modifications in entry portals are reported to have markedly decreased this problem.[52]

The most common complication after antegrade nailing is shoulder pain. The use of a lateral deltoid-splitting incision (**Fig. 12–19**) may result in a rotator cuff incision that is very posterior and that cuts across the insertion of the infraspinatus tendon. By contrast, an anterior incision leads directly to the supraspinatus insertion, which can be incised longitudinally and repaired (**Fig. 12–20**). In addition, the use of early physiotherapy is important.

Heterotopic ossification of the deltoid is a rare complication that we have reported in a patient with a severe

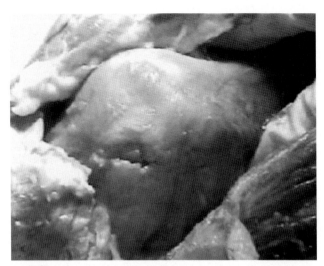

Figure 12–19 Rotator cuff damage associated with a lateral deltoid-splitting approach, as seen in a cadaver. The percutaneous incision was actually transversely oriented and cut across the fibers of the infraspinatus.

concomitant traumatic brain injury.[53] Thus, in head-injured patients who are treated with humeral nailing, consideration should be given to providing some form of prophylaxis against heterotopic bone. Nonunion after closed humeral nailing is frequently associated with distraction of the fracture. Avoiding such gaps is an extremely important concept that should be remembered whenever humeral nailing is performed.

Finally, radial nerve injury can occur during reaming or nail insertion. Although this is uncommon, whenever the opportunity arises (such as when nailing an open fracture), one should take care to be sure that the nerve is safe. It is not known if intramedullary nailing is indicated for patients with associated radial nerve palsies. Because the radial nerve may be displaced into the fracture site in this

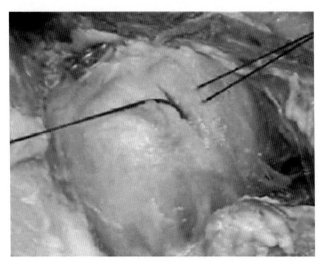

Figure 12–20 An anterior acromial approach leads to a less traumatic splitting of the supraspinatus tendon in line with its fibers.

instance, without a compelling reason to use a nail, nerve exploration and plating may be a more prudent alternative.

Retrograde Nailing

Due to the amount of bone that must be removed, the distal humerus is weakened and may be prone to fracture at the nail entry site. One biomechanical study indicated that 80% less energy in torque was required to fracture the humerus after creating retrograde portals.[54] In addition, there are clinical reports that describe iatrogenic fractures occurring at the entry site of nail insertion.[55] It is our observation that in humerus fractures with a narrow (< 10 mm) intramedullary canal, it is easy to inadvertently ream the anterior cortex of the distal humerus as the entry portal is being created, which further weakens the distal humerus (**Fig. 12–18**). At this time, the extent of remodeling that occurs after nail insertion is unknown.

Tips and Tricks

- During treatment of a humeral shaft fracture with a functional brace, it is important to tighten the two shells of the orthosis daily to compress the underlying soft tissues and create hydraulic compression of the fracture site to gain alignment. In addition, active shoulder and elbow motion is encouraged during fracture healing to avoid joint stiffness.
- One must be aware of distraction in transverse fracture patterns treated nonoperatively, which have an increased risk of nonunion.
- One must be careful to avoid injury to the lateral antebrachial cutaneous nerve in the distal portion of the incision when using the anterolateral approach to the humerus.

Pearls

- Radial nerve injuries are the most common nerve injury associated with humeral shaft fractures, with a reported incidence ranging from 1.8 to 34%.
- A common mistake during the evaluation of a patient with a humeral shaft fracture is to observe extension of the fingers as a sign of radial nerve function, which is instead a test of the intrinsic muscles of the hand and their innervation by the ulnar nerve. Evaluation of the radial nerve is performed by testing wrist extension with grading of the motor function.
- Radial nerve injuries that occur during attempted reduction of the fracture often resolve spontaneously and are not an absolute indication for exploration or other surgical treatment.
- Acceptable parameters for the alignment of humeral shaft fractures include angulation of up to 20 degrees in the anterior/posterior plane, 30 degrees in varus or valgus, and up to 3 cm of shortening.

On the DVDs

Video 12–1 (Disk 2) Posterior Plating Humerus Fracture
This video demonstrates posterior plating of a simple transverse fracture in a patient with a floating elbow injury.
Video 12–2 (Disk 2) Intramedullary Nailing of the Humerus
This video demonstrates the use of a cannulated intramedullary nail to treat a diaphyseal humerus fracture. The starting point, handling

the rotator cuff, and eliminating all gaps are critical steps demonstrated in this procedure.
Video 12–3 (Disk 2) Humerus Flexnail This video demonstrates the use of the flexible humerus nail. Proper start point and angle, as well as the function of the stiffening mechanism are demonstrated.

References

1. Sarmiento A, Kinman PB, Galvin EG, Schmitt RH, Phillips JG. Functional bracing of fractures of the shaft of the humerus. J Bone Joint Surg Am 1977;59:596–601
2. Sarmiento A, Horowitch A, Aboulafia A, Vangsness CT Jr. Functional bracing for comminuted extra-articular fractures of the distal one-third of the humerus. J Bone Joint Surg Br 1990;72:283–287
3. Sarmiento A, Zagorski JB, Zych GA, Latta LL, Capps CA. Functional bracing for the treatment of fractures of the humeral diaphysis. J Bone Joint Surg Am 2000;82:478–486
4. Castellá FB, Garcia FB, Berry EM, Perelló EB, Sánchez-Alepuz E, Gabarda R. Nonunion of the humeral shaft: long lateral butterfly fracture: a nonunion predictive pattern? Clin Orthop Relat Res 2004;424:227–230
5. Tscherne H, Gotzen L. Pathophysiology and classification of soft tissue injuries associated with fractures. In: Tscherne H, Gotzen L. Fractures with Soft Tissue Injuries. Berlin: Springer-Verlag; 1984
6. Gustilo RB, Anderson JT. Prevention of infection in the treatment of one thousand and twenty-five open fractures of long bones: retrospective and prospective analyses. J Bone Joint Surg Am 1976;58:453–458
7. Klenerman L. Fractures of the shaft of the humerus. J Bone Joint Surg Br 1966;48:105–111
8. Holstein A, Lewis GB. Fractures of the humerus with radial nerve paralysis. J Bone Joint Surg Am 1963;45:1382–1388
9. Mast JW, Spiegel PG, Harvey JP, Harrison C. Fracture of the humerus shaft: a retrospective study of 240 adult fractures. Clin Orthop Relat Res 1975;112:254–262
10. Pollock FH, Drake D, Bovill EG, Day L, Trafton PG. Treatment of radial neuropathy associated with fractures of the humerus. J Bone Joint Surg Am. 1981;63:239–243
11. Shah JJ, Bhatti NA. Radial nerve paralysis associated with fractures of the humerus: a review of 62 cases. Clin Orthop Relat Res 1983;172:171–176
12. Böstman O, Bakalim G, Vainionpaa S, Wilppula E, Patiala H, Rokkanen P. Immediate radial nerve palsy complicating fracture of the shaft of the humerus: when is early exploration justified? Injury 1985;16:499–502
13. Böstman O, Bakalim G, Vainionpaa S, Wilppula E, Patiala H, Rokkanen P. Radial palsy in shaft fracture of the humerus. Acta Orthop Scand 1986;57:316–319
14. Foster RJ, Swiontkowski MF, Bach AW, Sack JT. Radial nerve palsy caused by open humeral shaft fractures. J Hand Surg [Am] 1993;18:121–124
15. Seligson D, Ostermann PA, Henry SL, Wolley T. The management of open fractures associated with arterial injury requiring vascular repair. J Trauma 1994;37:938–940
16. Solomon HB, Zadnik M, Eglseder WA. A review of outcomes in 18 patients with floating elbow. J Orthop Trauma 2003;17:563–570
17. Yokoyama K, Itoman M, Kobayashi A, Shindo M, Futami T. Functional outcomes of "floating elbow" injuries in adult patients. J Orthop Trauma 1998;12:284–290
18. Frassica FJ, Frassica DA. Evaluation and treatment of metastases to the humerus. Clin Orthop Relat Res 2003;415(Suppl):S212–S218
19. Tingstad EM, Wolinsky PR, Shyr Y, Johnson KD. Effect of immediate weight-bearing on plated fractures of the humeral shaft. J Trauma 2000;49:278–280
20. Chapman JR, Henley MB, Agel J, Benca PJ. Randomized prospective study of humeral shaft fixation: intramedullary nails versus plates. J Orthop Trauma 2000;14:162–166
21. Flinkkila T, Hyvonen P, Siira P, et al. Recovery of shoulder joint function after humeral shaft fracture: a comparative study between antegrade intramedullary nailing and plate fixation. Arch Orthop Trauma Surg 2004;124:537–541
22. Gregory PR, Sanders R. Compression plating versus intramedullary fixation of humeral shaft fractures. J Am Acad Orthop Surg 1997;5:215–223
23. McCormack RG, Brien D, Buckley RE, McKee MD, Powell J, Schemitsch EH. Fixation of fractures of the shaft of the humerus by dynamic compression plate or intramedullary nail: a prospective, randomized trial. J Bone Joint Surg Br 2000;82:336–339
24. Uhl RL, Larosa JM, Sibeni T, Martino LJ. Posterior approaches to the humerus: when should you worry about the radial nerve? J Orthop Trauma 1996;10:338–340
25. Mills WJ, Hanel DP, Smith DG. Lateral approach to the humeral shaft: an alternative approach for fracture treatment. J Orthop Trauma 1996;10:81–86
26. Vander Griend, Tomasin J, Ward EF. Open reduction and internal fixation of humeral shaft fractures: results using AO plating techniques. J Bone Joint Surg Am 1986;68:430–433
27. Livani B, Belangero WD. Bridging plate osteosynthesis of humeral shaft fractures. Injury 2004;35:587–595
28. Apivatthakakul T, Arpornchayanona O, Bavornratanavech S. Minimally invasive plate osteosynthesis (MIPO) of the humeral shaft fracture: is it possible? A cadaveric study and preliminary report. Injury 2005;36:530–538
29. Chiu F-Y, Chen C-M, Lin C-FJ, et al. Closed humeral shaft fractures: a prospective evaluation of surgical treatment. J Trauma 1997;43:947–951
30. Lin J, Hou SM. Antegrade locked nailing for humeral shaft fractures. Clin Orthop Relat Res 1999;365:201–210
31. Ingman AM, Waters DA. Locked intramedullary nailing of humeral shaft fractures: implant design, surgical technique, and clinical results. J Bone Joint Surg Br 1994;76:23–29
32. Hall RF Jr, Pankovich AM. Ender nailing of acute fractures of the humerus: a study of closed fixation by intramedullary nails without reaming. J Bone Joint Surg Am 1987;69:558–567

33. Shazar N, Brumback RJ, Vanco B. Treatment of humeral fractures by closed reduction and retrograde intramedullary Ender nails. Orthopedics 1998;21:641–646

34. Henley MB, Chapman JR, Claudi BF. Closed retrograde Hackethal nail stabilization of humeral shaft fractures. J Orthop Trauma 1992;6:18–24

35. Qidwai SA. Treatment of humeral shaft fractures by closed fixation using multiple intramedullary Kirschner wires. J Trauma 2000; 49:81–85

36. Flinkkila T, Hyvonen P, Lakovaara M, Linden T, Ristiniemi J, Hamalainen M. Intramedullary nailing of humeral shaft fractures: a retrospective study of 126 cases. Acta Orthop Scand 1999;70:133–136

37. Farragos AF, Schemitsch EH, McKee MD. Complications of intramedullary nailing for fractures of the humeral shaft: a review. J Orthop Trauma 1999;13:258–267

38. Albritton MJ, Barnes CJ, Basamania CJ, Karas SG. Relationship of the axillary nerve to the proximal screws of a flexible humeral nail system: an anatomic study. J Orthop Trauma 2003;17:411–414

39. Moran MC. Distal interlocking during intramedullary nailing of the humerus. Clin Orthop Relat Res 1995;317:215–218

40. Crates J, Whittle AP. Antegrade interlocking nailing of acute humeral shaft fractures. Clin Orthop Relat Res 1998;350:40–50

41. Riemer BL, Butterfield SL, D'Ambrosia R, Kellam J. Seidel intramedullary nailing of humeral diaphyseal fractures: a preliminary report. Orthopedics 1991;14:239–246

42. Rommens PM, Blum J, Runkel M. Retrograde nailing of humeral shaft fractures. Clin Orthop Relat Res 1998;350:26–39

43. Blum J, Janzig H, Gahr R, Langendorff HS, Rommens PM. Clinical performance of a new medullary humeral nail: antegrade versus retrograde insertion. J Orthop Trauma 2001;15:342–349

44. Zinman C, Norman D, Hamoud K, Reis ND. External fixation for severe open fractures of the humerus caused by missiles. J Orthop Trauma 1997;11:536–539

45. Mostafavi HR, Tornetta P III. Open fractures of the humerus treated with external fixation. Clin Orthop Relat Res 1997;337: 187–197

46. Wisniewski TF, Radziejowski MJ. Gunshot fractures of the humeral shaft treated with external fixation. J Orthop Trauma 1996;10: 273–278

47. Marsh JL, Mahoney CR, Steinbronn D. External fixation of open humerus fractures. Iowa Orthop J 1999;19:35–42

48. Kamhin M, Michaelson M, Waisbrod H. The use of external skeletal fixation in the treatment of fractures of the humeral shaft. Injury 1978;9:245–248

49. Heim D, Herkert F, Hess P, Regazzoni P. Surgical treatment of humeral shaft fractures: the Basel experience. J Trauma 1993; 35: 226–232

50. Böstman O, Bakalim G, Vainionpää S, et al. Radial palsy in shaft fracture of the humerus. Acta Orthop Scand 1986;57:316–319

51. Ring D, Chin K, Jupiter JB. Radial nerve palsy associated with high-energy humeral shaft fractures. J Hand Surg [Am] 2004;29: 144–147

52. Riemer BL, D'Ambrosia R, Kellam JF, Butterfield SL, Burke CJ. The anterior acromial approach for antegrade intramedullary nailing of the humeral diaphysis. Orthopedics 1993;16:1219–1223

53. Schmidt AH, Templeman DC, Grabowski CM. Antegrade intramedullary nailing of the humerus complicated by heterotopic ossification of the deltoid: a case report. J Orthop Trauma 2001; 15:69–73

54. Strothman D, Templeman DC, Varecka T, Bechtold J. Retrograde nailing of humeral shaft fractures: a biomechanical study of its effects on the strength of the distal humerus. J Orthop Trauma 2000;14:101–104

55. Lin J, Hou SM, Hang YS, Chao EY. Treatment of humeral shaft fractures by retrograde locked nailing. Clin Orthop Relat Res 1997; 342:147–155

13 Distal Humeral Fractures

Lisa Cannada

Articular fractures of the distal humerus represent only ~2% of all fractures but always present a challenge to the treating orthopaedic surgeon. There are two distinct subgroups of patients in which these injuries occur.[1] The first group are the high-energy injuries that generally occur in younger patients **(Fig. 13–1A,B).** The second subgroup are the low-energy fractures that often result from a ground-level fall in the elderly and are often associated with osteoporosis. Most of these fractures present with marked displacement and significant comminution **(Fig. 13–2A,B).**

High-energy injuries differ from lower-energy injuries in terms of the proportion of open fractures and the incidence of injuries to more than one organ system. With the high-energy injury, there can be extensive comminution of the articular surface and metaphyseal region, and there can be bone loss in open injuries **(Fig. 13–1A,B).** In addition, the associated soft tissue injury needs to be considered in the planning and timing of treatment of these patients.

Lower-energy injuries may also have significant comminution that is due to the poor bone quality rather than the energy of the injury. These injuries represent a different challenge to the surgeon in terms of nonoperative and operative treatment. The elderly patient frequently has coexisting medical morbidities that may preclude surgery. In addition, the osteoporotic bone may make stable osteosynthesis difficult to achieve.

In the past it had been acceptable to treat this injury with conservative measures, partly because of the poor results reported in early series of internal fixation. Now, surgical repair of these fractures has become a fairly standard accepted treatment. A review of the literature documents that one can realistically expect 75% good or excellent results, with a range of 50 to 90%.[2–9]

The desired functional outcome after treatment of a fracture of the distal humerus is a painless elbow with satisfactory mobility. Achieving this requires careful surgical planning and execution to anatomically reconstruct the articular surface and restore the overall anatomy while providing stable fixation that allows early mobilization. In practice, realizing these goals is difficult in patients with osteoporotic bone, significant comminution, or soft tissue problems. There are many reported complications of treatment, including contractures, infection, nonunion, failure of fixation, symptomatic hardware (especially if an olecranon osteotomy is used), ulnar nerve dysfunction, and heterotopic ossification.

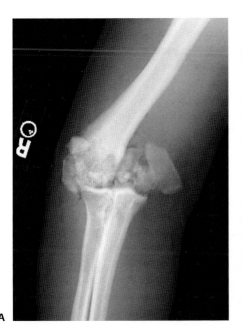
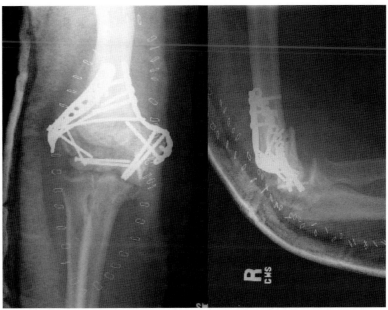

A   B

Figure 13–1 (A) A high-energy distal humerus fracture in a 24-year-old motorcyclist. **(B)** After open reduction and internal fixation.

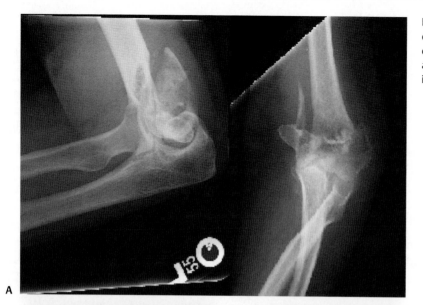

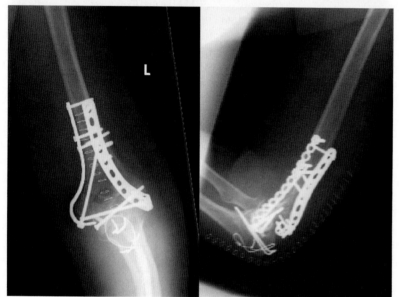

Figure 13–2 (A) A distal humerus fracture in an elderly woman. Note the osteoporosis and comminution. These injuries frequently occur after a low-energy fall. **(B)** After open reduction and internal fixation with an olecranon osteotomy.

Indications for Surgical Treatment

Physical Examination

The evaluation of a patient with a distal humerus fracture should include evaluation of the fracture, soft tissues, and neurovascular structures. Radiographs will provide further information regarding the bony injury. Many of these fractures are open, and the risk of an open injury is related to the mechanisms of injury. The posterior soft tissues especially should be carefully evaluated for the presence of an open wound. The wound most often is posterior and is created by the diaphyseal portion of the humeral shaft that compounds as the humeral shaft and condyles split. An open posterior wound indicates involvement of the extensor mechanism of the elbow and should be kept in mind during surgical planning.

There are several neurovascular structures that cross the elbow. Consideration of the deformity will help in assessing the vascular status. The brachial artery crosses the elbow anteriorly, and if there is significant anterior displacement, this may warrant a more careful evaluation of the brachial artery. The vascular status may be assessed with evaluation of the distal pulses and comparison to the opposite side. When discrepancies with the distal pulse or a compromised capillary refill are noted, further evaluation including angiography is warranted. There are three major peripheral nerves that cross the elbow joint: the median, radial, and ulnar nerves. The motor and sensory function of these nerves should be evaluated as part of the physical examination. Further evaluation includes examination of the joints above and below the injury in addition to a survey of the entire patient. In a patient with a high-energy injury, additional body system injuries may

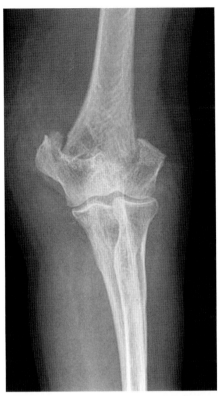

Figure 13–3 Anteroposterior x-ray of the distal humerus.

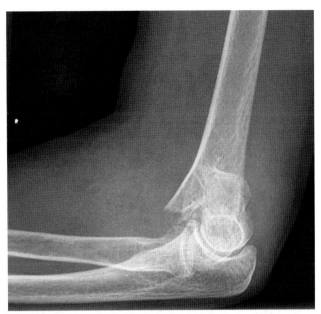

Figure 13–4 Lateral x-ray of the distal humerus.

ultimately impact the surgical decision making and affect the type of treatment and timing of surgery.

Radiographic Evaluation

With trauma to the elbow such as a distal humerus fracture, radiographs are routinely obtained in the anteroposterior (AP) and lateral projections. For the AP view of the elbow, the arm and forearm are positioned horizontally, resting on a radiolucent support, with the elbow joint fully extended and the fingers slightly flexed. The beam is directed perpendicular to the elbow joint. This view will demonstrate the distal humeral shaft, the elbow joint, and proximal portions of the radius and ulna in the coronal plane (**Fig. 13–3**).

For the lateral projection of the elbow, the forearm is resting on the ulnar side with the joint flexed 90 degrees, with the thumb pointing upward and the fingers slightly flexed. The beam is then directed vertically toward the radial head. The film in this projection demonstrates details regarding the distal humerus, the olecranon, and the radial head in the sagittal plane (**Fig. 13–4**).

Good-quality radiographs are necessary to assist with the surgical planning. However, because of the pain of the injury, it is often difficult to obtain true AP and lateral radiographs as described. With either or both appropriate pain medication and sedation, a traction radiograph may be of assistance in planning the surgical procedure. For this view, gentle longitudinal traction is applied to the

patient's arm in an extended position. In this way, a better AP view may be obtained. Similarly, it may be difficult to flex the injured elbow, and it may be necessary to obtain the lateral radiograph in an extended position.

For routine evaluation of distal humerus fractures, computed tomographic (CT) scanning is neither routinely necessary nor recommended because it is not likely to affect surgical decision making or alter the surgical approach.

Tips and Tricks
• Traction x-rays are valuable in preoperative planning.

Injury Classification

The goals of any fracture classification system are to provide a guide to treatment, indicate the prognosis of the injury, and provide a framework for surgeons and researchers to communicate with one another. As with any major fracture, there are several classification systems that have been proposed for distal humeral fractures. None has become universally accepted. Previous historical classifications regard fractures of the intercondylar region of the distal humerus as being T- or Y-type fractures.[10] However, understanding of the complex anatomy of these fractures has improved with the recognition that the distal humerus is best described by columns rather than by condyles, which allows the fractures to be more accu-rately described.

Riseborough and Radin proposed four types of fractures, including a nondisplaced fracture (type I), displaced T or Y fractures that separate the condyles from each other and from the shaft (type II), fractures with

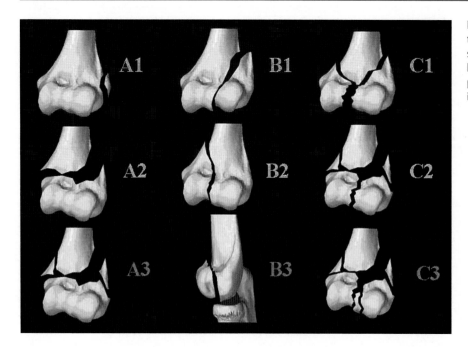

Figure 13–5 Arbeitsgemeinschaft für Osteosynthesefragen/Orthopaedic Trauma Association (AO/OTA) classification of distal humeral fractures. AO Dialogue 2/01 with permission. Copyright © 2001, AO Publishing, Zurich, Switzerland.)

rotational displacement of the condyles (type III), and displaced fractures with rotation and intra-articular comminution (type IV).[11] This is perhaps one of the simplest fracture classifications for the distal humerus; however, in this case the simplicity of this classification limits its usefulness in describing the types of distal humerus fractures.

As reported by Jupiter and Mehne, Mehne and Matta divided bicolumnar fractures of the distal humerus into six main types, including high T fracture, low T fracture, a Y fracture, an H fracture, and medial or lateral lambda fractures.[12] The classification system of Mehne and Matta is useful in the description of the low columnar fractures. Ring and Jupiter note that this classification does not account for fractures in multiple planes, including the coronal plane.[13] Coronal plane fractures are important to recognize and represent particularly difficult challenges to repair.

The Arbeitsgemeinschaft für Osteosynthesefragen/ Orthopaedic Trauma Association (AO/OTA) Comprehensive Fracture Classification organizes fractures of the distal humerus into three main groups, each with nine subtypes.[14] This classification system was developed to provide a comprehensive classification system adaptable to the entire skeletal system. The comprehensive classification of fractures organizes fractures into extra-articular (type A), partial articular (type B), and complete articular fractures (type C) and then further categorizes them based on the extent of the extra-articular and intra-articular fragmentation. This system provides more choices in the description of fractures but does not provide much useful information that serves as a guide to treatment and is difficult to use for

clinical decision making except in its most rudimentary form (A vs B vs C) **(Fig. 13–5)**.[15]

Ring et al described 21 patients with purely "articular" fractures of the distal humerus that were at or distal to the olecranon fossa, and noted that there were five potential articular fragments **(Fig. 13–6)**.[16] The standard classifications as already described do not recognize this pattern of injury, and it is best to simply describe these injuries anatomically **(Fig. 13–7A,B)**.

Nonoperative Treatment

Nonoperative treatment of distal humerus fractures is appropriate for some fracture types and population groups. Rarely, a patient may present a high operative risk or have systemic contraindications to surgery. Stable extra-articular distal humerus fractures (AO/OTA type A) can be treated nonoperatively as long as reasonable alignment can be maintained. The fracture may be reduced with gentle axial traction and neutral rotation and then placed in a posterior splint. If the soft tissue permits, this may be changed to a cast. To begin early range of motion, a hinged elbow brace or a cast should be applied after a 2-to 3-week period. In a multiple trauma patient, it may be difficult to obtain or maintain acceptable reduction, and in such a patient an otherwise stable distal humerus fracture may need to be treated operatively. Fixation of such fractures may be helpful in the care and mobilization of multiple trauma patients.

Another indication for nonoperative treatment would be a severely comminuted fracture in a patient with significant osteoporosis such that reconstruction is not

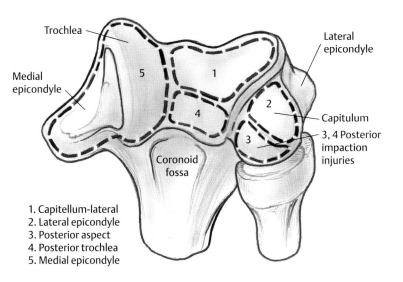

Trochlea

Medial epicondyle

Lateral epicondyle

Capitulum

3, 4 Posterior impaction injuries

Coronoid fossa

5

1

4

2

3

1. Capitellum-lateral
2. Lateral epicondyle
3. Posterior aspect
4. Posterior trochlea
5. Medial epicondyle

Figure 13–6 Illustration of the distal humeral articular surface, demonstrating the five possible components of an articular fracture.

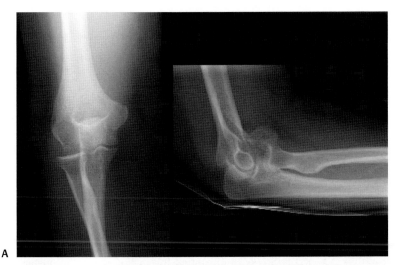

A

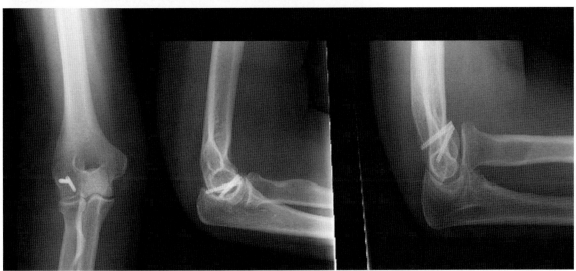

B

Figure 13–7 (A) Anteroposterior and lateral x-rays of a displaced capitellar fracture. **(B)** Postoperative views.

likely to succeed. This has been described as the "bag of bones" technique and consists of using a sling or collar and cuff immobilization using one of two methods: (1) immobilization between 100 and 125 degrees of flexion, increasing the amount of extension over the succeeding 3-week period; or (2) active motion initiated after a 2-week period of immobilization with the elbow at 90 degrees.[13] These patients may obtain an adequately mobile, pain-free elbow with limited morbidity, considering their systemic or local conditions. More recently, total elbow arthroplasty may be considered an option for such patients who are fit for surgery (see **Video 13–1, Disk 2**).[17,18]

If nonoperative management is chosen, the patient should be followed closely with serial radiographic assessment to ensure that the reduction is maintained. Generally, upright positioning and compression of the upper arm are all that is needed to maintain fracture reduction. However, there may need to be multiple adjustments to the splinting and repeat reductions if follow-up radiographs demonstrate loss of the reduction.

Tips and Tricks

- With all fractures of the distal humerus, rather than memorize a specific fracture classification, it is more valuable for the surgeon to recognize the multiplanar fracture lines and their relationship to the articular surface, determine whether there is comminution of the trochlea, and understand the extent of involvement of the medial and lateral columns and the olecranon fossa.

Surgical Treatment

General Concepts

Ultimately, the goals of fixation of distal humeral fractures are to provide a stable and mobile elbow joint, obtain union between the metaphyseal and diaphyseal bone, allow soft tissue healing, minimize the risk of infection, and allow the patient to rapidly regain functional use of the upper extremity. Cassebaum first described the principles of operative treatment of distal humerus intra-articular fractures in 1952.[19] He discussed five guidelines, of which the first was to reestablish the relationship of the condyles to each other and the relationship of the condyles to the ulna. The second principle is to keep the olecranon fossa open. His third principle was preservation and reestablishment of the forward tilt of the articular surface of the condyles. His fourth principle was fixation of condyles to the shaft, and his fifth principle was obtaining a secure fixation. He reported the results of nine cases with four excellent, four good, and one poor result by these criteria. These prin-

ciples remain valid today and provide the foundation for contemporary surgical management of these complex fractures (see **Video 13–2, Disk 2**).

Considerations in Planning Surgical Treatment

Distal humerus fractures involving the articular surface may occur from a high- or low-energy mechanism. Elderly patients may be injured from simple falls and yet sustain significantly comminuted distal humerus fractures due to their poor bone quality. The nature of these injuries is much different than that which occurs in falls from height, motor-vehicle collisions, or other high-energy mechanisms. These types of injuries occur in younger persons and still may result in fractures with significant comminution from the energy of the injury. It is important to remember that distal humeral fractures may be associated with a soft tissue injury that may affect surgical timing and planning. A fracture that has significant displacement with sharp fragments may "tent" the skin. This pressure on the skin from within may ultimately lead to skin breakdown. If surgery is to be delayed, this displacement should be corrected by closed reduction to minimize tension on the skin from the fracture. In addition, the soft tissues may have significant bruising and perhaps abrasions. Although incisions through areas of ecchymosis may not have significant implications in terms of rate of infection, incision through superficial abrasions or lacerations may result in problems with wound healing. Thus the skin should be examined closely, and the decision to pursue surgery should be made when the soft tissues will allow the incisions to be planned without increasing the patient's risk of infection or any skin necrosis from significant soft tissue injury.

Open distal humerus fractures occur as the result of a high- or low-energy injury. Like other open fractures, this type of injury warrants aggressive debridement, ideally within the first 6 to 8 hours of injury to minimize risk of infection. With any open fracture it is very important to perform a thorough debridement of the skin, subcutaneous tissue, muscle, and bone. Furthermore, the traumatic wound may not be in an area where the surgical incision was planned. Thus extension of the traumatic wound for debridement should take into account the exposure that is necessary for insertion of internal fixation, which is often performed at the same time. However, if the initial debridement is done in the middle of the night, without the appropriate operating room personnel and equipment, or if the patient is unstable, the upper limb may be placed in a splint or external fixator until a more appropriate time.

Preoperative and Intraoperative Planning

Surgical fixation of distal humerus fractures should be performed as soon as possible after injury, ideally within

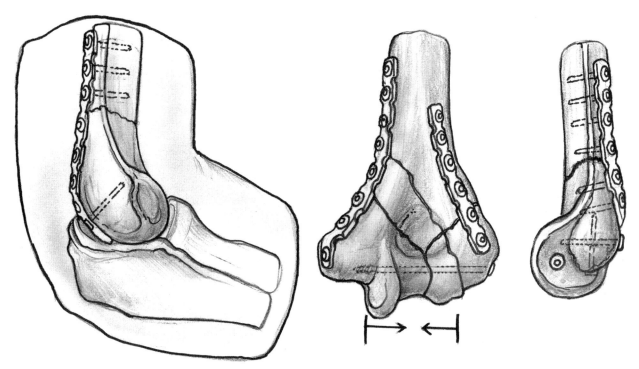

Figure 13–8 Drawing of double plating of the distal humerus. One plate is placed posteriorly along the lateral column, whereas the other plate is applied to the medial aspect of the medial column.

the first week. Early fixation minimizes the risk of skin breakdown from the splint, protects the soft tissues from the pressure of displaced bone fragments, and may decrease stiffness following an injury that is often complicated by decreased range of motion. If the patient has multiple injuries, special considerations may be required. For example, repair of the fracture may need to be delayed while more serious injuries are stabilized. If surgery must be delayed, the patient's arm may be splinted with a well-padded posterior splint with medial and lateral plaster reinforcements. If the patient is intubated, frequent evaluation of the skin prior to the surgery should be observed. Rarely, external fixation is considered for temporary management. External fixation is best chosen for provisional management of open fractures in multiply injured patients that cannot tolerate definitive surgery acutely.

Surgery should be planned based on careful radiographic assessment of the fracture type. Appropriate x-rays include an AP radiograph (preferably performed with traction) and a lateral radiograph (**Figs. 13–3** and **13–4**). When open reduction and internal fixation of distal humerus fractures are needed, plate fixation is the only practical option. Therefore, there are two primary considerations in preoperative planning: choosing the type, number, and length of plates to be used and deciding whether an olecranon osteotomy is necessary. With intra-articular distal humerus fractures, olecranon osteotomy

should be considered for access to the distal humeral articular surface. Preoperative planning with the use of templates should be done to have the appropriate equipment necessary. In addition, there should be an assortment of multiple screws of different sizes, K-wires, and reduction clamps. It is important not to forget consideration for iliac crest bone graft and the availability of a tourniquet.

For most distal humeral fractures, double plating of the distal humerus is recommended (**Fig. 13–8**). Rarely, one encounters unicondylar injuries that can be treated with plating of just the medial or lateral column. Standard plates are available that include small-fragment dynamic compression plates, reconstruction plates that can be more easily contoured to fit the distal humerus, and precontoured plates available from different manufacturers that are specifically designed for application to the distal humerus.

Patient Positioning

The patient's positioning needs to be considered because supine, lateral, and prone positions are all possible. The lateral decubitus position is the most versatile and also allows exposure of the iliac crest should bone grafting be necessary (see **Video 13–2, Disk 2**). With the patient in the lateral position, the elbow may be flexed over a tray or bolster. For the lateral decubitus position, a

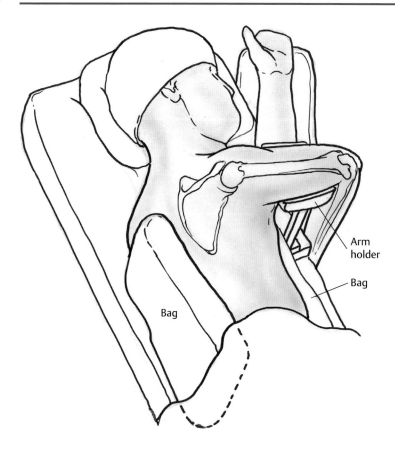

Figure 13–9 Patient positioning for surgery using the lateral decubitus position. Note the use of a beanbag and padding.

Arm holder

Bag

Bag

beanbag is preferred with an axillary roll and all bony prominences well padded (**Fig. 13–9**).

Prone positioning also works well for exposure of the distal humerus, but it may be a little more difficult to flex the elbow unless the arm is hung over the edge of a table. When the lateral decubitus or prone positions are contraindicated, the patient may be positioned supine. In this position, the shoulder has to be flexed and adducted and the arm pulled across the patient's chest by an assistant. Most often, the choice of position simply depends upon surgeon preferences.

Regardless of the position chosen, while the patient is being positioned it is recommended that the arm be suspended to prevent telescoping of the fragments and further damage to the soft tissues. The draping should be to the axillary region. After the prepping and draping commence, alcohol should be used to remove the Betadine prior to placement of the sterile tourniquet. Prophylactic antibiotics should be provided.

Intraoperative Imaging

With the exposures used to facilitate fixation of distal humerus fractures, there is normally full visualization of the fracture site and joint surface. However, intraoperative radiographs should be obtained in the AP and lateral planes to ensure adequate reduction of the joint surface, overall alignment of the limb, and positioning of the implants. Depending on the position of the patient during surgery, fluoroscopy may be of value to the physician in the evaluation of temporary fixation of the joint surface and plate placement. Placement of the C-arm may vary depending upon the position of the patient, and "practice" images should be taken before the final prepping and draping of the patient to be sure that adequate imaging is possible.

Approaches

Posterior Approach, Triceps Sparing or Splitting

A midline posterior incision is made over the distal humerus and then coursing around the tip of the olecranon and continuing distally. The incision should not be directly over the tip of the olecranon because this may cause wound problems and discomfort for the patient postoperatively. The incision should be performed sharply through the skin to the level of the triceps aponeurosis (**Fig. 13–10**). There are a few possible deep approaches once the skin incision is made. The triceps may be split through its fibers to bone, or a muscle-sparing approach may be done (**Fig. 13–11**). Alternatively, a triceps-sparing approach is described and utilizes mobile windows made

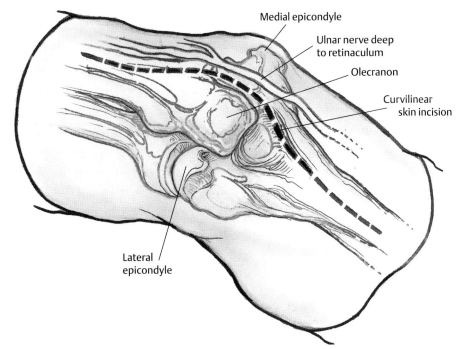

Medial epicondyle

Ulnar nerve deep
to retinaculum

Olecranon

Curvilinear
skin incision

Lateral
epicondyle

Figure 13–10 Recommended posterior skin incision. Note gentle curve around the elbow to minimize patient discomfort postoperatively.

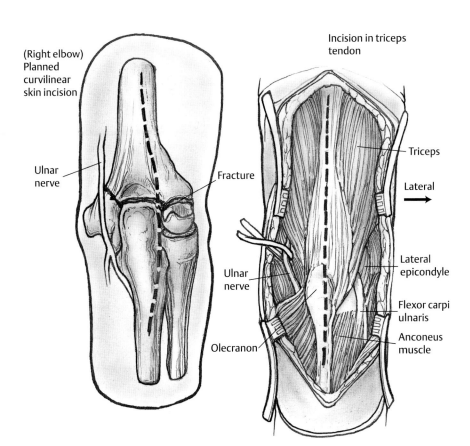

(Right elbow)
Planned
curvilinear
skin incision

Ulnar
nerve

Fracture

Incision in triceps
tendon

Triceps

Lateral

Ulnar
nerve

Lateral
epicondyle

Flexor carpi
ulnaris

Anconeus
muscle

Olecranon

Figure 13–11 Triceps-splitting exposure. Note protection around the ulnar nerve. FCU, flexor carpi ulnaris.

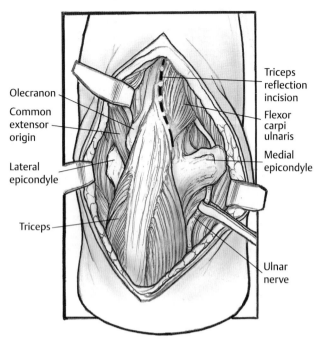

Figure 13–12 Alternative fracture exposure with reflection of the triceps muscle.

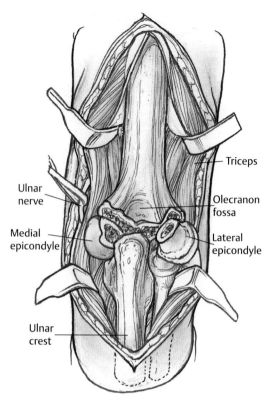

Figure 13–13 Exposure of the fracture with a triceps-splitting approach. Note the position of the retractors. This is the exposure of the fracture without (or prior to) olecranon osteotomy. Although the fractured epicondyles can be easily identified, full exposure of the joint surface is nearly impossible without the osteotomy.

on either side of the triceps while maintaining the triceps insertion (**Fig. 13–12**). This is done whenever possible to minimize soft tissue trauma. First, the distal humerus is approached laterally. As one dissects distally along the lateral aspect of the humerus, the posterior radial collateral arterial system is visualized. This arterial system should be protected. Sharp dissection continues further to elevate the triceps off the distal fragment at the level of the olecranon fossa. Proximally, along the lateral aspect of the arm, the radial nerve will be identified. The radial nerve may then be followed over the posterior aspect of the humerus.

At this point in time the tourniquet may need to be deflated and removed to allow further visualization if necessary. The triceps may then continue to be mobilized medially, with attention being paid to the radial nerve and its vena comitantes and the sensory nerve branches. Medially, the dissection along the humerus is sharply continued, and the ulnar nerve should be identified and followed down through the medial epicondyle. Once the ulnar and radial nerves have been identified, the olecranon osteotomy may be completed if desired. For some fractures with minimal or no articular involvement, mobilization of the triceps as described earlier may provide adequate exposure without further work. If visualization of the joint surface is needed, there are two options: formal olecranon osteotomy, or reflection of the triceps aponeurosis off the proximal ulna in continuity with the forearm fascia.

For the triceps-splitting approach, the same posterior incision is used. The ulnar nerve is identified and protected with a Penrose drain. The triceps is split in line with the incision to the bone (**Fig. 13–13**). The triceps may be split as far distal as the olecranon if needed. There should be a tendinous layer preserved medially and laterally to allow

for reattachment at the end of the procedure. In this manner, a triceps-splitting approach is advantageous in eliminating the need for an olecranon osteotomy if adequate visualization is obtained.

Posterior Approach, Olecranon Osteotomy

To perform an olecranon osteotomy, predrill the ulna with a 3.2 mm drill bit (**Fig. 13–14A,B**) (see **Video 13–2, Disk 2**). A power saw is then used to create a chevron osteotomy. The apex of the osteotomy should be distal so as to maintain as much bone in the proximal fragment as possible, and the osteotomy should be completed with the use of sharp osteotomes to avoid bone loss at the articular surface. The osteotomy should enter the articular surface at the bare area of the olecranon sigmoid fossa. Once the osteotomy is completed, the olecranon and attached triceps may be reflected proximally. Further mobilization of the ulnar nerve may be performed along with its collateral vascularity. This approach provides unimpeded visualization of the fracture and the distal humerus articular surface. Once the fracture is identified all bone ends should be thoroughly curetted and debrided. A dental pick may be needed to debride the fine fragments in a significantly comminuted fracture.

Several techniques have been described in the literature for fixation of the olecranon osteotomy. Malunion of the

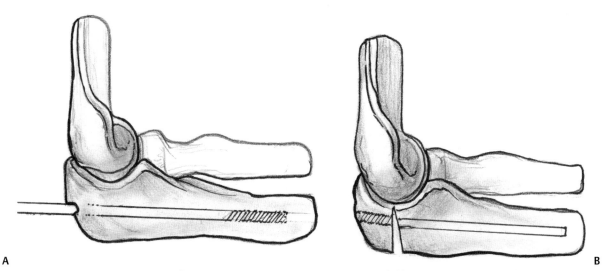

A

B

Figure 13–14 Olecranon osteotomy. **(A)** Predrilling of the osteotomy with a 3.5 mm drill bit. **(B)** Osteotomy completed. After screw fixation, the osteotomy should be in an anatomical position.

olecranon osteotomy could lead to pain and stiffness. Predrilling of the olecranon before the osteotomy is made is recommended to allow anatomical placement of a partially threaded 6.5 mm cancellous screw for fixation of the olecranon osteotomy **(Fig. 13–14A,B).** The length chosen is one that obtains purchase in the proximal to mid ulnar shaft. A washer is routinely used. Following placement of the screw, a tension-band wire is placed. A 2.0 mm drill bit should be used to drill a hole that is posterior to the 6.5 mm cancellous screw and just distal to the coronoid process. The figure-of-

eight tension-band wire is placed through the drill hole and crossed along the posterior aspect of the proximal ulna and then placed underneath the triceps. A 14- or 16-gauge angiocatheter can be used to pass the wire deep to the triceps tendon. The wires are twisted and tensioned appropriately. The washer is then tightened down with the 6.5 mm cancellous screw. Full range of motion and flexion and extension of the elbow should be completed to ensure that the tension-band wire is indeed allowing compression across the osteotomy site **(Fig. 13–15A,B).**

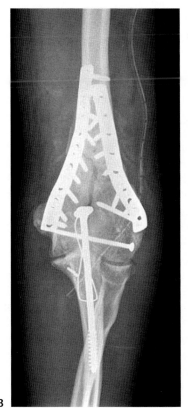

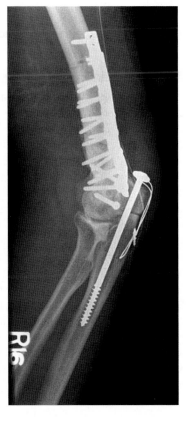

A,B

Figure 13–15 Photos of olecranon osteotomy fixation. **(A)** Anteroposterior x-ray. **(B)** Lateral x-ray.

An alternative technique to fix the osteotomy would be to use two parallel K-wires with a tension-band wire, as is commonly done for fixation of olecranon fractures (**Fig. 13–2B**). Following the standard fracture technique, the parallel K-wires should be drilled into the proximal aspect of the ulna in an oblique, posterior to anterior direction so that they engage the anterior cortex. The tension-band wire may then be placed as previously described, with the proximal wire placed underneath the two K-wires. Using this technique, Ring et al reported 98% union within 6 months, although 13% of the patients had symptomatic hardware that required removal.[20]

A final but rarely needed alternative to fixation of the olecranon osteotomy would be a plate. This would be necessary if there was a coexistent comminuted proximal ulna fracture, or if the osteotomy was inadvertently made too far distally. Either standard limited contact dynamic compression plates or precontoured proximal ulna places may be used.

Posterior Triceps-Reflecting Anconeus Pedicle Approach

The triceps-reflecting anconeus pedicle (TRAP) approach was described as an alternative approach for posterior fixation of distal humeral fractures.[21] The use of an olecranon osteotomy in the posterior approach is the exposure most often described for fixation of distal humerus intra-articular fractures. However, the olecranon osteotomy is known for complications, including malunion, nonunion, and need for additional surgery for removal of painful hardware. O'Driscoll felt that the olecranon osteotomy as usually performed denervates the anconeus muscle.[21] The anconeus muscle is innervated by a branch of the radial nerve, and this nerve is transected with the soft tissue dissection needed for an olecranon osteotomy. The anconeus muscle is a dynamic stabilizer of the elbow, and loss of its function may contribute to loss of elbow stability. However, following distal humerus fractures, instability has not been described as a significant complication, irrespective of whether olecranon osteotomy was performed; in fact, many distal humerus fractures are complicated by stiffness.

The TRAP approach for fixation of distal humerus fractures does not involve disruption of the proximal ulnar bony surface. In addition, should the patient require further surgery in the future, such as the need for a total elbow arthroplasty, the surgery can more easily be performed if there has not been an olecranon osteotomy. The disadvantage of this technique is visualization of the most distal part of the distal humerus. Extreme hyperflexion of the elbow is needed to visualize the distal surface with this approach. If a surgeon is not experienced with the repair of distal humerus fractures, the traditional posterior approach with olecranon osteotomy might be the easier alternative.

Patient Positioning

The patient may be positioned in either the lateral position or the supine position. O'Driscoll prefers the patient supine with a bolster under the scapula and arm.[21]

Exposure

A 15 cm long posterior approach is used. With any posterior approach at the tip of the olecranon, one should curve the incision medially or laterally to avoid skin wound healing problems in the future. Dissection is carried down to the level of the triceps tendon. The ulnar nerve is identified and dissected free. Anterior transposition of the ulnar nerve is performed if medial plating of the distal humerus is to be completed. The posterior approach is modified to develop the lateral aspect of the TRAP. The interval between the anconeus and extensor carpi ulnaris is identified and incised, starting ~10 cm distal to the olecranon and extending toward the lateral epicondyle, then carried proximally along the supracondylar ridge. The anconeus is dissected subperiosteally off the ulna and ultimately off the annular ligament and lateral collateral ligament complex. It is important that the annular ligaments and lateral collateral ligament of the elbow are preserved. The arthrotomy is made at the tip of the olecranon, and further dissection through the capsule is performed at that time.

The medial portion of the TRAP is similar to the triceps-reflecting approach as described by Bryan and Morrey.[22] This approach is started 10 cm distal to the olecranon and continued proximally along the border of the olecranon and along the edge of the flexor carpi ulnaris. Further exposure of the ulna continues subperiosteally. An important step at this point in the procedure is to place a marking suture in the periosteum where the triceps insert. This ensures that at the end of the procedure the tendon is reattached anatomically. Dissection is carried proximally, and ultimately the planes of dissection between the medial and lateral approach will meet on the humerus, beneath the triceps, and on the ulna beneath the anconeus. The attachments of the distal anconeus are released in the triceps, and the anconeus pedicle can then be reflected proximally. Flexion of the elbow will allow exposure to the distal humerus at this time. Plate fixation may then commence as described.

Triceps Reattachment

For the attachment of the triceps tendon, 2.0 mm drill holes are made in the proximal ulna criss-crossing the triceps insertion on the proximal surface of the olecranon. An additional drill hole should be made transversely just distal to the other two. Reinsertion of the triceps begins with a modified Mason-Allen locking suture using heavy, nonabsorbable suture. The suture is placed through the tendon and then through the drill holes that are in the bone. The tendon is secured to the bony surface. The suture is tied and then proximally woven in a Bunnell fashion for imbrication of the tendon. This also minimizes the tension on the reattachment side. The fascial sleeve is then closed with a running locking suture.

Completion of this approach with reattachment of the tendon allows immediate rehabilitation with full active and passive range of motion of the elbow with no resistive exercises.

Ulnar Nerve Management

Ulnar nerve dysfunction is a known complication of distal humerus fractures and their fixation. The nerve is at risk both from the original trauma and from the surgical procedure. The surgeon must make a decision whether to transpose the nerve, and the resulting choice may affect the outcome. The soft tissue damage associated with distal humerus fractures is extensive, and fibrosis about the bed of the nerve can be expected. Surgical trauma could possibly lead to further scarring; however, to transpose the ulnar nerve properly it must be released proximally and distally to lie tension free in its new bed. Thus, at times a complete release of the ulnar nerve for transposition would require substantially more surgical dissection than otherwise needed as part of the procedure. If the ulnar nerve does not contact hardware, the nerve may be placed back in its original bed as long as its nutritional supply is maintained by using only the minimal dissection needed for protection and by avoiding traction. However, if nerve transposition is necessary or desired, the nerve is released adequately proximally and distally to complete the transposition without tension. The nerve may then be placed submuscularly or subcutaneously, depending on surgeon preference.

Fracture Reduction and Fixation

Once adequate exposure of the fracture has been obtained, the next step is to proceed with reduction of the fracture (see **Video 13–2, Disk 2**). Distal humerus fractures with intra-articular extension often prove to be quite difficult to reduce for a few reasons. With loss of the medial and lateral columns, there is significant loss of stability. There is often significant comminution of either or both the metaphyseal and articular segments, and the bone fragments may be too small for screw fixation. In addition, the distal surface is composed primarily of cancellous bone, in which it is more difficult to gain stable fixation. Typically, the sequence of reduction and fixation is begun distally, first reconstructing the articular surface and then reducing the restored articular mass to the columns. In all but the most simple fracture patterns, fixation is performed first with K-wires to reconstruct the articular surface. Once the articular surface is provisionally reconstructed, definitive fixation may be completed with a combination of screws as necessary. It is important to avoid lag screw fixation across the distal humeral articular surface. In the presence of articular comminution, lag screw fixation across this surface may compress and alter the actual shape of the distal humerus. Following fixation of the articular fragments, the distal humerus is reduced and stabilized to the humeral shaft.

Biomechanical and clinical studies have shown that two plates placed at a 90 degree angle provide optimum fixation.[23–25] To accomplish this, it is convenient to place one plate on the posterior aspect of the lateral column and another on the medial aspect of the medial column. If standard plates are to be used, plate contouring will be necessary and templates should be used to assist in plate bending. The hardware must be fashioned to avoid the articular surfaces and to bend appropriately to obtain a mechanical advantage with fixation and also allow the patient to have a full range of motion postoperatively. Given that the medial plate must bend around the medial epicondyle, a reconstruction plate is usually used medially because it is easier to contour. After properly contouring the plate around the distal humerus, one can insert distal fixation with screws that are perpendicular to the articular surface, thus providing a stronger biomechanical advantage. The lateral plate requires less contouring and is recommended to be a limited contact dynamic compression plate; the size may vary depending on the patient's distal humerus anatomy. The plate should be placed as distally as possible while avoiding the articular surface. When possible, a long "home run screw" can be inserted from the most distal hole of the plate, up the column, and engage the opposite cortex of the humeral shaft. Precontoured plates are available from several manufacturers that obviate the need for plate contouring, which often requires repeated attempts.

Purely articular fragments are effectively repaired with headless screws.[16] Small osteochondral fragments are best stabilized with variable compression screws countersunk within the articular surface and placed perpendicular to the fracture line. The head of the screw is inserted to the level of the subchondral bone to maximize purchase and avoid prominence in case of cartilage loss. Alternatively, minifragment 2.0 or 2.7 mm screws can also be used and must also be countersunk through the articular surface, or small threaded wires can be placed and cut off flush with the cartilage surface **(Fig. 13–5)**.

Once the fracture and olecranon osteotomy (when performed) have been secured, radiographs are obtained and closure begins. Intraoperative radiographs or fluoroscopy should be used to confirm the reduction and fixation of the fracture. One should confirm that all screws are out of the joint surface and that the reduction of the fracture is acceptable. Normally, the capitellum bisects the anterior cortex of the distal humerus. The articular surface should be congruous. The radial head should be congruent with the capitellum, and the normal valgus carrying angle of the elbow should be restored. In addition, the range of motion of the patient's elbow should be evaluated to ensure that there is no impingement from the hardware. It is important to remember to evaluate forearm rotation as well as elbow flexion and extension. With a triceps-sparing approach as described, there are no muscular planes to close. If a triceps-splitting approach was done, the muscle can be loosely approximated. Subcuticular sutures are used for the deep layer. Sutures are preferred in the skin to avoid any friction or rubbing that may occur with a staple closure. Postoperatively, a well-padded splint is applied.

The position of elbow splinting is controversial. Most often, the elbow is splinted in some degree of flexion, so that an elbow sling can be comfortably used following surgery. However, elbow extension is difficult to achieve postoperatively, and splinting the elbow in full extension may minimize this problem. Additionally, splinting in extension minimizes tension on the incision. If the elbow is splinted in flexion, avoiding extreme flexion (more than 90 degrees) is recommended. The splint should be left in place to allow the soft tissues to heal, and then range of motion should commence as early as the first week after surgery with gentle active and active-assisted range of motion.

Tips and Tricks

- Do not hesitate to perform olecranon osteotomy when articular visualization is needed.
- Triceps-sparing approaches are associated with moderately better strength and motion but may be more difficult for surgeons unaccustomed to their use.
- Beware of inadvertently narrowing the trochlea when using lag screws across the articular surface.
- Use countersunk, headless screws for fixation of osteochondral fragments.

Postoperative Care

One of the goals of open reduction and internal fixation is to obtain rigid internal fixation so that early functional use of the injured limb is possible. With rigid internal fixation, one can mobilize the patient earlier and thus perhaps minimize complications. In those fractures with adequate soft tissue coverage treated with open reduction and internal fixation, a postoperative splint is applied. Postoperative splinting helps with the decrease of soft tissue swelling and pain management techniques in the immediate postoperative period. We recommend beginning active and active-assisted range of motion between postoperative days 7 and 10. Passive range of motion should be avoided because it places excessive stress on the hardware fixation and may lead to the formation of heterotopic ossification. Occupational therapy is useful in the early postoperative period for range of motion of the wrist, hands, and shoulder.

Heterotopic ossification may be a complication of elbow trauma. This is known to occur more frequently about the elbow in burn victims and head-injured patients, but distal humerus fractures may have this complication. Early fixation, within the first 48 hours, has been found to decrease this risk when patients who had heterotopic ossification were evaluated.[26] Possible methods of prophylaxis against heterotopic ossification include radiation and nonsteroidal anti-inflammatories.[27] There is evidence to support a single, low dose of radiation after surgery about the elbow.[27] At this time, prophylaxis against heterotopic ossification is not a standard of care for routine distal humeral fractures but should be considered if the patient also has a head injury.

Tips and Tricks

- Consider prophylaxis against heterotopic ossification.

Outcomes

There are many inadequacies in the literature regarding distal humerus fractures. Multiple studies exist, but comparisons between studies are difficult because of the diversity of the study populations in terms of fracture types, patient age, energy of injury, multiple surgical techniques used, and different scoring indices of functional outcome. The results of fixation of simple distal humeral fractures without significant intra-articular comminution (OTA C1) are going to be different than those of more severe fracture patterns with intra-articular comminution (OTA C2–3). Some studies include simple distal humerus fractures, whereas others focus only on those patients who have severe intra-articular fractures. It is not valid to directly compare studies with different proportions of fracture types because results may be biased.

A major problem with comparing studies is that there is a wide variation in patient's age among the studies. Because age is associated with osteoporosis, studies with a larger proportion of older patients may demonstrate worse results after internal fixation than do studies of predominantly younger persons. In fact, recent studies of patients over 65 demonstrate a much better outcome after total elbow arthroplasty compared with open reduction and internal fixation.[17] In patients with osteoporotic bone, a type C2 or C3 fracture may occur with much lower energy of injury. Younger patients often have additional injuries and their mechanism of injury may involve a high-energy trauma. The quality of their bone and any associated soft tissue injury accompanying the fracture may all influence outcome. By including patients of different ages and patients with different mechanisms of injury, it is difficult to compare functional outcomes among different studies.

A second problem with interpretation of the literature is that functional outcome is reported using a variety of measures. Ideally, a standardized method would be used to compare outcomes and treatment. A useful functional outcome assessment should include patient self-assessment as well as objective measures. One of the goals of outcome analyses is to understand how technical factors related to the specific technique that is used affect outcomes. Although there is general agreement about the use of dual plates for repair of these fractures, there are many possible fixation techniques reported for fixation of distal humerus fractures, and controversy exists regarding some of the surgical techniques as well as the type of exposure. Two of the big areas of controversy include the use of ulnar nerve transposition and the type of olecranon osteotomy fixation. One study specifically included a population of high-energy trauma patients. Henley et al reported on 33 patients treated at a level 1 trauma center, with 20 of these classified as high-energy injuries.[4] Sixty-seven percent of their patients were described as being multiply injured, with 27% having ipsilateral upper extremity trauma. There were open fractures in 42%. Final results were available in 25 patients, with 92% of these having an excellent or good result. However, the complication rate was 45%. Nine of the 29 olecranon osteotomies had complications. Eight of these complications occurred in patients who had parallel K-wires and a tension band for olecranon fixation. There was only one patient who had osteotomy fixation with a 6.5 mm cancellous screw and tension-band wire that developed a complication.

As mentioned before, one of the controversies in the treatment of distal humerus fractures is the management of the ulnar nerve. Wang et al reported on the treatment of intra-articular fractures of the distal humerus in 20 patients and performed routine anterior subcutaneous transposition of the ulnar nerve using a posterior operative approach.[8] The majority of patients had more complex OTA C2 and C3 fractures. Two plates were placed, with one plate medial and one plate posterolateral. According to the Cassebaum rating and subjective functional status, there were 15 excellent or good results, two fair results, and three poor results. There were no reports of postoperative ulnar nerve palsies.

McKee et al reported on the functional outcome following surgical treatment of intra-articular distal humerus fractures through a posterior approach.[6] This study is unique because, instead of using surgeon- and radiographically based outcome measures, a more functional outcome assessment was done, with objective testing of muscle strength and use of patient-based questionnaires, including the Disabilities of the Arm, Shoulder and Hand (DASH) form, the Short Form-36 (SF-36) general health status questionnaire, and objective muscle testing. There were 25 patients in this study with an average age of 47 years and isolated closed, displaced intra-articular fractures of the distal humerus. All fractures were approached posteriorly with fixation of both the medial and lateral columns. There were 11 patients who underwent olecranon osteotomy, whereas the remainder of the patients were treated with a triceps-splitting approach. The average follow-up was 37 months. The average arc of motion was 108 degrees. Objective strength evaluation found decreased strength with flexion at 90 degrees and extension at 45, 90, and 120 degrees. The DASH score average was 20, indicating a mild residual impairment. The SF-36 score indicated minor but significant decreases in physical function scores and no changes in the mental scores. Six patients required more surgery, and in three of these patients it was due to painful elbow hardware.

Gofton and colleagues reviewed the functional outcome of 23 AO type C (bicondylar) distal humeral fractures managed with dual orthogonal plate fixation at a mean of 45 months.[28] These investigators used a combination of patient-rated outcomes [DASH, Patient Rated Ulnar Nerve Evaluation (PRUNE), American Shoulder and Elbow Surgeons Elbow form (ASES-e), and SF-36], as well as clinical, radiographic, and objective evaluations to assess outcomes. In this study the patients had minimal subjective deficits, with a mean satisfaction of 93%. The elbow range of motion was decreased in flexion-extension (122 degrees relative to 138 degrees, $p < .01$), whereas strength was lower for both elbow flexion-extension and forearm rotation ($p < .05$). Although the overall complication rate was 48%, most were resolved without further surgery. Routine ulnar nerve transposition was done and there were no ulnar neuropathies identified at follow-up.[28]

Another study specifically evaluated distal humerus fractures in 24 women older than age 65 and compared osteosynthesis to elbow arthroplasty.[17] It can be inferred that these patients had osteoporotic bone; the injuries were low energy, and there were no open fractures and no neurovascular injuries. Half were treated with open reduction and internal fixation, and half were treated with a total elbow arthroplasty. In those patients treated with open reduction and internal fixation, four patients had excellent results, four had good results, one had a fair result, and three had poor results. The poor results were all related to failure of fixation, one in the immediate intraoperative time period and two in the postoperative period. These were all converted to total elbow arthroplasty. The average Mayo score was 87.7, with an average arc of motion of 30 to 110 degrees in the patients treated with open reduction and internal fixation. In contrast, those patients who were treated with total elbow arthroplasty had less operative time and less tourniquet time, and there were 11 excellent and one good result. There were no fair or poor results. In this study, women with intra-articular distal humerus fractures over age 65 treated with total elbow arthroplasty had better outcomes.[17] Total elbow arthroplasty should be considered a viable treatment for women older than 65, and particularly those women with associated comorbidities as demonstrated in this study, including rheumatoid arthritis, osteoporosis, and routine use of systemic steroids.

Complications

The trend in treatment of intra-articular distal humerus fractures has shifted toward operative fixation of these complex fractures. However, despite anatomical reduction and rigid fixation of intra-articular fractures of the distal humerus, a full functional recovery may be difficult to realize. Some degree of loss of motion, particularly elbow extension, is commonplace following such an injury. Other complications that may occur after operative fixation of intra-articular distal humerus fractures include failure of fixation, nonunion and malunion, heterotopic ossification, and infection.

Failure of Fixation

Intra-articular distal humerus fractures are difficult to repair. The complex anatomy of the distal humerus must be completely understood so that anatomical restoration is achieved. Fracture comminution and instability, combined with difficulties in surgical exposure, make osteosynthesis a challenge in every case. In the older patient, there may be a significant osteoporosis and further comminution that creates even more difficulties with achieving stable reduction and fixation. Failure of fixation most often results from technical problems related to inadequate methods of fixation.[29] Smooth pins or K-wires alone are not strong enough to secure the distal humerus. The choice of plates may affect results. Failure of fixation has been documented when one-third tubular plates are used; use of a semitubular plate is not recommended for fixation of intra-articular distal humerus fractures.[9,30] Failure of fixation may also result from failure to secure one of the columns. Bicolumnar fixation with plates at 90 degrees to one another is recommended for all intra-articular distal humerus fractures.

The patient with failure of fixation may present with pain, decreased motion, and radiographic evidence of screw or plate failure or breakage. In these instances revision surgery should be considered. Failure to treat mechanical problems with fixation can lead to nonunion. The initial fixation should be scrutinized for technical errors, and repeat fixation performed with a mechanically sound construct. One should give strong consideration to adding bone graft or providing some other method of biophysical stimulation of fracture healing in these instances.

Nonunion

Nonunion of distal humerus fractures is a topic that has been neglected in the literature. In most large published series, this complication is rare; occurring in 2 to 10% of fractures.[4,5,7,8,29,31,32] The patient clinically presents with pain and often has accompanying soft tissue problems, including decreased range of motion, ulnar neuropathy, and heterotopic ossification. Revision surgery in a patient with a nonunion of the distal humerus is technically quite demanding due to the often osteoporotic bone, distortion of the local anatomy, previously implanted hardware (which may or may not have failed mechanically), and extensive pericapsular fibrosis.

The goal of treatment of any nonunion is restoration of function, achieving a stable union, acceptable alignment, and a functional range of motion. There are several prerequisites to successful surgical management: the patient must have sufficient bone stock and be able to tolerate the surgery, ulnar nerve transposition and capsular releases are often needed, the fracture must be mobilized and reduced properly, and stable internal fixation must be achieved.[33] Patients who undergo revision open reduction and internal fixation for nonunions may require additional surgery for hardware removal, excision of heterotopic bone, ulnar neurolysis, and/or manipulation under anesthesia.[33] In the largest published series of the treatment of distal humeral nonunions, Helfet et al reported on 52 patients with a delayed or nonunion of the distal humerus.[33] It took 26 years to collect the patients for this study. Nonunion most often resulted from mechanical failure of the initial fixation, although many of the patients had high-energy injuries. Helfet at al found that open reduction through an extensile exposure with soft tissue releases and rigid internal fixation consistently resulted in healing of distal humeral fractures that had been complicated by delayed union or nonunion.[33] The elbow range of motion increased from 71 degrees preoperatively to 94 degrees postoperatively. It should be noted that 15 patients in their series (29%) needed additional surgery after the index procedure.[33]

For a patient who is older and has low physical demands or whose bone stock is deficient, total elbow arthroplasty may be a reasonable treatment alternative for nonunions and malunions. It is important that the patient be carefully evaluated to rule out infection. A semiconstrained prosthesis is recommended in these instances because the soft tissue or bony structures may be incompetent to support elbow stability.[2]

Malunion

Malunion is an even less common complication of distal humeral fractures that have been treated operatively. Just as is the cases for a nonunion, the surgeon must carefully evaluate the complaints, expectations, radiographs, alignment, range of motion, and neurovascular examination of patients with malunited distal humeral fractures. Extra-articular malunion may lead to angular deformity, typically cubitus varus. The functional implications of such angular deformity are slight. In contrast, intra-articular malunion may contribute to posttraumatic arthritis with pain and stiffness.

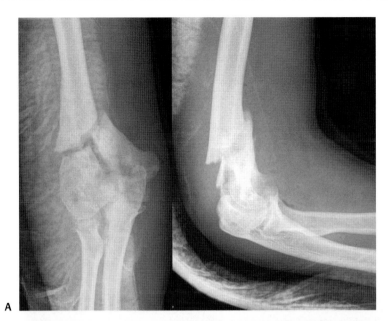

A

Figure 13–16 Infected distal humerus fracture. **(A)** Injury x-ray of open fracture. **(B)** Postoperative x-ray after plate fixation. (*Continued* p. 302)

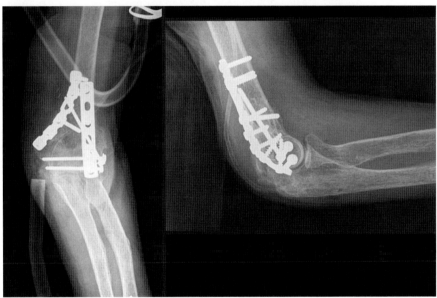

B

Surgical correction of selected patients with malunion would be expected to lead to improved results. In general, extra-articular malunion should be relatively straightforward to address with corrective supracondylar osteotomy, rigid fixation, and appropriate soft tissue releases, including ulnar neurolysis. Intra-articular malunion is much more difficult to address because of possible articular damage and the more difficult exposure. Although many such cases may be best managed with elbow arthroplasty, case reports suggest that corrective osteotomy in these difficult situations can lead to a good outcome.[34]

Infection

Fortunately, sepsis is rare following fixation of distal humeral fractures. One should be suspicious of infection when wound healing is disturbed or there are signs of sepsis such as purulent drainage or early fixation failure. When infection occurs, aggressive treatment is warranted. Serial wound debridements should be done, and both systemic as well as local antibiotics can be provided. Empirical antistaphylococcal antibiotics are typically provided until cultures are available. If the fixation is stable, the hardware may be maintained as long as the wound can be sterilized with just a few debridements **(Fig. 13–16A–D).** If the wound remains infected despite multiple debridements, hardware removal is indicated. Ring and colleagues used the Ilizarov fixator to salvage five patients with infected fractures of the distal humerus.[35] The fracture ultimately united in four of the five patients, and all five had greater than 85 degrees of elbow motion.

Figure 13–16 *(Continued)* Infected distal humerus fracture. **(C)** Clinical photograph of infected wound. **(D)** Debridement of the fracture site was performed with removal of bone graft. An olecranon osteotomy was performed for improved debridement. These x-rays demonstrate final healing after a 6-week course of intravenous antibiotics.

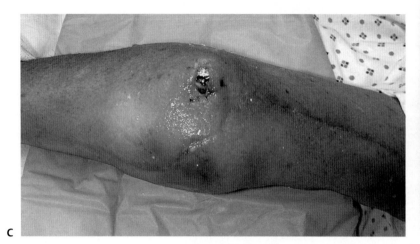

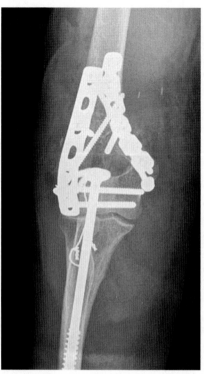

C

D

Ulnar Neuropathy

Ulnar nerve dysfunction is a known complication of distal humerus fractures. The nerve is at risk both from the original trauma and from the surgical procedure. The incidence of ulnar nerve palsy ranges in the literature is from 7 to 15% for ulnar nerve palsy.[3–5,8,13] A careful preoperative examination is of paramount importance in the evaluation of neurovascular function to identify nerve dysfunction prior to planned surgery. Most often, ulnar neuropathy results from surgical manipulation of the nerve, inadequate release of the nerve, and/or postoperative immobilization. These are all factors that may contribute to fibrosis about the nerve. At the time of surgical fixation, the surgeon is faced with the decision to transpose the nerve or not. Routine anterior subcutaneous transposition of the nerve has been recommended as a means of preventing the risk of ulnar nerve–related symptoms.[8,36] Wang et al transposed the ulnar nerve anteriorly in 20 patients and had no incidents of postoperative ulnar nerve complication.[8] Similarly, Gupta et al reported ulnar nerve neurapraxia in only one of 55 cases following treatment of intracondylar fractures of the distal humerus when an anterior transposition of the ulnar nerve was performed.[36] Important factors to consider are careful handling of the nerve at the time of surgery to minimize scarring and fibrosis, and if an anterior ulnar nerve transposition is completed, ensuring that there is adequate soft tissue release both proximally and distally

to allow the nerve to be transposed without tension in the tissues. Achievement of stable fixation to allow early range of motion may also minimize problems with ulnar nerve symptoms.

When a patient does present with ulnar nerve symptoms, good results are reported with ulnar nerve neurolysis. McKee et al reported on a series of 20 patients who had ulnar neurolysis for posttraumatic ulnar nerve symptoms at the time of reconstruction of the elbow; one had excellent, 17 had good, and two had poor results.[37] Poor results have been associated with failure of underlying elbow reconstruction.

Loss of Motion

The key to restoring a functional range of motion after surgical repair is early mobilization. The elbow is particularly prone to stiffness after prolonged immobilization; this tendency is even worse following a severe injury and extensive surgery. Thus it is important that surgical fixation achieves sufficient stability to allow early range of motion. Early mobilization with active and active-assisted flexion and extension is recommended. Supination and pronation are generally unaffected with distal humerus fractures, especially when treated with early mobilization.

Despite appropriate surgery, however, there are patients who develop severe stiffness and limitation of motion and are unable to perform their activities of daily living. The patient with severe stiffness can be treated with contracture release of the elbow, which may include an anterior and posterior capsular release and hardware removal. Often, the ulnar nerve may need to be transposed because there may be perineural fibrosis. Heterotopic ossification may contribute to decreased range of motion and stiffness and if present may need to be excised (see the following section).

Heterotopic Ossification

Heterotopic ossification is a recognized complication of distal humerus fractures that occurs in ~4% of cases, with a range of 3 to 49%.[5,32] Heterotopic ossification contributes to significant limitations of motion. It is thought to be more prevalent in those patients with head or spinal cord injuries and in burn patients. However, in patients suffering high-energy trauma, the original injury may play an important role in fibrosis and scarring. In the polytrauma patient there may be other contributing factors, including the difficulty of achieving early mobilization postoperatively because such patients may remain intubated or sedated for prolonged periods.

The problem of heterotopic ossification perhaps can be addressed with preventive measures initially. This has already been discussed in the section regarding the timing of surgery and the use of prophylaxis. The biggest dilemma about preventing heterotopic ossification is deciding whether prophylaxis should be offered, and if so, what method should be used. Because heterotopic ossification is not common in the absence of contributing factors such as head trauma, routine prophylaxis is not common. Low-dose radiation is effective when prophylaxis is warranted.[27]

Surgical excision of heterotopic bone should be considered when function is significantly impaired. Operative excision of heterotopic bone can be considered as early as 6 to 9 months after the injury. The surgical approach should be chosen depending on the location of the heterotopic bone and any other specific problems about the elbow. Excision of the bone should be completed along with any necessary capsular or ligamentous releases to restore mobility while maintaining stability. After excision of the bone, the patient should participate in a carefully controlled rehabilitation program. Postoperative prophylaxis with either or both indomethacin and a low dose of radiation should be considered.

Complications Related to the Olecranon Osteotomy

The olecranon osteotomy is valuable in providing excellent exposure of the articular surface of the distal humerus.

However, complications of this procedure have been reported, ranging from painful hardware to frank nonunion.[20] Jupiter el al reported up to 70% rate of hardware removal with fixation of distal humerus fractures, with most of these cases being related to the olecranon fixation.[5] Although the complication rate of olecranon osteotomy fixation with two parallel K-wires was high in the study by Henley et al,[4] Ring and colleagues more recently reported excellent union (98%) with use of a chevron osteotomy and secure fixation with K-wires anchored in the anterior cortex of the ulna and a figure-of-eight tension band.[20] Alternatively, use of a cancellous screw and tension-band wire may be used; advantages of this are the ability to predrill the screw and use it to achieve interfragmentary compression.

Prominent, painful hardware is the most common complication of olecranon osteotomy. Simple surgical removal of the offending hardware is typically effective. Healing complications are rare. When delayed union occurs, expectant management is often sufficient. Rarely, revision fixation might be necessary for symptomatic nonunion or loss of fixation.

New Techniques

With the same posterior approach, there are different techniques that can be used to visualize the articular surface of the distal humerus. These include olecranon osteotomy, the triceps-splitting approach, and the TRAP approach. Archdeacon described combining the olecranon osteotomy and a posterior triceps-splitting approach for complex fractures of the distal humerus.[38] This technique was used in his study in two patients with severe comminuted intra-articular fractures at the distal humerus with extension proximally to the midshaft of the humerus. By combining the two techniques, it allowed exposure of the distal humerus articular surface and the necessary exposure of the humeral shaft fracture to allow rigid fixation. There are no studies available that compare or provide outcomes regarding this combined approached.

Locking plates are now available that employ fixed-angle screws. Evidence indicates that these plates have improved fixation in osteoporotic bone in general.[39] However, when applied to a simulated distal humerus fracture, plate configuration (dorsal versus 90 degree) was more important than plate type (reconstruction plate vs locking compression plate).[25] The authors of this study did note that the bone–implant interface was less likely to fail during testing with locking compression plates, suggesting that there may be some improvement in fixation in osteoporotic individuals. The clinical significance of these findings is not yet known.

Pearls

- Distal humeral fractures have a bimodal age distribution: high-energy injuries generally occur in younger patients, whereas low-energy fractures predominate in the elderly and are often associated with osteoporosis.
- The trend in treatment of distal humerus fractures has shifted toward operative fixation.
- Operative fixation at best yields 75% good to excellent results.
- Postoperatively, the goal is early mobilization and return of function.
- The rates of nonunion (2%) and infection (0 to 6%) are low.
- Bicolumnar fixation is recommended for distal humerus fractures. Articular visualization may be improved with an olecranon osteotomy.
- Failure of fixation most often results from technical difficulties and inadequate methods of fixation.
- Ulnar nerve dysfunction is a known complication of distal humerus fractures, with a range of 7 to 15% for ulnar nerve palsy.

- Ulnar nerve transposition is controversial. The most important factors to consider at the time of surgery include careful handling of the nerve to minimize fibrosis and, if a transposition is completed, that an adequate release is done both proximally and distally.
- Heterotopic ossification occurs in ~4% of cases, with a range reported in the literature of 3 to 49%. The occurrence may increase with concomitant closed head injury, burns, or spinal cord injury.
- Hardware and nonunion problems may occur after an olecranon osteotomy. A chevron osteotomy and secure fixation (cancellous screw and tension-band wire) may lead to fewer problems.
- Total elbow arthroplasty may be beneficial in those patients over 65 years of age with significantly comminuted fractures and osteopenic bone. A semiconstrained prosthesis is recommended.

On the DVDs

Video 13–1 (Disk 2) Total Elbow Arthroplasty This video demonstrates the management of a comminuted distal humeral fracture in an elderly, osteoporotic patient with total elbow arthroplasty.
Video 13–2 (Disk 2) ORIF of the Distal Humerus This video shows the technique of internal fixation of a supracondylar/inter-

condylar (C2) fracture in a polytrauma patient. The video highlights the surgical exposure including olecranon osteotomy, fracture reduction, provisional fixation, and fixation of the medial and lateral column.

References

1. Robinson CM, Hill RM, Jacobs N, Dall G, Court-Brown CM. Adult distal humeral metaphyseal fractures: epidemiology and results of treatment. J Orthop Trauma 2003;17:38–47
2. Diana JN, Ramsey ML. Decision making in complex fractures of the distal humerus: current concepts and potential pitfalls. U Penn Orthop J 1998;11:12–18
3. Helfet DL, Schmeling GJ. Bicondylar intraarticular fractures of the distal humerus in adults. Clin Orthop Relat Res 1993;292:26–36
4. Henley MB, Bone LB, Parker B. Operative management of intra-articular fractures of the distal humerus. J Orthop Trauma 1987;1:24–35
5. Jupiter JB, Neff U, Holzach P, Allgower M. Intercondylar fractures of the humerus. J Bone Joint Surg Am 1985;67:226–239
6. McKee MD, Wilson TL, Winston L, Schemitsch EH, Richards RR. Functional outcome following surgical treatment of intra-articular distal humeral fractures through a posterior approach. J Bone Joint Surg Am 2000;82:1701–1707
7. Papaioannou N, Babis GC, Kalavritinos J, Pantazopoulos T. Operative treatment of type C intra-articular fractures of the distal humerus: the role of stability achieved at surgery on final outcome. Injury 1995;26:169–173
8. Wang K, Shih H, Shih C. Intercondylar fractures of the distal humerus: routine anterior subcutaneous transposition of the ulnar nerve in a posterior operative approach. J Trauma 1994;36:770–773

9. Wildburger R, Mahring M, Hofer HP. Supraintercondylar fractures of the distal humerus: results of internal fixation. J Orthop Trauma 1991;5:301–307
10. Cassebaum WH. Open reduction of T & Y fractures of the lower end of the humerus. J Trauma 1969;9:915–925
11. Riseborough EJ, Radin EL. Intercondylar T fractures of the humerus in the adult: a comparison of operative and non-operative treatment of twenty-nine cases. J Bone Joint Surg Am 1969;51:130–141
12. Jupiter JB, Mehne DK. Fractures of the distal humerus. In: Browner B, Jupiter J, Levine A, Trafton P, eds. Skeletal Trauma. Philadelphia: WB Saunders; 1991:1146–1176
13. Ring D, Jupiter JB. Complex fractures of the distal humerus and their complications. J Shoulder Elbow Surg 1999;8:85–97
14. Muller ME. The comprehensive classification of fractures of long bones. In: Muller ME, Allgower M, Schneider R, Willenegger H, eds. Manual of Internal Fixation: Techniques Recommended by the AO-ASIF Group. 3rd ed. Heidelberg: Springer-Verlag; 1991;p.
15. Wainwright AM, Williams JR, Carr AJ. Interobserver and intraobserver variation in classification systems for fractures of the distal humerus. J Bone Joint Surg Br. 2000;82:625–626
16. Ring D, Jupiter JB, Gulotta L. Articular fractures of the distal part of the humerus. J Bone Joint Surg Am 2003;85:232–238
17. Frankle MA, Herscovici D, DiPasquale TG, Vasey MB, Sanders RW. A comparison of open reduction and internal fixation and primary

total elbow arthroplasty in the treatment of intraarticular distal humerus fractures in women older than age 65. J Orthop Trauma 2003;17:473–480

18. Garcia JA, Mykula R, Stanley D. Complex fractures of the distal humerus in the elderly: the role of total elbow replacement as primary treatment. J Bone Joint Surg Br 2002;84:812–816

19. Cassebaum WH. Operative treatment of T and Y fractures of the lower end of the humerus. Am J Surg 1952;83:265–270

20. Ring D, Gulotta L, Chin K, et al. Olecranon osteotomy for exposure of fractures and nonunions of the distal humerus. J Orthop Trauma 2004;18:446–449

21. O'Driscoll SW. The triceps-reflecting anconeus pedicle (TRAP) approach for distal humeral fractures and nonunions. Orthop Clin North Am 2000;31:91–101

22. Bryan RS, Morrey BF. Extensive posterior exposure of the elbow: a triceps-sparing approach. Clin Orthop Relat Res 1982;166:188–192

23. Helfet DL, Hotchkiss RN. Internal fixation of the distal humerus: a biomechanical comparison of methods. J Orthop Trauma 1990;4:260–264

24. Schemitsch EH, Tencer AF, Henley MB. Biomechanical evaluation of methods of internal fixation of the distal humerus. J Orthop Trauma 1994;8:468–475

25. Korner J, Diederichs G, Arzdorf M, et al. A biomechanical evaluation of methods of distal humerus fracture fixation using locking compression plates versus conventional reconstruction plates. J Orthop Trauma 2004;18:286–293

26. Ilahi OA, Strausser DW, Gabel GT. Post-traumatic heterotopic ossification about the elbow. Orthopedics. 1998;21:265–268

27. Stein DA, Patel R, Egol KA, Kaplan FT, Tejwani NC, Koval KJ. Prevention of heterotopic ossification at the elbow following trauma using radiation therapy. Bull Hosp Jt Dis 2003;61: 51–154

28. Gofton WT, Macdermid JC, Patterson SD, Faber KJ, King GJ. Functional outcome of AO type C distal humeral fractures. J Hand Surg [Am] 2003;28:294–308

29. Sodergard J, Sandelin J, Bostman O. Mechanical failures of internal fixation in T and Y fractures of the distal humerus. J Trauma 1992;33:687–690

30. Gupta R. Intercondylar fractures of the distal humerus in adults. Injury 1996;27:569–572

31. Kinik H, Atalar H, Mergen E. Management of distal humerus fractures in adults. Arch Orthop Trauma Surg 1999;119:467–469

32. Kundel K, Braun W, Wieberneit J, Ruter A. Intraarticular distal humerus fractures: factors affecting outcome. Clin Orthop Relat Res 1996;332:200–208

33. Helfet DL, Kloen P, Anand N, Rosen HS. ORIF of delayed and nonunions of distal humerus fractures. J Bone Joint Surg Am 2003;85:33–40

34. Kazuki K, Miyamoto T, Ohzono K. Intra-articular corrective osteotomy for the malunited intercondylar humeral fracture: a case report. Osaka City Med J 2002;48:95–100

35. Ring D, Jupiter JB, Toh S. Salvage of contaminated fractures of the distal humerus with thin wire external fixation. Clin Orthop Relat Res 1999;359:203–208

36. Gupta R, Khanchandani P. Intercondylar fractures of the distal humerus in adults: a critical analysis of 55 cases. Injury 2002;33:511–515

37. McKee MD, Jupiter JB, Bosse G, Goodman L. Outcome of ulnar neurolysis during post-traumatic reconstruction of the elbow. J Bone Joint Surg Br 1998;80:100–105

38. Archdeacon MT. Combined olecranon osteotomy and posterior triceps splitting approach for complex fractures of the distal humerus. J Orthop Trauma 2003;17:368–373

39. Egol KA, Kubiak EN, Fulkerson E, Kummer FJ, Koval KJ. Biomechanics of locked plates and screws. J Orthop Trauma 2004;18:488–493

14 Elbow Trauma

David Ring and Neil Harness

The surgical treatment of trauma to the adult elbow, including most forms of traumatic elbow instability, has evolved rapidly in recent years because the problems have been better defined and many useful concepts and techniques have been established.[1] The lateral rather than the medial collateral ligament is now the focus of elbow stability, along with the coronoid process. Most simple elbow dislocations[2] and isolated partial radial head fractures[3] recover well without surgery, but the majority of other injuries to the proximal radius and ulna benefit from surgery. Each specific complex injury type is not very common. Surgeons must rely on a familiarity with normal and pathological anatomy of the elbow and a variety of repair techniques.

Anatomy

The olecranon and coronoid processes of the proximal ulna form the trochlear notch that articulates with the trochlea of the humerus. The trochlear notch has olecranon and coronoid articular facets separated by the relatively nonarticular transverse groove of the trochlear notch (**Fig. 14–1**). The trochlear notch prevents anterior-posterior translation of the ulna on the humerus and also provides varus, valgus, and rotational stability to the elbow. The amount of stability afforded the elbow from its bony architecture is greatest with the elbow in flexion and decreases with extension. It has been shown that the stability provided by the ulnohumeral articulation gradually decreases as the proximal ulna is incrementally resected.[4] The triceps inserts on the dorsal surface of the olecranon, blending with the periosteum and the forearm fascia.

The coronoid process is the anterior extension of the trochlear notch. It serves as the point of insertion of the anterior capsule and the anterior band of the medial collateral ligament, which inserts on the sublime tubercle of the anteromedial base of the coronoid process (**Fig. 14–1**).[5] The brachialis muscle extends slightly distal to the coronoid on the anterior surface of the ulna. The medial collateral ligament is made up of anterior, posterior, and transverse bands. The anterior band is the most discrete structure and the most important for valgus elbow stability.[6] It originates from the midportion of the undersurface of the medial epicondyle and also inserts on the sublime tubercle of the coronoid process. The lateral aspect of the coronoid is continuous with the radial (lesser sigmoid) notch of the ulna.

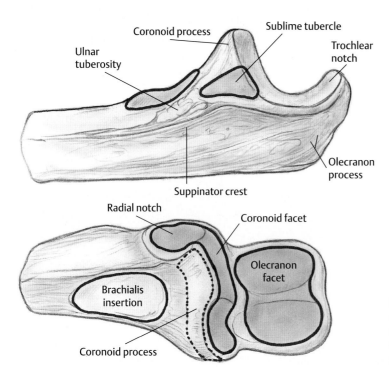

Figure 14–1 The trochlear notch has separate coronoid and olecranon articular facets. The brachialis has a broad attachment to the ulna that extends distal to the coronoid. The anterior band of the medial collateral ligament attaches to the medial aspect of the base of the coronoid.

The radial head articular surface is concave and articulates with the convex capitellum of the distal humerus. There is an angulation (~15 degrees) of the radial neck with respect to the radial shaft. Approximately 240 degrees of the outside circumference of the radial head articulates with the lesser sigmoid notch of the proximal ulna and is covered by hyaline cartilage.[7,8] The remaining anterolateral third is not covered by articular cartilage and is also the area most often fractured. The proximal radioulnar joint is stabilized by the annular and quadrate ligaments and the interosseous membrane.[9]

The lateral collateral ligament complex is probably the most important stabilizer of the elbow.[1] Its effect is most apparent when testing posterolateral rotatory (rather than varus) stability. Although some have emphasized the importance of the lateral ulnar collateral ligament itself,[10] others have found the contributions to posterolateral rotatory stability to be more complex, with contributions from the annular ligament and the fascia of the common extensor musculature.[11]

Handling of the skin around the elbow is fairly straightforward because there is an excellent blood supply with an extensive longitudinal collateral blood supply. A direct posterior skin incision allows access to nearly the entire elbow with the elevation of broad, full-thickness skin flaps.[12] It also limits the potential for injury to cutaneous nerves because these are kept in the flaps.[13] More limited lateral or medial incisions and simultaneous separate medial and lateral exposures can also be used.

Radial Head Fractures

The management of fractures of the radial head varies substantially depending upon whether the fracture is an isolated injury or part of a more complex injury that has compromised the stability of the elbow or forearm.[14] With isolated, nondisplaced, or minimally displaced fractures, the goal of treatment is to restore or maintain forearm rotation, which is nearly always possible with nonoperative treatment.[3,15] In more complex injuries, repair or replacement of the radial head is desirable for its contribution to elbow and forearm stability.[1,16]

Open reduction and internal fixation of comminuted radial head fractures is much less predictable than operative repair of simple fractures.[14,17] The risk of early fixation failure, eventual nonunion and collapse of the fracture, and restriction of forearm rotation[14] have made a metal prosthesis more appealing in the treatment of radial head fractures associated with destabilizing injuries of the forearm and elbow.[18]

Classification

Mason's classification of radial head fractures is popular but often misrepresented. He classified radial head fractures into three types: nondisplaced (type 1), displaced

partial articular (type 2), and displaced and comminuted fractures involving the entire head (type 3).[3] Johnston suggested a fourth category for radial head fractures associated with elbow dislocations;[19] however, this is not useful for two reasons: (1) there are several types of injury patterns that have an associated fracture of the radial head, all of which merit clear distinction from simple isolated fractures, and (2) regardless of the overall injury pattern, the specific characteristics of the fracture are important in determining management and prognosis. It is interesting to note that Mason did not account for fractures of the radial neck (those with the articular surface intact) in his system.

It is not uncommon to see Mason's system reported along with criteria for acceptable size and displacement of the fragments as measured on radiographs. There are little or no data to support these radiographic criteria, and the measurements themselves are likely to be unreliable based upon variations in patient positioning for radiographs and the measurement techniques used.

There are several additional injury factors that will affect management and prognosis of fractures of the radial head but are not consistently accounted for in classification systems. For both partial and complete articular fractures (Mason types 2 and 3), the number and size of fracture fragments is important. In many cases fragments are created that are either too small for internal fixation or are lost in the soft tissues. It is also common to encounter fragments with little or no subchondral bone, particularly in older osteoporotic individuals. These fragments will also be difficult or impossible to repair. There is often impaction of either fracture fragments or the entire radial head (**Fig. 14–2**). When central articular fragments are impacted, realignment can leave them with little support, and bone grafting may need to be considered in addition to internal fixation. It is not uncommon for major portions of the radial head to be impacted. This is often not apparent

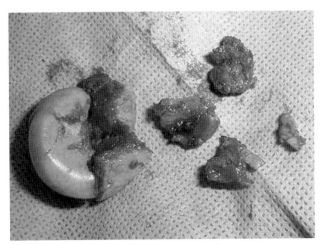

Figure 14–2 Fractures of the radial head often create impacted fragments and small fragments that cannot be repaired.

until it is noted that the smaller fragments cannot be repositioned accurately. Finally, there is occasionally a central impaction with expansion of the size of the radial head outward, which may be unsalvageable. All of these factors can be difficult to recognize and define. When the specific criterion of the number of fracture fragments is used, greater than three articular fragments (as suggested by Comprehensive Classification of Fractures, Muller et al[20]) has been associated with greater problems after operative fixation.[14]

It is important to distinguish fractures of the radial head associated with injury to the interosseous ligament of the forearm—the so-called Essex-Lopresti lesion.[21] Essex-Lopresti injuries are challenging to treat when recognized acutely but are associated with very poor and practically unsalvageable results when the forearm ligament injuries are initially overlooked.[22]

Radial head fractures are also an inherent part of posterior Monteggia fractures and posterior olecranon fracture-dislocations, present in over two thirds of patients.[23–26]

Nonoperative Treatment

Partial fractures of the radial head articular surface (Mason type 2) that are not associated with other fractures or ligament injuries usually do very well with nonoperative treatment in our experience, although at least one study has questioned this.[27] To our knowledge, there are no data to support the use of radiographic measurements (e.g., greater than 2 mm of articular surface incongruity, fragment involving greater than 30% of the joint) in deciding upon operative or nonoperative treatment. Because radiocapitellar arthritis is not a common sequela of this injury, the most important issue is whether the fracture limits forearm rotation by compromising the proximal radioulnar joint. Initially, patients may be too painful to demonstrate this; however, reexamination in a few weeks or aspiration and infiltration of the elbow joint with local anesthetic can help determine if there is a bony block to forearm rotation. Nonoperative treatment can be considered provided forearm motion is not restricted.

Comminuted fractures of the entire head are nearly always part of a complex injury to the forearm or elbow.[28] The treatment of Mason type 3 fractures of the radial head should be predicated on the high likelihood of associated ligament injury or fracture. For this reason, nonoperative treatment (or simple excision) of type 3 fractures should be considered with great caution. Type 3 fractures also have a high likelihood of restricting forearm rotation if treated nonoperatively.

The major risk when treating isolated fractures of the radial head that do not restrict forearm rotation is elbow stiffness. Although it is reasonable to apply a sling or splint to the elbow for comfort immediately after the injury, patients should realize that their recovery from the injury is directly dependent upon confident active use and motion exercises of the elbow as soon as possible after the injury.[3,15] Immobilization or failure to exercise the elbow within the first 2 weeks can cause permanent elbow stiffness. There should be little concern regarding fracture displacement or nonunion because nonunion of nonoperatively treated radial head fractures is uncommon and usually asymptomatic and inconsequential.[29,30]

Indications for Surgical Treatment

Excision of the radial head without replacement is a reasonable consideration in any patient that does not have either an Essex-Lopresti injury or a terrible triad fracture-dislocation of the elbow, but it should be used with great caution. When the stability of the forearm and elbow can be ensured, repair or replacement of the radial head has the relative advantages of supporting the elbow for vigorous activities such as throwing and heavy work and perhaps protecting the ulnohumeral joint from early arthrosis.[31] When the elbow is stable, excision of the radial head without prosthetic replacement is still a very useful treatment option in older patients with limited functional demands, and select younger patients. After excising the radial head, the elbow and forearm must be carefully tested for instability.[32]

Because the long-term performance of radial head prostheses is uncertain, it is preferable to repair the radial head when possible. The majority of partial (Mason type 2) fractures of the radial head are amenable to operative fixation; however, many of these partial head fractures consist of multiple small fragments, the repair of which is often tenuous. These complex partial radial head fractures should be considered for prosthetic replacement in the setting of troublesome injury patterns such as the Essex-Lopresti or terrible triad. Early failure of fixation in these injuries could compromise elbow or forearm stability and lead to substantial problems.

The results of the operative repair of fractures involving the entire radial head (Mason type 3) are much less predictable. When there are greater than three fragments, missing fragments, nonreconstructible fragments, or impacted fragments, operative fixation is much less likely to produce a good result,[14] and excision with or without prosthetic replacement is often preferable. Because most Mason type 3 fractures are associated with complex injury to the forearm or elbow, excision without replacement should be performed with caution and only in select patients.

Surgical Treatment

Surgical Anatomy

The posterior interosseous nerve (PIN) is at risk during approaches to the radial head due to its vulnerable location in the supinator muscle and its proximity to the radial neck. Pronation of the forearm translates the PIN away from the operative field approximately 1 cm anteromedially.[33] With the forearm in pronation, the proximal 38 mm of the lateral aspect of the radius may be safely exposed (average proximal safe zone 52.0 ± 7.8 mm). Supination decreases the safe zone to 22 mm (average 33.4 ± 5.7 mm).[34]

Surgical Technique

Operative Exposures

For isolated fractures Kocher's interval between the anconeus and extensor carpi ulnaris is useful; however, the surgeon should be careful not to incise the capsule posterior to the anterior margin of the anconeus because this can damage the lateral collateral ligament complex and lead to chronic posterolateral rotatory instability.[11] The capsular incision should be made obliquely, in line with the original muscle interval. A more anterior interval such as that described by Kaplan[35] and recently advocated by Hotchkiss[36] involves splitting the common extensors, roughly between the extensor digitorum communis and extensor carpi radialis brevis. Although this approach can better protect the lateral collateral ligament complex, it places the PIN at greater risk and can limit access to fragments that are displaced posteriorly in the elbow articulation.

When strict indications are applied, the majority of radial head fractures that are surgically treated will be part of a fracture-dislocation of the elbow. In this situation, the lateral collateral ligament complex is nearly always avulsed from the lateral epicondyle, as are some of the common extensor muscles **(Fig. 14–3)**. Furthermore, there is often a traumatic interval in the common extensor muscles that can be extended distally. In other words, it is

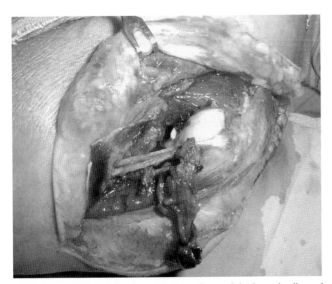

Figure 14–3 Elbow dislocations cause avulsion of the lateral collateral ligament from the lateral epicondyle. Although some of the musculotendinous tissues may remain attached to the epicondyle (as in this photo), the origin of the collateral ligament is nearly always avulsed.

easy to get excellent exposure of the radial head due to the associated ligament injury, and the interval to use is defined by the injury.

When treating a posterior olecranon fracture-dislocation, there is often a posterior muscle injury that can be used to expose the radial head, particularly when the olecranon fragment is mobilized proximally to access the coronoid (see **Video 14–1, Disk 2**). One should limit dissection between the proximal radius and ulna beyond what occurred due to the injury itself to limit the potential for radioulnar synostosis.

When distal exposure is needed for plate fixation, the forearm should be pronated to protect the PIN. Blunt dissection of the supinator and identification of the PIN may be advisable in particularly complex cases.

Radial Head Excision

Radial head excision is straightforward. The surgeon merely creates a safe and adequate exposure and removes the fragments. The level of resection is kept at the junction of the radial head and neck when possible in case a later reconstructive procedure is needed. If there is a lateral collateral ligament avulsion, it should be repaired.

Open Reduction and Internal Fixation

The techniques and prognosis of operative fixation of radial head fractures can vary substantially depending upon the type of fracture being treated. Most isolated partial articular (Mason type 2) fractures have limited displacement. Wide displacement is usually associated with fracture-dislocation of the elbow. The fractured area is rotated into the muscle interval (see **Video 14–1, Disk 2**). In most cases the fragment is impacted, and the periosteal sleeve is intact. The fragment can be repositioned by elevating it with a bone tamp. This technique preserves a measure of the inherent stability associated with impacted fracture fragments. Provisional fixation with 0.035 in. Kirschner wires is exchanged for 2.0 mm screws. Interfragmentary screws are used only if there is thick, good quality subchondral bone. Otherwise compression of the fragment is applied with a bone clamp or manually, and position screws are inserted. Alternatively, variable-pitch headless screws can be used to provide compression.

Partial articular fractures associated with fracture dislocation are more likely to be completely displaced with little or no soft tissue attachment. They are also more likely to be comminuted. If there are missing fragments, fragments too small to secure, fragments with little or no subchondral bone, or very osteoporotic fragments, operative fixation may be difficult or impossible. In the setting of a fracture-dislocation of the elbow or forearm, even a partial articular fracture of the radial head may be an important stabilizing element, and accepting tenuous fixation may be unwise. For this reason we have a relatively low threshold to resect the remaining radial head and replace it with a prosthesis rather than accept marginal fixation of a complex partial radial head fracture. If there are one or two large fragments with good quality subchondral bone, these can be realigned and secured with screws. In many cases one or more fragments are impacted. In addition, bone fragments are often missing or impacted between the radial head fragments and the radial neck. In both situations, it may be useful to use a plate to buttress the repair.

Fractures involving the entire head of the radius (Mason type 3) are nearly always associated with a fracture-dislocation of the forearm or elbow. When the fracture is associated with a complete posterior dislocation of the elbow, wide exposure of the radial head is facilitated by the avulsion of the lateral collateral ligament complex from the lateral epicondyle **(Fig. 14–3).** When the lateral collateral ligament is not ruptured (e.g., Essex-Lopresti injury, radial head fracture with medial collateral ligament injury), it may be necessary to detach the lateral collateral ligament origin and then repair it with a transosseous suture or suture anchors. Some surgeons prefer to perform an osteotomy of the lateral epicondyle and perform direct bone-to-bone repair at the time of closure.[37,38] In many cases it is easier to reassemble the articular fragments after they have been removed from the elbow wound and then replace the reconstructed radial head into the wound and secure it to the radial neck with a plate and screws. Small plates with 1.5 or 2.0 mm screws are used in most cases. In many cases a minicondylar or blade plate is used. Some newer plate designs feature screws that lock to the plate, forming fixed-angle buttress pins. Bone grafting should be considered if there are areas of the neck with significant bone loss.

Plates and screws placed upon the portion of the radial head that articulates with the sigmoid notch of the proximal ulna must be countersunk to limit the potential for impingement. A safe zone has been defined to allow insertion of hardware in the radial head. Based on anatomical studies, a 110 degree safe zone on the surface of the lateral aspect of the radial head may be mapped out during surgery.[7,8] A horizontal reference mark is made first with the forearm in neutral position. Two more horizontal marks are then made with the forearm in full pronation and supination. The most anterior limit is defined as two thirds the distance from the neutral to the fully supinated mark. The most posterior limit is one half the distance from the neutral to the fully pronated mark.

In general, if the safe zone is used, regular screws and plates should not impinge. In an anatomical study in which 2.0 or 2.7 mm T-plates were applied to the lateral aspect of the radial head with the forearm in neutral, there was no impingement with the sigmoid notch of the ulna.[39] Alternatively, the region between the radial styloid and Lister's tubercle is a useful guide for safe positioning of screws.[8]

A lag screw technique is ideal to provide compression and increased stability but is not always possible. In the case of an isolated radial head fracture, one or more variable pitch countersunk, headless screws may be used.

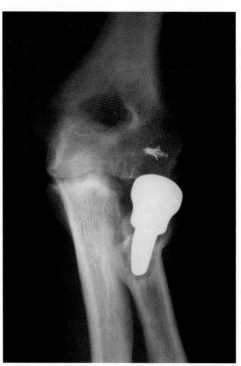

Figure 14–4 The major pitfall of prosthetic replacement of the radial head is insertion of a prosthesis that is too long, resulting in gapping of the lateral portion of the ulnohumeral joint and capitellar wear.

Prosthetic Replacement

The radial neck is prepared with small reamers. A tight fit is not necessary. The size of the prosthesis is selected based upon the resected fracture fragments. Prostheses that are too large can cause painful erosions of the capitellum and malalignment of the elbow **(Fig. 14–4).** Prostheses that are too small may provide inadequate stability. Oversizing of the prosthesis is more common, so it is safer to err toward a slightly smaller head. Using the largest fragment of the excised radial head as a template, a prosthesis with a slightly smaller diameter is selected. A prosthesis with a standard length is used in nearly every case. A pitfall is to measure the length of the head based on the largest radial head fragment. The prosthesis will sit on the proudest portion of the radial neck, equal to the shortest portion of the radial head. The level of resection should be the head–neck junction just as the neck begins to flare outward.

The radial head prosthesis acts as a stiff spacer. It does not need to have a tight fit in the intramedullary canal. It can be argued that a slightly undersized radial head and somewhat loose fit of the stem in the canal can accommodate for the imperfect anatomy of the radial head compared with the native radial head. Another way to try to account for this is by using a radial head prosthesis with a mobile, bipolar head. The bipolar prosthesis requires resection of the radial neck to the biceps tuberosity and cement fixation—both of which are likely to be more difficult to salvage if problems occur.

New Techniques

Several new plates and prostheses are in development. The plates incorporate locked buttress pins, which may help with support of the articular and metaphyseal fragments. The prostheses often incorporate a hinge for greater flexibility in anatomical contours.

Outcomes

Open Reduction and Internal Fixation

One retrospective review comparing open reduction and internal fixation versus nonoperative treatment of isolated Mason type 2 fractures of the radial head reported 90% good and excellent results for surgical treatment compared with 44% good and excellent results with nonoperative treatment. All of the fractures were Mason type 2 and were treated with screw fixation.[27] This is contrary to our experience in which the majority of Mason type 2 fractures recover very well without surgery, and long-term radiocapitellar arthritis is an uncommon source of problems or complaints in the office.

King et al reported a direct comparison of internal fixation of Mason type 2 and 3 fractures in 1991. They found that isolated noncomminuted Mason type 2 fractures had 100% good or excellent results. Type 3 fractures had only 33% good or excellent results, prompting the authors to recommend excision or arthroplasty in the setting of radial head comminution.[17]

Ring and colleagues found excellent results with operative treatment of isolated Mason type 2 fractures, but unsatisfactory results in four of 15 patients with Mason type 2 fractures associated with complex injuries. Among Mason type 3 fractures with fewer than three articular fragments, two had nonunions (one of which eventually healed over 2 years after the injury), and all had good forearm rotation. On the other hand, among patients with Mason type 3 fractures and greater than three articular fragments, only one of 14 achieved a satisfactory result (three early failures, six nonunions, four poor forearm rotation).[14]

Prosthetic Replacement

The use of a silicone prosthesis has lost favor due to fracture, dislocation, synovitis, lymphadenitis, and overall joint destruction.[40] Replacement of the radial head with a metal implant has been associated with good short- and medium-term results in 70 to 82% of patients in spite of the frequent complexity of the overall injury.[18,41,42] The long-term results are unknown. There is some concern that metal articulation with a radial head will cause problems. It is now well recognized that an oversized prosthesis will cause early changes on the capitellum with pain, synovitis, and limitation of motion.

Complications

Nonunion of radial head fractures can occur with both nonoperative and operative treatment. In both cases the nonunions are usually associated with limited or no symptoms, and late healing can occur. Crepitance and pain related to painful hardware often lead to a second surgery for radial head excision.

Loss of motion related to a malunited fracture of the radial head can often be salvaged with resection of the radial head.

Simple Elbow Dislocations

The elbow joint is inherently stable but dislocates at a rate second only to the shoulder, reflecting its vulnerability to injury.[43] Although most of the capsuloligamentous structures must be disrupted for a dislocation to occur,[44] the majority of patients do not experience a redislocation in the absence of associated fractures.[2,45] Dislocations of the elbow without associated fractures have been referred to as simple elbow dislocations, with fracture-dislocations representing complex dislocations.

Classification

The majority of elbow dislocations and fracture dislocations result in injury to all of the capsuloligamentous stabilizers of the elbow joint.[44,46–48] The exceptions include fracture-dislocations of the olecranon and other injuries with fractures of the coronoid involving nearly the entire coronoid process; these fractures are so unstable that elbow dislocation may occur despite less soft tissue injury.[1,16,26,49]

The progression of capsuloligamentous injury during elbow dislocation progresses from lateral to medial, and the elbow can completely dislocate with the anterior band of the medial collateral ligament intact (**Fig. 14–5A,B**).[44] There is also a variable degree of injury to the common flexor and extensor musculature.[46,47,50,51]

One recent study notes that the lateral collateral ligament complex fails by avulsion from the lateral epicondyle in over 75% of patients with elbow dislocations (**Fig. 14–3**).[52] In my personal observations treating over 60 fracture-dislocations of the elbow, I have found that the lateral collateral ligament is always avulsed from the lateral epicondyle. In many patients there are small pieces of the ligament or other long strands of musculotendinous tissue, which may lead the surgeon to misinterpret the situation (**Fig. 14–3**). Defined practically, reattachment of the soft tissue sleeve to the lateral epicondyle is nearly always sufficient.

Considerations of the direction of dislocation of the elbow are of limited value. Anterior dislocations are rare. Medial and lateral dislocations probably represent incompletely reduced posterior dislocations. Nearly all dislocations are posterior in direction. There is no established value to distinguishing posteromedial and posterolateral dislocations, although a posteromedial dislocation might be associated with a relative sparing of the medial soft tissues.[43,44]

O'Driscoll et al have described several stages of elbow instability.[44] Stage 1 involves partial or complete disruption of the lateral collateral ligament, which may result in slight posterior subluxation of the radial head with respect to the capitellum. Stage 2 involves an incomplete posterior dislocation with disruption of the lateral ligamentous complex and further injury to the osseous or ligamentous supporting structures either or both anteriorly and posteriorly. The medial edge of the ulna may be found to rest on the trochlea. This gives the appearance of the coronoid perched on the trochlea on a lateral radiograph.[44] Stage 3 is divided into three subgroups (A through C). Stage 3A involves injury to all the soft tissue support except the anterior band of the medial collateral ligament. The elbow dislocates in a posterolateral direction rotating about the intact anterior medial collateral ligament. Stage 3B involves injury to the entire medial ligamentous complex resulting in varus, valgus, and rotary instability. Stage 3C injuries are very unstable due to complete soft tissue disruption from the distal humerus with the ability to dislocate even when immobilized in a cast.[1]

Nonoperative Treatment

Nonoperative treatment is preferable for all simple elbow dislocations, with operative treatment reserved for the unusual patient with persistent instability after manipulative reduction and active exercise. Manipulative reduction can usually be obtained in the emergency room with conscious sedation. When the elbow has been dislocated for a long period of time, general anesthesia or regional block may be preferable. On occasion, very unstable dislocations that are seen acutely (for instance, an athlete on the playing field, or an older person with extensive muscle injury) may be reduced without anesthesia.

During manipulative reduction, it is important to keep the elbow in a relatively flexed position to limit the potential for entrapment of the median nerve and brachial artery within the joint. Usually, the alignment of the forearm in the medial-lateral plane is corrected first, and then the elbow is reduced with posteriorly directed pressure over the olecranon, supination of the forearm, and longitudinal traction. It can be helpful to perform the reduction with the patient in the lateral decubitus or prone position when an assistant is not available to provide countertraction on the upper arm.

Palpation of anatomical landmarks can be used to assess the alignment of the elbow prior to splinting and postreduction radiographs. The medial and lateral epicondyles and the dorsal point of the olecranon should form a triangle in the coronal plane. If the point of the olecranon is still posterior to the epicondyles, the elbow may not be concentrically reduced.

After manipulative reduction, testing of varus and valgus instability will not influence management. One should expect to find valgus instability unless this is one of the uncommon dislocations with incomplete medial collateral ligament injury. Varus instability is more difficult to isolate.[53] For the same reason, there is no point in performing a test for posterolateral rotatory instability (so-called pivot shift of the elbow[10]); one would expect it to be positive in 100% of adequately relaxed elbows, and it would not alter management.

It is more important to determine if there is a tendency for the elbow to subluxate or redislocate as the elbow is extended and at what point this occurs. If the elbow redislocates prior to ~30 degrees of flexion, retest it with the forearm in full pronation. Some surgeons have

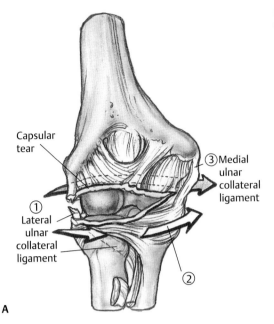

Capsular tear

③ Medial ulnar collateral ligament

① Lateral ulnar collateral ligament

②

A

Figure 14–5 (A) Soft tissue injury associated with elbow dislocation progresses from lateral to medial, with the anterior band of the medial collateral ligament the last structure to rupture. **(B)** There is a spectrum of posterolateral rotatory instability, with the final stage being complete dislocation. Complete dislocation can occur with the medial collateral ligament intact. (With permission from O'Driscoll SW, Morrey BF, Korinek S, An KN. Elbow subluxation and dislocation: a spectrum of instability. Clin Orthop 1992;280:186–197.)

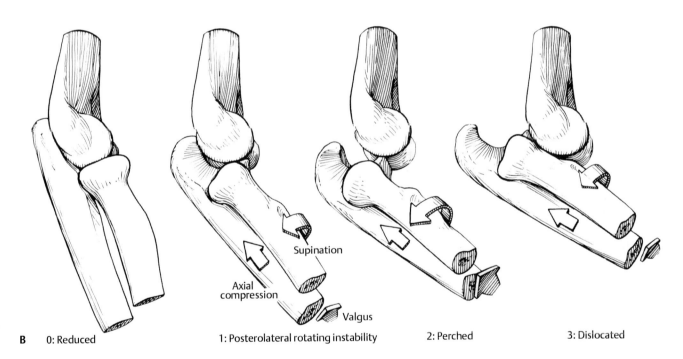

Supination

Axial compression

Valgus

B   0: Reduced   1: Posterolateral rotating instability   2: Perched   3: Dislocated

suggested that if this maneuver restores stability, a hinged brace that holds the forearm pronated may be useful.[54] Others recommend a hinged brace that prevents extension beyond the point of stability for a few weeks.[54] Our experience has been that an unstable elbow can dislocate in a cast,[55] and the patient may not be aware of it—therefore, we do not trust fracture braces and consider surgical treatment of elbows that redislocate prior to near terminal extension.

The patient is splinted for 1 or 2 weeks for comfort. The position of immobilization is usually 90 degrees of elbow flexion and neutral forearm rotation, although the forearm is pronated on occasion. Splinting for more than 2 weeks is associated with greater pain and stiffness.[2,45,50] In motivated patients it is not necessary to splint the elbow after dislocation.[56]

Patients should be seen by an orthopaedic surgeon within 2 weeks and encouraged to use their arm for light functional activity. They are taught exercises for regaining motion. Some patients will have a slight residual malalignment of the elbow on radiographs **(Fig. 14–6A,B)**.[47,57] Our preference is to treat this with a 1 week trial of confident active exercises because this often represents a type of "pseudosubluxation" related to muscle relaxation from

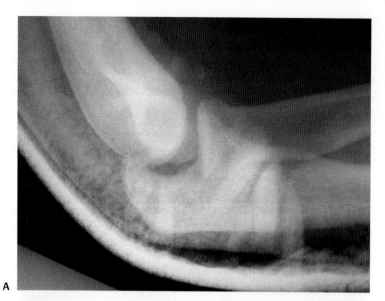

A

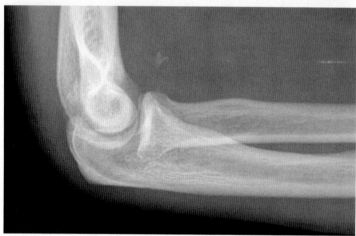

B

Figure 14–6 **(A)** Slight residual subluxation after dislocation or fracture dislocation is not uncommon. **(B)** Active exercises and use of the elbow add the contribution from the dynamic stabilizers of the elbow and usually restore a concentric reduction.

pain similar to that observed in shoulders. If addition of the dynamic muscular component of elbow stability fails to restore alignment, or if there is an associated coronoid fracture, surgical treatment may be necessary.

Indications for Surgical Treatment

In general, there are two types of patients in whom it may prove difficult or impossible to maintain a concentric reduction of a simple elbow dislocation: younger patients with very high-energy dislocations (such as a fall from several stories) and some older patients after simple falls. Both involve more extensive avulsion of the muscle origins along with the capsuloligamentous structures.[51]

Surgical Treatment

Surgical Anatomy

In some older patients, the medial muscular attachments to the humerus may be relatively spared, causing the elbow to hinge open due to more extensive disruption of the muscles and ligaments on the lateral side **(Fig. 14–7)**. The

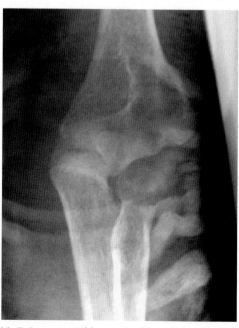

Figure 14–7 Some unstable simple elbow dislocations have relatively intact medial soft tissues, resulting in recurrent hinging open of the joint.

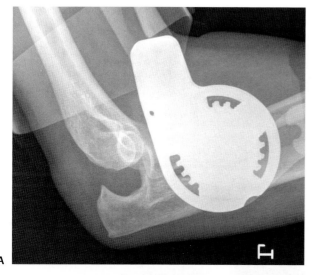

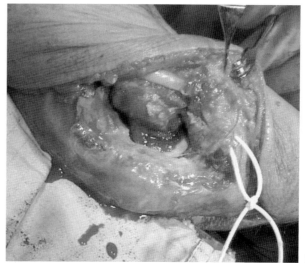

A

B

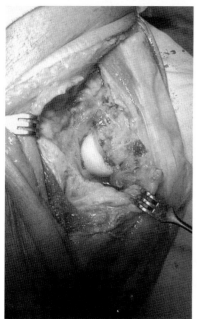

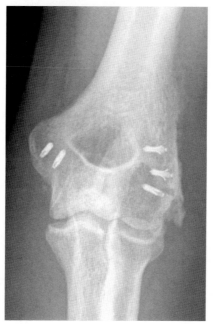

C,D

Figure 14–8 **(A)** Lateral elbow radiograph of a 38-year-old man immobilized in a hinged elbow brace after falling from a four-story height and sustaining an elbow dislocation treated with closed reduction. **(B)** The medial collateral ligament and a substantial portion of the flexor-pronator mass were avulsed from the medial epicondyle. **(C)** The lateral collateral ligament and most of the common extensor musculature were avulsed from the lateral epicondyle. **(D)** The medial and lateral soft tissues were reattached with suture anchors.

majority of patients with unstable simple elbow dislocations have extensive injury to the muscles that originates from the distal humerus.

Surgical Techniques

Soft Tissue Repair

Older patients with unstable simple elbow dislocations that seem to rotate out of joint on a relatively spared medial soft tissue hinge are usually easily stabilized by reattaching the lateral collateral ligaments and common extensor musculature to the lateral epicondyle **(Fig. 14–8A–D)**. If repair of the lateral soft tissue stabilizers alone proves insufficient, a medial exposure can be performed, the ulnar nerve subcutaneously transposed, and the medial collateral ligament and flexor-pronator muscle mass reattached to the medial epicondyle **(Fig. 14–8C,D)**. These repairs can be performed

either with suture anchors or with drill holes placed through bone. The origin of the lateral collateral ligament should be reattached as close as possible to its anatomical location at the center of rotation of the elbow—at the inferior point of a small tubercle on the lateral epicondyle. The origin of the medial collateral ligament should be reattached to the inferior surface of the medial epicondyle. The common flexor and extensor musculature is attached at these points and more proximal as needed.

Cross-Pinning of the Joint

In an older, infirm patient with limited demands and high anesthetic risks, a closed manipulation and cross-pinning of the elbow joint can be sufficient. Two stout, smooth Kirschner wires are used, avoiding the medial side of the elbow and the ulnar nerve. Some surgeons prefer to use screws due to concern that the Kirschner wires might not

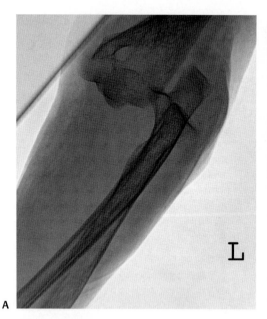

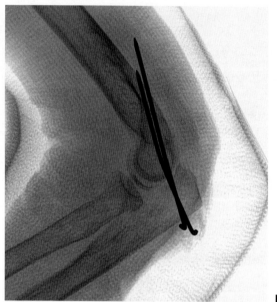

Figure 14–9 *(continued on page 317)*

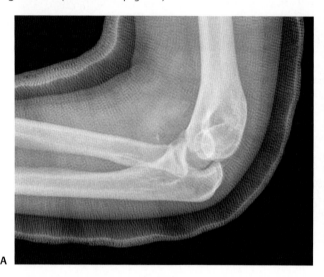

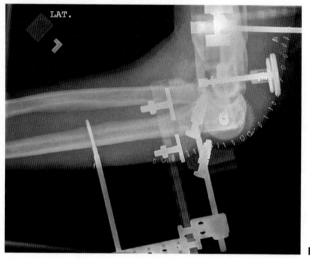

Figure 14–10 *(continued on page 317)*

be strong enough, but we have not had any problem with wires for this particular indication. The pins are protected with an above-elbow cast. The pins are removed and the cast discontinued 4 weeks later **(Fig. 14–9A–C).**

Hinged External Fixation

In younger patients with high-energy injuries, repair of the medial and lateral collateral ligaments is sometimes insufficient.[51] It is important to be prepared to either cross-pin the joint or apply a hinged external fixator **(Fig. 14–10A–C).** We prefer to use hinged external fixation and allow the patient to move because immobilizing the elbow may increase the already substantial risk of hetero-

topic ossification; however, stability always takes precedence over mobility in the treatment of elbow problems, and if a surgeon does not have the resources or technical ability to apply a hinged external fixator, cross-pinning may be used.

Determination of the isometric center of rotation at the elbow is critical to the use of a hinged external fixator. A temporary axis pin is placed in the distal humerus through the center of rotation. This roughly corresponds to a point on the medial aspect of the trochlea just anterior and inferior to the medial epicondyle and to the distalmost point of a small ridge on the lateral epicondyle in the center of the capitellum. Proper axis pin placement is confirmed with imaging. The frame is usually attached to the humerus first and then to the forearm.

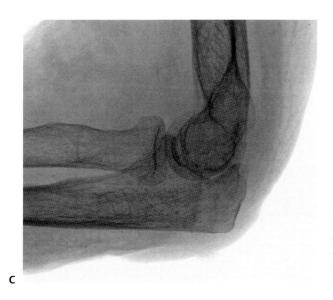

C

Figure 14–9 **(A)** An infirm 80-year-old woman sustained a simple elbow dislocation that could not be kept in a reduced position. **(B)** Under local anesthesia and sedation, two smooth, stout Kirschner wires were drilled across the joint with the elbow in 90 degrees of flexion. **(C)** The pins were removed 4 weeks later, and active motion was started. The elbow remained concentrically reduced and regained functional mobility.

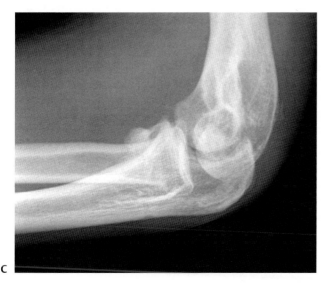

C

Figure 14–10 **(A)** A 30-year-old man with persistent subluxation of the elbow 3 weeks after a high-energy simple elbow dislocation. **(B)** Open reduction and hinged external fixation were performed. **(C)** Concentric reduction was achieved. Restoration of functional motion required a second procedure to remove heterotopic bone.

Several types of hinges are available. The Compass Hinge (Richards Inc., Memphis, Tennessee) may provide additional stability by virtue of both posteromedial and posterolateral pins. It also incorporates a worm gear that can be used to assist with motion during the initial painful postoperative period and can be used for static progressive stretch later on in the rehabilitation. The majority of other fixators are unilateral, although some can be used with transfixion pins if additional stability is desired. A lateral-only frame avoids the discomfort associated with a medial frame and pins, and this usually provides adequate stability. No matter what fixator is used, the lateral humerus pins must be placed with an open exposure adequate to protect the radial nerve.

Tips and Tricks

- Many surgeons repair the collateral ligaments and common flexor and extensor muscles using drill holes through bone. The potential advantages include broader contact between soft tissues and bone and more reliable fixation in poor quality bone. I believe that suture anchors simplify the repair and continue to use them in most patients.
- Application of a hinged external fixator is challenging. To simplify the procedure, stabilize the ulnohumeral joint in good alignment with one or two stout, smooth Kirschner wires while the hinge is applied.
- We always make a more substantial incision for the lateral humerus pins (at least 2 in.). We then dissect down to bone and use small Hohman retractors to ensure that the radial nerve is safe. We have yet to have a radial nerve palsy or injury in over 20 hinge applications.

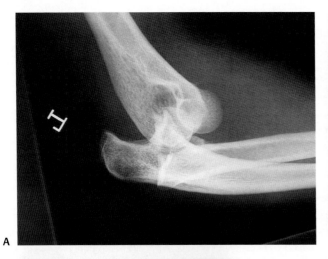

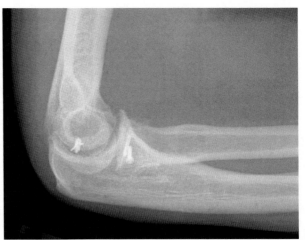

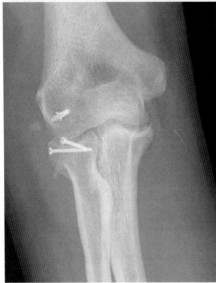

Figure 14–11 Posterior elbow dislocation with radial head fracture. **(A)** The most basic type of elbow fracture-dislocation is dislocation with fracture of the radial head only. **(B)** In this patient the radial head was repaired with screws, and the lateral collateral ligament was reattached with a suture anchor. **(C)** Concentric reduction and good elbow motion were obtained.

Outcomes

Closed treatment of simple elbow dislocations will result in a satisfactory outcome in the majority of patients. Terminal extension loss of 5 to 15 degrees is common.[57] The key to regaining elbow range of motion is avoidance of prolonged immobilization. In the study by Mehlhoff and colleagues, patients immobilized for more than 3 weeks had a significantly increased risk of stiffness and pain.[2]

Older patients with low-energy injuries usually do very well after operative treatment of an unstable elbow dislocation, even if the elbow has been immobilized for a month. Younger patients injured in high-energy injuries can be expected to have greater than average stiffness after operative treatment of an unstable elbow dislocation.

Pearls

- The progression of soft tissue injury in a simple elbow dislocation proceeds from lateral to medial and the elbow can dislocate with the anterior band of the medial collateral ligament intact.
- The elbow should be mobilized within 2 to 3 weeks after a simple elbow dislocation.
- The lateral collateral ligament nearly always fails by avulsion from its lateral epicondyle origin.

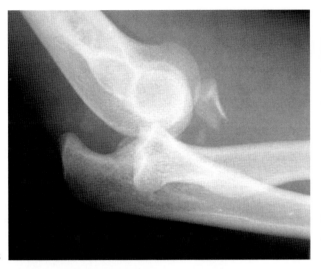
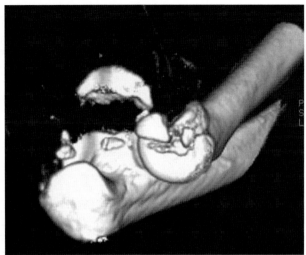

 A,B

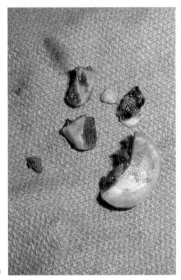
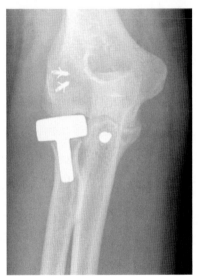

C,D

Figure 14–12 Terrible triad pattern of elbow fracture-dislocation. **(A)** The terrible triad refers to the elbow dislocation, fracture of the radial head, and fracture of the coronoid process (the triangular fragment in front of the trochlea). **(B)** This three-dimensional computed tomographic scan demonstrates a small transverse coronoid fracture and a complex partial radial head fracture. **(C)** The radial head fracture was complex and not reconstructible. **(D)** Prosthetic replacement of the radial head, screw and suture fixation of the coronoid, and lateral collateral repair kept the elbow reduced.

Complications

Simple elbow dislocations occasionally result in stiffness that is resistant to exercises and requires operative treatment. On occasion this is due to heterotopic bone formation. Ulnar neuropathy, instability or malalignment, and arthrosis are also seen after elbow dislocation.

Elbow Fracture-Dislocations: Elbow Dislocation with Fracture of the Radial Head

Elbow dislocations that are associated with one or more intra-articular fractures are at greater risk for recurrent or chronic instability.[16,48,58] Fracture-dislocations of the elbow usually occur in one of several distinct, recognizable injury patterns: (1) posterior dislocation with fracture of the radial head **(Fig. 14–11A–C)**; (2) posterior dislocation with fractures of the radial head and coronoid process—the so-called terrible triad injury **(Fig. 14–12A–D)**; (3) posteromedial varus rotational instability pattern injuries (anteromedial facet coronoid fracture and lateral collateral ligament avulsion from the lateral epicondyle) **(Fig. 14–13A–G)**; (4) anterior (trans-) olecranon fracture-dislocations **(Fig. 14–14A–D)**; and (5) posterior olecranon fracture-dislocations **(Fig. 14–15A–J)** (see **Video 14–1, Disk 2**). Each of these patterns is associated with characteristic injury components and fracture morphologies, the knowledge of which can help guide effective management.

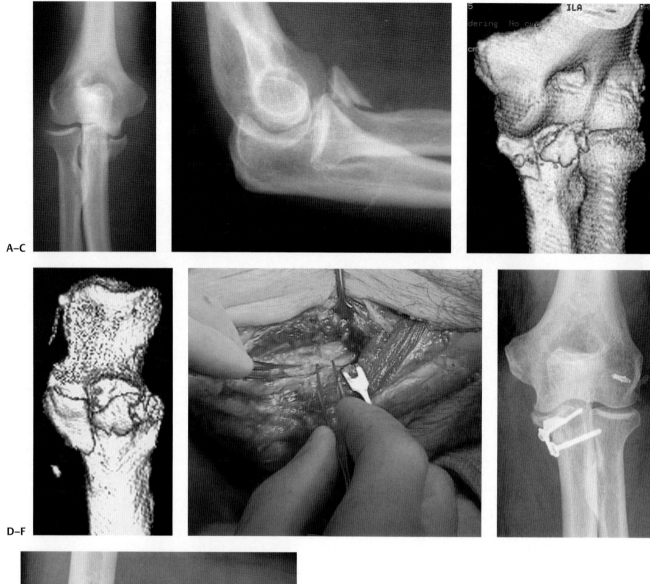

A–C

D–F

G

Figure 14–13 Varus posteromedial pattern injury. **(A)** A fracture of the anteromedial facet of the distal humerus is associated with this pattern of injury. Notice that there is hinging open of the radiocapitellar joint on the lateral side. **(B)** The appearance of the coronoid on the lateral radiograph suggests that it is a small tip fracture. **(C)** A three-dimensional computed tomographic scan demonstrates the external rotation of the humerus into the coronoid defect. **(D)** There are nearly always separate tip and antero-medial facet fragments. **(E)** A medial exposure between the heads of the flexor carpi ulnaris (after transposing the ulnar nerve) allows handling and fixation of the coronoid fracture while preserving the medial collateral lig-ament. **(F)** The coronoid is repaired with a plate and screws, and the lateral collateral ligament is reattached with a suture anchor. **(G)** Concentric ro-tation and excellent motion were achieved.

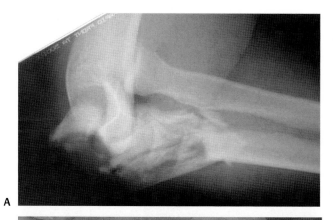

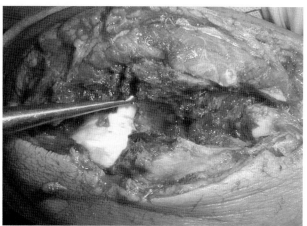

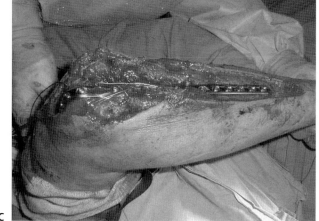

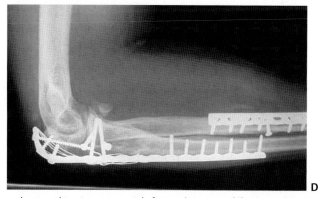

Figure 14–14 Anterior olecranon (or transolecranon) fracture-dislocation of the elbow. **(A)** Anterior fracture-dislocations resemble Monteggia injuries by virtue of the anterior radiocapitellar dislocation; however, they are ulnohumeral injuries with very little radioulnar disruption. **(B)** In this patient the coronoid is split in the sagittal plane, making it more straightforward to repair. **(C)** A long plate that bridges the metaphyseal comminution and tension wires that grab the triceps insertion are used for fixation. **(D)** Six months later the patients has a healed fracture, concentrically reduced elbow, and good elbow motion.

Posteromedial varus rotational instability pattern injuries and olecranon fracture-dislocations are not true dislocations in that apposition of the articular surfaces is not lost. Rather, they are fracture-subluxation injuries where the major problem is disruption of the trochlear notch. Fracture-dislocations of the olecranon will be considered along with olecranon fractures. Fracture-dislocations that are usually associated with small coronoid fractures will be considered together as coronoid fracture-dislocations.

Nonoperative Treatment

Dislocation of the elbow with fracture of the radial head alone can be treated nonoperatively; however, even a very small coronoid fracture increases the risks of nonoperative treatment substantially—if there is any doubt about the presence or absence of a coronoid fracture, a computed tomographic scan should be obtained. Broberg and Morrey[59] and Joseffson and colleagues[48] treated fracture-dislocations of the elbow either nonoperatively or with radial head excision and cast immobilization with fairly good results, but with two caveats: (1) an associated fracture of the coronoid was associated with problems keeping the elbow reduced, and (2) the fracture of the radial head was the ultimate determinant of the outcome, with many late radial head resections needed to restore forearm rotation.[59] In the absence of a coronoid fracture, stability and reasonably good mobility were achieved with either resection or neglect of the radial head and 4 weeks of cast immobilization. We have had a few patients with this injury pattern that either did not want operative treatment or did not want a radial head prosthesis (unreconstructible radial head) and we have used these methods; however, we advocate immediate

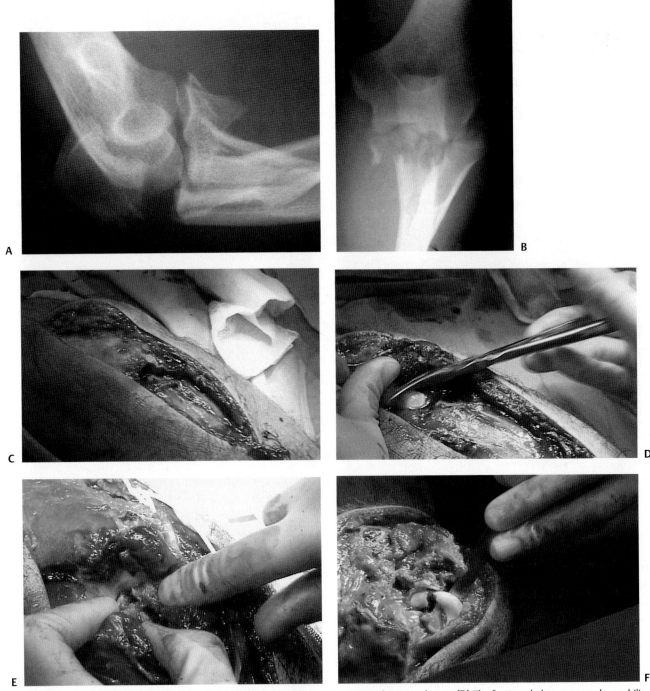

Figure 14–15 Posterior olecranon fracture-dislocation of the elbow. **(A)** Posterior olecranon fracture-dislocations can be considered part of the spectrum of posterior Monteggia injuries. There is an apex posterior deformity of the ulna, posterior dislocation and fracture of the radial head, and a large coronoid fracture. **(B)** The coronoid fracture is comminuted with three major articular fragments, including an anteromedial facet coronoid fragment. **(C)** Skin incision discloses a traumatic rent in the musculature. **(D)** The fractured olecranon can be mobilized proximally as one would do for an olecranon osteotomy. Removal of hematoma allows a good view of the coronoid and radial head. **(E)** This photograph demonstrates manual reduction of the coronoid fragments. **(F)** By re-creating the injury deformity, the radial head is delivered posteriorly into this wound, where fixation or resection and prosthetic replacement can be performed.

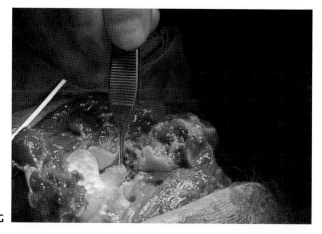

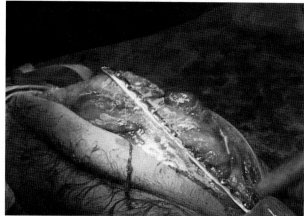

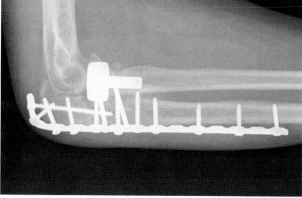

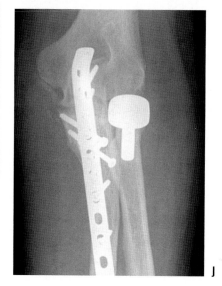

Figure 14–15 *(Continued)* **(G)** There are three large fragments of coronoid: anteromedial facet, lesser sigmoid notch, and a central fragment. **(H)** A long dorsal, contoured plate is applied. **(I)** A healed fracture and good elbow motion and function were achieved. **(J)** Separate screws help to secure the anteromedial facet of the coronoid.

active mobilization of the elbow and forearm as comfort allows. We have been impressed with the ability of these very motivated patients to regain good elbow function **(Fig. 14–16A–C).**

Indications for Surgical Treatment

We prefer operative treatment of elbow fractures with associated radial head fractures to confidently allow immediate active mobilization and thereby limit stiffness, to improve the outcome of the radial head fracture, and to optimize the long-term function of the elbow.

Surgical Treatment

Surgical Technique

Either a lateral or direct posterior skin incision can be used. The radial head is addressed as already described under radial head fractures. The lateral collateral ligament is repaired as already described under simple elbow dislocations. It would be extremely unusual for medial collateral ligament repair to be necessary.

> **Tips and Tricks**
>
> • The lateral collateral ligament is injured in every patient. This greatly facilitates exposure of the radial head.

Outcomes

Joseffson and colleagues reported no recurrent instability, an average 20 degree flexion contracture, and signs of arthritis in nearly all patients an average of 14 years after injury, with slightly worse arthrosis in patients that had radial head resection.[47] Sanchez-Sotelo and colleagues agree that absence of the radial head may increase the risk of arthritis after fracture-dislocation.[31]

Broberg and Morrey reported good or excellent results in 18 of 24 patients with an average follow-up of 10 years. They observed no instability. Poor results were associated with either immobilization for more than 4 weeks or nonoperative treatment of a comminuted radial head fracture (salvaged with a second operation for radial head excision). One drawback of this and other series is the failure to distinguish injuries with and without an associated coronoid fracture.[59,60]

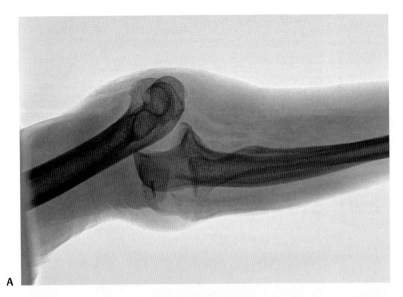

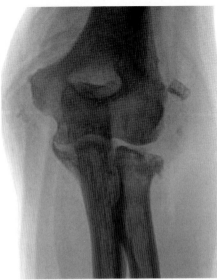

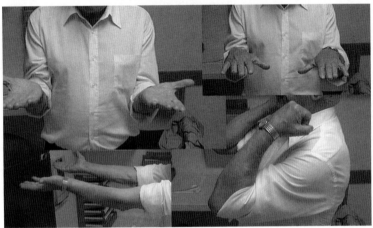

Figure 14–16 Some fracture-dislocations can be treated nonoperatively. **(A)** A 70-year-old man had a dislocation of the elbow and complex fracture of the radial head. He was extremely reluctant to have surgery and had full forearm rotation when seen a week after the injury. **(B)** I treated him with a sling and active use of the arm, and the elbow ligaments healed in good alignment. **(C)** He achieved an excellent functional result with no complaints of pain.

Elbow Fracture-Dislocations: Coronoid Fracture-Dislocations

Recent reports on elbow instability have emphasized the importance of the coronoid process.[1,16,55] The injuries that give surgeons the most trouble are the terrible triad, posteromedial varus, and olecranon fracture-dislocations with associated coronoid fractures.[1] In each case, the fracture of the coronoid is the most important and challenging part of the injury. Regan and Morrey[61] classified coronoid injuries based on the size of the fracture fragment, but it has become clear that the pattern of the overall injury and morphology of the fracture may be equally or more important. Consequently, our discussion of fracture-dislocations of the elbow will be organized according to the fracture of the coronoid process of the ulna. Injuries that are usually associated with small coronoid fractures will be considered as coronoid fracture-dislocations. Those associated with large coronoid fractures are usually part of an olecranon fracture-dislocation.

Classification

Regan and Morrey classified coronoid fractures based on the size of the fragment: type I, avulsion of the tip of the coronoid process; type II, a single or comminuted fragment involving 50% of the process or less; and type III, a single or comminuted fragment involving more than 50% of the process.[61] They also included a modifier to indicate the presence (type B) or absence (type A) of an elbow dislocation.

O'Driscoll et al proposed a new classification system for coronoid fractures based on the anatomical location of the fracture. Fractures may involve the tip, anteromedial, or basal aspect of the coronoid. The three groups are further divided into subtypes based on the severity of coronoid involvement. O'Driscoll's system considers the mechanism of injury along with the associated fractures and soft tissue injuries and helps to dictate treatment **(Fig. 14–17).**[1]

The first group of coronoid fractures involves the tip but does not extend medially past the sublime tubercle or into the body. Tip, subtype 1 fractures involve less than 2 mm of

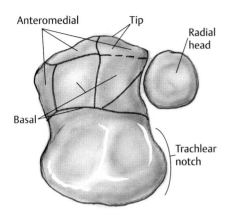

Figure 14–17 O'Driscoll's classification of coronoid fractures. Type 1 or tip fractures are associated with terrible triad lesions. Type 2 or anteromedial facet fractures are associated with varus posteromedial pattern injuries. Type 3 or basal fractures are associated with olecranon fracture-dislocations.

the coronoid and may be found in isolation or with a fracture dislocation. Tip, subtype 2 fractures involve greater than 2 mm and are largely associated with terrible triad injuries.

The second group of coronoid fractures involves the anteromedial aspect of the coronoid. Anteromedial subtype 1 fractures extend from just medial to the tip of the coronoid to the anterior half of the sublime tubercle (insertion of the anterior band of the medial collateral ligament). Anteromedial subtype 2 fractures are subtype 1 injuries with extension of the fracture line into the tip. Anteromedial sub type 3 fractures involve the anteromedial rim and the entire sublime tubercle with or without involvement of the tip of the coronoid. The mechanism of injury is usually a varus/ posteromedial rotation injury with axial loading. The lateral collateral ligamentous complex is generally disrupted unless the olecranon is also fractured. Radial head fractures may be seen in higher energy, subtype 3 injuries. Anteromedial coronoid fractures cause incongruent articulation of the ulnohumeral joint, which may lead to earlier onset of posttraumatic arthritis.

Basal coronoid fractures make up the third category and involve at least 50% of the height of the coronoid. Basal subtype 1 fractures involve the coronoid alone, whereas subtype 2 fractures are associated with fractures of the olecranon (see **Video 14–2, Disk 2**). In general, these fractures have less soft tissue disruption than those that involve only the tip of the coronoid.

We and others have made the following observations that may be useful in guiding treatment: (1) Terrible triad injuries nearly always have a small transverse fracture of the tip of the coronoid, including the anterior capsular attachment. Much less commonly, the coronoid fracture is either very large or involves the anteromedial facet of the coronoid preferentially. (2) Posteromedial varus rotational instability pattern injuries are defined by a fracture of the

anteromedial facet of the coronoid process. They also often have a fracture of the tip of the coronoid process and the sublime tubercle (insertion point of the anterior band of the medial collateral ligament). (3) In the setting of an olecranon fracture-dislocation, the coronoid fracture can be one simple large fragment; it can be fragmented into two or three large pieces (anteromedial facet, central, and lesser sigmoid notch) with or without a tip fragment as well, or it can be more comminuted.

Elbow Dislocation with Fractures of the Coronoid and Radial Head (Terrible Triad)

Nonoperative Treatment

Terrible triad fracture-dislocations are particularly prone to instability. Nonoperative treatment should be discouraged and undertaken only with great care. In our experience, patients that achieve good results with nonoperative treatment are comfortable, confident, and motivated. Cast immobilization cannot maintain reduction of the ulnohumeral joint. Confident active motion of the elbow adds the dynamic muscular component of stability and seems to be a critical component of nonoperative treatment.

Indications for Surgical Treatment

Patients with terrible triad fracture-dislocations of the elbow should be encouraged to undergo operative treatment.

Surgical Treatment

Surgical Technique

Either a posterior or lateral skin incision can be used (**Fig. 14–18A**). After development of skin flaps, one may find a relatively preserved fascia or a small rent in the common extensor area. Once a deep intramuscular interval is developed—usually in the interval created by the trauma, otherwise in Kocher's or Kaplan's interval—it becomes apparent that the lateral collateral ligament has been avulsed from the lateral epicondyle, along with variable amounts of the common extensor musculature (**Fig. 14–18B**).

An extensive medial skin flap is necessary only if the ulnar nerve is going to be released, the medial collateral ligament needs to be repaired, or there is an anteromedial facet fracture of the coronoid that needs to be repaired. Care must be taken to keep the flap full thickness to limit the potential for injury to the medial antebrachial cutaneous nerve. We have seen many patients with subacute and chronic ulnar nerve dysfunction after elbow trauma and now consider ulnar nerve release in every case—often done in situ, without transposition unless the nerve is unstable with flexion.

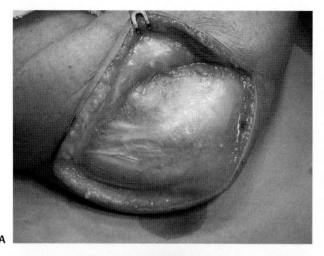

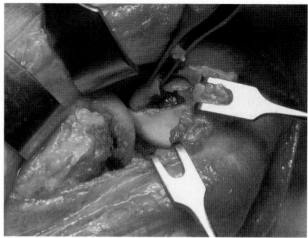

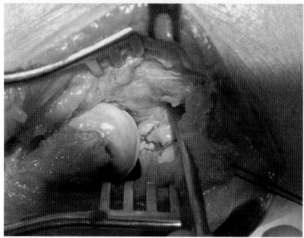

Figure 14–18 **(A)** The fascia over the lateral epicondyle is often intact upon initial elevation of a skin flap. **(B)** After incising the fascia, avulsion of the lateral collateral ligament origin and a variable amount of the common extensor muscles are apparent. Removal of the radial head fragments improves access to the coronoid. **(C)** The coronoid fracture is secured with a suture through drill holes. Replacement of the radial head and lateral collateral ligament was also performed.

The majority of patients with terrible triad injuries have a small, transverse fracture of the coronoid that can be repaired through the lateral exposure and will usually have a small single fragment **(Fig. 14–18C)**.[1,16] The ligament and muscle laceration created by the injury is extended by incising and elevating the origins of the radial wrist extensors along with the brachialis to expose the coronoid fragment. Removing the radial head fragments and splitting the annular ligament and the supinator distally affords additional exposure. When necessary the elbow can be subluxated to improve exposure.

Because radiocapitellar contact is critical to elbow stability in the setting of a terrible triad injury, even many partial radial head fractures (Mason type 2) will need to be considered for prosthetic replacement. Often these are comminuted, have small or lost fragments, or have poor quality bone. Resection of the radial head can improve exposure of the coronoid.

Transverse fractures of the tip of the coronoid are treated with sutures passed through drill holes in the ulna. If the fracture is very small, the suture is passed around the frag-

ment and through its capsular insertion. For larger transverse fragments the suture is passed through drill holes in the fracture fragment and is also passed through the capsule. Sutures provide more reliable fixation than screws. They restore the anterior buttress and capsular attachments, but the articular alignment is usually imperfect—in our opinion, this is of little consequence. For larger fragments the use of screw fixation in addition to suture fixation can be considered to improve the alignment, but the suture through the capsular attachment should be used as well because screw fixation of these small fragments is unreliable.

After fixation of the coronoid, replacement or repair of the radial head, and reattachment of the lateral collateral ligament and common extensor musculature, the elbow is tested for stability. This is done by allowing it to come into full gravity-assisted extension while supporting the humerus **(Fig. 14–19)**. The elbow should be stable enough that it does not dislocate with this maneuver. Under image intensification there may be slight subluxation. If the elbow dislocates or severely subluxates prior to 30 degrees short of full extension, additional repair should be consid-

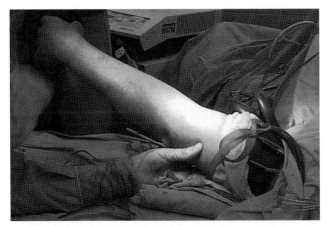

Figure 14–19 Stability is tested in full gravity extension. If there is a tendency to dislocation or subluxation, repair of the medial collateral ligament or hinged external fixation is considered.

ered. As described for unstable simple elbow dislocations, the medial collateral ligament and flexor-pronator muscles can be repaired, the elbow can be cross-pinned, or a hinged fixator can be applied.

Outcomes

The traditional thought that larger coronoid fractures faired worse than smaller fractures was based on a series of patients with isolated coronoid fractures and those associated with fracture dislocation of the elbow reported by Regan and Morrey in 1990.[61] They found that patients with large coronoid fracture fragments did poorer than those with small fragments; however, the majority of the patients were treated nonoperatively.[61] The current opinion is that smaller fracture fragments can be associated with more challenging injury patterns (e.g., the terrible triad) and can lead to recurrent instability and early arthrosis if inadequately treated.[1,16,55]

Terrible triad pattern injuries are prone to numerous complications. A recent series of 11 patients with posterior dislocation of the elbow and associated fractures of the coronoid process of the ulna and radial head was reported.[55] Seven elbows redislocated in a splint after manipulative reduction demonstrating the degree of instability of this fracture pattern. In all cases the coronoid fracture involved less than half of its height. None of the patients were treated with internal fixation of the coronoid. The radial head fracture was fixed in five and resected in four patients. The lateral collateral ligament was repaired in only three patients. Five of the patients, including all four with radial head resection, redislocated after surgery. The patients were followed for a minimum of 2 years. Based on the Broberg and Morrey functional score, there were two excellent, two good, three fair, and one poor result. Seven out of 11 patients had an unsatisfactory result overall. The patients who did better had retained

their radial head or undergone repair of the lateral collateral ligament or both.[55]

Data have been presented and will be published soon in support of routine fixation of the coronoid, radial head, and lateral collateral ligament in the setting of a terrible triad injury, documenting good results in most patients.

Complications

Instability, arthrosis, stiffness, heterotopic bone, and ulnar neuropathy are all commonplace after this injury—thus the label *terrible triad.*

Varus Posteromedial Rotational Instability Pattern Injuries

Fractures of the coronoid that preferentially involve the anteromedial facet have recently been recognized as a specific and potentially problematic pattern of injury.[1] This type of fracture is associated with lateral collateral ligament injury unless the fracture of the coronoid is very large or there is an associated fracture of the olecranon.

Nonoperative Treatment

Very little is known about these injuries, but nonoperative treatment is felt to be unwise.[1]

Indications for Surgical Treatment

Patients with varus posteromedial rotational instability pattern injuries should be encouraged to undergo operative treatment.

Surgical Treatment

Surgical Technique

The lateral collateral ligament is first exposed and repaired. Then a medial exposure of the coronoid is developed. The ulnar nerve is mobilized and transposed anteriorly into the subcutaneous tissues. The interval between the two heads of the flexor carpi ulnaris where the ulnar nerve usually lies provides a good access to the medial side of the coronoid.[1] The flexor pronator muscles are elevated off the anterior band of the medial collateral ligament. For even larger fragments the entire flexor pronator mass can be elevated off the medial ulna as described by Taylor and Scham.[62]

Alternatively, a more anterior interval, splitting the flexor-pronator muscles and elevating the anterior half along with the brachialis, can be used.[63] Both exposures can be used simultaneously.

The anteromedial facet fracture is stabilized with a medial buttress plate that stabilizes the medial fragment against the intact lateral coronoid. There is usually a tip fragment with the anterior capsular insertion attached. This can be difficult to secure with a plate or Kirschner wires and should be considered for suture stabilization when felt to be important for stability.

Outcomes

Anteromedial coronoid fractures with posteromedial rotary instability have only recently been described, and results of treatment are not yet available. It is possible to restore elbow stability by internal fixation of the coronoid fragment and repair of the lateral collateral ligament in most cases.[1,64]

Olecranon Fractures

Although fractures of the olecranon are intra-articular, they have relatively low rates of posttraumatic arthritis, probably because most fractures occur at the relatively nonarticular transverse groove of the trochlear notch. The goals of treatment of olecranon fractures are restoration of the normal contour and dimensions of the trochlear notch to restore stability, healing of the fracture to restore triceps function, and early mobilization of the elbow to limit stiffness. Operative treatment is required for most fractures. The specific operative technique is tailored to the characteristics of the injury: simple transverse fractures are treated with tension-band wiring (with an interfragmentary screw added for oblique fractures), and comminuted fractures and fracture-dislocations are repaired with a plate and screws.

Classification

Several classification systems have been described. Each has helped emphasize certain injury characteristics and management issues. Colton proposed a classification system based upon the displacement and character of the fracture.[65] According to this system, type I fractures are nondisplaced and stable. Type II fractures are displaced and may be divided into subgroups based on the fracture pattern: type IIA are avulsion fractures; type IIB are transverse or oblique fractures; type IIC are isolated comminuted fractures; and type IID are fracture-dislocations.[65] Within this system, a fracture is considered nondisplaced and stable if there are no more than 2 mm of displacement and no change in position of the fracture with gentle flexion and extension.

Schatzker and Tile suggested classification of olecranon fractures into five types: type A, a simple transverse fracture; type B, a complex transverse fracture with articular impaction centrally; type C, a simple oblique fracture; type D, a comminuted fracture; and type E, an oblique fracture distal to the midpoint of the trochlear notch.[66] Impaction is less important at the olecranon than in other articular fractures and probably does not need to be distinguished from other forms of comminution.

The Muller et al's classification of fractures groups olecranon fractures with those of the proximal radius and ulna.[20] The fractures are divided into types, groups, and subgroups. Type A fractures are extra-articular, type B fractures have intra-articular involvement of one bone, and type C intra-articular fractures involve both bones. The fractures are further divided into groups and subgroups based primarily upon the complexity of the fractures. Although inclusion of proximal ulna fractures along with proximal radius fractures is appealing for research purposes, in practice the characteristics important to treatment tend to get lost in the details.

The Mayo classification system for olecranon fractures evaluates displacement, stability, and comminution **(Fig. 14–20)**.[67] Type I is a stable, minimally displaced fracture (less than 2 mm of gap between the fracture fragments), type II is a displaced fracture, and type III fractures are associated with instability of the ulno-humeral articulation. The fractures are further subdivided into subgroups A and B, according to the absence or presence of comminution, respectively. This classifica-

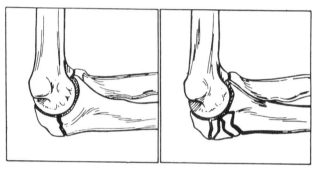

Type I: Undisplaced

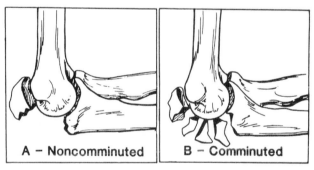

Type II: Displaced and stable

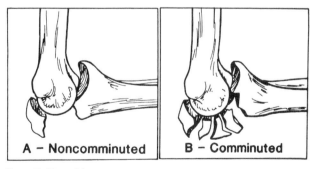

Type III: Unstable

Figure 14–20 The Mayo classification of olecranon fractures considers displacement, comminution, and joint subluxation. These subtypes relate closely to various treatment options. (With permission from Morrey BF. Fracture of the radial head. In: Morrey BF, ed. The Elbow and Its Disorders. 2nd ed. Philadelphia: WB Saunders; 1993:408.)

tion accounts for most of the important issues and helps guide treatment.

Nonoperative Treatment

Nondisplaced and minimally displaced fractures are treated nonoperatively. Standard treatment consists of 4 weeks of immobilization in a cast or splint with the elbow at 90 degrees and the forearm in neutral rotation. Immobilization in extension is not necessary for these stable fractures. Four weeks after the fracture, immobilization is discontinued, and gentle active-assisted range of motion is initiated. Resistive exercises are delayed until healing is established on radiographs, usually about 8 weeks after the injury.

Indications for Surgical Treatment

All displaced fractures of the olecranon merit operative fixation.

Surgical Treatment

Surgical Technique

Displaced Noncomminuted Fractures of the Olecranon

Displaced simple transverse fractures—the most common type of olecranon fracture[68,69]—are treated with tension-band wiring **(Fig. 14–21)** (see **Video 14–3, Disk 2**). Screw fixation alone does not provide rotational control, can distract the fracture, and does not always gain adequate hold of the distal fragment. Screw fixation combined with tension-wire fixation has been described. Problems associated with migration or prominence of the implants can be limited by the use of specific operative techniques.[70,71]

The tension-band principle converts the distractive force of the triceps into a compressive force across the fracture by applying fixation to resist distraction on the dorsal surface of the ulna.[66] Use of the tension-band principle requires an intact (or nearly intact) cortex opposite the implant—comminuted fractures are treated with plate fixation.

The patient can be positioned supine with the arm draped over the chest **(Fig. 14–22)**, in lateral decubitus with the arm supported by a bolster, or prone. Bone graft may be obtained from the iliac crest in all three positions but is rarely necessary. A sterile tourniquet may improve exposure and facilitate manipulation of the arm.

Although some authors recommend curving the skin incision to avoid the tip of the olecranon, we prefer a straight dorsal incision and have encountered few problems with it. The ulnar nerve is mobilized only if needed for exposure, if the nerve is injured, or if associated soft tissue injury risks compression or kinking of the nerve.

For simple, noncomminuted fractures, hematoma is removed from the fracture surfaces, and the periosteum is

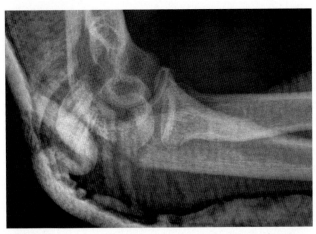

Figure 14–21 Tension-band wiring is most appropriate for olecranon fractures such as this with limited comminution and an intact articular surface that can be compressed together with active motion.

peeled back from the fracture edges to facilitate accurate repositioning.

The reduced fracture can be stabilized with a large pointed reduction forceps **(Fig. 14–23A)**. This may be facilitated by making a small drill hole in the distal fragment (the dorsal surface of the ulna diaphysis), allowing purchase of one tip of the pointed forceps. The other tip of the forceps grasps the olecranon and compresses the fracture.

Two parallel 0.045 in. Kirschner wires are then drilled across the fracture site **(Fig. 14–23B)**. The wires are directed slightly anterior to engage the anterior cortex of the distal fragment. A recent study suggested biomechanical advantages of this wire orientation as compared with intramedullary placement of the wires,[72] but the primary reason for engaging the anterior ulnar cortex is to attempt to limit the potential for migration of the wires. After drilling the wires through the anterior ulnar cortex, they are retracted several millimeters in anticipation of later impaction of the proximal end into the olecranon.

Two 2 mm transverse drill holes are placed through the apex of the diaphyseal ulna distal to the fracture site **(Fig. 14–23C)**. A 22-gauge stainless steel wire is passed through each hole, placed in a figure-of-eight configuration over the dorsum of the fracture site, and passed anteriorly to the Kirschner wires—under the triceps insertion—using a 14-gauge needle **(Fig. 14–23D)**. The wires are tensioned both medially and laterally until all slack is taken up in the wires and the twisted wire rests on the bone **(Fig. 14–23E)**. The wires are trimmed, and the ends are bent into the soft tissues. Using two 22-gauge wires rather than a single 18-gauge wire helps limit hardware prominence while providing adequate fixation strength **(Fig. 14–24A–C)**.

The proximal ends of the Kirschner wires are bent 180 degrees and impacted into the olecranon underneath the triceps insertion **(Fig. 14–23F and 14–24C)**. This decreases

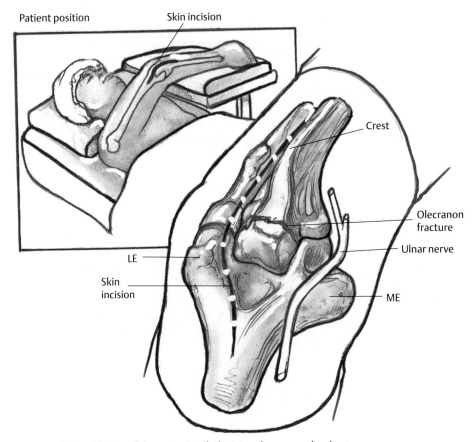

Patient position   Skin incision

Crest

Olecranon fracture

Ulnar nerve

LE

Skin incision

ME

Figure 14–22 Positioning of the patient with the injured arm over the chest.

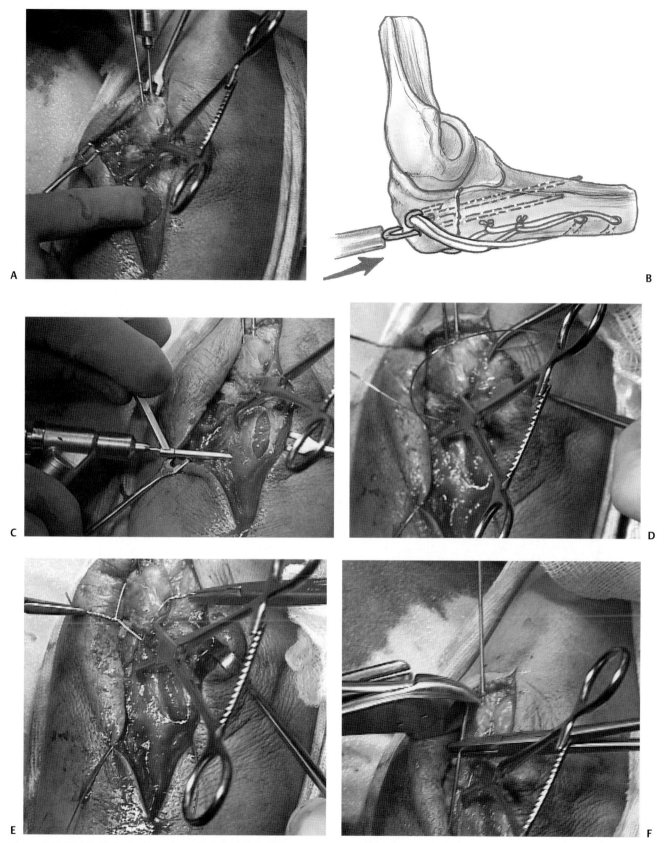

Figure 14–23 **(A)** With the fracture held reduced, two 0.045 in. Kirschner wires are drilled across the fracture obliquely, exiting the anterior ulnar cortex, just distal to the coronoid process. **(B)** This drawing depicts the important aspects of tension-band wiring. The Kirschner wires are drilled obliquely exiting the anterior ulnar cortex, and the proximal ends are bent 180 degrees and driven into the prox-imal olecranon (arrow) to limit wire prominence and the potential for wire migration. **(C)** Stainless steel tension-band wires (22 gauge) are passed through the ulna shaft, well distal to the fracture, each through its own drill hole. **(D)** Each wire is placed in a figure-of-eight orientation and passed through the insertion of the triceps onto the olecranon using a needle. **(E)** Each wire is tensioned on both sides, and the knots are bent into the soft tissues to limit prominence. **(F)** The pins are bent over and cut off.

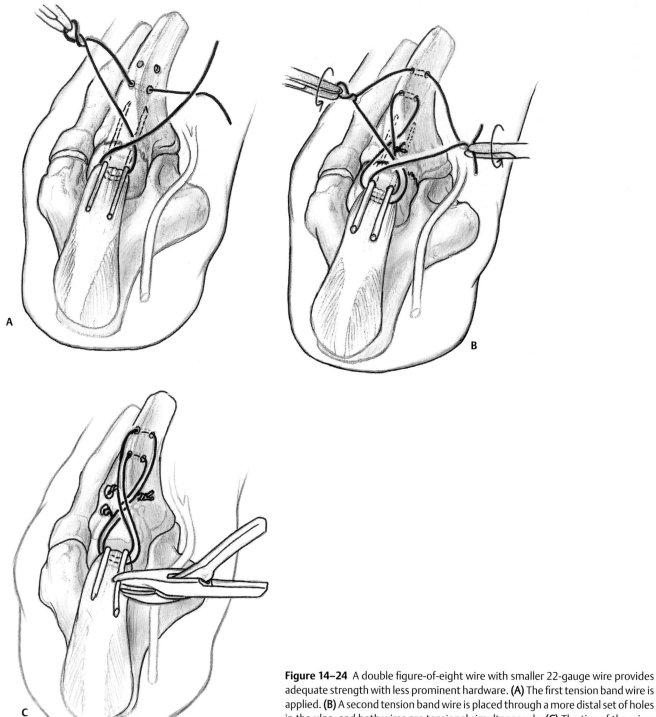

Figure 14–24 A double figure-of-eight wire with smaller 22-gauge wire provides adequate strength with less prominent hardware. **(A)** The first tension band wire is applied. **(B)** A second tension band wire is placed through a more distal set of holes in the ulna, and both wires are tensional simultaneously. **(C)** The tips of the wires are bent 180 degrees, cut off, and impacted into the olecranon.

the prominence of the wires and helps limit the potential for wire migration **(Fig. 14–25A,B)**.

Displaced Comminuted Fractures of the Olecranon

Operative Technique for Excision of Fragments and Advancement of the Triceps Displaced, comminuted fractures are treated with plate and screw fixation. Fragment excision

and triceps advancement are mostly of historical interest, although they may still be useful for patients with limited functional demands.[67] Fragment excision is not appropriate for fracture-dislocations.

When fragment excision and triceps advancement are elected, Morrey recommends limiting the resection to no more than half of the olecranon to maintain stability;[67] however, in an older infirm patient it may be reasonable to resect

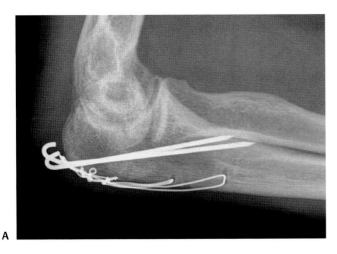

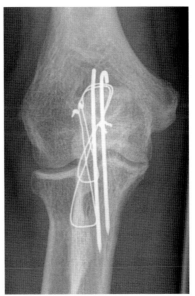

Figure 14–25 (A) The final fixation on lateral and **(B)** posteroanterior radiographs.

even more. It has been recommended that the triceps be reattached as close as possible to the articular surface to provide a smooth transition between joint and tendon as it glides over the trochlea. A recent biomechanical study demonstrated improved extensor strength with posterior attachment of the triceps.[73] Given the infirm and inactive patients in whom this technique would generally be used, these considerations are probably of limited importance. Stout nonabsorbable sutures are placed in the triceps insertion from which the bone fragments have been excised. A tendon-grasping stitch such as a Krackow stitch is used. These sutures are passed through drill holes initiated directly adjacent to the articular surface and exiting onto the dorsal surface of the ulna, where they are tensioned and tied.

Operative Technique for Plate and Screw Fixation For comminuted fractures there is no need to elevate periosteum or muscle attachments **(Fig. 14–26A).** Instead, the normal contour and dimensions of the trochlear notch are restored,

and the area of fragmentation is bridged with a plate and screws **(Fig. 14–26B).** For very unstable fractures it can be useful to temporarily stabilize the olecranon to the trochlea using a stout, smooth Kirschner wire (usually $\frac{5}{64}$ in.).

A 3.5 mm Limited Contact Dynamic Compression Plate (LC–DCP, Synthes, Paoli, Pennsylvania) contoured to wrap around the olecranon, or a precontoured 3.5 mm plate with 2.7 mm screws proximally (Zimmer, Inc., Warsaw, Indiana; Acumed LLC, Hillsboro, Oregon), is well suited to the olecranon. Proximally, the plate lies on the flat dorsal surface of the olecranon. Distally, it lies directly over the apex of the olecranon. This is unsettling to some surgeons, but stable fixation can be achieved, and very little muscle or periosteum need be elevated from the bone. The dorsal surface is the tension side of the olecranon and is the best surface for plating. Plates applied to the medial or lateral surface of the ulna are more likely to fail. The plate should extend well distal, particularly when comminution

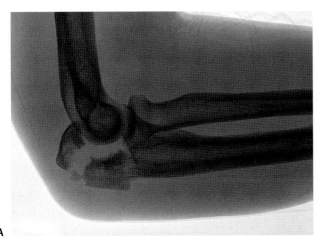

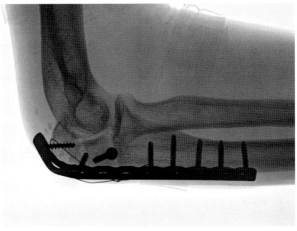

Figure 14–26 A comminuted fracture of the olecranon is treated with plate and screw fixation. **(A)** This lateral radiograph shows an olecranon fracture with a small proximal fragment and separate articular fragments. **(B)** A dorsal plate and screws are used to secure the fragments in correct position. A tension wire is used to improve fixation of the small proximal fragment by grabbing the triceps insertion.

is extensive. There are few disadvantages to a long plate in this area. If the proximal olecranon is small, osteoporotic, or extensively fragmented, the fixation can be reinforced using a tension-band wire passed through the triceps insertion (**Fig. 14–22**).

Tips and Tricks

- The key to limiting problems related to tension-band wires is to use techniques designed to limit prominence and prevent migration, to use smaller wires, and to use a bone tamp to flatten all of the prominent areas, the knots in particular. Placement of the drill holes in the shaft segment and passage of the wire through the ulna can be done prior to reduction of the fracture; this avoids problems with loss of fracture reduction while the tension-band wires are manipulated. A 14- or 16-gauge angiocatheter facilitates passage of the wire through the triceps tendon.

Outcomes

Simple Fractures

According to the experience at the Mayo Clinic, nonunion of simple olecranon fractures occurs in less than 1% of patients.[74] Most series report slight loss of flexion and extension in most patients, with severe stiffness uncommon.[69,75–78] The major problem has been symptoms related to prominent hardware.[70] Careful surgical technique can reduce this problem.[71]

Comminuted Fractures

Several series have reported predictable results with fragment excision and triceps advancement for comminuted fractures.[76,79] Although it is obvious that hardware complications and healing problems are less common, and motion is comparable, insufficient data are included to judge the performance of the elbow for more demanding functional tasks.

One-third tubular plates have been used successfully for relatively simple fractures but are too small for comminuted fractures and fracture-dislocations.[49] A 3.5 mm Limited Contact Dynamic Compression Plate (Synthes) is easily contoured and provides strong fixation of complex fractures and fracture-dislocations of the proximal ulna.

Bailey and colleagues reviewed the use of plate and screw fixation to treat 25 patients with complex fractures of the olecranon (11 fracture-dislocations). There were no significant differences in motion or strength between the injured and noninjured sides, and 22 patients achieved good or excellent results. Twenty percent of patients requested plate removal.[80]

Fracture-Dislocations of the Olecranon

When the olecranon process of the ulna is fractured, the proximal fragment usually displaces proximally, whereas the coronoid process and radial head remain in anatomical alignment with the trochlea of the distal humerus.[67] Fracture-dislocations of the olecranon are characterized by displacement or fracture of either the radial head or the coronoid process or both. The fracture of the proximal ulna associated with an olecranon fracture-dislocation is often complex and multifragmented.[26,49] Because the fragmentation of the proximal ulna often extends into the diaphysis or involves separation of the coronoid process, these injuries are often not identified as olecranon fractures.

Classification

Fracture-dislocations of the olecranon occur in either an anterior or posterior pattern of injury. The anterior olecranon-fracture dislocation has been described as a transolecranon fracture-dislocation of the elbow because the trochlea of the distal humerus appears to have driven through the olecranon process as the forearm is displaced anteriorly.[49] Anterior or transolecranon fracture-dislocations are usually the result of a high-energy direct blow. The olecranon fracture may be a simple oblique fracture but more often is a complex comminuted injury. Large (Regan and Morrey type 3) coronoid fractures are common in this pattern of injury. Fracture of the radial head is unusual. In a recent series, 29% of patients that presented with this fracture pattern had an associated wound.[49]

Distinction between anterior fracture-dislocations and posterior fracture-dislocations is straightforward because the radial head is displaced anteriorly rather than posteriorly relative to the capitellum; however, this anterior radiocapitellar dislocation often leads to misidentification of this injury as an anterior Monteggia fracture-dislocation.[26,49] Anterior fracture-dislocations of the olecranon threaten ulnohumeral stability and function, but the radioulnar relationships are usually preserved.[49] In contrast, anterior Monteggia fractures are fracture-dislocations of the forearm, with the ulnohumeral joint uninvolved.

The posterior olecranon fracture-dislocation represents the most proximal part of the spectrum of posterior Monteggia fractures. Posterior Monteggia injuries are characterized by an apex posterior fracture of the ulna, posterior dislocation of the radial head with respect to the capitellum, and, in about two thirds of injuries, fracture of the radial head.[23,24,26,81] Some authors have argued that the posterior olecranon fracture-dislocation does not represent a true Monteggia fracture because the radioulnar relationship is relatively spared when the apex posterior fracture of the ulna occurs at the level of the olecranon.[82] On the other hand, posterior olecranon fracture-dislocations, like more distal posterior Monteggia fractures, threaten both elbow and forearm function. Threats to elbow stability and function can include fracture of the olecranon, fracture of the coronoid process, fracture of the radial head, and injury to the lateral collateral ligament complex. Forearm function can be affected by the fracture or displacement of the radial head, malalignment of the ulna, or proximal radioulnar synostosis.

In some patients with complex fractures of the proximal ulna, the relationship between the radius and ulna and the trochlea may have been restored either spontaneously or by manipulative reduction. The displacement was probably posterior if the radial head is fractured, particularly if some of the fragments remain posterior. The distinction is important because anterior olecranon fracture-dislocations are stable once the alignment of the olecranon and coronoid is restored (see **Video 14–2, Disk 2**), and forearm function is rarely in jeopardy.[49] In contrast, ulnohumeral instability is common after posterior olecranon fracture-dislocations, and forearm function is often compromised.[25,26]

Surgical Treatment

Exposure of the ulna should preserve periosteal and muscle attachments. A contoured dorsal plate can be applied directly over the triceps insertion proximally and on the apex of the ulnar diaphysis distally without elevating muscle attachments. In spite of extensive fragmentation, bone grafts are rarely necessary if the soft tissue attachments are preserved.

The fractures of the radial head and coronoid process can be evaluated and often definitively treated through the exposure provided by the fracture of the olecranon process. Large coronoid fractures are best visualized and manipulated by mobilizing the olecranon fragments proximally as one would do for an olecranon osteotomy. If the coronoid is fractured into a few large fragments, it may be possible to secure these with screws. Separate anteromedial facet fragments often benefit from a second plate applied to the medial surface of the coronoid. If there is a separate tip fragment, a suture incorporating the capsular attachment should be used to secure it. Very comminuted fractures should be protected with hinged fixation.

Provisional fixation can be obtained with Kirschner wires to secure fragments to the distal ulnar metadiaphysis or trochlea of the humerus. The use of an external skeletal distractor can facilitate reduction and stabilize the fracture while plate fixation is obtained. Plate fixation of a complex fracture of the olecranon and proximal ulna is otherwise achieved using the techniques described for comminuted displaced fractures.

Outcomes

In a retrospective case series of 17 patients with transolecranon fracture dislocations, 88% had good or excellent results. Fourteen (82%) had a complex, comminuted fracture of the ulna. Even with extensive comminution of the

trochlear notch or a large coronoid fragment, results were good if alignment of the coronoid and olecranon facets was restored and stable internal fixation was obtained.[49] These results are surprisingly good, considering the complexity of many of these fractures. This may be due to several factors, including the relatively nonarticular area at the depths of the trochlear notch, the relative sparing of the collateral ligaments, and the excellent healing capacity at this site with preservation of muscle and periosteal attachments and bridge plating. The key is restoring the contour and dimensions of the trochlear notch with stable internal fixation, allowing early mobilization of the arm.

The experience with Monteggia fractures in adults was reviewed by the senior author, revealing more satisfactory results than were predicted by earlier studies. Posterior fracture dislocations of the olecranon may represent the most proximal fracture in the spectrum of Monteggia injuries. The posterior (Bado type II) fracture was found to be the most common (79%) and was associated with a fracture of the radial head in 68% and a fracture of the coronoid process in 25%. Several Bado type II fractures (24%) required reoperation within 3 months of the initial surgery. Complications secondary to loose hardware, wire prominence, and the need for radial head excision led to poor early results. However, after all reoperations and reconstructions had been performed, 83% of patients had a good/excellent result. Unsatisfactory results were associated with concomitant radial head fractures, malunion of the coronoid process or ulna, and proximal radioulnar synostosis.[26] Therefore, careful attention to stable anatomical fixation of associated coronoid and radial head injuries is crucial to successful treatment of these complex fractures.

Complications

Complications of olecranon fractures include failure of fixation, nonunion, elbow contracture, heterotopic ossification, ulnar neuropathy, and infection. Olecranon fracture-dislocations, particularly posterior Monteggia injuries, can have ulnohumeral instability. Implant prominence, although often included among complications, is probably better considered an inherent part of the treatment, which might require a second surgery.

Early failure of fixation is sometimes related to inappropriate forceful use of the arm by the patient, but usually reflects inadequate size or placement of a plate and screws for treatment of a complex fracture. One-third tubular and semitubular plates are too small for comminuted fractures or fracture-dislocations.[49] Early failure is usually straightforward to address with realignment and repeat internal fixation, although early repeat intervention may increase the risk of infection and heterotopic ossification.

Nonunion in simple olecranon fractures is now very uncommon. Papagelopoulos and Morrey stated that the rate of nonunion of simple olecranon fractures at the Mayo Clinic was less than 1%.[74] In two reports of nonunited fractures of the ulna, the majority of patients had fracture-dislocations of the elbow with complex comminuted fractures of the proximal ulna.[74,83] Union can be achieved and substantial function restored by debriding the nonunion site, providing stable fixation, and inserting autogenous bone grafts. Papagelopoulos and Morrey describe the use of corticocancellous bone plates.[74] We prefer to use a contoured 3.5 mm Limited Contact Dynamic Compression Plate and autogenous bone graft.[83]

Pearls

- Fractures of the olecranon with anterior dislocation of the forearm are usually associated with good forearm function and should not be confused with anterior Monteggia injuries.
- Fracture of the radial head is common in the setting of a posterior olecranon fracture-dislocation. The associated radial head fracture can contribute to limitation of forearm rotation and ulnohumeral instability.
- Large coronoid fractures are usually associated with olecranon fractures. Good results can be obtained with alignment and stable fixation.

Rehabilitation of Elbow Injuries

When stability has been restored and fracture fixation is secure, the elbow benefits from mobilization as soon as comfort allows, preferably within a few days of surgery. If stability is uncertain or fracture fixation is tenuous, application of a hinged external fixator may allow early protected mobilization of the elbow. In older patients with low-energy injuries and osteoporotic bone, tenuous fixation can be treated with immobilization for up to 4 weeks. Stability and healing should be emphasized over motion because a healed concentric joint can be reconstructed with capsular release, but nonunion or arthrosis may not be reconstructed.

Elbow exercises consist of active motion assisted by the other arm and by positioning of the shoulder so that gravity assists with elbow motion. It is important to avoid shoulder abduction after lateral collateral ligament repair—so-called varus stress precautions. Forceful passive manipulation of the elbow by the therapist is not useful and may cause loosening of implants or heterotopic bone.

Continuous passive motion comes in and out of fashion. It is difficult to construct a machine that consistently applies continuous motion and that doesn't require close inpatient monitoring for successful use. Furthermore, there does not seem to be any benefit of continuous passive motion over active exercise of the limb. In fact the converse may be true: patients that take a confident, active role in their rehabilitation seem to do the best.

Static progressive elbow splints (such as turnbuckle splints) and dynamic splints are often used to help regain motion.[84] These are usually initiated once it becomes clear that the patient is struggling to regain motion.

Complications

Neurapraxic nerve injuries are common with elbow fracture-dislocation, but nerve laceration is very uncommon. Brachial artery injury often occurs with open elbow dislocations and is treated with interposition vein grafting. Chronic ulnar nerve compression (cubital tunnel syndrome) is common after recovery from elbow trauma[85] and occasionally presents in the subacute setting and contributes to stiffness of the elbow.[86] We have had good results after release of posttraumatic ulnar neuropathy, although recovery may take years, particularly for motor function.[85]

Elbow stiffness is almost unavoidable after complex elbow trauma, particularly a slight flexion contracture. For flexion contractures greater than 30 degrees and lack of functional flexion that has not improved with exercises and splinting, operative elbow capsular release is considered.[63,87,88]

Heterotopic bone formation following elbow trauma is relatively common (seen in ~75% of patients) but does not restrict motion in most patients.[57] More substantial heterotopic bone can limit motion or cause complete ankylosis. Patients with central nervous system injury and elbow dislocation are at increased risk for heterotopic ossification,[89] and prophylaxis with radiation should be considered. We do not use routine prophylaxis in other patients, although we encourage most patients to use nonsteroidal anti-inflammatory medication as part of their pain control regimen.

Heterotopic bone that limits motion sufficient to merit operative treatment can be excised after it has matured on radiographs.[90] Although a waiting period of 12 to 18 months was common in the past, most elbow authorities now advocate excision of heterotopic bone as early as 4 months after injury provided that swelling is resolved, the scar is not adherent, and the heterotopic bone has well-defined margins and trabeculae. Although we have reported limited recurrence rates during a period when prophylactic radiation treatment was not available to us,[91] we now use it in most patients because its efficacy and safety are well established.[92,93]

Slight subluxation of the elbow after manipulative reduction or operative treatment of a dislocation or fracture-dislocation may be better treated with active motion than cast immobilization in confident patients because there is often an element of pseudosubluxation related to poor muscle tone (**Fig. 14–6A,B**). Persistent ulnohumeral instability is treated with restoration of radiocapitellar contact, lateral collateral ligament repair or reconstruction, restoration of the coronoid either by fixation or a bone graft when needed, and temporary hinged external fixation. Arthrosis is salvaged with fascial arthroplasty (healthy active patients) or total elbow arthroplasty (infirm older patients).

On the DVDs

Video 14–1   (Disk 2)   Trans-olecranon Elbow Fracture Dislocation   This video shows repair of a comminuted proximal ulnar fracture with associated radial head/neck fractures through a posterior incision. Repair of the radial head through the ulnar fracture and repair of the coronoid fragment are emphasized.

Video 14–2   (Disk 2)   ORIF of a Complex Elbow Injury   This video depicts open reduction and internal fixation of an olecranon fracture associated with a large coronoid process fracture. This prob-

ably represents a spontaneously reduced anterior olecranon fracture–dislocation. The patient also sustained a radius fracture treated with ORIF as well as pinning of the distal radial-ulnar joint.

Video 14–3   (Disk 2)   Tension Band Wiring of the Olecranon   This video demonstrates posterior tension band wiring of a displaced olecranon fracture. A revision fixation with a plate was necessary secondary to wire pullout from the cortex following the tension band wiring. Salvage reconstructive methods are shown.

References

1. O'Driscoll SW, Jupiter JB, Cohen M, Ring D, McKee MD. Difficult elbow fractures: pearls and pitfalls. Instr Course Lect 2003;52:113–134
2. Mehlhoff TL, Noble PC, Bennett JB, Tullos HS. Simple dislocation of the elbow in the adult: results after closed treatment. J Bone Joint Surg Am 1988;70:244–249
3. Mason ML. Some observations on fractures of the head of the radius with a review of one hundred cases. Br J Surg 1959;42:123–132
4. An KN, Morrey BF, Chao EYS. The effect of partial removal of proximal ulna on elbow constraint. Clin Orthop Relat Res 1986;209:270–279
5. Cage DJN, Abrams RA, Callahan JJ, Botte MJ. Soft tissue attachments of the ulnar coronoid process. Clin Orthop Relat Res 1995;320:154–158
6. Sojbjerg JO, Ovesen J, Nielsen S. Experimental elbow stability after transection of the medial collateral ligament. Clin Orthop Relat Res 1987;218:186–190
7. Smith GR, Hotchkiss RN. Radial head and neck fractures: anatomic guidelines for proper placement of internal fixation. J Shoulder Elbow Surg 1996;5:113–117
8. Caputo AE, Mazzocca AD, Santoro VM. The nonarticulating portion of the radial head: anatomic and clinical correlations for internal fixation. J Hand Surg [Am] 1998;23:1082–1090
9. Morrey BF. Anatomy of the elbow joint. In: Morrey BF, ed. The Elbow and Its Disorders. 2nd ed. Philadelphia: WB Saunders; 1995:16–52
10. Nestor BJ, O'Driscoll SW, Morrey BF. Ligamentous reconstruction for posterolateral rotatory instability of the elbow. J Bone Joint Surg am 1992;74:1235–1241
11. Cohen MS, Hastings H. Rotatory instability of the elbow: the anatomy and role of the lateral stabilizers. J Bone Joint Surg Am 1997;79:225–233
12. Patterson SD, Bain GI, Mehta JA. Surgical approaches to the elbow. Clin Orthop Relat Res 2000;370:19–33
13. Dowdy PA, Bain GI, King GJ, Patterson SD. The midline posterior elbow incision. J Bone Joint Surg Br 1995;77:696–699
14. Ring D, Quintero J, Jupiter JB. Open reduction and internal fixation of fractures of the radial head. J Bone Joint Surg Am 2002;84-A:1811–1815
15. Radin EL, Riseborough EJ. Fractures of the radial head. J Bone Joint Surg Am 1966;48:1055–1065
16. Ring D, Jupiter JB. Fracture-dislocation of the elbow. J Bone Joint Surg Am 1998;80:566–580
17. King GJW, Evans DC, Kellam JF. Open reduction and internal fixation of radial head fractures. J Orthop Trauma 1991;5:21–28
18. Moro JK, Werier J, MacDermid JC, Patterson SD, King GJW. Arthroplasty with a metal radial head for unreconstructible frac-

tures of the radial head. J Bone Joint Surg Am 2001;83:1201–1211
19. Johnston GW. A follow-up of one hundred cases of fracture of the head of the radius. Ulster Med J 1962;31:51–56
20. Muller ME, Nazarian S, Koch P, Schatzker J. The Comprehensive Classification of Fractures of Long Bones. Heidelberg: Springer-Verlag; 1990
21. Essex-Lopresti P. Fractures of the radial head with distal radioulnar dislocation. J Bone Joint Surg Br 1951;33B:244–247
22. Szabo RM, Hotchkiss RN, Slater RR. The use of frozen-allograft radial head replacement for treatment of established symptomatic proximal translation of the radius: preliminary experience in five cases. J Hand Surg [Am] 1997;22:269–278
23. Pavel A, Pittman JM, Lance EM, Wade PA. The posterior Monteggia fracture: a clinical study. J Trauma 1965;12:185–199
24. Penrose JH. The Monteggia fracture with posterior dislocation of the radial head. J Bone Joint Surg Br 1951;33-B:65–73
25. Jupiter JB, Leibovic SJ, Ribbans W, Wilk RM. The posterior Monteggia lesion. J Orthop Trauma 1991;5:395–402
26. Ring D, Jupiter JB, Simpson NS. Monteggia fractures in adults. J Bone Joint Surg Am 1998;80:1733–1744
27. Khalfayan EE, Culp RW, Alexander AH. Mason type II radial head fractures: operative versus nonoperative treatment. J Orthop Trauma 1992;6:283–289
28. Davidson PA, Moseley JB Jr, Tullos HS. Radial head fracture: a potentially complex injury. Clin Orthop Relat Res 1993;297:224–130
29. Ring D, Chin K, Jupiter JB. Nonunion of nonoperatively treated fractures of the radial head. Clin Orthop Relat Res 2002;398:235–238
30. Cobb TK, Beckenbaugh RD. Nonunion of the radial head and neck. Orthopedics 1998;21:364–368
31. Sanchez-Sotelo J, Romanillos O, Garay EG. Results of acute excision of the radial head in elbow radial head fracture-dislocations. J Orthop Trauma 2000;14:354–358
32. Smith AM, Urbanosky LR, Castle JA, Rushing JT. Radius pull test: predictor of longitudinal forearm instability. J Bone Joint Surg Am 2002;84-A:1970–1976
33. Strachan JC, Ellis BW. Vulnerability of the posterior interosseous nerve during radial head resection. J Bone Joint Surg Br 1971;53B:93–97
34. Diliberti T, Botte MJ, Abrams RA. Anatomical considerations regarding the posterior interosseous nerve during posterolateral approaches to the proximal part of the radius. J Bone Joint Surg Am 2000;82:809–813
35. Kaplan EB. Surgical approach to the proximal end of the radius and its use in fractures of the head and neck of the radious. Bone Joint Surg 1941;22:86–92
36. Hotchkiss RN. Displaced fractures of the radial head: internal fixation or excision. J Am Acad Orthop Surg 1997;5:1–10

37. Geel C. Fractures of the radial head. In: McQueen MM, Jupiter JB, eds. Radius and Ulna. Oxford: Butterworth-Heinemann; 1999:159–168

38. Heim U, Pfeiffer KM. Internal Fixation of Small Fractures. 3rd ed. Berlin: Springer-Verlag; 1988

39. Soyer AD, Nowotarski PJ, Kelso TB, Mighell MA. Optimal position for plate fixation of complex fractures of the proximal radius: a cadaver study. J Orthop Trauma 1998;12:291–293

40. Vanderwilde RS, Morrey BF, Melberg MW, Vinh TN. Inflammatory arthritis after failure of silicone rubber replacement of the radial head. J Bone Joint Surg Br 1994;76:78–81

41. Judet T, Garreau de Loubresse C, Piriou P, Charnley G. A floating prosthesis for radial head fractures. J Bone Joint Surg Br 1996; 78:244–249

42. Knight DJ, Rymaszewski LA, Amis AA, Miller JH. Primary replacement of the fractured radial head with a metal prosthesis. J Bone Joint Surg Br 1993;75:572–576

43. O'Driscoll SW. Classification and spectrum of elbow instability: recurrent instability. In: Morrey BF, ed. The Elbow and Its Disorders. 2nd ed. Philadelphia: WB Saunders; 1993:453–463

44. O'Driscoll SW, Morrey BF, Korinek S, An KN. Elbow subluxation and dislocation. A spectrum of instability. Clin Orthop Relat Res 1992; 280:186–197

45. Protzman RR. Dislocation of the elbow joint. J Bone Joint Surg Am 1978;60:539–541

46. Dürig M, Müller W, Rüedi TP, Ekkehard FG. The operative treatment of elbow dislocation in the adult. J Bone Joint Surg Am 1979; 61:239–244

47. Josefsson PO, Johnell O, Wendeberg B. Ligamentous injuries in dislocations of the elbow joint. Clin Orthop Relat Res 1987;221: 221–225

48. Josefsson PO, Gentz CF, Johnell O, Wendeberg B. Dislocations of the elbow and intraarticular fractures. Clin Orthop Relat Res 1989;246: 126–130

49. Ring D, Jupiter JB, Sanders RW, Mast J, Simpson NS. Transolecranon fracture-dislocation of the elbow. J Orthop Trauma 1997;11: 545–550

50. Josefsson PO, Gentz CF, Johnell O, Wendberg B. Surgical versus non-surgical treatment of ligamentous injuries following dislocation of the elbow joint. J Bone Joint Surg Am 1987;69:605–608

51. McKee MD, Bowden SH, King GJ, et al. Management of recurrent, complex instability of the elbow with a hinged external fixator. J Bone Joint Surg Br 1998;80:1031–1036

52. McKee MD, Schemitsch EH, Sala MJ, O'Driscoll SW. The pathoanatomy of lateral ligamentous disruption in complex elbow instability. J Shoulder Elbow Surg 2003;12:391–396

53. Morrey BF, An KN. Articular and ligamentous contributions to the stability of the elbow joint. Am J Sports Med 1983;11:315–320

54. Linscheid RL, O'Driscoll SW. Elbow dislocations. In: Morrey BF, ed. The Elbow and Its Disorders. 2nd ed. Philadelphia: WB Saunders; 1993:441–452

55. Ring D, Jupiter JB, Zilberfarb J. Posterior dislocation of the elbow with fractures of the coronoid and radial head. J Bone Joint Surg Am 2002;84:547–551

56. Ross G, McDevitt ER, Chronister R, Ove PN. Treatment of simple elbow dislocation using and immediate motion protocol. Am J Sports Med 1999;27:308–311

57. Josefsson PO, Johnell O, Gentz CF. Long-term sequelae of simple dislocation of the elbow. J Bone Joint Surg Am 1984;66:927–930

58. Heim U. Combined fractures of the radius and the ulna at the elbow level in the adult: analysis of 120 cases after more than 1 year [in French]. Rev Chir Orthop Reparatrice Appar Mot. 1998;84: 142–153

59. Broberg MA, Morrey BF. Results of treatment of fracture-dislocations of the elbow. Clin Orthop Relat Res 1987;216:109–119

60. Frankle MA, Koval KJ, Sanders RW, Zuckerman JD. Radial head fractures associated with elbow dislocations treated by immediate stabilization and early motion. J Shoulder Elbow Surg 1999;8:355–360

61. Regan W, Morrey BF. Fractures of the coronoid process of the ulna. J Bone Joint Surg Am 1989;71A:1348–1354

62. Taylor TKF, Scham SM. A posteromedial approach to the proximal end of the ulna for the internal fixation of olecranon fractures. J Trauma 1969;9:594–602

63. Hotchkiss RN. Elbow contracture. In: Green DP, Hotchkiss RN, Pederson WC, eds. Green's Operative Hand Surgery. Philadelphia: Churchill-Livingstone; 1999:667–682

64. Ring D, Jupiter JB. Surgical exposure of coronoid fractures. Tech Should Elb Surg 2002;3:48–56

65. Colton CL. Fractures of the olecranon in adults: classification and management. Injury 1973;5:121–129

66. Schatzker J, Tile M. The Rationale of Operative Fracture Care. 2nd ed. New York: Springer-Verlag; 1996

67. Morrey BF. Current concepts in the treatment of fractures of the radial head, the olecranon, and the coronoid. J Bone Joint Surg am 1995;77:316–327

68. Cabanela M, Morrey B. Fractures of the olecranon. In: Morrey B, ed. The Elbow and Its Disorders. 3rd ed. Philadelphia: WB Saunders; 1999:365–379

69. Murphy D, Greene W, Dameron T Jr. Displaced olecranon fractures in adults. Clinical evaluation. Clin Orthop Relat Res 1987;224:215–223

70. Macko D, Szabo RM. Complications of tension-band wiring of olecranon fractures. J Bone Joint Surg Am 1985;67:1396–1401

71. Chin KR, Ring D, Jupiter JB. Double tension-band fixation of the olecranon. Tech Shoulder and Elb Surgery 2000;1:61–66

72. Mullett JH, Shannon F, Noel J, Lawlor G, Lee TC, O'Rourke SK. K-wire position in tension band wiring of the olecranon: a comparison of two techniques. Injury 2000;31:427–431

73. Didonna ML, Fernandez JJ, Lim TH, Hastings H 2nd, Cohen MS. Partial olecranon excision: the relationship between triceps insertion site and extension strength of the elbow. J Hand Surg [Am] 2003; 28:117–122

74. Papagelopoulos PJ, Morrey BF. Treatment of nonunion of olecranon fractures. J Bone Joint Surg Br 1994;76:627–635

75. Horne J, Tanzer T. Olecranon fractures: a review of 100 cases. J Trauma 1981;21:469–472

76. Inhofe P, Howard T. The treatment of olecranon fractures by excision of fragments and repair of extensor mechanism: historical review and report of 12 fractures. Orthopedics 1993;16:1313–1317

77. Johnson R, Roetker A, Schwab J. Olecranon fractures treated with AO screw and tension bands. Orthopedics 1986;9:66–68

78. Wolfgang G, Burke F, Bush D. Surgical treatment of displaced olecranon fractures by tension band wiring technique. Clin Orthop Relat Res 1987;224:192–204

79. Gartsman GM, Scales JC, Otis JC. Operative treatment of olecranon fractures. J Bone Joint Surg Am 1981;63:718–721

80. Bailey CS, MacDermid J, Patterson SD, King GJ. Outcome of plate fixation of olecranon fractures. J Orthop Trauma 2001;15:542–548

81. Jupiter JB. Heterotopic ossification about the elbow. Instructional Course Lectures, In Wilkins KE, Morrey BF, Kobe FL et al. The American Academy of Orthopaedic Surgeons 1991;40:41–44

82. Bruce HE, Harvey JP, Wilson JC. Monteggia fractures. J Bone Joint Surg Am 1974;56:1563–1576

83. Ring D, Jupiter JB, Gulotta L. Atrophic nonunions of the proximal ulna. Clin Orthop Relat Res 2003;409:268–274

84. Green DP, McCoy H. Turnbuckle orthotic correction of elbow-flexion contractures after acute injuries. J Bone Joint Surg Am 1979;61: 1092–1095

85. McKee MD, Jupiter JB, Bosse G, Goodman L. Outcome of ulnar neurolysis during post-traumatic reconstruction of the elbow. J Bone Joint Surg Br 1998;80:100–105

86. Faierman E, Wang J, Jupiter JB. Secondary ulnar nerve palsy in adults after elbow trauma: a report of two cases. J Hand Surg [Am] 2001;26:675–678

87. Cohen MS, Hastings H. Post-traumatic contracture of the elbow: operative release using a lateral collateral ligament sparing approach. J Bone Joint Surg Br 1998;80:805–812

88. Mansat P, Morrey BF. The column procedure: a limited lateral approach for extrinsic contracture of the elbow. J Bone Joint Surg Am 1998;80:1603–1615

89. Garland DE, Blum CE, Waters RL. Periarticular heterotopic ossification in head-injured adults: incidence and location. J Bone Joint Surg Am 1980;62:1143–1146

90. Viola RW, Hastings H. Treatment of ectopic ossification about the elbow. Clin Orthop Relat Res 2000;370:65–86

91. Jupiter JB, Ring D. Operative treatment of post-traumatic proximal radioulnar synostosis. J Bone Joint Surg Am 1998;80:248–257

92. McAuliffe JA, Wolfson AH. Early excision of heterotopic ossification about the elbow followed by radiation therapy. J Bone Joint Surg Am 1997;79:749–755

93. Ring D, Jupiter J. The operative release of complete ankylosis of the elbow due to heterotopic bone in patients without severe injury of the central nervous system. J Bone Joint Surg Am 2003;85: 849–857

15 Forearm Fractures
Rena L. Stewart

Fractures of the radius and ulna are common injuries, with over 644,000 such fractures in the United States alone in 1998.[1] Falls constitute the most common mechanism, and 26% occur in children under 15 years of age.[1] Four major variants of forearm fractures exist: concomitant diaphyseal fractures of the radius and ulna (most common), fracture of the ulna with radial head dislocation (Monteggia fracture), fractures of the radius with distal radial ulnar joint (DRUJ) dislocation (Galeazzi fracture), and isolated fractures of the ulna. The unique feature of the forearm is that, unlike the other long bones of the body, the two bones of the forearm should be considered a "joint," rather than a pair of "long bones." In other long bones, anatomical restoration of the diaphysis is unnecessary, and, instead, simply reconstituting length, angulation, and rotation is the surgical goal. Because pronation and supination are achieved by rotation of the radius about the ulna, both the curvature of the radius and the integrity of the interosseous space must be anatomically re-created if the forearm is to return to full function (**Fig. 15–1A–C**).[2,3] Because the radius and ulna articulate with one another at both the distal and proximal ends, the integrity of these joints is a further essential ingredient in achieving excellent long-term results after injury.

With the exception of some isolated ulnar shaft fractures, operative management is the cornerstone of treatment of forearm fractures. Attention to surgical detail yields excellent rates of healing (98% in the radius and 96% in the ulna) and high levels of patient satisfaction.[4–6] The complex anatomy of the forearm and the need for anatomical reduction make the forearm both a demanding and a satisfying surgical challenge.

Classification

Like many diaphyseal fractures, radius and ulna fractures are not described by a common or universally accepted classification system. Because the surgical approach to the radius varies depending on what portion of the shaft is fractured, fractures of the radial diaphysis (and the adjacent ulna) are frequently divided simply into proximal, middle, and distal thirds. Galeazzi fractures are similarly described by which third of the radius is fractured. Isolated ulnar shaft fractures are generally classified simply as displaced and nondisplaced depending on if the fracture is displaced more or less than 50%, respectively.[7] Monteggia fractures are most commonly described using the Bado classification.[8] This classification describes the direction of the dislocation of the radial head, which is the same as the apex of the ulna fracture, and is either anterior (type I), posterior (II), or lateral (III). Type IV fractures involve anterior dislocation of the radial head with fracture of both the radius and ulna at the proximal third of the forearm (**Fig. 15–2A–D**).

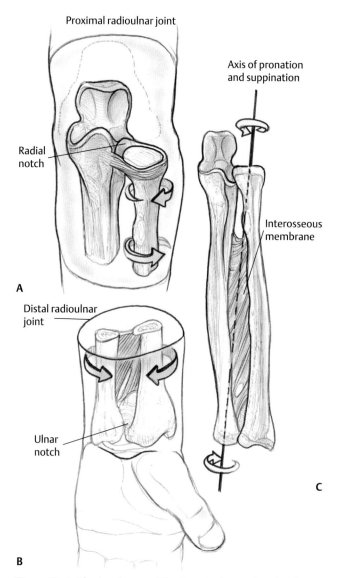

A

B

C

Figure 15–1 The two bones of the forearm form a functional unit, with the axis of rotation extending from the radiocapitellar joint to the distal radioulnar joint. **(A)** The proximal radioulnar joint. **(B)** The distal radioulnar joint. **(C)** The axis of forearm rotation.

Figure labels: Proximal radioulnar joint; Axis of pronation and suppination; Radial notch; Interosseous membrane; Distal radioulnar joint; Ulnar notch

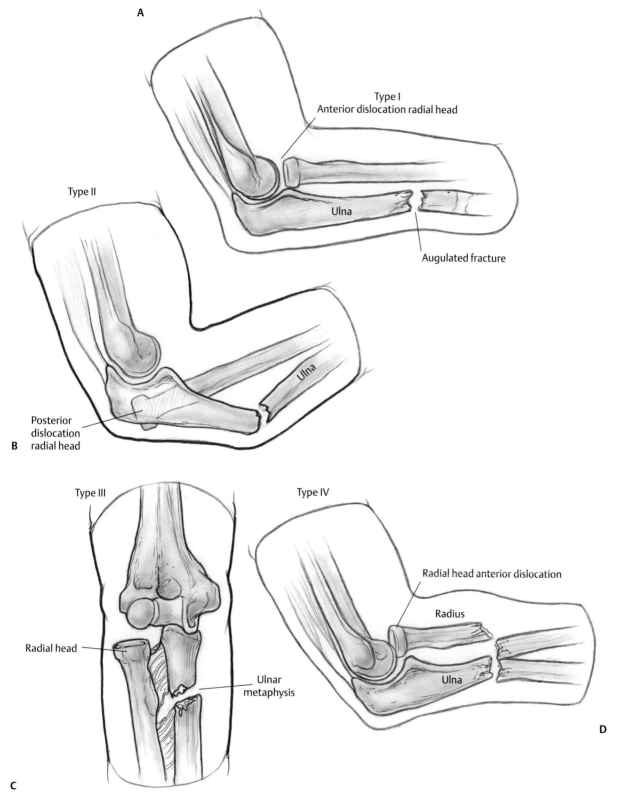

Figure 15–2 The Bado classification of Monteggia fractures. **(A)** A Bado type I injury with anterior dislocation of the radial head. **(B)** A Bado type II injury with posterior dislocation of the radial head. **(C)** A Bado type III injury is characterized by lateral dislocation of the radial head, typically associated with an ulna fracture just distal to the coronoid process. **(D)** A Bado type IV injury is characterized by an anterior dislocation of the radial head and fractures of both the radious and ulna.

Nonoperative Treatment

Indications for Nonoperative Treatment

In the forearm, there are two indications for nonoperative management. One indication is fractures involving skeletally immature children, the discussion of which is beyond the scope of this text. The other indication is isolated ulna shaft fractures caused by a direct blow, the so-called nightstick fracture. The accepted criteria for nonoperative management of the ulnar shaft is displacement less than 50% of the diaphyseal width and angulation less than 10 degrees.[7,9,10] Fracture of the ulna in the proximal third of the diaphysis has been shown to be associated with a greater loss of pronation (average 12 degrees) compared with distal third fractures (5 degrees) following nonoperative management.[2] Therefore, it has been suggested that proximal ulna fractures should be treated with operative management. It should be emphasized that the same principles do not hold true for the radius. It is exceedingly rare to find a truly isolated fracture of the radius because a direct blow is far less likely to land on the radial side of the arm. Vigilance must be maintained to look for concomitant DRUJ injury in cases of apparently "isolated" radius fractures because the DRUJ may have spontaneously reduced. Remember that the forearm is a ring, and it is "exceedingly difficult to break a Cheerio in only one place."

Reduction and Casting Techniques

Isolated ulnar shaft fractures that are treated nonoperatively do not require closed reduction because the indications for nonoperative management (less than 50% displacement and 10 degrees angulation) are the same as the criteria for acceptable fracture position.[7,9–13] Because both the interosseous membrane and the radius remain intact, such fractures are also considered stable and do not require rigid immobilization.[7,14,15] For this reason, below-elbow casting, splinting, and elastic bandages are frequently used to treat these fractures, with good results.[16–18] Above-elbow casting has been shown to significantly reduce the number of good or excellent results and is discouraged.[19]

Displaced fractures of the radius are associated with shortening, angulation, and some degree of injury to the distal radioulnar joint. Such fractures are essentially impossible to reduce and in the adult, are treated surgically.

Displaced fractures of both the radius and the ulna are very unstable. Although it is recommended that these injuries be treated surgically, provisional splinting is necessary. Typically, a well-padded dorsal-volar plaster splint is used with an interosseous mold to maintain alignment and provide some measure of stability while surgery is planned.

Functional Bracing

Functional bracing relies on the principle that a column of liquid (the fluid within the forearm) contained within a rigid boundary (the functional brace) is incompressible and therefore provides resistance to deformation. In the largest series of isolated ulnar shaft fractures published, Sarmiento et al showed a 99% union rate and 96% good or excellent functional result with functional brace treatment.[13] Functional braces allow free range of motion of both the elbow and the wrist and are lightweight and reasonably inexpensive; several studies have reproduced excellent results (**Figs. 15–3** and **15–4**).[10,12,13,20,21] In patients whose fluid status is frequently changing, such as severe congestive heart failure (CHF) or patients requiring large-volume resuscitation, functional bracing may not be effective.

Despite the good results achieved with functional bracing, there is also evidence that good results are possible with early mobilization. Cadaveric studies have shown that fractures with less than 50% displacement are stable to rotation.[7] Several authors have recommended early mobilization with either an elastic compression bandage or complete freedom following 1 to 2 weeks of below-elbow splinting.[7,19,22,23] Meta-analysis revealed that time to union was more rapid in patients treated by early mobilization than with functional braces, whereas the numbers of good and excellent results were similar.[18]

Rehabilitation

Isolated ulna shaft fractures treated with any of the previously described nonoperative methods generally have excellent results if early range of motion is instituted. Active range of motion of both elbow and wrist, including supination/pronation, should begin almost immediately as pain allows, certainly no later than 2 weeks following injury. Range of motion of the shoulder should also be emphasized. Patients should use the affected limb for activities of daily living such as grooming and eating. We restrict lifting to no more than 2 lb (1 kg) for the first 4 weeks and then increase as tolerated. Weight bearing (on regular crutches) is not allowed until 6 weeks, but the patient can use a platform crutch immediately as pain allows.

Indications for Surgical Treatment

All adult diaphyseal fractures of the forearm, with the exception of the minimally displaced, isolated ulna fracture described previously, are best treated by operative management.[4,24,25] Recall that the goals of treatment are twofold: anatomical restoration of length, rotation, and curvature of both bones as well as the interosseous space, and also to provide sufficient stability to allow early range of motion. These goals can only be achieved by operative means.[26]

Surgical Treatment

General Principles

Rigid internal fixation of forearm fractures is best achieved by following the traditional principles of fracture fixation.

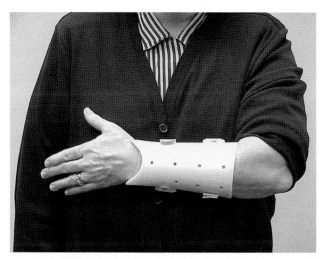

Figure 15–3 Photograph of a patient with an isolated ulnar shaft fracture treated in a functional brace.

When possible, interfragmentary compression, either via a lag screw with a neutralization plate (oblique or spiral fractures) or a compression plate (transverse fractures), is utilized. To apply these techniques, the fracture site must be fully exposed. One must also keep in mind that modern principles of fracture fixation emphasize the need to preserve blood supply to both soft tissues and bone by careful soft tissue handling and gentle reduction techniques. One of the challenges of fixation of forearm fractures is achieving a balance between adequate visualization of the fracture and soft tissue preservation.

Preoperative Planning

The importance of a thorough, well thought out preoperative plan cannot be overemphasized. Preoperative planning ensures that all equipment, personnel, special tools, and imaging will be ready and available. A small investment of time in preoperative planning should eliminate the frustration, wasted time, and danger associated with "unforeseen" intraoperative problems.

Preoperative planning for forearm fractures is relatively simple and will require good quality anteroposterior (AP) and lateral x-rays, tracing paper, a set of transparent templates of all implants to correct scale, and several marking pens. With digital images, the magnification is variable, but such x-rays usually include a marker or scale that can be used to calculate the correct size. Computerized templates are now available that allow preoperative planning to be performed directly on the digital images, eliminating the pen-and-paper method.

The preoperative plan should consist of two key elements: the drawing of the fracture fragments with the appropriate implants applied and also a "surgical plan," which lists all of the steps necessary for the procedure. The plan should be all encompassing, including positioning, draping, tourniquet, anesthetic, surgical approach, steps for fracture reduction and implant application, closure, dressing, and splinting. **Fig. 15–5A–C** shows a preoperative

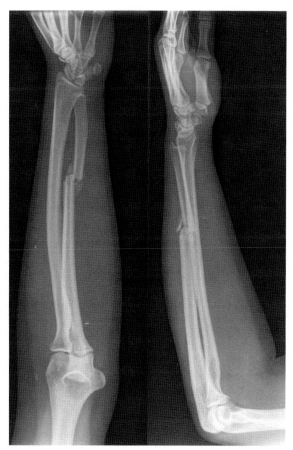

Figure 15–4 Isolated ulnar shaft fracture at 8 weeks treated with early motion. There has been no change in fracture displacement or angulation, and early callus is visible.

plan of a radius and ulna fracture. Comparison of the postoperative x-rays with the plan should show a final result that looks remarkably similar to the preoperative sketch.

Positioning and Draping

All radius and ulna fractures can be approached easily with the patient supine and the arm abducted perpendicular to the body on a radiolucent arm table. The arm can then be supinated or pronated to allow a volar or dorsal approach. The elbow is generally flexed to 90 degrees to approach the ulna. This setup will allow the surgeon and assistant to sit on either side of the arm table. A tourniquet should be applied to the upper arm, as far proximal as possible, and draping should leave the elbow within the surgical field with enough room to flex and extend fully. If a patient is positioned prone or lateral for repair of another fracture, it is well worth the time of repositioning to supine prior to addressing the forearm fracture.

Imaging

It is imperative that intraoperative imaging of the entire forearm can be obtained. Although the "mini C-arm"

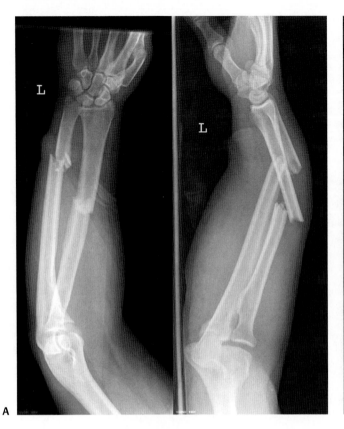

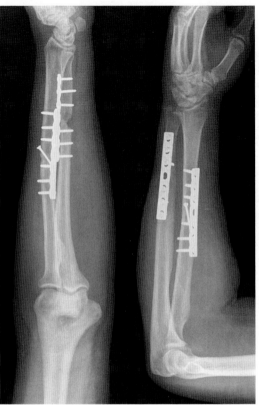

A

C

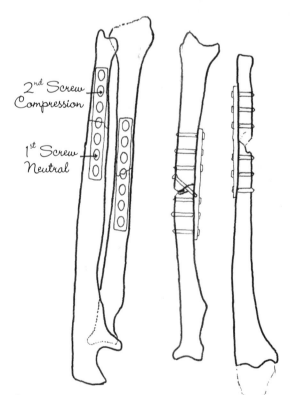

B

Pre-Op Plan

1. Supine/Arm table / Tourniquet *No Exsanguination
2. "Henry's" (Anterior) Approach to Radius
3. Expose fx Ø stripping *Specials : Dental pick
4. Reduce → Interfragmentary screw
5. Neutralization plate - 7 hole LCDC plate
    (leave central hole open)
6. Ulnar - approach to ulna : ECU/FCU interval
7. Reduce *Make sure no comminution on
    interosseous membrane!
8. Compression Plate
    Screw #1 - Hole 6 (proximal) in neutral
    Screw #2 - Hole 2 (distal) in compression
    Fill holes 1/3/5/7 neutral
9. ✔ Flouro + full ROM
10. Close subcut d̄ skin (Drain *if* needed)
11. No splint

2ⁿᵈ Screw
Compression

1ˢᵗ Screw
Neutral

Figure 15–5 Example of preoperative planning. **(A)** Anteroposterior and lateral radiographs of a displaced radius and ulna fracture. **(B)** Illustration of actual preoperative plan detailing the operative steps, implants, and equipment. **(C)** Postoperative x-rays. Note how close the actual fixation resembles that drawn on the preoperative plan.

reduces radiation and may be controlled by the surgeon, the small field of view limits its usefulness in assessing forearm fractures. Recall that one of the essential goals of surgery is the anatomical restoration of radial curvature. This requires imaging that will include the entire length of the radius on a single view, which is only possible with a regular-sized fluoroscope or plain x-ray.

Surgical Anatomy and Choice of Surgical Approach

The surgical anatomy of the forearm is complex, and all approaches to the radius present dangers for intraoperative injury to neurovascular structures. To conceptualize surgical anatomy of the forearm, it may be easiest to focus on the three main muscle groups, each supplied by a different nerve or nerves **(Fig. 15–6)**. A surgical incision made between any two muscle groups proceeds through an internervous plane. Once these internervous planes are understood, the location of neurovascular structures encountered during each approach can be learned safely. The first muscle group is the "mobile wad of three," which forms the proximal, lateral border of the forearm in supination. These three muscles are the brachioradialis and the extensor carpi radialis longus (ECRL) and brevis (ECRB). The radial nerve innervates the brachioradialis and ECRL, whereas the posterior interosseous nerve (PIN), also known as the deep posterior branch of the radial nerve,

supplies the ECRB. Despite the fact that this muscle group is innervated by two nerves, the mobile wad should be thought of as a single group because no surgical approach divides these muscles. Instead, the approaches enter the forearm on either side of this group. Traveling ulnarward across the anterior surface of the forearm, the next group of muscles is the flexor-pronator group. Again, though this group of eight muscles is supplied by two different nerves (median and ulnar), it should be conceptualized as a single group from a surgical perspective because none of the approaches to the radius pass between or divide muscles in this group. The flexor-pronator group consists of three layers: superficial [pronator teres, flexor carpi radialis (FCR), palmaris longus, and flexor carpi ulnaris (FCU)], middle [flexor digitorum superficialis (FDS)], and deep [flexor digitorum profundus (FDP), flexor pollicis longus (FPL), and pronator quadratus]. Continuing to move clockwise around the forearm, the next muscle group encountered is the extensors. Once again, despite this group having more than one innervation (radial and PIN), no approaches transect this group, and the internervous planes are formed on either side of the extensors.

Having established three muscle groups in the forearm, it is now much easier to understand the three approaches that lie between each of the groups. The approach to the ulna is directly along its subcutaneous border, between the extensor and flexor-pronator groups. The dorsal approach to the radius lies between the extensors and the mobile

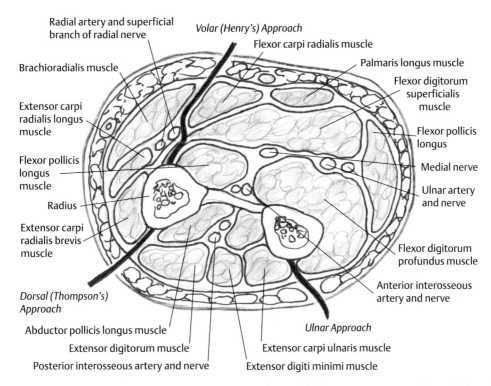

Figure 15–6 The muscle "groups" or "blocks" showing the internervous planes of the forearm. One group is the "mobile wad," another group is the flexor-pronator muscles, and the third group is the extensors.

wad. The volar approach to the radius lies between the opposite edge of the mobile wad and the flexor-pronators. Now that the internervous planes have been defined, the surgical dangers of each approach can be more easily understood.

The ulna lies subcutaneously and can be approached safely and easily between the extensor and flexor-pronator groups **(Fig. 15–7A,B).** This approach enters between the extensor carpi ulnaris (ECU) and FCU muscles, both of which attach to the ulnar border by a shared aponeurosis. This is an internervous plane between the PIN (to ECU) and the ulnar nerve (to FCU). Protection of these nerves is accomplished by careful subperiosteal stripping of the muscles. The ulnar nerve travels volar to the FCU, between the FDP and FDS, and caution must be taken to ensure that dissection does not stray into the substance of the muscle, endangering the nerve. At the most distal extent of the

approach to the ulna, the dorsal cutaneous branch of the ulnar nerve may be endangered. The dorsal branch arises ~5 cm proximal to the wrist joint and crosses dorsally, superficial to the extensor retinaculum. Care must be taken to identify and dorsally retract this branch when the most distal aspect of the ulna and the ulnar styloid are exposed. The ulnar artery travels with the ulnar nerve and is similarly protected if dissection of the FCU remains subperiosteal.

The radius may be approached from either the volar/anterior side using the classic extensile approach of Henry[27] **(Fig. 15–8A,B)** (see **Videos 15–1, 15–2, Disk 2**) or dorsal side using the approach described by Thompson **(Fig. 15–9A–C).**[28] Each approach has advantages and surgical dangers. There are several considerations in choosing either the volar or the dorsal approach. The first is the position of the plate in relation to the bending forces on the

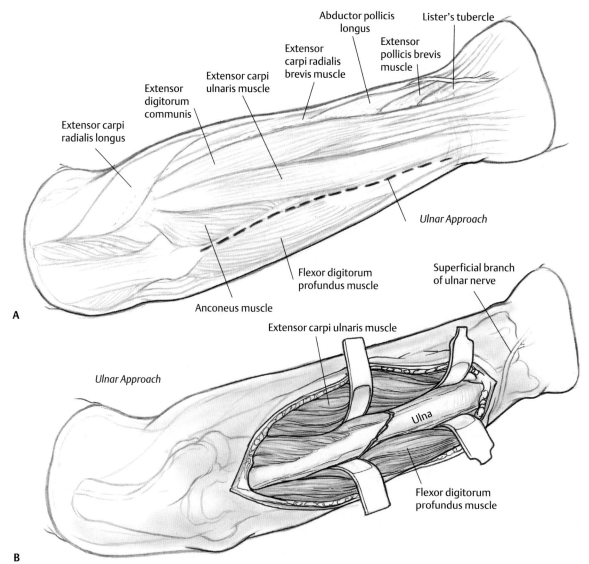

Figure 15–7 The approach to the ulnar shaft. **(A)** The superficial dissection is between the extensor carpi ulnaris and the flexor carpi ulnaris. **(B)** Appearance of the completed approach to the ulna.

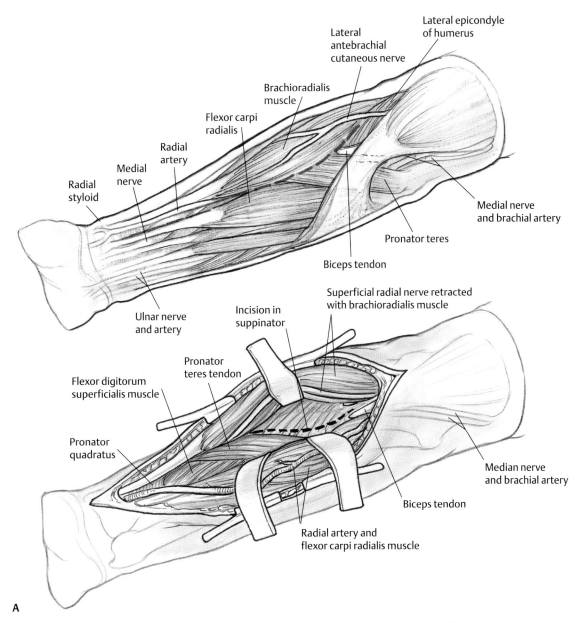

Figure 15–8 The volar approach to the forearm. **(A)** Superficial approach. *(continued on page 348)*

fracture. A plate placed on the dorsal or dorsoradial surface (via the dorsal approach) will be applied on the "tension" side of the fracture, which is advantageous.[29] However, the dorsal approach also positions the surgical scar on the most visible surface of the forearm. The aesthetics of this scar may be a consideration, especially in patients with a tendency toward hypertrophic or keloid scars. Most important is to choose an approach that allows adequate visualization and manipulation of the fracture with minimal danger to neurological and vascular structures. The two most important structures that influence the choice of approach are the PIN and the branches of the radial artery. The PIN supplies innervation to all of the extensor musculature of the forearm, and damage will result in a severe functional deficit.[30] The PIN is at risk during both volar and dorsal approaches to the proximal third of the forearm.

The PIN branches off from the radial nerve anterior to the lateral epicondyle of the humerus in the cubital fossa.[31] The PIN then pierces the supinator muscle, diving between the two heads of the muscle to wind around the posterior surface of the radius. In 25% of individuals, the PIN will come into direct contact with the radial neck, placing it in danger if retractors are placed around the proximal radius. The PIN continues distally within the body of the supinator muscle and emerges dorsally ~1 cm proximal to the distal border of this muscle. The volar approach does not allow direct visualization of the PIN. Protection of the nerve relies on first displacing the nerve as far away from the surgical field as possible by fully supinating the forearm (which displaces the nerve posteriorly and laterally). The supinator muscle is then incised along its insertion, which is on the medial side of the radius, away from the nerve.

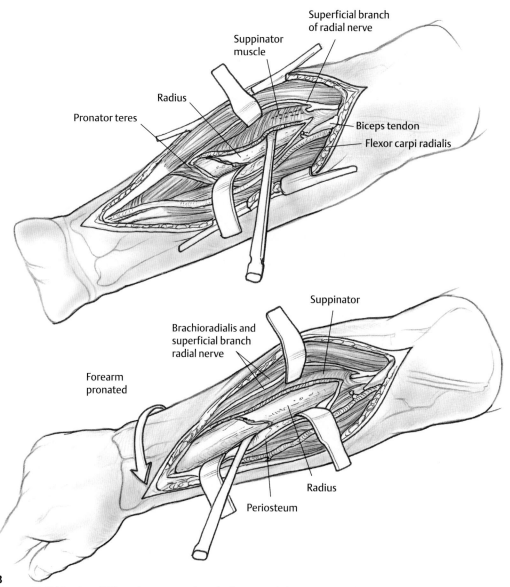

Figure 15–8 *(Continued)* The volnar approach to the forearm. **(B)** Deep approach. Note the relation to the posterior interosseous nerve.

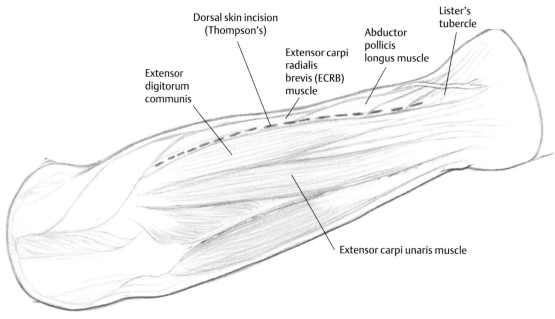

Figure 15–9 The dorsal approach to the forearm. **(A)** Skin incision.

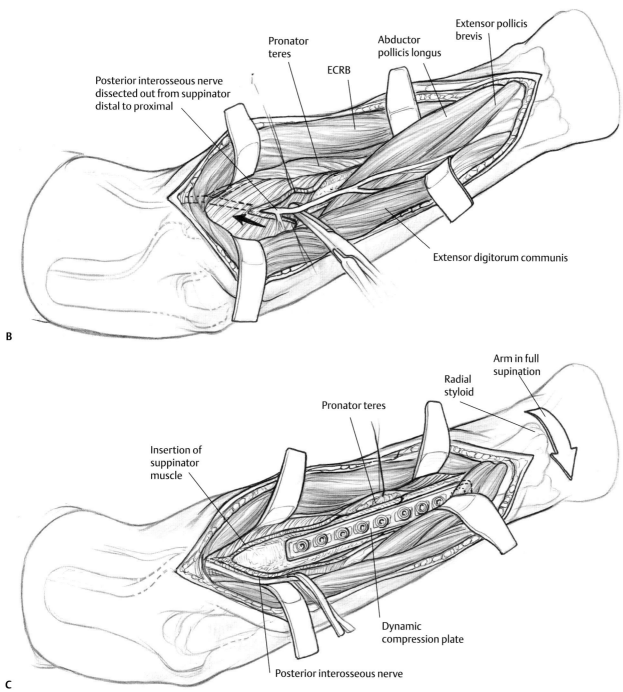

Figure 15–9 *(Continued)* The dorsal approach to the forearm. **(B)** Midlevel dissection. **(C)** Deep dissection. Note the relation to the posterior interosseous nerve.

Careful subperiosteal stripping of the supinator protects the PIN as the muscle lies between the bone and the nerve as it is lifted off the radius.

In contrast, the dorsal approach allows, and in fact demands, direct visualization of the PIN. Here the interval between the forearm extensors and the mobile wad is employed, and dissection between the ECRB and the extensor digitorum communis (EDC) leads down onto the supinator muscle. The PIN can be found in one of two ways. The nerve can be dissected from the midsubstance of the supinator, working proximal to distal. It is generally

easier to identify the most distal border of the supinator and then find the PIN as it emerges dorsally ~1 cm proximal to this border. Once the PIN has been identified, follow the nerve into the supinator muscle from distal to proximal.

The second anatomical consideration in the choice of volar versus dorsal approach to the radius is the branches of the radial artery. In the proximal forearm, the radial artery arises from the bifurcation of the brachial artery just below the bend of the elbow at the level of the neck of the radius. It gives off several branches near the elbow. The radial recurrent artery arises immediately below the elbow and immediately turns back to ascend into the arm. Initially it lies on the supinator muscle and then between the brachioradialis and the brachialis. It is this initial length of the radial recurrent artery as it lies on the volar surface of the supinator muscle that presents a surgical danger during the volar approach to the radius. The radial recurrent artery gives several muscular branches to the brachioradialis in this region that traverse across the surgical plane for the volar approach. Therefore, these branches must be identified and ligated before the supinator muscle can be visualized. Particularly in a muscular forearm, the surgical wound is quite deep at this point, and identification and ligation of these arteries prove quite at the bottom of a deep surgical approach. Thus our suggestions for choice of surgical approach to the radius would be as follows:

- Proximal third: dorsal approach unless high probability of hypertrophic or keloid scar or very thin forearm (in which case use volar approach)
- Middle third: volar approach
- Distal third: volar approach

The rest of the surgical anatomy of the forearm is relatively simple. The superficial radial nerve runs along the undersurface of the brachioradialis muscle and can be retracted quite safely along with the muscle. The radial artery is covered by the medial edge of the brachioradialis muscle proximally, lying between the brachioradialis and the pronator teres. It then becomes superficial, lying between the brachioradialis and the FCR, covered by the superficial and deep fascia. The artery is accompanied by two venae comitantes along its entire course, and these may aid in the identification of the artery. The artery is generally retracted medially with the FCR muscle during the volar approach to the radius.

Surgical Techniques

Ulna

The patient should be positioned supine as previously discussed. The incision is straight along the subcutaneous border of the ulna, which can be identified along its length by palpation (see **Video 15–2, Disk 2**). The length of the incision is determined by the fracture pattern, generally extending 3 to 5 cm on either side of the fracture. One may begin with a relatively shorter incision and extend either end as needed when the fracture site is exposed. When repairing a fracture of both bones of the forearm, it may be advantageous to delay inflation of the tourniquet until approaching the radius because the approach to the ulna can be performed quite easily without tourniquet control. This may save valuable tourniquet time for later in the operation when it is most needed for the radius. There is also evidence that patients in whom a tourniquet is not used have less

postoperative pain.[32] Once the skin is incised, the common aponeurosis of the FCU and ECU will be visible. Palpate along the aponeurosis to identify the area where this layer is thinnest and the ulna is most easily felt, which will correspond to the interval between the FCU and ECU. Beginning distally, sharply incise this deep fascia in line with the skin incision. More proximally, some of the fibers of the ECU extend across the ulna and may need to be incised to reach the bone. Minimize the transection of muscle fibers whenever possible. Now carefully examine the area adjacent to the fracture to determine whether the trauma caused more stripping of periosteum from the dorsal or volar surface of the ulna. The plate can be placed on either the volar or dorsal surface of the ulna **(Fig. 15–10A,B)**. The fracture characteristics may dictate which surface is optimal. However, if the fracture configuration allows the plate to be positioned on either side, it should be placed on the surface that has already endured the most periosteal stripping. This avoids circumferential stripping of the bone.

The fracture ends must be thoroughly but gently cleaned of all intervening clot, periosteum, and muscle. The fracture ends must then be reduced, using an atraumatic technique. Use of a "lion jaw" or "alligator" clamp creates further periosteal stripping and crush injury to the periosteum beneath the clamp and should be reserved as a last measure. Gentle reduction of the fragments may often be accomplished with longitudinal traction of the forearm (usually by means of an assistant) and gentle manipulation with the aid of a dental pick, a piercing reduction clamp, and the surgeon's fingers. When a perfect reduction is achieved, a pointed reduction clamp should be placed with the points oriented perpendicular to the fracture line and clamped tightly. This will only be possible in oblique or spiral fractures; transverse fractures cannot be clamped in place.

Oblique and Spiral Fractures

Both oblique and spiral fractures should have an interfragmentary lag screw placed to maximize compression across the fracture. The fracture must remain anatomically reduced and tightly clamped during screw insertion. The interfragmentary screw should be placed perpendicular to the fracture line in the standard lag screw fashion.[29] To lessen the risk of propagating a fracture line from the screw hole to the fracture edge, the screw must be placed a minimum of two outer diameters away from the edge (2×3.5 mm = 7 mm from the edge for 3.5 mm screws). The use of smaller screws is advantageous because the heads of 2.0 mm and 2.4 mm screws are flat, and the plate can be positioned over the top of them if needed. Also, the use of smaller screws may allow the placement of two interfragmentary screws across the fracture, which increases rotational stability without compromising pullout strength (Stewart, unpublished data) **(Fig. 15–11A,B)**.

Once the interfragmentary screws are in place, a "neutralization" plate is applied. Because the fracture is

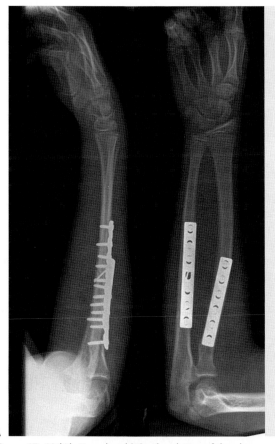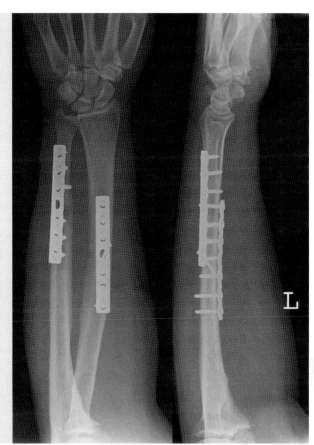

A   B

Figure 15–10 (A) Dorsal and **(B)** volar plating of the ulna.

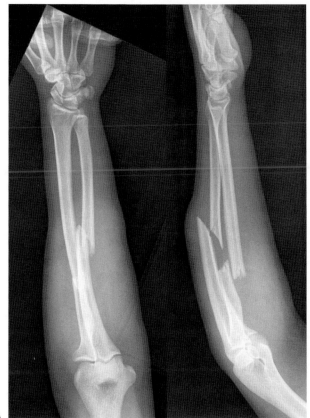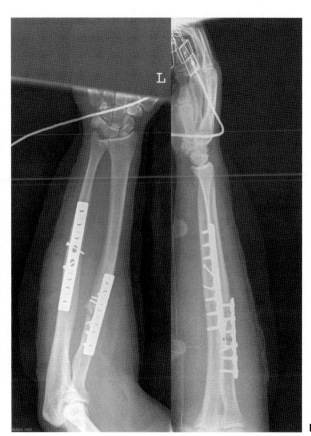

A   B

Figure 15–11 Example of the use of lag screws and a neutralization plate. **(A)** Anteroposterior and lateral radiographs of the forearm showing an oblique fracture of the ulna with a nondisplaced butterfly fragment, and a more transverse fracture of the radius. **(B)** Postoperative radiographs show fixation of the ulna with two interfragmentary lag screws and an eight-hole dorsal neutralization plate.

already compressed by the lag screws, no further compression can be accomplished, and the plate should be placed with all screws in the "neutral" position. There is no need to contour the neutralization plate (except at the most distal or proximal end of the bone) because the ulna is straight. For fractures of the mid- and proximal ulna, the ideal plate is a 3.5 mm dynamic compression plate (DCP, Synthes, Paoli, Pennsylvania).[29,33] Larger plates create a detrimental stress riser (see discussion of 4.5 mm plates in Complications), whereas one-third tubular plates do not provide adequate strength in fixation of the bones of the forearm.[6] A smaller 2.7 mm plate works well for fractures of the distal ulna. It is generally accepted that in nonosteoporotic bone with good screw purchase, six cortices (three bicortical screws) above and below the fracture provide adequate fixation. When possible, an interfragmentary lag screw can be placed through a hole in the plate, after overdrilling the near cortex. The author's preferred method is to use a single 3.5 mm interfragmentary screw or two 2.0 mm screws and apply a neutralization plate separately along the volar or dorsal

surface where periosteal stripping has already occurred **(Fig. 15–12A,B)**.

Transverse Fractures

With transverse fractures, compression is achieved with the plate because a lag screw cannot be used. The plate should be "precontoured" with a slight bend so that the apex of the concave surface sits ~1 mm off the bone at the level of the fracture. The precontoured plate will ensure that when compression is applied, the side of the bone farthest away from the plate is also brought under compression. It is quite acceptable to first position the plate while the fracture is reduced to ensure that the fit and contour are right. Then the plate may be held in place with the surgeon's hand while the first screw is placed through the plate in neutral position. The fracture can then be reduced with the plate in place and the opposite end of the plate held against the bone either with the surgeon's fingers or with a clamp. As before, the use of clamps is minimized to avoid periosteal stripping or crushing. Once the fracture is reduced, a

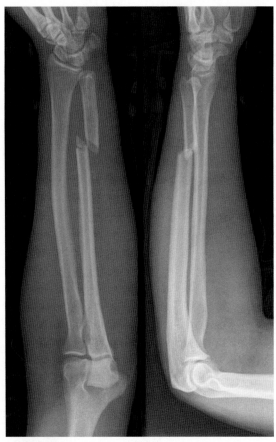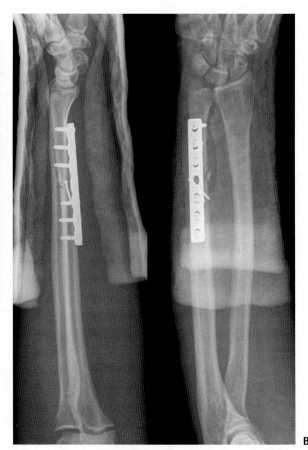

Figure 15–12 Fixation of an isolated, displaced ulnar fracture. **(A)** Anteroposterior and lateral radiographs of the forearm showing a displaced, short oblique fracture of the ulna with a small butterfly fragment. **(B)** Postoperative radiograph showing fixation of the ulna with minifragment 2.0 mm lag screws and a seven-hole volar 3.5 mm neutralization plate.

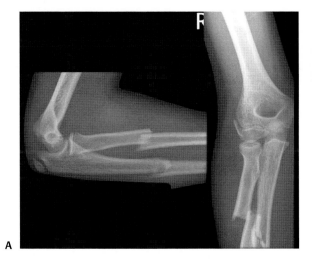

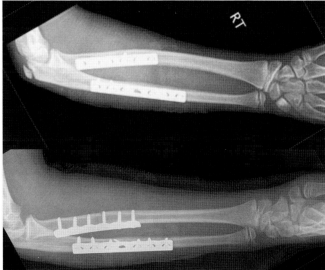

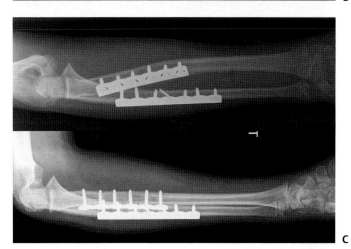

Figure 15–13 Compression plating to stabilize a transverse fracture. **(A)** Anteroposterior and lateral radiographs of the forearm showing displaced, transverse fractures of the radius and ulna in a teenage patient. **(B)** Postoperative radiographs show anatomical reduction and fixation of both bones with compression plates. Note that there are no interfragmentary screws in this case. **(C)** Final radiographs.

"compression" screw should be placed in the eccentric hole position on the side of the fracture opposite the first screw. The rest of the plate holes are filled with screws in neutral position, although it is possible to insert multiple compression screws if needed. Again, six cortices above and below the fracture are necessary **(Fig. 15–13A–C).**

Comminuted Fractures

Comminuted fractures present a greater challenge because the more severe damage to the bone's blood supply increases the risk of nonunion. Therefore, the avoidance of periosteal stripping is of even greater importance. Also, in comminuted fractures, it may be impossible to line the fragments up, and there may be no way to determine if the correct length or alignment has been achieved. As a general rule, if there are more than two intercalary fragments, it is better to simply restore length and alignment while spanning the fracture with a long plate. Remember that the forearm is well vascularized and

that small fragments of bone will frequently heal so long as some blood supply is left intact.

If the intermediate fragments are large enough for reconstruction, each piece of bone will need to have the edges cleaned of all clot and soft tissue. It is also imperative to see the fracture edge clearly during reduction to fit together small notches or "keys" along the bone edge. It is therefore necessary to clean back the periosteum ~1 mm from the fracture edge, which is easily done with a sharp scalpel. If any undisplaced fractures exist, these should be secured first with interfragmentary screws. This will ensure that these do not break off and become displaced fragments during manipulation of the bone. The use of small screws (2.0 or 2.4 mm) allows very small fragments to be secured. Secure each free fragment in turn to the remaining intact shaft. It is ideal to place two interfragmentary screws across each fracture line to prevent rotation, and this is most easily accomplished using 2.0 mm screws, all placed in interfragmentary compression mode. Methodically fitting small fragments of bone back together will ensure that proper length and alignment of the bone are achieved. When all of the fragments have been secured with screws, a long plate should be selected to span across the entire fracture (**Fig. 15–14A,B**). The plate should be long enough to allow a minimum of eight cortices above and below the fracture. Because early motion is always the goal of treatment of forearm fractures, the fracture stability should be tested at the conclusion of the fixation to ensure that adequate stability has been achieved.

If the fracture is grossly comminuted and anatomical reconstruction of each fragment is not possible, then a "bridge plating" technique should be used. In this instance, the entire fracture envelope is left intact (**Fig. 15–15A,B**). The application of a bridge plate requires cleaning the bone surface to accommodate the plate only on the proximal and distal intact cortex and allowing the plate to lie over the fracture fragments and hematoma. Fluoroscopic guidance is often needed to determine appropriate fracture length. Either the distal or the proximal radioulnar joints can be pinned in position and the plate applied to maintain this length.[34] Length can also be determined by measuring the patient's contralateral uninjured ulna or radius preoperatively and using this as a template.

Dorsal Approach to the Radius

With the patient supine, the arm is exsanguinated and the tourniquet inflated. Palpate the lateral epicondyle of the humerus proximally and Lister's tubercle of the radius distally. The incision should be a straight or gentle curve beginning just anterior to the lateral epicondyle and extending distally to the ulnar side of Lister's tubercle. To avoid making an overly long incision, begin with an incision that extends 3 to 5 cm on either side of the fracture. Clear the subcutaneous fat from the underlying fascia so that the interval between the ECRB and the EDC can be seen. Both muscles will have fibers running longitudinally, and it is sometimes difficult to identify the interval between them. The interval is more easily distinguished distally. Incise the superficial fascia between the ECRB and EDC, and spread the two muscles apart by blunt dissection. If it is difficult to separate the muscles, it is possible that the dissection has strayed from the intermuscular plane and is instead within the belly of one or the other muscles. If this occurs, go back to the superficial layer, clear off the fascia, and search again for the true interval. More distally, the abductor pollicis longus (APL) and extensor pollicis brevis (EPB) muscles (sometimes referred to as "the outcroppers") cross the surgical field. To extend the approach more distally, the interval between the ECRB and the proximal edge of the APL should be developed using blunt dissection. The APL and EPB can then be lifted and retracted proximally or distally to allow the radius beneath them to be exposed.

Once the ECRB and EDC are spread apart, the supinator muscle is draped over the proximal third of the radial shaft.

As discussed, the PIN lies within the supinator muscle and must now be identified. The nerve can be identified in two ways. Working proximal to distal, the origin of ECRB and a portion of the origin of ECRL are detached from the lateral epicondyle and then retracted laterally. The PIN is then palpated within the proximal portion of the supinator muscle and is carefully dissected free from the substance of the muscle. This method is generally more difficult and involves greater destruction of muscle. Also, in any patient in whom a tourniquet cannot be used, this approach is impossible due to muscle bleeding obscuring the safe view of the nerve. A simpler method is to locate the PIN at the distal edge of the supinator muscle where it emerges 1 cm proximal to the distal edge of the muscle. The nerve can then be dissected from the supinator moving proximally. Care should be taken to preserve the muscular branches of the PIN to the supinator. When the nerve is fully identified, the arm should be fully supinated to move the PIN as far away from the radius as possible. The supinator muscle should then be sharply incised along its origin on the anterior surface of the radius. Always be aware of the exact position of the PIN as the supinator is detached. The supinator muscle can then be elevated from the radial shaft by subperiosteal elevation, which will leave the substance of the muscle between the bone and the PIN.

In the central third of the forearm, the APL and EPB drape across the radius as described. In addition to incising the fascia along the proximal border of the APL, the fascia along the distal border of the EPB will need to be released so that the two muscles can be lifted free of the radius and retracted distally or proximally as needed. Recall that this incision is not well suited to fixation of fractures in the distal third of the radius due to the prominence of dorsally positioned plates and interference with the extensor tendons near the wrist.[35] However, if required, the distal aspect of the dorsal radius can be exposed by simply separating the ECRB and EPL and subperiosteal lifting of these muscles from the bone.

Volar Approach to the Radius

The volar or anterior approach of Henry is the workhorse approach to the upper extremity and is extensile from the shoulder to the carpal tunnel. It is the approach of choice for distal and middle third fractures of the radius and can also be used for proximal third fractures. The patient should be positioned in the same manner described previously and a tourniquet applied. For this approach, the arm should not be exsanguinated prior to tourniquet inflation. This will engorge the two venae comitantes that run parallel to the radial artery, making this structure much easier to identify. The landmarks for the incision are the biceps tendon at the level of the elbow crease and the radial styloid. The incision is straight or gently curved beginning just lateral to the biceps tendon and to the radial styloid. The incision is centered over the fracture and

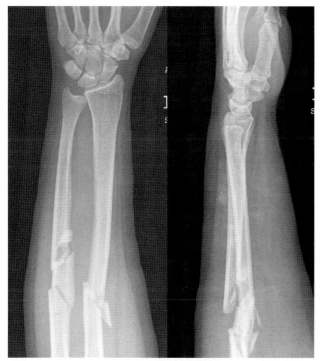

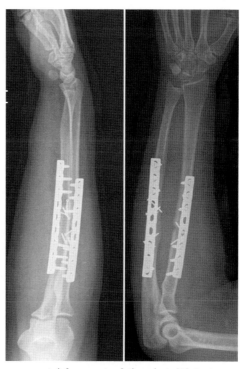

A

B

Figure 15–14 Fixation of a very comminuted fracture of the radius and ulna. **(A)** Anteroposterior and lateral radiographs of the forearm showing comminuted fractures of the radius and ulna. Note the short

segmental fragment of the ulna. **(B)** Postoperative radiographs showing reduction and fixation of the ulna with several smaller interfragmentary lag screws and a long nine-hole neutralization

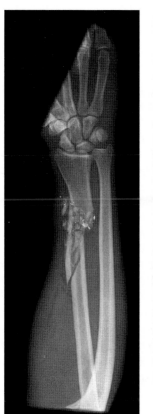

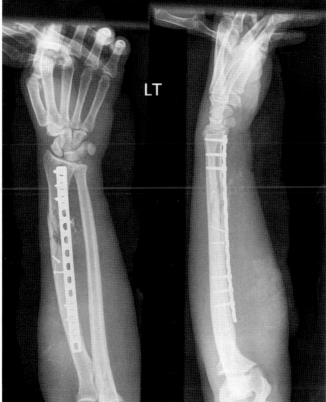

LT

A

B

Figure 15–15 Bridge plating. **(A)** Anteroposterior radiograph of the forearm showing a displaced, comminuted fracture of the distal third of the radius due to a gunshot. Note the shortening of the radius related to the ulna. **(B)** Postoperative anteroposterior and lateral radiographs of the forearm after fixation of the radius with a bridging

plate. The length and alignment of the radius have been restored while the comminuted zone is simply spanned by the plate. No attempt is made to anatomically reduce all comminuted fragments, although two minifragment (2.7 mm) lag screws were used to stabilize one of the larger butterfly fragments.

extended as required. Clear the subcutaneous fat so that the interval between the brachioradialis and the FCR can be identified. The interval is more easily seen distally. In the most proximal aspect of the forearm, the superficial interval will be between the brachioradialis and the pronator teres. The brachioradialis muscle drapes across the forearm, and its medial border is frequently more than halfway across the forearm. Carefully incise the fascia between the brachioradialis and the FCR. The radial artery lies directly below the medial edge of the brachioradialis in the middle of the forearm and will be quite near when the muscular interval is opened. It should be identified, along with the two engorged venae comitantes, and freed along its length. The artery should be mobilized to allow it to be retracted medially. Occasionally, there will be several muscular branches arising from the radial artery that make its retraction medially difficult. In this case, it is acceptable to retract the artery to the lateral side of the wound, so long as it is protected. The superficial radial nerve lies beneath the brachioradialis and should be identified; damage to it may result in a bothersome neuroma.

The deep dissection differs depending upon location. In the distal forearm, the pronator quadratus and FPL arise from the radius. With the forearm supinated, the periosteum of the radius may be incised lateral to these muscles, with additional exposure obtained by medial elevation and retraction. In the middle third of the forearm, the radius is covered by the pronator teres and FDS muscles. With the forearm pronated, the insertion of the pronator teres onto the lateral radius is visible, and it may be detached and reflected medially. In the proximal third of the forearm, the PIN is at risk. To safely expose the proximal radius, the forearm should be supinated to move the PIN laterally away from the radius; the same maneuver exposes the insertion of the supinator on the anterior aspect of the radius. The supinator muscle may be incised along its broad insertion and carefully retracted laterally. Excessive traction must be avoided.

Plate Application to the Radius

The principles of plate application on the radius are identical to those described for the ulna. There is one complicating factor, however, due to the geometry of the radius. The ulna is essentially a straight bone, so that a plate placed on either the volar or dorsal surface will lie parallel to the bone (**Fig. 15–16**). This means that even in highly comminuted fractures, the alignment of the ulna will be very close to anatomical if the bone is simply aligned with the plate.

In contrast, the radius is a curved bone, with an apex radial bow. This curvature allows the radius to rotate about the ulna in pronation and supination. Failure to re-create this radial bow will result in impairment of pronation and supination. For every 5 degrees of radial curvature that is not restored, the patient will lose 15 degrees of rotational motion.[2,36,37] For this reason, when a plate is applied to the radius on either the dorsal or the volar surface, the radius should not be parallel to the plate. Instead, there should be

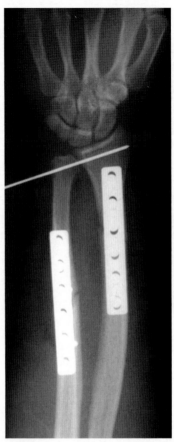

Figure 15–16 Plate positioning on the forearm. Because of the relatively straight shape of the ulna, straight plates applied to the ulna restore alignment. In contrast, because of the normal bow of the radius, a straight plate applied on the volar or dorsal surface of the radius must be eccentric at its proximal and distal ends.

an unequal amount of bone visible on either side of the plate. At either end of the plate, there should be more bone visible on the concave side of the radius (the ulnar border of the radius). At the center of the plate, there should be more bone visible on the convex side of the radial border of the bone (**Fig. 15–16**). This is an important radiographic clue that the radial bow has been appropriately restored and should be carefully noted when intraoperative images are obtained. Because a standard compression plate cannot be bent sideways, there is tendency of the bone to be straightened by the plate when repairing a fracture that spans a long segment of the radius. In such a circumstance, a gentle bow can be contoured into the plate, which is then applied to the radial side of the bone, thereby restoring the normal bow.

Monteggia Fractures

Fractures of the ulna with accompanying dislocation of the radial head are a relatively uncommon injury, accounting for 1 to 16% of forearm fractures, depending on the series (**Fig. 15–17**).[25] Monteggia fractures, as these are known, have also been associated with notoriously poor results compared with other forearm fractures, frequently with

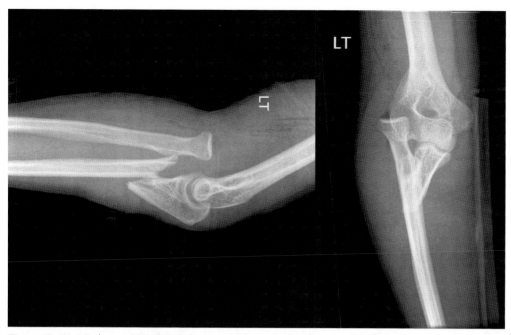

Figure 15–17 A Bado type I Monteggia fracture, with an angulated proximal third ulna fracture and anterior dislocation of the radial head.

more than 50% of patients reporting fair, poor, or unsatisfactory results.[38,39] Multiple complications were reported, including nonunions, redislocation of the radial head, synostosis, nerve injury, and poor motion, with particularly poor results and frequent complication in the Bado type II or posterior Monteggia lesions.[38,40-44] It appears that some improvement in these dismal results has been achieved with increasing attention to the need for absolute stability of the ulna fracture fixation and to associated fractures, including the coronoid process.[45-47]

All Monteggia fractures in adults should be treated with operative fixation to allow early range of motion (Fig. 15–18A,B). Stable internal fixation of the ulna fracture should be performed as described previously using interfragmentary screws wherever possible and a 3.5 mm plate. If the fracture is comminuted (a frequent finding in Monteggia fractures) and there is no stable cortical contact, bone grafting should be used.[46] It is important to remember that the method of tension-band wiring of olecranon fractures can only be used in purely transverse, noncomminuted fractures, which is very seldom the case in a Monteggia-type injury. Therefore, even with very proximal ulna fractures, stable fixation using a plate should be the goal.

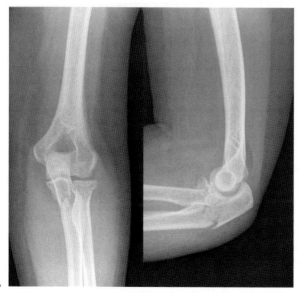
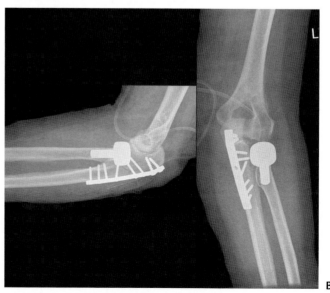

A   B

Figure 15–18 (A,B) A "Monteggia equivalent" injury, with a posteriorly angulated proximal ulna fracture and an impacted radial neck with similar angulation. In this case, the ulna was plated, and the radial head was excised and replaced with a radial head prosthesis.

To extend the surgical incision to the most proximal tip of the ulna, the incision will continue along the subcutaneous ulnar border and should curve as it crosses the tip of the olecranon. It is generally best to curve the incision to the lateral side of the olecranon so the ulnar nerve will not be endangered; this also avoids having a scar directly over the area where a patient will rest the elbow. It is not absolutely necessary to dissect the ulnar nerve free of its cubital tunnel when approaching the olecranon. If care is taken to be vigilant about the location of the nerve, it can be left within the tunnel. We prefer to place plates on the ulnar side of the olecranon so that drilling is performed in an ulnar to radial direction, ensuring the safety of the ulnar nerve. It is also possible to place the plate directly along the dorsal surface of the ulna; however, this frequently results in prominent hardware requiring removal. The exception is the posterior Monteggia lesion, when the plate must be placed on the dorsal surface because this will be the tension surface for this fracture and is required for maximal biomechanical stability **(Fig. 15–18A,B)**. Because the goal is to achieve at least six cortices of screw purchase above and below the ulna fracture, a 3.5 mm plate may not allow enough screws to be placed in a small proximal fragment. The use of a 2.7 mm reconstruction plate may be helpful in this situation and will still provide excellent resistance to bending. Periarticular plates are now available designed especially for the proximal ulna. Whatever plate is used, the elbow must be taken through a full range of motion at the conclusion of fixation to ensure that stability has been achieved and range of motion can be begun. Indirect methods to restore anatomical length of a shortened, comminuted ulna fracture are preferable to extensive periosteal stripping. A distracter or the plate-tensioning device both work well. Periosteal stripping must be kept to a minimum to avoid the frequent complications of nonunion and synostosis with the radius.

With anatomical alignment of the ulna fracture, reduction of the radial head is usually achieved. On rare occasions, the radial head may "buttonhole" through the capsule or anconeus muscle. If the radial head is irreducible, a separate incision should be made to approach the radial head and perform open reduction (see Chapter 14). Never attempt to expose the radial head through the ulnar incision because this will greatly increase the risk of synostosis. Careful observation of the elbow through a full range of motion under fluoroscopy should be made with particular attention to the possibility of a coronoid fracture. If a coronoid fracture exists and the elbow remains unstable, repair of the coronoid is required, which is beyond the scope of this chapter.

Galeazzi Fractures

Like Monteggia fractures, Galeazzi fractures are uncommon, representing only 3 to 6% of forearm fractures.[48,49]

This fracture pattern combines a fracture of the radius, most commonly at the junction of the distal and middle third, with a disruption of the DRUJ **(Fig. 15–19A,B)** (see **Video 15–3, Disk 2**).[50] It is exceedingly rare to find an isolated fracture of the radius, and a high index of suspicion must be maintained so as not to overlook the DRUJ injury. Several radiographic clues exist to identify disruption of the DRUJ: (1) widening of the DRUJ space on AP view, (2) dorsal translation of the ulna relative to the radius seen on the lateral view, (3) fracture of the ulnar styloid base, and (4) radial shortening greater than 5 mm relative to the distal ulna.[48,51] The most common pattern of the radius injury is a shortened, oblique, or transverse fracture with apex dorsal angulation.[52–54] Careful neurological examination is also necessary for these injuries.

The treatment of Galeazzi fractures in adults should be operative **(Fig. 15–19A,B)** (see **Video 15–3, Disk 2**). Multiple authors have reported unsatisfactory results with closed reduction and casting, likely due to the strongly deforming forces of the brachioradialis, the pronator quadratus, and the thumb extensors.[48,53,54] The radius fracture should be anatomically reduced and stability fixed as previously described via the volar (Henry's) approach. Once the radius has been anatomically fixed, the ulna will frequently reduce within the DRUJ. This must be checked carefully with intraoperative radiographs or fluoroscopy. The stability of the DRUJ must then be assessed by rotation of the forearm through a full range of supination and pronation. If the DRUJ remains reduced through this range, particularly in pronation, no further treatment is required, and early postoperative range of motion exercises can be begun. If the DRUJ is unstable in pronation but stable in supination, the arm should be immobilized in supination. Initial splinting should be followed by a hinged elbow brace or hinged cast that will allow elbow flexion and extension while the arm remains in full supination. This should be worn for 4 to 6 weeks to allow soft tissue healing of the DRUJ capsule. Finally, if the DRUJ is unstable in both pronation and supination, the joint must be stabilized with percutaneous Kirschner wires. Two wires should always be used, and they should be placed ~1 to 2 cm apart, with the most distal pin placed just proximal to the proximal edge of the DRUJ. Pins should not be placed through the DRUJ itself because this is a cartilaginous joint. To avoid pin breakage, slightly larger pins, such as 2 mm K-wires, should be used and should be placed while the arm is supinated. Pins should start in the ulna and traverse across to engage both cortices of the radius. The arm should then be immobilized in supination in hinged brace to allow elbow flexion and extension as already described.

There has recently been some interest in repair of the DRUJ capsule. The joint may be approached dorsally and the capsular tissue reattached via drill holes in the ulna styloid or by suture anchors.[52] Similarly, if the DRUJ is irreducible, it should be opened dorsally to remove intervening soft tissue, most commonly the ECU or extensor digiti minimi tendons.[55–60] If opening the joint is necessary, several

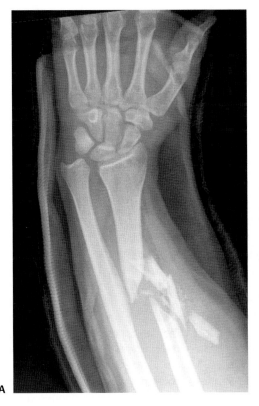

A

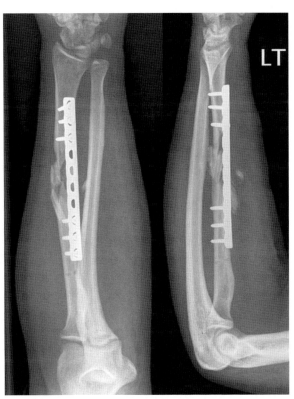

B

Figure 15–19 A Galeazzi fracture. **(A)** Anteroposterior radiograph of the forearm showing a comminuted radial shaft fracture and obvious widening of the distal radioulnar joint (DRUJ). **(B)** Anteroposterior and lateral radiographs after open reduction and internal fixation of the radius. The DRUJ was stable after fixation.

authors suggest repair of the triangular fibrocartilage complex (TFCC) at that time, but no data comparing outcomes with the procedure exist.[52,59] After repair of the DRUJ capsule or the TFCC or both, the joint should be pinned as described. It may be safe to pin the DRUJ in neutral position rather than full supination to reduce loss of pronation (increasingly important because many patients require keyboard use as a daily function). Finally, an unstable DRUJ with an ulna styloid fracture at the styloid base may require fixation of the ulna fragment. The TFCC, which has been shown to play a major role in stabilization of the DRUJ, attaches to this fragment, and stability of the DRUJ can be achieved with open reduction and internal fixation (ORIF) of the styloid fragment by either a 2.0 or a 2.4 mm interfragmentary screw or a tension band.[52]

The results for Galeazzi fractures are quite good when treated with rigid compression plating and appropriate evaluation of the DRUJ stability.[48,58] A significantly high complication rate has been noted in several studies, including intraoperative radial nerve injury (most commonly the dorsal interosseous nerve), which was injured in 7 to 19% of cases reported.[48,55]

Bone Grafting

Traditionally, bone grafting of forearm fractures was recommended whenever comminution of the radius or ulna exceeded 50% of the diameter of the bone or in open fractures.[4] Union rates following routine autogenous bone grafting of such injuries was reported to be 98%.[4] However, Wright et al[61] and Wei et al[62] found exactly the same union rate (98%) in forearm fractures treated with ORIF without bone grafting. Currently, routine bone grafting of acute forearm fractures does not seem necessary but may still be considered for cases of segmental bone loss or in patients with factors that might contribute to delayed union, such as smoking. Delayed bone grafting is a predictably successful procedure in those few patients with nonunions or bone loss.[63,64]

Intramedullary Nailing

As in other long bones, intramedullary nailing of forearm fractures is theoretically attractive because it might limit the invasiveness of surgery and be associated with better functional and cosmetic outcomes.[65] Despite these theoretical advantages, nailing of adult forearm fractures has not really become accepted and seems to be associated with inferior results compared with plating.[65,66] The angular and rotational stability of intramedullary fixation of the adult forearm is considered insufficient for safe, early mobilization. Nevertheless, there is a role for intramedullary fixation of the radius or ulna in certain instances, such as pathological fractures or those associated with severe soft tissue injuries.[67] Although interlocking nails exist for the forearm, their use is difficult, and restoring the anatomical bow of the radius can be difficult. The use of intramedullary devices is easiest in the ulna because of its straight medullary canal and the easily accessible entry point at the olecranon.[67] In contrast, intramedullary fixation of the radius requires an eccentric entry point in the dorsal aspect of the distal radius. Interlocking nails may provide better stability, but the use of interlocking screws may endanger the posterior interosseous nerve when used in the proximal radius.[68] When used, such screws should be inserted using small open incisions with the arm in neutral rotation.[68]

New Techniques

Locking plates have been recently introduced, and some have reported their use in the forearm.[69–71] One of the main advantages of locking plates is the fact that they are not compressed against the bone and may better maintain bone vascularity compared with traditional plates.[69–71] In confirmation of this, Hofer et al found better formation of callus with the use of the Point-Contact Fixator (PC-Fix, Stratec, Winterthur, Switzerland).[71] In an animal model, fractures repaired with the PC-Fix were more resistant to infection than fractures treated with standard plates.[72] However, routine use of locking plates in the forearm may lead to certain complications, primarily related to malunion. Locking plates do not themselves contribute to fracture reduction and will fix the fracture in situ.[73] This may result in inadvertent residual bowing of the ulna that could contribute to radial head instability or insufficient restoration of the radial bow. There are so few complications from the use of standard small fragment plates in the forearm that these implants should still be considered the treatment of choice. One clinical, prospective, randomized trial compared the PC-Fix to traditional plating with the limited contact dynamic compression plate (LC-DCP, Synthes, Paoli, Pennsylvania) and found equal clinical results regarding operative time, time to union, callus formation, pain, or functional outcome.[74]

Outcomes

The outcomes after forearm fractures in adults has been poorly documented because most series report small numbers of patients with insufficient follow-up and have not utilized validated general or specific outcomes assessment tools. Goldfarb et al recently described the functional assessment of forearm fractures in adults.[75] Twenty-four fractures in 23 patients were comprehensively assessed with a combination of objective clinical and radiological outcomes at a mean of 34 months after surgery. Clinical outcome measures included the Disabilities of the Arm, Shoulder and Hand (DASH) and Musculoskeletal Functional Assessment (MFA) questionnaires, as well as measurement

of range of motion of the forearm and wrist, grip, and pinch strength. Despite the patient self-reported good overall function based on the DASH and MFA scores, measurement of forearm motion demonstrated significant losses of pronation, grip, and pinch strength. These deficiencies were associated with poorer subjective outcomes.[75]

Complications

There are numerous general and treatment-specific complications that can occur following fractures of the forearm; one classic review documented complications occurring in 28% of patients treated operatively with plate fixation.[76] General complications include soft tissue and neurovascular injury, including compartment syndrome, peripheral nerve lesions, and musculotendinous injury. Malreduction and poor function are so common with nonoperative treatment of forearm fractures in adults that surgery should nearly always be performed. Radioulnar synostosis can occur following operative or nonsurgical management and is particularly problematic in patients with head injuries.[76]

Following surgery, other complications such as infection, iatrogenic nerve injury, malunion, nonunion, and hardware-related problems can occur. Nonunion after plating is often due to inadequate fixation; Stern and Drury found nonunion in 17% of fractures fixed with three screws compared with 4% when five or more screws were used.[76] Range of motion correlates with restoration of the normal bow of the radius; operative methods provide sufficient means to restore anatomy.[3]

Radioulnar synostosis is a rare complication following forearm shaft fractures. Jupiter and Ring reported their experience with simple excision of the synostosis in 18 cases and recognized three anatomical variations: type A is a synostosis occurring at or distal to the bicipital tuberosity, type B indicates a synostosis involving the radial head and proximal radioulnar joint, and type C represents a synostosis that extends across the elbow to include the distal humerus.[77] After an average follow-up of 34 months, the synostosis recurred in only one patient, who happened to be the only patient in the series who had also suffered a closed head injury at the time of the initial injury. The other 17 limbs regained an average 139 degrees of forearm rotation. Earlier resection of the synostosis led to better results.[77]

A frequently discussed complication of forearm fractures is the risk of refracture after plate removal, which has been reported in 4 to 20% of cases.[33,78] The risk of refracture is related to the amount of callus, the duration since implant removal, and the size of the hardware that was used. Most reports that document high rates of refracture include patients that had 4.5 mm DCPs, which were relatively oversized and caused significant osteopenia because of stress shielding and avascularity. Rates of refracture appear to be much lower following removal of 3.5 mm plates.

The volar compartment of the forearm is the second most common site for compartment syndrome, after the anterior compartment of the leg.[79] One should remember that acute compartment syndrome can occur following fractures of the radius and ulnar shafts, distal radius fracture, and isolated fracture of the proximal ulna.[80] As elsewhere, treatment of acute compartment syndrome requires immediate fasciotomy of the volar and sometimes dorsal compartments. For a detailed description of the management of compartment syndromes of the forearm, the reader is referred to Chapter 3.

Pearls

- Acceptable criteria for nonoperative management of isolated ulna fracture: 50% displacement and 10 degrees angulation
- Radial bow: every 5 degree loss of radial curvature equals a 15 degree loss of supination/pronation.
- Always use 3.5 mm DCPs or LC-DCPs (never 4.5 mm)
- Incidence of refracture after hardware removal with 4.5 mm plates > 20%
- *No contact sports after plate removal for 6 months*
- Bone graft: only if no cortical contact
- Percent of patients with PIN in direct contact with radial neck equals 25%.

On the DVDs

Video 15–1 (Disk 2) ORIF of an Isolated Radius Fracture This video demonstrates compression plating of a displaced radius fracture using Henry's anterior approach, with an evaluation of the DRUJ following stabilization of the radius.

Video 15–2 (Disk 2) ORIF of a "Both Bone Forearm Fracture" This video demonstrates plate fixation of a forearm fracture involving both the radius and ulna in an adult. A detailed explanation of

Henry's approach as well as the appropriate order of fixation of the radius and ulna are demonstrated.

Video 15–3 (Same as Video 14–2, Disk 2) Radius Fracture with Pinning of the Distal Radial-Ulnar Joint (Galeazzi Fracture, Part of ORIF of a Complex Elbow Injury) This video depicts open reduction and internal fixation of an olecranon fracture as well as a large coronoid fracture. The patient also sustained a radius fracture treated with ORIF as well as pinning of the distal radial-ulnar joint.

References

1. Chung KC, Spilson SV. The frequency and epidemiology of hand and forearm fractures in the United States: abstract. J Hand Surg [Am] 2001;26:908–915
2. Schemitsch EH, Richards R. The effect of malunion on functional outcome after plate fixation of fractures of both bones of the forearm in adults. J Bone Joint Surg Am 1992;74:1068–1078
3. Schemitsch EH, Jones D, Henley MB, Tencer AF. A comparison of malreduction after plate and intramedullary nail fixation of forearm fractures. J Orthop Trauma 1995;9:8–16
4. Chapman MW, Gordon JE, Zissimos AG. Compression-plate fixation of acute fractures of the diaphyses of the radius and ulna. J Bone Joint Surg Am 1989;71:159–169
5. Grace TG, Eversmann WW Jr. Forearm fractures treatment by rigid fixation with early motion. J Bone Joint Surg Am 1980;62:433–438
6. Ross ERS, Gourevitch D, Hastings GW, Wynn-Jones CE, Ali S. Retrospective analysis of plate fixation of diaphyseal fractures of the forearm bones. Injury 1989;20:211–214
7. Dymond IW. The treatment of isolated fractures of the distal ulna. J Bone Joint Surg Br 1984;66:408–410
8. Bado JL, Springfield T. The Monteggia lesion. Clin Orthop Relat Res 1967;50:71–86
9. Brakenbury PH, Corea JR, Blakemore ME. Non-union of the isolated fracture of the ulnar shaft in adults. Injury 1981;12:371–375
10. Zych GA, Latta LL, Zagorski JB. Treatment of isolated ulnar shaft fractures with prefabricated functional fracture braces. Clin Orthop Relat Res 1987;219:194–200
11. Tynan MC, Fornalski S, McMahon PJ, Utkan A, Green S, Lee TQ. The effects of ulnar axial malalignment on supination and pronation. J Bone Joint Surg Am 2000;82-A:1726–1731

12. Sarmiento A, Latta LL, Zych G, McKeever P, Zagorski JP. Isolated ulnar shaft fractures treated with functional braces. J Orthop Trauma 1998;12:420–423
13. Sarmiento A, Cooper JS, Sinclair WF. Forearm fractures early functional bracing: a preliminary report. J Bone Joint Surg Am 1975;57:297–304
14. Failla JM, Jacobson J, Van Holsbeeck M. Ultrasound diagnosis and surgical pathology of the torn interosseous membrane in forearm fractures/dislocations. J Hand Surg [Am] 1999;24:257–266
15. McHenry TP, Pierce WA, Lais RL, Schacherer TG. Effect of displacement of ulna-shaft fractures on forearm rotation: a cadaveric model. Am J Orthop 2002;31:420–424
16. De Boeck H, Haentjens P, Casteleyn PP, Opdecam P. Treatment of isolated distal ulnar shaft fractures with below-elbow plaster cast: a prospective study. Arch Orthop Trauma Surg 1996;115:316–320
17. Pearce PK, Der Tavetain A, Handoll HH. Interventions for isolated diaphyseal fractures of the ulna in adults: abstract. Cochrane Database Syst Rev 2004(2):CD000523
18. Mackay D, Wood L, Rangan A. The treatment of isolated ulnar fractures in adults: a systemic review. Injury 2000;31:565–570
19. Gebuhr P, Holmich P, Orsnes T. Isolated ulnar shaft fractures: comparison of treatment by functional brace and long arm cast. J Bone Joint Surg Br 1992;74:757–759
20. Oberlander MA, Seidman GD, Whitelaw GP. Treatment of isolated ulnar shaft fractures with functional bracing. Orthopedics 1993;16:29–32
21. Ostermann PA, Ekkernkamp A, Henry SL. Bracing of stable shaft fractures of the ulna. J Orthop Trauma 1994;8:245–248

22. Atkin DM, Bohay DR, Slabaugh P, Smith BW. Treatment of ulnar shaft fractures: a prospective, randomized study. Orthopedics. 1995;18:543–547

23. Pollock FH, Pankovich AM, Prieto JJ, Lorenz M. The isolated fracture of the ulnar shaft: treatment without immobilization. J Bone Joint Surg Am 1983;65:339–342

24. Moed BR, Kellam JF, Foster JR, et al. Immediate internal fixation of open fractures of the diaphysis of the forearm. J Bone Joint Surg Am 1986;68:1008–1017

25. Burwell HN, Charnley AD. Treatment of forearm fractures in adults with particular reference to plate fixation. J Bone Joint Surg Br 1964;46:404–425

26. Perren SM. Evolution of the internal fixation of long bone fractures: review article. J Bone Joint Surg Br 2002;84:1093–1110

27. Henry AK. Extensile Exposure. 2nd ed. Edinburgh: Churchill Livingstone; 1973:100–107

28. Thompson JE. Anatomical methods of approach in operations on the long bones of the extremities. Am Surg 1918;68:309–329

29. Muller ME, Allgower M, Schneider R, Willenegger H. Manual of Internal Fixation. Corrected 3rd printing. New York: Springer-Verlag; 1995

30. Hirachi K, Kato H, Minami A, Kasashima T, Kaneda K. Clinical features and management of traumatic posterior interosseous nerve palsy. J Hand Surg [Br] 1998;23:413–417

31. Diliberti T, Botte MJ, Abrams RA. Anatomical considerations regarding the posterior interosseous nerve during posterolateral approaches to the proximal part of the radius. J Bone Joint Surg Am 2000;82:809–813

32. Omeroglu H, Ucaner A, Tabak AY, Guney O, Bicimoglu A, Gunel U. The effect of using a tourniquet on the intensity of postoperative pain in forearm fractures: a randomized study in 32 surgically treated patients. Int Orthop 1998;22:369–373

33. Deluca PA, Lindsey RW, Ruwe PA. Refracture of bones of the forearm after the removal of compression plates. J Bone Joint Surg Am 1988;70:1372–1376

34. Ebraheim NA, Elgafy H, Georgiadis GM. Comminuted Monteggia fracture-dislocation: a technique for restoration of ulnar length: case reports. Am J Orthop 2000;29:960–963

35. Keogh P, Khan H, Cooke E, Mc Coy G. Loss of flexor pollicis longus function after plating of the radius: report of six cases. J Hand Surg [Br] 1997;22:375–376

36. Tarr RR, Garfinkel AI, Sarmiento A. The effects of angular and rotational deformities of both bones of the forearm: an in-vitro study. J Bone Joint Surg Am 1984;66:65–70

37. Yasutomi T, Nakatsuchi Y, Koike H, Uchiyama S. Mechanism of limitation of pronation/supination of the forearm in geometric models of deformities of the forearm bone. Clin Biomech (Bristol, Avon) 2002;17:456–463

38. Llusa Perez M, Lamas C, Martinez I, Pidemunt G, Mir X. Monteggia fractures in adults: review of 54 cases. Chir Main 2002;21:293–297

39. Reynders P, De Groote W, Rondia J, Govaerts K, Stoffelen D, Broos PL. Monteggia lesions in adults: a multicenter BOTA study. Acta Orthop Belg 1996;62(Suppl 1):78–83

40. Arenas AJ, Artazcoz FJ, Tejero A, Arias C. Anterior interosseous nerve injury associated with a Monteggia fracture-dislocation: case report. Acta Orthop Belg 2001;67:77–80

41. Biyani A, Olscamp AJ, Ebraheim NA. Complications in the management of complex Monteggia-equivalent fractures in adults: abstract. Am J Orthop 2000;29:115–118

42. Givon U, Pritsch M, Levy O, Yosepovitch A, Amit Y, Horoszowski H. Monteggia and equivalent lesions: a study of 41 cases. Clin Orthop Relat Res 1997;337:208–215

43. Preston C, Chen AL, Wolinsky P, Tejwani NC. Posterior dislocation of the elbow with concomitant fracture of the proximal ulnar diaphysis and radial head: a complex variant of the posterior Monteggia lesion. J Orthop Trauma 2003;17:530–533

44. Ring D, Jupiter JB, Gulotta L. Atrophic nonunions of the proximal ulna: abstract. Clin Orthop Relat Res 2003;409:268–274

45. Jupiter JB, Leibovic SJ, Ribbans W, Wilk RM. The posterior Monteggia lesion. J Orthop Trauma 1991;5:395–402

46. Ring D, Jupiter JB, Simpson S. Monteggia fractures in adults. J Bone Joint Surg Am 1998;80:1733–1744

47. Simpson NS, Goodman LA, Jupiter JB. Contoured LCDC plating of the proximal ulna. Injury 1996;27:411–417

48. Moore TM, Klein JP, Patzakis MJ, Harvey JP Jr. Results of compression-plating of closed Galeazzi fractures. J Bone Joint Surg Am 1985;67:1015–1021

49. Moore TM, Lester DK, Sarmiento A. The stabilizing effect of soft-tissue constraints in artificial Galeazzi fractures. Clin Orthop Relat Res 1985;194:189–194

50. Galeazzi R. Ueber ein besonderes Syndrom bei Verletzungen im Bereich der Unterarmknocken. Arch Orthop Unfallchir 1934;35:557–562

51. Bruckner JD, Lichtman DM, Alexander AH. Complex dislocations of the distal radioulnar joint: recognition and management. Clin Orthop Relat Res 1992;275:90–103

52. Morgan WJ, Breen TF. Complex fractures of the forearm. Hand Clin 1994;10:375–390

53. Kraus B, Horne G. Galeazzi fractures. J Trauma 1985;25:1093–1095

54. Mikic ZD, Galeazzi fracture-dislocations. J Bone Joint Surg Am 1975;57A:1071–1080

55. Alexander AH, Lichtman DM. Irreducible distal radioulnar joint occurring in a Galeazzi fracture: case report. J Hand Surg [Am] 1981;6:258–261

56. Cetti NE. An unusual cause of blocked reduction of Galeazzi injury. Injury 1977;9:59–61

57. Rettig ME, Raskin KB. Galeazzi fracture-dislocation: a new treatment-oriented classification. J Hand Surg [Am] 2001;26:228–235

58. Beneyto MF, Renu AJM, Claramunt FA, Soler RR. Treatment of Galeazzi fracture-dislocations. J Trauma 1994;36:352–355

59. Strehle J, Gerber C. Distal radioulnar joint function after Galeazzi fracture-dislocations treated by open reduction and internal plate fixation. Clin Orthop Relat Res 1993;293:240–245

60. Mohan K, Gupta AK, Sharma J, Singh AK, Jain AK. Internal fixation in 50 cases of Galeazzi fracture. Acta Orthop Scand 1988;59:318–320

61. Wright R, Schmeling GJ, Schwab JP. The necessity of acute bone grafting in diaphyseal forearm fractures: a retrospective review. J Orthop Trauma 1997;11:288–294

62. Wei SY, Born CT, Abene A, Ong A, Hayda R, DeLong WG Jr. Diaphyseal forearm fractures treated with and without bone graft. J Trauma 1999;46:1045–1048

63. Barbieri CH, Mazzer MR. Use of a delayed cortical bone graft to treat diaphyseal defects in the forearm. Int Orthop 1999;23:295–301

64. Davey PA, Simonis RB. Modification of the Nicoll bone-grafting technique for nonunion of the radius and/or ulna: abstract. J Bone Joint Surg Br 2002;84:30–33

65. Street DM. Intramedullary forearm nailing. Clin Orthop Relat Res 1986;212:219–230

66. Salai M, Segal E, Amit Y, Chechick A. Closed intramedullary nailing of forearm fractures in young patients. Harefuah 1998;134:106–108,158–159

67. Boriani S, Lefevre C, Malingue E, Bettelli G. The Lefevre ulnar nail. Chir Organi Mov 1991;76:151–155

68. Tabor OB, Bosse MJ, Sims SH, Kellam JF. Iatrogenic posterior interosseous nerve injury: is transosseous static locked nailing of the radius feasible? J Orthop Trauma 1995;9:427–429

69. Fernandez Dell'Oca AA, Tepic S, Frigg R, Meisser A, Haas N, Perren SM. Treating forearm fractures using an internal fixator: a prospective study. Clin Orthop Relat Res 2001;389:196–205

70. Haas N, Hauke C, Schutz M, Kaab M, Perren SM. Treatment of diaphyseal fractures of the forearm using the Point Contact Fixator (PC-Fix): results of 387 fractures of a prospective multicentric study (PC-Fix II). Injury 2001;32(Suppl 2):B51–B62

71. Hofer HP, Wildburger R, Szyszkowitz R. Observations concerning different patterns of bone healing using the Point Contact Fixator (PC-Fix) as a new technique for fracture fixation. Injury 2001;32(Suppl 2):B15–B25

72. Eijer H, Hauke C, Arens S, Printzen G, Schlegel U, Perren SM. PC-Fix and local infection resistance: influence of implant design on postoperative infection development, clinical and experimental results. Injury 2001;32(Suppl 2):B38–B43

73. Hertel R, Eijer H, Meisser C, Hauke C, Perren SM. Biomechanical and biological considerations relating to the clinical use of the Point Contact-Fixator: evaluation of the device handling test in the treatment of diaphyseal fractures of the radius and/or ulna. Injury 2001;32(Suppl 2):B10–B14

74. Leung F, Chow SP. A prospective, randomized trial comparing the limited contact dynamic compression plate with the point contact fixator for forearm fractures: abstract. J Bone Joint Surg Am 2003;85:2343–2348

75. Goldfarb CA, Ricci WM, Tull F, Ray D, Borrelli J Jr. Functional outcome after fracture of both bones of the forearm. J Bone Joint Surg Br 2005;87:374–379

76. Stern PJ, Drury WJ. Complications of plate fixation of forearm fractures. Clin Orthop Relat Res 1983;175:25–29

77. Jupiter JB, Ring D. Operative treatment of post-traumatic proximal radioulnar synostosis. J Bone Joint Surg Am 1998;80:248–257

78. Hidaka S, Gustilo RB. Refracture of bones of the forearm after plate removal. J Bone Joint Surg Am 1984;66:1241–1243

79. McQueen MM, Gaston P, Court-Brown CM. Acute compartment syndrome: who is at risk? J Bone Joint Surg Br 2000;82: 200–203

80. Ghobrial TF, Eglseder WA Jr, Bleckner SA. Proximal ulna shaft fractures and associated compartment syndromes. Am J Orthop 2001;30:703–707

16 Distal Radius Fractures

Paul M. Simic and Jeffrey D. Placzek

Many fractures of the distal radius are relatively uncomplicated and are effectively treated by closed reduction and casting. However, fractures that are either or both unstable and involve the articular surfaces can jeopardize the congruence of the wrist and distal radioulnar joints and the kinematics of these articulations. The goal of the treating physician is to restore the functional anatomy of the distal radius by a method that does not compromise hand function. The fracture pattern, the degree of displacement, the stability of the fracture, and the age and physical demands of the patient determine the best treatment option.

Nearly 20% of all fractures treated in emergency departments in the United States involve the distal end of the radius, and these have a bimodal age distribution, with the adolescent/young adult and elderly populations being the most affected.[1] Distal radial metaphyseal fractures involve the radiocarpal and/or the distal radioulnar joint (DRUJ) in ~50% of cases.[2]

Over the past 20 years, more sophisticated internal and external fixation techniques and devices have been developed for the treatment of displaced fractures of the distal radius. Specifically, the use of percutaneous pin fixation, external fixation devices that permit distraction and palmar translation, low-profile internal fixation plates with locking screws, and arthroscopically assisted reduction have improved the management of these fractures. Furthermore, the increased use of bone grafting and improved bone graft substitutes has contributed to improving fracture stability and outcome.

Anatomy

The distal radius functions as a foundation for the wrist joint. Integrity of the bony, articular, and ligamentous structures is needed to maintain motion and transmit load. At the metaphyseal flare of the distal radius, the thickness of the cortical bone decreases and the amount of cancellous bone increases, forming a zone predisposed to fracture.[3] The dorsal aspect of the distal radius is somewhat convex and acts as a fulcrum for extensor tendon function. The dorsal cortical surface of the radius thickens to form Lister's tubercle as well as osseous prominences that support the extensors of the wrist.[4] Supporting ligaments arising from the dorsal surface include the radioscaphoid and radiotriquetral ligaments. The palmar radial aspect of the radius is flat, and from this surface originate the major

radial supporting ligaments of the wrist: the radial collateral, radiocapite, and radiotriquetral ligaments.[5,6]

The distal radius has three concave articular surfaces— the scaphoid fossa, the lunate fossa, and the sigmoid notch. A central anterior/posterior ridge divides the scaphoid facet from the lunate facet, with each facet concave in both the anteroposterior and radioulnar directions. The areas of thickened metaphyseal cortex provide segments of bone that reliably resist fracture, causing predictable fracture patterns that often propagate between the scaphoid and lunate facets of the distal aspect of the radius.[4,6,7]

The sigmoid notch of the distal radius is semicylindrical in shape and articulates with the ulnar head. During rotation of the radius about the ulna, there is translation of the distal ulna volarly with forearm supination and dorsally with forearm pronation. The triangular fibrocartilage complex (TFCC) originates from the ulnar aspect of the radius and attaches to the base of the ulnar styloid. The thickened dorsal and volar margins of the triangular fibrocartilage become the dorsal and volar radioulnar ligaments.[8,9] Radial deformity, especially radial shortening, can alter the kinematics of both the DRUJ and the TFCC.[5,10,11]

Both the extrinsic and interosseous ligaments of the wrist maintain dynamic and static stability. The scapholunate and lunotriquetral interosseous ligaments stabilize the scaphoid, lunate, and triquetrum complex that articulates with the distal aspect of the radius and the TFCC. The flexor and extensor tendons of the wrist pass across the distal aspect of the radius to insert onto the carpal bones or the bases of the metacarpals. Only the brachioradialis tendon inserts onto the distal aspect of the radius. It is often a deforming force upon the fracture fragments.[2,6]

Wrist function is dependent on the integrity and alignment of the radius with its carpal and ulnar articulations. Loss of this association can significantly affect wrist and hand function.

Classification

A classification system should communicate the relative severity of the fracture and describe the corresponding treatment options. Although the Mayo classification has demonstrated moderate intraobserver reliability, the Frykman and Melone classifications have only fair interobserver agreement.[12] The Arbeitsgemeinschaft für Osteosynthesefragen (AO) classification system is the most detailed and inclusive. We find it useful for broad anatomical categorization of large numbers of fractures for trauma registries. Significant interobserver agreement ($p < .05$) with use of the AO system was achieved after the classification was reduced from 27 detailed descriptions of fractures to three major fracture types (extra-articular, intra-articular with part of the metaphysis intact, and intra-articular fractures with complete disruption of the metaphysis).[6,12,13]

AO type A fractures (extra-articular) are usually bending injuries through the metaphysis and affect neither the articular surface of the radiocarpal nor the radioulnar joints. AO type B fractures (partial intra-articular) result from shear or impaction injuries, causing fractures of the volar/dorsal rim, radial styloid, or medial corner, or causing a central articular surface die-punch fracture. A portion of the articular surface remains in continuity with the metaphysis, which adds greatly to the stability of the fracture. AO type C fractures (complex articular) are generally high-energy fractures, often involving a combination of shear and impaction. None of the articular surface remains in continuity with the metaphysis. Comminution of the distal radial metaphysis can be present in many of these injuries. It is defined as involvement of more than 50% of the diameter of the metaphysis as seen on any radiograph, comminution of at least two cortices of the metaphysis, or more than 2.0 mm of shortening of the radius.[2,6]

Radiographic Evaluation

Preoperative planning is of vital importance to successful surgery, and adequate radiographic views of the wrist are required.[14] The initial posteroanterior, lateral, and oblique radiographs of the distal radial fracture are very important because they show the extent and direction of the initial displacement. The oblique radiograph is particularly helpful in identifying displacement of fractures of the lunate facet. Postreduction radiographs help to identify any residual deformity and the degree of comminution. Standard posteroanterior traction radiographs help in determining whether the fracture is intra-articular or extra-articular and may also demonstrate the presence of associated intracapsular or interosseous carpal ligament injuries. Disruption of the smooth congruent lines of the radiocarpal and midcarpal rows would suggest either or both interosseous and intracapsular ligament pathology.[15] The important radiological relationships (given as average values) are radial inclination (23 degrees), radial height (12 mm), volar tilt (11 degrees), DRUJ reduction, and radial width (normally within 1 mm of the contralateral side).[16]

With fracture comminution, displacement, or complex intra-articular extension, standard radiography may not be sufficient. Computed tomography (CT) allows for more accurate and in-depth assessment of the complexity of the injury. CT should be performed if conventional radiographs provide insufficient detail and, specifically, when a detailed evaluation is needed of radiocarpal articular step-off and gap displacement: factors crucial in predicting the development of radiocarpal osteoarthritis.[17,18] CT can provide a more accurate diagnosis of the displacement pattern, number of fragments, and degree of involvement at both the radiocarpal and radioulnar joints.[19] CT is also helpful in determining the surgical approach by identifying volar or dorsal displacement that may not be evident on plain radiographs.

Indications for Treatment

The fracture pattern, degree of displacement of the fracture fragments, and stability of the fracture determine whether surgical treatment rather than immobilization with a cast is needed. Both clinical and biomechanical research has determined that even fractures with 1 to 2 mm of intra-articular displacement can result in degeneration of the joint, causing pain and stiffness of the wrist.[5,6,20–22]

Shortening of the distal end of the radius by amounts as small as 2.5 mm or any residual dorsal tilt of the distal radial articular surface results in a significant increase in the axial load transmitted to the ulnar shaft.[23] Biomechanical studies have shown that as the distal radius tilts dorsally, the contact area of the distal articular surface with the scaphoid and the lunate decreases in size and shifts dorsally.[23,24] Furthermore, increased dorsal tilt produces DRUJ incongruency and tightens the interosseous membrane, thereby limiting forearm rotation.[10,25] These findings theoretically suggest that malunion of extra-articular fractures is biomechanically unsound and can lead to posttraumatic arthritis, midcarpal instability, and pain.[26–28] Furthermore, patients with malunited extra-articular fractures can develop posttraumatic arthritis of the radiocarpal and radioulnar joints, decreased wrist motion, reduced grip strength, and carpal subluxation with wrist instability.[2,29,30]

In a now classic study, Knirk and Jupiter reported that 2 mm or more of displacement of the distal radial articular surface resulted in posttraumatic osteoarthrosis.[22] Other investigators have found, however, that displacement of even 1 mm resulted in pain and stiffness of the wrist.[21,31] It is well known that intra-articular malreduction contributes to rapid degenerative changes of the wrist joint.[20,22,26] In particular, the importance of anatomical reduction of the lunate fossa has now been demonstrated.[32,33]

A large body of clinical and experimental evidence supports the premise that achieving anatomical reduction of the distal radius is of paramount importance. Fractures with loss of 2 mm or more of radial height, change in radial inclination of 5 degrees or more, loss of volar tilt of 10 degrees or more, loss of DRUJ reduction, and/or with more than 1 to 2 mm of intra-articular step-off should be reduced. Surgical intervention is considered if an acceptable reduction cannot be achieved or maintained by closed means.

The deleterious effects of prolonged immobilization on articular cartilage and the surrounding soft tissue structures have been demonstrated both clinically and experimentally.[34] Establishing stable fixation to allow early motion and rehabilitation should also be a goal. A realistic balance between achieving anatomical reduction, securing stable fixation, minimizing soft tissue disruption, and allowing early rehabilitation can be realized with knowledge and application of current techniques and technology.

Nonoperative Treatment

Closed reduction and cast immobilization are still the appropriate treatment for nondisplaced, stable fractures. These fractures are characterized by minimal radial metaphyseal comminution, little or no loss of height, and no significant displacement or angulation. A well-padded splint with the wrist in neutral position, the metacarpalphalangeal joints completely unobstructed, and the overlying wrap loosely approximated will provide adequate immobilization to a truly stable and nondisplaced fracture, without contributing to hand swelling and stiffness.

To prevent displacement of the reduced fracture during immobilization, the position of acute wrist flexion, extreme forearm pronation, and ulnar deviation (the Cotton-Loder position) has been utilized in the past. However, excessive wrist flexion compromises the carpal tunnel and interferes with normal flexor tendon function. This position of immobilization is no longer popular because of the problems encountered with median nerve compression and finger/wrist stiffness.[35,36]

Nondisplaced fractures are kept immobilized until adequate bone healing has occurred, typically in 6 to 8 weeks. At this point, the cast may be replaced with a removable volar splint and active wrist exercises begun. During the entire treatment period, metacarpophalangeal motion and digit function should be emphasized.

Surgical Treatment

Surgical Approaches

General Concepts

In general, fracture configuration determines the surgical approach to be utilized. In the past, dorsally angulated fractures were approached dorsally so that the plate would serve to buttress the comminuted zone and prevent recurrent dorsal displacement. Today, many dorsally displaced extra-articular fractures are fixed through a volar approach. With the wide variety of volar locking plates currently available, even the most distal fractures can usually be corrected by this method.[37,38] Although extra-articular

volarly displaced fractures can generally be fixed through a volar approach utilizing a simple buttress plate, application of a locking plate in this situation may provide increased stability and allow a more vigorous rehabilitation protocol to ensue.

Intra-articular fractures leave the surgeon with one of several options to pursue. The most direct solution to this problem is to do an open dorsal approach to the distal radius with a capsulotomy to allow direct visualization of the intra-articular reduction. This allows direct plating of the distal radius and bone grafting to support the articular surface with unobstructed access. In other cases, the surgeon may opt for arthroscopically assisted reduction aided by percutaneous pinning. Here, bone graft may be added for articular support through a mini dorsal incision. Intra-articular fractures that have large fragments may also be approached from the volar side of the wrist. In this case, an extended flexor carpi radialis (FCR) approach is utilized.[39] By releasing the first extensor compartment and the insertion of the brachioradialis, pronation of the proximal fragment out of the wound allows for exposure of the distal fracture fragments and dorsal bone grafting if necessary. This method is aided by intraoperative fluoroscopic assessment of the articular reduction. Regardless of the operative tactic that is chosen, final reduction should be verified by at least the use of intraoperative fluoroscopy, and preferably by direct visualization of the joint surface if possible.

Volar Approaches

Extended FCR Approach

The most common approach to the volar aspect of the distal radius is through the tendon sheath of the FCR (**Fig. 16–1A–F**) (see **Video 16–1, Disk 2**). A longitudinal incision ~8 cm in length is centered over the FCR tendon sheath. A zigzag extension of the distal end of the incision across the volar wrist flexor crease may be used to assist in gaining further access to the radial styloid fragment. Dissection is carried through the subcutaneous tissue, and the tendon sheath of the FCR is identified and incised. The FCR tendon is retracted ulnarly, and the dorsal aspect of the FCR sheath is sharply incised. The muscle belly and tendon of the flexor pollicis longus (FPL) is retracted ulnarly, and the pronator quadratus is visualized. The pronator quadratus is sharply incised off its radial attachment, leaving a small sleeve for later repair if deemed appropriate. The pronator quadratus is then elevated off the anterior radius using a Freer or other small elevator, thus exposing the entire anterior distal radius. Care is taken to avoid injury to the volar carpal ligaments. Improved mobilization and visualization of the fracture fragments can be obtained by "extending" this approach.[39] To extend this approach, the insertions of the brachioradialis, the first dorsal compartment, and the distal portion of the FCR

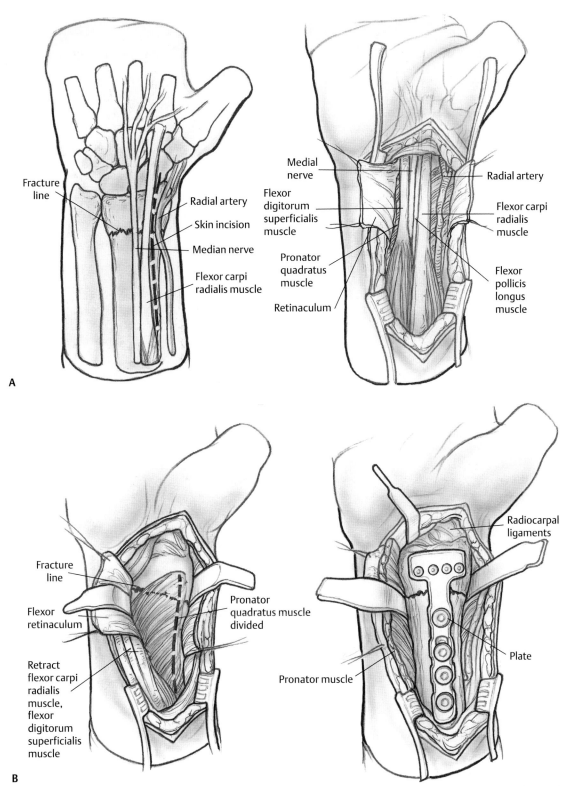

Figure 16–1 Extended flexor carpi radialis (FCR) approach. The most common approach to the volar aspect of the distal radius is through the tendon sheath of the FCR tendon. **(A)** After retracting the flexor carpi radialis and flexor digitorum superficialis muscles ulnarwards, the pronator quadratus is incised along the dotted line. **(B)** The volar surface of the distal radius is exposed after retraction of the pronator quadratus. *(Continued on page 368)*

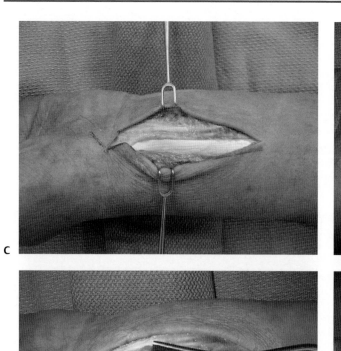

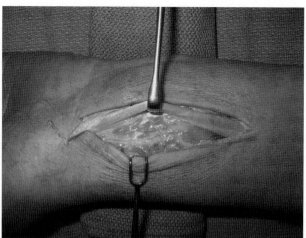

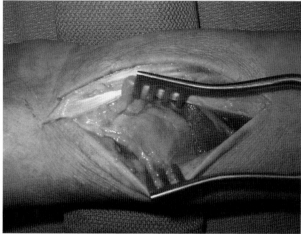

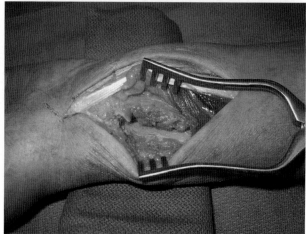

Figure 16–1 *(Continued)* Extended flexor carpi radialis (FCR) approach. **(C)** Expose and incise the FCR tendon sheath, dissecting distally to the level of the superficial radial artery. **(D)** Retract the FCR ulnarly, protecting the median nerve. Incise the floor of the sheath, continuing dis-tally to the level of the scaphoid tubercle. **(E)** Develop the plane between the flexor pollicis longus and radial septum to expose the pronator quadratus. **(F)** Release the pronator quadratus muscle from the radial insertion to expose the volar surface of the radius.

tendon sheath is sharply elevated off of the radial styloid. This allows for pronation of the proximal fragment out of the wound and thus improved exposure for reduction and bone grafting **(Fig. 16–2A–C).** In a recent cadaveric india ink injection study (Placzek et al[39a]), we found robust blood flow remaining to the distal radial shaft and metaphyseal segment after an extended FCR approach was undertaken. Branches from the anterior interosseous artery entering the ulnar aspect of the radius remained undisturbed during this approach.

Central (Extensile) Palmar Approach

For fractures involving the lunate facet, volar carpal ligaments, DRUJ, or those requiring concomitant release of the transverse carpal ligament, an extended approach based on a carpal tunnel incision may be utilized. The incision begins where Kaplan's cardinal line transects the axis of the fourth metacarpal. The incision follows the curve of the thenar crease, is angled slightly ulnarly at the wrist crease, and then continues proximally over the required distance. The carpal tunnel may be released in the standard fashion followed by continued release of the distal deep forearm fascia. The flexor tendons and the median nerve may be retracted radially to visualize the floor of the carpal tunnel. The pronator quadratus can then be lifted as previously described to reveal the extent of the distal radius. The plane of dissection leaves the ulnar neurovascular bundle retracted ulnarly while the contents of the carpal canal (i.e., median nerve and flexor digitorum superficialis, flexor digitorum profundus, and flexor pollicis longus muscles) are retracted radially.

Dorsal Approaches

Through the Floor of the Third Compartment

The dorsal aspect of the distal radius is most commonly approached through the floor of the third dorsal compartment

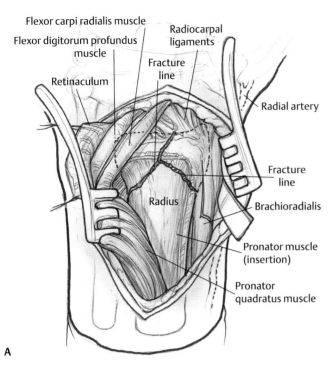

Flexor carpi radialis muscle
Flexor digitorum profundus muscle
Retinaculum
Radiocarpal ligaments
Fracture line
Radial artery
Fracture line
Radius
Brachioradialis
Pronator muscle (insertion)
Pronator quadratus muscle

A

Figure 16–2 Improved mobilization and visualization of the fracture fragments can be obtained by "extending" the volar approach. **(A)** Illustration of the volar approach to the distal radius. **(B)** The insertions of the brachioradialis, the first dorsal compartment, and the distal portion of the flexor carpi radialis tendon sheath are sharply elevated off the radial styloid. **(C)** This allows for pronation of the proximal fragment out of the wound and thus improved exposure for reduction and bone grafting.

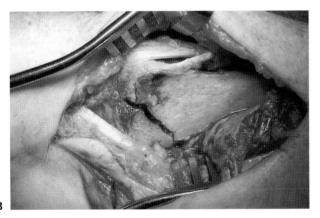

B

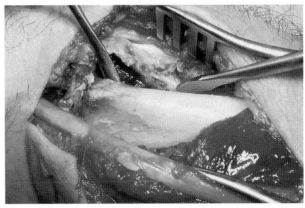

C

(Fig. 16–3A–D). This approach allows complete exposure of the dorsal radius from the radial styloid to the DRUJ. Its distal extent allows for capsulotomy and direct visualization of the articular surface as well as examination of the scapholunate ligament. A longitudinal incision of 8 to 10 cm is made on the dorsal aspect of the wrist just ulnar to Lister's tubercle. Dissection is carried down through the subcutaneous tissue, with care taken to protect small cutaneous nerve branches. Incision is made into the third dorsal extensor compartment, and the extensor pollicis longus is lifted and retracted radially. The fourth compartment can then be elevated subperiosteally and retracted ulnarly, with care being taken to avoid direct entrance into the compartment itself. Similarly, the first and second compartments can be lifted subperiosteally as a group and retracted radially. A longitudinal incision through the dorsal capsule/dorsal radiocarpal ligament allows for

exposure of the proximal carpal row and the articular surface of the distal radius.

Between the First and Second Dorsal Compartments

When fixation is needed of a large radial styloid fragment, an approach between the first and second dorsal compartments may be utilized. A longitudinal incision is made just radial to Lister's tubercle. Dissection is carried down through the subcutaneous tissue, with care taken to protect branches of the superficial radial nerve and lateral antebrachial cutaneous nerve. Incision is made between the first and second compartments, which are subperiosteally elevated and retracted in a radial and ulnar direction, respectively. At the distal end of the incision, care must be taken to avoid injury to the radial artery as it

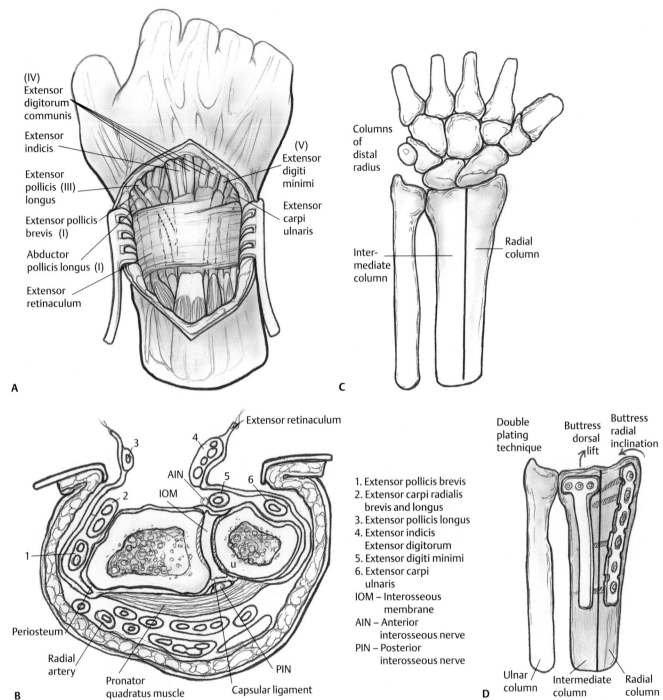

(IV) Extensor digitorum communis

Extensor indicis

Extensor pollicis (III) longus

Extensor pollicis brevis (I)

Abductor pollicis longus (I)

Extensor retinaculum

(V) Extensor digiti minimi

Extensor carpi ulnaris

A

Columns of distal radius

Intermediate column

Radial column

C

Extensor retinaculum

AIN

IOM

Periosteum

Radial artery

Pronator quadratus muscle

Capsular ligament

PIN

B

1. Extensor pollicis brevis
2. Extensor carpi radialis brevis and longus
3. Extensor pollicis longus
4. Extensor indicis
   Extensor digitorum
5. Extensor digiti minimi
6. Extensor carpi ulnaris
IOM – Interosseous membrane
AIN – Anterior interosseous nerve
PIN – Posterior interosseous nerve

Double plating technique

Buttress dorsal lift

Buttress radial inclination

Ulnar column

Intermediate column

Radial column

D

Figure 16–3 The dorsal approach: the dorsal aspect of the distal radius is most commonly approached through the floor of the third dorsal compartment. This approach allows complete exposure of the dorsal radius from the radial styloid to the distal radioulnar joint, allowing fracture reduction and fixation of the involved columns. **(A)** Illustration of the superficial exposure, showing the extensor retinac- ulum and the underlying tendons. **(B)** The columns of the distal radius. **(C)** Cross-sectional anatomy of the dorsal approach showing elevation of the various extensor compartments. **(D)** Illustration of the use of small, "fragment-specific implants to the radial and intermediate columns of the distal radius.

courses beneath the first dorsal compartment. Dorsal capsulotomy is made to view the articular reduction.

Through the Floor of the Fifth Dorsal Compartment

When the fracture involves an isolated die-punch fracture of the lunate fossa, exposure of the distal radius may best

be achieved by an approach through the fifth dorsal compartment. A longitudinal incision is made centered over the DRUJ. Dissection is carried down through the subcutaneous tissues, with care taken to avoid branches of both the superficial radial nerve and the dorsal cutaneous branch of the ulnar nerve. The fifth dorsal compartment is opened, and the tendon of the extensor digiti minimi is elevated and retracted ulnarly. The fourth dorsal compartment can then be elevated subperiosteally for exposure of the fracture fragments.

Specific Procedures

Open Reduction and Internal Fixation

Open reduction and internal fixation is being used more frequently in the treatment of distal radius fractures. Both limited open reduction and more formal extended open reduction procedures provide a variety of options. Newer designs in low-profile plating systems and other internal fixation devices allow for improved fracture fixation without leading to soft tissue complications.

Open Reduction Internal Fixation of Intra-Articular Distal Radius Fractures

For intra-articular fractures of the distal radius, particularly those that are comminuted and need to be reconstructed with the aid of direct visualization, we prefer the dorsal approach through the floor of the third dorsal compartment and reconstruction with either a single low-profile T-type plate or a double plating technique as popularized by Rikli et al.[40–42] For fractures without significant comminution and with fragments that can be captured with a single plate, we prefer the dorsal Locon-T plate (Wright Medical Technology, Inc., Arlington, Tennessee), which has been shown to provide stable fixation without extensor tendon irritation as seen with other dorsal plates[42a] (Simic et al, in review). For fractures with multiple fragments that are difficult to stabilize with a single large T-plate, two minifragment (2 mm or similar) "fragment-specific" plates are fashioned along the radial and intermediate columns of the radius, with the plates angled at 50 to 70 degrees to one another. This method of fixation has been shown to provide superior stiffness in all bending modes as compared with other thicker plates such as an AO 3.5 mm T-plate or a Synthes π-plate.[43] Furthermore, the double plating technique demonstrated decreased angle of deformation and decreased gap formation at the fracture site when compared with other plating techniques, although this does not reach statistical significance. Although an individual 2 mm titanium plate is not as rigid as other plates, the combination of two plates placed at ~60 degrees from one another allows for rigid fixation while maintaining a low profile and a low incidence of extensor tendon irritation.[42,43] Furthermore, the newly available Synthes 2.4 mm locking compression plates (LCPs) allow for the same advantages of the 2.0 mm titanium plates from the modular hand set while offering increased rigidity and the benefits of a rigid fixed-angle device.

A dorsal approach through the floor of the third dorsal compartment is undertaken as already described (**Fig. 16–3A–D**). Retraction is maintained with the use of mini Hohman retractors. The fracture fragments that are often impacted are mobilized with the use of a Freer elevator and debrided. The radial styloid fragment is usually reduced first, aided by traction placed along the thumb or the index and long fingers. Provisional fixation can be obtained with the use of a 0.062 in. K-wire placed obliquely from the tip of the radial styloid. For fractures amenable to fixation with a single large T-plate, an appropriate plate such as the Locon-T is precontoured and secured to the radial shaft. Individual fracture fragments are then captured, with the screws placed distally (**Fig. 16–4A–F**).

Alternatively, two smaller 2 mm plates can be used (**Fig. 16–5A–D**). Based on the size of the fragment, an appropriate plate (i.e., T-shaped, L-shaped, straight) of the necessary length (usually six to nine holes) is precontoured for the radial styloid fragment. With the appropriate length maintained, this plate is first attached to the radial shaft at the hole just proximal to the fracture site using a standard AO technique. All of the distal screws are then placed because fixation in this metaphyseal bone may be tenuous. Finally, the rest of the screws are inserted into the proximal part of the plate along the radial shaft.

The remaining fragments of the intermediate columns are then reduced. The resulting metaphyseal defect is filled with crushed cancellous bone graft or other bone graft substitute, which will help buttress the articular surface and speed union. An appropriate plate is then fashioned to control the fragments of the intermediate column. This will usually be a T-plate with two or three distal horizontal screws. This plate is applied as already described. After osteosynthesis is completed, the subperiosteally elevated retinacular flaps are sutured over the plate using 3–0

Tips and Tricks

- Maintain thick subperiosteal retinacular flaps to avoid tendon irritation.
- Provisional fixation may be aided by the use of 0.062 in. K-wires. An obliquely placed K-wire through the radial styloid as well as a transversely placed K-wire under the subchondral surface will help stabilize the radial and intermediate columns, respectively.
- Precontour the plates such that they aid in compression of smaller distal bony fragments and help maintain the normal anatomical 10 degrees of palmar tilt.
- Be cautious to avoid screw penetration into the DRUJ when stabilizing the intermediate column.
- 2.4 mm plates may be utilized in larger patients.
- Always ensure reduction intraoperatively with the use of anatomical views[44] obtained with the image intensifier.

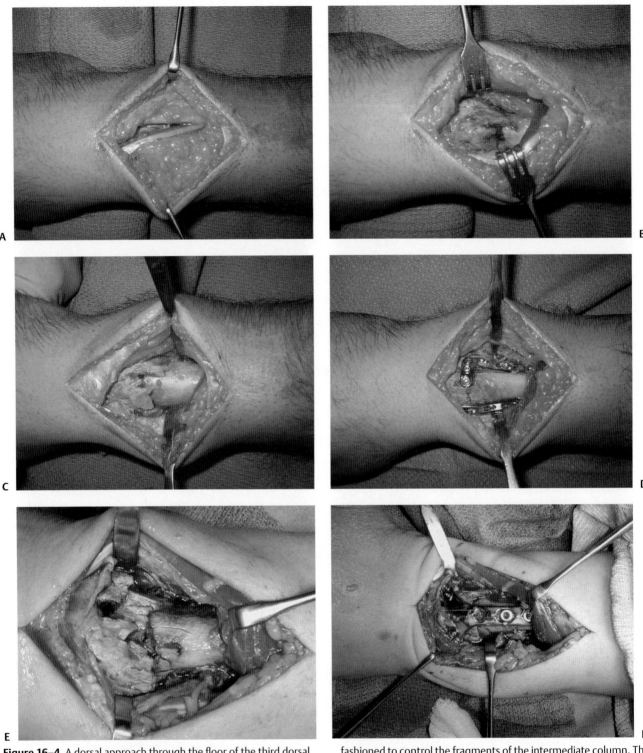

Figure 16–4 A dorsal approach through the floor of the third dorsal compartment is utilized, providing excellent exposure to the fracture site. Intraoperative photographs of the **(A)** superficial and **(B)** deep exposure. **(C)** Fracture is reduced with both direct and indirect means. **(D)**. Based on the size of the fragment, an appropriate plate (i.e., T-shaped, L-shaped, straight) of the necessary length is precontoured for the radial styloid fragment. An appropriate plate is then fashioned to control the fragments of the intermediate column. This will usually be a T-plate with two or three distal horizontal screws. **(E)** Intraoperative photograph of a different fracture that is amendable to fixation with a single, large T-plate. **(F)** For fractures amenable to fixation with a single large T-plate, an appropriate plate such as the Locon-T is precontoured and secured to the radial shaft. Individual fracture fragments are then captured with the screws placed distally.

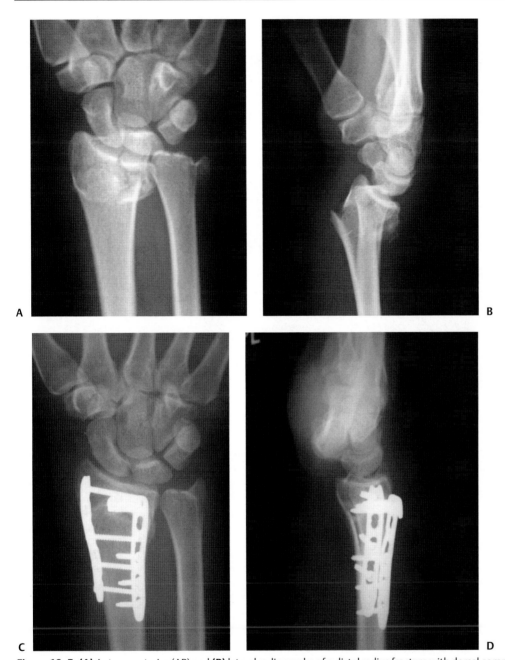

Figure 16–5 **(A)** Anteroposterior (AP) and **(B)** lateral radiographs of a distal radius fracture with dorsal comminution and intra-articular gapping and step-off > 2 mm. Postoperative **(C)** AP and **(D)** lateral radiographs following open reduction and internal fixation with dorsal approach utilizing two smaller, low-contour locking dorsal plates.

Vicryl (Ethicon, Inc., Somerville, New Jersey) or equivalent suture such that no tendon is in contact with the plate itself. The capsular defect is closed with interrupted 3–0 nonabsorbable braided suture in a figure-of-eight fashion. A suction drain is utilized for 24 hours when deemed necessary. A short-arm volar splint is applied with the metacarpal-phalangel (MCP) joints and fingers free to allow range of motion. A thermoplastic splint is fabricated at the patient's first follow-up visit, and a range of motion exercise program is started.

Open Reduction Internal Fixation of Extra-Articular Distal Radius Fractures

Although volarly displaced fractures have long been fixed through a volar approach, it was not until the recent advent of locking and fixed-angle distal radius plates that volar fixation of dorsally displaced distal radius fractures became popular.[37–39,45] Many volar locking plates have recently been introduced to the market; two of the most popular fixed-angle distal radius plates are the Avanta SCS/V plate

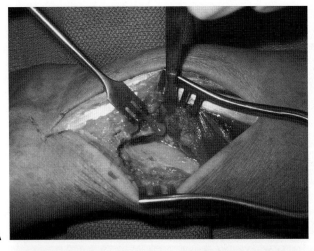

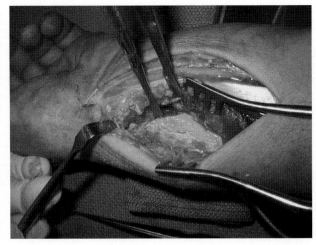

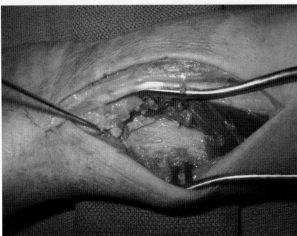

Figure 16–6 Sequential steps in the repair of a distal radius fracture using the volar approach. **(A)** Initial exposure. The fracture line is visible. **(B)** A blunt elevator is used to debride the fracture site. **(C)** Provisional reduction and fixation with a 0.062-inch K-wire. *(Continued)*

(Avanta Orthopaedics, San Diego, California) and the Hand Innovations DVR plate (Hand Innovations, Miami, Florida). Both of these plates have performed extremely well in our hands, and each has its own unique advantages. The anatomical design of the Avanta SCS/V plate, with its pegs placed at the most distal aspect of the plate, allows for rigid fixation of fractures that are extremely distal such that little bone is available for purchase in the distal fragment. Furthermore, the fact that all drill holes are placed at one time and individual screws are not needed speeds the application of this plate. The Hand Innovations DVR plate allows for the placement of multiple screws placed out of plane to one another. This screw configuration gives this plate a theoretical advantage of increased pullout strength from the distal fragment. The system also allows for the use of threaded pins if one wishes to capture the dorsal cortex with the distal fragment screws.

An extended FCR approach is utilized as already described **(Fig. 16–1A–F)** (see **Video 16–1, Disk 2**). Traction by

the use of finger traps or manual traction may be used to help assist in reduction and regain length. Fracture fragments are mobilized with the use of a Freer elevator and debrided **(Fig. 16–6A–E)**. Reduction is obtained aided by traction, prying with a Freer elevator, or direct pressure over the fracture fragments. Care is taken to obtain not only the appropriate length, radial inclination, and volar tilt but also the appropriate rotation (i.e., the distal fragment should not be pronated or supinated in relationship to the proximal fragment). Provisional fixation may be held with 0.062 in. K-wires, often with one through the radial styloid directed proximally as well as one started proximal-radial and directed into the ulnar aspect of the distal fragment. The locking plate of one's choice is then applied according to the manufacturer's recommended technique.

In the case of the Avanta plate, the drill guide will first be applied at the oblong hole and the guidewires placed in the middle guidewire holes distally. For difficult-to-reduce fractures, these plates can be applied distally first and utilized

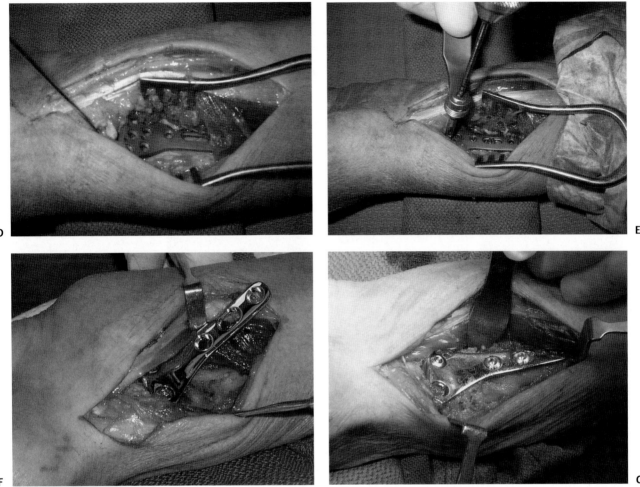

Figure 16–6 *(Continued)* Sequential steps in the repair of a distal radius fracture using the volnar approach. **(D)** If anatomical reduction is obtained, the volar locking plate is positioned and **(E)** secured distally with the locking screw or peg technique. Proximally, standard cortical screw technique is utilized. **(F)** For difficult-to-reduce fractures, the plate can be applied distally first and utilized to help gain reduction **(G)**.

to help gain reduction (**Fig. 16–6F,G**). The plate and guidewire position is then verified with fluoroscopy. If good reduction and plate position are obtained, the distal peg holes are drilled. The plate inserter is utilized to assist in application of the plate. The plate is then reduced to the shaft; a screw is inserted into the oblong hole, and reduction is once again checked with fluoroscopy. If the reduction is deemed appropriate, the remainder of the shaft screws are placed.

When utilizing the Hand Innovations DVR plate, after reduction is obtained, the plate may be provisionally held with the use of K-wires. As with the Avanta plate, the plate is first secured to the shaft at the oblong hole. This allows the plate to be shifted proximally or distally, should realignment be necessary. Again, for difficult-to-reduce fractures, the plate can be applied distally first and utilized to help gain reduction. Next, using the 2 mm drill bit, the proximal-row pegs at the distal end of the plate are placed. The distal-row pegs may then be placed if there is severe comminution or osteoporosis that demands extra fixation (**Fig. 16–7A,B**).

Percutaneous Pinning

For some displaced fractures of the radius, the use of percutaneous pins has been an accepted practice either alone or in conjunction with external fixation (see **Video 16–2, Disk 2**). Percutaneous pin fixation is an excellent technique, provided the distal radius is not severely comminuted or osteoporotic, because the trabecular bone of the metaphysis provides little inherent stability. It is especially useful for unstable fractures, both extra-articular and intra-articular, and is useful in combination with other modes of fixation.

A variety of different techniques have been described in the literature, depending on the fracture pattern. Kirschner wires (K-wires), 0.045 to 0.0625 in. diameter, can be placed through the radial styloid (transstyloid), within the fracture site (intrafocal), into distal fragments

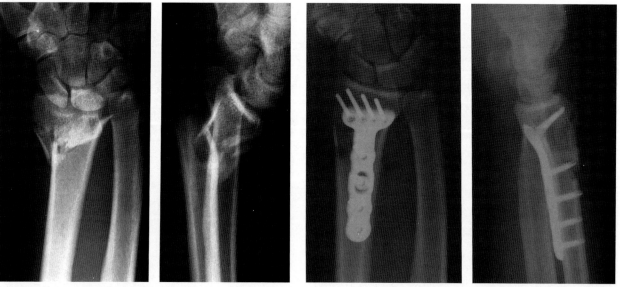

Figure 16–7 (A) Distal radius fracture with significant comminution, shortening, dorsal tilt, and instability. **(B)** Open reduction and internal fixation with a volar locking plate.

Tips and Tricks

- Releasing the insertion of the brachioradialis, the first dorsal extensor compartment, and the distal FCR tendon sheath allows for decreased tension across the fracture site and increased ease of reduction **(Fig. 16–2A–C)**.
- The extended FCR approach described earlier allows for access to dorsally displaced fracture fragments as well as bone grafting to the dorsal side of fracture.
- For difficult-to-reduce fractures, the plate can be applied distally first and utilized to help gain reduction **(Fig. 16–6F,G)**.
- When unable to fully restore palmar tilt, the distal end of the plate may be applied first, leaving the proximal portion of the plate sitting up volar to the radius. When the proximal plate is then secured to the shaft, the anatomical palmar tilt will be restored.
- When unable to fully restore radial inclination, the distal end of the plate may be applied first, leaving the proximal portion of the plate sitting ulnar to the radial shaft. When the proximal plate is then secured to the central shaft, radial inclination will be restored.
- When unable to fully restore radial length, the distal end of the plate may be applied first and then a lamina spreader or Freer elevator utilized in the fracture gap to restore length before the proximal plate is secured to the shaft.
- Consider the use of a drain because the median nerve has little tolerance for swelling or hematoma in the postoperative period. This may assist in minimizing finger stiffness and reflex sympathetic dystrophy symptoms associated with median nerve compression.

to aid in reduction, and across the DRUJ for gross DRUJ instability. Fluoroscopy throughout the procedure is invaluable to evaluate reduction and fixation.[16,46–51]

In the case of AO type B1 fractures, the radial styloid is fractured with differing amounts of displacement. Reduction not only restores the articular congruence but also realigns the support for the volar capsular ligaments of the wrist. After closed reduction with the aid of traction and fluoroscopic imaging, two K-wires are passed through the radial styloid until they penetrate the intact cortex of the shaft proximally **(Fig. 16–8A,B)**. The radial styloid lies anterior to the mid axis of the radius and is surrounded by several branches of the radial sensory nerve. Percutaneously placed wires or screws should be introduced through a drill guide and directed in a proximal, ulnarward, and dorsal direction. Ideally, the fixation should be perpendicular to the fracture line.[2,52]

Another method of percutaneous pin fixation is the intrafocal pin technique of Kapandji, which is best reserved for noncomminuted extra-articular fractures (AO type A2). In this technique, the Kirschner wires are introduced into the fracture site itself, rather than through the distal fracture fragment. The K-wire can be used to wedge open the fracture reduction and then be advanced through the far cortex to prevent the distal fragments from redisplacement. This procedure is performed first in the radio to ulnar direction, and then 90 degrees from the first wire in a dorsal to palmar direction, allowing reduction and maintenance of radial inclination and palmar tilt, respectively.[2,53]

Percutaneous pins can also aid the reduction and fixation of smaller, intra-articular fracture fragments. In AO type C fractures, with multiple intra-articular fragments, K-wires can be used to "joystick" bony fragments into

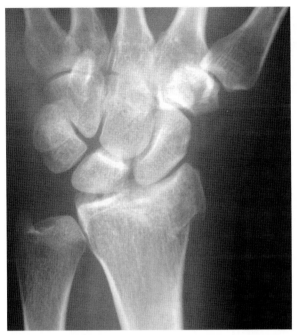
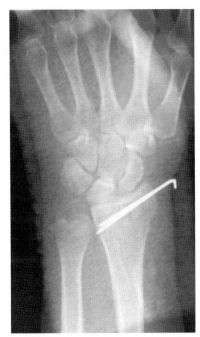

A   B

Figure 16–8 (A) Example of a displaced radial styloid fracture. **(B)** After closed reduction with the aid of traction and fluoroscopic imaging, two K-wires are passed through the radial styloid until they penetrate the intact cortex of the shaft proximally.

reduced positions. A pointed tenaculum clamp can be applied through external puncture wounds to aid in compression of the fragments. After reduction, the pins are then advanced across the fracture lines into adjacent subchondral metaphyseal bone. Also, the fracture site can be opened through a mini incision and the K-wire driven in under direct visualization to capture the small bone fragments after elevation and reduction of the small pieces. With severe comminution of both the articular and metaphyseal regions, a combination of percutaneous pins, internal fixation, and external fixation is frequently required to maintain reduction.[5,16,21]

External Fixation

External fixation devices are an excellent means of overcoming the deforming forces of the forearm muscles that pull comminuted distal radial fractures into a collapsed, shortened position. With severe comminution of the metaphysis, it may be difficult to stabilize the reconstructed articular surface to the shaft of the radius. An external fixator can restore stability when both volar and dorsal cortices are comminuted.[16,54–64] External fixation should only be used when the fracture pattern does not allow for stable internal fixation and early motion, or there are other contraindications to open surgery.

There has been a constant evolution in technique and device design since the original idea in 1944, by Anderson and O'Neil,[65] of using skeletal traction held with an external frame. Much has been learned and improved upon since then. The initial practices of excessive distraction,

extreme wrist flexion and ulna deviation, and long periods of wrist immobilization (over 8 weeks) created frequent problems with postoperative pain, wrist and hand stiffness, disuse atrophy, nonunion, and reflex sympathetic dystrophy.[66] With increased experience and understanding of physiological and biomechanical principles, these complications are much less common.[2,67]

The realization that ligamentotaxis does not always accomplish anatomical reduction of all intra- and extra-articular fracture components spurred the development of new techniques and improvements in external fixation devices. In the case of unstable fracture fragments, the addition of percutaneous pinning or internal fixation techniques allows for external fixation with minimal distraction to prevent metaphyseal shortening and to neutralize the extensor and flexor forces across the fracture site. The need for positioning the wrist in extreme flexion and ulnar deviation to provide reduction was also diminished or eliminated.[66–68] The wrist may initially be overdistracted to aid in reduction, but the amount of distraction must subsequently be decreased to an acceptable amount following fixation.[16]

A large variety of devices are available for external fixation of fractures of the distal aspect of the radius. All involve distraction across the wrist joint with placement of pins in the radius and the metacarpals. Newer external fixation devices are lighter, easier to assemble and implant, radiolucent, and adjustable in multiple planes once the device is secured.

The observation that longitudinal distraction alone does not restore palmar tilt has led to improvements in

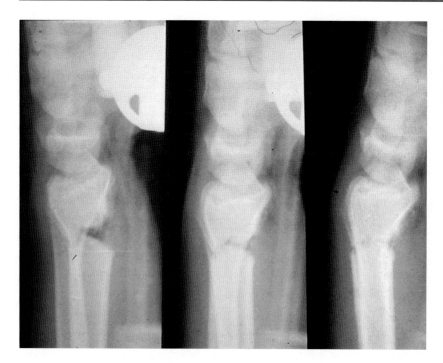

Figure 16–9 The observation that longitudinal distraction alone does not restore palmar tilt has led to improvements in external fixation devices and their application. Palmar translation in addition to longitudinal distraction can often restore the palmar tilt as well as maintain radial height.

devices and their application. Palmar translation in addition to longitudinal distraction can often restore the palmar tilt as well as maintain radial height **(Fig. 16–9)**. The ability to position and adjust the amount of palmar translation across the fracture site with use of more sophisticated external fixation devices provides improved reduction and allows placement of the wrist in the optimal physiological position of extension **(Fig. 16–10A,B)**.[67,69]

Overdistraction of the wrist is assessed by observing the distance between the capitate and lunate. A gap greater than 2 to 3 mm indicates that too much force is being used. Also, the fingers should be able to be passively flexed easily. Excessive flexion or ulnar deviation must be avoided because either position increases the risk of compression of the median nerve, reflex sympathetic dystrophy, and extrinsic tightness, causing stiffness of the fingers.[16] The external fixation device should usually be removed after 5 to 6 weeks and wrist motion initiated.

Technique of External Fixation

Although a wide variety of external fixators are currently available, the most commonly used external fixator in our practice is the Synthes small external fixator set. Steps for application include the following:

- A dorsal radial incision is made over the radius ~5 cm proximal to the fracture site. The superficial branch of the radial nerve is identified and carefully protected.

- A 2 mm drill bit with soft tissue protector sleeve is then used to drill the radius to accept 3 mm partially threaded pins. The pins may be drilled such that they are parallel or approximate a 45 degree angle to one another.

- Next, incisions are made over the dorsal radial second metacarpal in the region of the metaphyseal diaphyseal flares. These pins are inserted at a 30 degree angle from dorsal to volar. This prevents encroachment on the thumb while allowing for unobstructed views on the lateral radiographs. These pins may also be inserted parallel or at a 45 degree angle in relation to

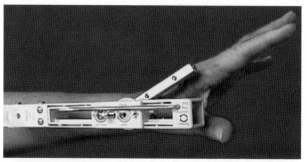

A

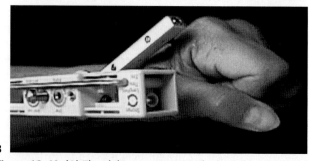

B

Figure 16–10 (A) The ability to position and adjust the amount of palmar translation across the fracture site with use of more sophisticated external fixation devices provides improved reduction and allows placement of the wrist in the optimal physiological position of extension. **(B)** The patient also has full finger function and can easily make a fist.

one another. The 2.5 mm AO partially threaded half pins are then inserted. These pins should be inserted with the index finger held in flexion to avoid tethering of the dorsal extensor mechanism. For ease of closure, the wounds are closed before the frame is assembled.

- A bar-to-bar clamp is placed on connecting bars, which are then placed between the two half pins. At this point, traction is applied, a closed reduction undertaken, and a long graphite bar placed between the two bar-to-bar clamps and secured.

- Because longitudinal distraction and palmar translation are often inadequate to provide optimal reduction, mini dorsal incision and bone grafting are now used to buttress the joint surface into near anatomical position. Bone grafting through a mini dorsal incision hastens healing, allows for increased fracture stability and direct visualization of the joint surface, and ultimately shortens the patient's time spent in the fixator.

- At this point, supplemental percutaneous K-wire fixation adds stability to the fixation configuration and allows for the overdistraction to be removed from the fixator. The fixator can then be double-stacked with a second carbon fiber rod to increase fixator stability.

Utilizing this technique followed by functional bracing, the fixator may be removed as early as 3 weeks, with few complications and little to no settling.[70] Although nonbridging external fixation has been recommended for fixation of displaced distal radius fractures,[71–75] it is our contention that fracture patterns that allow for nonbridging external fixation can usually undergo internal fixation and early motion, thus avoiding the inconvenience and complications associated with external fixation devices. In light of this, we believe there is little role for nonbridging external fixation in the treatment of distal radius fractures.

Although external fixation devices may maintain radial length, individual fracture fragments may still heal in a displaced or angulated position. As mentioned, supplementation with percutaneous pinning can often provide sufficient stability (see **Video 16–2, Disk 2**).[76,77] The external fixator that is utilized should allow pin insertion and frame application prior to fracture fragment reduction. The device can then facilitate fracture alignment and reduction. Manipulation and fixation of intra-articular fragments with K-wires may then be accomplished after the frame is applied (**Fig. 16–11A–D**).[16]

K-wire augmentation can significantly improve the stability of an unstable extra-articular distal radius fracture regardless of the type of external fixator that is used.[77] The addition of a dorsal pin in combination with an external fixation device can easily correct the dorsal tilt found in many fractures of the distal radius.[78,79]

For a dorsally displaced fracture, a limited dorsal incision can be used while distracting the wrist with an external fixator. A nerve hook, Freer elevator, or percutaneously placed pins can be used to elevate the joint fracture fragments. If there is more than 4 to 5 mm of impaction, iliac crest bone graft, bone graft substitute, or allograft is recommended to fill the metaphyseal defect.[16,80]

Combined Internal and External Fixation

Complex fractures involving metaphyseal comminution of both the volar and the dorsal cortices, as well as possible articular comminution, may preclude use of traditional internal fixation techniques alone. Likewise, external fixation alone will not reduce depressed articular fragments. Often a combination of internal and external fixation is required to manage these complex fractures. External fixation devices may maintain radial length, but individual fracture fragments need additional fixation. When supplementation with percutaneous pinning cannot provide sufficient stability, a combination of K-wires, plates, screws, external fixation, and bone grafting is frequently required to guarantee maintenance of reduction and healing. Dorsal and volar approaches may be required to obtain reduction and fixation.[2,16,81,82] The development of both volar and dorsal locking plating systems, however, lessens the need to combine internal and external fixation techniques.

Arthroscopically Assisted Reduction

Standardized techniques of performing wrist arthroscopy have been developed to evaluate various wrist disorders and can be applied to intra-articular distal radius fractures. These techniques require less surgical dissection, cause less postoperative pain, and are associated with a shorter recovery time and an earlier return to work for the patient.[83] Wrist arthroscopy provides the ability to directly assess the articular surface for step-offs or gaps and ligaments for tears. The volar aspect of the wrist and the TFCC are easily visualized with the arthroscope compared with open techniques. Surgical treatment of intra-articular distal radius fractures solely under fluoroscopic visualization appears in some instances to be inadequate to reestablish articular congruency.[16,81,84–88]

Arthroscopic examination of an intra-articular fracture to the distal radius should be delayed for approximately 5 to 7 days following injury to allow bony and soft tissue bleeding to resolve and swelling to begin to subside. During the procedure, the joint is irrigated to remove most debris, the fracture and amount of displacement are evaluated, and the scapholunate and lunotriquetral ligaments as well as the TFCC are inspected. K-wires can then be used to joystick bony fragments into a reduced position, and then to fix fragments together and to the metaphysis. Also, a mini–open approach with reduction of intra-articular fragments with a Freer elevator or small bone tamp and placement of bone graft for support is often necessary. The direct arthroscopic visualization of the articular surface during reduction and fixation helps to ensure a stable, congruent joint surface (**Fig. 16–12A–F**).[16,88]

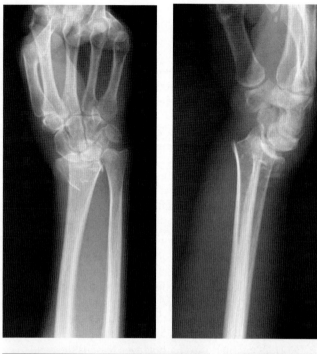

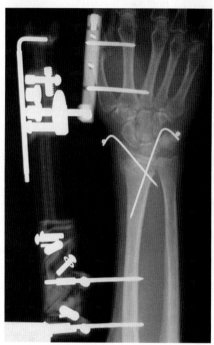

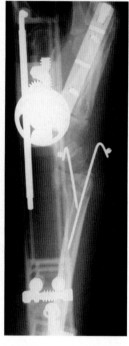

A

B

Figure 16–11 Example of a completely displaced distal radius fracture. **(A)** Preoperative anteroposterior and lateral radiographs of the injury. Although external fixation devices may maintain radial length, individual fracture fragments may still heal in a displaced or angulated position. **(B)** Postoperative radiographs following external fixation supplemented with percutaneous pinning can often provide sufficient stability.

Wrist arthroscopy must be performed quickly because the hand, wrist, and forearm rapidly fill with fluid, which can result in an iatrogenic compartment syndrome. Keeping the distal forearm and hand wrapped with the Esmarch bandage reduces the amount of extravasated fluid.[16]

Bone Graft

Both extra- and intra-articular distal radius fractures often involve significant cortical comminution and loss of cancellous bone in the metaphyseal region. During the healing process, collapse of the distal fragments into the cancellous defects in the metaphyseal and subchondral regions can lead to secondary displacement and loss of reduction.

As described with various fixation techniques, bone graft provides mechanical internal support of articular fragments, accelerates bone healing, and provides osteoconductive and osteoinductive potential to the remaining partially devitalized bone. This is true not only when performing open reduction and internal fixation, which necessitates a more extensive exposure, but also for more limited open reduction and fixation with screws or percutaneous pins.

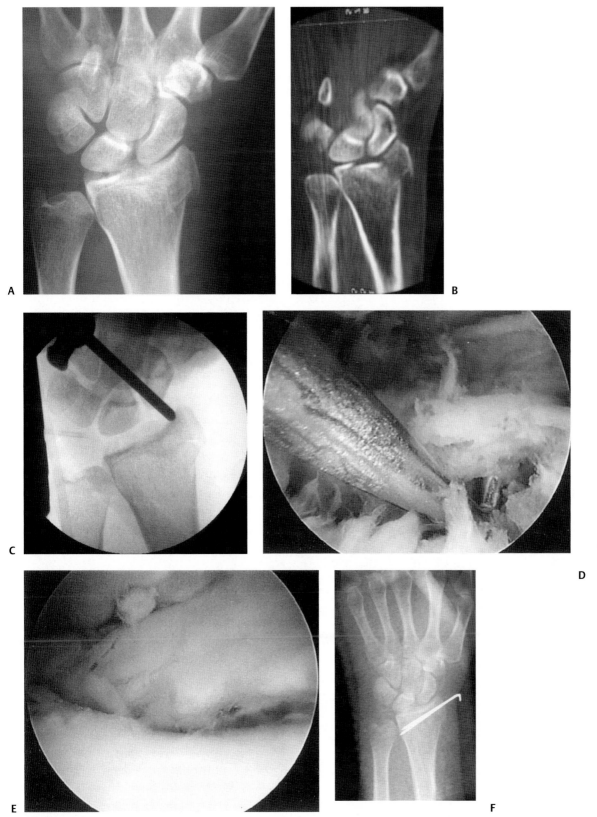

Figure 16–12 Example of a radial styloid fracture with articular incongruity and impaction. Wrist arthroscopy provides the ability to directly assess the articular surface for step-offs or gaps and ligaments for tears. K-wires can then be used to joystick bony fragments into a reduced position, and then to fix fragments together and to the metaphysis. The direct arthroscopic visualization of the articular surface during reduction and fixation helps to ensure a stable, congruent joint surface. **(A)** Radiograph of the injury, with an obvious radial styloid fracture and suggestion of additional articular impaction. **(B)** A CT scan confirms the impacted articular surface. **(C)** Intraoperative fluoroscopic picture showing introduction of a small arthroscope into the radiocarpal joint. **(D)** The articular impaction is well seen. **(E)** Appearance after elevation of the impacted articular surface. **(F)** Postoperative radiograph showing articular reconstruction and fixation with two K-wires.

Early data and collective experience suggest that bone graft substitutes can also provide improved treatment methods and outcomes, without the morbidity of autogenous bone or the risks of allograft.[89] Coralline hydroxyapatite has been effective at maintaining articular surface reduction when used in combination with external fixation and K-wires and has a safety profile comparable to other forms of treatment.[77]

An injectable bone grout has been developed to fill fracture voids and to maintain internal fixation in stable fractures and in displaced fractures that are reducible and stable. This bone grout has chemical, crystalline, and structural characteristics very similar to bone. The substance is reported to be gradually replaced by host bone after the fracture has healed.[90]

Advances in Rehabilitation

Ideally, patients should start an active and passive rehabilitation therapy program for motion of the digits, elbow, and shoulder, and rotation of the forearm within 24 hours following surgery. Stiffness of the digits usually develops from lack of early motion. Early motion decreases tendon adhesions and reduces soft tissue swelling.[16,34] Splints and casts must allow full MPJ range of motion by not extending beyond the distal palmar crease.

If only K-wire fixation was performed, a sugar-tong splint or short arm cast is used for 6 to 8 weeks. Then a removable forearm-based Thermoplastic wrist splint is used for another 4 weeks. When external fixation is used, a soft dressing with an arm sling is sufficient, and forearm rotation is begun early with emphasis on supination. Bone grafting with additional percutaneous pins may allow for removal of the fixator as early as 3 weeks when used in conjunction with functional bracing. If traditional nonlocking plate fixation is able to provide stable fixation, treatment involves a short arm cast or splint, with active wrist range of motion begun after 3 to 4 weeks.[16] If stable fixation is achieved through the use of locked or fixed-angled devices, however, then range of motion may begin at the first postoperative visit **(Fig. 16–13A–D).**

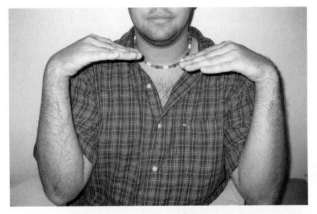
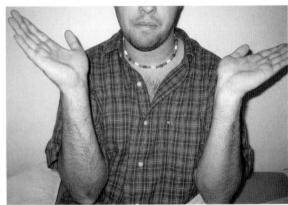
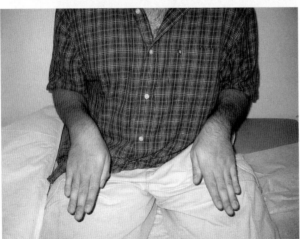
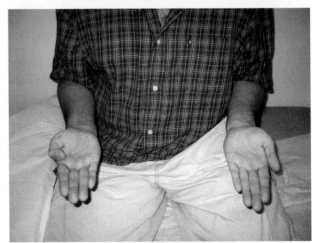

Figure 16–13 When stable fixation is achieved through the use of locked or fixed-angled devices, range of motion exercises can be initiated within 1 week postoperatively. This patient has achieved excellent range of motion just 6 weeks following open reduction and internal fixation of the right distal radius fracture with a dorsal locking plate system.

Complications

As mentioned in the introduction of this chapter, historically many surgeons believed that most patients with distal radius fractures did relatively well, regardless of treatment. However, distal radius fractures are often associated with poor results and high complication rates. High-energy fractures, especially those involving an intra-articular component, are especially susceptible to poor outcomes. Though much progress has been made in minimizing complications and poor outcomes, significant room for improvement remains.

Median nerve injury is one of the most commonly observed complications in distal radius fractures. A thorough prereduction neurovascular exam must be done and documented. Mild sensory impairment can usually be followed clinically. If symptoms of acute carpal tunnel syndrome are present, emergent reduction of the fracture must be done to decompress the median nerve. If median nerve compromise persists after reduction, then immediate carpal tunnel release is recommended.[35] If a nerve deficit is present in a patient requiring operative intervention for a fracture, a carpal tunnel release is indicated.[16,91] Prophylactic release in the absence of symptoms is not justified,[92] nor is it necessary if the symptoms of acute carpal tunnel syndrome resolve following closed reduction.

Mild forms of reflex sympathetic dystrophy (RSD) are quite common with distal radius fractures. Patients with increasing pain, swelling, joint stiffness, and paresthesias during fracture healing require early attention. Acute median nerve compression may play a role in the causation of RSD, but the relationship is not completely understood.[36,93,94] Excessive joint distraction during treatment with external fixation has been implicated as a potential cause of RSD.

Tendon ruptures due to irritation by an underlying plate occur but are infrequent. The extensor pollicis longus (EPL) and common extensor tendons are most commonly affected. Prominent dorsal plates or screws may cause tendon irritation and synovitis, which leads to late rupture. New low-profile plating systems should reduce the risk of tendon complications.

Distal radius malunion affects the biomechanics of both the radiocarpal and radioulnar joints. Abnormal biomechanics in the wrist leads to pain in the radiocarpal, radioulnar, and/or ulnocarpal joints, decreased range of motion, and/or midcarpal instability.[26] Corrective radial osteotomy for extra-articular malunion is indicated for younger patients with 15 degrees or more of dorsal angulation and in older patients if the radius deformity is causing radial-sided wrist pain. Intra-articular malunions with a step-off greater than 2 mm are advocated by some as indications for surgical correction.[30,95] Restoration of DRUJ anatomy is also important for successful outcome. Nonunion, though rare, is related to patient smoking, inadequate immobilization, and overdistraction.[16]

Posttraumatic arthritis can occur following intra-articular fractures of the distal radius. Although restoration of the joint by early articular reconstruction is thought to lessen the risk of later degenerative change, subsequent traumatic arthritis can result even in patients with excellent reductions.[96] For severe, posttraumatic arthritis, wrist fusion or, in a few patients, wrist arthroplasty, will be indicated.[16]

Pearls

- The important radiological relationships (given as average values) are radial inclination (23 degrees), radial height (12 mm), and volar tilt (11 degrees).
- Fractures with loss of 2 mm or more of radial height, change in radial inclination of 5 degrees or more, loss of volar tilt of 10 degrees or more, loss of DRUJ reduction, and/or with more than 1 to 2 mm of intra-articular step-off should be reduced.
- Closed reduction and cast immobilization are still the appropriate treatment for nondisplaced, stable fractures. A well-padded splint with the wrist in neutral position, the metacarpal-phalangeal joints completely unobstructed, and the overlying wrap loosely approximated will provide adequate immobilization to a truly stable and nondisplaced fracture, without contributing to hand swelling and stiffness.

New Technologies

The techniques of fracture fixation are continuously being modified and improved, in part by the development of new, and sometimes better, technologies. The recent advent of locking-plate designs has demonstrated increasing utility in many types of fracture patterns and locations. Both dorsal and volar locking plates for fractures of the distal radius have shown tremendous usefulness, as depicted in this chapter. Competition in this implant market has led to the design of locking plates that utilize variable-angle positioning for the locked screws and pegs. Further advances are likely to come.

Fragment-specific fixation systems utilizing smaller plates and fixed-angle devices for each fracture fragment have also been developed (see **Video 16–1, Disk 2**). Similar to the technique of using two smaller plates with a dorsal approach, these systems can help establish more direct fixation of smaller individual fragments in severely comminuted intra-articular fracture patterns.

An intramedullary nail for the distal radius is available that purports to provide stable fixed-angle support with a minimally invasive technique (see **Video 16–3, Disk 2**). Through a radial styloid insertion point, the nail is introduced and then secured, with the ability to lock several screws or pegs or both distally at fixed angles to buttress and support the distal fragments.

On the DVDs

Video 16–1   (Disk 2)   ORIF Distal Radius Fracture with Volar Plate   This video demonstrates open reduction and internal fixation of a distal radius fracture through a volar approach to the distal radius. The fracture is stabilized with a volar plate designed for the distal radius. A fragment-specific radial styloid plate is also used.

Video 16–2   (Disk 2)   External Fixation and Pinning of a Distal Radius   This patient sustained a distal radius fracture treated with

closed reduction and external fixation of the distal radius, combined with percutaneous pinning with Kirschner wires.

Video 16–3   (Disk 2)   Stabilization of a Distal Radius Fracture Using a Dorsal Intramedullary Plate   This video demonstrates an innovative device that combines intramedullary fixation with dorsal plate fixation to treat a distal radius fracture.

References

1. Owen RA, Melton LJI, Johnson KA, Ilstrup DM, Riggs BL. Incidence of Colles' fracture in a North American community. Am J Public Health 1982;72:605–607
2. Fernandez DL, Palmer AK. Fractures of the distal radius. In: Green DP, Hotchkiss RN, Pederson WC, eds. Green's Operative Hand Surgery. 4th ed. New York: Churchill Livingstone; 1999: 929–985
3. Dobyn JH, Linschied RL. Fractures and dislocations of the wrist. In: Rockwood CA, Green DP, eds. Fractures in Adults. 2nd ed. Philadelphia: JB Lippincott; 1984:411–509
4. Melone CPJ. Distal radius fractures: patterns of articular fragmentation. Orthop Clin North Am 1993;24:239–253
5. Jupiter JB, Fernandez DL, Whipple TL, Richards RR. Intra-articular fractures of the distal radius: contemporary perspectives. In: Cannon WDJ, ed. Instructional Course Lectures. Vol 47. Rosemont, IL: American Academy of Orthopaedic Surgeons; 1998:191–202
6. Trumble TE, Culp RW, Hanel DP, Geissler WB, Berger RAC. Intra-articular fractures of the distal aspect of the radius. In: Zuckerman JD, ed. Instructional Course Lectures. Vol 48. Rosemont, IL: American Academy of Orthopaedic Surgeons; 1999:465–480
7. Lewis OJ, Hamshere RJ, Bucknill TM. The anatomy of the wrist joint. J Anat 1970;106:539–552
8. Palmer AK, Werner FW. The triangular fibrocartilage complex of the wrist—anatomy and function. J Hand Surg [Am] 1981;6:153–162
9. King GJ, McMurtry RY, Rubenstein JD. Kinematics of the distal radioulnar joint. J Hand Surg [Am] 1986;11:798–804
10. Adams BD. Effects of radial deformity on distal radioulnar joint mechanics. J Hand Surg [Am] 1993;18:492–498
11. Palmer AK, Werner FW. Biomechanics of the distal radioulnar joint. Clin Orthop Relat Res 1984;187:26–35
12. Andersen DJ, Blair WF, Steyers CMJ, Adams BD, el Khouri GY, Brandser EA. Classification of distal radius fractures: an analysis of interobserver reliability and intraobserver reproducibility. J Hand Surg [Am] 1996;21:574–582
13. Lichtenhahn P, Fernandez DL, Schatzker J. Analysis of the "user friendliness" of the AO classification of fractures. Helv Chir Acta 1992;58:919–924
14. Zanetti M, Gilula LA, Jacob HA, Hodler J. Palmar tilt of the distal radius: influence of off-lateral projection initial observations. Radiology 2001;220:594–600
15. Gilula LA, ed. The Traumatized Hand and Wrist: Radiographic and Anatomic Correlation. Philadelphia: WB Saunders; 1992
16. Duncan SF, Weiland AJ. Minimally invasive reduction and osteosynthesis of articular fractures of the distal radius. Injury 2001;32(Suppl 1):SA14–24
17. Pruitt DL, Gilula LA, Manske PR, Vannier MW. Computed tomography scanning with image reconstruction in evaluation of distal radius fractures. J Hand Surg [Am] 1994;19:720–727
18. Rozental TD, Bozentka DJ, Katz MA, Steinberg DR, Beredjiklian PK. Evaluation of the sigmoid notch with computed tomography following intra-articular distal radius fracture. J Hand Surg [Am] 2001;26:244–251
19. Katz MA, Beredjiklian PK, Bozentka DJ, Steinberg DR. Computed tomography scanning of intra-articular distal radius fractures: does it influence treatment. J Hand Surg [Am] 2001;26:415–421
20. Catalano LWI, Cole RJ, Gelberman RH, Evanoff BA, Gilula LA, Borrelli JJ. Displaced intra-articular fractures of the distal aspect of the radius: long-term results in young adults after open reduction and internal fixation. J Bone Joint Surg Am 1997;79: 1290–1302
21. Fernandez DL, Geissler WB. Treatment of displaced articular fractures of the radius. J Hand Surg [Am] 1991;16:375–384
22. Knirk JL, Jupiter JB. Intra-articular fractures of the distal end of the radius in young adults. J Bone Joint Surg Am 1986;68:647–659
23. Short WH, Palmer AK, Werner FW, Murphy DJ. A biomechanical study of distal radial fractures. J Hand Surg [Am] 1987; 12: 529–534
24. Pogue DJ, Viegas SF, Patterson RM, et al. Effects of distal radius fracture malunion on wrist joint mechanics. J Hand Surg [Am] 1990;15:721–727
25. Kihara H, Palmer AK, Werner FW, Short WH, Fortino MD. The effect of dorsally angulated distal radius fractures on distal radioulnar joint congruency and forearm rotation. J Hand Surg [Am] 1996; 21:40–47
26. Martini AK. Secondary arthrosis of the wrist joint in malposition of healed and uncorrected fracture of the distal radius [in German]. Aktuelle Traumatol 1986;16:143–148
27. Miyake T, Hashizume H, Inoue H, Shi Q, Nagayama N. Malunited Colles' fracture: analysis of stress distribution. J Hand Surg [Br] 1994;19:737–742
28. Taleisnik J, Watson HK. Midcarpal instability caused by malunited fractures of the distal radius. J Hand Surg [Am] 1984;9:350–357
29. Amadio PC, Botte MJ. Treatment of malunion of the distal radius. Hand Clin 1987;3:541–559
30. McMurtry RY, Axelrod T, Paley D. Distal radial osteotomy. Orthopedics 1989;12:149–155
31. Trumble TE, Schmitt SR, Vedder NB. Factors affecting functional outcome of displaced intra-articular distal radius fractures. J Hand Surg [Am] 1994;19:325–340
32. Mekhail AO, Ebraheim NA, McCreath WA, Jackson WT, Yeasting RA. Anatomic and x-ray film studies of the distal articular surface of the radius. J Hand Surg [Am] 1996;21:567–573
33. Wagner WFJ, Tencer AF, Kiser P, Trumble TE. Effects of intra-articular distal radius depression on wrist joint contact characteristic. J Hand Surg [Am] 1996;21:554–560

34. Dias JJ, Wray CC, Jones JM, Gregg PH. The value of early mobilization in the treatment of Colles' fractures. J Bone Joint Surg Br 1987;69:463–467

35. Cooney WP, Dobyns JH, Linscheid RL. Complications of Colles' fractures. J. Bone Joint Surg Am 1980;62:613–619

36. Grundberg AB, Reagan DS. Compression syndromes in reflex sympathetic dystrophy. J Hand Surg [Am] 1991;16:731–736

37. Orbay JL. The treatment of unstable distal radius fractures with volar fixation. Hand Surg 2000;5:103–112

38. Constantine KJ, Clawson MC, Stern PJ. Volar neutralization plate fixation of dorsally displaced distal radius fractures. Orthopedics 2002;25:125–128

39. Orbay JL, Fernandez DL. Volar fixed-angle plate fixation for unstable distal radius fractures in the elderly patient. J Hand Surg [Am] 2004;29:96–102

39a. Placzek JD, Sobel GV, Arnocsky SP, Quinn M, Magnell T. The effect of an extended flexor carpi radialis approach on a blood flow to the distal radius: a cadaveric study. Orthopedics 2005;28:1364–1367

40. Rikli DA, Regazzoni P. Fractures of the distal end of the radius treated by internal fixation and early function: a preliminary report of 20 cases. J Bone Joint Surg Br 1996;78:588–592

41. Rikli DA, Regazzoni P, Babst R. Dorsal double plating for fractures of the distal radius: a biomechanical concept and clinical experience [in German]. Zentralbl Chir 2003;128:1003–1007

42. Jakob M, Rikli DA, Regazzoni P. Fractures of the distal radius treated by internal fixation and early function: a prospective study of 73 consecutive patients. J Bone Joint Surg Br 2000;82:340–344

42a. Simic PM, Robison J, Gardner MJ, Gelberman RH, Weil AJ, Boye MI. Treatment of distal radius fractures with a low-profile dorsal plating system: an outcomes assessment. J Hand Surg Am 2006; 31:382–386

43. Peine R, Rikli DA, Hoffmann R, Duda G, Regazzoni P. Comparison of three different plating techniques for the dorsum of the distal radius: a biomechanical study. J Hand Surg [Am] 2000;25:29–33

44. Boyer MI, Korcek KJ, Gelberman RH, Gilula LA, Ditsios K, Evanoff BA. Anatomic tilt x-rays of the distal radius: an ex vivo analysis of surgical fixation. J Hand Surg [Am] 2004;29:116–122

45. Lee HC, Wong YS, Chan BK, Low CO. Fixation of distal radius fractures using AO titanium volar distal radius plate. Hand Surg 2003; 8:7–15

46. Habernek H, Weinstabl R, Fialka C, Schmid L. Unstable distal radius fractures treated by modified Kirschner wire pinning: anatomic consideration, technique, and results. J Trauma 1994;36:83–88

47. Munson GO, Gainor BJ. Percutaneous pinning of distal radius fractures. J Trauma 1981;21:1032–1035

48. Naidu SH, Capo JT, Moulton M, Ciccone WI, Radin A. Percutaneous pinning of distal radius fractures: a biomechanical study. J Hand Surg [Am] 1997;22:252–257

49. Rayhack JM. The history and evolution of percutaneous pinning of displaced distal radius fractures. Orthop Clin North Am 1993;24: 287–300

50. Ring D, Jupiter JB. Percutaneous and limited open fixation of fractures of the distal radius. Clin Orthop Relat Res 2000;37:105–115

51. Rodriguez-Merchan EC. Plaster cast versus percutaneous pin fixation for comminuted fractures of the distal radius in patients between 46 and 65 years of age. J Orthop Trauma 1997;11:212–217

52. Gupta R, Raheja A, Modi U. Colles' fracture: management by percutaneous crossed-pin fixation versus plaster of Paris cast immobilization. Orthopedics 1999;22:680–682

53. Trumble TE, Wagner W, Hanel DP, Vedder NB, Gilbert M. Intrafocal (Kapandji) pinning of distal radius fractures with and without external fixation. J Hand Surg [Am] 1998;23:381–394

54. Graff S, Jupiter J. Fracture of the distal radius: classification of treatment and indications for external fixation. Injury 1994;25 (Suppl 4):S-D14–25

55. Huch K, Hunerbein M, Meeder PJ. External fixation of intra-articular fracture of the distal radius in young and old adults. Arch Orthop Trauma Surg 1996;115:38–42

56. Jakim I, Pieterse HS, Sweet MB. External fixation for intra-articular fractures of the distal radius. J Bone Joint Surg Br 1991;73:302–306

57. Pennig D, Gausepohl T. External fixation of the wrist. Injury 1996;27:1–15

58. Riggs SA, Cooney WPI. External fixation of complex hand and wrist fractures. J Trauma 1983;23:332–336

59. Rikli DA, Kupfer K, Bodoky A. Long-term results of the external fixation of distal radius fractures. J Trauma 1998;44:970–976

60. Schuind F, Donkerwolke M, Rasquin C, Burny F. External fixation of fractures of the distal radius: a study of 225 cases. J Hand Surg [Am] 1989;14:404–407

61. Seitz WH, Froimson AI, Leb R, Shapiro JD. Augmented external fixation of unstable distal radius fractures. J Hand Surg [Am] 1991;16: 1010–1016

62. Seitz WH Jr. External fixation of distal radius fractures: indications and technical principles. Orthop Clin North Am 1993;24:255–264

63. Simpson NS, Wilkinson R, Barbenel JC, Kinninmonth AW. External fixation of the distal radius: a biomechanical study. J Hand Surg [Br] 1994;19:188–192

64. Weiland AJ. External fixation, not ORIF, as the treatment of choice for fractures of the distal radius. J Orthop Trauma 1999;13:570–572

65. Anderson R, O'Neil G. Comminuted fractures of the distal end of the radius. Surg Gynecol Obstet 1944;78:434–440

66. Combalia A. Over-distraction of the radio-carpal and mid-carpal joints with external fixation of comminuted distal radial fractures. J Hand Surg [Br] 1995;20:566–567

67. Agee JM. External fixation: technical advances based upon multiplanar ligamentotaxis. Orthop Clin North Am 1993;24:265–274

68. Kaempffe FA, Wheeler DR, Peimer CA, Hvisdak KS, Ceravolo J, Senall J. Severe fractures of the distal radius: effect of amount and duration of external fixator distraction on outcome. J Hand Surg [Am] 1993;18:33–41

69. Agee JM, Szabo RM, Chidgey LK, King FC, Kerfoot C. Treatment of comminuted distal radius fractures: an approach based on pathomechanics. Orthopedics 1994;17:1115–1122

70. Leung KS, Shen WY, Tsang HK, Chiu KH, Leung PC, Hung LK. An effective treatment of comminuted fractures of the distal radius. J Hand Surg [Am] 1990;15:11–17

71. Krishnan J, Wigg AE, Walker RW, Slavotinek J. Intra-articular fractures of the distal radius: a prospective randomised controlled trial comparing static bridging and dynamic non-bridging external fixation. J Hand Surg [Br] 2003;28:417–421

72. McQueen MM. Redisplaced unstable fractures of the distal radius: a randomised, prospective study of bridging versus non-bridging external fixation. J Bone Joint Surg Br 1998;80:665–669

73. McQueen MM, Simpson D, Court-Brown CM. Use of the Hoffman 2 compact external fixator in the treatment of redisplaced unstable distal radial fractures. J Orthop Trauma 1999;13:501–505

74. Flinkkila T, Ristiniemi J, Hyvonen P, Hamalainen M. Nonbridging external fixation in the treatment of unstable fractures of the distal forearm. Arch Orthop Trauma Surg 2003;123:349–352

75. Franck WM, Dahlen C, Amlang M, Friese F, Zwipp H. Distal radius fracture: s non-bridging articular external fixator a therapeutic alternative? A prospective randomized study [in German]. Unfallchirurg 2000;103:826–833

76. Dunning CE, Lindsay CS, Bicknell RT, Patterson SD, Johnson JA, King GJ. Supplemental pinning improves the stability of external fixation in distal radius fractures during simulated finger and forearm motion. J Hand Surg [Am] 1999;24:992–1000

77. Wolfe SW, Austin G, Lorenze M, Swigart CR, Panjabi MM. A biomechanical comparison of different wrist external fixators with and without K-wire augmentation. J Hand Surg [Am] 1999; 24: 516–524

78. Markiewitz AD, Gellman H. Five-pin external fixation and early range of motion for distal radius fractures. Orthop Clin North Am 2001;32:329–335

79. Braun RM, Gellman H. Dorsal pin placement and external fixation for correction of dorsal tilt in fractures of the distal radius. J Hand Surg [Am] 1994;19:653–655

80. Swigart CR, Wolfe SW. Limited incision open techniques for distal radius fracture management. Orthop Clin North Am 2001;32:317–327

81. Cooney WP, Berger RA. Treatment of complex fractures of the distal radius: combined use of internal and external fixation and arthroscopic reduction. Hand Clin 1993;9:603–612

82. Ring D, Prommersberger K, Jupiter JB. Combined dorsal and volar plate fixation of complex fractures of the distal part of the radius. J Bone Joint Surg Am 2004;86-A:1646–1652

83. Gupta R, Bozentka DJ, Osterman AL. Wrist arthroscopy: principles and clinical applications. J Am Acad Orthop Surg 2001; 9: 200–209

84. Auge WKI, Velazquez PA. The application of indirect reduction techniques in the distal radius: the role of adjuvant arthroscopy. Arthroscopy 2000;16:830–835

85. Geissler WB. Arthroscopically assisted reduction of intra-articular fractures of the distal radius. Hand Clin 1995;11:19–29

86. Geissler WB, Freeland AE. Arthroscopic management of intra-articular distal radius fractures. Hand Clin 1999;15:455–465

87. Hanker GJ. Diagnostic and operative arthroscopy of the wrist. Clin Orthop Relat Res 1991;26:165–174

88. Wolfe SW, Easterlling KJ, Yoo HH. Arthroscopic-assisted reduction of distal radius fractures. Arthroscopy 1995;11:706–714

89. Ladd AL, Pliam NB. The role of bone graft and alternatives in unstable distal radius fracture treatment. Orthop Clin North Am 2001; 32:337–351

90. Cassidy C, Jupiter JB, Cohen M, et al. Norian SRS cement compared with conventional fixation in distal radial fractures: a randomized study. J Bone Joint Surg Am 2003;85-A:2127–2137

91. Paley D, McMurty RY. Median nerve compression by volarly displaced fragments of the distal radius. Clin Orthop Relat Res 1987; 21:139–147

92. Odumala O, Ayekoloye C, Packer G. Prophylactic carpal tunnel decompression during buttress plating of the distal radius: is it justified? Injury 2001;32:577–579

93. Hove LM. Nerve entrapment and reflex sympathetic dystrophy after fractures of the distal radius. Scand J Plast Reconstr Surg Hand Surg 1995;29:53–58

94. Monsivais JJ, Baker J, Monsivais D. The association of peripheral nerve compression and reflex sympathetic dystrophy. J Hand Surg [Br] 1993;18:337–338

95. Marx RG, Axelrod TS. Intra-articular osteotomy of distal radial malunions. Clin Orthop Relat Res 1996;327:152–157

96. Jupiter JB, Fernandez DL, Toh CL, Fellman T, Ring D. Operative treatment of volar intra-articular fractures of the distal end of the radius. J Bone Joint Surg Am 1996;78:1817–1828

17 Carpus Fractures and Dislocations

Jeffry Todd Watson and Martin I. Boyer

Carpal Instability

Carpal instability, literally defined, occurs when the wrist demonstrates symptomatic malalignment, is unable to bear loads, and has abnormal kinematics during any portion of its arc of motion. This can occur as an acute condition following injury or as a chronic, ongoing process as seen in patients with inherent excessive ligamentous laxity or ligament attenuation from inflammatory arthropathy. Because the obvious focus of this text is on traumatic conditions, this chapter focuses on carpal instability as a result of acute injury to osseous and key ligamentous components of the wrist. Such conditions are often referred to as "perilunate injuries."

Prior to any discussion of carpal instability, a brief review of the key anatomical components of the wrist required for stable, coordinated motion is in order. After all, surgical management for these conditions is aimed at restoring the functional integrity of these structures. For simplicity, the carpal bones are traditionally organized into proximal (scaphoid, lunate, triquetrum, and pisiform) and distal (trapezium, trapezoid, capitate, and hamate) rows. The static and dynamic relationship between these bones is maintained by those ligaments within (intrinsic) and those spanning (extrinsic) each row.

Extrinsic ligaments arise from the dorsal and volar aspects of the distal ulna and radius to insert on the proximal and distal carpal rows. The stout palmar ligaments (**Fig. 17–1**),

from radial to ulnar, consist of the radioscaphocapitate (RSC), the long radiolunate (LRL), the short radiolunate (SRL), and the ulnocarpal ligaments. The RSC spans across the volar waist of the scaphoid before inserting on the capitate and acts as a fulcrum for the scaphoid as it flexes and extends with radioulnar deviation. It and the adjacent LRL, which joins the volar rim of the radius and the volar lip of the lunate, suspend the radial side of the carpus and prevent it from "sagging" or palmarly subluxing relative to the radius. The SRL extends from the volar rim of the lunate fossa to the lunate, inserting just ulnar to the LRL. The ulnocarpal ligaments originate from the volar periphery of the triangular fibrocartilage complex to insert on the lunate and triquetrum. They function to support the ulnar carpus and prevent it from sagging palmarly or subluxing relative to the distal ulna.

On the dorsum of the wrist, the dorsal radiocarpal (DRC) ligament spans from the central dorsal distal radius with the joint capsule to attach to the dorsal aspect of the triquetrum. The dorsal intercarpal (DIC) ligament connects the dorsal triquetrum to the dorsal surfaces of the scaphoid and trapezium (**Fig. 17–2**).

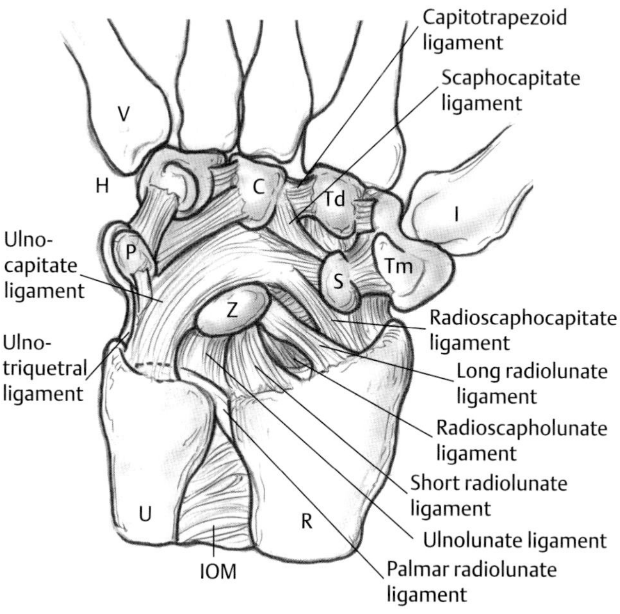

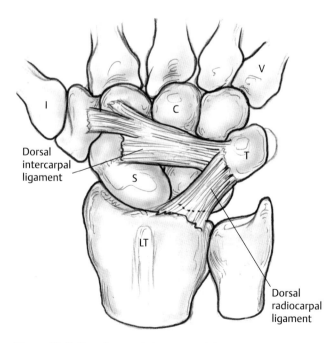

Figure 17–1 Volar extrinsic ligaments of the wrist radioscaphocapitate, long radiolunate, short radiolunate, and ulnocarpal.

Figure 17–2 Dorsal extrinsic ligaments of the wrist, which actually blend in with the joint capsule. The dorsal radiocarpal ligament spans from the central portion of the dorsal radial joint margin to attach to the dorsal aspect of the triquetrum. The dorsal intercarpal ligament, not truly extrinsic to the carpus, links the dorsal triquetrum and the dorsal scaphoid and trapezium.

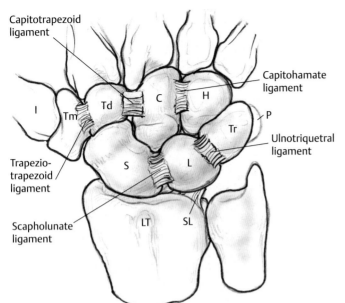

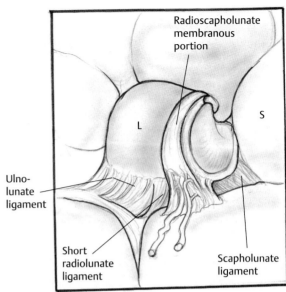

Figure 17–3 Intrinsic ligaments of the proximal carpal row, which provide the contiguous mechanical link among the carpal bones to allow coordinated, reciprocal motion between the proximal and distal rows. Note that, whereas the scapholunate ligament has a crescent shape, the dorsal (ligamentous) portion is stouter and mechanically more significant than the central (membranous) portion. Conversely, the volar portion of the lunatotriquetral ligament is stronger than the dorsal aspect.

The intrinsic ligaments link the scaphoid, lunate, and triquetrum to allow flexion and extension of the proximal carpal row simultaneous with wrist radial and ulnar deviation (**Fig. 17–3**). The scapholunate ligament is noted to have three morphologically distinct regions, the dorsal aspect being the thickest.[1,2] Conversely, the lunatotriquetral ligament is more stout on the palmar side.[3]

Various theories have been proposed to explain the kinematics of wrist motion, and there is no need to cover the full details in this text. The key is to understand that the proximal and distal carpal rows rely on a contiguous, stable ligament and osseous link among and between them to provide reciprocating motion relative to each other (**Fig. 17–4A–C**). This is often referred to as the "ring" concept.[4] With ulnar deviation, the proximal row extends as the distal row flexes. The opposite occurs with ulnar deviation. Structural failure of any bone or ligament portion of this linkage within the proximal row results in loss of coordinated motion of the carpus with the possibility of progressive collapse, painful arthrosis, and disability. The goal of surgical management is restoration of this linkage.

Classification

Not all injuries resulting in carpal instability are readily apparent on plain x-rays. Static instability refers to those injuries visible in standard radiographs. This may take the form of a carpal fracture, widening of scapholunate or lunatotriquetral joints, or excessive scapholunate angle on the lateral view. Dynamic instability requires stress maneuvers such as clenched fist or ulnar deviation to demonstrate pathology on plain films or fluoroscopy.[1]

Perhaps the most widely shared classification of perilunate injury that links injury mechanism and sequential failure of anatomical components is that described by Mayfield and colleagues.[5] When the wrist is loaded during a fall, it is often in a position of extension and ulnar deviation, resulting in progressive supination of the carpus relative to the radius. As the loaded wrist continues to supinate, osseous or ligamentous failure begins with the radial aspect, proceeds through the carpus, and exits the ulnar side of the wrist. Therefore, Mayfield proposed four stages of progressive perilunar instability as follows:

- *Stage I* Rupture of scapholunate and palmar radioscaphocapitate ligaments. This would appear as widening of the scapholunate interval on normal or stress views of the wrist, with perhaps an increased scapholunate angle on the lateral x-ray (**Fig. 17–5**).

- *Stage II* Dislocation of the capitolunate joint.

- *Stage III* Disruption of the lunatotriquetral and ulnocarpal ligaments, as seen in a perilunate dislocation, in which the lunate remains in the lunate fossa of the radius while the remainder of the carpus displaces dorsally (**Fig. 17–6A,B**).

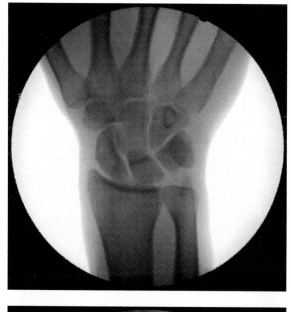
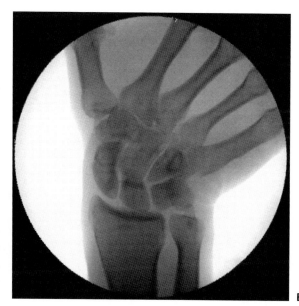

A

B

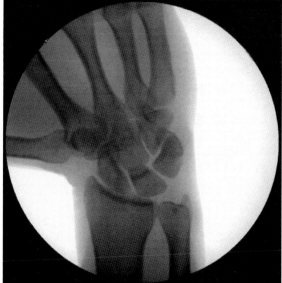

C

Figure 17–4 (A) Neutral posteroanterior (PA) radiograph of the wrist. **(B)** During ulnar deviation of the wrist, the proximal row extends, as evidenced by the scaphoid having a more elongated profile on the PA view. **(C)** Conversely, during radial deviation, the proximal flexes and the "cortical ring" of the scaphoid are seen. Continuity of the intercarpal ligament and osseous linkages within the proximal row is essential for this coordinated interaction.

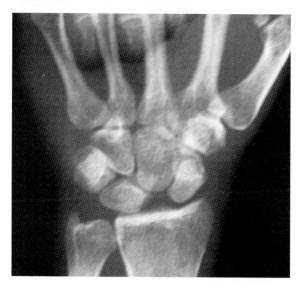

Figure 17–5 Mayfield stage I x-ray. The scapholunate interval is widened (> 3 mm) on the posteroanterior view, and the scapholunate angle is increased (beyond 60 degrees) on the lateral view, indicating disruption of the scapholunate joint.

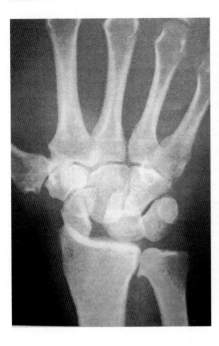
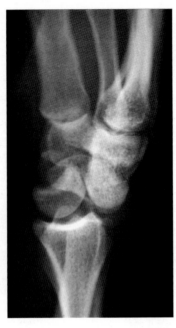

Figure 17–6 Mayfield stage III x-ray. With progression of force around the lunate toward the ulnar aspect of the wrist, the lunatotriquetral ligament has failed, and the carpus no longer has any mechanical link to the lunate. As the remainder of the carpus (and hand) dislocates dorsally, the lunate remains in the lunate fossa of the radius, making this a perilunate dislocation. Note that the dislocation does not always have to be present upon presentation for the actual ligamentous injuries to have occurred.

- *Stage IV* Lunate dislocation, during which the dorsal radiocarpal ligament and capsule has torn to allow the lunate to displace palmarly into the carpal canal. It is usually still tethered palmarly by the stout radiolunate ligaments, resulting in the "spilled teacup" appearance on the lateral x-ray **(Fig. 17–7A,B).** The remainder of the carpus is usually collinear with the radius, as opposed to being dorsal to it in perilunate dislocations seen in stage III.

Note that the foregoing classification only addresses ligamentous disruption, which does not always occur in isolation as the force passes through the carpus. Beginning with the radial side, fractures of the radial styloid, scaphoid, capitate, triquetrum, and ulnar styloid may occur with force transmission **(Fig. 17–8).** Greater arc injuries are fracture patterns in which the force takes a wider, transosseous path through the carpus. Lesser arc injuries are those that involve a more narrow pathway of soft tissue ligamentous failure

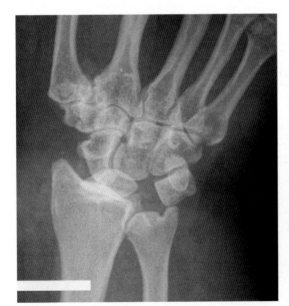
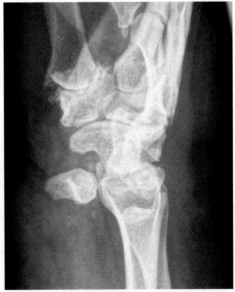

Figure 17–7 Mayfield stage IV x-ray. The dorsal radiocarpal ligament has failed, and the lunate has now dislocated palmarly out of the lunate fossa of the radius. Because the strong radiolunate ligaments often remain intact, the palmar portion of the bone remains approximated to the radius, resulting in the "spilled teacup" appearance of the lunate often seen on the lateral radiographs of lunate dislocations.

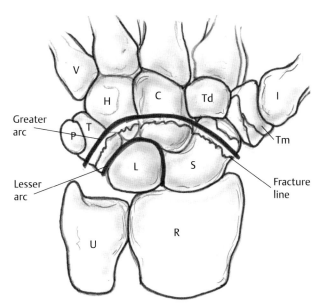

Figure 17–8 Lesser arc injury patterns are mainly ligamentous, involving tears of the scapholunate and lunatotriquetral ligaments as the force moves from radial to ulnar through the carpus. Greater arc injuries, however, traverse osseous components as the force follows a wider path around the lunate. Mixed patterns involving components of both (transscaphoid perilunate dislocation) are not uncommon.

around the lunate, as described by Mayfield above. Inferior arc injuries result from forces passing proximal to the lunate, resulting in disruption of radiocarpal and ulnocarpal ligaments with or without radial or ulnar styloid fractures. Acute carpal instability frequently involves both bony and ligamentous components, such as those seen in the stage III transscaphoid-perilunate dislocation **(Fig. 17–9A,B)**. These injuries frequently result in fractures of the carpal bones themselves as the force passes over and around the lunate.

Isolated lunatotriquetral instability, also referred to as a reverse perilunate injury, is thought to occur as a result of a fall on the radially deviated outstretched hand (recall that the hand is typically in ulnar deviation during perilunate injuries). Failure of the dorsal and central portions of the LT ligament is insufficient to result in altered carpal mechanics. However, failure of the palmar portion of the ligament, combined with loss of secondary dorsal capsular (radiotriquetral and scaphotriquetral) ligaments, results in progressive static volar intercalated segmental instability (VISI) deformity (see later discussion).

The proximal carpal row, without the scaphoid acting as a stable link or strut bridging against compressive forces across the wrist, would simply collapse into flexion or extension as the distal row migrated proximally. A dorsal intercalated segmental instability (DISI) deformity occurs when the lunate assumes an *extended* position on the lateral radiograph relative to the radius as the capitate migrates proximally. Likewise, a VISI deformity occurs when the lunate appears *flexed* relative to the radius as the capitate moves proximally.

Nonoperative Treatment

Load transmission across the carpus traverses the two mobile carpal rows that must be able to maintain a stable relationship in any posture. This relies on the integrity of the scaphoid, acting as a rigid strut or link between the two rows, and the intrinsic ligaments joining the scaphoid, lunate, and triquetrum. Failure of any of these components results in progressive carpal collapse from baseline compressive forces of the musculotendinous units crossing the wrist and the bony anatomy of the distal radius and carpus itself. Vigorous external loads are not required to cause

Figure 17–9 Transscaphoid perilunate fracture-dislocation. Bony overlap on plain films can hinder determination of injury pattern. Traction views offer a better profile of injured components. **(A)** Injury films. **(B)** Traction view.

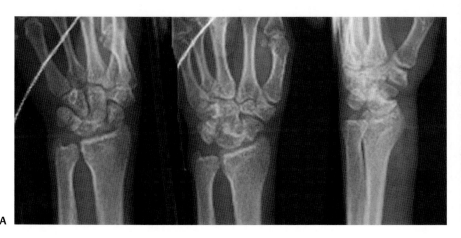
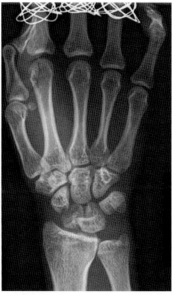

A   B

progressive collapse of the proximal row with subsequent proximal migration of the distal row and secondary arthritic changes. Therefore, there is no logic in the nonoperative treatment of these injuries. With the exception of a truly nondisplaced, stable scaphoid waist fracture or partial ligament tear, these injuries simply do not heal reliably with immobilization alone.

Although surgical stabilization is the definitive treatment for these injuries, a provisional reduction in the acute ambulatory setting is often necessary. In both perilunate and lunate dislocations, there may be considerable pressure on the median nerve from the lunate. Patients often have median nerve sensory deficits, and allowing the wrist to remain in an unreduced position with ongoing pressure on the nerve may have deleterious effects. A closed reduction with minimal anesthesia can usually be performed at the initial presentation in a manner similar to that of dorsally displaced distal radius fractures.

With or without adjunctive intravenous sedation, traction is applied through the digits either through the use of fingertraps or manually with countertraction on the arm proximally. While applying volar pressure on the lunate with a thumb, the capitate is initially extended and then translated palmarly to engage the distal articular surface of the lunate (**Fig. 17–10A,B**). With reduction, an audible or palpable "clunk" might not occur. Fluoroscopy or plain x-rays are needed to verify the reduction. A sugar tong splint molded to keep the wrist from extending should be applied until the time of definitive surgical treatment.

Occasionally, closed reduction of a perilunate or lunate dislocation is not possible. In ligamentous injuries in which the lunate alone is separated from the remainder of the carpal bones, the lunate may buttonhole through the

stout volar capsule (**Fig. 17–11**). With traction applied during the reduction maneuver, the capsular rent merely tightens further to prevent the lunate from returning to its anatomical position relative to the carpus. In these situations, open reduction must be performed. In addition, some transosseous perilunate injuries are so unstable that the reduction cannot be maintained following the release of traction, despite the application of a well-molded splint.

Although surgery remains the definitive, necessary treatment to restore stability in these injuries, failure of closed reduction does not always mandate immediate operative treatment. If swelling is minimal and there are no or mild subjective sensory deficits in a closed injury, it is permissible to leave the irreducible dislocation in that position until a more convenient scheduling time. However, should the patient develop progressive sensory loss with marked swelling, nerve decompression through a carpal tunnel release and open reduction becomes more emergent.

Indications for Surgical Treatment

As already emphasized, all of these injuries are quite unstable, rendering closed treatment and external immobilization rather ineffective. Although a closed reduction may be achieved through manipulation and traction, carpal collapse and proximal migration tend to occur in both transosseous and transligamentous varieties. In general, operative treatment is best performed within 2 weeks of injury. Beyond this interval, capsular scarring ensues and requires significant bone and soft tissue stripping to mobilize the bones adequately to obtain reduction (see **Video 17–1, Disk 2**). Vascular compromise of the carpal bones becomes a concern.

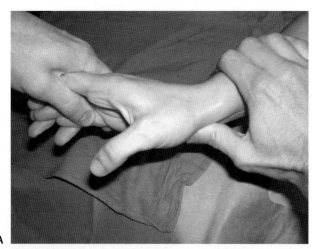
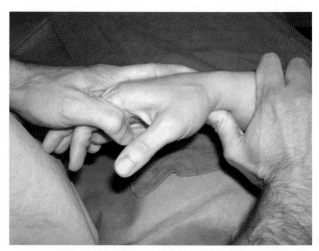

A   **B**

Figure 17–10 (A) Technique for provisional closed reduction of lunate and perilunate dislocations. The distal forearm is held with one hand with the thumb over the carpal canal with pressure on the lunate. If the lunate is dislocated within the carpal canal, it is "milked" from proximal to distal in an effort to flip it back up into the lunate fossa. **(B)** With the other hand, traction is applied as the hand and remaining carpus are maneuvered volarly, back in line with the lunate. Fingertraps with countertraction can be quite helpful.

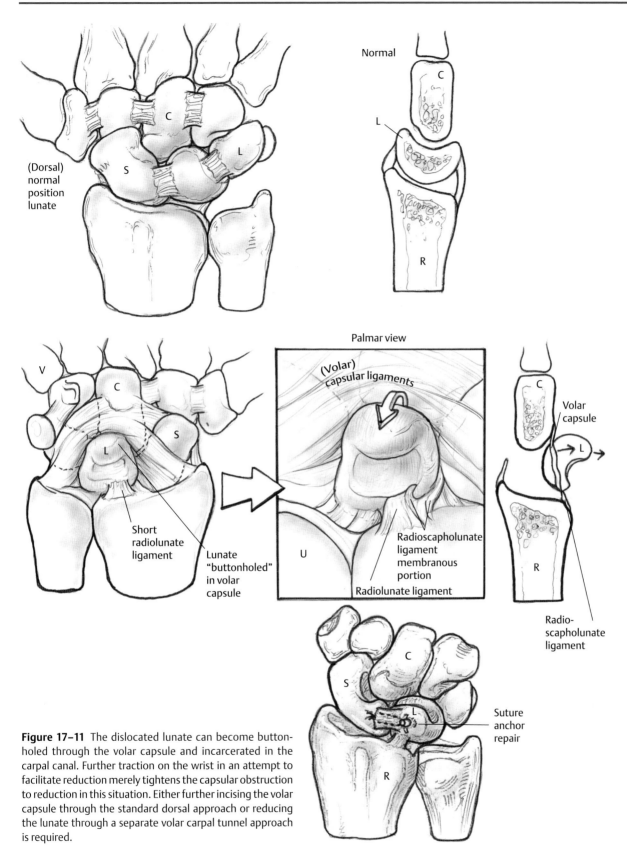

Figure 17–11 The dislocated lunate can become buttonholed through the volar capsule and incarcerated in the carpal canal. Further traction on the wrist in an attempt to facilitate reduction merely tightens the capsular obstruction to reduction in this situation. Either further incising the volar capsule through the standard dorsal approach or reducing the lunate through a separate volar carpal tunnel approach is required.

Also, as suggested in the preceding section, emergent carpal tunnel release should be performed in the setting of significant swelling with progressive numbness or motor deficit.

Surgical Treatment

Surgical Anatomy and Options for Treatment

Preoperative planning begins with an appreciation for the nature and full extent of the injury. Recall that carpal instability represents a spectrum of structural failure as the deforming load passes through the wrist. All components of injury may not be apparent on initial plain films. For example, a small radial styloid fracture noted on initial films may be the only suggestion of the more problematic and significant scapholunate tear or scaphoid fracture. The need for meticulous physical examination (tenderness over scapholunate or lunatotriquetral ligaments) and perhaps further radiographic stress views cannot be overemphasized. Traction films taken at the time of initial assessment can be quite helpful **(Fig. 17–9A,B)**.

A strategy for exposure and repair can be derived following recognition of injured components. Larger radial styloid fractures should be repaired to restore articular congruity as well as the suspensory role of the radioscaphocapitate ligament. Fractures of the scaphoid or disruptions of the scapholunate ligament require open reduction and rigid fixation or direct ligamentous repair. Capitate or triquetrum fractures also require open reduction and rigid fixation. There is some debate regarding the need for direct repair of the lunatotriquetral ligament. Many surgeons feel that restoration of the anatomical relationship of the lunatotriquetral (LT) joint with K-wire fixation alone is sufficient without performing direct repair of the ligament through bone tunnels or anchors. Others, however, may recommend using a combined dorsal and volar approach to allow direct repair of the more significant palmar portion of the lunatotriquetral ligament (see **Video 17–1, Disk 2**). An ulnar styloid fracture that is large enough to involve the entire insertion of the deep portion of the triangular fibrocartilage should be repaired. Nevertheless, the presence of an ulnar styloid fracture in the setting of a bony or ligamentous radial-sided wrist injury should alert the examiner to the likelihood of more subtle injuries within the carpus.

Surgical Techniques

Proper room setup and equipment preparation are essential (see **Video 17–1, Disk 2**). The patient is supine on a standard table with a stable arm board attached. Either standard or mini C-arm fluoroscopy with accompanying sterile draping will be needed, but the arm board does not have to be radiolucent. Many surgeons prefer to tilt the mini C-arm parallel to the floor, avoiding the need to image through the table. K-wires (0.045 and 0.062 in.) and a

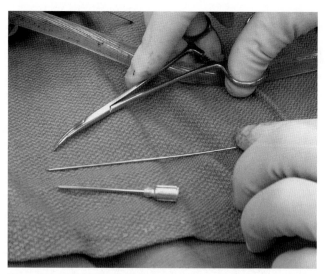

Figure 17–12 A 0.045 in. wire and blunt-tipped metal 14 gauge needle to act as soft tissue sleeve.

drill with appropriate size attachment will be needed. A chuck and accompanying chuck attachment for the drill will be needed for placement of compression screws. Our current preference for placement of compression screws is the standard-size Accutrak (Acumed LLC, Hillsboro, Oregon) screw, although other compression screw systems are also available. Whichever screw system is used, the screw needs to be cannulated to allow accurate placement of a guide pin prior to insertion. If ligament repair is to be performed, we prefer to use small (2 to 4 mm) suture anchors. Finally, a 14 gauge metal cannula or catheter **(Fig. 17–12)** will facilitate accurate placement of percutaneous wires while minimizing the risk of entangling surrounding soft tissues (a painful superficial radial nerve or dorsal sensory ulnar nerve neuroma can undermine an otherwise successful skeletal result). Use of a tourniquet is mandatory. Maintaining reduction while passing fixation wires or screws usually requires all four hands of the surgeon and assistant, making it difficult to repeatedly stop and apply suction to the wound for visualization. Most of these procedures can be performed within 2 hours of tourniquet time.

With the exception of larger radial styloid or ulnar fractures, a single dorsal incision is usually sufficient. A palmar incision will also be needed in the setting of an acute carpal tunnel syndrome or dislocated lunate that cannot be reduced through capsular release via the dorsal approach.

Whether a longitudinal or transverse dorsal incision is used is a matter of personal preference. The transverse incision allows for exposure of the entire carpus along with the radial and ulnar styloids. The transverse scar is also less noticeable than a longitudinal one. However, access to the radial or ulnar metaphysis, should it become necessary, is limited. Our preference is a longitudinal dorsal incision passing directly over Lister's tubercle. Exposure for fixation of radial and ulnar styloids is accomplished

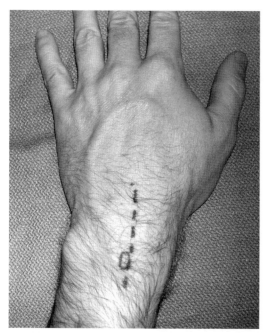

Figure 17–13 Dorsal longitudinal wrist incision beginning just proximal to the dorsal radial (Lister's) tubercle and extending to the carpometacarpal (CMC) joint level usually offers adequate exposure for osseous and ligamentous repair.

through separate longitudinal incisions over each with little risk for flap necrosis **(Fig. 17–13).**

For the longitudinal dorsal incision, incise the skin 4 to 6 cm in line with Lister's tubercle centered over the proximal carpal row, creating full-thickness flaps down to the level of the extensor retinaculum. Incise the distal portion of the retinaculum in line with the extensor pollicis tendon. Releasing a portion of the septum between the third and fourth compartments facilitates broader exposure of the dorsal capsule with a self-retaining retractor, reflecting the second- and third-compartment tendons radially and the fourth compartment ulnarly. If an existing posttraumatic tear is present in the dorsal capsule, try to incorporate it into the dorsal capsulotomy. Otherwise, make a full-thickness incision in the capsule in line with Lister's tubercle for 2 to 3 cm. If the scapholunate ligament is intact, overzealous penetration with the blade during this incision may result in an iatrogenic division of the ligament. Therefore, once through the capsule, lay the blade flat to elevate it from its dorsal attachments on the carpal bones. Avoid excessive dorsal stripping distally on the scaphoid because this may interrupt its main vascular supply along the dorsal ridge. This should provide adequate exposure to the dorsal carpus from the dorsal pole of the scaphoid to the radial margin of the triquetrum. Applicable reduction and stabilization techniques will, of course, depend on the degree and components of the individual injury.

Transscaphoid injury patterns traverse either the waist or the proximal pole of the bone. Placement of temporary 0.045 in. K-wires dorsally in both fragments to serve as

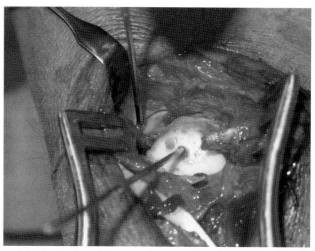

Figure 17–14 Placement of 0.045 in. K-wire "joysticks" in the proximal and distal fragments of the scaphoid facilitates obtaining and maintaining reduction as fixation K-wires or guide pins for cannulated screws are placed for stabilization.

joysticks for fragment manipulation and reduction is beneficial **(Fig. 17–14).** Gently debride the hematoma from the fracture site with a dental pick and irrigation. While one surgeon obtains and maintains the reduction by using the wire joysticks, the other passes a guidewire from the cannulated compression screw set across the fracture site down the central third of the scaphoid **(Fig. 17–15).** Correct position of this pin is critical. The starting point is generally at the dorsal ulnar "corner" of the scaphoid. Use the sterile-draped C-arm to help with correct placement of the pin down the central third axis, stopping intermittently to verify position on posteroanterior (PA) and lateral views. When checking the PA view, avoid the tendency to extend the wrist to the point where the dorsal rim of the radius impinges on and bends the wire. The distal tip of the wire should not enter the distal cortex of the scaphoid. Once

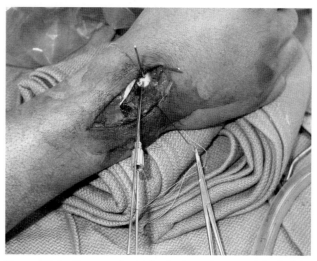

Figure 17–15 Passage of a guide pin down the central third of the scaphoid for fixation of a scaphoid fracture.

satisfactory depth and position of the guide pin are verified, measure the depth of the pin with either the accompanying depth gauge from the set or an equal-length pin in the set. The selected screw size needs to be ~4 mm less than the measured depth of the guide pin. Selecting a screw size that is too long is a common error.

Once the screw length has been determined, pass the guide pin across the scaphotrapezial joint, seating it in the trapezium to avoid inadvertent withdrawal of the wire when using the cannulated drill. To avoid rotational displacement that tends to occur with drill and subsequent screw passage, pass a supplemental 0.045 in. K-wire across the fracture in a line that will not obstruct the other instruments. Using the cannulated hand drill, drill down to a depth 2 mm longer than the selected screw size, observing the markings on the side of the drill (**Fig. 17–16**). Closely observe the fracture site and use the joysticks to resist any displacement that may occur with passage of the drill or screw. As the screw is advanced over the guide pin, compression and increasing resistance occur as it nears the end of the drill tunnel. Remove the guide pin and the derotation wire during the final stages of seating the screw to facilitate fracture site compression. The proximal end of the screw must be countersunk beneath the proximal cortex. If it is prominent, replace the guide pin and change the screw out for the next shorter size.

Capitate fractures are managed using cannulated compression screw techniques similar to those already described for the scaphoid. Fixing a capitate fracture prior to a coexisting scaphoid fracture facilitates access for reduction and accurate screw placement in the proximal capitate fragment. At times, the proximal pole of the capitate may flip a full 180 degrees, with the cartilaginous dome facing distally. Reduction can be performed either using a K-wire joystick or simply with a dental pick because the distal fragment is immobile. Once the fracture is reduced, pass

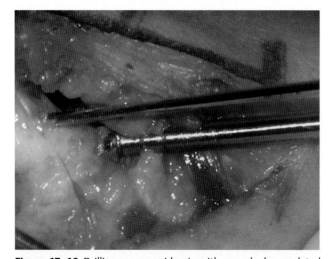

Figure 17–16 Drilling over a guide pin with a marked cannulated hand drill. One surgeon maintains reduction with the joysticks as the drill is passed. A temporary derotational K-wire across the fracture site can also resist displacement during drilling and screw placement.

the guide pin and follow the remaining fixation steps as already outlined for scaphoid fractures (**Fig. 17–17**).

In the case of a complete lunate dislocation (Mayfield stage IV), the unreduced lunate rests in the palmar canal. As mentioned earlier, the palmar capsule may impede closed reduction. In such cases, the palmar rent in the palmar capsule may be extended through the dorsal exposure to allow the lunate to be "flipped up" back into the lunate fossa. If this cannot be accomplished through the dorsal approach, or if the patient has a progressive acute carpal tunnel syndrome, a separate palmar approach will be required.

Once the lunate rests in the lunate fossa, formal scapholunate reduction and stabilization may proceed. Again, placement of K-wire joysticks dorsally in the lunate and proximal pole of the scaphoid facilitates reduction. Typically, the lunate tends to rest in an extended position relative to the scaphoid with disruption of the scapholunate ligament. Therefore, place the joysticks in such an orientation to allow some flexion of the lunate and extension of the scaphoid with reduction. Direct observation is the best method to tell if the scapholunate joint is reduced because subtle rotational offset is difficult to determine with reliance on fluoroscopy alone. A Freer elevator placed in the radioscapholunate interval should assist in adequate visualization for this determination.

Prior to actually performing the reduction, preparations are made for accurate placement of the 0.045 in. fixation wires while avoiding injury to the sensory branches of the radial nerve and the radial artery. To determine the approximate level of skin entry for the wire, simply hold it superficial to the wound to determine the angle needed to traverse the scapholunate joint while staying out of the scaphocapitate interval (**Fig. 17–18A,B**). A small stab wound is then made with a knife through the dermis only at the appropriate entry point. Use a small-tipped hemostat to spread down to the joint capsule overlying the appropriate entry level of the distal scaphoid. While holding the tips of the hemostat open, place a 14 gauge metal cannula up against the scaphoid. Use the fluoroscope to determine the correct tilt of the cannula for accurate passage across the scapholunate interval while the assisting surgeon maintains the reduction. Keeping the cannula firmly seated against bone, drill the K-wire through it across the scapholunate interval. Pass the wire far enough for good purchase in the lunate while avoiding penetration into the radiocarpal joint. Pass a second 0.045 in. K-wire across the joint into the lunate for better stability using the same method. A third wire is then placed across the scaphocapitate joint.

Now that the scapholunate interval is reduced and stabilized, repair the ligament using small anchors with 4–0 braided suture. Usually, the tear is more off one bone, while the majority of the ligament remains attached to the other. Use a small rongeur or curet to debride a small area of the bone in preparation for ligament reattachment (**Fig. 17–19**). Two or three anchors are placed in the proximal pole of the bone to which the ligament is to be repaired.

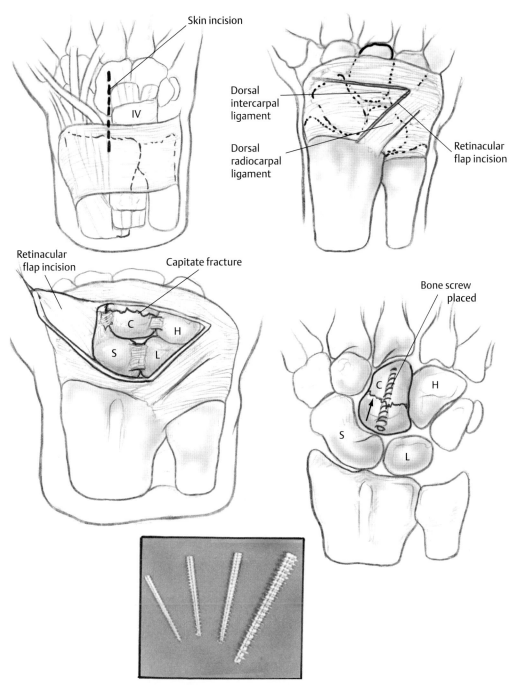

Figure 17–17 Capitate fracture stabilized with compression screw using techniques similar to those of scaphoid fracture fixation.

The attached 4–0 suture is then passed through the ligament in a horizontal mattress fashion and tied down to secure the ligament to the bed of prepared bone **(Fig. 17–20).**

In some instances (often seen in more subacute presentations several weeks following injury), there may not be sufficient ligament tissue to offer a substantial primary repair. Many authors have advocated dorsal capsulodesis using a flap of proximally based dorsal capsule to augment the ligament repair.[6] The distal portion of the tongue of the dorsal capsule is attached to the dorsal portion of the distal pole of the scaphoid (after it has been restored to anatomical position relative to the lunate) through the use of either drill tunnels or suture anchors. Following the 8 to 12 weeks of immobilization, this may help resist the tendency of the scaphoid to drift into flexion, should a weak scapholunate ligament repair be inadequate.

As already mentioned, some surgeons perform pin fixation alone of the lunatotriquetral joint without performing formal repair of the ligament. Should ligament repair be desired, it can be done using the steps outlined earlier for repair of the scapholunate ligament. The triquetrum tends to rest slightly dorsal relative to the lunate with tears of this

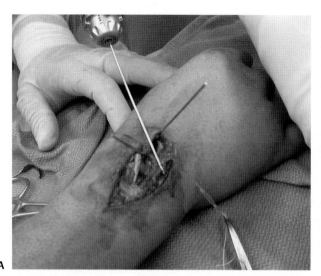
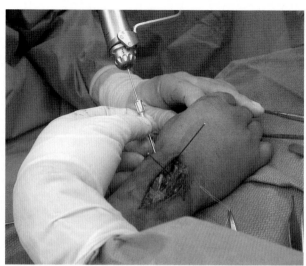

A   **B**

Figure 17–18 **(A)** Prior to actually drilling the wire, holding it over the wound facilitates determining the correct angle and entry point of the wire through the skin. **(B)** Drilling wire across scapholunate joint with blunt-tipped needle soft tissue sleeve.

ligament, and dorsal pressure against the triquetrum for reduction should be performed when passing the wires across the joint. Again, use of the 14 gauge metal sleeve will minimize the risk of injury to the dorsal sensory branches of the ulnar nerve. If a reparable flap of the lunatotriquetral ligament is visible, a direct repair using small suture anchors or bone tunnels may be utilized. However, recall that the dorsal portion of the lunatotriquetral ligament is less substantial than the palmar portion. Therefore, some surgeons employ a separate palmar approach through the floor of the carpal canal to perform a direct palmar ligamentous repair.

Once the carpus has been stabilized, the pins are either cut short beneath the skin or bent down and capped outside the skin. Should they be cut beneath the skin, ensure they are cut short enough. Prominent pins beneath the skin may eventually erode through and result in an infection underneath the cast.

If a radial styloid fracture is large enough to involve the radioscaphocapitate ligament or to create a significant deformity in the scaphoid fossa, it should be reduced and stabilized. If a transverse skin incision has been employed to address the carpal instability, it can be extended radially to expose the radial styloid underneath the first dorsal compartment tendons. If a longitudinal dorsal incision was used, make a second longitudinal incision centered over the radial styloid (**Fig. 17–21**). With either approach, take a moment to identify and gently retract the sensory branches of the radial nerve. Failure to do so will result in a painful neuroma or an anesthetic area on the dorsoradial aspect of the hand that consumes the patient's attention despite a perhaps otherwise good outcome. Once nerve branches have been identified and reflected, divide the extensor retinaculum over the first dorsal compartment and reflect the underlying tendons to expose the radial styloid and brachioradialis insertion. The

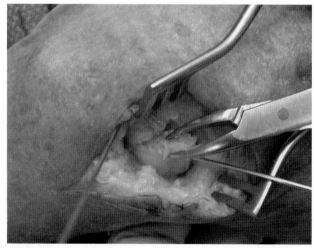

Figure 17–19 Prior to placing suture anchors and repairing ligament, debride the bed of the ligament detachment down to bleeding bone surfaces using either a small rongeur or a bur.

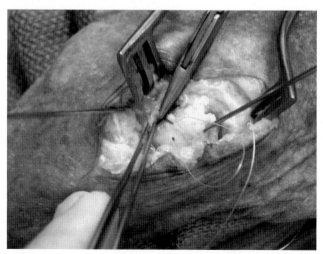

Figure 17–20 Passing of suture through avulsed ligament stumps after placement of the anchor in prepared bone site.

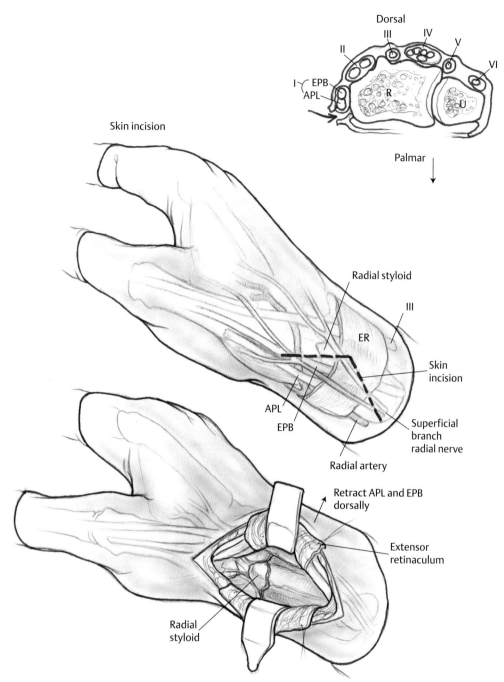

Figure 17–21 Radial wrist approach for reduction and fixation of a radial styloid fracture. Immediately after incising the dermis with a knife, use fine scissors to spread down to the first dorsal compartment retinaculum to avoid injury to the sensory branches of the radial nerve. Open the first compartment along its dorsal margin to avoid potential palmar subluxation of the first compartment tendons.

radial artery can be found lying deep to the tendons just beyond the radial styloid and should be protected. Although the styloid fragment may appear reduced along the radial metaphysis, it is important to confirm reduction of the joint surface by fluoroscopy or direct visualization. Subtle rotational deformities of the fragment often result in significant joint incongruity. Once reduction is confirmed, a compression screw is placed across the fracture into the radial metaphysis. A cannulated 4.0 mm screw or regular 3.5 mm screw

placed over a washer using lag technique is sufficient. A cannulated compression screw also works quite well and avoids the issue of prominent screw heads **(Fig. 17–22).**

Clearly, not all ulnar styloid fractures need to be stabilized. Only those ulnar styloid fragments that encompass the deep insertion of the triangular fibrocartilage require fixation **(Fig. 17–23).** This may be assessed by simply stressing the distal radioulnar joint in the sagittal plane after other distal radius and carpal injuries have been stabilized. If

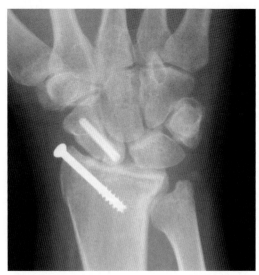

Figure 17–22 Postoperative x-ray of a repaired radial styloid fracture (following concomitant repair of the proximal pole of a scaphoid fracture through a dorsal incision).

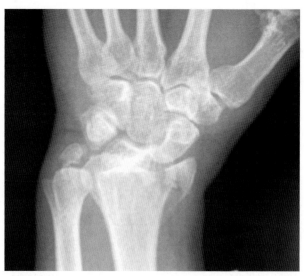

Figure 17–23 A larger ulnar styloid fracture necessitating repair, as the insertion of the triangular fibrocartilage resides at the base of the unstable fracture fragment.

the joint is unstable, then the ulnar styloid should be fixed to restore the insertion of the triangular fibrocartilage into the ulna. We find a combination K-wire and tension-band technique provides stable, low-profile fixation.

The approach to the distal ulna is made through a longitudinal incision beginning ~4 cm proximal to the styloid along the ulnar subcutaneous border. Distally, the dorsal sensory branch of the ulnar nerve traverses the incision around the tip of the styloid and should be protected. Release the ulnar extent of the extensor retinaculum to expose the fracture. Use either a knife or an elevator to expose the ulnar aspect of the cortex for a distance of 2 to 3 cm proximally. After obtaining the reduction with a dental pick, pass a 0.045 in. K-wire through the tip of the styloid into the cortex of the ulnar metaphysis proximally **(Fig. 17–24A,B)**. A 24 gauge K-wire is used to establish the tension-band construct. Passing the cerclage wire around the base of the styloid is facilitated by using a bent 18 gauge needle passed around the base. The wire is then inserted into the protruding sharp tip of the needle and pushed through it. If the wire becomes incarcerated and will not pass through the needle, simply withdrawing the needle will usually result in the wire being pulled through with it. After crossing the wire over the cortex of the ulna, pass it through a transverse drill hole in the ulna 2 to 3 cm proximal to the styloid. The cerclage wire is then twisted together to provide compression of the fracture through a tension-band effect. The K-wire is bent, cut, and advanced down to the tip of the styloid **(Fig. 17–25)**.

A palmar approach may be required for an urgent carpal tunnel release or reduction of an incarcerated lunate dislocation. This is performed through a more extensile incision than that traditionally used for a routine carpal tunnel release. Beginning at the level of Kaplan's

cardinal line **(Fig. 17–26)**, the incision courses proximally between the thenar crease and the hook of the hamate. The incision ends ~2 cm proximal to the wrist flexion crease. Dissection proceeds down to the level of the transverse carpal ligament, which is divided sharply along its full length while avoiding injury to the underlying median nerve. Following evacuation of the hematoma, an incarcerated lunate may be exposed by retracting the carpal canal contents. Avoid placing retractors along the radial aspect of the median nerve with this maneuver because this may result in injury to the recurrent motor branch. If the lunate is stuck in the canal, make a relaxing incision in the palmar capsule to allow reduction back into the lunate fossa.

Tips and Tricks

- Palpation of the entire wrist [distal radius, distal radial ulnar joint (DRUJ), radial and ulnar styloids, specific carpal bones and joints] with attention to each component is the mainstay of a competent assessment for perilunate injuries. Even in the acute setting, patients are more focally tender over specific fracture or ligament injuries than elsewhere in the wrist. This is the key to not missing more subtle injury presentations.
- Traction radiographs in the acute setting are helpful to delineate the injury pattern.
- Clenched fist view with ulnar deviation can reveal an otherwise normal-appearing scapholunate gap or scaphoid fracture on plain film.
- Carefully evaluate the joint for presence of bone or loose cartilage fragments that could become problematic later.

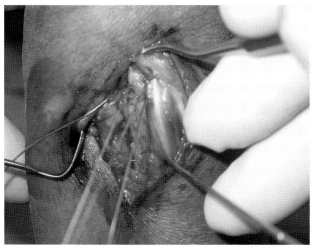 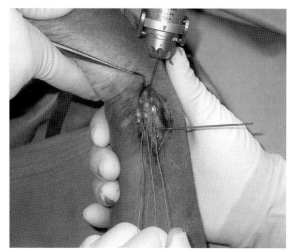

A   B

Figure 17–24 **(A)** The ulnar styloid fragment, with the attached triangular fibrocartilage complex, is reduced and held in place **(B)** a 0.045 in. K-wire is placed at the tip and drilled across the fracture into the ulnar cortex.

Rehabilitation

Postoperatively, the wrist is placed in a sugar tong spica splint in neutral position. At 4 to 6 weeks, this is converted to either a long arm or Muenster cast. Pins may be removed at 8 weeks, but immobilization is continued in a short arm cast until 12 weeks. Beginning immediately after surgery, active digital motion is encouraged. The patient may then be placed in a removable wrist splint for comfort as strengthening and range of motion exercises begin.

New Techniques

For some time, wrist arthroscopy has been used effectively as both a diagnostic measure and a treatment modality for soft tissue problems in the wrist, particularly along the ulnar aspect (triangular fibrocartilage tears). As experience with this technology has grown, some surgeons find it useful for management of both fractures and incomplete ligamentous injuries in the carpus.[7,8]

For acute partial ruptures of the scapholunate ligament, scapholunate widening or increased scapholunate

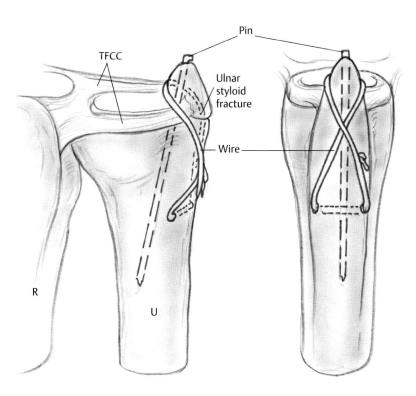

R

U

Figure 17–25 After the wire has been passed around the base of the styloid and through the transverse drill hole in the ulnar metaphysis, it is tightened with a needle driver to create a tension-band effect to provide compression at and further stabilize the fracture site. TFCC, triangular fibrocartilage complex.

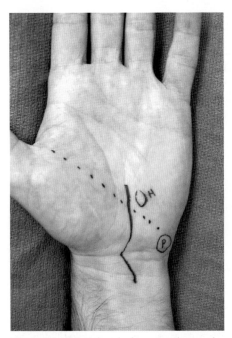

Figure 17–26 Landmarks for extensile carpal tunnel release incision (skin marking), which lies between the thenar crease and the hook of the hamate. Kaplan's line extends from the fully extended thumb to the distal pisiform and serves as an estimate of the level of the superficial palmar vascular arch.

angulation that is evident on plain films in complete injuries is often lacking. If a patient has swelling, localized tenderness, pain with scapholunate shift test, and a mechanism consistent with a scapholunate injury, arthroscopy is an excellent tool to assess the amount of soft tissue injury and subtle degrees of scapholunate incongruity. The only suggestion of such incongruity may be the dorsal lip of the scaphoid being rotated distally relative to the dorsal lip of the lunate, as viewed with the scope in the midcarpal joint. Furthermore, slight widening of the joint can better be defined using the scope and probe from within the midcarpal portal.

Definitive management of partial scapholunate injuries has been performed with arthroscopically assisted pin fixation. Arthroscopy can offer more accurate reduction and pin placement assessment and has been reported as effective definitive management for acute injuries.[7,8]

Outcomes

Any discussion of treatment outcomes for these injuries must begin with an appreciation for the poor results associated with missed or untreated perilunate injuries. With the exception of perhaps partial tears of the interosseous ligaments with no subsequent separation or disconjugate motion, splinting or immobilization alone is usually inadequate and may progress to the progressive collapse and instability patterns seen in untreated injuries.[9]

Despite significant advances in understanding the pathomechanics and diagnosis of carpal instability, reliable data on treatment outcomes for these injuries are surprisingly sparse. This is likely due to the difficulty in comparing such a variety of injury patterns and treatment options. Nonetheless, treatment delays, open injuries, fracture malunion (shortened, flexed scaphoid), and articular damage appear to be associated with poor results.[10]

Closed treatment of acute scapholunate injuries with or without pin fixation is associated with poor long-term satisfaction and maintenance of alignment.[9,11] Restoration of normal intercarpal relationships through open reduction and K-wire fixation accompanied by ligamentous repair is clearly recommended by most surgeons. Arthroscopically assisted reduction and pinning, however (see earlier discussion), has been effectively employed. Satisfactory outcomes have been reported by multiple authors employing either dorsal or combined dorsal-volar approaches for reduction and stabilization.[11–13]

All salvage procedures for established separations or dislocations with secondary degenerative changes are associated with some loss of motion and incomplete pain relief. Four-corner arthrodesis and proximal row carpectomy are probably the most commonly utilized salvage techniques. One study suggests that range of motion and grip are slightly better in the proximal row carpectomy group, although a more recent study found minimal subjective or objective differences in short-term follow-up.[14,15]

Complications

Perhaps the most common complication of injuries resulting in carpal instability is failure to promptly recognize and diagnose the condition. Recall that initial plain films may appear normal despite the presence of a scaphoid fracture or significant ligamentous injury. Undetected, these conditions are notorious for progressing toward carpal collapse with secondary painful arthrosis and disability. As suggested earlier, if operative treatment is delayed beyond 3 weeks, callous will be present and fracture mobilization is significantly more difficult, requiring extensive soft tissue stripping and difficulty with anatomical reduction. This may account for the suboptimal results documented with such delay in treatment.

Progressive arthrosis may occur secondary to persistent malalignment or due to osteochondral damage incurred at the time of injury. One multicenter study documented a posttraumatic arthritis incidence of 56% following surgical treatment.[10] Attention to quality of reduction, especially in the presence of comminution of scaphoid or capitate fractures, will help avoid malunion and nonunion. Use of compression screw fixation for a comminuted fracture may result in significant shortening, collapse, and deformity. Malunited scaphoid fractures with a secondary humpback deformity can be addressed with traditional palmar opening wedge reduction and cortical bone grafting through a palmar approach.[16] Aside from degenerative arthrosis, stiffness often occurs following these injuries, probably as a result of the scarring inherent to healing of torn ligaments and joint capsule.[17]

Median nerve dysfunction may occur due to prolonged pressure on the nerve secondary to posttraumatic swelling (acute carpal tunnel syndrome) or as a result of nerve contusion at the time of injury. Obviously, recognition and prompt decompression of an ongoing acute carpal tunnel syndrome is the best way to avoid prolonged or permanent median motor and sensory deficits due to pressure. In general, neurapraxia sustained from the inciting trauma should resolve with observation.

Technique-related complications are frequently due to pin insertion. Percutaneous insertion of pins without protection of soft tissues places the superficial branches of the radial nerve and dorsal sensory branches of the ulnar nerve at risk. The radial artery, lying just distal to the radial styloid, is also vulnerable to injury during pin placement. Use of a soft tissue protection sleeve and gentle spreading to clear a path to the joint capsule can minimize the danger to these nerves.

Finally, despite good operative technique, ligament repair may attenuate or fail with subsequent progression to secondary arthritic changes. Keeping pins in a minimum of 8 weeks while maintaining cast immobilization until 12 weeks may decrease the likelihood of this occurring.

Pearls

- Recall radiographic parameters for static scapholunate instability:
  - Increased scapholunate angle on lateral x-ray (range 30 to 60 degrees)
  - > 3 mm gap at scapholunate joint
  - Scaphoid cortical "ring" sign on PA film with < 7 mm distance from the ring to the proximal cortex of the scaphoid (suggesting excessive scaphoid flexion)
- Open reduction and pin fixation with direct ligament repair is the standard for acute scapholunate ligament separations. For perilunate fracture-dislocations, rigid bone fixation combined with repair of associated ligament injuries should be performed.
- Delayed treatment of perilunate fractures or dislocations is associated with poorer outcomes.
- The natural history of scapholunate advanced collapse (SLAC) follows a predictable sequence of arthritic involvement of the radial styloid, scaphoid fossa, scaphocapitate joint, capitolunate joint, and finally pancarpal arthrosis with sparing of the lunate fossa.
- Scaphoid nonunion advanced collapse (SNAC) also typically follows a sequential pattern beginning with the radial styloid and then progressing to the scaphocapitate joint, capitolunate joint, and perhaps eventually pancarpal arthrosis. Again, the lunate fossa is generally spared.

Scaphoid Fractures

In the preceding section, scaphoid fractures were discussed as a component of the greater spectrum of perilunate injury. However, scaphoid fractures usually occur without accompanying injuries within the carpus and represent the most common isolated carpal fracture. Unfortunately, scaphoid fractures also represent a notorious cause of morbidity because symptomatic nonunions and malunions are known to have an incidence of up to 50% in displaced patterns managed nonoperatively.[18] Furthermore, because these injuries often have a fairly innocuous presentation and are frequently dismissed as sprains, they are often undertreated until they present later as painful nonunions. This section focuses on the diagnosis, management (nonoperative and operative), complications, and outcomes of scaphoid fractures as an isolated entity.

Some of the relevant anatomy and the mechanical role of the scaphoid was covered in the preceding section on dislocations and carpal instability. However, a few more points merit emphasis. As mentioned, the scaphoid is the most radial element of the proximal carpal row and serves as a rigid strut between the proximal and distal rows. Absence or structural failure of the scaphoid results in proximal migration of the distal row with gradual collapse and secondary arthritic changes, similar to that seen following untreated perilunate ligamentous injuries.

The scaphoid resides adjacent to the lunate and articulates proximally with the scaphoid fossa of the distal radius. A subtle ridge on the radius usually separates the scaphoid fossa from the lunate fossa. The scaphoid and lunate are joined by the scapholunate ligament (**Fig. 17–3**), which is a crucial functional link between the two bones and is required for stable, congruous motion of the proximal carpal row. The distal concavity of the scaphoid rests against the proximal pole of the capitate. Distally, the trapezium and trapezoid form what is know as the "triscaphe" or scaphotrapeziotrapezoid joint with the scaphoid.

The scaphoid is traditionally divided into three main regions: the distal pole, the waist, and the proximal pole. This designation is largely a result of the different prognosis for fractures in each region. Fractures of the distal pole usually heal with little difficulty. Waist fractures with the slightest degree of displacement demonstrate a significant decline in union rate with traditional immobilization techniques.[18] Displaced proximal pole fractures seem to exhibit the highest nonunion rate.

The basis for this distinct difference in regional fracture behavior resides in the peculiar blood supply to the scaphoid. Gelberman and Menon confirmed previous studies suggesting that the majority of the blood supply arrives as radial artery branches entering the dorsal ridge. This supplies 70 to 80% of the total vascularity to the bone and 100% to the proximal pole, which is completely covered by cartilage and has no independent blood supply. A lesser vascular contribution comes from another radial artery branch entering at the distal scaphoid tubercle, supplying only the distal 30% of the bone.[19] Therefore, any displaced fracture involving the proximal half of the scaphoid severely jeopardizes the retrograde vascularity of the proximal fragment and may result in increased healing time and avascular necrosis of that portion of the bone.

Key ligaments about the scaphoid are the aforementioned scapholunate ligament and radioscaphocapitate ligament. The radioscaphocapitate ligament (**Fig. 17–1**) originates on the volar rim of the radius ~4 mm from the radial styloid and spans across the waist of the scaphoid to insert on the volar surface of the capitate. This ligament functions to suspend the radial side of the carpus and acts as a fulcrum for the scaphoid as it flexes and extends with radial and ulnar deviation, respectively.

Diagnosis

As with perilunate injuries, the key to diagnosis in scaphoid fractures is to maintain a high index of suspicion in the patient who has seemingly mild radial-sided wrist pain following a fall or load with the wrist extended. The scaphoid fails as the proximal pole is fixed in the scaphoid fossa of the radius as the hyperextension force is transmitted to the remainder of the bone. Another less common mechanism is seen in the "puncher's fracture," during which the scaphoid experiences a direct axial load.

Whatever the mechanism, the patient will present with radial-sided wrist pain and swelling, depending on the timing of presentation. In the first few days following injury, the patient may have diffuse radial-sided wrist pain and swelling, making the focal point of tenderness difficult to localize. Waist fractures will usually have tenderness to palpation in the anatomical snuffbox. Proximal and distal pole fractures will have more tenderness along the dorsal or palmar scaphoid surfaces, respectively. Patients who have an identical mechanism but have sustained a scapholunate ligament tear instead of a scaphoid fracture will generally be more tender dorsally, just distal to Lister's tubercle.

Standard radiographs should include PA, lateral, oblique (45 degrees pronated), and ulnar deviated "clenched fist" PA views. Initially, the fracture may not be visible on plain radiographs. If no fracture is visible and the patient has a history and exam strongly suggestive of an injury, one option is to treat this as a nondisplaced fracture with cast immobilization initially and reevaluate the patient in 2 to 3 weeks with a series of repeat plain films. By then, the bone has had a chance to undergo visible resorptive changes in response to the fracture, making the fracture visible on x-ray.

Because a 2 to 3 week period of immobilization without the certainty of a diagnosed fracture may represent a problem for some patients, other modalities are available for earlier diagnosis. Bone scan has traditionally been used to screen for scaphoid fractures when initial x-rays are inconclusive. Increased uptake on bone scan may occur starting 24 hours after injury. Unfortunately, associated soft tissue injury, synovitis, or concomitant arthrosis can result in false-positive findings on bone scan. Furthermore, the bone scan does not demonstrate the anatomical features of the fracture.

Given the foregoing bone scintigraphy shortcomings and continued progress in resolution and applications of magnetic resonance imaging (MRI), the latter is seeing an increasing role in diagnosis of occult scaphoid fractures. Bone edema from the fracture can be detected readily with MRI, and it has been shown to have greater sensitivity and specificity than bone scintigraphy.[20] Aside from no radiation exposure, MRI offers the further advantages of providing more anatomical detail of the fracture along with the vascular status of the proximal fragment. Specifically, early and late stages of avascular necrosis demonstrate characteristic changes on T1- and T2-weighted images, which has a significant impact on planning treatment.

Ultrasound offers another radiation-free modality for early diagnosis of occult scaphoid fractures at a lower cost than MRI, but results are clearly dependent on the experience and skill of the individual radiologist. Furthermore, it offers little of the anatomical and vascular detail found with MRI.

Computed tomography (CT) can also be used as a diagnostic tool, but it will be less sensitive than MRI at detecting subtle edema changes in the bone with little cortical disruption, which may be the only findings in an occult injury. However, CT is very useful in defining the actual anatomy and deformity of the fractured scaphoid. A "humpback" deformity may not be apparent on plain x-rays, but CT slices taken in the sagittal plane of the scaphoid will demonstrate the angulation of the bone, which would usually be addressed surgically. Because determination of actual union of a scaphoid fracture can be difficult clinically and on plain films, CT is useful at providing slices in multiple orientations to the fracture site to detect bridging bone formation.

Nonoperative Treatment

Multiple factors unique to both the patient (age, occupation, activity level, associated injuries) and the fracture (location within the bone, displacement, stability, vascularity) require consideration when determining whether a scaphoid fracture can be treated better with cast immobilization versus operative fixation. A truly nondisplaced, stable scaphoid waist or distal pole acute fracture can be managed safely with cast immobilization. Displacement of 1 mm or more on plain films is known to have a significantly higher rate of nonunion if treated nonoperatively.[18] Furthermore, plain films have been suggested to underestimate the degree of displacement, and some advocate the use of CT to better visualize the fracture pattern before planning treatment.

Exactly what form of immobilization is most conducive to healing of these fractures remains controversial. A commonly debated issue is whether long versus short arm casting is better. One study by Gellman et al comparing long versus short arm casting for nondisplaced scaphoid fractures suggested a slightly higher union rate and shorter period of immobilization for waist and proximal pole nondisplaced fractures initially treated with 6 weeks of long arm casting followed by short arm casting as opposed to those treated immediately with short arm casting.[21] Clay et al compared short arm against short arm thumb spica casting for nondisplaced fractures, and concluded that inclusion of the thumb made no difference.[22] Such findings were echoed in a 2001 series of 262 patients by Burge, who also found no difference in union rates with thumb spica compared with short arm casting.[23] Perhaps such ambiguity in defining the optimal position and type of cast for these fractures is due to the fact that these are stable patterns that will heal simply with adequate protection against loading or extreme positioning.

Indications for Surgical Treatment

As already suggested, factors inherent to both the patient and the fracture influence the decision of operative versus nonoperative treatment. Patient activity requirements, fracture stability, fracture location, and associated injuries must all be considered.

Although cast immobilization is a safe, time-tested treatment method for acute, truly nondisplaced scaphoid waist fractures, percutaneous screw fixation (through either dorsal or volar approach) has been demonstrated to result in union while allowing earlier return to preinjury activity level.[24] Proposed advantages over casting alone include decreased period of cast immobilization, faster recovery time, and earlier return to contact sports or labor while still maintaining a low complication rate compared with formal open reduction and internal fixation (ORIF).[25-27]

There is little room for nonoperative treatment of scaphoid fractures exhibiting any displacement. Nonunion rates of acute displaced fractures treated nonoperatively are known to approach 50%.[18] ORIF with headless compression screws allows for restoration of anatomy while improving the ability of the bone to heal. Furthermore, rigid fixation may decrease immobilization time and allow early motion. Union rates up to 93% have been reported using either dorsal or volar approaches.[28] Aside from being prone to nonunion, displaced fractures that do heal in a malaligned position may result in carpal instability with stiffness and posttraumatic arthritis. Comminution at the fracture site also represents an unstable pattern that merits rigid operative fixation.

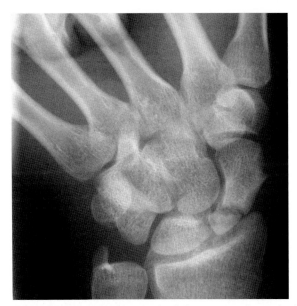

Figure 17–27 Scaphoid proximal pole fracture, initially nondisplaced, that progressed to nonunion despite immediate cast immobilization.

Fractures of the proximal pole, due to their tenuous blood supply, are also at risk for the development of symptomatic nonunion (**Fig. 17–27**). Accordingly, there is a growing trend toward early surgical intervention in even nondisplaced proximal pole fractures to avoid the gradual fracture displacement seen as union time is prolonged. Cannulated compression screw fixation can be accomplished through a dorsal approach with minimal complications.[25]

Finally, scaphoid fractures occurring as a component of any perilunate injury pattern, as covered in the previous section on acute carpal instability, require open reduction and rigid fixation. Such injuries are markedly unstable, and closed anatomical reduction without rigid fixation is likely to result in nonunion, persistent instability, and collapse. The scaphoid fracture component of such injuries is usually addressed through the same dorsal incision employed to reduce the remainder of the carpus.

Surgical Treatment

Surgical Anatomy and Options for Treatment

Either dorsal or volar open approaches can be used for scaphoid fixation. Percutaneous fixation, with or without the assistance of the arthroscope, can also be performed from either the dorsal or the volar aspect. Which approach to use is determined by location of the fracture, associated injuries, degree of deformity or comminution, and comfort of the surgeon with the particular technique. Displaced fractures of the distal pole are clearly best managed using an open or percutaneous volar approach because this provides easy access to the fragment for reduction and fixation. Likewise, proximal pole fractures are best managed from the dorsal aspect of the wrist. Scaphoid waist fractures have been successfully managed using dorsal or volar approaches. Earlier noncannulated compression screws relied on volar placement of a jig for measurement and drilling, so management of some waist and more proximal pole fractures was quite tedious. Modern cannulated screw fixation allows accurate placement and measurement of screws from either direction, depending on surgeon preference. A "humpback" deformity or typical volar comminution of the waist would be better managed with a volar approach, which allows distraction of the volar cortex and accurate placement of potential bone graft. If there are associated perilunar osseous or ligamentous injuries to be addressed, scaphoid reduction and fixation can be accomplished through the same dorsal exposure (refer to the technique described in the previous carpal instability section). The dorsal approach allows slightly more consistent placement of the screw down the central axis of the bone. Some concern is raised about placing such a defect in the articular surface of the proximal pole, but no deleterious effect from this has ever been shown. The use of arthroscopically assisted reduction and percutaneous fixation techniques is receiving growing interest. Familiarity with this technique and difficulty of fracture reduction should dictate its application to a particular injury pattern.

In acute scaphoid fractures, bone grafting is generally employed when comminution and collapse are evident at the fracture site. Adequate autograft quantity can be obtained through volar or dorsal metaphyseal windows created in the distal radius with a small osteotome. Because there has not been adequate time for bone resorption or cyst formation in acute fractures, iliac crest bone grafting is usually unnecessary.

Surgical Techniques

The open volar approach employs an oblique incision traversing the scaphotrapezial joint and coursing proximally over the flexor carpi radialis tendon at the level of the wrist flexion crease (**Fig. 17–28**). The superficial branch from the radial artery courses through the midportion of the wound and should be cauterized or ligated. The flexor carpi radialis sheath is incised and the tendon is reflected with a self-retaining retractor. Cutting through the floor of the flexor tendon sheath and volar joint capsule at the volar margin of the distal radius exposes the scaphoid close to the waist. The capsular incision is extended over the distal pole across the scaphotrapezial joint. The capsule is adherent to the distal pole and will need to be sharply reflected with the knife. Note that cutting the joint capsule at this level results in division of the radioscaphocapitate ligament, which will need to be repaired at the conclusion of the procedure.

K-wires (0.045 in.) placed as joysticks in each fragment assist in reduction. As the reduction is held with the

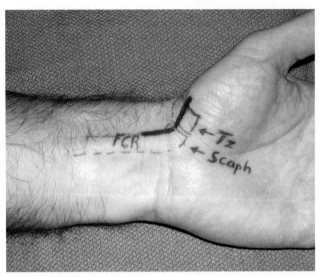

Figure 17–28 Incision line for a volar approach courses across the trapeziometacarpal joint (outlined in photo) down to the intersection of the flexor carpi radialis tendon with the wrist flexion crease. At that point, the incision proceeds proximally over the sheath for ~3 cm.

K-wire joysticks, a guide pin from the cannulated compression screw set is passed from the distal pole across the fracture into the proximal pole down the central third of the bone (**Fig. 17–29**). At times, the proximal portion of the trapezium overhangs the distal portion of the scaphoid, obscuring the ideal starting point for the guidewire. In this situation, the overhanging portion of the trapezium can be removed with a rongeur with no untoward effect. Hyperextending the wrist over a towel roll also helps in exposing the distal pole starting point. The wire position should be verified in multiplanar fluoroscope views during passage.

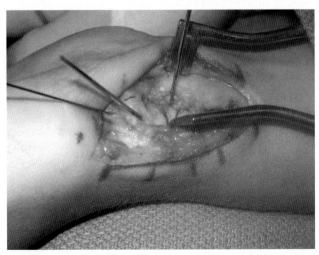

Figure 17–29 Placement of a central guide pin in the scaphoid during a volar approach. An assistant maintains reduction with K-wire joysticks placed in both fragments.

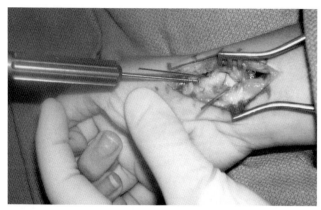

Figure 17–30 After placement of a derotation pin across the fracture site, overdrill the guide pin ~2 mm longer than the measured depth over the guide pin, using depth markings on the drill for guidance.

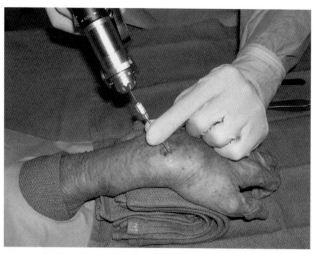

Figure 17–31 Placement of a dorsal percutaneous pin across a scaphoid fracture using a blunt-tipped needle to protect the soft tissues. The fourth dorsal compartment tendons are particularly vulnerable to injury during drilling and screw placement, so exercise caution with appropriate retraction.

The wire can be seated in the proximal pole cortex but should not penetrate into the radiocarpal joint.

The included depth gauge or an equal-length guide pin is used to determine depth of the wire. The selected screw length needs to be about 4 mm less than the measured depth of the guide pin. Again, it is better to err on placing a screw slightly shorter than anticipated as opposed to having an excessively long screw protruding either proximally or distally.

The remaining steps for placing an accessory derotation K-wire, drilling with the depth-metered cannulated drill (**Fig. 17–30**), and placing the screw are identical to those outlined for dorsal fracture fixation in the foregoing carpal instability section. Note that repair of the sectioned radioscaphocapitate ligament is key during closure of the joint capsule.

Fixation of proximal pole and waist fractures from the dorsal approach is performed in the same manner as described in the carpal instability section. The transverse skin incision, however, does not typically need to be as broad as that used in lunate or perilunate fracture-dislocations.

Percutaneous screw fixation is also an option for nondisplaced or minimally displaced scaphoid fractures. Proposed advantages of percutaneous fixation include avoidance of section and repair of ligaments, decreased potential stripping or devascularization of fracture fragments, earlier recovery of motion, and perhaps faster return to normal activities or work.

Percutaneous fixation can be accomplished through either dorsal (**Fig. 17–31**) or volar approaches. For proximal pole fragments, the dorsal approach allows better placement of the screw in the smaller fragment. Although either approach can be used for waist fractures, one recent cadaveric study compared the approaches and found that the dorsal-proximal approach allowed for a more central placement of the screw into the distal pole, but there was little difference in screw position at the waist.[29]

For volar percutaneous screw placement, the wrist is hyperextended and ulnarly deviated over a towel roll, similar to the open volar technique (**Fig. 17–32**). The starting point for guidewire placement is at the distal scaphoid tubercle, aiming proximally, ulnarly, and dorsally. Fluoroscopy is needed to confirm that the pin trajectory appears down the central third of the scaphoid toward the proximal ulnar corner of the bone. Wrist hyperextension is

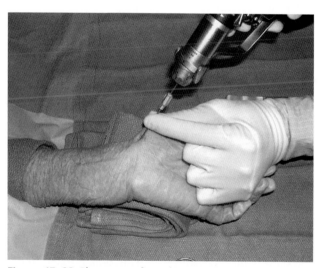

Figure 17–32 Placement of a volar percutaneous pin across a scaphoid fracture requires a short longitudinal (1 to 2 cm) incision over the trapeziometacarpal joint. Obtaining the correct angle for guide pin placement requires placing the drill quite flat against the thenar eminence and metacarpal, so a blunt-tipped needle can be quite helpful in maintaining the pin angle while also protecting the soft tissues.

key to allow the foot of the trapezium to retract and expose as much of the central area of the distal scaphoid pole as possible. Again, resection of a small portion of an overhanging trapezial foot may be required. Following acceptable positioning of the guide pin, a derotation 0.045 in. K-wire is placed across the fracture, avoiding passage so close to the guide pin that it could interfere with cannulated drill or screw placement. Screw length determination, drilling, and screw placement follow the same guidelines used in open placement. A 3 to 4 mm incision is needed around the guide pin for overdrilling and screw placement.

Tips and Tricks

- More than 1 mm of displacement of any scaphoid fracture is an indication for operative fixation. Plain radiographs frequently underestimate the amount of displacement, and CT is a useful adjunct for more accurate assessment.
- MRI is gradually replacing bone scan in diagnosis of occult scaphoid fractures with normal plain films, demonstrating greater sensitivity and specificity.

Rehabilitation

The stability of the scaphoid fracture dictates the pace of mobilization and return to activity. Mobilization of nondisplaced fractures treated with percutaneous screw fixation can begin within 1 to 2 weeks at the time of postoperative splint removal. The patient can be given a removable thumb spica splint to be removed for daily mobilization and even gentle strengthening exercises. Impact loading and contact sports are to be avoided for at least 6 weeks.

For patients with displaced fractures, comminution, or proximal pole involvement, mobilization may need to progress at a slower pace. Digital motion should begin immediately in the postoperative dressing. Active and passive wrist motion, however, should be delayed until some early callus begins to form. This may not occur until the 6 week point or later. Documentation of union (perhaps with CT scan) should occur prior to return to contact sports.

New Techniques

Most of the recent advances in management of scaphoid fractures are in the form of better diagnostics through MRI (see earlier discussion) and better screw fixation devices. Specifically, low-profile, cannulated compression screws allow for accurate placement relative to the fracture using minimally invasive techniques.

As wrist arthroscopy has found a role in management of carpal instability, it has also been effectively employed for reduction and percutaneous fixation of scaphoid fractures. Slade and colleagues reported on a series of 27 fractures treated with this technique with a 100% union rate at an average of 12 weeks (those treated earlier healed within 8 weeks).[27] Proposed advantages of arthroscopy were confirmation of fracture alignment and assessment for concomitant soft tissue injuries.

Complications

Perhaps the most notorious complication of scaphoid fractures is nonunion. The true incidence of this is unknown because not all patients with nonunions ever present to a physician. However, the prognosis for untreated scaphoid nonunions is widely accepted as being poor, with progressive collapse and arthrosis almost a certainty.[30,31] A contributing factor is the fragile vascularity of the bone with obvious negative implications for fracture healing, as already discussed. However, one avoidable cause is simply failure to diagnose and adequately treat these often innocuous-appearing injuries, a problem to be addressed through greater vigilance upon evaluation. Attention to fracture features indicating patterns at risk for nonunion through nonoperative treatment (comminution, proximal pole fractures, associated carpal osseous and ligamentous injuries) can minimize the incidence of undertreatment of at-risk patterns.

Despite recognition and indicated screw stabilization of scaphoid fractures, nonunion and other complications may still occur. Meticulous placement of the guide pin into the central third of the scaphoid and care to avoid rotatory displacement or distraction during screw placement may help to minimize delayed union or nonunion. Likewise, placement of an excessively long screw may result in prominent, painful hardware protruding into the radiocarpal or scaphotrapezial joints. Furthermore, premature unprotected full contact or loading activities may also contribute to failure of union. CT evaluation of fracture healing is superior to plain radiographs in determination of whether union healing has occurred.

One criticism of the open dorsal approach to displaced waist fractures is the vulnerability of the scaphoid vascularity entering the dorsoradial ridge of the bone. Vigorous exposure or reckless instrument placement in this region may result in a nonviable proximal fragment with little chance of healing.

Fractures that have volar waist comminution or have had some delay in treatment may have assumed a humpback deformity with an intrascaphoid angle of greater than 35 degrees. Such a deformity may be better assessed with preoperative CT scans. If the fracture is fixed or allowed to heal in this position, the malunion may result in chronic pain, decreased motion, and eventually posttraumatic arthritis.[18]

Stiffness is often seen following both operative and nonoperative treatment approaches to scaphoid fractures, especially in the flexion-extension arc. One argument for more aggressive treatment of these fractures with rigid screw fixation is to allow for earlier range of motion exercises to shorten immobilization and minimize stiffness. However, although early range of motion at 4 months may be better, one randomized study suggests that grip strength and motion at 2 years were similar for nondisplaced fractures treated with either cast immobilization or percutaneous screw fixation.[24]

Other recognized complications are those inherent to dorsal or radial approaches to the carpus. Painful neuromas can be avoided through recognition and careful handling of the sensory branches of the radial nerve and terminal branches of the lateral antebrachial cutaneous nerve. Infection rates are relatively low, but careless sterile technique can always change that.

Outcomes

Evaluation of scaphoid fracture treatment outcomes must take the fracture type into consideration. Clearly, nondisplaced, stable fracture patterns will fare better than displaced patterns with cast immobilization. Multiple studies have suggested higher nonunion rates with nonoperative treatment of displaced or unstable patterns.

Cast immobilization remains the standby and an effective treatment for nondisplaced fractures of the waist and distal pole. Union rates greater than 95% have been reported with nondisplaced fractures promptly diagnosed and immobilized.[32,33] The key is to be certain that the fracture is truly nondisplaced and not initiate an inappropriate course of immobilization for an unstable fracture pattern.

Operative treatment of stable or nondisplaced patterns has also begun to receive some attention. The goal is to provide stable fixation that allows earlier return of motion and return to activity. However, as already mentioned, ultimate motion and grip strength at 2 year follow-up has been shown to be similar in cast immobilization and percutaneous fixation groups.[24]

Open reduction internal fixation of acute displaced scaphoid fractures with cannulated compression screws has been shown to be effective in multiple studies, with union rates greater than 90%.[25] Volar and dorsal approaches have been used effectively. With either approach, perhaps the most important element is accurate reduction and stable bone fragment apposition upon screw placement.

Fractures of the proximal pole are known to have difficulty healing due to the precarious retrograde vascularity of this portion of the bone. Immobilization times of 6 months with nonunions occurring in up to one third of cases presents a vexing problem for the surgeon.[34,35] Accordingly, there is growing interest in primary screw fixation through a dorsal approach. One series of 17 patients with acute unstable proximal pole fractures treated with primary surgical fixation resulted in a 100% union rate with an average healing time of 10 weeks.[25] Although this is only one series, other reports are promising in comparison with nonoperative treatment.

Other Carpal Fractures

Because the scaphoid is the most common carpal fracture and has demonstrated a proclivity to not heal well, it deservedly receives the most attention in discussions on the topic. When other carpal fractures occur, it is often in the setting of a perilunate injury with some greater arc component, as discussed previously in the carpal instability segment of this chapter. However, isolated fractures of other carpal bones do occur and can be rather debilitating. Like the scaphoid, these bones are largely covered with cartilage and have limited vascularity. Furthermore, odd shapes of the bones and irregular orientation of the fracture patterns can make diagnosis on plain films exceedingly difficult. CT scan is recommended for accurate assessment of these injuries, when suspected.

Triquetral fractures usually occur in the form of capsular avulsions from the dorsal ridge. Smaller dorsal chip or avulsion fractures are usually adequately treated with 4 to 6 weeks of cast immobilization. Larger chip avulsions may suggest a significant degree of carpal instability because the insertion of the DRC and DIC ligament has been rendered incompetent. Recall that isolated disruption of the lunatotriquetral ligament does not result in a VISI deformity. However, when combined with dorsal capsular avulsion, a VISI posture may result and require surgical treatment.

Minimally displaced triquetral body fractures from dorsal- or ulnar-sided impact usually heal uneventfully with cast immobilization. However, when triquetral body fractures occur as a greater arc component of a perilunate injury, surgical stabilization with K-wires or compression screws is recommended.

Trapezium fractures usually occur as a load is imparted to the joint through the metacarpal base. This may result in a variety of fracture patterns, including vertical split, horizontal, comminuted, and anterior ridge (encompassing the transverse carpal ligament origin) fractures.[36] Depending on the degree of displacement of the bone and articular surface, most of these fractures will heal with a 4 to 6 week course of cast immobilization. Large articular gaps or step-offs may require 1.5 or 2.0 mm screw immobilization. Accompanying fractures of the first metacarpal base may result in excessive axial instability, and operative fixation is also preferred in such a case. Comminuted fractures may be best treated with distraction fixation through the first metacarpal. Specifically, fixing the first metacarpal to the second metacarpal with 0.062 in. K-wires while maintaining distraction may allow the smaller comminuted fragments of the trapezium to consolidate without collapse. Some fractures of the anteromedial ridge, caused by avulsion from the transverse carpal ligament following crush injuries, may develop nonunion and require excision.

There are two main types of hamate fractures: hook and body fractures. Hook fractures usually result from either a single direct blow (striking the hard ground during a golf swing) or multiple contusions (tennis, baseball batting). They are also seen following direct carpal crush injuries, in which the transverse carpal ligament may avulse its insertion. The patient will have point tenderness in the palm to palpation over the hook. Pain with motion of the small finger flexor tendons may also be noted. Proximity to the ulnar neurovascular bundle can result in numbness in the palmar distribution of the ulnar nerve. Untreated, hook fractures can result in persistent palmar pain, weakness of grip, and attritional ruptures of small and ring flexor tendons. Diagnosis with plain films is difficult, and CT is recommended.

Nondisplaced hook fractures are treated with cast immobilization. The waist of the hook represents a watershed zone of vascularity and is the region most at risk for developing nonunion. Should this occur (as evidenced by chronic pain and sclerotic fracture margins on CT), excision of the fragment through a palmar approach is recommended.[37]

Hamate body fractures may result as a component of a carpal fracture-dislocation, direct ulnar-sided blow, crush injury, or longitudinal load through the fifth metacarpal while punching with a fist. Minimally or nondisplaced fractures are treated with cast immobilization with or without inclusion of the ulnar two metacarpophalangeal joints. Larger displaced fragments may require ORIF. If there is a large dorsally displaced fragment as a result of a dorsal fourth or fifth carpometacarpal (CMC) joint dislocation, the joint will require reduction through axial traction. The hamate fragment may require pin or screw stabilization, depending on the fragment size, to prevent recurrent CMC joint subluxation. Pinning the base of the unstable metacarpals to the adjacent stable third metacarpal base can reduce the deforming load.

Lunate fractures without a clear underlying injury should be viewed with some skepticism. Idiopathic avascular necrosis (Kienbock's disease) may be the culprit in

such a setting and will not likely respond to measures directed at treating fractures of healthy, vascularized bone. Although the lunate usually receives bountiful blood supply from dorsal and volar sources, 20% of lunates only have a single palmar nutrient artery.[38] Fractures through such regions of marginal vascularity are prone to nonunion and collapse.

Five types of lunate fractures have been described based on vascularity and location of the fracture within the bone.[39] It is safe to assume that any displaced fracture through the lunate body merits operative fixation with either wires or screws. Thin osteochondral fractures of the proximal articular surface are often small enough to treat with temporary immobilization. If pain persists, resection of the unstable fragment can be palliative.

Capitate fractures usually result from an extreme hyperextension force through the carpus and may occur alone or as a component of a perilunate fracture-dislocation. Given the mechanism, accompanying scaphoid fractures are quite common and should always be ruled out with adequate imaging. Similarly, if a scaphoid waist fracture is the presenting injury, an occult capitate fracture may also be present. Nondisplaced capitate fractures may occur in about any plane, and may be visible only on CT or MRI.

The proximal portion of the capitate is intra-articular and has no independent vascular source.[40] Therefore, transverse fractures through the waist of the bone render this portion avascular with any degree of displacement. As a result, painful nonunions may develop from seemingly innocuous, minimally displaced fractures. ORIF is the treatment mainstay for displaced fractures. If avascular necrosis is evident on plain films or MRI, bone grafting should also be considered.

Trapezoid fractures are the rarest of all isolated carpal fractures and usually result from an axial load imparted down the second metacarpal. Simple cracks in the bone may be treated with cast immobilization. Any displacement or proximal migration of the index metacarpal may require operative treatment. Specifically, larger fractures through the body may require stabilization with 1.5 or 2.0 mm screws. If comminution is present, the axial deforming force may need to be minimized through longitudinal distraction of the index metacarpal and pinning of the metacarpal to the third metacarpal base. If collapse and arthrosis result, arthrodesis of the trapezoid-metacarpal joint may be indicated.

On the DVDs

Video 17–1   (Disk 2)   Repair of Perilunate Dislocation   This video of a 6-week-old lunate dislocation demonstrates the surgical repair of this injury. A precise reduction is necessary, and in this case mandates both a volar and dorsal approach. Stabilization is provided by temporary wire fixation and scapholunate ligament reconstruction.

References

1. Linscheid RL, Dobyns JH, Beabout JW, Bryan RS. Traumatic instability of the wrist: diagnosis, classification, and pathomechanics. J Bone Joint Surg Am 1972;54:1612–1632
2. Berger RA, Blair WF, Crowninshield RD, Flatt AE. The scapholunate ligament. J Hand Surg [Am] 1982;7:87–91
3. Ritt MJ, Linscheid RI, Cooney WP III, Berger RA, An KN. Lunotriquetral ligament properties: a comparison of three anatomic subregions. J Hand Surg [Am] 1998;23:425–431
4. Lichtman DM, Schneider JR, Swafford AR, Mack GR. Ulnar midcarpal instability–clinical and laboratory analysis. J Hand Surg [Am] 1981;6:515–523
5. Mayfield JK, Johnson RP, Kilcoyne RK. Carpal dislocations: pathomechanics and progressive perilunar instability. J Hand Surg [Am] 1980;5:226–241
6. Lavernia CJ, Cohen MS, Taleisnik J. Treatment of scapholunate dissociation by ligamentous repair and capsulodesis. J Hand Surg [Am] 1992;17:354–359
7. Ruch DS, Poehling GG. Arthroscopic management of partial scapholunate and lunatotriquetral injuries of the wrist. J Hand Surg [Am] 1996;21:412–417
8. Whipple TC. Role of arthroscopy in treatment of scapholunate instability. Hand Clin 1995;11:37–40
9. Adkison JW, Chapman MW. Treatment of acute lunate and perilunate dislocations. Clin Orthop Relat Res 1982;164:199–207
10. Herzberg G, Comtet JJ, Linscheid RL, Amadio PC, Cooney WP, Stadler J. Perilunate dislocations and fracture-dislocations: a multicenter study. J Hand Surg [Am] 1993;18:768–779
11. Apergis E, Maris J, Theodoratos G, Pavlakis D, Antionou N. Perilunate dislocations and fracture-dislocations: closed and early open reduction compared in 28 cases. Acta Orthop Scand Suppl 1997;275:55–59
12. Kozin SH. Perilunate injuries: diagnosis and treatment. J Am Acad Orthop Surg 1998;6:114–120
13. Minami A, Ogino T, Oishio I, Minami M. Correlation between clinical results and carpal instabilities in patients after reduction of lunate and perilunar dislocations. J Hand Surg [Br] 1986;11:213–220
14. Wyrick JD, Stern PJ, Kiefhaber TR. Motion-preserving procedures in the treatment of scapholunate advanced collapse wrist: proximal row carpectomy versus four-corner arthrodesis. J Hand Surg [Am] 1995;20:965–970
15. Cohen MS, Kozin SH. Degenerative arthritis of the wrist: proximal row carpectomy versus scaphoid excision and four-corner arthrodesis. J Hand Surg [Am] 2001;26:94–104
16. Tomaino MM, King J, Pizillo M. Correction of lunate malalignment when bone grafting scaphoid nonunion with humpback deformity: rationale and results of a technique revisited. J Hand Surg [Am] 2000;25:322–329
17. Cooney WP, Bussey R, Dobyns JH, Linscheid RL. Difficult wrist fractures: perilunate fracture-dislocations of the wrist. Clin Orthop Relat Res 1987;214:136–147
18. Cooney WP, Dobyns JH, Linscheid RL. Fractures of the scaphoid: a rational approach to management. Clin Orthop Relat Res 1980;149:90–97
19. Gelberman RH, Menon J. The vascularity of the scaphoid bone. J Hand Surg [Am] 1980;5:508–513
20. Fowler C, Sullivan B, Williams LA, McCarthy G, Savage R, Palmer A. A comparison of bone scintigraphy and MRI in the early diagnosis of the occult scaphoid waist fracture. Skeletal Radiol 1998;27:683–687
21. Gellman H, Caputo RJ, Carter V, Aboulafia A, McKay M. Comparison of short and long thumb-spica casts for non-displaced fractures of the carpal scaphoid. J Bone Joint Surg Am 1989;71:354–357
22. Clay NR, Costigan PS, Gregg PJ, Barton NJ. Need the thumb be immobilised in scaphoid fractures? A randomised prospective trial. J Bone Joint Surg Br 1991;73:828–832
23. Burge P. Closed cast treatment of scaphoid fractures. Hand Clin 2001;17:541–552
24. Bond CD, Shin AY, McBride M, Dao KD. Percutaneous screw fixation or cast immobilization for nondisplaced scaphoid fractures. J Bone Joint Surg Am 2001;83:483–488
25. Rettig M, Raskin K. Retrograde compression screw fixation of acute proximal pole scaphoid fractures. J Hand Surg [Am] 1999;24:1206–1210
26. Slade JF III, Jaskwhich D. Percutaneous fixation of scaphoid fractures. Hand Clin 2001;17:553–574
27. Slade JF III, Gutow AP, Geissler WB. Percutaneous internal fixation of scaphoid fractures via an arthroscopically assisted dorsal approach. J Bone Joint Surg Am 2002;84A(Suppl 2):S21–S36
28. Rettig ME, Kozin SH, Cooney WP. Open reduction and internal fixation of acute displaced scaphoid waist fractures. J Hand Surg [Am] 2001;26:271–276
29. Chan KA, McAdams TA. Central screw placement in percutaneous screw scaphoid fixation: a cadaveric comparison of proximal and distal techniques. J Hand Surg 2004;29:74–79
30. Ruby LK, Stinson J, Belsky MR. The natural history of scaphoid non-union: a review of fifty-five cases. J Bone Joint Surg Am 1985;67:428–432
31. Mack GR, Bosse MJ, Gelberman RH, Yu E. The natural history of scaphoid non-union. J Bone Joint Surg Am 1984;66:504–509
32. Eddeland A, Eiken O, Hellgren E, Ohlsson N-M. Fractures of the scaphoid. Scand J Plast and Reconstr Surg. 1975;9:234–239
33. Russe O. Fracture of the carpal navicular: diagnosis, nonoperative treatment, and operative treatment. J Bone Joint Surg Am 1960;42:759–768
34. Dickison JC, Shannon JG. Fractures of the carpal scaphoid in the Canadian army. Surg Gynecol Obstet 1944;79:225–239
35. Barton N. Twenty questions about scaphoid fractures. J Hand Surg [Br] 1992;17B:239–310
36. Tracy CA. Transverse carpal ligament disruption associated with simultaneous fractures of the trapezium, trapezial ridge, and hook of hamate: a case report. J Hand Surg [Am] 1999;24:152–155
37. Walsh J, Bishop AT. Diagnosis and management of hamate hook fractures. Hand Clin 2000;16:397–403 viii.
38. Gelberman RH, Bauman TD, Menon J, Akeson WH. The vascularity of the lunate bone and Kienbock's disease. J Hand Surg [Am] 1980;5:272–278
39. Teisen H, Hjarbaek J. Classification of fresh fractures of the lunate. J Hand Surg [Br] 1988;13:458–462
40. Vander Grend R, Dell PC, Glowczewski F, Leslie B, Ruby LK. Intraosseous blood supply of the capitate and its correlation with aseptic necrosis. J Hand Surg [Am] 1984;9:677–683

18 Hand Fractures and Dislocations

James P. Higgins and Thomas J. Graham

Fractures of the tubular bones of the hand are common because the hand and upper extremity are used in almost every endeavor of commerce, socialization, vocational pursuit, and athletic activity. In general, the majority of these fractures can be treated by closed methods. However, there is a subset of hand fractures for which advanced surgical methods should be considered to optimize outcome.

Complex hand fractures pose intellectual and technical challenges that set them apart from those injuries in which conventional closed fracture management is adequate. Because of the extreme dexterity demands of the hand, small losses in motion can result in large functional deficits. The acral location of the hand in the bony skeleton results in a high proportion of crushing injuries as the mechanism of fracture.

The hand has a complex skeletal structure, delicate muscles, intimate neurovascular structures, and a relatively immobile soft tissue envelope. As a result, soft tissue coverage issues, nerve compression, compartment syndrome, and digit perfusion are important considerations in hand fracture management. Finally, the complexity and intimate relationship of the tendon mechanisms and the bony infrastructure can result in limited functional results despite optimal bony reduction, fixation, and healing.

This chapter addresses the operative treatment of fractures of the tubular bones distal to the carpus, the metacarpals and phalanges, and dislocations of their intervening joints. In the treatment of these injuries, it must be emphasized that there are no absolute indications for open management or primacy of a single method of fixation. Individual patient circumstances and fracture personality must be considered on a case-by-case basis. Optimal outcomes will be achieved if the treatment method is tailored to the unique clinical situation, and the surgeon is facile with the technical aspects of the surgery and the integrated rehabilitation plan.

The surgical decision-making algorithms and technical recommendations are covered for selected fractures and dislocations. These include:

1. Open fractures
2. Combined injuries—associated bone, tendon, nerve, vessel, soft tissue injuries
3. Fractures not permitting closed reduction
4. Juxta-articular or intra-articular fractures
5. Multiple adjacent fractures
6. Metadiaphyseal fractures
7. Fractures with rotational deformity, particularly spiral oblique fractures

The specific considerations and indications for surgical management of these fractures are described, starting with the most distal structures and proceeding proximally.

Fractures of the Distal Phalanx

For the purpose of this chapter, three fractures of the distal phalanx have been identified: extra-articular tuft and shaft fractures, extensor tendon avulsion fractures, and flexor tendon avulsion fractures. The management of these three entities is discussed in this section.

Extra-articular fractures of the distal phalanx are often crush injuries resulting in comminuted tuft or midshaft fractures. These require an assessment of the soft tissue as well as bony injuries because one may often influence the management of the other. This is especially true when considering the intimate relationship between the specialized nail elements and the distal phalanx.

Intra-articular distal interphalangeal (DIP) joint fractures are either extensions of a comminuted shaft fracture or are fractures with associated flexor tendon (jersey finger) or extensor tendon (mallet finger) avulsions **(Fig. 18–1).** Flexor digitorum profundus (FDP) avulsion

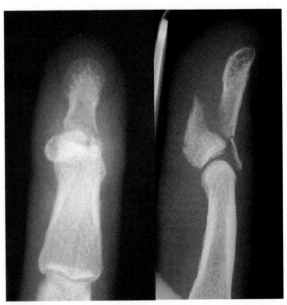

Figure 18–1 Anteroposterior and lateral projections of a comminuted intra-articular fracture of the P3 phalanx. Flexion of the volar fragment reflects the pull of the intact flexor digitorum profundus insertion.

occurs with forceful extension against a flexed DIP joint as may occur when a football player grasps an opponent's jersey during a tackle. Conversely, the majority of terminal extensor mallet avulsions usually occur when an axial load forcibly flexes an extended finger. This relationship of mechanism and fracture pattern exists in all but the largest mallet fractures, which can instead be the result of hyperextension and impaction forces. These particular fractures often demonstrate disruption of the majority of the articular surface, causing volar subluxation of the distal phalanx.

Nonoperative Treatment

Extra-articular Distal Phalanx Fractures

Extra-articular crush injuries to the distal phalangeal tuft are often highly comminuted and demonstrate very small fragments. Associated nailbed injuries often require operative management because they represent true open fractures, and inadequate reapproximation of the sterile matrix may result in delayed nail plate "lift off."

Open fractures with fragments penetrating the nailbed may require only irrigation, debridement, reduction, and splinting. A well-reduced comminuted tuft or midshaft fracture is often adequately controlled by repair of the soft tissue envelope and immobilization. If the fracture pattern will permit fixation, longitudinal K-wires may be used to stabilize some of the fragments while providing a foundation for the sterile matrix repair. Care must be exercised to extract all soft tissue/nail bed elements from the fractured phalanx. For the first few days immobilization using a short arm splint minimizes discomfort and swelling. This is then replaced with a digital splint with the DIP extended and the proximal interphalangeal (PIP) joint free to prevent excessive loss of motion.

Mallet Fractures

Mallet finger avulsion fractures are most often treated in a closed fashion with an extended splinting regimen. Relative indications for operative management of mallet fractures have been described according to the percentage of the articular surface involved, subluxation of the DIP joint, or overall influence of the loss of extensor continuity on the digital posture (i.e., development of swan neck deformity).[1–3]

The more important determinant of mallet fracture management is the stability of the joint relationship. If the distal phalanx demonstrates any volar subluxation, even when placed in an extension splint, fixation of the fragment to which the terminal tendon is attached may be required. If no subluxation exists, the mallet finger can be treated with 6 to 8 weeks of DIP extension splinting followed by gradually resuming active flexion over the following 2 weeks.

Intra-articular Distal Phalanx Fractures: Flexor Digitorum Profundus Avulsion Injuries

Avulsion injuries of the FDP tendon, with or without associated fractures, are always considered to be surgical problems because of the predictably poor finger function that is the result of nonoperative management. There is no accepted role for the nonoperative management of these injuries, except in patients who are unable to comply with postoperative rehabilitation or are not functional, or for whom the medical risks of surgery outweigh the advantages.

Surgical Treatment

Extra-articular Distal Phalanx Fractures

Surgical Anatomy

The extensor mechanism insertion is at the dorsal lip of the distal phalangeal epiphysis. The germinal nail matrix (combination of the nail growth elements made up of the dorsal and intermediate matrices) lies just distal to this insertion. The volar plate inserts onto the epiphysis and proximal metaphysis of the distal phalanx, whereas the FDP insertion flares out at the metaphyseal region. The volar cortical margin demonstrates a much more significant metaphyseal flare than the dorsal cortex, making the medullary canal significantly dorsal to the midaxis of the finger.

Surgical Technique

All distal phalanx fractures require an assessment of the nailbed. If a nailbed laceration is suspected, the nail plate should be removed and the nail matrix repaired. In the absence of a substantial nailbed injury or when only a minor subungual hematoma is present, the nailplate can be maintained as an assistant or substitute for fixation because it stabilizes some of the more minor distal phalangeal fractures.

Use of fixation in distal tuft fractures is indicated for injuries demonstrating displaced fragments large enough to provide purchase for a Kirschner wire. Although outcomes of nonoperative management are generally good for simple distal phalanx fractures, fixation of these more complicated injuries can reduce the risk of symptomatic nonunion, nail deformity, and unstable digital pulp pads.[4] Fixation is usually performed percutaneously by retrograde insertion of a 0.045 or 0.062 in. smooth wire under fluoroscopic guidance. Single pin fixation is often adequate, although two caveats are provided. First, a single longitudinal pin may keep the fracture fragment aligned but not coapted with the phalangeal base; efforts should be made to compress the fragments together to improve the bony contact and stability. The second potential problem is that even well-reduced fractures may easily distract or rotate along the shaft of the pin postoperatively. For this reason a second antiparallel pin should be utilized whenever the fracture and the patient's anatomy will accommodate it.

Tips and Tricks

- These fractures are slow to heal, and ideally the surgeon may maintain the wire fixation for 6 to 8 weeks if possible; yet most patients snag their pin or develop some sensitivity to the implant, requiring removal before that time.
- Despite the exposed location, the wires have a remarkably low rate of infection yet may aseptically loosen from lack of purchase or repeated microtrauma. To minimize this risk of inadvertent pin loss or excessive motion, the surgeon should not hesitate to pass the wire across the extended DIP. This provides greater purchase as well as soft tissue stabilization, which is more likely to promote bony healing. The risk of stiffness at the DIP joint level is legitimate but has been minor in our experience with this technique.
- Passage of the longitudinal pin is more challenging than it may at first appear. The medullary canal is very dorsal to the midlateral line of the digit, requiring the pin to be introduced just volar to the sterile matrix in the center of the hyponychium. If difficulty is encountered, the surgeon should resort to fluoroscopic assistance before several attempts result in loss of adequate bone purchase for accurate alignment.

Intra-articular Distal Phalanx Fractures: Flexor Digitorum Profundus Avulsion Fractures

The FDP tendon may rupture at its insertion, with or without an associated bony fracture fragment. These most commonly occur in the ring finger, although such injuries have been reported in all digits. Leddy and Packer described a well-accepted classification system.[5] Type 1 injuries are nonbony FDP avulsions that retract into the palm. Type 2 avulsions contain a small fragment that retracts to the PIP joint level, with the A3 pulley preventing the fragment from further passage proximally in the tendon sheath. Type 3 avulsions are less common large fragment avulsions that are able to retract only to the A4 pulley level just proximal to the DIP joint. All of these injuries have been considered surgical problems due to the predictable loss of active DIP flexion. Particular attention is paid to timing of surgical reconstruction due to the tendon biology and the risk of extensive musculotendinous shortening over time.

Type 1 avulsions are best treated as acutely as possible. Retracted tendons have complete disruption of the normal dorsal vincula and their blood supply. Repair should be pursued within 7 to 10 days of the injury to avoid degeneration and contraction of the tendon stump.

Type 2 and type 3 avulsions may be repaired at a remote time, although repair is easiest within 7 to 10 days after injury. Several considerations mitigate for early intervention. Although the position of the bony fragment may be determined radiographically, a tendon detachment may also have occurred at the fragment–tendon interface, leaving the fragment in the finger while the tendon has retracted to the palm. Although unusual, this condition warrants the urgency of the type 1 nonbony avulsion in the setting of a fracture/avulsion. Furthermore, the benefits of delayed repair (decreased swelling, joint mobilization) are difficult to obtain with the continuous presence of a fracture fragment within the flexor tendon sheath. There is no specific time limit on the viability of primary repair in these injuries, which it may be feasible for a matter of weeks to months.

Surgical Technique

The surgical approach is via a midaxial or volar zigzag incision. Care is taken to minimize trauma to the sheath and its contents. In a type 1 avulsion a counterincision is made in the palm over the A1 pulley, and a pediatric feeding tube is passed from distal to proximal through the tendon sheath. The retracted tendon should be readily located in the palm because more proximal migration is prevented by the muscular origin of the lumbricals. The feeding tube is used to escort the tendon through the intact sheath. A distally based periosteal flap is raised at the site of the avulsion, and the cortex is roughened to create an inflammatory nidus for adherence of the reattached stump. Using a stout, double-armed monofilament suture, the tendon may be reattached though predrilled holes from the reattachment site to the dorsum of the nail at the level of the lunula and secured over a bolster and a button. The periosteal flap is sutured volarly over the inset tendon for additional security. The monofilament suture is cut and removed with the button 4 weeks later after adequate strength of the repair is established. More commonly a buried anchor may be used under the same periosteal window to provide fixation to the insertion site without the need for an exterior button. This provides the security of long-term support of the repair while healing. These anchors must be placed obliquely and with care to obtain good purchase while not violating the dorsal cortex/nailbed.

Type 2 fracture fragments are often very small and can be treated similarly to type 1 avulsions after either resection of the small fragment or simultaneous fixation of the fragment and tendon reinsertion achieved by sutures woven through the tendon–fragment interface. The anchor or button repair may securely maintain excellent reduction of these smaller fragments.

Type 3 fractures are large enough to require fixation of the bony fragment with Kirschner wires. Attention should

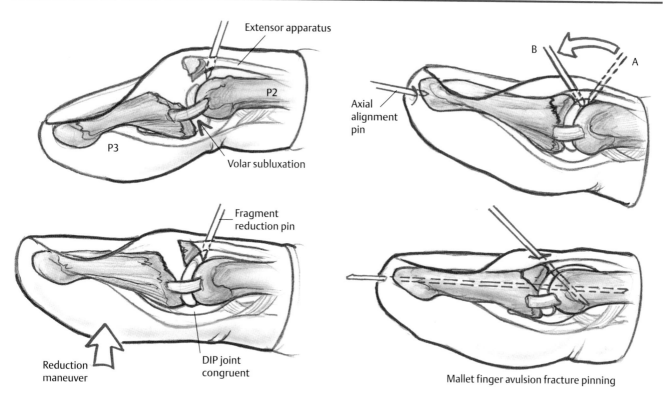

Figure 18–2 Technique of reduction and stabilization of a displaced mallet fracture with volar subluxation. The dorsal pin "levers" the avulsion fragment attached to the terminal tendon into place. The body of the phalanx is reduced and secured with a transarticular pin. DIP, distal intraphalangeal joint.

be paid to accurate alignment of the articular surface. These fragments may contain the majority of the joint surface, and instability may exist without anatomical reduction. Fixation with K-wires with at least a single wire holding the DIP joint in extension is usually necessary.

Extensor Tendon Avulsion Fractures

The vast majority of mallet fractures do not require operative fixation. These fractures can be treated like their nonbony mallet counterparts with extension splinting. Even if these small fragments are not well reduced radiographically, the DIP articular surface remodels well, and adequate DIP extension results.

Rarely, a combination of injury to the extensor apparatus, oblique retinacular ligaments, collateral ligaments, and the dorsal fracture can cause or permit volar subluxation of the distal phalanx. In these most severe of mallet finger deformities, operative intervention is required.

There are two options for treatment of the subluxated mallet finger: combination closed pinning or open repair, both of which are usually augmented with DIP stabilization.

Because tenuous skin coverage, potential nail deformity, and terminal sensory nerve branch division are very real challenges of any open procedure about the distal phalanx, we have preferred to attempt closed treatment initially. The surgeon should not lose sight of the basic goal of reducing the DIP joint by focusing on the relationship

between the dorsal epiphyseal fragment and the remainder of the phalanx; however, it is logical and attractive to attempt both joint and fracture reduction.

An innovative method to accomplish both goals is a dual pinning technique that relies on indirect pinning or "levering" to reduce the displaced dorsal rim while the relationship is stabilized by a longitudinal pin (**Fig. 18–2**).[6] The levering pin is inserted through the skin at an acute angle to the dorsum of the middle phalanx; its tip pierces the terminal tendon and comes to rest on the juxta-articular margin of the dorsal middle phalanx condyles, therefore volar to the displaced distal phalanx fragment. The pin is then manipulated to lever the distal phalanx fragment into a nearly anatomical position and driven into the head of the middle phalanx. With the dorsal rim fracture and its attached terminal tendon now in a better position, the distal phalanx is aligned and secured with a longitudinal pin.

We have even found that developing a tensioning relationship between the two wires, either through a rubber band construct or special bending that associates the two pins, has improved the stability of the construct. The major advantages of this maneuver are the ability to perform adequate reduction and stabilization through closed methods and avoiding further comminution or potential terminal tendon avulsion by instrumenting the small dorsal fragment.

As with any complex fracture, closed methods or percutaneous techniques may fail to deliver the desired outcome.

In the very small subset of mallet injuries in which all closed methods have failed, and those manifesting considerable volar distal phalanx subluxation, an open approach can be employed. A zigzag incision is centered over a transverse limb along the DIP extension crease. Great care is taken to remove all soft tissue and callus blocking perfect manual reduction of both the joint and the fracture line. Multiple attempts at fixation of this fracture will inevitably lead to comminution or deformity of the fracture fragment and make a good result unobtainable.

Several steps are carefully executed to maximize results. A 0.045 in. K-wire is driven from the distal phalanx articular surface volar to the fracture line to the fingertip and withdrawn to the articular surface for passage across the DIP joint after fracture reduction. Care is taken to avoid placement of this wire within the fracture site to avoid creating an obstacle for complete reduction. With the DIP joint openly flexed, the PIP in extension, and the metacarpophalangeal (MCP) in hyperextension, the fracture fragment is reduced.

A second wire is then driven through the extensor tendon proximal to the bone fragment through the head of the middle phalanx at a 45 degree angle to the coronal plane. This acts as a blocking pin to proximal migration of the fragment. The pin should also be oriented from the midline to lateral on the sagittal plane. This provides ample midline space for passage of the longitudinal pin across the DIP joint after the joint is returned to the extended position and the fracture is reduced. A third pin may then be introduced perpendicular to the fracture plane through the fragment if it is large enough to accommodate additional fixation.

Other methods may be employed for fixation of these fractures, including K-wire fixation without blocking pins, tension-band wiring, and pullout suture/button or anchor fixation. In all cases, however, the goal is to avoid further compromise of the terminal tendon while reducing the DIP joint. A final caution is added against pinning the DIP joint in extreme (greater than 20 degrees) hyperextension. Although the DIP joint that is splinted in hyperextension tends to regain excellent flexion, those pinned in this position have a proclivity to remain stiff and less functional.

Extra-articular Proximal and Middle Phalanx Fractures

Nonoperative Treatment

The anatomy of the proximal and middle phalanges is similar. They are both tubular bones with articular surfaces at both ends, the distal of each being nearly identical bicondylar morphology. The distal extents of both phalanges are also notable for a subcondylar fossa region that accommodates the distal member in flexion. Although the proximal

articulations differ, both are concave and supported by a flared metaphyseal region.

There are slight differences in the soft tissue relationships that must be recalled and respected when considering injuries and subsequent treatments in these bones. Collateral ligaments support both the MCP and the PIP joint, yet the proximal stabilizers have both epiphyseal and metaphyseal insertions, whereas the PIP joint collaterals are almost exclusively attached to the epiphysis. The extensor tendon central slip inserts on the dorsal epiphysis of the middle phalanx. The proximal phalanx has no flexor insertions, whereas the flexor digitorum superficialis inserts on volar ridges over the central 60% of the middle phalanx.

Extra-articular fractures of the proximal and middle phalanges can thus be subdivided by region but are still considered together because their behavior and management are quite similar.

Phalangeal Neck Fractures

Phalangeal neck fractures are almost exclusively seen in children but can present in the adult as a result of sporting or occupational trauma. These may be treated by closed methods if nondisplaced but usually require open reduction and internal fixation (ORIF). The displaced phalangeal neck fracture is usually dorsally displaced and rotated 90 degrees so that the articular surface of the phalangeal head faces dorsally (**Fig. 18–3**).

Fractures of the Phalangeal Shaft

Phalangeal shaft fractures may be of a simple identifiable pattern (transverse, oblique, spiral) or comminuted, with

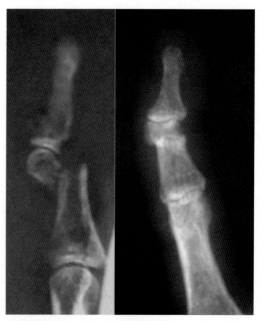

Figure 18–3 Subcondylar or neck fracture of the P2 phalanx, with extended distal articular fragment.

or without bone deficits. These fractures must be assessed for their reducibility and subsequent stability. Nondisplaced fractures may be treated in a closed fashion if great care is taken to ensure proper rotation, and unstable patterns are closely monitored for later displacement. Spiral oblique fractures are rarely treated nonoperatively due to their tendency to shorten and rotate. Transverse midshaft fractures that require closed reduction are also to be closely observed because they tend to angulate over time. Proximal phalangeal shaft fractures assume an apex volar position because of the strong pull of the interosseous muscles on the proximal fragment. Middle phalangeal fractures may display angulation in either apex volar or dorsal positions depending on the mechanism of the injury and the relationship of the fracture line to the superficialis and central slip insertional forces.

Phalangeal base fractures of the proximal phalanx are amenable to closed treatment if nondisplaced or stable after closed reduction. The reduction is performed by flexion of the proximal fragment and MCP joint first, then flexion of the distal fragment to obtain reduction. This reduction must be viewed critically. Malrotation is common and difficult to assess without the benefit of being able to bring the digit through a range of motion to detect scissoring. Minimal degrees of volar angulation and shortening can yield poor functional results. Acceptable closed reductions are held in the safe position (MCP joints maximally flexed, PIP joint extended) for 3 to 4 weeks before beginning gentle motion under the guidance of a therapist.

Surgical Treatment

Indications for surgical management of these phalangeal fractures include open fractures, failure of closed reduction, unstable fracture patterns (particularly spiral oblique fractures), and malrotation. The challenge is successfully balancing the concepts of stability and mobility while matching the appropriate fixation device to the fracture pattern, all in the setting of extreme emphasis on dexterity and ultimate motion recovery. Surgical management of these fractures will be addressed by fracture pattern.

Transverse Shaft Fractures

The realistic choices for treatment of transverse fracture of tubular bones are pins or plates; simple interfragmentary screws are not useful because of the fracture orientation. The decision on whether to pin or plate will be based upon the behavior of the fracture and the potential for optimizing outcome by striking the optimal balance between surgical morbidity (favoring closed pinning) and potential for an accelerated rehabilitation program (favoring plating).

One of the most effective, yet technically challenging, methods of closed treatment is collateral recess pinning. Using this technique, one or two pins are introduced from the phalangeal head region in a retrograde direction, crossing the fracture plane and penetrating the subchondral bone or opposite endosteum of the proximal fragment. When two pins can be accommodated in the canal, this crossing construct provides rotational control. Pins are kept extra-articular in the distal aspect of the phalanx in an effort to minimize joint stiffness. The collateral ligaments of the interphalangeal (IP) joints originate dorsal to the axis of rotation of the phalangeal head. Here the collateral recess provides a bony landmark for palpation. This surface irregularity in the phalangeal shaft offers purchase for the introduction of the very obliquely oriented pins, preventing extracortical deflection **(Fig. 18–4A,B)**.

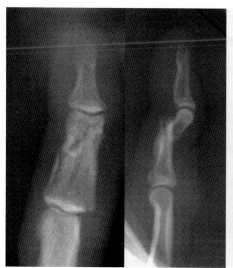
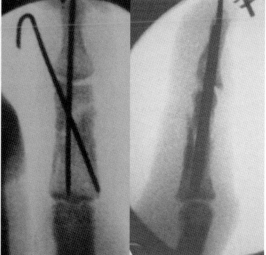

A   B

Figure 18–4 (A) Anteroposterior and lateral views of an extra-articular P2 fracture with longitudinal diaphyseal extension. **(B)** Postoperative series demonstrating a combination of collateral recess pinning and transarticular pinning.

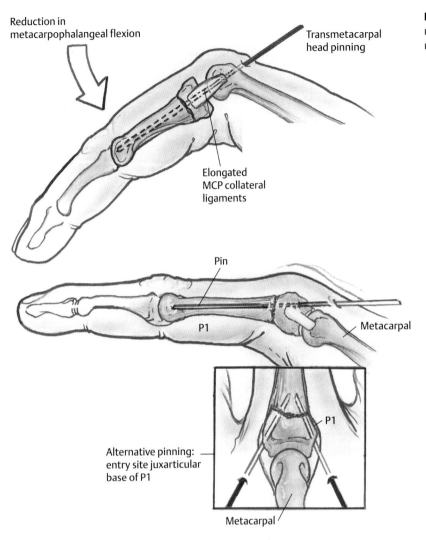

Reduction in metacarpophalangeal flexion

Transmetacarpal head pinning

Elongated MCP collateral ligaments

Pin

P1

Metacarpal

Alternative pinning: entry site juxarticular base of P1

P1

Metacarpal

Figure 18–5 Intramedullary (Eaton-Belsky) pinning of proximal phalangeal base fractures. MCP, metacarpophalangeal.

Tips and Tricks

- When utilizing the collateral recess pinning technique, two technical tricks should be employed. The two pins should initially be placed only up to the fracture plane. One pin may then be used as a joystick to aid in reduction under fluoroscopic control while the second pin achieves initial fixation. The rotation is then assessed prior to passage of the second pin. The most difficult part of this technique is the oblique introduction of the pins. This should be achieved first so that the required manipulation does not disrupt an initial reduction or single pin fixation. The second technical consideration is soft tissue management. Introduction of the pins should be attempted with the finger in the intrinsic plus position (IP extended). This will prevent the percutaneous pins from both tethering the soft tissue and mechanically blocking IP joint extension.

- For selected extra-articular transverse fractures of the proximal phalangeal base that are unstable and may not be amenable to the use of a condylar blade plate, a specific transarticular pinning method provides both fracture stability and internal splinting of the MCP joint in flexion, the lengthened position for the collateral ligaments. As described by

Belsky et al,7 this technique is simpler than collateral recess pinning and avoids manipulation of the soft tissue envelope of the PIP joint **(Fig. 18–5)**. The fractures are reduced with distraction and MCP flexion. A Kirschner wire is introduced through the head of the metacarpal and into the base fragment of the flexed proximal phalanx. The wire is driven to the level of the fracture line. This first maneuver stabilizes the small proximal fragment and makes an accurate reduction under image intensifier more easily obtainable.

- Distraction and flexion across the fracture plane provide reduction that can be secured by driving the wire across the fracture line and down the medullary canal. After the first wire is in place, meticulous assessment of digital rotation provides an opportunity to adjust the final reduction prior to passage of a second antiparallel wire to hold rotation **(Fig. 18–6)**. This second wire may be driven through the metacarpal head or may alternatively be introduced via the lateral cortical margin of the phalangeal base—a technique that is particularly well suited for the radial border of the index digit and the ulnar border of the small digit.

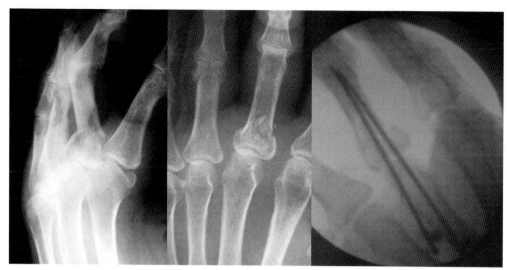

Figure 18–6 For selected fractures of the proximal phalanx, a single or dual pinning Eaton-Belsky technique can be employed. A clinical example of a displaced metadiaphyseal proximal phalanx fracture treated with two 0.045 in. smooth wires used to stabilize the fracture in a reduced position.

Spiral Oblique Fractures

In our experience, these fractures are best treated with interfragmentary screw fixation **(Fig. 18–7)**. This provides the rigidity and early motion benefits of internal fixation without the prominence and excessive tendon contact of plating. Most often seen in the proximal phalanx, these fractures can be approached via a gentle curvilinear incision over the proximal phalanx. This incision should sweep volar to the finger's midaxis at the PIP level to maximize exposure. Although longitudinal splitting of the extensor tendon is commonly employed, we prefer one of several other extensor handling options to provide exposure with minimal postoperative adhesions.

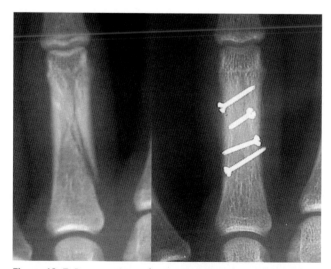

Figure 18–7 Preoperative and postoperative radiographs of oblique midshaft proximal phalanx fracture with interfragmentary screws.

Wide exposure may be achieved by excision of one of the oblique bands of the extensor hood distal to the MP joint sagittal bands and lateral to the central extensor tendon **(Fig. 18–8)**. Excising this triangle of extensor on the radial aspect of the digit also minimizes the chance of postoperative intrinsic adhesions.[8]

An alternative deep exposure that is used when a fracture line extends over the entire diaphysis, or even enters the PIP joint, is the Chamay exposure.[9] In this seldom-needed but useful technique, the extensor apparatus is incised as a distally based V, with the central slip insertion on the middle phalanx as the base of this tendon flap **(Fig. 18–9)**.

Thorough clearance of debris in the fracture plane, meticulous reduction, provisional wire fixation, and attention to proper technique are the ingredients of a successful result with these fractures. As with all applications of interfragmentary screw fixation, care should be taken to introduce the screws out of plane in relation to each other and sufficiently distant from each other and the fracture line to prevent iatrogenic fragmentation.

Comminuted Phalangeal Shaft Fractures

These fractures usually result from higher energy mechanisms, so the soft tissue envelope is often compromised; in addition to assessment of skin integrity and fracture pattern, determination of neurovascular status is important. The results are predictably poorer than noncomminuted phalangeal shaft fractures, and fixation can be more challenging. If the comminution is minimal, percutaneous pinning may provide adequate control of the major fragments and maintain alignment during the healing phase.

Moderately or severely comminuted phalanx fractures often display an intact base and head with primarily central

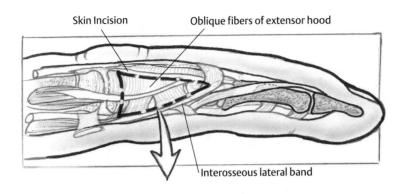

Skin Incision

Oblique fibers of extensor hood

Interosseous lateral band

Figure 18–8 Surgical exposure of the proximal phalanx with minimal disruption of the dorsal extensor mechanism can be done by excision of the lateral band "triangle" component of the extensor hood. This provides access to the midlateral aspect of the proximal phalanx.

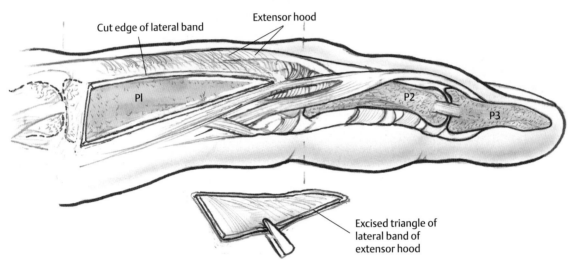

Cut edge of lateral band

Extensor hood

Pl

P2

P3

Excised triangle of lateral band of extensor hood

diaphyseal destruction. These fractures may best be addressed with minicondylar blade plating **(Fig. 18–10A,B).** This technique provides a rigid construct to prevent shortening and malrotation. A 1.5 mm minifragmentary system should be used on the proximal or middle phalanx. The blade may be placed proximally or distally and should be used on the end with less length of intact bone (i.e., where the greatest need for the stability of the blade construct exists).

The ideal position for the plate placement is subject to several key factors: purchase of the blade and juxta-articular screw, maximization of cortical contact when the fracture is reduced, and purchase of the screws into diaphyseal fragments. These factors can usually be addressed while also placing the plate along one of the lateral margins of

the phalanx, thus minimizing its contact with the extensor mechanism.

After one of the appropriate extensor-side exposures is obtained, the blade is introduced first. We have typically employed a smooth 0.045 in. wire for provisional reduction; the wire can later be exchanged for the screw that accompanies the blade, so it is placed in a slightly eccentric position. The location of the blade is then determined by direct visualization using the selected implant.

The hole for the blade is predrilled parallel to the articular surface with the 1.5 mm drill bit. The plate's blade is cut to match the measured depth. Although most commercially available systems have precontoured their plates to accommodate the metaphyseal flare, additional plate bending may be desired. The advantage of leaving in the

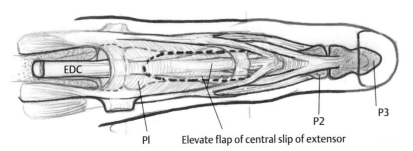

EDC

Pl

Elevate flap of central slip of extensor

P2

P3

Figure 18–9 The dorsal Chamay approach to the dorsal aspect of the proximal phalanx and proximal interphalangeal joint. This approach is based on a distally based flap of the central slip, which is elevated off the proximal phalanx while maintaining its insertion into the middle phalanx. The lateral bands are left intact. EDC, extensor digitorum communes tendon.

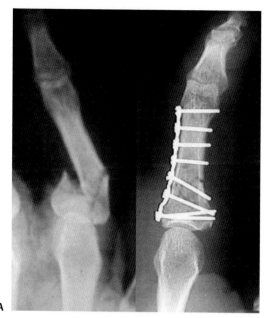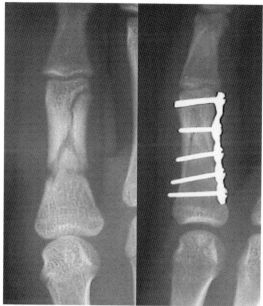

A   **B**

Figure 18–10 Preoperative and postoperative radiographs of comminuted proximal phalanx fractures treated with minicondylar blade plate technique. Note that the blade component can be utilized both proximally and distally to stabilize the more comminuted segments. **(A)** Blade placed proximally to treat MCP joint comminution. **(B)** Blade placed distally to treat PIP joint comminution.

provisional wire is now apparent because the screw hole aperture in the plate adjacent to the blade can be slipped over the pin to guide the plate into position.

Often, we have found it useful to employ a reduction clamp or other compression device to firmly seat the blade in position. After confirming reduction and length/position of hardware the parallel screw is applied at the base of the plate locking the plate into position. The rest of the screws are then applied along the available cortical bone across the fracture site.

In some of the most severely comminuted phalangeal fractures, there is not available purchase for plate or wire

fixation. In this setting external fixation is an option that needs to be considered. These can be constructed with K-wires and elastics, or commercially available fixators may be used. The specifics of the use and applications of external fixation devices on the phalanges will be discussed in greater detail in the section to follow on PIP fractures. The fixators can be joint spanning or nonspanning **(Fig. 18–11)**, fixed or dynamic.

Periarticular or intra-articular fractures may require spanning fixators to get adequate purchase for the half-pins or K-wires. If a joint needs to be spanned, two considerations must be entertained to minimize potential

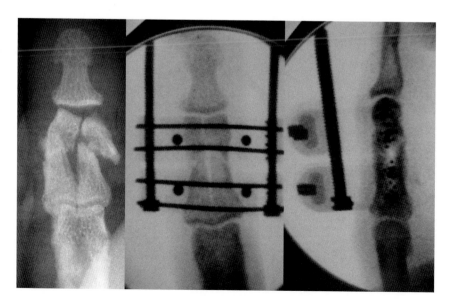

Figure 18–11 Preoperative and postoperative radiographs of a comminuted middle phalanx fracture treated with nonspanning external fixation.

joint stiffness as a result of the prolonged distraction. If spanning the PIP joint to treat a comminuted middle phalanx fracture, efforts should be made to use dynamic fixation using a laterally mounted fixator with proximal pin through the axis of rotation of the head of the proximal phalanx. This construct is less often utilized at the MCP level because of the inaccessible location of the metacarpal head in nonborder digits.

The second consideration is positioning of nondynamic spanning fixators. If the spanned joint cannot be mobilized, efforts should be made to distract the joint in the intrinsic plus position (MCPs flexed, IPs extended). This is more easily achieved at the IP joints than at the MCP.

Regardless of the selected method of fixation of these comminuted fractures, always consider the need for bone graft. These fractures are often impacted and demonstrate poor bony contact of fragments. Small portions of cancellous bone can readily be harvested from the dorsal distal radius through a corticotomy created on the floor of the second extensor compartment immediately proximal to Lister's tubercle. Alternatively, some surgeons prefer harvesting graft from the volar approach under the pronator teres—this site can yield excellent corticocancellous graft for spanning large intercalary defects. Exposure is provided through a minimal incision between the long digital flexors and the radial artery (volar approach of Henry). A third option in the setting of multiple digital trauma is bone graft from other amputated digits if applicable and available.

The Proximal Interphalangeal Joint

The PIP joint has rightly been the focus of extraordinary attention in our surgical specialty. It has been described as the "epicenter of the hand" and has been the subject of exhaustive mathematical (Fibonacci) as well as anatomical and surgical study.

Anatomy

The same qualities that make PIP motion vital to almost all dexterous hand function also place the joint in a vulnerable position for injury. Its bicondylar hinge joint design offers 110 degrees of flexion arc and will allow only 7 to 10 degrees of lateral motion in its midrange of flexion.[10] Several anatomical features afford this stability. The matched bony architecture of the condylar heads of the proximal phalanx and the concave facets of the base of the middle phalanx provide a stable infrastructure. This is reinforced by the intrinsic capsular supports of a stout volar plate and collateral ligaments. The extensor tendon inserting at the dorsal base of the middle phalanx and the long flexors of the digits provide secondary extrinsic stabilizers along with the oblique and transverse retinacular ligaments. Axial, extension, rotational, and lateral bending forces challenge this

combination of bony, intrinsic, and extrinsic ligament restraints to maintain joint function and integrity.

The bony architecture of the proximal phalangeal head articulates with 110 degrees of joint surface of the base of the proximal phalanx. Because it permits 100 to 110 degrees of motion, the proximal phalangeal head provides 210 to 220 degrees of articular surface for normal motion. Unlike the cam-shaped MCP joint, the PIP joint's axis of rotation is equidistant from the articular surface throughout the arc of the curvature. To accommodate this requirement, the neck of the proximal phalanx is a narrow bony isthmus with a subcondylar fossa to accommodate the volar lip of the middle phalanx in maximal flexion. These architectural relationships make the joint both vulnerable to injury and intolerant of even minor derangement.

Examination of the relative anatomy of the PIP collateral ligaments and the volar plate is a requirement for a thorough understanding of PIP dislocations, fracture-dislocation of the base of the middle phalanx, and fractures of the proximal phalangeal head. The collateral ligaments originate from the collateral recesses. These are bony depressions located dorsal to the axis of rotation of the proximal phalangeal head. Two components of the collaterals extend distally and volarly. The primary collateral ligament (PCL) is the larger of the two, inserting on the most volar three quarters of the base of the middle phalanx and distal margin of the volar plate. The accessory collateral ligament (ACL) inserts primarily into the volar plate and dorsal aspect of the flexor sheath. The ACL acts as a support sling for the flexor sheath, maintaining a constant moment arm throughout the joint's range of motion. On the joint's flexor surface is the stout fibrous volar plate (VP). Its distal insertion is strongest at the lateral margins of the base of the middle phalanx. This is also the site of insertion of the ACL. The volar plate's fibrocartilage matrix is oriented transversely here, making this distal insertion susceptible to the dorsal longitudinal stress forces that result in PIP dislocations.

Dorsal Dislocation of the Proximal Interphalangeal Joint

The PIP joint can dislocate dorsally, laterally, and volarly. These terms describe the position of the middle phalanx as related to the articular head of the proximal phalanx.

Dorsal dislocations are the most common form of PIP dislocation and are created by a hyperextension and axial loading force. These demonstrate predictable failure patterns of the intrinsic support system, with avulsion of the volar plate insertion occurring first. This injury alone can result in a hyperextended subluxation of the joint. When the injurious forces are of sufficient magnitude and direction, the pathology extends as a rent between the accessory and proper collateral ligaments. In this situation the middle phalanx can completely dislocate dorsally, with the PCL adhering to the base of the middle phalanx.[10]

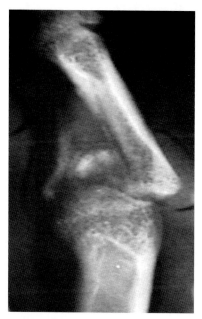

Figure 18–12 Oblique view of a pilon fracture of the base of the middle phalanx. Note the depressed central fragment of the articular surface.

Biomechanical studies have shown that one third of dorsally directed stress injuries applied to PIP joints will result in fracture-dislocations of the "conventional" type.[11] In this situation the volar plate is avulsed with a portion of the weak trabecular bone on the volar central lip of the middle phalanx. Injuries of greater magnitude, with slightly greater axial force application vectors, can lead to central impaction of the base of the middle phalanx. These are also known as pilon fractures. The signature of the pilon fracture is a compressed central articular base fracture of the middle phalanx **(Fig. 18–12)**. The volar lip (site of volar plate attachment) and the dorsal lip (site of central slip attachment) may be intact or are often "splayed out" as the trabecular bone fails in compression.

Perhaps the most important characteristic of dorsal dislocations or fracture-dislocations is whether they can be reduced by closed methods, and whether that reduction can be maintained in a concentric relationship. Therefore, these injuries can be categorized into stable and unstable groups, as determined by their maintenance of reduction when brought into extension.

A fracture fragment encompassing greater than 40% of the middle phalangeal joint surface will likely result in an unstable reduction due to the loss of the buttressing articulating support provided by the volar lip of the middle phalanx **(Fig. 18–13)**.

Closed Treatment

Dorsal dislocations can be readily reduced with manipulation under digital block anesthesia. Longitudinal distraction combined with dorsal pressure applied to the proximal phalangeal head results in a satisfying reduction. X-rays are taken to confirm concentric reduction. Four days of dorsal block splinting is provided. Joint motion is then vigorously pursued to avoid permanent joint stiffness.

Fracture-dislocations are reduced similarly and tested for stability in extension with the benefit of digital block anesthesia. Those that are stable in extension are started on a dorsal block splinting regimen, popularized by McElfresh et al.[12] Once it has been determined that a reduction is stable to about the 30 to 45 degree range, a dorsal splint is fabricated that excludes the last 45 degrees of extension while permitting flexion to the level of comfort or ability to move the usually swollen digit.

After 5 to 7 days, a 30 degree blocker is substituted, followed 1 week later with either a final 10 to 15 degree blocker or, more often, simple buddy taping. The result is a minimally swollen digit with greater than 95 to 100 degrees

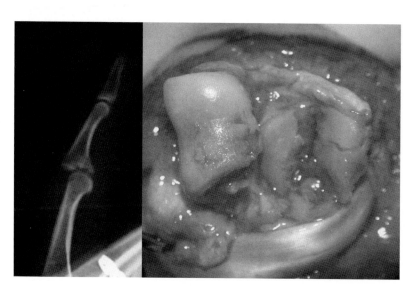

Figure 18–13 Unstable proximal interphalangeal (PIP) fracture dislocation. Note the depressed and comminuted volar articular surface evident radiographically and upon exploration of the joint. Opposing PIP joint surfaces are "shotgunned" open to demonstrate.

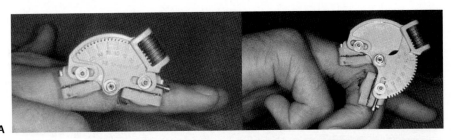

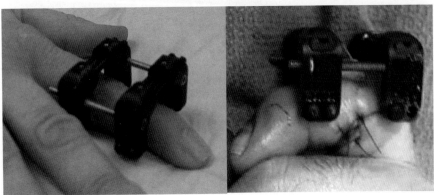

Figure 18–14 Examples of commercially available dynamic proximal interphalangeal external fixators. **(A)** The unilateral Compass Hinge (Smith-Nephew Richards, Memphis, Tennessee). **(B)** BioSymMetRic Fixator (Biomet, Warsaw, Indiana).

of flexion and near full extension (perhaps lacking 10 degrees) at the third postinjury week. More advanced specific rehabilitation techniques are then employed to gain the residual arc of motion.

Rarely, unstable fracture-dislocations will be difficult to reduce and demonstrate persistent dorsal subluxation with midrange extension. These require surgical treatment to obtain joint reduction, restore articular congruity, and maintain reduction.

Surgical Treatment of Unstable Proximal Interphalangeal Fracture-Dislocations

Once the determination of irreducibility and/or recurrent instability is made, the surgeon must select from a variety of options for surgical management. Unstable fracture-dislocations that demonstrate adequate reduction and articular congruity with distraction and volar force applied to the base of the middle phalanx are candidates for ORIF, dynamic external fixation, or both. Those fractures that do not demonstrate adequate articular congruity with manipulation will likely require ORIF with pins or screws, or a volar plate arthroplasty.

Dynamic External Fixation

The dynamic external fixator is a method of neutralization of the deforming injury forces that may act on a compromised skeletal foundation or a joint. It should be used to protect reduction and other means of fixation but should not be considered as a primary means of reduction and fixation or a panacea that obviates the need for sound primary treatment of PIP fracture-dislocations.

A distinct advantage of the advanced PIP fixators is that they enable the patient to start mobilization early in the postoperative course. If the distraction maintains reduction through a range of motion, the minimal dissection required for fixator placement is preferable to extensive exposure of a comminuted fracture. Frames may be unilateral or bilateral, constructed by the surgeon, or commercially produced (**Fig. 18–14A,B**). In our experience, unilateral fixators provide less stability than bilateral frames. Asymmetric impaction and extensive soft tissue disruption typically require the control afforded by bilateral frames. Unilateral fixation is probably best reserved for contracture releases or other minor PIP injuries when there is little or no compromise to the basic skeleton.

Of the commercially available frames, only one affords bilateral control, the BioSymMetRic Fixator (Biomet, Warsaw, Indiana). This design can be used as a static or dynamic frame, allows for variable distraction, and the box configuration is biomechanically strong. The radiolucent frame does not obscure the PIP joint, permitting easy visualization of the joint reduction at the time of surgery and during follow-up. It can be placed in a static fashion or a dynamic mode and easily converted. This enables it to be used as a miniexternal fixator for complex fractures and then be converted to a dynamic distraction frame to allow early motion.

A commonly used unilateral commercially available frame, the Compass Hinge (Smith-Nephew Richards, Inc. Memphis, Tennessee) allows for very facile conversion from static to dynamic modes. However, some elements of the frame and the worm gear are not radiolucent and often obscure visualization of the joint. The Compass Hinge's ability to control the extremely complex fracture-dislocations is limited because of its unilateral design. It is anchored to the phalanges with smooth wires that tend to deform or loosen with time. The passive motion advancement feature is unique and clever but can be duplicated by cooperative patients who pursue a supervised rehabilitation regimen. Nevertheless, the ability to incrementally advance the PIP joint through this passive means is a singular option available only with the Compass Hinge.

Application of a Bilateral Dynamic External Fixator

Regardless of fixator model choice, the most integral step in the application is the identification and instrumentation of the PIP axis of rotation. The axis of rotation for the PIP joint is a single point that is equidistant from the distal, palmar, and dorsal surfaces of the head of the proximal phalanx.

Under fluoroscopic guidance, care must be exercised to obtain a lateral view where the proximal phalanx condyles completely overlap; this is a perfect lateral view. The tip of one of the external fixator pins is placed in the center of the head under the fluoroscopic image.

On gross examination the axis of rotation can be determined by locating the point of intersection between the flexion crease line and the midaxial line with the PIP joint flexed. The wire driver is brought into the plane of the fluoroscopy beam, and the pin is driven across the axis. If the pin is placed correctly, it appears as a single dot on a perfect lateral of the proximal phalanx.

After accurate placement of the axis of rotation pins, two parallel pins are placed in the midaxis of the middle phalanx. The frame of the external fixator has radiographic markers that can be used as a guide to pin placement. Prior to pin insertion through the frame, it is important to ensure that room has been left for eventual distraction. The two pins in the middle phalanx should pass transversely through the axis in a parallel orientation to each other. This will maintain a linear relationship between the proximal and middle phalanges when the frame is applied. The frame is quadrangular in shape, controlling the PIP joint from both sides, and affords the potential for differential distraction of the joint on the side of asymmetrical depression.

The radial and ulnar sides of the fixator are connected and stabilized dorsally by two transverse rails. These set the width of the frame to accommodate swelling and prevent irritation. The screw mechanism for distraction is located at the distal aspect of the frame so it can be accessed for later adjustment in an office setting. Both the radial and ulnar sides of the frame have a distraction mechanism. This allows for differential distraction and correction of radial/ulnar deviation that may be an issue in more comminuted pilon fractures or for protection of tenuous fixation or incompetent soft tissues.

In selected circumstances (bone loss, extensive comminution with tenuous fixation, some children's PIP injuries, midshaft fractures), the frame may be applied as a static fixator. This is achieved by placing a fourth pin through the frame in the proximal phalanx parallel to the previous pins in the midaxial plane.

When the surgeon is ready to allow the patient to begin motion, the fixator can be converted from the static to the dynamic mode in the office by removal of this pin without releasing the distraction of the fixator.

Bent Wire Fixation

Bent wire fixators are of lower cost and are made from readily available materials **(Fig. 18–15).** These are a good option if cost is a factor or a commercial fixator is not available. Having some facility with the application of one or more of these frames is essential for any surgeon treating complex hand trauma. There has been substantial interest in developing "homemade" bent wire fixators in the last half decade. Agee, Slade, and others have reported their innovative designs for these devices.[13–17]

The majority of these fixators can be used in a dynamic fashion and provide longitudinal distraction only. The Agee force-couple bent wire fixator has an additional component of volar translation force to the base of the middle phalanx that can be employed if longitudinal distraction alone results in any dorsal translation or loss of reduction during range of motion under fluoroscopy.

A basic bent wire fixator design is obtained by placing an axis of rotation pin in the head of the proximal phalanx, as already described. A second parallel pin is placed along the shaft of the middle phalanx. On each side of the digit, the axis of rotation pin is bent 90 degrees in the direction of the fingertip. The wire should be long enough to extend beyond the fingertip. The distalmost aspect of the pin is bent into an S configuration. The second middle phalanx

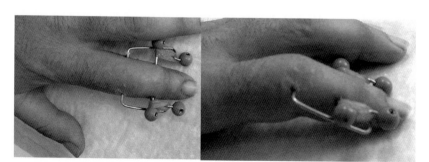

Figure 18–15 Bent wire proximal interphalangeal external fixator with rubber band distraction.

pin is bent into a U configuration. This provides a housing for elastic bands to pull the two constructs together, thereby distracting across the PIP joint. To provide more stability to the construct, a third parallel pin is placed more proximally in the midaxis of the middle phalanx. The ends of this pin are bent around the shaft of the longitudinal arm of the axis of rotation pin in an "eye hook" pattern. This maintains the longitudinal arm in alignment with the digit throughout a range of motion. The distraction can be altered by increasing or decreasing the number of elastic bands applied and can easily be adjusted in the office postoperatively.

A second substantially different design requires mention. The Agee force-couple design provides a simultaneous palmar translation force on the base of the middle phalanx and a dorsal translation force on the head of the proximal phalanx.[13] Through an ingenious use of a lever and elastic tension, this simply constructed fixator provides a continuous reduction force throughout a range of motion of the PIP joint.

The Agee force-couple fixator utilizes three pins. The first is a transverse pin through the axis of rotation of the proximal phalangeal head, executed similarly to those for the fixators mentioned earlier. This pin serves as a fulcrum for leverage of the second pin. The second pin is inserted in the base of the middle phalanx, distal to the fracture line, and dorsal to the midaxis of the phalanx. Both ends of the second pin are bent 90 degrees and oriented proximally, passing volar to the first (axis of rotation) pin. A second bend is then made in the pin, orienting the ends to point dorsally.

The third pin should be a terminally threaded 0.062 in. wire driven perpendicular to the digit through the dorsum of the middle phalanx, approximately 1 cm distal to the insertion of the central slip. Elastic bands are then applied between the central distal pin and the two vertical arms of the proximally bent pin. This force translates into a joint-reducing force as already described through the leverage of the distal bent pin around the axis of the rotation pin. This is maintained throughout active motion of the digit.

Postoperative Management for Fixation Devices

Active range of motion exercises and edema control are begun under the guidance of a hand therapist 3 to 5 days after surgery. Radiographs should be checked at 2 week intervals. Removal of the frame may be performed in the office at 4 weeks or when radiographs show fracture healing. The patient continues active and passive range of motion exercises and starts a progressive strengthening program.

Open Treatment of Proximal Interphalangeal Fracture-Dislocations

If distraction across the PIP joint cannot obtain congruity of the PIP joint surface, open reduction with or without external fixation needs to be pursued. The cost of widely open management of these fractures is a significant loss of motion, so minimally invasive techniques should be employed when feasible. Fracture fragments can often be manipulated with percutaneous joystick pins to set the stage for percutaneous pinning (often in conjunction with external fixation).

A centrally depressed pilon fracture with a well-reduced volar margin of the middle phalanx is another example of a fracture that will not reduce with distraction but can often be addressed in a minimally invasive fashion (**Fig. 18–16A–E**). For these fractures a small dorsal incision can be made over the middle phalanx. The triangular ligament distal to the central slip insertion is incised, providing access to the dorsal cortex. A small corticotomy is fashioned to allow access to the medullary canal. Bone graft can then be introduced and densely packed down into the base of the middle phalanx. This can often permit the surgeon to tamp down the centrally depressed fragment and obtain articular congruity assessed under magnified fluoroscopic view. These fractures should always be protected by external fixation to neutralize the compressive forces across the PIP joint postoperatively (**Fig. 18–17**).

If the foregoing methods fail, a more invasive approach is made via a midaxial or volar Brunner incision and exposure of the flexor sheath over the PIP joint. If the fragments can be reduced and pinned or screwed without violating the flexor sheath, this should be attempted. In the most severe unstable fracture dislocations, the volar base will be too comminuted to permit congruous reduction of the joint surface. In this case a volar plate arthroplasty is a reasonable option.[18] This procedure provides a soft tissue arthroplasty of the volar half of the base of the middle phalanx for articulation with the proximal phalangeal head. The exposure of the volar plate requires opening the flexor tendon sheath between the A2 and A4 pulleys. The flexor tendons are retracted laterally as atraumatically as possible. The distal margin of the volar plate is liberated from fragments of the destroyed volar margin fracture. The fracture site is cleared of debris, and a smooth transverse margin of intact dorsal cartilage is created. This is meticulously performed so that the advanced volar plate will abut the intact dorsal cartilage evenly across the entire width of the phalanx and provide a smooth, gliding surface for the head of the proximal phalanx. Adequate advancement of the volar plate is achieved by collateral ligament resection. The distal end of the volar plate is secured in position adjacent to the dorsal cartilage with pullout sutures. These are usually secured to the lateral margins of the volar plate, passed through drilled bone tunnels to be tied over the dorsum of the middle phalanx distal to the central slip insertion within the substance of the triangular ligament.

Postoperative Management for Open Treatment of Proximal Interphalangeal Fracture-Dislocations

Rehabilitation after open treatment of PIP fracture-dislocations varies according to the individual patient's

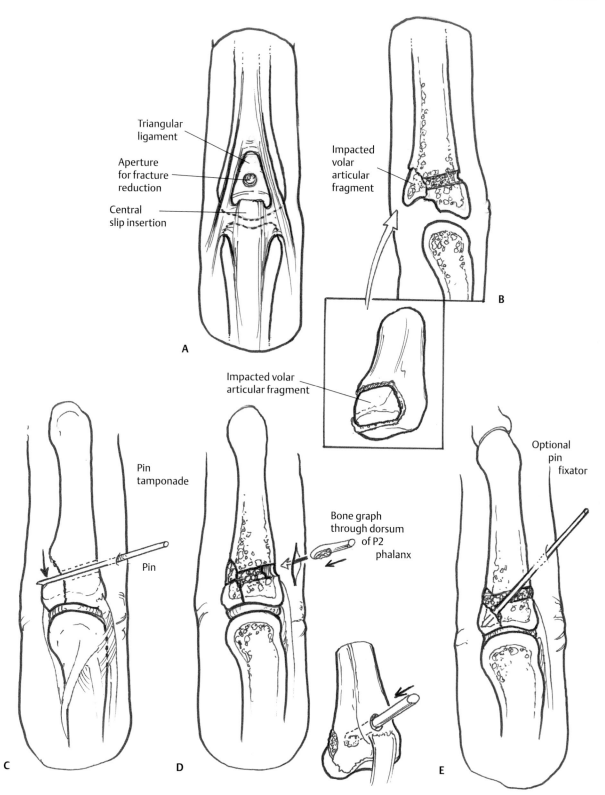

Figure 18–16 Technique of reduction and bone grafting of depressed proximal interphalangeal fracture dislocations performed via a corticotomy on the dorsum of the middle phalanx. Note that the corticotomy is made in the region of the triangular ligament in an attempt to leave the rest of the extensor mechanism undisturbed. **(A)** Corticotomy created at dorsal base of proximal phalanx in location of triangular ligament, distal to central slip insertion. **(B)** Corticotomy allows access to impacted volar lip fragment. **(C)** Kirshner wire introduced via corticotomy is employed to obtain fracture reduction. **(D)** Reduced fragment may be supported with bone graft introduced through same aperture. **(E)** Reduced fracture fragments are then maintained with Kirshner wires and external fixation.

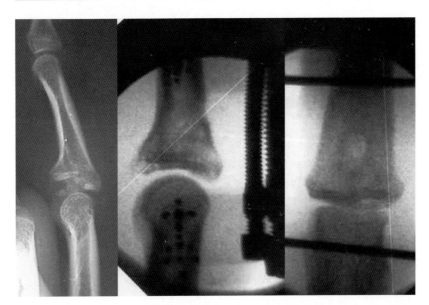

Figure 18–17 Preoperative and postoperative radiographs demonstrating depressed proximal interphalangeal fracture dislocation treated with reduction and bone grafting via a dorsal cortico-tomy of the middle phalanx. After the joint space is reduced and supported with bone graft, the reduction is protected with an external fixator.

circumstances and surgeon's comfort with the stability of fixation. However, there is a premium on early active motion to take advantage of the anatomical reduction and fracture stability.

Certainly, few fractures in the hand are as unforgiving as an openly treated PIP fracture with a long delay in postoperative mobilization. Most injury patterns and fixation constructs will be protected from subluxation or impaction by external fixation to provide dynamic rehabilitation while controlling dorsal subluxation forces and neutralizing longitudinal loading or compressive forces. In these cases the rehabilitation protocol will follow that outlined in the preceding section on external fixation.

The volar plate arthroplasty procedure is maintained in a flexed posture to take tension off the joint surface–volar plate interface while protecting the joint from the dorsal subluxation force exerted when the joint is in extension. Many surgeons will supplement the volar plate arthroplasty with a protective Kirschner wire through the flexed PIP joint, or through the head of the proximal phalanx as a blocking pin maintaining PIP flexion. These pins are removed at 3 weeks and replaced with a dorsal blocking splint. By the fourth week unrestricted active extension is permitted. Dynamic extension splinting is commenced at the fifth week if full extension is not achieved.

New Techniques

In the setting of severely comminuted and impacted fracture-dislocations of the base of the middle phalanx, investigators have pursued joint surface allografting using the distal articular surface of the hamate.[19] This aspect of the hamate has a dual facet surface for articulation with the fourth and fifth metacarpal bases. This surface demonstrates many of the same surface characteristics of the base of the proximal phalanx **(Fig. 18–18).** The technique

is technically demanding, utilizing wide exposure and mini-screw fixation, but early investigations are showing promise.

Lateral and Volar Dislocations of the Proximal Interphalangeal Joint

Two other fracture-dislocation patterns are encountered with less frequency. Lateral dislocations of the PIP joint result from torsional and/or lateral stress forces and result in a predictable sequence of disruption of the soft tissue stabilizers of the joint. Typically, the origin of the PCL first ruptures from the collateral recess of the proximal phalanx.

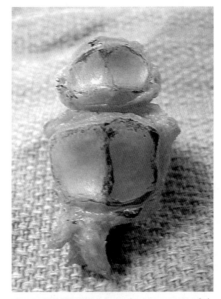

Figure 18–18 Anatomical comparison of the morphology of the P2 articular base (top) and the metacarpal facets of the hamate (bottom, note the hamulus).

This rupture extends into the junction of the ACL and PCL and can culminate in a distal volar plate rupture from its insertion on the middle phalanx.[10] The dislocation alone does not require surgical intervention except in rare cases. Indications for surgical management include instability due to complete collateral tears that fail closed management, or inability to obtain congruent reduction due to entrapment of the collateral ligament in the joint.[20] In these cases the joint will demonstrate an unbalanced articulation on anteroposterior (AP) radiograph, and no closed manipulation can affect or maintain reduction.

These collateral ligament avulsions can also present as fracture-dislocations with avulsed bony segments from either the origin or the insertion of the PCL. These injuries should be treated with a similar stepwise approach of the volar lip fracture-dislocations already described. Articular congruity should be established and maintained using any combination of closed treatment, pinning, external fixation, or open screw fixation.

Volar dislocations are the most unusual and distinctive of the three patterns. These are created from a volar translation or rotational force and are usually readily reducible. Two important points need to be remembered when these injuries are encountered. First, the dorsal tenting of the proximal phalangeal head against the extensor mechanism may enable one condyle to protrude through a rent between the central slip and the lateral band. If the reduction is attempted with the MCP joint in extension, distraction of the PIP may tighten the extensor mechanism around the condyle, making reduction impossible. Reduction attempts should be made with the MCP and PIP in flexion to decrease the tension on the volarly displaced lateral band. Should this not succeed, open reduction may be required.

The second caveat is the risk of central slip avulsion or marginal fracture avulsion in this setting. All volar dislocations should be evaluated after closed reduction or during open reduction for central slip integrity. After closed reduction this may best be evaluated as described by Elson.[21] The test is performed with the examiner maintaining the PIP joint in passive flexion over a 90 degree rigid surface, like a table top. The patient is asked to attempt to actively extend the DIP joint against resistance. When the central slip is intact, the lateral bands will be drawn distally with the intact central slip as it spans the flexed PIP joint. The lateral bands are kept in slack and are unable to extend the DIP. If the central slip insertion is completely disrupted, the lateral bands are untethered and have the ability to migrate proximally and actively extend the DIP joint.

Central slip avulsions may also occur with an associated fracture of the dorsal lip of the middle phalangeal base in axial load injuries. These fragments are usually quite small; however, they portend a significant central slip injury that can result in boutonniere deformity if left untreated.

Central slip avulsions or fracture avulsions should be treated surgically to reestablish the insertion's integrity.

Large fragments may be treated with 1.5 mm screw or Kirschner wire fixation. Smaller fragments or tendon avulsions may be treated with sure anchor fixation introduced dorsally and oriented distally and volarly to provide resistance to the vector of pull of the central slip. Regardless of fixation method, the surgeon must be meticulous in re-creating the normal anatomical position of the central slip mechanism. Overzealous reefing of the central slip distally will unbalance the complex relationships of the extensor mechanism and result in a DIP extensor lag. It is wise to protect the repair with a Kirschner wire crossing the PIP joint in extension for 3 weeks prior to starting protected motion under the supervision of a therapist with extension splinting.

Condylar Fractures of the Proximal Interphalangeal Joint

Condylar fractures of the head of the proximal phalanx are another commonly encountered subtype of intra-articular PIP fractures. These can occur on the coronal or sagittal plane and can involve one or both condyles. These fractures do not represent an avulsion injury but are rather sustained from axial loading of the joint with variable degrees of angulation. These are very difficult to manage because of the unstable nature of the fractures and their importance to congruent motion of the PIP joint. Closed treatment of nondisplaced condylar fractures often results in displacement, requiring delayed intervention. These fractures are best managed with operative fixation. Although multiple pin fixation may stabilize a well-reduced fragment, open reduction and interfragmentary screw fixation provides benefits of earlier rehabilitation (**Fig. 18–19**). Fragment size and configuration will dictate the feasibility of screw fixation. Bicondylar fractures are a particularly

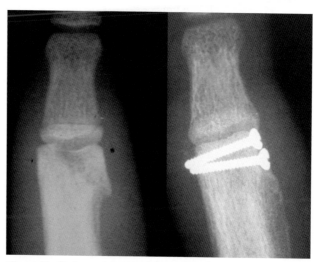

Figure 18–19 Preoperative and postoperative radiographs of a unicondylar fracture of the head of the proximal phalanx treated with interfragmentary screw fixation.

difficult variant that may be treated with minicondylar blade plate fixation or a combination of wire fixation and external fixation spanning the PIP joint.

Metacarpophalangeal Joint Dislocations

MCP joint dislocation is much less common in the adult than its PIP counterpart because of the relatively sturdy ligamentous housing of the MCP joint. The volar plate and collateral ligaments provide similar volar and lateral support without significant dorsal stabilizing capsular ligaments. The MCP construct is made significantly more stable, however, by the presence of stout intermetacarpal ligaments. These interconnect the volar plates of the second through fifth digits, creating a linked chain of intrinsic stabilizers. These structures, as well as the surrounding soft tissue envelope, make the MCP joints less exposed and prone to dislocation than the PIP joints.

When these dislocations occur, they most commonly involve the vulnerable border digits, with the index being most common. The vast majority are dorsal dislocations; volar MCP dislocations are very rare. Dorsal MCP dislocations are the result of a hyperextension force. Patients present with pain and inability to flex the MCP joint. The MCP joint is held in a mild hyperextension posture, with slight flexion at the distal joints.

There is characteristic skin puckering seen in the palm at the level of the joint, and the metacarpal head is prominent and palpable volarly. Radiographs may demonstrate an osteochondral shear fracture typically seen on the dorsal metacarpal head.[22]

Nonoperative Treatment

Nonoperative treatment is possible for subluxated MCP joints. In this case the volar plate has become disrupted proximally and is draped in hyperextension over (i.e., dorsal to) the metacarpal head. Reduction can be affected by application of a volar force applied to the dorsal base of the proximal phalanx, usually after insufflating the area of the joint with anesthetic medication. Attempts at longitudinal distraction or exaggeration of the hyperextension deformity will convert the reducible subluxation into an irreducible MCP dislocation by permitting the volar plate to fall dorsally between the metacarpal head and the base of the proximal phalanx. If a subluxated MCP joint is successfully reduced, the patient may be placed in a dorsal blocking splint, preventing hyperextension beyond neutral. Early active motion is started with the supervision of a therapist within a week of injury.

True dorsal dislocations, in contrast to subluxations, are rarely amenable to closed reduction. The volar plate becomes entrapped dorsal to the metacarpal head. The A1 pulley and flexor tendons remain attached to the volar plate, placing the flexor tendons dorsal to the metacarpal

head. In the case of index MCP dislocations, the flexors fall to the ulnar side of the metacarpal, whereas the lumbrical lies radial to the metacarpal. This creates a musculotendinous noose that tightens around the metacarpal neck with attempts at closed reduction via longitudinal distraction. This same anatomical relationship holds true for the rare central ray (long and ring) MCP dislocations. A slight variation occurs in small finger MCP dislocation where flexor tendons form the radial side of the noose, with the hypothenar muscles wrapping around the ulnar side of the metacarpal head. The surgeon must identify this anatomical obstacle and avoid numerous forceful reduction attempts to prevent undue damage to the articular surface of the metacarpal head.

Surgical Treatment

The approach to the irreducible MCP dislocation is determined by surgical preference. Both volar and dorsal exposures are feasible and safe in experienced hands. Delivering the desired result with the greatest margin of safety is the key, which is why there is general bias to choosing the dorsal approach. The dorsal approach is made via a gentle, curved, longitudinal incision. The extensor tendon and capsule are split longitudinally, or the sagittal bands are divided alongside the extensor. This provides ease of access to the former joint by inspecting the dorsally subluxated proximal phalanx. The interposed volar plate is typically found draped over the metacarpal head. Most often, the volar plate can simply be extricated from the joint by "pushing" it volarward with a blunt instrument such as a Freer elevator. Longitudinally splitting the volar plate may facilitate its extrusion from the joint in the rare instance that simple, direct manipulation is inadequate. The dorsal approach also provides excellent access for fixation for the occasional osteochondral shear fracture of the metacarpal head.

The volar approach provides access to the intrinsic and extrinsic flexors of the joint that often serve a secondary role in preventing reduction, as already described. Its disadvantages are the inaccessibility of dorsal shear fractures and relatively difficult access to the volar plate. The volar approach does, however, provide visualization of all of the other involved structures and offers the surgeon more of an ability to assess the joint when initial reduction attempts are hindered.

The volar approach is performed via a chevron or zigzag incision over the palpably prominent MCP head. Caution is required during dissection due to the immediate subdermal position of the tented digital nerve in the field (radial digital nerve in index dislocations and ulnar digital nerve in small finger dislocations). Soft tissue dissection is performed to permit the metacarpal head to project out of the wound while the proximal phalanx falls further dorsally. The A1 pulley is longitudinally released. These maneuvers relieve tension on the musculotendinous noose and permit the joint to be further hyperextended and the volar plate visualized. The volar plate and musculotendinous noose are then escorted volar to the metacarpal head, taking great care not to damage the cartilage surface of the joint. No soft tissue reconstruction is required because the wound is closed without suture of the volar plate. A dorsal blocking splint is used for 2 weeks and followed by active and passive range of motion exercises under the supervision of a therapist.

Metacarpal Fractures

The metacarpals are also frequently fractured tubular bones of the hand, but they possess different inherent osteology, surrounding soft tissue envelopes, and adjacent joint relationships when compared with the phalanges. For these reasons, the fracture patterns that affect the metacarpals, and the techniques employed to treat them, differ from those used in phalangeal fracture management.

It is logical to approach metacarpal fracture fixation by dividing the topic into the following anatomical subsections: (1) base fractures and carpometacarpal (CMC) dislocations, (2) fractures of the diaphysis, and (3) fractures of the metacarpal neck, or "boxer's" fractures. An interesting characteristic of metacarpal fracture management is that differing fracture types can often be managed by the same fixation technique.

Pertinent examples of the treatment commonality include the use of collateral recess pinning for stabilization of neck fractures, middiaphyseal fractures, and even CMC fracture-dislocations. We have had success managing a variety of fractures, even combination neck and head splitting fractures, with intramedullary ("bouquet") pinning. Therefore, we will describe in detail the techniques that are adaptable to metacarpal fracture fixation while also discussing the behavior of selected fracture types.

Base Fractures and Carpometacarpal Fracture-Dislocations

Distinct anatomical relationships exist at the base of the metacarpals. Because no extrinsic musculotendinous units insert on the carpus, the metacarpals are the initial site for distal anchoring of several tendon systems. The trabecular bone of the base is vulnerable to fracture from a variety of forces; this is especially true of the border digits. The relationships at the CMC joints are extremely stable in the radial rays, yet very mobile on the ulnar side.

Base Fractures

It is more logical to concentrate on selected fracture types of the metacarpal base, although almost any form of fracture pattern can manifest there. Avulsion fractures of the wrist flexor or extensor insertions and extra-articular

compression/impaction fractures can be seen and typically do not present management challenges.

Difficult fractures of the metacarpal base that warrant expanded discussion are the family of thumb base fractures, particularly the Bennett's and Rolando's variants, and the "reverse Bennett's" intra-articular fracture of the small ray.

Thumb Carpometacarpal Fracture-Dislocations

Bennett's Fracture

Fractures of the thumb metacarpal base, known as Bennett's fractures, require specific mention due to the unique anatomy of this joint and the specific demands of this fracture. Fractures of the thumb metacarpal base are produced by an axial load sustained by the flexed joint. The fracture line splits the articular surface, leaving a reduced smaller fragment on the volar ulnar surface attached to the anterior oblique ligament of the CMC joint. The larger portion of the articular surface, which actually includes the remainder of the thumb ray, is displaced dorsally, proximally, and radially with the intact metacarpal shaft. The unstable fracture pattern is further destabilized by the deforming forces of the insertion of the abductor pollicis longus muscle on the metacarpal base and the adductor pollicis muscle on the distal metacarpal.

Inadequate articular reduction leads to unsatisfactory results radiographically and functionally. It is rare for a Bennett's fracture to go on to nonunion; however, malunions are seen in those fractures in which anatomical reduction was not achieved early and maintained through healing.

Due to the difficulty in achieving and maintaining articular congruity in a closed fashion, these fractures are best treated with closed reduction and percutaneous pinning or ORIF. Percutaneous pinning is pursued if the volar-ulnar fragment is too small to provide purchase for screw fixation and anatomical closed reduction can be achieved. If adequate closed reduction cannot be performed, or if the fracture fragment is greater than about one third of the articular surface, open reduction and screw fixation is employed. With the advent of exceedingly small implants and the employment of smooth wires, even very small unstable fractures can be adequately secured.

Closed reduction is performed by providing a combination of longitudinal distraction and pronation to the thumb while applying volar-ulnar pressure on the metacarpal base. If this successfully reduces the articular surface, oblique 0.045 in. Kirschner wires are driven from the radial base of the thumb metacarpal into the trapezium and/or into the adjacent index metacarpal base. Including the smaller volar-ulnar metacarpal fragment in the construct is not essential because the major fragment is relocated and stabilized back to the trapezium and will unite with the nondisplaced minor fragment. These pins

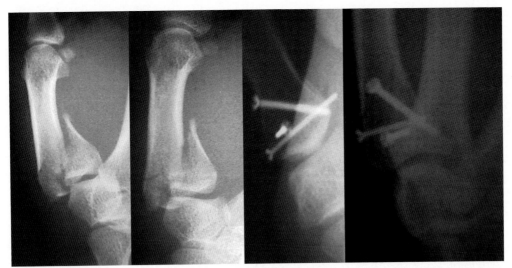

Figure 18–20 Preoperative and postoperative radiographs of a Rolando's fracture treated with interfragmentary screw fixation.

are left in position for 5 to 6 weeks with thumb spica splint protection.

Pinning is effective in accomplishing most goals of fracture fixation, except permitting early mobilization. Either the fracture pattern itself or the nature of the patient's needs (athlete, surgeon, etc.) may mitigate for more aggressive fracture fixation. Therefore, if open reduction is required or desired, the CMC joint is approached via a curvilinear volar Wagner incision along the glabrous border of the volar skin. Proximally, the incision is not extended ulnar to the flexor carpi radialis (FCR) to avoid injury to the palmar cutaneous sensory branch of the median nerve. The dissection is sharply taken down to the radial border of the thenar musculature, which is elevated ulnarward, permitting access to the CMC joint capsule. The capsule is incised in such a way that later repair or reefing can be conducted, and the fracture line is visualized on the volar aspect of the joint. The articular surface is reduced and held with a provisional intraoperative wire or the use of a dental pick. The reduction is best secured with two 1.5 or 2.0 mm lag screws introduced from the dorsum to engage the smaller fragment with the leading threads of the screws. Because of the protected position of the smaller fragment, screws cannot be introduced from the fragment into the metacarpal. The position and placement of these screws should be meticulously determined and confirmed by intraoperative fluoroscopy to obtain an excellent result.

Rolando's Fracture

An even more challenging variant of the metacarpal base fracture is the comminuted intra-articular fracture, known as a Rolando fracture. These can vary from a three-part intra-articular T fracture to a severely comminuted variant that defies fragment characterization.

Because articular congruity is the most important goal in treatment of these fractures, they are almost always best treated in an open fashion **(Fig. 18–20).** However, it should be mentioned that in selected cases of extensive comminution or in elderly patients or those refusing surgery, an early motion program can be instituted. This treatment can result in a functional, if not anatomically perfect, joint.

Three-part fractures are often amenable to 2 mm T-plate fixation or minicondylar blade plating. Open reduction with K-wire fixation is performed if articular fragments are too small to accommodate screws. In less common cases of very severe comminution where K-wires cannot obtain control of the articular fragments, a spanning external fixator may be used with proximal pins in the trapezium and distal pins in the distal metacarpal. With any of these techniques, the same open volar approach should be utilized to facilitate the articular reduction.

If plating or screw fixation is achieved, patients are started in supervised motion 1 week after surgery. Pin fixation cases require 5 to 6 weeks of thumb spica splinting. External fixation should be maintained for 6 weeks, given the severity and comminution of the fractures requiring its use. Radiographic follow-up provides the surgeon with a guideline for duration of external fixation, but the mobility of the MCP and IP joints should be pursued during the time that the fixator is in place.

Fracture-Dislocations of the CMC Joints of the Index through Small Rays

Fracture-dislocations of the CMC joints are the result of an axial loading force sustained along the axis of the metacarpals. CMC fracture-dislocations of the radial two rays rarely occur in isolation but can be seen in high-energy injuries involving all four CMC joints.

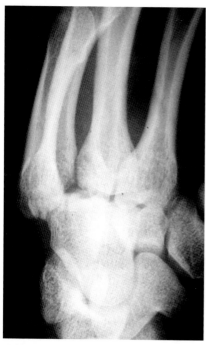

Figure 18–21 Oblique radiograph demonstrating fourth and fifth carpometacarpal fracture dislocations.

Far more commonly encountered are fracture dislocations of the fifth (small) and/or fourth (ring) rays **(Fig. 18–21).** The metacarpal bases articulate with steeply oriented hamate articular facets. Most commonly, the fifth metacarpal base will fracture, leaving a fragment of its volar, radial margin reduced, while the shaft and ulnar base displace dorsally and ulnarly. Associated dorsal rim fractures of the hamate are not uncommon. Despite this

level of disruption, these injuries are difficult to diagnose on standard x-rays because of the significant overlap of the hamate and fifth metacarpal base on normal AP radiographs.

The clinical sine qua non of CMC injury is the "balloon hand": when there is significant dorsal swelling, it usually belies a CMC disruption **(Fig. 18–22).** Interestingly, this tumescence is not as tense as the examiner may anticipate simply from the appearance. The areolar tissues of the dorsum accommodate significant fluid volume, and the swelling is hematoma that has collected in the suprafascial space.

Two things can be done to confirm the diagnosis: direct examination and special radiographs (semipronated, semisupinated, or distraction films). Prominence or step-off at the CMC joint, especially when accompanied by overt instability, is the most telling indicator of the nature and extent of the injury, including its reducibility.

Views obtained with the hand 30 degrees pronated from a fully supinated position will optimize visualization of this fracture-dislocation. A semisupinated view may allow visualization of the index and long rays. Distraction views can reveal a disorganized series of CMC relationships, irregular joint spaces, and avulsion/impaction fractures. If examination and plain radiographs are equivocal, computed tomographic (CT) scan can provide detailed images displaying degree of displacement and comminution as well as extent of hamate involvement.

Nonoperative Treatment

Closed treatment of these injuries merits a degree of caution. When evaluated acutely, the fragments may be

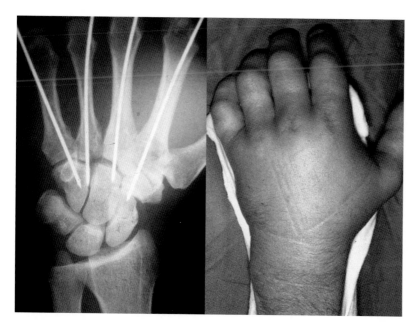

Figure 18–22 Carpometacarpal dislocations of digits 2 through 5 treated with collateral recess pinning, shown on left. Typical "balloon hand" presentation is shown on the right.

mobile enough to achieve a good reduction but may not be stable. Loss of reduction is difficult to detect due to the significant soft tissue swelling as well as the difficulty of radiographic assessment. The inherently unstable nature of these fracture-dislocations and the difficulty in identifying loss of reduction lead most surgeons to employ closed reduction and percutaneous pinning to provide stability.

Operative Treatment

This is best performed with the assistance of intraoperative fluoroscopy to confirm accurate reduction. Pins are then driven across the CMC joint to hold reduction. Pinning is achieved either by using a longitudinal collateral recess technique or by entering from the ulnar border of the fifth metacarpal base into the hamate and the adjacent fourth metacarpal base (if uninjured). These pins are maintained for 6 weeks while digital motion is permitted.

Open reduction and collateral recess pinning offers many advantages in treatment of these fracture-dislocations. Direct visualization of the small fragments enables accurate reduction of the articular surface. Many of these fragments are displaced 180 degrees and incarcerated in the joint or fracture line. Furthermore, an evolving compartment syndrome accompanies many of these injuries. Simultaneous release of the intraosseous compartments (both volar and dorsal) is easily achievable through the same incisions used to judge and affect CMC reduction. In a minority of cases, compressed dorsal fractures of the hamate often need to be elevated to realign the articular surface. Bone graft can be packed behind these compression fractures to provide support for the articular surface. In rare situations of severe comminution and joint surface destruction, acute CMC arthrodesis can be performed with bone graft. This is better tolerated in the index and long finger CMC joints than in the more mobile ulnar digit CMC joints.

Surgical Technique

Collateral recess pinning was discussed previously in the context of PIP fracture management, but it is at the metacarpal level that the technique has its greatest utility. The palpable "shoulders" of the collateral recess on the dorsolateral aspect of the MCP head provide a perfect point of entry for unilateral or crossing Kirschner wires directed proximally and obliquely across the fracture sites from the neck to the CMC joints **(Fig. 18–23)**. Inserting the pin by hand allows the surgeon to feel the most prominent aspect of the collateral recess. Power is then employed to machine a cortical aperture that permits direction (and possible redirection) of the pin. The advancing point contacts

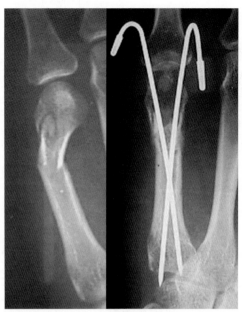

Figure 18–23 Metacarpal metadiaphyseal fracture treated with collateral recess pinning.

the thick middiaphyseal cortex tangentially and then follows the intramedullary route to the base. Ideally, proximal fixation is obtained with cortical purchase in the subchondral plate of the metacarpal base. The CMC joint is spanned when stabilizing the CMC fracture-dislocations. Two crossing wires are used to control rotation whenever they can be accommodated. The index, long, and small rays are most amenable to this technique. The ring digit is most challenging because of the smaller collateral shoulders and the gracile medullary canal.

Finally, introduction of the pins should be attempted with the digit in the intrinsic plus position (MCP joint maximally flexed). This will prevent the percutaneous pins from tethering the soft tissue, including the skin, while the hand is positioned for splinting. Additionally, the collateral ligament is at its greatest length in this position.

Metacarpal Neck Fractures

Metacarpal neck fractures are very common injuries sustained from the longitudinal impact of the flexed metacarpal head against an unyielding object. This mechanism results in a predictable apex dorsal position. Controversy exists around the surgical indications for these fractures because historical accounts and perpetuated dogma eschew operative treatment in even severely displaced fractures. Furthermore, nonunion is rare, and malunion is often asymptomatic.[23] Most surgeons would agree on some general surgical indications, including persistent rotational deformity despite closed reduction, extension lag due to excessive metacarpal head flexion, multiple fractures, or excessive displacement (greater

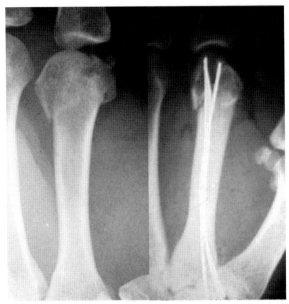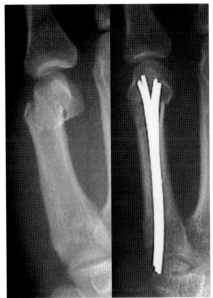

Figure 18–24 Preoperative and postoperative radiographs of **(A)** index and **(B)** fifth digit metacarpal neck fractures treated with bouquet pinning.

than 50 to 60 degrees). Displacement (volar angulation) is compensated by CMC motion and MCP hyperextension to achieve digital positioning in extension. Because of the relatively minimal range of motion at the index and long finger CMC joints, neck fractures demonstrating greater than 15 to 20 degrees of angulation will result in extension lag at the MCP and will be more strongly considered for surgery. The ulnar two rays are capable of 20 to 30 degrees of motion at the CMC joint and can therefore tolerate 20 to 30 degrees of apex dorsal angulation of the neck fractures without demonstrating effective extension lag.[24]

Beyond these functional guidelines, the surgeon should tailor the surgical indications to the needs of each patient. Consideration should be given to the predictable sequelae of closed (palpability of the metacarpal head in the palm, visible absence of the dorsal prominence of the MCP joint) and open treatment (scarring, potential for loss of motion).

The Jahss maneuver for closed reduction of the metacarpal neck fractures is performed with the MCP joint positioned in flexion, and reduction is achieved by applying a dorsally directed force to the metacarpal head through pressure on the proximal phalanx. Care is taken to assess rotation by comparison of the nail plate position to that of its adjacent digit. Splinting with the MCP flexed and the PIP extended is maintained for 2 to 3 weeks. Later in the treatment course, the splint can be converted to free the PIP joint and start motion at that level. The MCP joint is freed from the splint at 4 to 5 weeks, and the patient is given a protective gutter thermoplastic splint for 2 more weeks while motion is permitted at the wrist and MCP joints.

Open Treatment of Metacarpal Neck Fractures

The surgeon's portfolio of operative techniques for the open treatment of metacarpal neck fractures should include intramedullary ("bouquet") pinning and collateral recess pinning **(Fig. 18–24A,B)**. The latter has been extensively covered in this chapter. The determining factor as to whether it will be useful resides in the integrity of the collateral recess shoulders. This is usually easily determined from conventional radiographs but can be imaged on live fluoroscopy or with a Brewerton view, which is the best radiographic technique for assessing this region of the metacarpal head. The Brewerton view is obtained by positioning the supinated hand in 65 degrees of MCP flexion, with IP joints extended. With the digits flat on the x-ray plate and the metacarpals off the surface of the plate, the x-ray tube is positioned 15 degrees ulnar to the midline of the hand. This provides excellent visualization of the metacarpal head articular surface.

Bouquet pinning is most appropriate for border digit neck fractures, whereas collateral recess pinning may be utilized for any digit.

Technique of Metacarpal Bouquet Pinning (Special Reference to the Fifth and Second Rays)[25]

Bouquet Pinning of the Fifth Ray

A 2 to 3 cm incision is created at the glabrous border of the hand at the level of the extensor carpi ulnaris (ECU)

BOUQUET PINNING

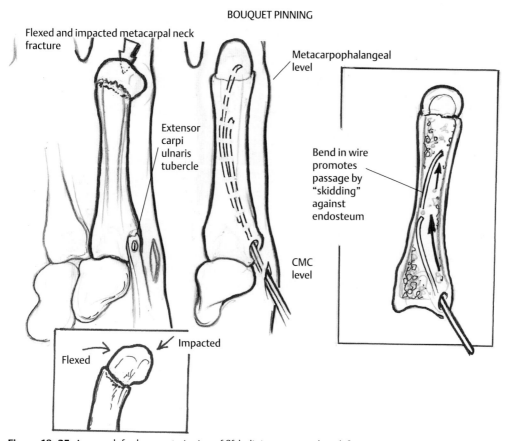

Figure 18–25 Approach for bouquet pinning of fifth digit metacarpal neck fractures. CMC, carpometa carpal.

tendon (**Fig. 18–25**). Care must be exercised to protect branches of the dorsal sensory branch of the ulnar nerve. Dissection continues to the ulnar border of the ECU tendon insertion. This tendon may be longitudinally split or reflected dorsally. A small area of prominence, or "shoulder," at the ulnar border of the metacarpal base becomes readily visible. The oblique cortical surface that lies between this shoulder and the CMC joint is the area that will provide access to the medullary canal. Use of fluoroscopy to locate the entry site is recommended to avoid potential pitfalls. A cortical window is made on this surface using hand tools or power drills. After initial opening of the canal, the entry site may be enlarged with curets. The portal of entry must be large enough to accommodate the desired number of pins (usually three). The size of the hole is ~4 to 6 mm in diameter.

Two technical steps are helpful to remember. The K-wire tips should be cut to make them blunt. Leaving the sharp tip may create a second perforation in the cortex and make it difficult to deflect off the wall of the medullary canal. Second, the pins should be contoured with a gentle bend along their entire length. The wires will more firmly control the distal fragments if this contour places the pin tips against the endosteum in its final position.

As the pin is introduced in an antegrade fashion, it is best controlled with two large needle holders. This will allow for controlled progression of the pin and optimize its position in the metacarpal head. While one needle holder is used to advance the pin, the second is applied closer to the insertion site. This tends to "stiffen" the implant and permit easier passage. The hand should be radially deviated to enable the pin to be passed more readily. Before passing the leading edge of the pin across the fracture site, a manual reduction maneuver should be performed. A typical difficulty is passage of the pin through the fracture site and out of the medullary canal. If this occurs, the pin should be withdrawn to the fracture plane and rotated to redirect the tip before reduction of the fracture and pin readvancement. Once the fracture has been reduced and the pins placed, the ends are cut as close to the canal as possible. The pins can be advanced slightly with a bone tamp, leaving the proximal ends within the canal. Three pins are usually utilized to provide multiplanar stability. Passage of additional pins is often limited by the narrowing medullary canal at the midshaft level.

Bouquet Pinning of the Index Finger Metacarpal

Index finger metacarpal bouquet pinning is very similar to that of fifth ray fixation. After exposure of the metacarpal base, the fibers of the extensor carpi radialis longus (ECRL) are elevated or split at the radial aspect of the metacarpal base. The remainder of the steps reflect those already described. In this setting, ulnar deviation of the wrist can help facilitate passage of the pin.

Postoperative Care

Following bouquet pinning, a program of active and active-assisted motion commences as comfort permits, usually about 3 to 7 days after surgery. In fact, we have refrained from rigid immobilization in favor of a bulky dressing that initially allows digital motion at all levels, including the MCP. A removable, short arm, safe-position orthosis is furnished to immobilize the hand during the intervals between exercise sessions, although the patient is encouraged to pursue motion vigorously and often. It is logical to begin strengthening when motion recovery exceeds 50 to 75% of normal. The majority of patients are able to return to heavy labor vocations at the eighth postoperative week.

Patients undergoing collateral recess pinning follow a supervised therapy program. Because pin stability and pin tract infections are concerns, appropriate immobilization is required while the pins are indwelling. This is usually accomplished with an initial 3 to 4 weeks of rigid immobilization followed by interval splinting. Careful motion of adjacent digits and even other digital segments of the operated ray can be pursued. At 1 month postop after pin removal, an active and active-assisted motion protocol of the DIP, PIP, and MCP joints is initiated. The patient is maintained in an orthosis for an additional 2 weeks. With clinical and radiographic signs of healing, the splint is gradually weaned.

Diaphyseal Metacarpal Fractures

Metacarpal shaft fractures can be classified into transverse, spiral oblique, and comminuted fractures. Certain conditions exist as indications for operative intervention that apply to all metacarpal shaft fractures, whereas specific concerns should be addressed according to fracture pattern.

Multiple metacarpal fractures, open fractures, malrotation, and instability after reduction are general indications for ORIF. Knowledge of determinants of acceptable reduction and predictors of fracture stability enables the experienced hand surgeon to identify more subtle surgical indications. Small degrees of dorsal angulation at the midshaft level are functionally well tolerated. Up to 30 degrees of dorsal angulation of the small finger and 20 degrees of the ring are acceptable. The index and middle metacarpals require more anatomical reduction because their ability to accommodate deformity with CMC mobility is minimal.

Malrotation of any digit after reduction is unacceptable because even small degrees of malrotation can result in significant scissoring of the digits in the flexed posture. Central metacarpals are stabilized by stout intermetacarpal ligaments distally that prevent excessive foreshortening when protected by intact neighboring rays.

Border digit metacarpal fractures are not afforded the same scaffold of stability and are therefore more apt to be treated open if unstable. Fracture pattern characteristics also influence management decisions because they can aid the surgeon in predicting stability of reduction over time. Spiral oblique fractures are a good example. These fractures are unstable with axial loading and tolerate only a minimal degree of malreduction before significant malrotation is manifested. These fractures are only treated in a closed fashion if conditions are optimal (i.e., nondisplaced, central ray, greenstick fractures) with vigilant radiographic and clinical follow-up.

Those fractures treated closed are generally treated in 3 to 4 weeks of short arm casting with MCP joints in flexion and IP joints free. The cast is then removed, and motion is initiated. Removable splinting with the MCP joints free is usually maintained for an additional 2 weeks; buddy taping is also surprisingly effective in maintaining stability while allowing motion. Duration of immobilization and timing of return to unrestricted use of the hand are altered around this framework according to the fracture characteristics and the age and activities of the patient.

Open Treatment of Metacarpal Diaphyseal Fractures

As with all fractures, metacarpal shaft fracture treatment requires the surgeon to be familiar with multiple fixation techniques. Judgment must be utilized to select the method that will achieve the most rigid fixation while maximizing functional outcomes.

Transverse midshaft fractures are not amenable to interfragmentary screw fixation. Intramedullary bouquet pinning techniques (as described earlier) are used by some surgeons in this setting,[26,27] but the technique is most amenable to metacarpal neck fracture fixation and frequently results in fracture gapping when applied to midshaft fractures, in the authors' experience.

The gold standard for transverse metacarpal fracture management is probably plating. It provides an opportunity for anatomical restoration and rigid fixation with fracture compression in these situations. The risk of tendon adhesion and loss of motion is balanced by the opportunity for early aggressive rehabilitation.

The standard approach to open metacarpal fixation is via longitudinal or gently curvilinear dorsal incisions. These may be directly over the involved metacarpal or in the intermetacarpal spaces, if adjacent fractures are to be fixed. Care is taken to preserve the dorsal hand sensory fibers of the radial and ulnar nerves during this approach.

Extensor tendons are retracted to permit access to the fracture plane. Care should be taken to expose the fractures while maintaining a layer of periosteum and

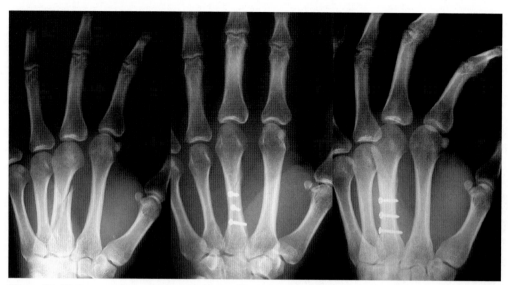

Figure 18–26 Preoperative and postoperative radiographs of middle digit spiral oblique metacarpal fracture treated with interfragmentary screw fixation.

interosseous muscle fascia for closure over the hardware as much as possible. This will serve as a protective buffer between the hardware and extensor tendons postoperatively, and theoretically will provide an enhanced biological environment for healing.

Subperiosteal dissection is performed around the fracture line itself, but further periosteal stripping is to be minimized. After removing callus and fracture debris, anatomical reduction may be provisionally maintained using longitudinal K-wire fixation. Most metacarpal fractures can be treated with 2.0 or 2.4 mm plates placed either dorsally or laterally. Compression may be achieved with dynamic compression plates (DCP) plates using standard Arbeitsgemeinschaft für Osteosynthesefragen (AO) technique. The plating technique should obtain at least four cortices of screw purchase on each side of the fracture. Interfragmentary screws placed through the plate will increase the stability of the construct, but this is not achievable in transverse midshaft fractures. Clinical and radiographic reduction are confirmed during and after fixation. The subtlest challenge of metacarpal fracture care is avoiding malrotation.

In noncomminuted fractures the interlocking fragments can provide accurate guidance; however, fractures with even minimal comminution can be misleading in this regard. Clinical assessment of the position of the digit and rotation as brought through a range of motion should be performed frequently during fixation to ensure that reduction is maintained.

After successful fixation, the fascia and periosteum are closed over the plate, and the skin is closed. Patients are splinted for edema control for less than a week after surgery. Motion and edema control therapy is then begun under the supervision of a hand therapist.

Spiral oblique fractures are generally treated with Kirschner wire or interfragmentary screw fixation. The surgeon should strive for perfect reduction because minimal rotation will result in significant scissoring. For this reason, wire fixation has a minimal role.

If the fracture requires open reduction, the surgeon should employ screw fixation to deliver the benefit of anatomical restoration, fracture compression, and early motion (**Fig. 18–26**). The obliquity of the fracture line may also determine fixation method because interfragmentary screw fixation requires that the longitudinal length of the fracture should be two to three times the diameter of the metacarpal shaft. A ratio of less than 2 would indicate that the fracture is not oblique enough to accommodate interfragmentary screw technique. Such fractures require plating to provide adequate protection from torsional and bending forces. When interfragmentary screw fixation is appropriate, the surgeon should strive for fixation with at least two screws, and the screws should be placed a distance of at least twice the screw diameter apart to avoid splitting the cortices.[28]

The surgical approach for interfragmentary screw fixation is similar to that described above. The often-extreme oblique nature of these fractures requires somewhat more extensive fracture line management because periosteum and debris within the fracture line should be meticulously cleared throughout the length of the fracture. Attempts should be made to directly visualize as much of the fracture as possible to achieve perfect reduction and avoid the pitfall of slight malrotation.

Provisional intraoperative fixation with wires may be employed as mentioned earlier. To achieve maximal resistance axial compressive forces, screw placement should be perpendicular to the metacarpal shaft. Screws placed

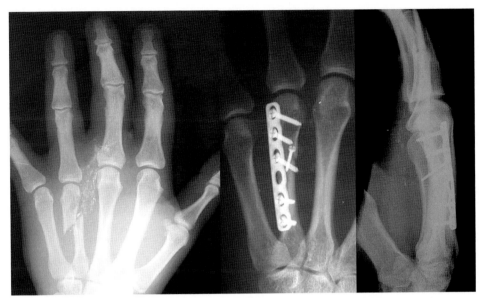

Figure 18–27 Preoperative and postoperative radiographs of an open comminuted ring finger metacarpal fracture from a gunshot wound treated with plate fixation. Note the additional interfragmentary screw fixation.

perpendicular to the fracture plane provide resistance to torsional deforming forces. It is best to have at least one screw in each of these planes, if possible. Two or three 2.4 mm screws are typically achievable.

Caution should be exercised when selecting the screw technique. A lag screw technique offers the appeal of fracture compression but also risks the loss of reduction due to the oblique nature of these fractures. If the surgeon accepts imprecise reduction before lag screw fixation, the compressive force of the engaged distal cortex will further displace the fracture by sliding the fragment along the oblique fracture line.

Comminuted metacarpal shaft fractures are best treated with plating and screw technique. This provides the best method of maintaining the fracture out to length while obtaining optimal reduction and fixation of any rotational displacement (**Fig. 18–27**). Often these fractures occur in the metaphyseal region and leave the surgeon with minimal purchase on the metacarpal base.

In these situations 2.0 mm blade or T plating can obtain adequate proximal stability. Severely comminuted fractures may be augmented with cancellous bone graft unless contamination from open injuries is prohibitive. In the setting of segmental bone loss in open injuries, the soft tissue envelope will often dictate the management. If soft tissue coverage is adequate, plating can be used to stabilize and bridge the defect, while bone graft is pursued acutely or in a delayed fashion.

In the setting of open wounds with significant soft tissue loss, plating may be pursued if adequate debridement and immediate flap coverage are provided. If the coverage

is marginal, or is provided in a delayed fashion, bridging external fixation provides a means of maintaining length and stabilizing soft tissue prior to definitive coverage. The use of a simple bent wire that is inserted into the distal and proximal stable units, spanning the diaphyseal comminution, is effective in providing provisional fixation. In this setting, external fixation can be exchanged for rigid internal fixation at the time of flap coverage; intercalary bone grafting can also be performed when tissue stability is assured.

Some surgeons advocate intermetacarpal Kirschner wire fixation in the setting of metacarpal comminution or segmental loss to maintain length.[29] Although this method of transfixation pinning has the appeal of ease of application, it has many disadvantages. When applied between a fractured metacarpal and a single adjacent metacarpal, transfixion pins provide minimal stability, particularly in the flexion/extension plane. If the transfixion pins span the fractured metacarpal and two adjacent metacarpals in an effort to increase stability, they serve to flatten the natural arch of the metacarpals. If placed very distally in the metacarpal heads, they increase the likelihood of adjacent MCP stiffness. Finally, this method requires prolonged immobilization in a hand with significant soft tissue and bony ("combined") injury, precisely when the hand requires enough stability to start early rehabilitation and salvage functional losses. This stability could be supplied by rigid internal fixation spanning the defect. Ultimately, we do not recommend this cross-pinning technique for any of the aforementioned fractures unless the more logical solutions are exhausted.

Pearls

- The most important determinant of mallet fracture management is the stability of the joint relationship. Joint subluxation is an indication for surgical intervention, not the size or position of the fracture fragment.
- Flexor tendon avulsion classification:
  - **Type 1:** nonbony FDP avulsions that retract into the palm
  - **Type 2:** small avulsion fragment retracts to the PIP joint level, with the A3 pulley preventing the fragment from further passage proximally in the tendon sheath
  - **Type 3:** large avulsion fragments that retract just proximal to the DIP joint
- Proximal phalangeal shaft fractures assume an apex volar position because of the strong pull of the interosseous muscles on the proximal fragment. Middle phalangeal shaft fractures may display angulation in either apex volar or dorsal positions, depending on the mechanism of the injury and the relationship of the fracture line to the superficialis and central slip insertional forces.
- Common bone graft harvest sites for small bone fracture fixation in the hand:
  - Dorsal distal radius via floor of second compartment
  - Volar distal radius beneath pronator teres
  - Salvage from other amputated parts in the multiply traumatized hand
- A PIP fracture/dislocation fragment encompassing greater than 40% of the middle phalangeal joint surface will likely result in an unstable reduction due to the loss of the buttressing articulating support provided by the volar lip of the middle phalanx.
- Digital external fixation subtypes:
  - Fixed versus dynamic
  - Joint spanning versus nonspanning
  - Unilateral versus bilateral
  - Commercially produced versus wire fixators
- Surgical options for the unstable PIP fracture dislocation with greater than 40% destruction of volar base of middle phalanx:
  - Volar plate arthroplasty

- Hemihamate autograft reconstruction
- Salvage procedures–arthrodesis/implant arthroplasty
- Irreducible PIP dislocations are usually the less common volar subtype due to incarceration of one condyle between the central slip and lateral band. In contrast, irreducible MCP dislocations are the more common dorsal subtype due to incarceration of the metacarpal head between the intrinsic and extrinsic muscles.
- Elson's test for central slip integrity: With the PIP in passive flexion, inability to actively extend the DIP joint indicates that a complete central slip avulsion has not occurred.
- Reduction of a subluxated MCP joint is performed by application of a volar force applied to the dorsal base of the proximal phalanx. Attempts at longitudinal distraction or exaggeration of the hyperextension deformity will convert the reducible subluxation into an irreducible MCP dislocation by permitting the volar plate to fall dorsally between the metacarpal head and the base of the proximal phalanx.
- Destabilizing forces acting on the Bennett's fracture:
  - Abductor pollicis longus
  - Flexor pollicis longus
  - Adductor pollicis
- Closed reduction of a Bennett's fracture is performed by providing:
  - Longitudinal distraction of the thumb
  - Pronation to the thumb
  - Volar-ulnar pressure on the metacarpal base.
- Surgical indications for metacarpal neck fractures:
  - Rotational deformity despite closed reduction
  - Extension lag due to excessive metacarpal head flexion
  - Multiple fractures
  - Excessive angulation
- Positioning for Brewerton view (for radiographic visualization of the metacarpal head): Position the supinated hand in 65 degrees of MCP flexion, with IP joints extended. With the digits flat on the x-ray plate and the metacarpals off the surface of the plate, the x-ray tube is positioned 15 degrees ulnar to the midline of the hand.

References

1. Kronlage SC, Faust D. Open reduction and screw fixation of mallet fractures. J Hand Surg [Br] 2004;29:135–138
2. Pegoli L, Toh S, Arai K, Fukuda A, Nishikawa S, Vallejo IG. The Ishiguro extension block technique for the treatment of mallet finger fracture: indications and clinical results. J Hand Surg [Br] 2003;28:15–17
3. Takami H, Takahashi S, Ando M. Operative treatment of mallet finger due to intra-articular fracture of the distal phalanx. Arch Orthop Trauma Surg 2000;120:9–13
4. Zook EG, Guy RJ, Russell RC. A study of nail bed injuries: causes, treatment and prognosis. J Hand Surg [Am] 1984;9:247–252
5. Leddy JP, Packer JW. Avulsion of the profundus tendon insertion in athletes. J Hand Surg [Am] 1977;2:66–69

6. Hofmeister EP, Mazurek MT, Shin AY, Bishop AT. Extension block pinning for large mallet fractures. J Hand Surg [Am] 2003;28:453–459
7. Belsky MR, Eaton RG, Lane LB. Closed reduction and internal fixation of proximal phalangeal fractures. J Hand Surg [Am] 1984;9:725–729
8. Freeland AE, Sud V, Lindley SG. Unilateral intrinsic resection of the lateral band and oblique fibers of the metacarpophalangeal joint for proximal phalangeal fracture. Tech Hand Up Extrem Surg 2001;5:85–90
9. Chamay A. A distally based dorsal and triangular tendinous flap for direct access to the proximal interphalangeal joint. Ann Chir Main 1988;7:179–183

10. Kiefhaber TR, Stern PJ, Grood ES. Lateral stability of the proximal interphalangeal joint. J Hand Surg [Am] 1986;11:661–669

11. Rhee RY, Reading G, Wray RC. A biomechanical study of the collateral ligaments of the proximal interphalangeal joint. J Hand Surg [Am] 1992;17:157–163

12. McElfresh EC, Dobyns JH, O'Brien ET. Management of fracture-dislocation of the proximal interphalangeal joints by extension-block splinting. J Bone Joint Surg Am 1972;54:1705–1711

13. Agee JM. Unstable fracture-dislocations of the proximal interphalangeal joint: treatment with the force couple splint. Clin Orthop Relat Res 1987;214:101–112

14. Hastings H, Ernst JM. Dynamic external fixation for fractures of the proximal interphalangeal joint. Hand Clin 1993;4:659–674

15. Inanami H, Ninomiya S, Okutsu I, Tarui T. Dynamic external finger fixator for fracture-dislocation of the proximal interphalangeal joint. J Hand Surg [Am] 1993;18:160–164

16. Suzuki Y, Matsunaga T, Sato S, Yokoi T. The pins and rubbers traction system for treatment of comminuted intra-articular fractures and fracture-dislocations of the hand. J Hand Surg [Br] 1994;19:98–107

17. Slade JF, Baxamusa TH, Wolfe SW, Gutow A. External fixation of proximal interphalangeal joint fracture-dislocations. Atlas of Hand Clinics 2000;5:1–29

18. Eaton RG, Malerich MM. Volar plate arthroplasty of the proximal interphalangeal joint: a review of ten years' experience. J Hand Surg [Am] 1980;5:260–268

19. Williams RM, Kiefhaber TR, Sommerkamp TG, Stern PJ. Treatment of unstable dorsal proximal interphalangeal fracture/dislocations using a hemi-hamate autograft. J Hand Surg [Am] 2003;28:856–865

20. Kato H, Minami A, Takahara M, Oshio I, Hirachi K, Kotaki H. Surgical repair of acute collateral ligament injuries in digits with the Mitek bone suture anchor. J Hand Surg [Br] 1999;24:70–75

21. Elson RA. Rupture of the central slip of the extensor hood of the finger: a test for early diagnosis. J Bone Joint Surg Br 1986;68:229–231

22. Green DP, Terry GC. Complex dislocation of the metacarpophalangeal joint: correlative pathological anatomy. J Bone Joint Surg Am 1973;55:1480–1486

23. Statius Muller MG, Poolman RW, van Hoogstraten MJ, Steller EP. Immediate mobilization gives good results in boxer's fractures with volar angulation up to 70 degrees: a prospective randomized trial comparing immediate mobilization with cast immobilization. Arch Orthop Trauma Surg 2003;123:534–537

24. Amadio PC, Beckenbaugh RD, Bishop AT, et al. Fractures of the hand and wrist. In: Jupiter JB, ed. Flynn's Hand Surgery. Baltimore: Williams & Wilkins; 1991:122–185

25. Rettig LA, Graham TJ. Closed pinning and bouquet pinning of fractures of the metacarpals. In: Strickland JW, Graham TJ, eds. Master Techniques in Orthopaedic Surgery: The Hand. Philadelphia: Lippincott Williams & Wilkins, 2005:27–46

26. Gonzalez MH, Hall RF Jr. Intramedullary fixation of metacarpal and proximal phalangeal fractures of the hand. Clin Orthop Relat Res 1996;327:47–54

27. Gonzalez MH, Igram CM, Hall RF Jr. Flexible intramedullary nailing for metacarpal fractures. J Hand Surg [Am] 1995;20:382–387

28. Kozin SH, Thoder JJ, Leiberman G. Operative treatment of metacarpal shaft fractures. J Am Acad Orthop Surg 2000;8:111–121

29. Galanakis I, Aligizakis A, Katonis P, Papadokostakis G, Stergiopoulos K, Hadjipavlou A. Treatment of closed unstable metacarpal fractures using percutaneous transverse fixation with Kirschner wires. J Trauma 2003;55:509–513

19 Pelvic Ring Injuries

Kyle F. Dickson

Pelvic ring disruptions are typically part of a complex set of injuries to both the axial skeleton and the contents of the pelvis, including the gastrointestinal tract, the bladder and lower genitourinary tract, and the pelvic floor structures. Pelvic ring injuries can be life threatening in the acute phase. Surviving patients may have chronic problems due to associated neurovascular injury, pelvic ring deformity or instability, and the sequelae of associated injuries to the surrounding soft tissues or visceral structures. These factors can lead to persistent pain, sitting imbalance, limb-length discrepancy, sexual/reproductive dysfunction, or bowel/bladder dysfunction. Clearly, the decisions about the management of pelvic ring injuries must consider all of these factors, and these injuries can be very difficult to treat successfully. Low-energy pelvic injuries due to minor falls rarely require surgical intervention. Conversely, patients with high-energy pelvic injuries often require operative treatment to save their life and prevent complications related to instability or deformity of the pelvis. Patients with high-energy pelvic injuries are often hemodynamically unstable with significant associated injuries. Their survival relies on the acute management of the associated injuries as well as the pelvic injury. The acute management of pelvic injuries is beyond the scope of this chapter.

This chapter deals primarily with the operative techniques used in pelvic injury management, including placement of external fixators, as well as definitive open reduction internal fixation of the various types of pelvic injuries. The complex three-dimensional bony and soft tissue structure of the pelvis is unfamiliar to many orthopaedic surgeons and complicates successful treatment of injuries to the pelvis. Classification systems include components of anatomy, stability and deformity, and injury vector force. These classification systems may aid in the treatment of potential associated injuries.[1] When making decisions about the definitive fixation of pelvic injuries, however, it is critical to understand the stability and deformity of the pelvis. Once the vector of deformity is discovered, the vector of reduction can then be planned using various combinations of closed and open reduction techniques. Of secondary importance is the type of fixation. In general, among the higher energy pelvic injuries, internal fixation is mechanically superior to external fixation.[2] The external fixator is used more commonly during the initial stabilization of the patient, prior to definitive internal fixation. The exception to this generality is the use of definitive external fixation in injuries that are stable posteriorly (i.e., internal rotation deformity of the pelvis or an open book pelvis) where an anterior external fixator can be used for definitive fixation. This chapter briefly reviews the classification system that is useful for determining indications for surgical treatment and choosing appropriate definitive fixation. Emphasis will be placed on surgical treatment by initially describing the deformities that are common and the specific techniques regarding approach and reduction of the pelvic injury.

Classification and Anatomy

Prior to the orthopaedic surgeon being able to classify a pelvic injury, the anatomy of the pelvic injury must be understood. The inherent bony stability of the pelvis is very limited. **Fig. 19–1** demonstrates the key role that ligaments

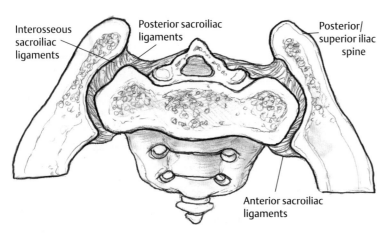

Interosseous sacroiliac ligaments

Posterior sacroiliac ligaments

Posterior/ superior iliac spine

Anterior sacroiliac ligaments

Figure 19–1 Illustration of an inlet view of the pelvis with the spine removed showing the sacroiliac joint. The joint is stabilized by the anterior sacroiliac joint ligaments, the interosseous ligaments, and the strong posterior sacroiliac joint ligaments.

Table 19–1   Classification of Pelvic Ring Injuries[8]

	Type	Feature	Stability
Anteroposterior compression, external rotation	APC-I	Pubic diastasis < 2.5 cm or isolated pubic fracture	Stable
	APC-II	Pubic diastasis > 2.5 cm, widening of anterior sacroiliac (SI) joint	Rotationally unstable, vertically stable
	APC-III	Pubic diastasis > 2.5 cm with complete SI joint disruption	Rotationally and vertically unstable
Lateral compression, internal rotation	LC-I	Anterior sacral impaction, horizontal pubic ramus fracture	Stable
	LC-II	Anterior sacral impaction, posterior iliac wing (crescent) fracture, or posterior SI joint disruption	Rotationally unstable, vertically stable
	LC-III	LC-II with external rotation of opposite hemipelvis	Rotationally and vertically unstable
Vertical shear		Vertical displacement	Unstable
Combined		Complex deformity	Unstable

deformity, tilting of the patient while the radiograph is taken, or both.

Understanding the mechanism of injury allows the surgeon to predict the type of deformity. Burgess et al. proposed a classification of pelvic ring injuries that is based on the underlying mechanism of injury.[8] Pelvic ring injuries are divided into anterior-posterior compression, lateral compression, vertical shear, or combined patterns **(Table 19–1)**. The anterior-posterior and lateral compression injuries are each divided into three subtypes with increasing degrees of instability. This scheme has proven valuable because it allows one to predict instability and consider reduction and fixation strategies that are appropriate for a particular case. For example, a patient that is hit from the side in a motor vehicle accident often has a lateral compression type of injury causing an internal rotation, flexion, and adduction deformity of the hemipelvis[6,7] **(Figs.**

19–6 and 19–7A,B)**. Likewise, patients that fall on their back or are crushed from the front often have an open book pelvic injury with an external rotation and abduction deformity **(Figs. 19–8A,B; 19–9; and 19–10)**.

Nonoperative Treatment

A pelvic fracture that is classified as a Bucholz type I pelvic injury is stable and should be treated using nonoperative techniques. Another type of pelvic ring injury that can be managed nonoperatively is the lateral compression injury with impaction of the sacrum and minimal displacement of the anterior ring **(Figs. 19–6 and 19–11)**. Additionally, fractures that involve the pubic rami without a clear injury posteriorly also do not require surgical treatment. Rarely avulsion of the ischium, anterior-superior iliac spine, or anterior-inferior iliac spine does occur. In these cases the pelvic ring is stable; however, there can be significant displacement of the avulsed fragment. No literature gives definitive recommendations on operative versus nonoperative treatment of displaced avulsion fractures, and decision making should occur on an individual case-by-case basis. The author uses greater than 1 cm of displacement as an indication to operate on these avulsions. Minimally displaced or impacted injuries of the pelvis are both radiographically and mechanically stable. These injuries can be treated by touch-down weight bearing for 6 to 8 weeks. Initial weekly x-rays should be performed to ensure that no additional deformity occurs. After 6 to 8 weeks, more aggressive exercise and range of motion ambulation training with physical therapy is recommended.

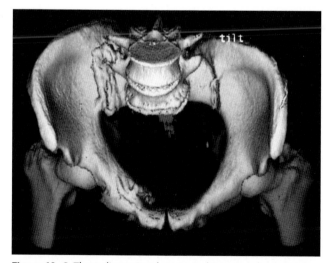

Figure 19–6 Three-dimensional computed tomography showing an injury as a result of a T-bone motor vehicle collision causing a mild internal rotation and flexion deformity to the right hemipelvis. This is a lateral compression type I injury according to the Young and Burgess classification, with a stable impaction fracture of the anterior sacral ala.

Indications for Surgical Treatment

The indications for surgical treatment of pelvic ring injuries include those patients that fail nonoperative treatment as well as those pelvic injuries that are unstable or that have

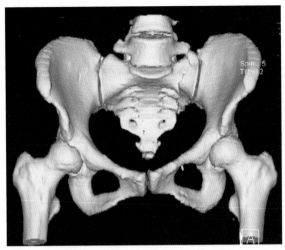

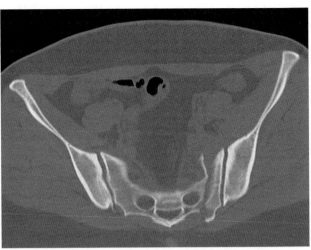

A   B

Figure 19–7 Example of an unstable lateral compression type II injury. **(A)** As shown by three-dimensional computed tomography (CT), there is an internal rotation deformity of the pelvis, associated with a disimpacted, complete fracture of the sacrum. **(B)** Axial CT through the sacrum, which clearly shows the unstable fracture of the sacrum.

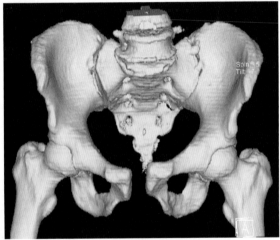

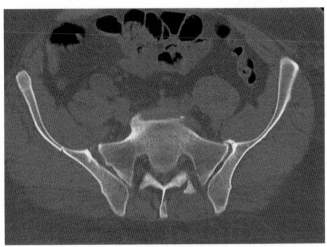

A   B

Figure 19–8 Example of an anteriorposterior compression type II (APC-II) injury of the pelvis. **(A)** This injury is characterized by widening of the pubic symphysis of greater than 2.5 cm and widening of the right anterior sacroiliac joint. **(B)** Axial computed tomographic cuts confirm that the posterior sacroiliac ligaments are intact.

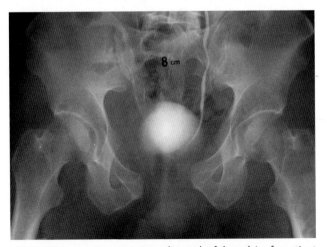

Figure 19–9 Anterior posterior radiograph of the pelvis of a patient who had a horse rear back and fall on him, causing an open book injury with 8 cm diastasis of the symphysis with posterior stability.

unacceptable deformity. As mentioned in the nonoperative section, avulsion fractures should be reviewed on a case-by-case basis. In general, avulsion with displacement greater than 1 cm leads to significant pain and weakness of the involved muscle that is attached, and therefore the author recommends operative fixation of these injuries. An additional indication for surgery includes pelvic injuries that may be stable but have significant deformity. An example of this may include an internal rotation deformity as a result of a lateral compression type of injury in which there is greater than 20 degrees of internal rotation of the hemipelvis, or greater than 1 cm leg length discrepancy **(Fig. 19–12)**.[6,7] Additionally, these internal rotational deformities can cause a ramus fracture that pierces the bladder or vagina. In these cases it is necessary to externally rotate the hemipelvis to remove the bone from the bladder or vagina. Because these are stable injuries, a simple external

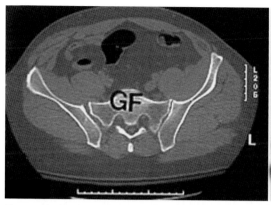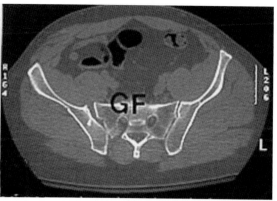

Figure 19–10 Same patient as from **Fig. 19–9.** With greater than 6 cm of symphysis diastasis, a complete disruption of the sacroiliac (SI) joint may exist. The left panel shows a superior cut from a computed tomographic scan indicating a complete disruption of the SI joint both anteriorly and posteriorly. However, a more inferior cut (right panel) shows that the more important posterior-inferior sacroiliac ligaments are intact.

fixator can be used to externally rotate the pelvis and restore the normal pelvic anatomy. Unfortunately, if the deformity persists, an osteotomy is required prior to performing the external rotation[7] **(Figs. 19–12** and **19–13).** However, in most cases ramus fractures do not require fixation whether there is an isolated anterior injury or a combined anterior and posterior injury. In cases where there is greater than 15 mm of displacement associated with a posterior injury, the very strong pectineal fascia may be disrupted, and therefore open reduction and internal fixation of the ramus fracture is indicated.[9] In external rotation deformities or open book pelvic injuries, the indication for surgery is greater than 2.5 cm of diastasis of the pubic symphysis. Widening of less than 2.5 cm may require surgical fixation if there is an associated posterior injury. Disruptions of the posterior sacroiliac ligaments of the pelvis begin to occur with more than 2.5 cm of displacement. There are pelvic injuries that appear as simple symphysis diastasis that actually include a complete disruption of the posterior part of the pelvis. In these injuries, reduction of the diastasis with an anterior external fixation frame will widen the posterior complex and demonstrate posterior instability **(Fig. 19–14A,B).**

The majority of pelvic injuries that require operative treatment are those that have complete instability of the hemipelvis. This may occur through the sacroiliac joint,

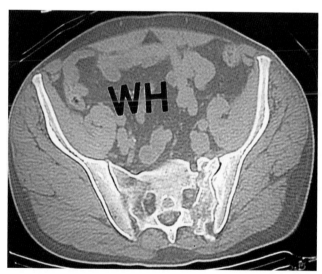

Figure 19–11 A computed tomographic scan shows a stable sacral impaction injury. The surgeon must assess the severity of the deformity and perform follow-up x-rays to ensure no further worsening of the deformity occurs.

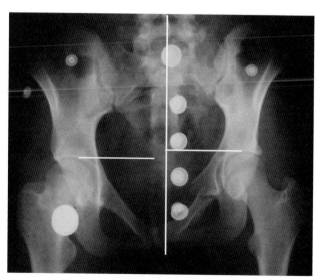

Figure 19–12 An anteroposterior radiograph of a young female patient with a significant internal rotation deformity of the left hemipelvis. The initial deformity was minimal but progressed over several weeks. She had limb length inequality and visible asymmetry of her anterior iliac crest. Note the medialization of the left hip and shortening of the left leg, as indicated by the white reference lines.

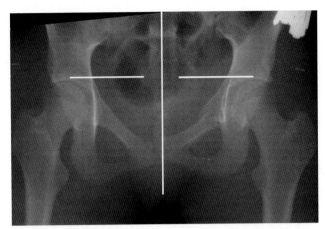

Figure 19–13 An intraoperative anteroposterior radiograph of the patient in **Fig. 19–12** after correction of the internal rotation deformity with an external fixator. The fixator was applied with an oblique vector to push the left hemipelvis laterally and distally. Note that the offset of the left hip has been restored and the leg lengths equalized, as shown by the white reference lines.

or with a combination fracture-dislocation involving either the sacrum or the iliac wing (crescent fracture). Alternatively, injuries can involve just the sacrum or just the iliac wing posteriorly. Instability is determined by a combination of physical examination and radiographic analysis. The radiographic signs of instability were defined in the classification section and include either or both greater than 5 mm of displacement of the sacroiliac joint and a fracture gap versus a fracture impaction. Additionally, a mobile hemipelvis during physical examination is an indication for surgical treatment. The surgical treatment of a pelvis fracture involves three steps: the approach,

the reduction, and the fixation. In high-energy pelvic injuries, patients can have significant associated morbidity. While performing acute stabilization of the pelvis, orthopaedic surgeons have the ability to control the reduction and prevent complications. A thorough understanding of the anatomy of the pelvis, as well as the deformity of the fracture, will optimize these two areas of control.

Surgical Treatment

Anterior Ring Injuries

Pubic Symphysis Diastasis (see Video 19–1, Disk 2)

As already mentioned, symphysis pubis displacement of greater than 2.5 cm is an indication for surgical treatment. The method of fixation can be either an external fixator or internal fixation with a plate. External fixation can be successful but is associated with the risk that a missed posterior disruption will lead to posterior pelvic deformity **(Fig. 19–14A,B)**. Another problem with external fixation is pin tract infections and skin necrosis in obese patients. Finally, patient acceptance of external fixation is not good. External fixation can be implemented with either an anterior or a posterior frame. As mentioned earlier, placement of most external fixators occurs in the acute setting to stabilize the hemipelvis in a hemodynamically unstable patient (systolic blood pressure less than 90 mm Hg) who has a mechanically unstable fracture. The technique for placing an anterior and a posterior frame will be described. Placement of the anterior frame is safer, and most orthopaedic

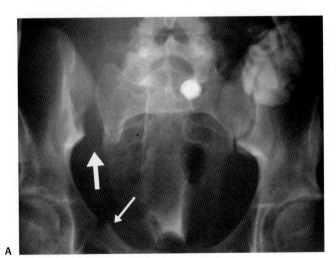

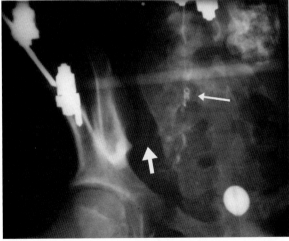

A   B

Figure 19–14 Example of the failure of an anterior pelvic fixator to stabilize the posterior pelvic ring. **(A)** An initial anteroposterior radiograph shows an unstable right hemipelvis with wide displacement of the right sacroiliac joint (broad white arrow). There were also minimally displaced fractures of the pubic rami, barely visible in the lower portion of the image (narrow white arrow). The patient was hemodynamically

unstable, and an anterior external fixator was applied, despite the fact that there was not significant displacement of the anterior pelvic ring. **(B)** Radiograph of the patient after placement of the anterior external fixator still shows signs of posterior instability with even greater widening of the right sacroiliac joint (broad white arrow). Note the embolization coils in the right internal iliac artery (narrow white arrow).

surgeons are more comfortable with the anterior technique. However, an anterior external fixator may not provide adequate support in a completely unstable pelvic fracture. In general, a four-pin external fixator is used. Understanding the deformity can allow the surgeon to better place the incisions for the pin placement. For example, if there is an external rotation deformity, the surgeon should place the incision medial to the iliac crest to reduce tenting of the skin with the pins following reduction. The gluteus medius tubercle is the ideal placement for the anterior pins.

A stab incision is made 2.0 to 2.5 cm posterior to the anterior superior iliac spine. This incision is taken down to the crest of the iliac wing. Laterally, the iliac wing often has a shelf. However, medially or internally the iliac wing is confluent with the crest. Therefore, placing a K-wire along the inner cortex helps define the angle of the gluteus medius tubercle and helps the surgeon place a longer fixator pin within the bone. The author's preference for pin placement is two pins separated by ~4 cm. Initially, a pilot drill hole is placed through the cortex on the top of the iliac crest. A Schanz pin is then placed into the drill hole and driven between the two tables of cortical bone in the iliac wing. If the pin exits the pelvis, it still has a good bicortical bite. The other pin is placed using the same technique. After two pins are placed on each side, they are attached to each other with a bar after manipulating the two hemipelves together to obtain a reduction. These two bars are then attached to a third bar once reduction is obtained. In the acute setting in a hemodynamically unstable patient, the surgeon must understand the vectors required to obtain a reduced pelvis.[6] Frequently, in completely unstable pelvis injuries, reduction of the posterior pelvis is important to controlling bleeding and obtaining hemodynamic stability. A combination of traction either in full extension or with hip flexion to approximately 45 degrees along with compression in the posterior part of the pelvis will usually accomplish a very acceptable reduction of the hemipelvis. A frequent mistake occurs when surgeons try to compress the diastasis anteriorly, causing a flexion internal rotation deformity of the hemi-pelvis, often opening up the posterior part of the pelvis (**Fig. 19–14A,B**).

In the acute setting, the stabilization and reduction of the posterior part of the pelvis are more important than decreasing the volume of the pelvis.[10] Once the reduction is performed, tightening of the external fixator clamps will allow the surgeon to obtain relative stability of the hemipelvis. The skin is released around the pins, preventing later maceration and infection, and a second level of bars is added for stability. Alternatively, a two-pin fixation can be used with the pin placed between the anterior superior iliac spine and the anterior inferior iliac spine. These pins yield excellent purchase in the supra-acetabular bone and can be incorporated into an anterior frame or used bilaterally to compress the posterior injury. One dis-

advantage of the two-pin technique is that an adduction-abduction rotational deformity is harder to correct with a single pin on each side of the pelvis.

The posterior external fixation frame (C-clamp) is used for the same indications as the anterior fixator, with the additional advantage of posterior stabilization. The contraindication for placement of the posterior clamp is an iliac wing fracture anterior to the sacroiliac joint because compression of the joint will not help the reduction of the iliac wing fracture. Comminution of the sacrum requires special consideration because overcompression can be harmful to the patient. The technique for placement of the posterior clamp is as follows. With the patient in the supine position, an imaginary line is drawn from the anterior superior iliac spine to the posterior superior iliac spine along the side of the patient. This line is divided into thirds, and a longitudinal stab incision is made at the interval between the posterior third and the middle third (**Fig. 19–15**). This site should be roughly in line with the greater trochanter of the femur. A long clamp is then introduced through the stab wound down to the bone. The bone is palpated with the clamp, and the flare of the iliac wing is located. This flare is at the level of the anterior end of the sacroiliac joint; thus pin insertion anterior to this risks penetration of the peritoneal cavity if the pin traverses the ilium. Immediately posterior to the flare is the area where the pin should be placed. This corresponds to the area of the iliac wing outside the sacroiliac joint. Once this area is determined, a pin is placed on both sides and hammered into the iliac wing. A clamp is then placed over the pins, and the surgeon manually compresses the clamp to fit snugly against the pins. The clamp has a cannulated, threaded bolt that slides over the pins and is tightened with a wrench, providing additional compression of the posterior pelvic injury. Traction is helpful in reducing the

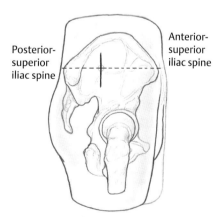

Figure 19–15 The ideal position of the site for insertion of the pin for a posterior C-clamp is the point that lies at the intersection of a line from the anterior-superior iliac spine (ASIS) to the posterior superior iliac spine (PSIS) and the line represented by the border of the middle third and posterior third on the lateral aspect of the pelvis.

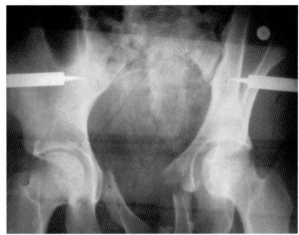

A

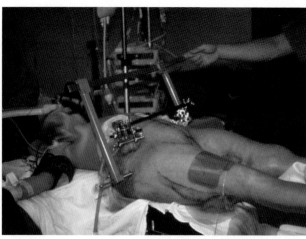

B

Figure 19–16 Example of the use of a posterior C-clamp. The patient was crushed by machinery and was hemodynamically unstable. **(A)** Anteroposterior radiograph of the pelvis taken during resuscitation showing placement of the C-clamp pins in the posterior ilium. **(B)** Clinical photograph of the patient during a later operative procedure, showing the pelvic C-clamp. Because of severe posterior pelvic skin loss, definitive posterior stabilization was not felt to be safe. An anterior fixator was later used to supplement the posterior C-clamp, as shown in this photograph.

completely unstable pelvic injury prior to initiating compression (**Fig. 19–16A,B**).

As mentioned, overcompression is a potential complication, and therefore radiographic evaluation is required following application of the frame. One concern is that the posterior pins of the C-clamp may lead to a subsequent infection when iliosacral screws are placed for the definitive treatment of the posterior pelvic injury. In the author's series of more than 20 staged cases using the above protocol, there have been no secondary infections of the iliosacral screws. However, the concern remains.

Symphyseal disruptions are more commonly treated using open reduction and internal fixation of the symphysis. There are two approaches commonly used: either a midline incision or the Pfannenstiel approach. The midline incision is most frequently used as an extension of an exploratory laparotomy performed by the general surgeons to treat intra-abdominal pathology. More commonly, a Pfannenstiel approach is performed. The incision for the Pfannenstiel approach begins 1 cm above the symphysis pubis and is ~10 cm in length (**Fig. 19–17A,B**). A critical component of the exposure is to maintain the rectus abdominis attachment to the rami anteriorly. Adequate visualization and reduction of the fracture can be performed with the rectus attached. If the muscle insertion is detached during the approach, patients may have postoperative pain. Frequently, one head of the rectus is traumatically disrupted and requires repair to the remaining rectus as well as reattachment to the distal insertion. Deep to the skin layer, the fascia covering the two heads of the rectus is identified. The midline can be identified by noting a chevron V pattern of the muscle fibers. The crossing of the two sides of the fibers guides the surgeon to the midline between the two heads of the rectus. If muscle is seen, then the incision is angled to try and stay between the two heads of the rectus.

Once these are separated, the rectus can be cleared from the superior portion of the rami while maintaining its attachment anteriorly. The superior ramus attachment of the rectus is released initially with an electrocautery medially and then using a periosteal elevator laterally. The superior portion of the rectus insertion is released on each side of the symphysis pubis. Hohman retractors are used beneath the rectus to help improve the exposure. A malleable retractor is used to hold back the bladder for exposure and to prevent injury (**Fig. 19–18**).

Alternatively, laparotomy sponges can be packed between the symphysis pubis and the bladder, providing both retraction and protection of the bladder. Once the superior portions of the rami are cleared, reduction is performed using a Weber clamp. The skin is separated from the rectus, and the Weber clamp is usually placed through the anterior insertions of the rectus onto the pubic tubercles, as demonstrated in **Fig. 19–19**. Small pilot holes may be drilled into the bone to allow more secure purchase of the bone by the Weber clamp. Often, in addition to the external rotation injury, there may be an associated flexion-extension deformity in the pelvis. By manipulating the clamps, both deformities can be corrected, and a perfect anatomical reduction can be achieved. The cartilage between the two pubic bones is maintained and not debrided. If more force is required to achieve reduction, a Farabeuf or Jungbluth clamp can be used anteriorly with either a 4.5 or 3.5 mm reduction screw (**Fig. 19–20A,B**). In complete pelvic ring disruptions with posterior translation of one side of the pelvis, the displaced hemipelvis must be "pulled" anteriorly. Application of this type of vector usually requires the use of a Jungbluth clamp. Rarely, a reduction screw may pull out when large reduction forces are needed; in this circumstance a nut can be placed on the far side of the

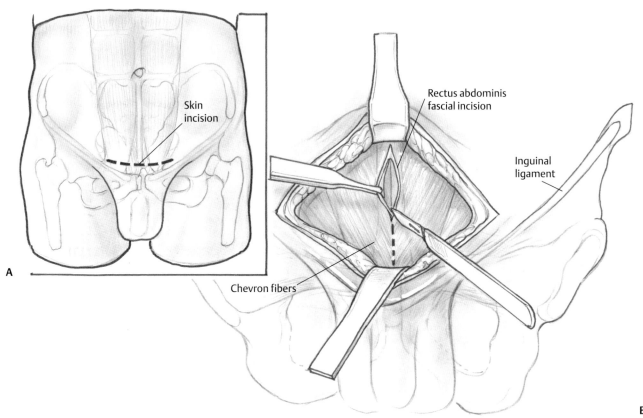

Figure 19–17 The approach for plating of the symphysis pubis. **(A)** The Pfannenstiel skin incision is made one fingerbreadth above the symphysis pubis. **(B)** The two bodies of the rectus muscle are separated by identifying the chevron V pattern in the fascia.

screw to help maintain fixation during reduction. The additional dissection of the anterior pubis needed for these maneuvers can cause further disruption of the insertion of the rectus as well as damage to the suspensory ligaments to the penis. These additional steps should only be used if the initial reduction attempts fail.

Once an acceptable reduction is achieved, the surgeon confirms that no posterior widening has occurred and there is posterior stability. Various options that are available for symphyseal plating include a two-hole plate with either 6.5 or 4.5 mm screws, or a four- or six-hole plate with smaller (3.5 or 4.5 mm) screws. The author prefers a six-hole curved

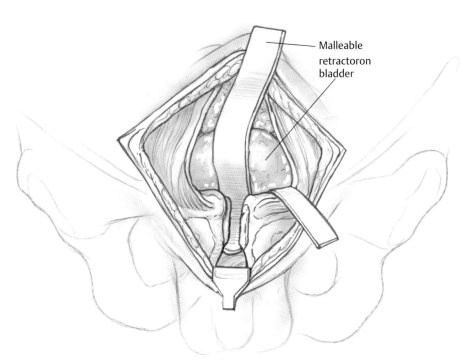

Figure 19–18 Usually one side is exposed at a time, with a Hohman used to raise the rectus off the cephalad surface of the rami and a malleable retractor used to protect the bladder.

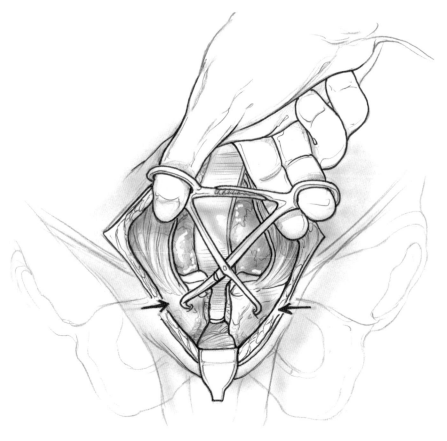

Figure 19–19 A Weber clamp is placed superficial to the rectus, compressing the symphysis.

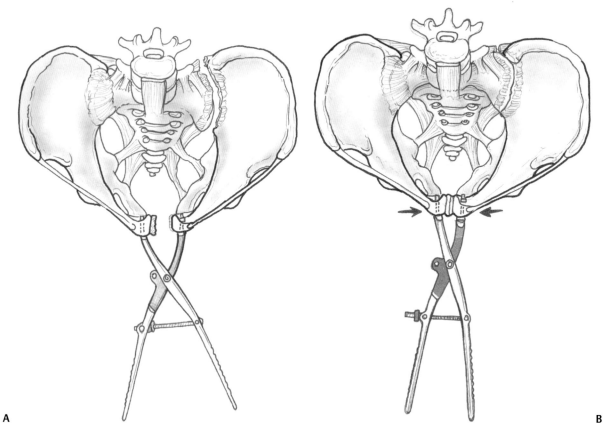

A   B

Figure 19–20 (A) The placement of a Jungbluth clamp for reduction of posterior translation caused by a combination of displacement of the symphysis pubis and sacroiliac joint. **(B)** Reduction of the posterior displacement and symphysis diastasis with the Jungbluth clamp.

plate with either 3.5 or 4.5 mm screws. The plate is placed on the superior aspect of the rami. Additionally, a second plate can be placed anteriorly for a more rigid 90/90 degree construct. This two-plate construct is not required in the acute setting.[9] In malunion cases, double-plating is occasionally required.[5] The surgeon bends the superior plate down ~15 degrees before the last hole on each side of the plate where the pubis bone connects with the rami. This anatomical sloping of the rami occurs over the obturator foramen. Screws inserted in the plane of the pubis can be up to 90 mm in length, and average 60 to 70 mm in length. Screws over the obturator foramen are significantly shorter, usually in the 20 to 30 mm range.

The timing of the repair of an associated genital urinary disruption is controversial. Frequently, urologists do not like to repair urethral injuries until several months after the initial disruption. In these cases a suprapubic catheter is required; however, this is associated with a high risk of infection. Tunneling the suprapubic catheter away from the symphysis disruption is helpful to prevent contamination of an anterior wound. However, in most cases ureterocystoscopy is possible with realignment of the urethra over a Foley catheter. This is the preferred approach and should be performed whenever possible. Delaying open reduction and internal fixation until the urine is no longer leaking into the pelvic area is indicated to prevent infection. The author usually waits 3 to 5 days after a urethral injury prior to plating the symphysis. Bladder ruptures should be repaired at the time of fixation of the symphysis regardless of whether it is an intra- or an extraperitoneal rupture.

Pubic Ramus Fractures (see Video 19–2, Disk 2)

As previously mentioned, most pubic ramus fractures are treated nonsurgically. Additionally, those that occur in conjunction with posterior pelvic instability can be treated nonsurgically without any loss of reduction.[9,11] Although fixing the rami fractures may increase the stability of the pelvis, this is usually not necessary. Operative intervention is indicated in the following situations: when the pubic rami are impinging upon the bladder or vagina due to an internal rotation injury of the hemipelvis, when there is greater than 20 degrees of internal rotation of the hemipelvis, and when there is an associated leg length discrepancy of greater than 1 cm. In these cases, external fixation offers a simple method to externally rotate the hemipelvis and remove the ramus fracture from the bladder or vagina (**Figs. 19–12** and **19–13**). Alternatively, the Pfannenstiel incision can be extended into a modified Stoppa approach as needed to apply a plate across even high ramus fractures.[12] Using the modified Stoppa approach, a plate can be placed from one sacroiliac joint all the way around the symphysis to the opposite sacroiliac joint. The difference between using the Stoppa approach and conventional symphyseal plating is that the plate runs along the inside of the pelvis as opposed to the superior aspect

of the ramus. This technique is used when there is a posterior injury with greater than 1.5 cm of diastasis of the ramus fracture, indicating that the iliopectineal fascia has been disrupted. Disruption of the iliopectineal fascia leads to greater instability of the ramus fracture, and therefore surgical stabilization is indicated.

Alternatively, a ramus screw can be placed from the pubic tubercle into the supra-acetabular bone as a method of fixation.[13] Placement of this intramedullary screw requires experience with fluoroscopy to ensure that this rami screw does not penetrate the joint. An obturator oblique with a cephalad tilt allows the corridor of bone to be visualized where the screw can be placed safely.

The timing of fixation is controversial and needs to be planned on a case-by-case basis. Performing initial fixation as early as possible often makes it easier to achieve reduction by either closed or open techniques. Initial stabilization with either or both external fixation and percutaneous iliosacral screws can achieve excellent success. However, if anatomical reduction is not achieved by closed methods, performing open reduction prior to achieving hemodynamic stability and allowing the initial bleeding to cease can lead to significant blood loss and potential mortality to the patient. In general, the author's preference in a hemodynamically unstable patient with a mechanically unstable pelvis is to stabilize the pelvis with a pelvic sheet or external fixator in the emergency room. If the patient is going to the operating room due to another emergency condition, the external fixator can be placed in the operating room. Additionally, closed reduction and percutaneous fixation of posterior disruptions can be undertaken at the same time. Anatomical closed reductions become progressively more difficult to achieve after 24 hours. Occasionally, symphyseal plating is used in combination with an exploratory laparotomy to give the pelvis some anterior stability. However, only a few degrees of a malunion anteriorly can translate into more than a centimeter of displacement posteriorly. Ideally, definitive fixation is undertaken when the patient has stabilized and is in positive fluid balance (5 to 7 days from the injury).

Posterior Ring Injuries (see Video 19–3, Disk 2)

Sacroiliac Joint Dislocations (see Video 19–4, Disk 2)

Good radiographic evaluation is required for accomplishing either an anterior or a posterior approach to the posterior pelvic injury. Therefore, the surgeon must position the pelvis to ensure that good AP, lateral, inlet, and outlet views can be obtained to evaluate the reduction and perform the fixation of the pelvis.

With all pelvic injuries, reduction of the sacroiliac joint or the posterior pelvic injury is critical prior to inserting fixation. During the initial period (less than 48 hours) following injury, closed reduction and fixation can potentially be achieved. Closed reduction techniques include traction and manipulation using traction, as well as manipulation of the reduction using the external fixator or half pins (in the anterior-inferior iliac crest region) as reduction aids. Definitive fixation of the sacroiliac joint is often accomplished using iliosacral lag screws. Anterior sacroiliac plating and transiliac bars or plating are also acceptable options. If closed reduction fails to achieve an anatomical reduction, or if more than 48 hours has elapsed since the injury occurred, open reduction and internal fixation of the posterior pelvic injury is indicated. The approach to sacroiliac joint disruptions can be undertaken either anteriorly or posteriorly. Benefits of the anterior approach include better visualization of the joint, the ability to keep the patient in the supine position (often preferred due to associated injuries in multiple trauma patients), and sparing the more damaged posterior soft tissue. The major problem associated with the anterior approach is achieving reduction of a posteriorly displaced hemipelvis. Posterior displacement is very difficult to reduce and hold from the anterior approach while placing definitive fixation. Often the reduction has to be held manually while fixation is being placed. Additional problems occur if there is a sacral fracture. Such injuries cannot be fixed with anterior plating, and reduction of a sacral fracture is very difficult from the front. Finally, the L5 nerve root is in significant danger with the anterior approach **(Fig. 19–21)**. The anterior approach is indicated if there is a posterior crush injury to the soft tissue that prevents a posterior approach, if the patient has multiple trauma that cannot be placed in the prone position, and if there is an iliac wing fracture that is anterior to the sacroiliac joint.

The posterior approach facilitates reduction of the posterior pelvis using clamping techniques as opposed to the

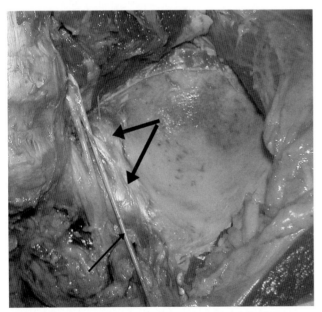

Figure 19–21 The L5 nerve root (thin arrow) runs along the anterior sacrum just 2 cm medial to the sacroiliac joint, identifiable by the shiny anterior capsule (broad arrows).

anterior approach. The surgeon can debride the joint with less risk of damaging the L5 nerve root. The ability to more easily achieve reduction using clamping techniques with a posterior approach is beneficial in patients that have had a long time interval from the injury to their definitive fixation. The surgeon also has more options for the types of fixation of the posterior pelvis when using a posterior approach (iliosacral screws, transiliac bars or plate, or lumbopelvic fixation). The primary problem with the posterior approach is that damage to the soft tissue from the injury may prevent this approach from being used safely. Another disadvantage is that the surgeon does not have the same visualization of the sacroiliac joint that is available from an anterior approach. The posterior approach is indicated in sacral fractures and in crescent fractures (fractures of the iliac wing) where the fracture line is primarily posterior to the sacroiliac joint, as well as when decompression of nerve roots is required.

The anterior approach is performed with the patient in the supine position. The leg is draped free to enable the surgeon to flex the hip and relax the psoas muscle and to manipulate the leg with traction and rotation to help reduce the injury. The surgical incision utilized is the iliac portion or upper window of the ilioinguinal incision. This incision is placed from the anterior-superior iliac spine to the point where the crest begins to fall away posteriorly and can no longer be easily palpated. The dissection is taken down to the iliac crest. The tendinous portion between the abdominal musculature and the abductors is incised. No muscle should be cut during this approach. Often there is abdominal muscle overhang that will be transected if the surgeon cuts straight to the crest. It is better to approach the crest somewhat laterally and inferiorly through the insertion between the abductors of the hip and the abdominal muscles that attach on the iliac crest. Using this technique, the muscle is not damaged, and the closure can more easily and securely be performed. This is especially important in very thin patients who will complain if they have a prominent iliac wing and their "love handles" have not been properly restored. Once the crest is exposed, the iliacus and iliopsoas are raised from the inner table of the ilium from the crest to the sacroiliac joint. Once the sacroiliac joint is palpated anteriorly, careful dissection is required to cross over the remaining ligaments of the sacroiliac joint and gain access to the sacrum. The L5 nerve root is ~2 to 3 cm medial to the sacroiliac joint superiorly. As one moves inferiorly on the sacrum, the L5 nerve root crosses the sacroiliac joint **(Fig. 19–21)**.

As a result of these anatomical relationships, careful dissection on the sacrum is required to prevent damage to the L5 nerve root. Once 2 cm of the sacrum is exposed, a sharp Hohman retractor can be gently hammered into the sacrum, allowing retraction and excellent visualization of the sacroiliac joint. Retraction of the L5 nerve root must be minimized to prevent an L5 nerve palsy. As already mentioned, reduction of the sacroiliac joint can be problematic. An occasionally helpful technique when the symphysis is disrupted is manipulation of the symphysis with the Jung-bluth clamp (**Fig. 19–20A,B**). Additionally, use of a Farabeuf clamp on the iliac wing to manipulate the rotation of the hemipelvis as well as compress the sacroiliac joint is often useful. This can also be done with an external fixator or a pin placed into the crest and used as a joystick. Clamp placement in this area can be very difficult. Occasionally, in a thin person, flexion of the hip to relax the psoas muscle combined with a Farabeuf or Jungbluth clamp placed across the sacroiliac joint can complete the reduction.

Once anatomical reduction of the sacroiliac joint is achieved, many types of fixation can be used. Although technically demanding, iliosacral screws can be placed from the anterior approach. This is aided by elevation of the pelvic region with blankets utilized to elevate the patient off the radiolucent operating table. Because the sacroiliac joint is exposed, another option is placement of two plates. Either 4.5 or 3.5 mm plates can be used and should be positioned at ~90 degrees to each other. The best bone in this region is along the pelvic brim, and a three-hole plate with one screw in the sacrum and the other two in the ilium along the brim achieves the best fixation. The surgeon has to remember that the sacroiliac joint is oriented obliquely in a medial direction ~10 degrees. Therefore, to prevent the screws from going into the joint, the angle of the screws has to be adjusted appropriately. Once the anterior-inferior plate is in place, a second plate can be added in a more posterior-superior location. This plate is oriented in a plane ~90 degrees to the first plate.

Again, one screw should be placed in the sacrum and two in the ilium. There are special plates that have been developed for this area; however, their clinical usefulness over the foregoing construct has not been proven.

For the posterior approach, the patient should be placed in the prone position on a radiolucent table. The pelvis should be positioned so that appropriate inlet and outlet views can be performed. This often requires 6 in. of blankets or sheets under the thighs to prevent flexion of the pelvis and allow a good AP view of the pelvis. These blankets are in addition to chest rolls that improve ventilation in a prone patient. A critical aspect prior to embarking on a posterior approach is the assessment of the soft tissues. A common soft tissue problem is the Morel-Lavallée lesion, which can become infected in greater than one third of cases.[14] This soft tissue degloving injury requires a thorough debridement prior to definitive fixation. Therefore, if the patient has one of these lesions, the author will do a thorough debridement with cultures prior to definitive fixation. If at the time of debridement the hematoma does not appear infected, then the patient will undergo a re-prep and drape, and definitive fixation will be performed during the same surgical procedure. Prior to prepping the patient, radiographic evaluation is performed with the C-arm to ensure that good inlet, outlet, lateral, and AP views can be obtained.

The incision is made 1 cm lateral to the posterior-superior iliac spine and is carried inferiorly or caudal in a straight line going from just above the crest to the midbuttocks area (**Fig. 19–22A,B**). The dissection is carried down

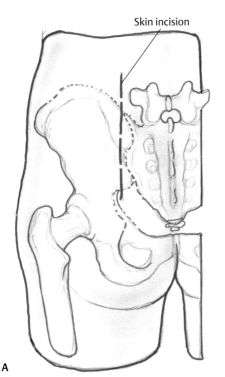 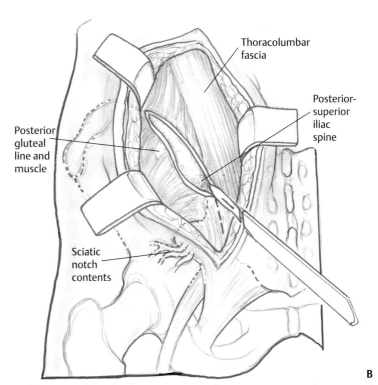

A **B**

Figure 19–22 (A) The posterior approach to the pelvis skin incision begins 1 cm lateral and 2 cm superior to the posterior-superior iliac spine and passes to the midbuttocks. **(B)** The skin is elevated off the gluteus fascia, followed by the gluteus maximus being elevated off the lumbodorsal fascia.

through the skin to the fascia of the gluteus maximus. This fascia is somewhat tenuous and therefore may be somewhat difficult to maintain after raising a skin flap medially. The key to this approach is to elevate a full-thickness skin flap. The gluteus maximus originates from both the iliac crest superiorly and the lumbodorsal fascia inferiorly. An incision straight down to the posterior-superior iliac spine will cut through muscle of the gluteus maximus. If the muscle is incised, coverage of the posterior-superior iliac spine is more difficult, and there may be a higher incidence of wound dehiscence. A critical step in the approach to the posterior pelvis is to elevate the gluteus maximus muscle flap off the lumbodorsal fascia. This allows easier and more secure coverage of the posterior sacroiliac joint and decreases the risk of infection.[15] Inferiorly, the origin of the gluteus maximus is close if not at the midline spinous process.

After exposing the entire origin of the gluteus maximus, the muscle is elevated from the crest as well as the lumbodorsal fascia, providing exposure to the sacrum and the sciatic notch. At the elbow or bend of the sacrum where the coccyx begins, the lateral origin of the piriformis is taken down from the lateral border of the sacrum. The release of the piriformis starts distally and extends proximally, allowing the contents of the sciatic notch to fall away and preventing iatrogenic damage to these structures.[16] The piriformis still has an origin on the anterior sacrum, but the lateral border is released, allowing placement of clamps through the notch. The gluteus maximus is

also taken off the lateral and posterior aspect of the iliac wing. Debris is removed from the joint, and a laminar spreader is often used to help with visualization and debris removal. Careful use of the lamina spreader is required because excessive widening of the sacroiliac joint can stretch and damage the lumbosacral plexus. The articular cartilage of the sacroiliac is never debrided, but loose pieces of articular cartilage are discarded. Once the sacroiliac joint is debrided posteriorly, a small portion of the joint is visualized and is used to guide reduction. There is a concave surface on the sacrum that fits into the convex surface of the ilium. The sacroiliac joint forms somewhat of an L shape, with the bottom end of the L visualized posteriorly and the long part of the L visualized anteriorly.

Reduction of the sacroiliac joint is the most difficult step in treating these injuries. The clamps that are used for reduction include an angled Matta clamp that is placed through the sciatic notch, with one prong on the sacral ala and the other on the outer side of the iliac wing. This helps reduce external rotation deformities as well as diastasis of the sacroiliac joint. Additionally, a Weber clamp is placed from the posterior-superior iliac spine to the sacral spinous process and reduces cephalad displacement and internal rotation deformities of the hemipelvis. Combinations of these two clamps in the proper position and order of tightening will usually achieve anatomical reduction (**Figs. 19–23** and **19–24**). With sacral fractures, placement of the angled Matta clamp on the S1 body can aid in reduction.[13] To

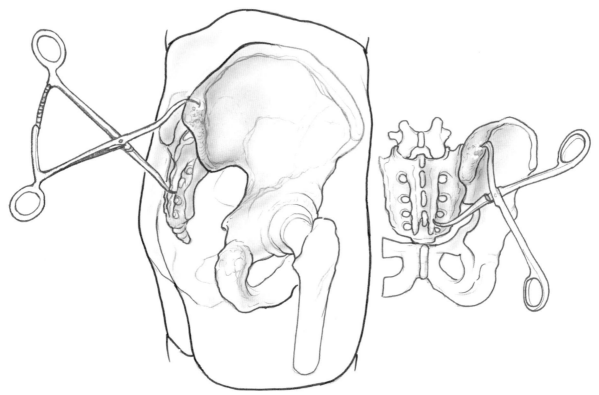

Figure 19–23 Reduction clamp placement to correct cephalad displacement of the hemipelvis. This method can be used in treatment of a sacroiliac joint disruption or sacral fracture.

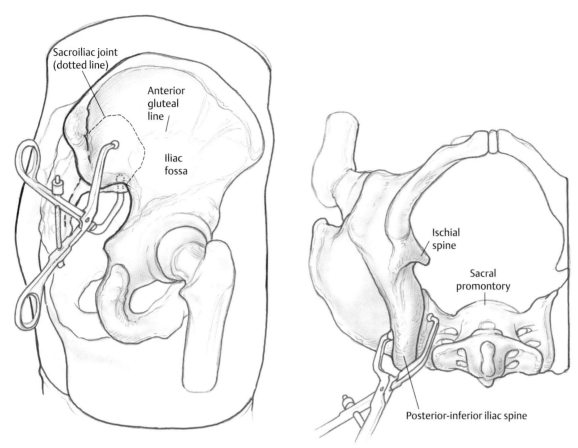

Figure 19–24 Two views showing safe placement of reduction clamps to correct diastasis of the joint and external rotation of the hemipelvis in reduction of a sacroiliac joint disruption. This method can be used in treatment of a sacroiliac joint disruption or sacral fracture.

perform this safely, the anterior aspect of the sacrum is palpated medial to the fracture site and between the S1 and S2 nerve roots. The clamp should be placed along the inside of the surgeon's finger, placing the point into the sacral body while avoiding the risk of clamping any neurovascular structures. The key to reduction is to create the appropriate reduction vector using a combination of clamps. The most common deformities seen in operative posterior pelvic injuries include cephalad and posterior translation, diastasis, and rotational injuries (abduction/adduction, internal rotation/external rotation).[6] Often, translational deformities are corrected, but rotational deformities persist. Awareness of the bony landmarks helps the surgeon recognize and correct residual rotational deformities. Subtle manipulation of clamp placement will often correct the deformity.

Once anatomical reduction is achieved on the inlet, outlet, AP, and lateral views, iliosacral screws are the primary form of fixation **(Fig. 19–25A–M)**. Posterior tension-band plating (see sacral fracture section) can be performed as well using a 14- to 16-hole reconstruction plate placed at the superior portion of the sciatic notch below the posterior-superior iliac spine **(Fig. 19–26A,B)**. Tension-band plates are used in cases of significant comminution of the sacrum or severe osteoporosis and may be used as an adjunct to iliosacral screws. As mentioned, the mainstay for fixation

posteriorly is iliosacral screws. Placement of iliosacral screws requires a thorough understanding of the anatomy of the posterior pelvis and an appreciation of the dangers of incorrect placement of the screws. Significant morbidity and mortality, including amputations, have been attributed to poor placement of iliosacral screws **(Fig. 19–27)**. The exact placement of iliosacral screws can be variable and is constrained by the bony anatomy (i.e., sacral dysmorphism–lumbarization of S1 vertebrae or a significantly slanted sacral ala). Some authors believe that a more posterior to anterior approach is beneficial because it stays out of the more anterior articular surface of the sacroiliac joint. This may be beneficial in sacroiliac joint injuries; however, the screws may be shorter and have most of their purchase in the sacral ala, which is significantly weaker than S1 vertebrae bone. The author prefers placing a longer screw into S1 body knowing that the strongest bone is in the superior end plate of S1. These often penetrate the articular cartilage but are usually removed 1 year after they are placed. The use of cannulated screws enhances the surgeon's ability to put the screws in percutaneously. The drawback with cannulated screws is the lack of tactile response in placement of threaded K-wires. The use of percutaneous screws may be more difficult if an anatomical reduction of the sacroiliac joint has not been achieved because malreduction can

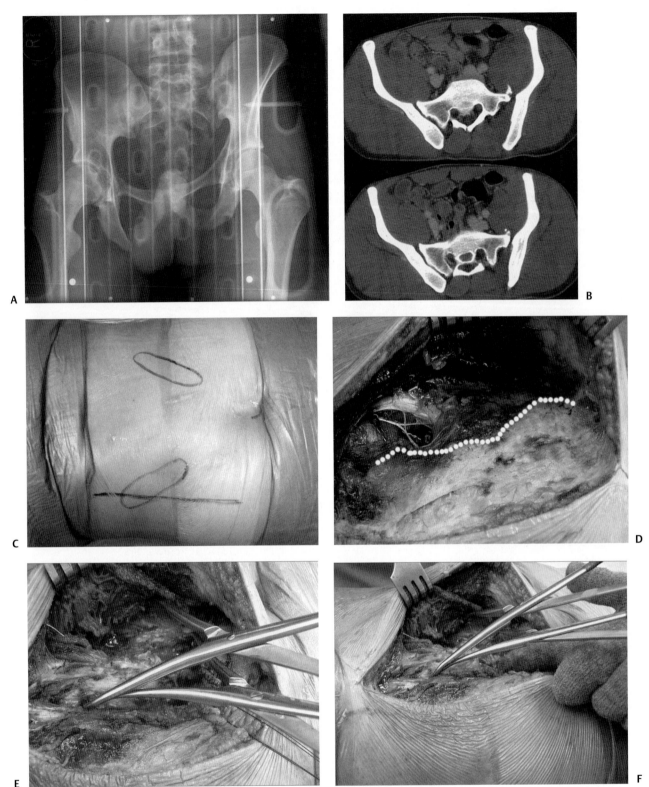

Figure 19–25 Example of the posterior approach to the sacroiliac joint for reduction and fixation of a complete sacroiliac joint disruption. **(A)** Anteroposterior (AP) radiograph of the injured pelvis demonstrating mild right sacroiliac joint widening, right pubic root fracture, complete disruption of the left sacroiliac joint, and cephalad translation of the left hemipelvis. **(B)** Computed tomographic scan confirming the observations made from the AP radiograph of the pelvis. **(C)** A posterior approach to the left sacroiliac joint was chosen. The viewpoint is that of the surgeon standing on the left side of the patient. The patient is prone on a radiolucent table, with the patient's head toward the left. Note the cephalad translation of the left posterior iliac crest. The skin incision is drawn. Normally the skin incision is slightly more lateral. **(D)** An incision down to the muscle fascia is performed. In this case, there is a mild degloving injury. The gluteus maximus will be reflected laterally to expose the sacroiliac joint. The gluteus maximus originates from the lumbodorsal fascia over the sacrum and from the iliac crest. Its origin is outlined by the dotted line. **(E)** In this case, two pointed-reduction clamps are utilized for the reduction. Normally, a clamp is also placed from the posterior iliac crest to the anterior aspect of the sacrum. **(F)** The reduction anteriorly along the sacroiliac joint is palpated with the surgeon's index finger.

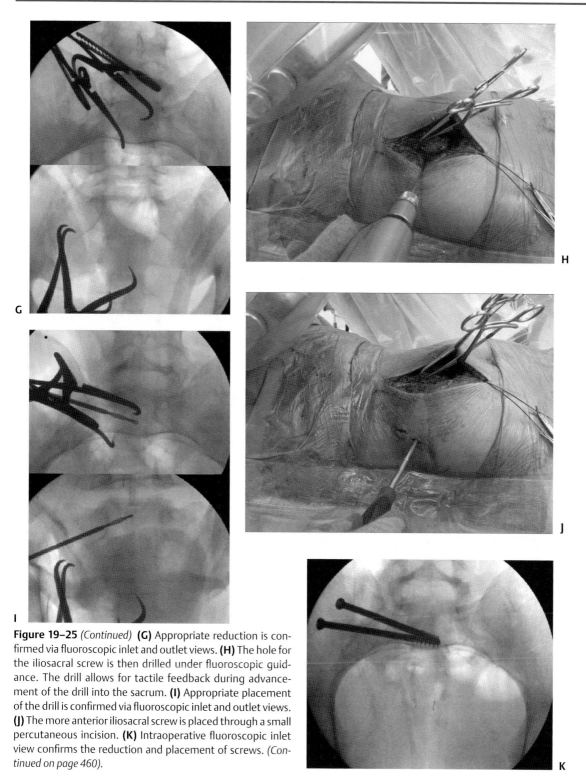

Figure 19–25 *(Continued)* **(G)** Appropriate reduction is confirmed via fluoroscopic inlet and outlet views. **(H)** The hole for the iliosacral screw is then drilled under fluoroscopic guidance. The drill allows for tactile feedback during advancement of the drill into the sacrum. **(I)** Appropriate placement of the drill is confirmed via fluoroscopic inlet and outlet views. **(J)** The more anterior iliosacral screw is placed through a small percutaneous incision. **(K)** Intraoperative fluoroscopic inlet view confirms the reduction and placement of screws. *(Continued on page 460).*

further reduce the narrow corridor of bone in which iliosacral screws can be safely placed.

Quality fluoroscopic views demonstrating the AP, inlet, outlet, and lateral projections are critical to ensure iliosacral screws can be placed safely **(Fig. 19–28A–C).** The author's preferred starting point for iliosacral screws is the intersection between a line drawn cephalad from the posterior border of the sciatic notch to a line where the flare of the iliac wing begins (end of the sacroiliac joint). At this intersection point, move a few millimeters posteriorly (into the sacroiliac joint area) onto the flatter part of the iliac wing and drill the first of two iliosacral screws under fluoroscopic guidance. Once this starting hole is checked on the inlet, outlet, and AP views, drilling commences using an oscillating drill to improve the tactile feel and to ensure that only three out of four cortices are penetrated. The author

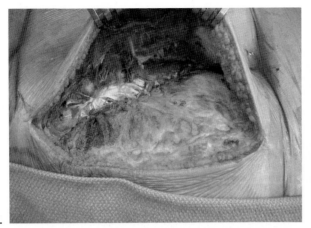

L

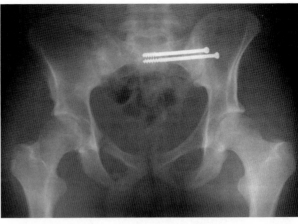

M

Figure 19–25 *(Continued)* Example of the posterior approach to the sacroiliac joint for reduction and fixation of a complete sacroiliac joint disruption. **(L)** The gluteus maximus flap is closed utilizing multiple absorbable sutures. Closure is completed over suction drainage.

(M) Postoperative AP radiograph of the pelvis. The right sacroiliac joint was not addressed because it was felt to have minimal displacement. (Case courtesy of Philip J. Kregor, MD.)

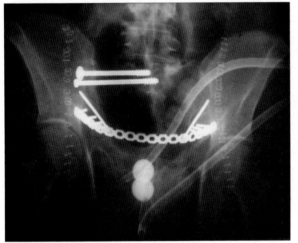

A

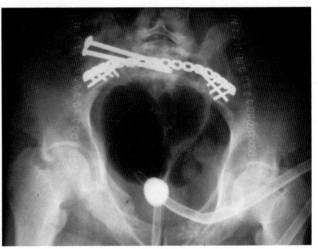

B

Figure 19–26 Example of a posterior pelvic tension-band plate. **(A)** An anteroposterior radiograph of the pelvis showing both a tension plate placed over the posterior pelvis and iliosacral screws. In general, the two iliosacral screws are used for sacral fractures. **(B)** Inlet radiograph

of the pelvis showing the fixation achieved. There is slight residual internal rotation of the hemipelvis that may be difficult to perfectly assess and correct from the posterior approach. (Case courtesy of Dave Templeman, MD, and Andrew Schmidt, MD.)

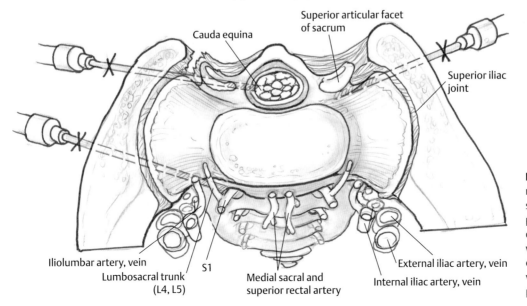

Figure 19–27 Errors in placement of a guide pin, drill, or screw can have disastrous complications. Posterior placement can cause nerve root damage, whereas anterior placement can cause nerve injury (L5) or vascular injury (sacral venous plexus, iliac vein or artery).

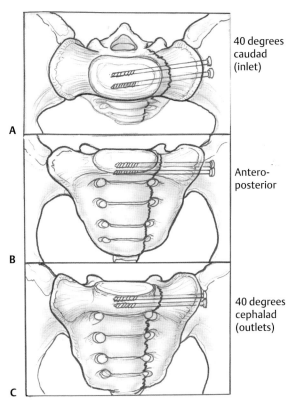

A

40 degrees
caudad
(inlet)

B

Antero-
posterior

C

40 degrees
cephalad
(outlets)

Figure 19–28 (A) Inlet, **(B)** anteroposterior view with two safely placed iliosacral screws in a sacral fracture and **(C)** outlet.

uses a 3.2 mm oscillating drill, feels each of the three cortices penetrated by the drilling, and ensures the drill remains in bone at all times. These three cortices that should be penetrated are the outer and inner cortex of the iliac wing and the inner cortex of the sacrum. The drill is gently advanced with an in-and-out motion to feel the bone and to ensure that, after the third cortex is penetrated, the drill remains in bone and does not penetrate the fourth cortex. As the drill progresses, inlet, outlet, and AP views are continuously checked.

Once the drill is well into the S1 body, the drill is left in place, and a lateral view is used to ensure the precise location of the drill bit. The lateral view is a critical step that can prevent serious complications during the placement of iliosacral screws. A free drill bit of the same size is used to measure the length of the screw off the drill bit that is left in place. The drill bit is left in place while the second drill is used to place a second iliosacral screw safely. The ideal location of the second screw is a little anterior and cephalad to the first screw. Various screw options include cannulated versus solid, and fully threaded versus partially threaded screws. The author in most cases uses a solid partially threaded screw with minimal thread length. The weakest point of the screw is the junction between the thread and the shank of the screw. Placing this junction as far away as possible from the sacroiliac joint (or sacral fracture) yields the greatest strength to the construct and diminishes the

risk of breakage. A theoretical disadvantage to using a partially threaded screw is overcompression of a sacral fracture with subsequent nerve palsy. In the author's experience of more than 100 sacral fractures treated with iliosacral screws, no iatrogenic nerve palsies have occurred. A washer can be used with the screw to prevent the screw from penetrating the outer cortex of the iliac wing. Additionally, a transsacral screw can be placed through the S1 body from one iliac wing to the other. Very thorough attention to the foregoing principles is required to implant this screw safely. A transsacral screw may give increased resistance to vertical migration and therefore prevent loss of reduction in comminuted sacral fractures.[16] An S2 iliosacral screw can be used and, in some cases of sacral dysmorphism, must be used. The placement of an S2 iliosacral screw is much more technically demanding as a result of the smaller corridor of bone available for safe placement of the iliosacral screw. AP, inlet, outlet, and lateral views are performed prior to closure to ensure anatomical reduction and safe placement of the screws.

In general, in completely unstable pelvic injuries, the posterior hemipelvis requires reduction prior to the anterior pelvis. This principle holds true even if there is an associated acetabular fracture. Reduction of the pelvis posteriorly will facilitate the reduction of the acetabulum. Occasionally, stabilization may occur anteriorly, but even a few millimeters of rotation anteriorly can translate into more than a centimeter posteriorly. Therefore, posterior reduction and fixation are critical prior to anterior reduction and fixation.

The main potential complication that needs to be avoided when placing iliosacral screws is damage to the L5 nerve root. Without careful technique, a guide pin, drill, or screw can be placed in a manner in which it starts in bone, exits in the area of the sacral ala (in the area of the L5 nerve root), and then reenters the bone into the S1 body. Having a good tactile feel ensuring the pin or drill remains in bone through three cortices, as well as good radiographic evaluation, can prevent this complication from occurring.

Crescent Fracture—Sacroiliac Joint Dislocation

Crescent fractures can be approached from the anterior approach; however, in most of these cases, the fracture will be difficult to visualize (i.e., the sacral fracture is more medial or the crescent fracture is posterior to the sacroiliac joint). In these cases the author prefers a posterior approach if the condition of the soft tissue will allow it. This allows a direct visualization of the fracture site, which either is posterior to the sacroiliac joint or enters the posterior part of the sacroiliac joint. Occasionally the posterior fractured piece of ilium remains attached to the sacrum through the sacroiliac joint ligaments, and the injury is stable once the fracture is reduced and fixed **(Fig. 19–29A–F)**. The difficulty with crescent fractures is obtaining an acceptable reduction. The deformity that is most problematic is the internal/external rotation of the hemipelvis, which is difficult to manipulate

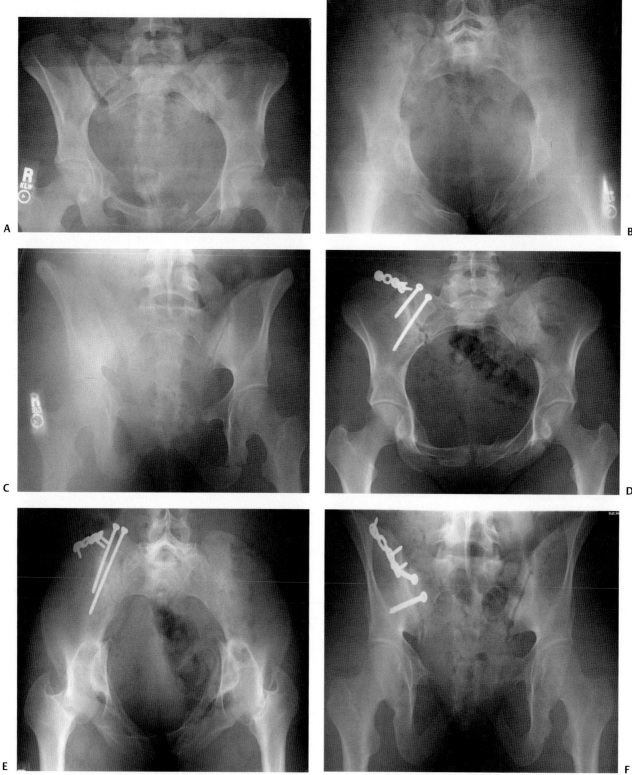

Figure 19–29 Example of a sacroiliac fracture-dislocation due to a lateral compression injury. **(A)** Anteroposterior (AP) view of the injury. Note that the posterior iliac wing (crescent) fracture may be difficult to appreciate on this view. The right hemipelvis is internally rotated and slightly flexed, and there are fractures of all four pubic rami. **(B)** Inlet and **(C)** outlet views of the injury. The crescent fracture is readily seen on the inlet view. **(D)** AP, **(E)** inlet, and **(F)** outlet views of the pelvis taken several months after reduction and fixation of the posterior ilium with a four-hole reconstruction plate and two lag screws. Note that the anterior ring fractures did not require fixation.

from the posterior approach. Reduction techniques using clamps and a half pin as a joystick can allow reduction of the sacroiliac joint and the fracture.

The surgeon starts with the reduction of the posterior crescent fracture of the iliac wing. The bone of the posterior iliac wing is weaker more superiorly. Therefore, a commonly used reduction method is to use small screw-holding clamps (Farabeuf or Jungbluth) placed just cephalad to the top border of the sciatic notch to allow fixation above and below the clamp in bone strong enough that the reduction screw will withstand the forces required to obtain an anatomical reduction. The superior portion of the sciatic notch is excellent bone and allows good fixation of these crescent fractures. Depending on the size of the crescent fracture and the mechanics of the injury, the sacroiliac joint may be either stable or unstable after fixation of the crescent fracture. Initial reduction techniques include two Farabeuf clamps, one placed close to the crest and one close to the sciatic notch. A 3.5 mm screw is placed on both sides of the fracture line and should be offset so that when they are aligned, the crescent fracture is reduced. After careful debridement of the fracture, the Farabeuf clamp is manipulated until anatomical reduction is achieved. If difficulty is encountered in reducing the fracture, an angled Matta reduction clamp is placed through the notch with one point on the sacral ala and the other point on the iliac wing. The clamp can internally or externally rotate the hemipelvis depending on its position. Careful planning of the placement of the Farabeuf clamps prevents the surgeon from blocking potential key areas for fixation. In general, the author places the Farabeuf clamp more superiorly than the superior border of the sciatic notch so that a plate can be placed along the border of the notch in good strong bone. The other clamp is placed more superiorly but not quite at the top of the crest to allow another plate along the crest if required. In placing the reduction screws, the surgeon must be aware of the obliquity of the fracture line and not block reduction with the screws. After anatomical reduction is achieved, lag screw fixation secures the reduction followed by definitive plate fixation. Occasionally plates are used as reduction aids, pulling or pushing fractured bone. The lag screws are placed from the posterior-superior iliac spine toward the anterior iliac spine and can range up to 130 mm in length.

The lag screws are usually supported with two plates. The plates vary in length depending on the size of the crescent fracture. The most posterior hole of the plate is bent 90 degrees over the posterior border of the ilium. A lag screw can be placed in this hole running between the inner and outer cortical tables of the ilium, supplementing the fixation. Careful attention is required not to block additional screw placement within the plate. Once this lag screw is placed, the plate is seated down, and additional screws can be placed on both sides of the fracture. The author's preference is 3.5 mm screws and a 3.5–4.5 mm reconstruction plate. Once the crescent fracture is reduced, the sacroiliac joint is evaluated for instability. In many cases there is adequate stability with repair of the crescent fracture, and the sacroiliac joint does not require stabilization (**Fig. 19–29A–F**).

Sacral Fractures (see Video 19–5, Disk 2)

Like the previous two posterior injuries discussed, sacral fractures can be quite difficult to reduce (**Fig. 19–30A–F**). Using the techniques described, anatomical reduction of sacral fractures can be achieved. The incidence of neurological injuries increases with a sacral fracture. Some authors believe that placement of a partially threaded screw can compress the sacrum and cause a neurological injury. In more than 100 patients treated with iliosacral screws for sacral fractures, the author has had no iatrogenic nerve injuries with use of partially threaded screws. The approach for sacral fractures is similar to the approach for sacroiliac disruption previously described. The sacral fracture line is debrided, with careful attention to the nerve roots. The combination of a Weber clamp posteriorly and the angled Matta clamp through the notch allows anatomical reduction (**Fig. 19–24**).[6,16] In sacral fractures, the angled Matta clamp point needs to be medial to the fracture of the sacrum. The surgeon's index finger is placed between the S1 and S2 nerve roots onto the S1 body. The backside of one side of the clamp is slid along the index finger until the point is sitting on the S1 body, ensuring safe placement and subsequent reduction. Similar to sacroiliac joint disruptions, the surgeon must use a combination of the two camps, slightly moving the tips and alternating the pressure placed until anatomical reduction is achieved. Sacral fractures associated with significant comminution may require support in addition to the iliosacral screws. In these cases, the author uses a posterior tension-band plate spanning from one iliac wing to the other. As mentioned, a 14- to 16-hole plate is placed caudad to the posterior-superior iliac spine (just cephalad to the superior border of the sciatic notch), between spinous processes of the sacrum so that the plate will not be prominent, yet allows three screws of fixation into both iliac wings. The plate is slid underneath the back musculature with a bend at each end. Generally, the author uses a plate with three holes lateral to the sacroiliac joint bilaterally. The third screw from the end on each side is placed between the two tables of cortical bone of the iliac wing. These screws can be longer than 130 mm. The plate is bent between the second and third hole on each side so the last two screws traverse the iliac wing. The plate is usually bent slightly in the midline, conforming to the slight anterior sloping of the sacrum along its posterior surface.

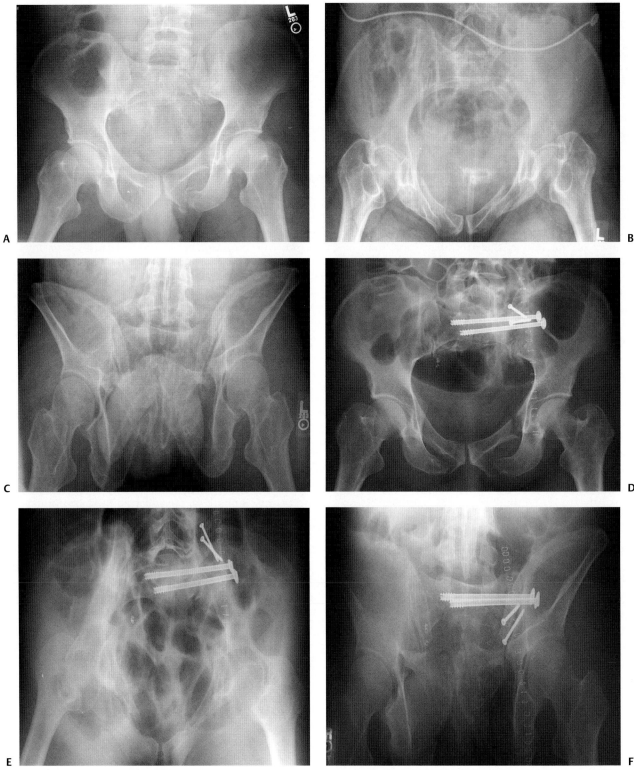

Figure 19–30 (A) Anteroposterior (AP) radiograph of an injured pelvis showing an unstable-appearing (disimpacted) left sacral fracture with evidence of vertical and lateral translation of the left hemipelvis. There does not appear to be a significant rotational deformity. **(B)** The inlet view does not show significant deformity. **(C)** The outlet view confirms that there is significant cranial displacement of the left pelvis, as indicated by the difference in the height of the ischial tuberosity. **(D)** AP, **(E)** inlet, and **(F)** outlet views after stabilization of the left hemipelvis by open reduction of the left sacral fracture, insertion of two iliosacral screws, and repair of a small associated crescent fracture of the posterior iliac wing.

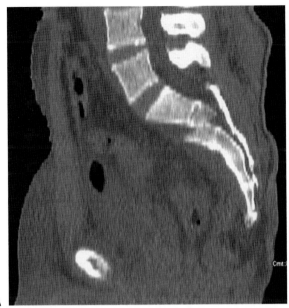
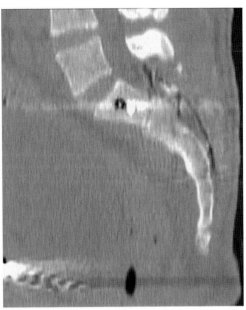

A   B

Figure 19–31 (A) A sagittal computed tomographic (CT) reconstruction of an H-type bilateral sacral fracture that shows the typical kyphotic deformity of the sacrum. **(B)** A sagittal CT reconstruction of the H-type bilateral sacral fracture in **(A)** after reduction and fixation with bilateral iliosacral screws.

An additional sacral fracture that is problematic is the H- or U-type fracture of the sacrum. These bilateral fractures of the sacrum are often seen in jumpers and are a complete disassociation of the lower extremities and the caudad part of the sacrum from the spine. These patients can have significant deformity with kyphosis of the sacrum. The reduction of these injuries is problematic due to the fact that the entire pelvis requires distraction **(Fig. 19–31A,B)**. The technique the author has used in this rare pattern is placement of pedicle screws in L5 (occasionally in L4 as well) down to the posterior-superior iliac spine. This allows traction between the intact portion of S1 (attached to the spine) and the iliac wing (and caudad part of the sacrum). Traction and hyperextension of the pelvis and lower extremities are required to obtain reduction. This should be the positioning of the patient prior to opening the fracture. Traction with the foregoing construct deforms the pelvis by pushing the pelvis laterally, distally, and into flexion. By bending the spinal rods appropriately, the surgeon can rotate the rods after distraction to reduce these deformities. Once an anatomical reduction is achieved, iliosacral screws are placed to fix both of the hemipelves to the S1 body. Additionally, a tension plate can be placed posteriorly for added stability.

After fixation the spinal instrumentation is removed. Some surgeons may retain the pedicle fixation for additional stability. They claim a more rapid recovery due to immediate weight bearing as tolerated compared with 8 weeks of touch-down weight bearing. However, there are disadvantages with leaving the lumbopelvic fixation. An additional surgery is required to remove the implants, and this type of fixation may cause permanent morbidity with pain and deformity (angulation at the S1–L5 junction). In the author's experience, the lumbopelvic fixation can be removed without any loss of reduction and without the added morbidity of the added fixation. Although the rehabilitation is slower, the long-term outcome is the same or better without the lumbopelvic fixation. The main problem with these fractures is the failure to diagnose the fracture pattern so the kyphotic deformity is not reduced. This leads to significant morbidity to the patient and is very difficult to correct later after the fracture heals.

Another difficult fracture to reduce is the windswept deformity **(Fig. 19–32A–D)**. This bilateral pelvic injury involves one hemipelvis in internal rotation and the other hemipelvis in external rotation. Adhering to the principles previously described in this chapter, this deformity can be reduced anatomically during the acute period. Often, anterior external fixation is used to correct the rotational deformities prior to definitive posterior fixation with iliosacral screws.

Rehabilitation

The rehabilitation of patients with completely unstable pelvic injuries involves touch-down weight bearing for 8 weeks. After 8 weeks, the patient may begin weight bearing as tolerated with range of motion and resistance

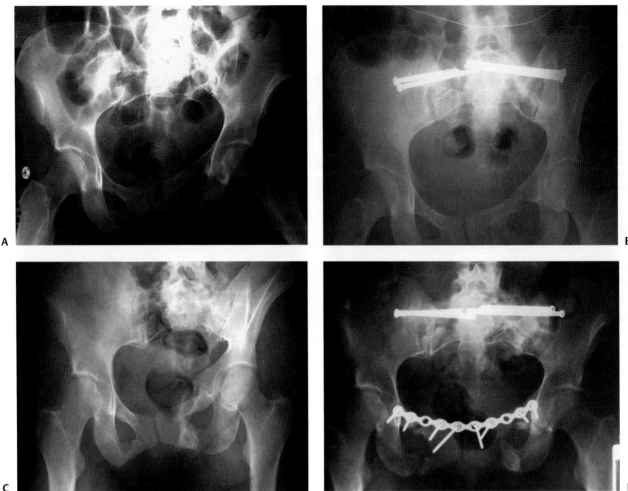

Figure 19–32 **(A)** Anteroposterior (AP) radiograph of the pelvis of a patient with a windswept deformity of the pelvis with external rotation of the right hemipelvis and internal rotation of the left hemipelvis. **(B)** An AP radiograph of the pelvis after fixation with iliosacral screws with the same deformity. **(C)** An AP radiograph of the pelvis after removal of the iliosacral screws and before a three-stage pelvic reconstruction involving release of the anterior and posterior ligaments, osteotomies of both sides of the sacrum and bilateral superior and inferior rami, and reduction and fixation of the pelvis. **(D)** An AP radiograph of the pelvis after the three-stage pelvic reconstruction correcting the windswept deformity of the pelvis. Although the deformity is improved, it required an extremely large surgery. Initial appropriate reduction and fixation would have been much better for the patient.

Tips and Tricks

- External fixation pins are placed through a pilot hole in the iliac crest and driven between the inner and outer tables of bone.
- A reasonable reduction of an unstable posterior pelvis may be obtained by a combination of traction, either in full extension or flexed up to ~45 degrees, along with compression in the posterior part of the pelvis.
- Contraindication for placement of the C (posterior) clamp is an iliac wing fracture anterior to the sacroiliac joint.
- Maintain the rectus attachment to the rami anteriorly during the Pfannenstiel approach.
- When placing intramedullary ramus screws, an obturator oblique fluoroscopic view with a cephalad tilt allows the corridor of bone to be visualized where the screw can be placed safely.

- The anterior approach for posterior pelvic instability is indicated if there is a posterior crush injury to the soft tissue that prevents a posterior approach, if the patient has multiple trauma and cannot be placed in the prone position, and if there is an iliac wing fracture that is anterior to the sacroiliac joint.
- The posterior approach for posterior pelvic instability is indicated in sacral fractures and in crescent fractures where the fracture line is primarily posterior to the sacroiliac joint, as well as if decompression of nerve roots is required.
- An occasionally helpful technique for reduction of the sacroiliac joint when the symphysis is disrupted is manipulation of the symphysis with the Jungbluth clamp.

(continued)

- Another trick is using a Farabeuf clamp on the iliac wing to manipulate the rotation of the hemipelvis as well as compress the sacroiliac joint.
- There is a concave surface on the sacrum that fits into the convex surface of the ilium, helping guide reduction of the sacroiliac joint from posterior.
- The lateral fluoroscopic view is a critical step that can prevent serious complications during the placement of iliosacral screws.
- In performing the posterior approach, expose the origin of the gluteus maximus on the lumbodorsal fascia. Do not cut straight down onto the posterior-superior iliac spine (PSIS) because damage to the gluteus maximus will occur. Never debride the cartilage of the sacroiliac joint. However, loose pieces of cartilage are discarded.
- In general, reduction of the posterior pelvic injury should precede reduction of an acetabular fracture or the anterior pelvic injury. Starting the reduction anteriorly, the surgeon must be aware that a few millimeters or degrees of malreduction anteriorly can lead to more than a centimeter displacement posteriorly.

exercises. Patients with bilateral injuries are limited to wheelchair transfers for 8 weeks. Most patients mobilize on the intact side and use crutches or a walker.

New Techniques

Future techniques that will help the treatment of pelvic injuries include the newer computer-assisted, minimally invasive navigation of both the reduction and the fixation of the pelvis. The technology is improving rapidly and soon will allow surgeons to measure the deformity and the reduction more accurately prior to placing screws using a minimally invasive technique. The difficulty in treating pelvic fractures has always been with the reduction. Fixation using computer technology and minimally invasive surgery already exists. However, additional clamps and reduction techniques need to be developed to enable the minimally invasive reduction and fixation techniques to display their true benefits.

Outcomes

Multiple studies have shown no difference in the outcome of pelvic injuries despite the level of injury. Often in these studies, completely unstable pelvis injuries are treated conservatively or with external fixators only.

However, other studies have shown that the degree of displacement of the hemipelvis affects the patient outcome.[17,18] Return to work outcomes have varied from 40 to 100% following pelvic fractures. In summarizing the outcome studies, the associated injuries seem to be more important than the pelvic injury in determining patient outcomes. The most significant factor in outcome is the degree of neurological injury. Neurological injury leads to significant impairment for the patients. In general, the surgeon should anatomically reduce the pelvis to restore function to the patient and prevent long-term deformities.[5] In one study most patients returned to work and had an excellent result if anatomical reduction was achieved.[16]

Complications

The two roles for the orthopaedic surgeon in patients with pelvic fractures are to anatomically reduce the pelvis and prevent complications. Complications that occur from the injury are not preventable. However, iatrogenic injuries can be prevented. Kellam et al reported a 25% infection rate with a posterior approach to the pelvis.[15] This high infection rate is due to operating through damaged soft tissue and cutting straight down to the bone (not elevating the gluteus maximus flap). Careful consideration of the soft tissue, as well as an anatomical approach, can reduce this rate of infection to 2.8%.[11] If the posterior soft tissue has sustained too much damage, an anterior approach should be chosen. Careful evaluation and treatment of Morel-Lavallée lesions can also decrease the rate of infection.

Although, injury-related nerve damage can occur, the surgeon must work to prevent iatrogenic nerve injury. Careful understanding of the anatomy, as well as proper reduction and fixation techniques, can prevent damage to nerves that may already be slightly injured secondary to the accident. Somatosensory evoked potentials as well as other nerve monitoring can be used in an attempt to decrease the rate of nerve injury. However, the benefits of nerve monitoring in the acute setting have been controversial. The author's use of nerve monitoring has been limited to correction of chronic malunions that require significant reductions.[5] In the author's opinion, nerve monitoring in the acute setting is not indicated. Finally, because of the complexity of pelvic fractures and the associated injuries, the absolute correlation between reduction and function has not been demonstrated definitively. However, it is the author's strong opinion, which is supported in the literature and by personal experience with more than 1000 pelvic injuries, that the more anatomical the reduction is, the better the functional outcome for the patient.[11,17,18] Therefore, the goal of every surgeon is to anatomically reduce and fix the pelvis and avoid complications.

Pearls

- Unstable posterior injuries require internal fixation.
- External fixators can be used in the hemodynamically and mechanically unstable pelvic injury patient as a temporary life-saving device.
- External fixators can be used with relatively stable (i.e., no vertical migration) posterior injuries (i.e., open book pelvis), although the author prefers a symphyseal plate. It is the treatment of choice when an internal rotation deformity of the hemipelvis causes greater than a 20 degree internal rotation deformity or greater than 1 cm leg length discrepancy, or when a rami fractured piece protrudes into the bladder or vagina.
- Stability by physical exam is determined by the compression test.
- Radiographic instability is diagnosed when there is greater than 5 mm of displacement of the sacroiliac joint, iliac fracture, or sacral fracture (a gap rather than impaction). Remember, the pelvic injury can be minimally displaced but can be grossly unstable, so a combination of physical and radiographic exams needs to be performed to determine stability.
- The inferior sacroiliac ligaments are most important for stability and should be viewed on the CT scan prior to determining instability (i.e., superior cuts of the CT scan can show widening of the sacroiliac joint; however, inferior cuts show an anatomically reduced sacroiliac joint).
- Nonoperative treatment for pelvic injuries includes sacral impaction injuries, isolated rami fractures, or avulsions with less than 1 cm of displacement. A weekly AP x-ray exam for 4 weeks is indicated to ensure no further increase in deformity.
- Operative indication for symphysis diastasis is 2.5 cm of widening. Widening less than this may be fixed if there is a posterior injury. Be aware of a missed completely unstable posterior pelvic injury.
- A posterior external fixation frame (C-clamp) may give better compression posteriorly but is contraindicated in cases where the iliac fracture is anterior to the sacroiliac joint.
- Leave the rectus abdominis attached to the pelvis when plating the symphysis pubis. Never debride the symphyseal cartilage.
- If stable pelvic fractures have greater than 20 degrees internal rotation of the hemipelvis or greater than 1 cm of leg length discrepancy, or if the rami fracture is impinging on the bladder or vagina (tilt fracture), operative fixation is indicated.
- Most rami fractures are treated conservatively. Those with greater than 1.5 cm of displacement with an unstable posterior injury are treated operatively due to disruption of the iliopectineal fascia.
- The main complication of iliosacral screw placement is an L5 nerve root injury due to the guide pin, drill bit, or screw being placed too anteriorly so the pin exits and reenters the sacrum in the sacral ala area, damaging the L5 nerve root.
- Bilateral sacral fractures and U- or H-type fracture patterns are frequently misdiagnosed as simple sacral fractures and can cause significant morbidity from nerve injuries. These injuries completely disassociate the pelvis and the lower extremities from the spine. They frequently have a kyphotic deformity. They can best be seen on a lateral sacral view or lateral sacral CT reconstruction.
- The most important component to the outcome of pelvic injuries is the preoperative nerve exam. Secondarily associated injuries and quality of reduction are also important.

On the DVDs

Video 19–1 (Disk 2)   ORIF of Pubic Symphysis Iliosacral Lag Screws Placement Pubic symphysis plate fixation and percutaneous iliosacral screw fixation are demonstrated. The Phannensteil approach, symphysis reduction techniques, and plate application are emphasized.

Video 19–2 (Disk 2)   ORIF of a "Tilt" Fracture Variant of the Pelvis This video is a malunion of the anterior pelvis in a young female with dyspareunia. A Pfannensteil approach is used to expose the malunion, and an osteotomy with open reduction and internal fixation is used to treat this deformity.

Video 19–3 (Disk 2)   Iliosacral Lag Screws This video reviews the anatomy of the posterior pelvis, the risks involved in placement of iliosacral screws, and the technique to safely implement this technique.

Video 19–4 (Disk 2)   ORIF of a Left Sacroiliac Joint Fracture-Dislocation A fracture-dislocation of the sacroiliac joint is openly reduced after being exposed through the posterior approach. Stabilization is provided through iliosacral screws.

Video 19–5 (Disk 2)   ORIF of a Left Sacral Fracture The posterior approach to the sacrum is demonstrated for open reduction and internal fixation of a Denis II left sacral fracture with significant displacement. Open reduction techniques and iliosacral screw fixation are shown.

References

1. Dalal SA, Burgess AR, Siegel JH, et al. Pelvic fracture in multiple trauma: classification by mechanism is key to pattern of organ injury, resuscitative requirements, and outcome. J Trauma 1989;29:981–1000

2. Kellam J. The role of external fixation in pelvic disruptions. Clin Orthop Relat Res 1989;241:66–82

3. Reilly MC, Bono CM, Litkouhi B, Sirkin M, Behrens FF. The effect of sacral fracture malreduction on the safe placement of iliosacral screws. J Orthop Trauma 2003;17:88–94

4. Bucholz RW. The pathological anatomy of Malgaigne fracture-dislocation of the pelvis. J Bone Joint Surg Am 1981;63:400–404

5. Matta JM, Dickson KF, Markovich GD. Surgical treatment of pelvic nonunions and malunions. Clin Orthop Relat Res 1996;329:199–206

6. Dickson KF, Matta JM. Skeletal deformity following external fixation of the pelvis. J Orthop Trauma 2006; In press

7. Dickson KF, Frigon VA. Open reduction internal fixation of a pelvic malunion through an anterior approach: a case report. J Orthop Trauma 2001;15:519–524

8. Burgess A, Eastridge BJ, Young JWR, et al. Pelvic ring disruptions: effective classification system and treatment protocols. J Trauma 1990;30:848–856

9. Matta JM. Anterior fixation of rami fractures. Clin Orthop Relat Res 1996;329:88–96

10. Grimm MR, Vrahas MS, Thomas KA. Volume characteristics of the intact and disrupted pelvic retroperitoneum. J Trauma 1998;44:454–459

11. Matta JM, Tornetta P III. Internal fixation of unstable pelvic ring injuries. Clin Orthop Relat Res 1996;329:129–140

12. Cole JD, Bolhofner BR. Acetabular fracture fixation via a modified Stoppa limited intrapelvic approach: description of operative technique and preliminary treatment results. Clin Orthop Relat Res 1994;305:112–123

13. Rout ML Jr, Simonian PT, Grujic L. The retrograde medullary superior ramus screw for the treatment of anterior pelvic ring disruptions. J Orthop Trauma 1995;9:35–44

14. Hak DJ, Olson SA, Matta JM. Diagnosis and management of closed degloving injuries associated with pelvic and acetabular fractures: the Morel-Lavallée lesion. J Trauma 1997;42:1046–1051

15. Kellam J, McMurtry R, Paley D, Tile M. The unstable pelvic fracture: operative treatment. Orthop Clin North Am 1987;18:25–41

16. Dickson KF, Hsu J, DiFusco J. Sacral fractures: new technique for reduction and results. Presented at the Annual Meeting, American Academy of Orthopedic Surgeons, Washington D.C., February 2005

17. Semba R, Yasukawa K, Gustilo R. Critical analysis of results of 53 Malgaigne fractures of the pelvis. J Trauma 1983;23:535–537

18. Tile M. Pelvic ring fractures: should they be fixed? J Bone Joint Surg Br 1988;70:1–12

20 Acetabular Fractures

Philip J. Kregor and Michael Stover

The acetabulum is a socket of bone formed from the fusion of the ilium, ischium, and pubis at the triradiate cartilage. It articulates with the femoral head in a highly constrained joint. Judet and colleagues and Letournel defined the socket as being supported from the sciatic buttress by two columns of bone: the anterior column (made up of the ilium and pubis) and the posterior column (made up of the ischium) (**Fig. 20–1**).[1,2] Fractures of the acetabulum that are displaced and result in a loss of congruence between the femoral head and the remaining intact portion of the superior articular surface typically have a poor prognosis. When such injuries are treated surgically, hip joint preservation and maintenance of hip function typically result if operative complications are avoided.[3] Increased experience with the treatment of these types of injuries improves the treating physician's ability to correctly evaluate radiographs, determine the appropriate surgical approach, perform adequate reductions, and understand the impact of associated injuries on treatment. Due to the relative rarity of acetabular fractures and their typically higher energy mechanisms, treatment of these injuries is ideally performed by surgeons with advanced training working at specialized hospitals interested in the care of multiply injured patients. However, all orthopaedic surgeons should be comfortable with the diagnosis and initial management of these injuries. Because the initial management of acetabular fractures often impacts their definitive treatment, optimum initial treatment requires some knowledge of the eventual management of the injury as well.

The initial radiographic evaluation of an acetabular fracture typically includes an anteroposterior (AP) x-ray of the pelvis obtained in a patient complaining of inguinal ("groin") or lateral hip pain following injury or as part of a trauma imaging protocol in a multiply injured or obtunded patient. From this initial radiograph, fractures involving the acetabulum are usually identified by evaluating the six radiographic "lines" as described by Judet and colleagues and Letournel (**Fig. 20–2; Table 20–1**). Although not specific anatomical structures, these lines represent areas of bone tangent to the radiographic beam and define the supporting columns or walls of the acetabulum. Thorough assessment of these lines is a critical step toward understanding the two-dimensional radiographic representation of the complex three-dimensional innominate bone. Additionally, the AP pelvis radiograph allows for the potential comparison to the contralateral normal hip to determine if there is a change in the relationship of the femoral head to the "radiographic roof." When reviewing an AP radiograph of the pelvis, the coccyx and the pubic symphysis should align with one another on the intact side of the pelvis. If they do not, the image is malrotated, and this fact should be considered when assessing any deformity of the pelvis.

Although some fractures of the acetabulum are obvious and associated with wide displacement of the bone, subluxation, and/or dislocations of the femoral head, others are associated with less displacement evident on the AP pelvic radiograph. Oblique radiographs or Judet views,

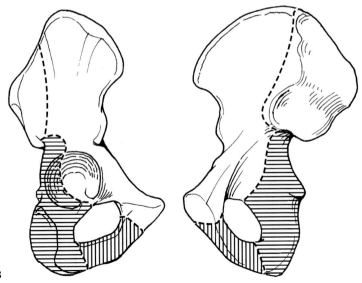

Figure 20–1 The acetabulum, as defined by Judet and colleagues and Letournel, consists of an anterior column and posterior column. The anterior column (white) consists of the iliac crest, iliac wing, pelvic brim, anterior wall, and pubic ramus. The posterior column (crosshatched) consists of the posterior column, posterior wall, and the ischium. **(A)** The outer view of the innominate bone. **(B)** The inner view of the innominate bone.

A,B

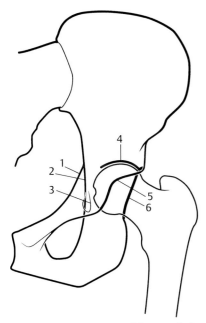

Figure 20–2 The six lines of the acetabulum visible on an anteroposterior radiograph of the hip. Note that the anterior wall at the lateral edge of the acetabulum is slightly lateral to the edge of the posterior wall. 1. Iliopectineal line. 2. Ilioischial line. 3. Radiographic teardrop. 4. Radiographic roof. 5. Anterior wall. 6. Posterior wall.

Table 20—1   The Six Acetabular Lines Visible on an Anteroposterior Hip Radiograph

1. Iliopectineal line
2. Ilioischial line
3. Radiographic teardrop
4. Radiographic roof
5. Anterior wall
6. Posterior wall

mechanism, groin pain, and no obvious finding on the AP pelvic radiograph. It nicely depicts subtle fractures of the posterior wall, femoral neck, or femoral head. The opposite iliac oblique view is commonly inadequately rotated due to the need for positioning the patient partially on the injured side. This view is used to evaluate the posterior column, anterior wall, and iliac wing. Sufficient pain control is mandatory to obtain radiographs with adequate rotation that will provide reliable information. Adequate rotation is usually present on the radiographs when the medial extent of the femoral head meets the tip of the coccyx. When standard Judet views are inadequate or cannot be obtained, corresponding computed tomographically (CT) reconstructed Judet images can be reconstructed from axial CT data but are suboptimal.

Classification

A systematic approach to evaluating the plain radiographs can reliably result in the appropriate diagnosis of the injury to the bone. The importance of this lies in the

taken with the patient rolled 45 degrees in either direction, allow for orthogonal evaluation of the innominate bone **(Fig. 20–3A–C).** The easier of the views to obtain is the obturator oblique view because the patient is rotated off the affected side. Named because it profiles the obturator ring, this view allows evaluation of the anterior column, posterior wall, and ischial ramus. It is an important film in the evaluation of a patient with a high-energy

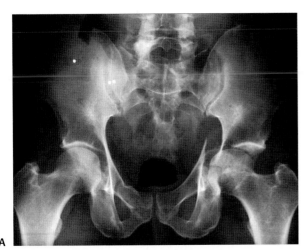

A

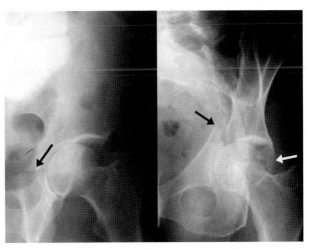

B,C

Figure 20–3 Example of radiographic assessment of a transverse/posterior wall acetabular fracture. **(A)** Anteroposterior radiograph demonstrating disruption of the iliopectineal and ilioischial lines, with medial displacement of the femoral head relative to the acetabular roof. **(B)** The iliac oblique radiograph reveals the posterior

column fracture (black arrow) and the medial subluxation of the femoral head. **(C)** Obturator oblique radiograph shows significant displacement of the anterior aspect of the fracture (black arrow) with the previously described subluxation of the femoral head. A posterior wall fracture is subtle (white arrow).

Elementary Patterns

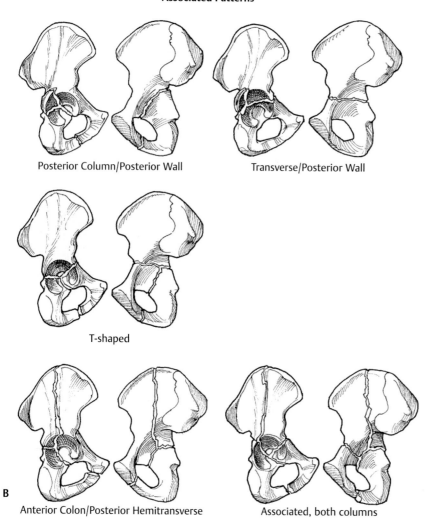

Figure 20–4 (A,B) The Judet–Letournel classification of acetabular fractures. The individual patterns are described in the text and in **Table 20–2.** These are five **(A)** elementary and five associated patterns **(B).**

Posterior Wall   Posterior Column

Anterior Wall   Anterior Column   Transverse

A

Associated Patterns

Posterior Column/Posterior Wall   Transverse/Posterior Wall

T-shaped

B

Anterior Colon/Posterior Hemitransverse   Associated, both columns

Table 20–2   The Acetabular Fracture Classification of Letournel and Judet

Elementary patterns
    Posterior wall
    Posterior column
    Anterior wall
    Anterior column
    Transverse
Associated patterns
    Posterior column/posterior wall
    Transverse/posterior wall
    T-shaped
    Anterior column (wall)/posterior hemitransverse
    Associated both column

subsequent treatment decisions for the patient. Based on the radiographic analysis of cadaveric bone and injury films, Judet and colleagues and Letournel developed a classification system for fractures of the acetabulum.[1,2] Their classification consists of five elementary and five associated fracture patterns, and allows for transitional forms to exist (**Fig. 20–4A,B; Table 20–2**). The Letournel classification is not only descriptive in nature; its primary importance lies in its ability to direct the most appropriate surgical approach to the acetabulum.[2,3,4] Accurate radiographic diagnosis of the injury will enable the surgeon to determine the best surgical approach and improve the chances of achieving an adequate reduction.

It is beyond the scope of this chapter to discuss in detail the classification of acetabular fractures utilizing the Letournel classification. Any surgeon who is contemplating operatively addressing an acetabular fracture should be well versed in the classification. This knowledge is challenging to obtain but is thoroughly discussed in the classic book by Letournel and Judet.[4] This chapter assumes a working knowledge of the Letournel classification. A concise yet thorough description of the classification and surgical approaches has also been written by Letournel.[2] However, some fundamental aspects of the Letournel classification system are important to review. These include[4,5]

- Five elementary fracture patterns are defined: posterior wall, posterior column, anterior wall, anterior column, and transverse fractures. Letournel termed each of these fractures elementary, secondary to the "purity" of the fracture line.
- Five associated fracture patterns are described: transverse with posterior wall, posterior column/posterior wall, anterior column or wall/posterior hemitransverse, T-shaped, and associated both-column fractures. As noted later, classification of an acetabular fracture is relatively reproducible from one surgeon to another. However, there are transitional fractures that do not fall neatly into one category, particularly between a T-shaped, anterior column/posterior hemitransverse, and a both-column fracture.
- Column fractures separate an entire column from the innominate bone, whereas wall fractures separate only a portion of the articular surface. Column fractures have a fracture line that enters the obturator foramen and a fracture in the ischiopubic (inferior) ramus.
- Anterior column fractures can exit the anterior aspect of the innominate bone either at a high (iliac crest), intermediate (anterior-superior iliac spine), low (psoas gutter at the level of the anterior-inferior iliac spine), or very low pectineal eminence) position.
- Anterior column fractures commonly involve a portion of the quadrilateral surface. This feature, combined with the typical external rotation of the anterior column, allows for medialization of the femoral head to occur.
- Transverse acetabular fractures involve both columns of the innominate bone. However, they are not described as both-column fractures, which is instead a term that applies to a specific type of associated fracture. Transverse acetabular fractures are an elementary fracture secondary to the purity of the fracture line. They separate a portion of the superior innominate bone with a portion of the dome from the lower ischiopubic segment. The ischiopubic segment rotates in two ways. First, it rotates around a vertical axis passing through the pubic symphysis, which allows the acetabulum to appear to be displaced inward. Second, a rotation occurs about a horizontal axis from the posterior aspect of the fracture to the pubic symphysis. Transverse fractures can be classified further with regard to where they involve the articular surface of the dome: through the roof (transtectal), through the high point of the cotyloid fossa (juxtatectal), and through the cotyloid fossa and involving the inferior portions of the anterior and posterior walls (infratectal).
- Fractures that involve the iliac crest are anterior column, anterior column/posterior hemitransverse fractures, and both-column fractures.
- Anterior column/posterior hemitransverse fractures may be thought of as a combination of an anterior column fracture with the posterior half of a transverse fracture. The posterior column fracture tends to be low and minimally displaced. This is in distinction to posterior column involvement in associated both column fractures.
- Elderly patients with low-energy falls tend to have anterior column or anterior column/posterior hemitransverse acetabular fractures. Both fractures can have quadrilateral surface involvement (**Fig. 20–5**), medial articular dome impaction ("gull wing sign") (**Fig. 20–6**), or posterior wall impaction.

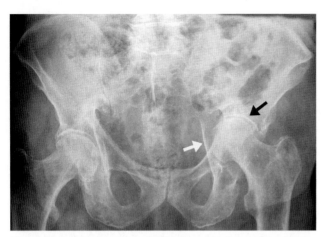

Figure 20–5 Anteroposterior (AP) radiograph of the pelvis, showing a left acetabular fracture. There is a fracture line into the iliac crest not well appreciated on the AP pelvis film. There is significant disruption and displacement of the ilioischial line, and the angulation of this landmark signifies disruption of the quadrilateral surface (white arrow). Finally, medial displacement of the femoral head and superior displacement and angulation of the acetabular roof are seen (black arrow). The latter findings suggest impaction and comminution of the cancellous bone above the acetabulum.

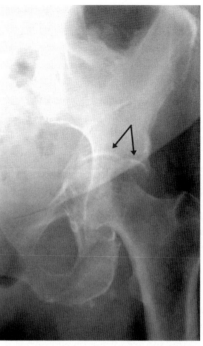

Figure 20–6 Example of the "gull wing" sign (arrows) in an elderly woman with an anterior column fracture, representing impaction of the acetabular dome. Note that the medial aspect of the femoral head is medial to the ilioischial line. The intact articular dome is the lateral aspect of the gull sign. The medial aspect of the gull sign represents the impacted and/or displaced articular surface of the anterior column.

• The associated both-column fracture has a distinguishing feature of having no portion of the articular dome in continuity with the intact ilium **(Fig. 20–7A–G).** In addition, there is a fracture line separating the anterior column (which itself has been separated from the intact ilium) and the posterior column. The femoral head usually medializes, the anterior column externally rotates, and the posterior column internally rotates. The labrum usually remains intact to all the fragments, and thus the femoral head remains congruent to the acetabulum, which is termed secondary congruence. The radiographic "spur sign," if present, is pathognomonic for an associated both-column fracture. It is best seen on the obturator oblique view and represents the outer aspect of the inferior aspect of the innominate bone, which is separated from the articular dome fragments.

Beaule et al have confirmed that the Letournel classification has significant interobserver and intraobserver reliability among surgeons involved in a high volume of acetabular fracture surgeries per year (> 40 cases/year).[5] CT scans have not proven helpful in determining the classification of the acetabular fracture.[5] However, CT does provide valuable information regarding the number of fracture fragments (comminution), orientation of fracture lines, displacement of the fracture, direction and rotation of fracture displacement, and whether there is marginal

impaction or incarcerated fragments in the hip joint. The CT scan is therefore essential for appropriate preoperative planning.

Whether a fracture line and its displacement may have an impact on the eventual outcome of the hip joint is likely determined by the fracture location, the amount of displacement, and its effect on hip joint stability. Initially it was recognized that fractures involving the superior articular surface had an increased risk of posttraumatic arthrosis. Matta et al subsequently attempted to define the superior articular surface using roof arc angles.[6] These angles are defined by a vertical line drawn through the center of the femoral head and another from the center of the femoral head to the point where the fracture enters the articular surface on each of the three pelvic radiographs, with the leg out of traction **(Fig. 20–8A,B).** Measurement of roof arc angles requires that the femoral head is not subluxed, and these arcs cannot be used to evaluate either the both-column fracture pattern (because usually the acetabulum medializes along with the subluxated femoral head, referred to as secondary congruency) or

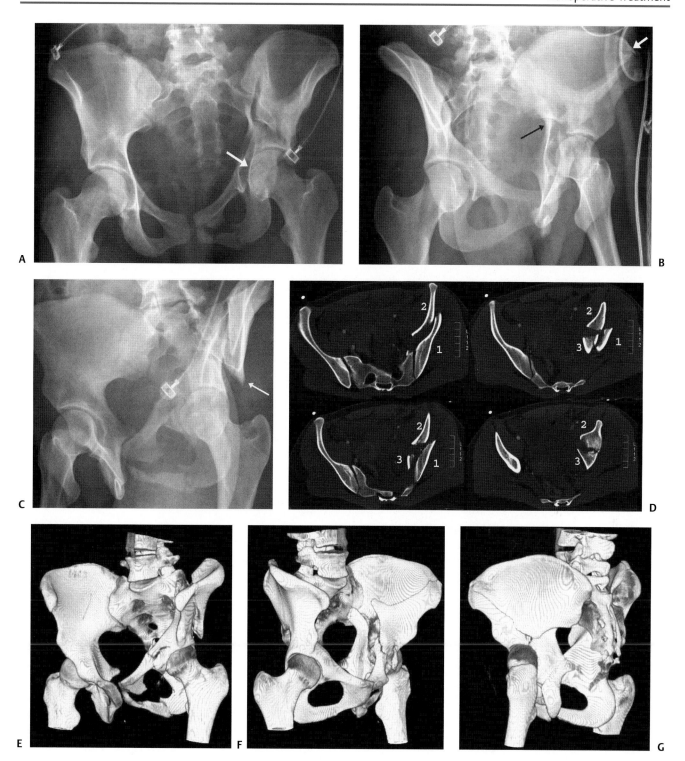

Figure 20–7 Example of an associated both-column acetabular fracture. **(A)** The anteroposterior pelvic radiograph reveals that the femoral head overlies the ilioischial line, indicating medialization of the hip (arrow). **(B)** The iliac oblique view demonstrates fracture line extension to the iliac crest ~2.5 cm from the anterosuperior iliac spine (white arrow). Significant displacement of the posterior column is also seen (black arrow). **(C)** The obturator oblique view demonstrates the "spur sign" (arrow), which represents the inferior/lateral aspect of the innominate bone. Thus there is no compo-nent of the articular surface that is in continuity with the intact ilium. **(D)** Several computed tomographic axial cuts of the fracture. The intact ilium is designated as fragment 1, the anterior column as fragment 2, and the posterior column as fragment 3. The inferior aspect of fragment 1 represents the bone that makes up the spur sign. **(E)** Three-dimensional reconstruction views of the fracture: the obturator oblique and **(F)** iliac oblique views, and **(G)** an outer "en face" view of the iliac wing.

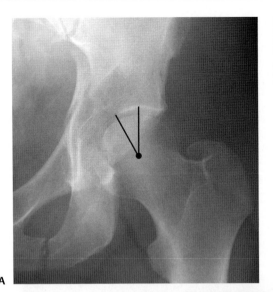

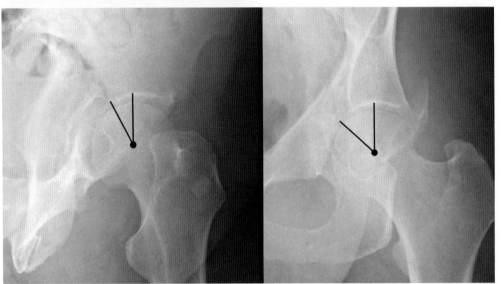

Figure 20–8 The roof arc angles are determined for the **(A)** anteroposterior and **(B)** iliac oblique, and **(C)** obturator oblique radiographs. A point is placed in the center of the femoral head. A line is drawn vertically from this point. Another line is drawn from the center of the femoral head to the fracture line in all three acetabular views. The angle is then determined.

posterior wall fractures (because these fractures rarely disrupt the superior articular surface on any view). Although the precise definition has changed since initial publications, currently a fracture is felt to be within the superior articular surface if it enters the joint at an angle less than 45 degrees. Using a mathematical model, this definition has been extrapolated to CT, where if a fracture line enters the articular surface in a CT cut less than 1 cm from the cranial subchondral condensation of the acetabulum, it is felt to involve the weight-bearing dome.[7] Vrahas et al attempted to provide an objective measure of the fractures' impact on stability using a cadaveric model.[8] Fractures of the anterior column entering above the anterior-inferior iliac spine (obturator oblique roof arc angle of ~30 degrees) and fractures of the posterior column

entering above the ischial spine (iliac oblique roof arc of ~70 degrees) resulted in femoral head subluxation in a single-leg stance model. This possibly demonstrates a greater relative importance of the posterior column to stability. This is likely due to the inclination of the pelvis and the relatively posterior vector of force to the hip during simulated single-leg stance. This may have implications regarding fracture stability and safe hip range of motion arcs during subsequent treatment.

Fractures that involve the superior aspect of the articular dome have been shown in cadaveric testing to be associated with altered contact pressures in several situations.[9] Step malreduction of a transtectal (high) transverse acetabular fracture resulted in increased peak contact pressures in the superior acetabular articular surface, as shown by pressure-sensitive film in cadaveric testing. Gap malreductions of a transtectal transverse fracture and gap and step malreductions of a juxtatectal transverse fracture did not result in increased contact pressures in the hip. This information, along with the amount of fracture displacement, may have clinical importance in determining the likelihood of arthritis in operatively or nonoperatively treated acetabular fractures.

Nonoperative Treatment

Nonoperative treatment of acetabular fractures is currently indicated for the following types of fractures:

- Those that do not involve the weight-bearing articular surface as defined by roof arc angles on plain radiographs or by CT
- Those that are displaced less than 2 mm within the superior articular surface and maintain congruence between the femoral head and acetabulum with the involved leg out of traction
- Fractures of the posterior wall with less than 20% involvement of the articular surface and no incarcerated fragments
- Those that have secondary congruence following an associated both-column fracture

Due to the changes in articular stress patterns seen with concentric both-column fractures and the associated medialization of the joint, it is recommended that the majority of both-column fractures should be surgically treated unless medically contraindicated. Fractures with minimal displacement are at times difficult to classify, but if the displacement is truly minimal and the femoral head is concentrically reduced, classification of the fracture serves little purpose. If possible, with respect to associated injuries, these patients should be mobilized with 30 lb (10 to 15 kg) weight bearing on the affected limb as soon as possible. The authors do not recommend routine stress evaluation of the acetabulum unless the injury pattern includes a marginal-size posterior wall fragment in a cephalad location or if the acetabular fracture is associated with a contiguous injury to the pelvic ring. Adherence to these selection criteria may allow successful nonoperative treatment of certain fractures. Additionally, a nonoperative course of treatment may be necessary if surgical treatment is contraindicated due to a patient's medical condition, preexisting arthrosis within the joint, severe comminution, poor bone quality, skin lesions over the proposed incision, or infection.

The surgeon must exercise caution when treating a posterior wall fracture nonoperatively. The location as well as the size of the fracture must be considered. Fractures in-

volving less than 20% of the articular surface may still cause instability of the hip, especially if the fracture is involving the superior aspect of the posterior wall **(Fig. 20–9A–E).** If a question remains regarding subtle instability of the hip joint following initial radiographic evaluation, dynamic stress views can be used to further evaluate. Tornetta described the use of dynamic stress views in fractures that met nonoperative criteria to demonstrate the ability of the femoral head to maintain congruence with the acetabulum prior to patient mobilization.[10] He defined nonoperative criteria as roof arc measurements in all three acetabular views > 45 degrees, a subchondral CT arc of 10 mm, displacement of less than 50% of the posterior wall, and congruence on all three acetabular views. Forty-one patients with 41 fractures underwent dynamic stress views to assess loss of congruency between the femoral head and acetabular roof. The mean displacement of the fractures was 7 mm. In 12 patients, the dynamic fluoroscopic stress views showed some movement of the displaced fragments, but the congruency was altered in only three (one transverse fracture—also with an associated pubic diastasis; two posterior wall fractures). These three patients underwent operative fixation, and the other 38 fractures were treated nonoperatively. Results of the patients were good or excellent in 91% of the patients treated nonoperatively.

Indications for Surgical Treatment

The benefits of operative treatment of acetabular fractures can be both long and short term. The short-term benefits are associated with stable reconstruction of the joint to allow for early mobilization of the patient. The long-term benefit is to avoid or delay the onset of posttraumatic arthrosis and thereby preserve the function of the hip joint for many years to come. Such benefits are realized in the majority of operatively treated acetabulum fractures as long as complications can be avoided.[3]

Surgery is indicated for all acetabulum fractures that result in subluxation of the femoral head or loss of congruence with the acetabular articular surface. This can occur secondary to fracture displacement or retained fragments within the joint. If the hip remains concentric, but the fracture involves the superior articular surface and is displaced greater than 2 mm, surgical treatment should be strongly considered. In this circumstance, patient factors must be taken into account to individualize treatment. For example, surgery is more likely to be considered in a 20-year-old with an isolated injury than in a debilitated, minimally functional person of advanced age. If surgery on the acetabulum is contemplated, the fracture pattern and the impact that any associated injuries may have on treatment should be thoroughly understood, and the surgeon should determine whether he or she has enough experience in caring for the injury, that the

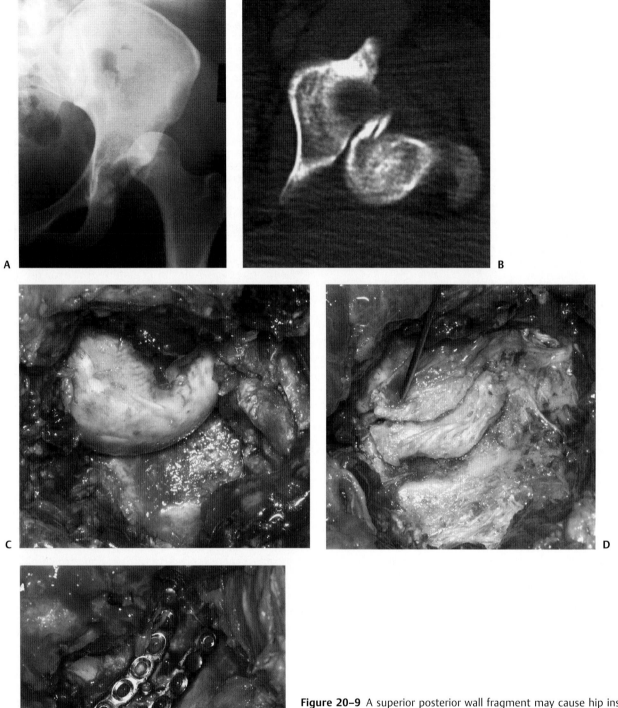

Figure 20–9 A superior posterior wall fragment may cause hip instability even if it is quite small. **(A)** Anteroposterior radiograph of the dislocated hip. **(B)** Computed tomographic cut through the hip joint at the level of the articular dome. The patient had recurrent instability of the femoral head after an open reduction without fixation of the small superior posterior wall fracture. The patient then was referred for further care. **(C)** Intraoperative photo demonstrates significant wear of the femoral head. **(D)** Intraoperative view of a relatively small but superior posterior wall acetabular fracture. **(E)** Plate fixation of the small superior posterior wall fracture.

appropriate team is available, and that the patient is stable enough to undergo operative intervention. If any of these conditions are not met, then the surgery should be delayed or the patient should be transferred to a center that may have individuals with subspecialty training in this area.

Surgical Treatment

Surgical Anatomy and Approaches

Understanding the mechanism of injury for each fracture type and where the displaced fracture lines are located for each individual fracture will greatly assist in understanding the pathoanatomy of the acetabulum following injury. The acetabulum ("hip socket") is disrupted by the femoral head secondary to forces applied indirectly to differing parts of the femur. Depending on the resultant force vector, the head is driven into the socket, resulting in bone failure. The typical resultant displacement (final position of the fracture fragments taking into account all possible linear and rotational displacements) is determined by the remaining tissue attachments to the fracture fragment and the final position of the femoral head after injury. The fragments will tend to rotate around the femoral head as it is driven through the bone. Reduction of the femoral head with traction close to its anatomical position will result in a possible decrease in displacement but will rarely realign fragments to an acceptable position or provide fracture stability (**Fig. 20–10**). Therefore, initial relocation of the femoral head relative to the intact articular surface prior to attempting surgical repositioning of the fracture fragments will facilitate subsequent reduction maneuvers by removing the deforming force of the femoral head. This is one of the main reasons that traction tables have been advocated for the surgical treatment of acetabular fractures.[3,11] Understanding residual displacement will allow the surgeon to develop reliable reduction maneuvers so that successful reconstructions can be performed.

Skin Preparation and Antibiotics

Postoperative infection following fixation of an acetabular fracture is a devastating complication. As such, the skin prepping and draping should be done with meticulous detail, and perioperative antibiotics should be administered before the skin incision is made. Plastic drapes are used to isolate the surgical wound from the rest of the patient. This is especially important in trauma patients, who may have abrasions or other open wounds. The skin is cleansed with a combination of Betadine/alcohol or a mixture of alcohol/iodophor (DuraPrep, 3M Corporation, St. Paul, Minnesota). The incisional site is covered with Ioban (3M Corporation). A first-generation cephalosporin (cefazolin) or Vancomycin is given within

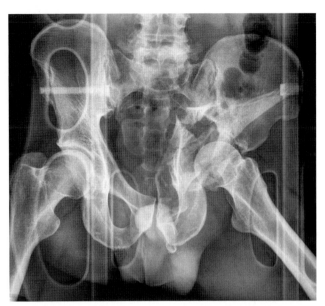

Figure 20–10 Example of an associated both-column fracture with significant medialization of the femoral head. The surgeon cannot anticipate reduction of such a fracture with skeletal traction.

30 minutes prior to skin incision and is routinely continued for 48 hours. If there is concern regarding gram-negative infection (e.g., urinary tract infection, polytrauma patient), an aminoglycoside is added preoperatively and for 48 hours postoperatively (gentamicin 300 mg IV q 24 hours).

Kocher-Langenbeck Approach (see Video 20–1, Disk 2)

The Kocher-Langenbeck approach is the preferred approach for a posterior wall fracture, posterior column fracture, posterior column/posterior wall fracture, most transverse fractures, most transverse with posterior wall fractures, and certain T-shaped fractures. The patient may be positioned either prone or laterally, preferably on a radiolucent table. In most cases, the prone position on a specially designed fracture table is preferred. Use of the prone position on a specialized table has several advantages:

- The prone position facilitates palpation of the reduction of the ischiopubic segment along the quadrilateral surface.
- It eases clamp placement through the greater sciatic notch onto the anterior column/pelvic brim area.
- It helps to maintain the involved limb in a position of hip extension and knee flexion to relax the sciatic nerve.
- Both prone positioning and gentle traction can alleviate the deforming force of the femoral head on the fracture, which may facilitate reduction.
- Having the patient prone with the hip extended and the knee flexed allows for safe, controlled distraction of the hip joint for removal of intra-articular fragments or to assess fracture reduction.

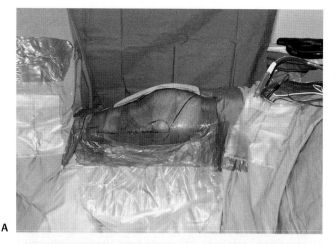

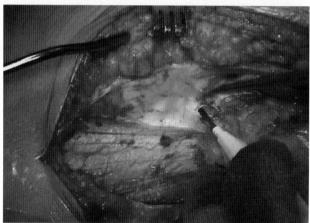

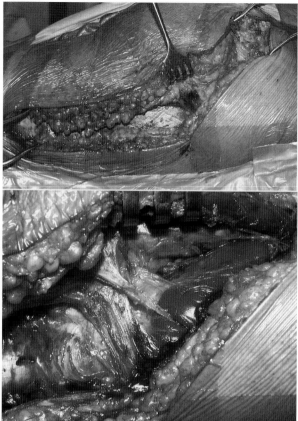

C

B

Figure 20–11 Example of prone positioning for Kocher-Langenbeck incision. **(A)** Skin incision. The lower limb of the incisions extends from the tip of the greater trochanter approximately half the length of the femur. The upper limb creates an angle of ~110 degrees with the horizontal limb and heads for the posterior-superior iliac spine. **(B)** Dissection through the subcutaneous tissue and through the iliotibial band and fascia of the gluteus maximus (upper panel) uncovers the greater trochanteric bursa (lower panel). **(C)** The gluteus maximus is released from its insertion on the posterolateral border of the femur ~1.5 cm from its insertion. On the undersurface of this tendon, ~1.5 cm from the top of the insertion, is a branch of the first perforating vessel.

- It allows improved isolation of the surgical limb for easier skin preparation and draping.

The advantages of the lateral position include the ability to perform a trochanteric flip osteotomy with surgical dislocation of the hip if necessary. In addition, such positioning requires no special table or setup.

The Kocher-Langenbeck approach allows for complete direct visualization of the area of the greater sciatic notch, supra-acetabular region, posterior column, and subcotyloid groove area. It allows for digital palpation and clamp application of the quadrilateral surface area.

Patient positioning is important in the prone position on the acetabular fracture table. Care must be taken to ensure that the patient is level on the table, that the boot is securely placed on the operative and nonoperative legs/feet, and that there is not undue stretch on the brachial plexuses. This latter factor can be ensured by keeping an angle of ~70 degrees between the torso and the patient's arms. The operative leg is kept in slight hip extension with the knee flexed 60 degrees. Hip flexion during surgery will relax the anterior iliofemoral ligament, easing distraction of the hip to facilitate assessment of fracture reduction and retrieval of loose bodies inside the hip joint. All retractors should be removed from the sciatic notch during this maneuver to avoid undue tension on the nerve.

The surgical approach begins ~5 cm from the posterior-superior iliac spine, aims toward the tip of the greater trochanter, and then continues down the midlateral aspect of the femur (**Figs. 20–11A–G** and **20–12A,B**).[2,12] Sharp dissection is carried down to the fascia of the gluteus maximus, which is in continuity with the iliotibial band. The iliotibial band is then divided along the midlateral aspect of the proximal femur working from a distal to cephalad direction. Care must be taken not to divide the iliotibial band too posteriorly because this will encroach upon the insertion of the gluteus maximus on the posterolateral border of the proximal femur. After dividing

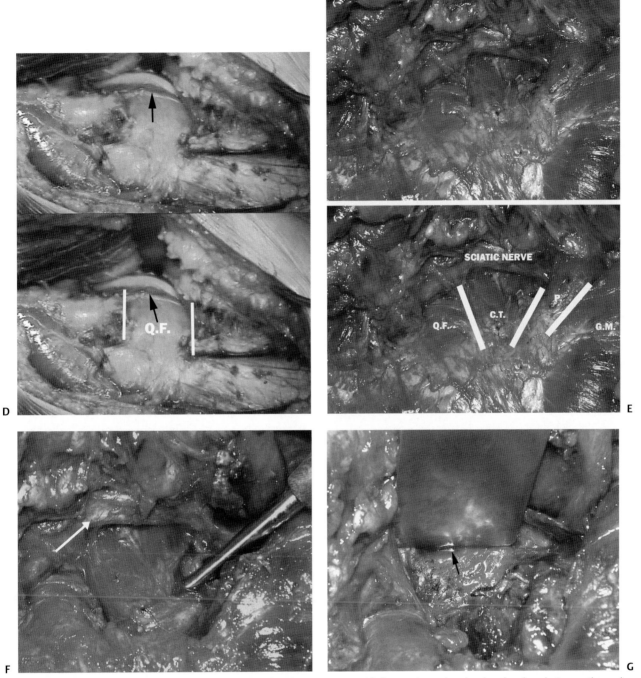

Figure 20–11 *(Continued)* **(D)** The sciatic nerve (arrow) is best found on the posterior border of the quadratus femoris (Q.F.), a broad, fleshy, muscular belly just cephalad to the gluteus maximus insertion. **(E)** Anatomy of the short external rotators and sciatic nerve. The sciatic nerve in most cases is found posterior to the quadratus femoris (Q.F.) posterior to the conjoint tendon (C.T.) and anterior to the piriformis (P.) The gluteus medius (G.M.) can be retracted cephalad to expose the gluteus minimus. **(F)** A wood-handled, curved elevator is used to develop the plane between the undersurface of the conjoint tendon and the hip capsule. The sciatic nerve is seen on the posterior border of the conjoint tendon (arrow). **(G)** A sciatic nerve retractor is placed in the lesser sciatic notch (arrow) for protection of the sciatic nerve. An assistant on the opposite side of the table holds this retractor as well as the tagged end of the obturator internus/gemelli muscle bellies. This helps protect the sciatic nerve from the sciatic nerve retractor.

the fibers of the iliotibial band to the level of the greater trochanter, palpation of the muscle fibers of the gluteus maximus is done to define the raphe between the superior one third and the inferior two thirds of the gluteus maximus. This delineates the intervascular interval between the superior gluteal artery (superior one third of the gluteus maximus) and the inferior gluteal artery (inferior two thirds of the gluteus maximus). When this

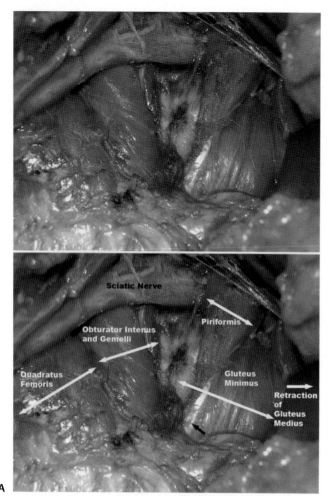

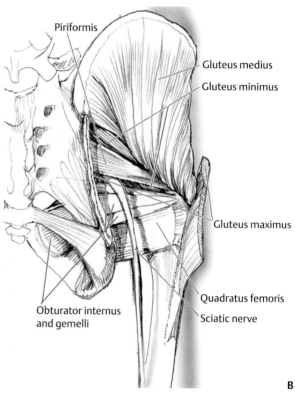

Figure 20–12 The Kocher-Langenbeck approach from the prone or lateral position. The sciatic nerve is best found on the posterior border of the quadratus femoris. It runs posterior to the conjoint tendon (obturator internus/superior and inferior gemelli) and in most cases passes anterior to the piriformis muscle belly. Note that the gluteus minimus extends inferior and deep to the piriformis muscle belly. **(A)** Intraoperative photographs—the black arrow points to the piriformis tendon. **(B)** Schematic.

division is palpated with the surgeon's index finger, the fascia over this area can be divided. The gluteus maximus is then released from the proximal femur approximately 1.5 cm from its insertion because this allows for easier retraction of the posterior flap. Two common errors in the initial phases of the exposure are not extending the Kocher-Langenbeck incision far enough distally and not releasing the gluteus maximus fibers completely. Either one of these two factors can lead to difficulty in retracting the posterior flap. The Charnley retractor may then be placed at the level of the greater trochanter, retracting the fascia of the gluteus maximus posteriorly and the iliotibial band anteriorly.

The next key maneuver is the identification and protection of the sciatic nerve. In elective hip reconstruction cases, the sciatic nerve is often found around the piriformis muscle belly. However, in cases of acetabular fractures, the anatomy of this area is significantly disturbed. The best place to find the sciatic nerve is on the posterior

border of the quadratus femoris. After the sciatic nerve is identified, it may be freed from its surrounding areolar fatty tissue. In most cases, the sciatic nerve is posterior to the obturator internus tendon and anterior to the piriformis tendon; however, there can be some variability.[13] The interval between the quadratus femoris and the gemelli is then identified. The conjoint tendon consists of the inferior gemellus, obturator internus, and superior gemellus. The surgeon needs to develop the interval between the hip capsule and the undersurface of the conjoint tendon. While doing so, one feels a thick tendinous band at the superior aspect of the undersurface of the conjoint tendon, which is the tendon of the obturator internus. The conjoint tendon, including the obturator internus tendon and the surrounding inferior and superior gemellus muscles, is transected ~1.5 cm from its insertion on the posterior aspect of the greater trochanter. The release of the conjoint tendon 1.5 cm from the greater trochanter relies upon knowledge of the nearby deep branch of the medial femoral circumflex artery, which lies anterior to the obturator internus tendon and quite close to the proximal femur at this level.[14] For the same reason, after the obturator internus/conjoint tendon is divided, the piriformis tendon is then divided proximally 1.5 cm from its insertion. After identifying and releasing the obturator internus tendon, the surgeon can follow the muscle belly/tendon to the lesser sciatic notch. The piriformis can be followed back to the greater sciatic notch. A natural frenulum occurs between the undersurface of the obturator internus and the joint capsule/posterior column. This may be divided back to the level of the lesser sciatic notch, and the multipennate (multifingered) tendon of the obturator internus, as it exits from the lesser sciatic notch, is then visualized. There is a bursa between the undersurface of the obturator internus tendon and the lesser sciatic notch that facilitates identification of the latter. Finally, the gluteus minimus may be elevated as needed from an inferior to superior direction, depending upon how much exposure is needed for a given fracture pattern. The retroacetabular surface is thus exposed.

After the exposure of the retroacetabular surface is completed, fracture reduction for the given fracture pattern is performed as described in the following sections on surgical techniques. If needed during reduction of the fracture, the medial wall of the acetabulum (the quadrilateral plate) can be palpated through the greater sciatic notch. To accomplish this, the short external rotators are elevated off the quadralateral surface with a curved elevator placed through the greater sciatic arch. The muscular belly of the piriformis muscle, as well as the short external rotators, is elevated off the surface of the quadrilateral surface through the greater sciatic notch with a curved elevator.

Following surgical reduction of the acetabular fracture, the wound is copiously irrigated with 6 L of sterile saline using a high-pressure irrigation system. The tendon of the piriformis and the conjoint tendon are repaired with a no. 1 resorbable suture (while taking care to protect the medial circumflex vessel), and the tendon of the gluteus maximus is repaired with a no. 5 suture. Two $\frac{1}{8}$ in. suction drains are placed below the fascial level. The fascia is then closed utilizing no. 1 suture, and subcutaneous tissue is once again irrigated. The subcutaneous tissue is then closed utilizing nonabsorbable suture, with the skin closed with skin staples.

Ilioinguinal Approach (see Video 20–2, Disk 2)

The ilioinguinal approach was developed by Letournel to access the entire anterior pelvic ring from the pubic symphysis to the sacroiliac joint.[2,3,12,15] Previous anterior approaches provided limited access to the pelvis medial to the psoas gutter (such as the extended Smith-Peterson approach) and poor visualization of the quadrilateral surface.

The ilioinguinal approach takes advantage of three "windows" to provide visualization of the entire aspect of the internal iliac fossa, anterior column, pelvic brim, parasymphyseal region, and quadrilateral surface. The windows are defined by, and require mobilization of, the iliopsoas muscle and the external iliac vessels. The lateral window exposes the iliac fossa and upper part of the pelvic brim. The middle window, between the iliopsoas and the vascular bundle, allows one to see the quadrilateral plate and iliopectineal eminence. The medial window supplies access to the superior ramus, symphysis, and retropubic space.

The ilioinguinal approach is the preferred approach for an anterior column fracture, anterior column/posterior hemitransverse fracture, and an associated both-column fracture. It may be utilized for anterior wall fractures and transverse fractures in which the major displacement is anterior. This approach is best suited for surgical reconstruction of fractures involving the pubic bone from the pubic symphysis to the iliopectineal eminence, and those fractures extending to the anterior ilium or iliac crest. The major limitation of the ilioinguinal approach is lack of direct joint access, necessitating indirect reduction of the intra-articular fractures. With anterior column/posterior hemitransverse and associated both-column injuries, a lateral soft tissue hinge (the labrum) is maintained between the posterior fracture fragment and intact or fractured (associated both column) rim, respectively, that can facilitate indirect reduction of the posterior column component of the fracture.

The patient is positioned supine with the hip in slight flexion to relax the iliopsoas. Paralysis during the procedure can be beneficial for retraction of the abdominal/hip musculature. The patient can be positioned on a fracture table or with the leg free and prepped into the field. The classic ilioinguinal approach (**Fig. 20–13A–G**) begins with a skin incision 1 to 2 cm above the pubic symphysis, gently curving up to a point just below the anterior-superior iliac spine, proceeding along, but just below, the iliac crest past its lateralmost convexity. Once the skin and subcutaneous tissue are divided, the external oblique fascia is identified over the abdomen, and the interval between the abdominal and hip abductor muscles is identified at the iliac crest. The lateral window is developed by releasing the abdominal muscle insertion from the iliac crest and the iliacus insertion from the internal aspect of the ilium. The iliopsoas is elevated from the internal iliac fossa to the pelvic brim anteriorly and the sacroiliac joint posteriorly. Control of the nutrient artery of the ilium is necessary. This can cause significant bleeding unless bone wax is placed over the nutrient artery foramen, which is located approximately 1.5 cm lateral and 1.5 cm anterior to the sacroiliac joint. This area is now packed with a moist sponge.

Anteriorly, after identifying the external inguinal ring, the external oblique fascia is split just above the ring from the lateral aspect of the rectus abdominis to a point just above the anterior-superior iliac spine. Reflecting the

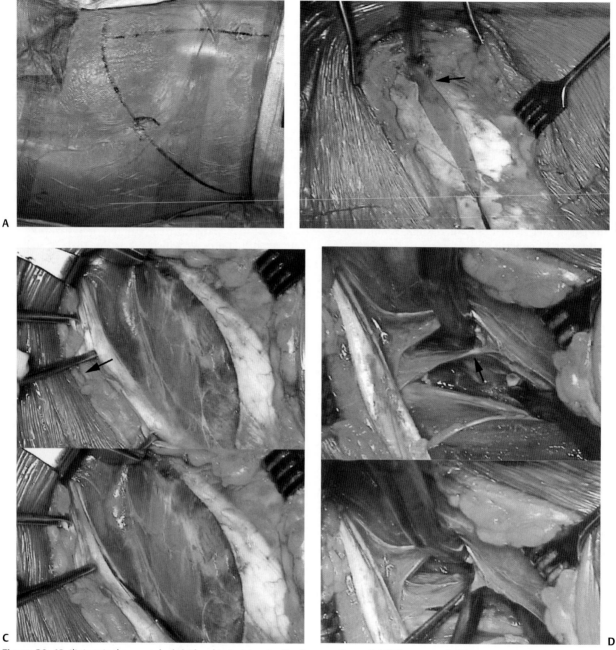

Figure 20–13 Ilioinguinal approach. **(A)** The skin incision for the ilioinguinal approach begins ~2 cm superior to the pubic symphysis and curves for the outer aspect of the anterior-superior iliac spine (marked) and along the lateral aspect of the iliac crest. The proposed incision is drawn, along with the midline of the abdomen, indicating the linea alba. Note that the patient is viewed from the side. **(B)** After dissection through the subcutaneous tissue, the external inguinal ring is found (arrow). Division of the external oblique is then performed. **(C)** The external oblique aponeurosis is then reflected distally (arrow), and the inguinal ligament (floor of the inguinal canal) is divided, leaving ~3 to 4 mm of fibers on the cephalad edge of the inguinal ligament. **(D)** After division of the inguinal ligament, the iliopectineal fascia (arrow) is defined (upper view). The fascia is then often divided (lower view) down to the pectineal eminence and back toward the sacroiliac joint.

external oblique distally, the contents of the inguinal canal (spermatic cord, ilioinguinal nerve) are identified and isolated with a Penrose drain. The floor of the inguinal canal is formed by the conjoint tendon of the internal oblique and transversus abdominis muscles. The distalmost edge is defined by the inguinal ligament. The ligament is more de-

veloped and better defined laterally, thinning medially toward its insertion at the pubic tubercle. The true pelvis is accessed by incising the ligament 2 to 3 mm proximal to its reflection to the external oblique fascia. Care should be exercised when dividing this ligament laterally because in the majority of individuals the lateral femoral cutaneous

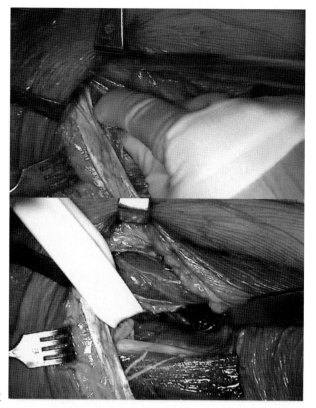

E

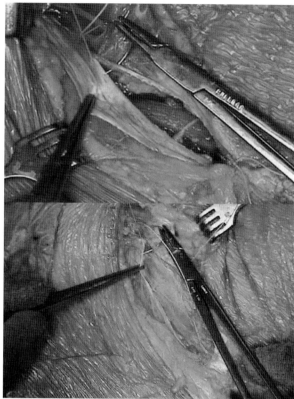

G

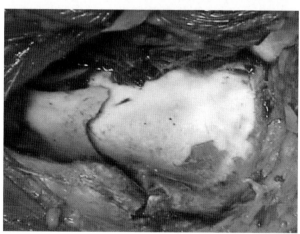

F

Figure 20–13 *(Continued)* **(E)** The external iliac artery and vein are palpated and isolated with a Penrose drain. Shown in the bottom photo is the "middle window" where the surgeon can delineate and visualize the quadrilateral surface with the aid of a curved retractor placed in the area of the ischial spine. **(F)** Intraoperative view of the "lateral window" with exposure of the internal iliac fossa. The anterior column fracture is seen. This window can be used to visualize and reduce the sacroiliac joint if necessary. **(G)** At the end of the ilioinguinal approach, the floor of the inguinal canal (upper view) is repaired utilizing a running suture, and the external oblique aponeurosis is closed (lower view).

nerve is directly under the ligament and should be spared. Generally, the nerve is 1 to 2 cm medial to the anterior-superior iliac spine, but this is variable. As the conjoint tendon is released laterally from the anterior-superior iliac crest, the more anterior iliopsoas can be elevated from the interspinous area and from the enveloping fascia of the tensor fascia lata distally. Additional flexion of the hip will allow elevation of the iliopsoas medially to the iliopectineal eminence and anterior pelvic brim. Medial dissection over the brim and onto the quadrilateral surface at this point is limited by the iliopectineal fascia.

Blunt dissection performed from lateral to medial over the anterior aspect of the psoas will help define the femoral nerve on the medial aspect of the iliopsoas muscle belly. To gain access to the true pelvis, the iliopectineal fascia on the medial aspect of the iliopsoas muscle must be divided. The iliopectineal fascia separates the iliopsoas muscle and femoral nerve from the adjacent external iliac vessels, so division of this structure must be done with great care. There are often small vascular connecting branches between the muscle belly of the iliopsoas and the external iliac artery that should be ligated. The arterial pulse in the external iliac/femoral artery is palpated just medial to the iliopectineal fascia. Next, the iliopectineal fascia is defined on both its medial and lateral aspects and is cut from anterior to posterior and excised. The femoral nerve and psoas muscle are isolated with a Penrose drain. This will facilitate lateral retraction of the muscle and protection of the femoral nerve while working in the middle window. Placement of retractors through the middle window onto the quadrilateral surface to retract the vessels medially and the iliopsoas and femoral nerve laterally will improve visualization in this area. Care must be taken not to prolong medial retraction on the external iliac artery and vein and to periodically check the pulse distal to the retractors because occlusion of the femoral artery can complicate work through the middle window.

An option prior to elevating the tissues from the superior ramus and quadrilateral surface within the middle window is to develop the medial window. In the midline of the abdominal wall, underneath the arcuate line, the fascial elements of the abdominal muscles coalesce into a single layer located anterior to the rectus. To develop the medial window, the incision previously made through the external oblique aponeurosis is extended to the midline over the rectus abdominis. This layer of fascia is elevated from the rectus muscle distally, while maintaining its insertion to the anterior pelvic ring, allowing for repair at the completion of the case. The rectus is split transversely from the superior ramus. The retropubic space of Retzius is entered and the bladder swept from the posterior aspect of the pubic body. Superficial dissection lateral to the rectus is not recommended so that the lymphatics are not disrupted. A finger is then swept along the posterior aspect of the ramus from both the middle and medial windows to identify and palpate any retropubic vascular anastomosis.[16] Once controlled with vascular clips or cautery, subperiosteal exposure of the superior ramus and quadrilateral plate can be completed safely. To utilize the lateral window for access to the quadrilateral surface, 50 to 60 degrees of hip flexion is needed. This cannot be accomplished with the fracture table. Therefore, use of the fracture table will usually require more extensive use of the second (middle) window for visualization and indirect reduction of the posterior column.

Modifications of the ilioinguinal approach have been developed to improve access to specific areas of the innominate bone and the hip joint for specific indications. Weber and Mast defined a posterior extension to provide access to the posterolateral ilium for fractures involving the sacroiliac joint.[17] Kloen et al described incorporation of the Smith-Peterson interval anteriorly to facilitate exposure of the anterior rim and to gain intra-articular access while using the ilioinguinal approach.[18] Elimination of the medial window in favor of a midline split of the rectus abdominis and development of the Stoppa exposure as part of the ilioinguinal approach can also improve visualization and allow clamp and implant access to the quadrilateral surface and posterior column.[19]

Extended Approaches

Extended approaches have been developed to provide direct access to both the anterior and posterior columns as well as the joint surface for complex reconstructions. Therefore, by definition, they are laterally based, and all involve elevation of the abductor muscle mass from the lateral ilium. These include the triradiate,[20] T-extensile,[21] and extended iliofemoral approaches.[2,12] These approaches are usually indicated for fractures involving both the anterior and posterior columns having a specific injury pattern that does not reliably allow for reduction of the opposite column from the Kocher-Langenbeck or ilioinguinal approach. Indications for an extended approach include

- Associated both-column fractures with extension into the sacroiliac joint, with associated fragmentation of the posterior column or significant displacement or fragmentation of the posterior wall
- An associated both-column fracture in which the peripheral rims of the anterior and posterior column components do not maintain an intimate relationship following displacement (indicating capsulolabral dissociation of the anterior and posterior columns, making indirect reduction of the posterior column difficult)
- High (transtectal) transverse, transverse plus posterior wall and T-shaped fractures, especially if associated with anterior injuries to the pelvic ring (symphysis dislocation or rami fractures).
- Fractures involving both columns greater than 3 weeks old. Bone resorption at the fracture lines combined with callus formation makes adequate reconstruction difficult without direct visualization of the articular surface reduction.

Relative contraindications to an extended approach include advanced physiological age (> 50 years), soft tissue degloving injuries, morbid obesity, occlusion of the internal iliac vascular pedicle, and traumatic brain injury. Inherent to the surgeon's decision to use an extensile approach is the balance between improved exposure versus increased morbidity commonly associated with these approaches.[3,22]

The authors' preference for an extensile approach is the extended iliofemoral. The next section discusses this approach in detail and provides references for descriptions of alternate extensile approaches.

Extended Iliofemoral Approach

The extended iliofemoral approach gives direct access to the entire outer aspect of the innominate bone, the greater sciatic notch area, the sacroiliac joint region, and the pelvic brim down to the level of the pectineal eminence. Letournel described an expanded exposure of the extended Smith-Peterson approach, allowing for access

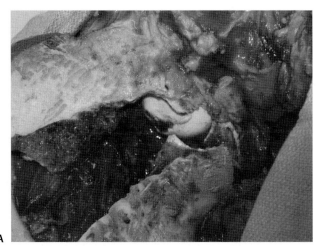

A

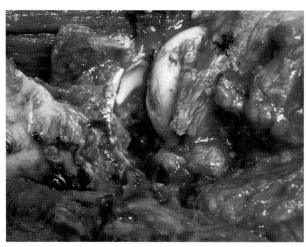

B

Figure 20–14 The extended iliofemoral approach. **(A)** Outer exposure of the innominate bone afforded by the extended iliofemoral approach. **(B)** Distraction of the hip joint with the extended ilio- femoral approach with capsulotomy (if necessary) allows for direct visualization of the articular surface of the acetabulum.

to the retroacetabular surface and caudally to the ischial ramus.[2] The patient is positioned lateral, with the leg in distal femoral traction and with the hip in neutral flexion and the knee flexed to relax the sciatic nerve. The approach can be broken down into four potential stages **(Fig. 20–14A,B)**. The skin incision begins just beyond the posterior-superior iliac spine, curving along the crest to the anterior-superior iliac spine. This should be performed slightly below the palpable crest and then turn distally just posterior to the anterior-superior iliac spine, continuing over the belly of the tensor muscle toward the lateral aspect of the patella. First, the interval between the abdominal muscles and hip abductors is identified at the iliac crest. The origins of the gluteus medius and maximus are released from the iliac crest, and they, along with the gluteus minimus, are elevated from the lateral ilium to the cranial aspect of the greater sciatic notch and the supra-acetabular region. The gluteus maximus origin from the cristae glutae of the ilium should be completely released posteriorly.

Next, the leg portion of the incision should continue caudally approximately half the length of the leg, just past the distal end of the tensor fascia muscle belly insertion into the iliotibial band. The fascia over the tensor fascia lata is split, and the muscle elevated from its origin on the anterior lateral ilium and mobilized posteriorly with the abductor flap. Distally, the posterior portion of the enveloping tensor fascia is incised, the tensor fascia is retracted laterally, and an additional fascial layer overlying the rectus femoris is identified. Care should be taken when incising this next fascial layer because the ascending branches of the lateral femoral circumflex vessels lie directly beneath this layer. The vessels are then isolated and ligated to allow for adequate flap mobility. Then, one can easily identify the rectus femoris and vastus lateralis in the distal portions of the wound. Next, the proximal abductor

flap can be further mobilized caudally and posteriorly, and the reflected head of the rectus tendon followed to the supra-acetabular region. The superior gluteal pedicle is elevated from the anterior aspect of the greater sciatic notch. The anterior trochanter is easily palpated in the wound but is deep to very dense retinacular tissue. The gluteus minimus tendon is usually found in the supra-acetabular region and can be followed to the tip of the trochanter. Distally, a finger can be swept laterally along the vastus lateralis muscle to its insertion on the vastus ridge of the trochanter. These two landmarks can guide dissection through the retinacular tissue, usually performed with heavy scissors, to the insertion of the minimus on the anterolateral trochanter.

The gluteus minimus tendon is released from the trochanter. A finger can then be passed posteriorly from proximal and distal to isolate the oblique insertion of the gluteus medius. The gluteus medius tendon can then be tenotomized from the trochanter or released by an osteotomy of the greater trochanter. If a tenotomy is performed, small sections of the tendon should be released at a time, placing sutures along its length to maintain the orientation and position of the tendon for subsequent repair. If an osteotomy is performed, it should be done lateral to the piriformis insertion to protect the vascular supply to the femoral head.[14] Finally, the posterior column and greater sciatic notch can be exposed in a manner similar to that described for the Kocher-Langenbeck approach. The piriformis and obturator internus tendons are released from the trochanter and elevated from the retroacetabular surface to the greater and lesser notches. An anterior and superior capsulotomy can be performed to directly visualize the articular surface. Digital access to the quadrilateral surface and internal aspect of the true pelvis can be accomplished through the greater sciatic notch. Care should be taken as to how the internal aspect of the pelvis is accessed superiorly or anteriorly. If the fracture line exits along the crest, attachments to the anterior-superior iliac crest and anterior-inferior iliac crest should be maintained to provide vascularity to the anterior column fragment. Clamp and digital access to the pelvic brim can also be accomplished through the intraspinous area. For transverse or T-shaped fractures, soft tissue attachments should be maintained along the iliac crest to maintain vascularity to the anterior ilium. In this situation, the rectus femoris insertion can be released to visualize the anterior limb of a transversely oriented fracture line to the anterior rim of the acetabulum. The iliopsoas can be elevated from the pelvic brim to visualize the reduction and for anterior clamp placement while maintaining abdominal muscle origins attached to the iliac crest.

Surgical Techniques

Treatment of Posterior Wall Fractures through the Kocher-Langenbeck Approach (see Video 20–1, Disk 2)

The important questions to ask in the preoperative assessment of a posterior wall fracture are

- How far does the posterior wall fragment extend anteriorly? The surgeon should determine preoperatively whether the fracture can be visualized and reduced through the exposure afforded by the Kocher-Langenbeck approach. In certain cases, the "posterior wall" fracture will extend quite superiorly and the gluteus medius and minimus will not allow the surgeon to adequately visualize the posterior wall, or the musculature will be significantly devitalized in an attempt to see this fracture. Neither one of these situations is desirable. If the fracture extends quite superior or anterior, the Ganz trochanteric flip osteotomy may be desirable.[23]
- A characterization of the posterior wall, in terms of its size and how many fragments it has, can be best assessed on the AP radiograph of the pelvis and the obturator oblique radiographs, and is then confirmed via CT scan.
- The presence of intra-articular fragments is noted. If there are intra-articular fragments, the quantity and size of these fragments must be assessed.
- The presence of marginal impaction, its size, and its location should be noted.
- The surgeon should ask if there is an incomplete or minimally displaced transverse fracture.
- The surgeon must ask if there is an associated femoral head fracture or femoral head injury or both.

The surgical tactics/sequence for a posterior wall fracture begins with the Kocher-Langenbeck approach, as noted earlier. Care is taken to avoid devitalization of the abductor muscles. Once exposed, the edges of the fracture

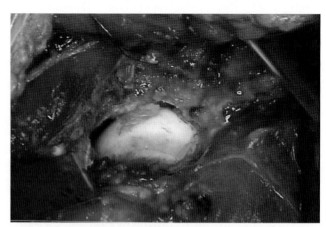

Figure 20–15 Distraction of the hip joint seen from the Kocher-Langenbeck approach performed in the prone position with the aid of an acetabular fracture table.

as well as the cancellous surfaces of both the posterior wall fragment and the recipient bed are debrided. The surgeon should "memorize" the original position of small, separate osteochondral fragments, which will facilitate reducing the posterior wall into the appropriate position. Distraction of the hip joint for complete visualization and debridement of the joint is then performed. This can be performed with the fracture table if the patient is in the prone position (with the knee flexed), or a femoral distractor may be utilized if the patient is in the lateral position **(Figs. 20–15 and 20–16).** Headlight visualization, Frazier-tip suction, and pituitary rongeurs are helpful for identification and removal of fragments from the hip joint. In most cases, the ligamentum teres has been avulsed. The ligamentum teres is debrided because often there are small chondral or osteochondral fragments

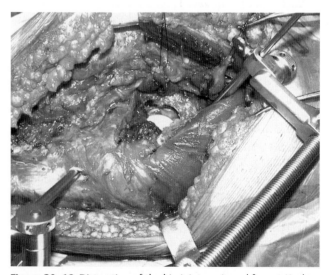

Figure 20–16 Distraction of the hip joint as viewed from a Kocher-Langenbeck approach with the patient in the lateral position and with the aid of a femoral distractor.

in the substance of the ligamentum teres. Occasionally, there may be fragments that are anterior to the femoral head, which can be retrieved with a right-angle clamp. The surgeon should make note of any cartilage damage to the femoral head. The femoral head is then brought back into position by releasing the traction afforded either by the fracture table or the femoral distractor. Reduction of the posterior wall is performed with the joint reduced to utilize the femoral head as a template.

Marginal impaction can be present in the form of osteochondral fragments that have been displaced and rotated 70 to 90 degrees and driven into the cancellous bone of the posterior column. Marginal impaction is present in 11 to 23% of cases.[2,3,24] If there is marginal impaction present, the impacted fragments are reduced back into position (**Fig. 20–17A–C**). A bone graft may be obtained from the greater trochanter through a 1.5 cm rectangular cortical defect to place bone graft behind the elevated marginal impaction. Small, separate osteochondral fragments are reduced into position and held by minifragment screws, if necessary (2.0 or 2.7 mm lag screws). The posterior wall is then reduced into position. The common displacement of the posterior wall is cephalad and peripheral displacement. One or two ball-spike pushers are then utilized for the reduction. Interfragmentary lag screws may be placed through the posterior wall if it is large enough. The direction of such lag screws should be anticipated before the posterior wall is reduced into position because this allows the surgeon to avoid intra-articular placement of the lag screw. The screws should not be overtightened, which may cause displacement of the fragment prior to plate placement. Finally, an appropriately undercontoured 3.5 mm reconstruction plate is then placed across the posterior wall, providing compression and a buttressing effect across the fracture (**Fig. 20–18A–C**). The shape of the plate is critical to its function. The outer cortical surface of the posterior wall is convex. The plate is contoured with a sharp angle distally between the first and second holes. This allows a long screw (typically 50 to 70 mm) to be placed into the ischium. The lower half of the plate has a slight curve (concave anteriorly) to accommodate the curvature of the posterior wall. The upper portion of the plate is slightly undercontoured so that it lies off the bone in the upper portion of the plate but is touching the posterior wall in its middle area.

Then, using a ball spike in one of the upper holes, the upper plate is pushed against the bone. This maneuver exerts a tremendous compressive force against the convexity of the posterior wall fragment. The plate should be long enough so that two screws can be placed superiorly in the ilium. Lag screws are placed, if necessary, through the plate. Confirmation of appropriate reduction and fixation of the posterior wall is then assessed via digital palpation and visualization of the fracture lines, and the screws are confirmed to be extra-articular with

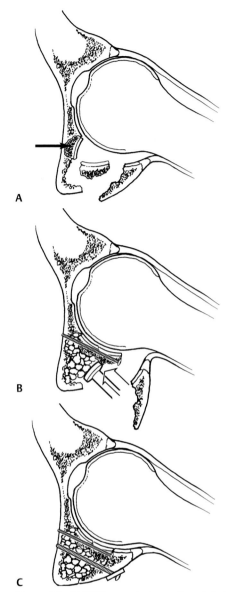

Figure 20–17 With a posterior wall acetabular fracture, marginal impaction and free osteochondral fragments may be seen. **(A)** The marginal (arrow) impaction is seen rotated ~70 degrees from its normal position. It is driven back into cancellous bone. In addition, there is a free osteochondral fragment. The posterior wall is left attached to the capsule. **(B)** Utilizing the femoral head as a template, the marginal impaction is derotated into position, and the osteochondral fragment is also placed into its appropriate position. Bone graft or bone graft substitute is then placed behind these fragments. Supplementary minifragment screws (2.0 or 2.7 mm) may be placed through these fragments for further support. **(C)** The posterior wall is then reduced into position, and a posterior wall plate is placed.

fluoroscopy.[25] The obturator oblique view may also be utilized for assessment of the reduction, though it must be understood that this is only accurate to ~2 mm, and that direct visualization of the fracture reduction is better for assessment (**Fig. 20–19A–D**).

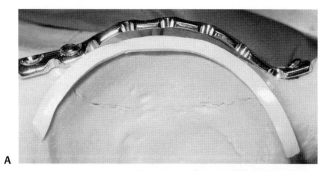

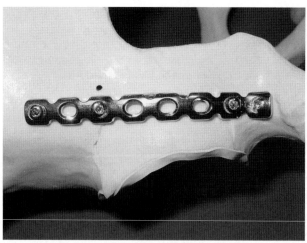

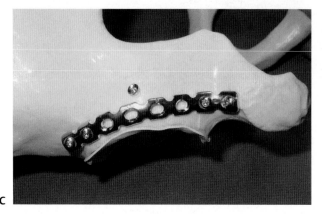

Figure 20–18 Direct contouring and positioning of the posterior wall plate is critical. **(A)** Overcontouring of the plate does not allow for appropriate buttressing of the posterior wall. **(B)** Another common error is to not bend the plate "on the flat," and thus the plate does not lie over the major portion of the posterior wall. In addition, bringing the plate straight up on the posterior column and going more cephalad than the greater sciatic notch will place the superior gluteal neurovascular bundle at risk. **(C)** Appropriate contouring of a posterior wall plate.

Common errors with the surgical sequence or reduction include devitalization of the abductors, poor visualization of the superior-posterior wall fracture, and inadequate handling of intra-articular fragments. Attempts at cranial and anterior access to the supra-acetabular bone will stretch the abductors and superior gluteal nerve, increasing local injury. Hip abduction will help to relax the muscles, but if more access is needed, a trochanteric osteotomy may be indicated. The vascularity of the posterior wall, as with any fracture, should be preserved. With a posterior wall fracture, this is usually achieved through maintenance of the capsular and labral attachments. Another possible error is inadequate debridement of intra-articular bony fragments. A preoperative cataloging of the intra-articular fragments is helpful in avoiding this. Poor reduction or poor support of the impacted fragments can be minimized by utilizing the femoral head as a template, and also by aggressive use of bone graft behind the marginal impaction.

Common errors with posterior wall fixation include overcontouring of the plate so that the superior and inferior aspects of the plate contact the bone, but the plate over the midsubstance is not sufficiently buttressing the posterior wall (**Fig. 20–18A**). Two other common errors with plate contouring include not bringing the plate peripheral enough on the acetabulum so the posterior wall is not adequately buttressed, as well as not bending the plate "on the flat" so that the plate instead goes straight up the posterior column rather than curving more anteri-

orly above the acetabulum. Posterior plate placement above the greater sciatic notch (when the plate goes directly up the posterior column) will place the superior gluteal nerve and artery at risk (**Fig. 20–18B**).

Treatment of a Posterior Column Fracture through a Kocher-Langenbeck Approach

The posterior column fracture is, in all cases, addressed through the Kocher-Langenbeck approach. The patient should be positioned prone because it is critical to assess the rotational displacement of the posterior column through the greater sciatic notch. The reduction is very difficult to obtain. The common deformity of the posterior column is slightly gapping superiorly with cephalic translation, or malrotation. This can best be appreciated by palpating the superior aspect of the posterior column through the greater sciatic notch. A useful reduction strategy for a posterior column fracture is to use a short angled-jaw forceps or an asymmetrical Verbrugge or Weber clamp through the greater sciatic notch. A Shanz pin in the ischium may be helpful for rotational control. An initial lag screw is usually placed from the posterior column into the intact ilium. In obese patients, this lag screw may be difficult to place, and therefore a two-hole plate in the area of the greater sciatic notch can also be utilized for provisional fixation. A six-hole plate is then placed along the posterior column. Because this plate functions less as a buttress, it is not necessary to place this along the acetabular rim as is

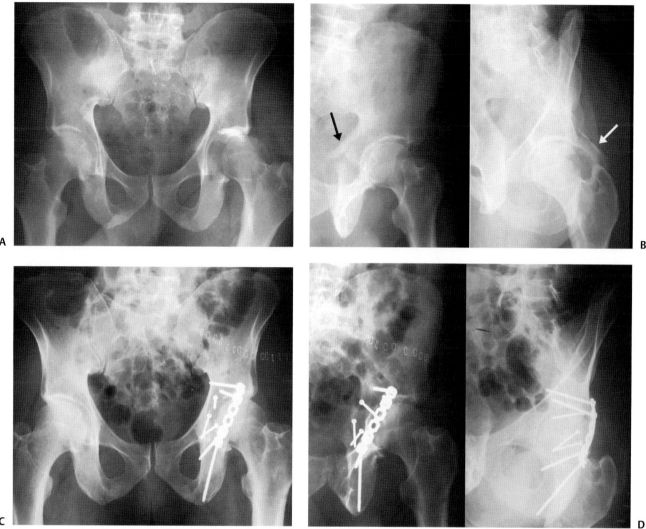

Figure 20–19 Example of a posterior wall acetabular fracture. **(A)** Anteroposterior (AP) radiograph demonstrating a probable intra-articular fragment with widening of the medial joint space. **(B)** Judet view of the injury. The obturator oblique view (right panel) clearly shows the displaced posterior wall (white arrow). Note that in the iliac oblique view (left panel) there is a separate cortical fragment along the greater sciatic notch (black arrow). This is an extended posterior wall. **(C)** Postoperative AP pelvic radiograph. Separate interfragmentary screws were used to fix the extended posterior wall, and a posterior buttress plate was applied. The radiographic landmarks have been restored. **(D)** Postoperative Judet radiographs.

the case with the posterior wall. An additional lag screw may be placed more peripherally across the posterior column fracture.

Treatment of the Transverse Fracture through the Kocher-Langenbeck Approach

For the reasons already noted, transverse fractures are addressed in most cases via the prone approach. Useful tools for reduction of a transverse fracture include distal femoral traction, an ischial tuberosity Shanz pin for rotational control of the ischiopubic segment, an angled-jaw clamp, a Weber or an asymmetrical Verbrugge clamp placed through the greater sciatic notch, or a Farabeuf clamp or small pelvic reduction clamp placed along the

posterior column **(Figs. 20–20A–C** and **20–21A,B).** Often, the posterior column component of a transverse fracture may appear to be perfectly reduced. However, palpation of the anterior component of the fracture through the greater sciatic notch will reveal either or both malrotation and gapping. This can be corrected by rotation of the ischial fragment using the Shanz pin in the ischial tuberosity, and/or clamp application through the greater sciatic notch onto the anterior column component of the fracture. After the fracture is reduced, a lag screw from the posterior column into the anterior column may be placed, as well as a lag screw across the posterior column component of the fracture. The clamps may then be removed because the fracture is now reduced, and a plate can be placed across the posterior column. In most transverse fractures, one plate is sufficient.

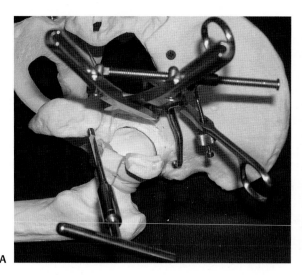

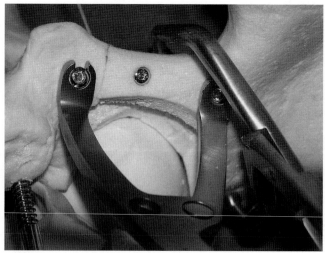

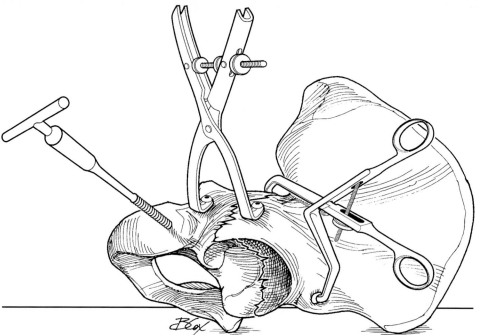

Figure 20–20 Multiple reduction maneuvers and clamps are often necessary for reduction of the transverse fracture. **(A)** A short angled-jaw forceps is placed through the greater sciatic notch onto the anterior column. A pelvic reduction clamp is placed across the posterior column with one screw on each side of the fracture. An ischial tuberosity Shanz pin is placed for derotation of the ischial pubic segment. **(B)** Close-up view of the reduction maneuver of this transverse fracture. A lag screw has been placed from the intact ilium into the ischiopubic segment. **(C)** Schematic of the aforementioned reduction techniques.

Treatment of the Transverse with Posterior Wall Fracture through the Kocher-Langenbeck Approach (see Video 20–1, Disk 2)

The key concepts in treating an associated transverse with posterior wall acetabular fracture are, first, addressing the transverse component of the fracture and, second, repairing the posterior wall component of the fracture **(Figs. 20–22A–D** and **20–23A–H).** By doing so, the surgeon converts a complex transverse/posterior wall fracture into two simpler fractures: 1. a transverse fracture that has undergone reduction and fixation, and 2. a remaining poste-

rior wall fracture. During the initial approach, a suture may be placed in the posterior wall fragment to reflect it out of the way as the surgeon addresses the transverse component of the fracture. In most cases, a lag screw is placed in the posterior column across the transverse component of the fracture. Additionally, a lag screw may be placed from the posterior to anterior column. If the posterior wall fragment is large, and the transverse fracture is horizontally oriented, a plate along the greater sciatic notch can substitute for a posterior interfragmentary screw. At this point, the posterior wall fragment is debrided and reduced as previously described. An appropriately sized plate is

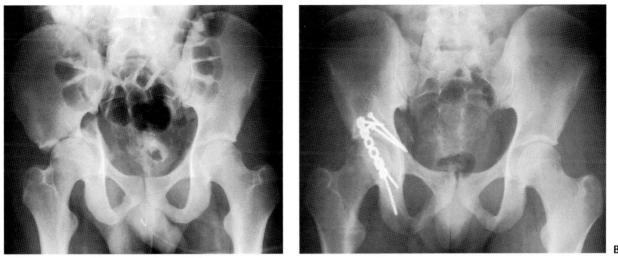

A   B

Figure 20–21 A transtectal transverse acetabular fracture in an 18-year-old male in which the Kocher-Langenbeck approach is utilized for reduction. **(A)** Anteroposterior (AP) injury pelvic radiograph. **(B)** Follow-up AP radiograph at 2 years postoperative.

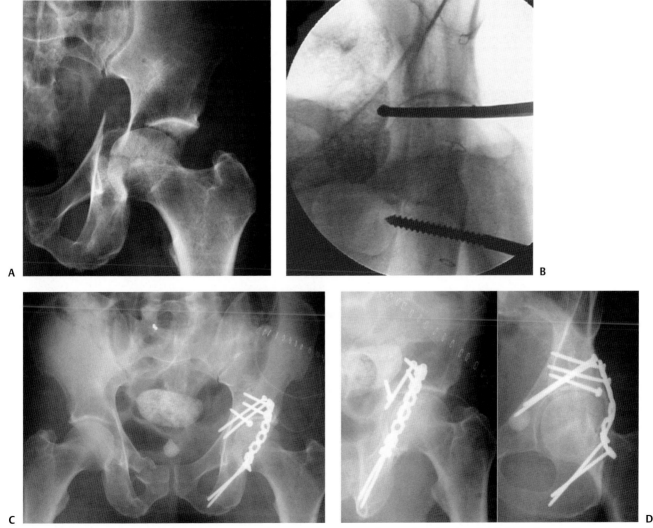

A   B

C   D

Figure 20–22 Reduction and fixation of a transverse with posterior wall acetabular fracture through a Kocher-Langenbeck approach with the patient in the prone position. **(A)** Injury radiograph. **(B)** A short angled-jaw forceps is placed through the greater sciatic notch onto the anterior column, and an ischial tuberosity Shanz pin is placed for rotational control. **(C)** Postoperative radiograph of the pelvis. **(D)** Postoperative Judet films.

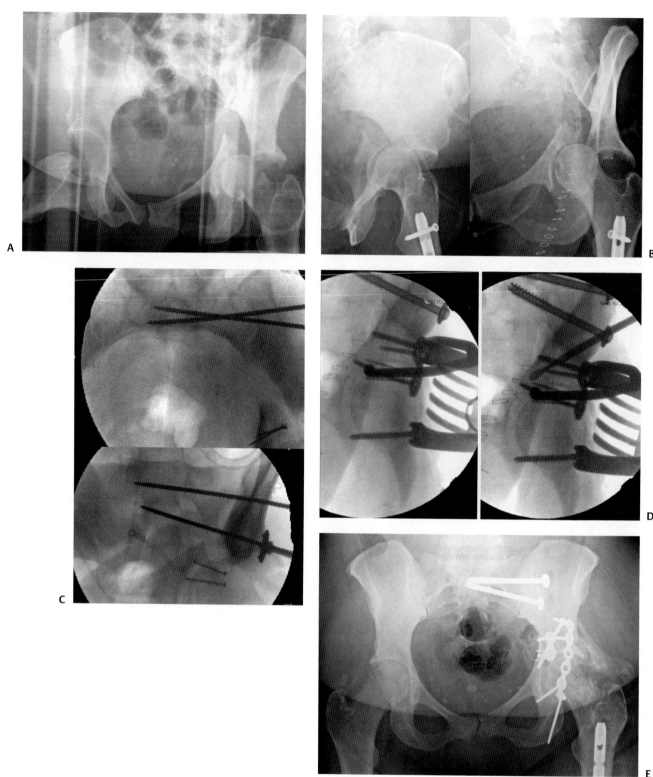

Figure 20–23 Transverse with posterior wall acetabular fracture and associated pelvic ring pathology in a 63-year-old diabetic female. **(A)** The left transverse with posterior wall acetabular fracture is associated with a left sacroiliac joint disruption with mild abduction/external rotation of the left hemipelvis. The patient also has a right inferior/anterior hip dislocation and a left femoral shaft fracture. **(B)** Judet views of the same injury. **(C)** A Kocher-Langenbeck approach to the left hip was made, and minifragment screws were placed in a separate osteochondral fragment. The transverse component of the fracture was not reducible, however. Therefore, a percutaneous screw fixation of the left sacroiliac joint was performed. Note the use of a ball-spike pusher with a disk on the sciatic buttress region to correct the abduction/external rotation deformity of the left hemipelvis. **(D)** Intraoperative obturator oblique views showing reduction of the transverse component of the fracture. In this case, this was accomplished by short angled-jaw forceps through the greater sciatic notch and a pelvic reduction clamp along the posterior column. A lag screw is being placed from the posterior column into the anterior column. **(E)** Anteroposterior (AP) pelvic radiograph at 6 months. The patient developed Brooker stage III heterotopic ossification.

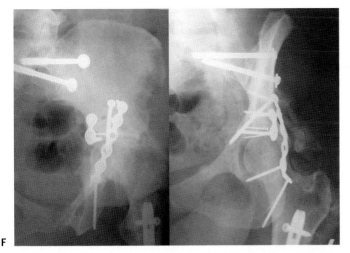

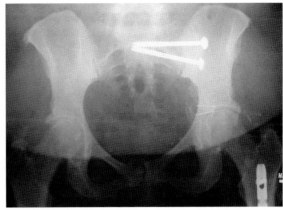

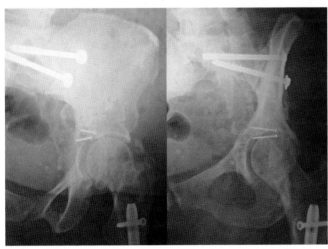

Figure 20–23 *(Coninued)* **(F)** Judet radiographs at 6 months. **(G)** The patient underwent removal of the heterotopic ossification and hardware about her left hip. AP radiograph at 2 years. **(H)** Judet views at 2 years. The patient had minimal pain. (5/5/5 with modified d'Aubigne and Postel scale.[3])

then placed across the posterior wall. If the posterior wall is extremely small or peripheral, two plates may be necessary. In this case, a shorter plate is used to repair the transverse fracture that is placed more posteriorly (closer to the sciatic buttress), and a second plate is used to address the posterior wall **(Fig. 20–23).**

Treatment of the T-Type Acetabular Fracture through the Kocher-Langenbeck Approach

A key feature of a T-type fracture is that the anterior column component and the posterior column component of the ischiopubic (inferior) fragment are separate. The T-type fracture may be addressed through an extended iliofemoral approach, a sequential combined approach, or the Kocher-Langenbeck approach. This latter approach is most suitable if the patient is relatively elderly (greater than 55 years of age), or the anterior column component of the fracture is low or minimally displaced. When approaching this fracture through a Kocher-Langenbeck approach, the surgeon may have difficulty with reduction of the anterior column component of the fracture.

The three possible strategies used in open reduction internal fixation of the T-type fracture from the Kocher-Langenbeck approach would be (1) reduction of the anterior column followed by reduction of the posterior column; (2) reduction of the posterior column followed by reduction of the anterior column; and (3) creation of an intact ischiopubic segment, followed by reduction of this inferior ischiopubic segment to the intact ilium. The latter tactic may be utilized in the case of the ischial T fracture, where the vertical limb of the fracture goes into the ischium. The most common tactic used with the Kocher-Langenbeck approach in the prone position would be reduction of the anterior column component of the fracture first, followed by reduction and fixation of the posterior column component of the fracture. In most of these cases, the posterior column component of the fracture can be displaced by use of a lamina spreader between the intact ilium and the posterior column. The femoral head may then be distracted by use of the fracture table, and a clamp can be placed onto the anterior column. Occasionally, a bone hook or rotational reduction aid such as a Shanz pin may be placed into the anterior column. A lag screw may then be placed from the posterior

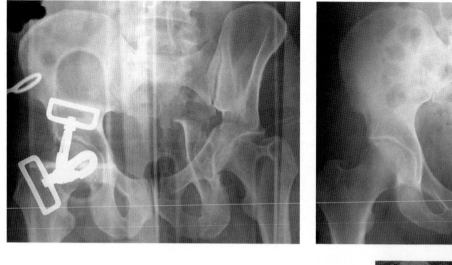

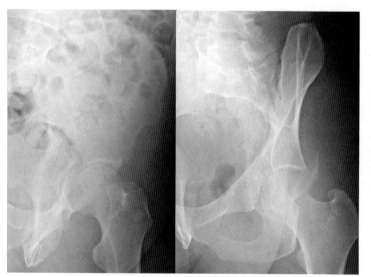

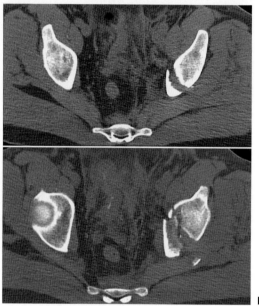

Figure 20–24 T-type with posterior wall acetabular fracture in a 42-year-old male. **(A)** Anteroposterior (AP) pelvic radiograph with posterior dislocation of the femoral head. Note the wide displacement of the posterior column and minimal displacement of the anterior column. **(B)** AP pelvic radiograph taken after closed reduction of the left hip. **(C)** Judet views of the same hip taken after re-duction of the femoral head. Note the high involvement of the posterior column into the greater sciatic notch, minimal displacement of the anterior column, and posterior wall fracture. **(D)** Computed tomographic (CT) scan of the pelvis demonstrating what appears to be a typical anterior to posterior transverse acetabular fracture.

column into the anterior column, and the posterior column component of the fracture is then reduced into position. If the posterior wall is also fractured, it is reduced and internally fixed, as already noted for a posterior wall. Alternatively, the posterior column may be addressed first, followed by the anterior column **(Fig. 20–24A–H).**

Treatment of the Anterior Column Utilizing the Ilioinguinal Approach (see Video 20–2, Disk 2)

The fractures that are commonly indicated for the ilioinguinal exposures are fractures of the anterior column, anterior plus posterior hemitransverse, the associated both-column, and less commonly the transverse or T-shaped fracture. The first step in the reduction of each of these three fractures is to reduce the anterior column component of the fracture. After exposure of the inner aspects of the ilium through the three windows of the ilioinguinal approach, it is very common to also incise portions of the abductor origin along the iliac crest adjacent to the fracture line (either anterior or posterior to the gluteus medius tubercle) to palpate the reduction of the fracture on the outer aspect of the ilium. This generally involves elevating the tissues for 2 to 3 cm off the external aspect of the innominate bone. The reduction usually begins from posterior to anterior as well as from cranial to

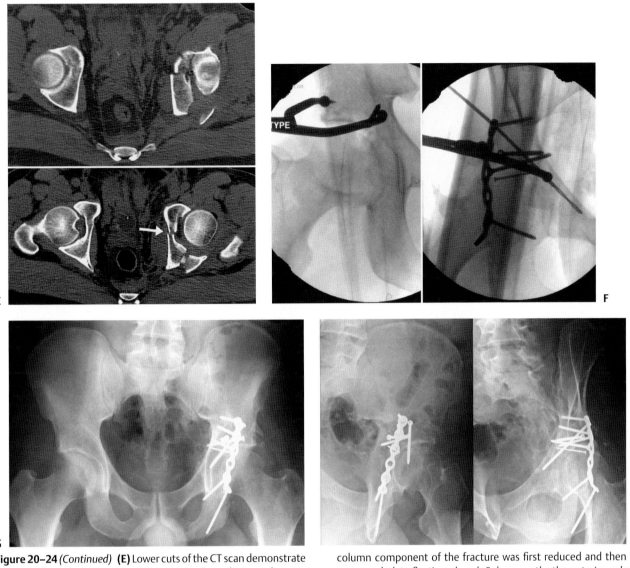

Figure 20–24 *(Continued)* **(E)** Lower cuts of the CT scan demonstrate a frontal plane dissociation between an anterior column and posterior column (arrow), confirming the diagnosis of a T-type with posterior wall acetabular fracture. **(F)** Intraoperative fluoroscopic views demonstrating reduction and fixation. In this case the posterior column component of the fracture was first reduced and then lag screw and plate fixation placed. Subsequently, the anterior column component of the fracture was then reduced and a lag screw placed from posterior to anterior. **(G)** AP radiograph at 1 year. **(H)** Judet films of the left hip at 1 year.

caudal. With anterior column fractures, various instruments are used to control the internal and external rotation deformities. Clamps are used to help lateralize the fragment as well as to control flexion and extension in the sagittal plane. Therefore, a common scenario is to use a Farabeuf clamp on the anterior aspect of the iliac wing (either in the interspinous notch or along the iliac crest) for rotational control **(Fig. 20–25A,B)**. One could also use a Shanz pin placed in the area of the anterior-superior spine. Reduction of the anterior column then proceeds with initial longitudinal traction of the lower extremity to obtain length, followed by rotational repositioning of the anterior column fragments to reduce the fracture at the iliac crest and pelvic brim. A clamp can then be placed at the iliac crest to maintain the reduction. This can be in the

form of a pointed reduction forceps or an angled-jaw clamp. The "King Tong," three prong, or angled-jaw clamp can then be placed at the outer aspect of the intact ilium and to the pelvic brim to help control lateralization and flexion **(Figs. 20–25, 20–26)**.

Palpation of the outer aspect of the ilium can confirm the appropriate lateralization and rotation of the anterior column, and the reduction can be visualized along the internal aspect of the ilium and the pelvic brim **(Fig. 20–27)**. Often, the anterior column component of the fracture includes a pie-shaped wedge of the ilium. If this is the case, the wedge fragment should be reduced first to the intact ilium above the posterior iliac spine. This is secured with an interfragmentary screw, and commonly a plate is used to neutralize the forces of reduction that are subsequently

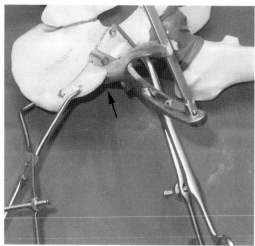

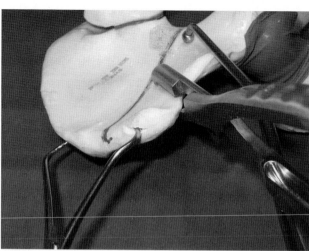

A

B

Figure 20–25 The reduction of an anterior column component of an anterior column fracture, associated both-column fracture, or anterior column with posterior hemitransverse acetabular fracture. **(A)** Common reduction aids include a Weber clamp (pointed reduction clamp) on the iliac crest and a large angled-jaw clamp (or King Tong clamp) from the anterior column to the intact ilium on the outer aspect of the innominate bone. In addition, a Farabeuf clamp or Schanz pin can be placed in the interspinous notch for rotational control of the anterior column (arrow). **(B)** Close-up view.

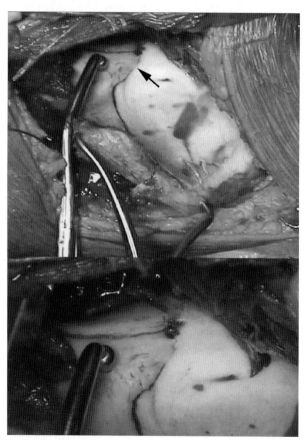

Figure 20–26 Intraoperative view of the reduction of an anterior column component of a fracture in a manner similar to that shown in **Fig. 20–25**. An angled-jaw forceps is utilized to reduce the anterior column to the intact ilium in the upper view (arrow). Appropriate reduction is confirmed by interdigitation of the fracture. In this use, the reduction was not perfect. It was corrected by the use of another clamp.

used for the anterior column. It is also very common that a small cortical fracture fragment will be displaced from the posterior aspect of the pelvic brim. This is anatomically reduced because it can serve as a key for reduction of the anterior column.

There is often also a fragment of the superior surface of the sciatic buttress adjacent to the ipsilateral sacroiliac joint **(Fig. 20–28)**. Appropriate debridement and cleaning of the bed as well as anatomical reduction of this cortical fragment are paramount because the sciatic buttress is the cornerstone of the anterior reconstruction. Once the main component of the anterior column is in position and the reduction is held by clamps, interfragmentary fixation is placed. An interfragmentary screw at the iliac crest as well as another one from the anterior-inferior spine along the corridor of the supra-acetabular bone into the posterior superior spine will help to maintain the position of the anterior column. If possible, a screw placed just lateral to the brim in the anterior column and placed into the sciatic buttress will help to maintain the reduced position at the pelvic brim. Next, a buttress plate is placed along the pelvic brim from the intact ilium to the superior ramus. Typically, a 10- to 14-hole plate would be utilized to span the entire pelvic brim to the pubic tubercle. This plate is placed just lateral to the pelvic brim and curved around to lie on the superior-posterior edge of the pubic ramus and onto the pubic body. Bringing the plate more laterally will increase the complexity of the plate's contour by placing it over the iliopectineal eminence and into the concavity of the superior-anterior surface of the pubic ramus.

The plate is slightly underbent to facilitate a push onto the anterior column as the plate is secured. The plate is initially secured to the intact ilium just lateral to the sacroiliac

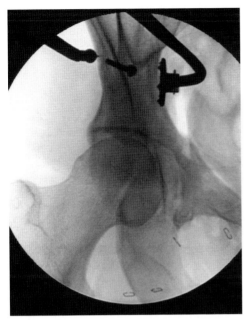

Figure 20–27 Intraoperative fluoroscopic view of reduction of the anterior column to the intact ilium. This is performed in the setting of an anterior column, anterior column/posterior hemitransverse, and associated both-column acetabular fractures. The fracture plane between the anterior column and the intact ilium is in the frontal plane, and therefore after the reduction is achieved, lag screws are placed from anterior to posterior, as seen here.

joint. This allows fixation into the area of the posterior iliac spine. The plate is next secured along the superior aspect of the pubic ramus, usually from the medial window. This plate is utilized to neutralize flexion and adduction rotational forces on the anterior column fragment. At times, a shorter plate can be utilized that spans from the intact ilium to the iliopectineal eminence, particularly if the patient has poor bone quality where screw-only fixation is insufficient and there is no significant fragmentation of the anterior column

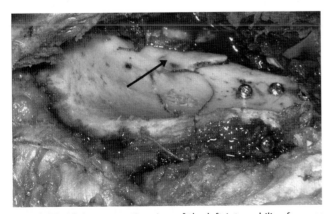

Figure 20–28 Intraoperative view of the left internal iliac fossa as viewed from the lateral window of an ilioinguinal approach. Here the anterior column is reduced to the intact ilium. There is often a separate cortical fragment in the area of the sciatic buttress (arrow), which is important to reconstruct to judge reduction of the anterior column to the intact ilium.

at the level of the superior ramus. This so-called push plate will help maintain the position of the anterior column as well as act as a washer for subsequent placement of screws into the posterior column. Image intensification, including an AP and an obturator oblique view, will help to evaluate the position of the anterior column after reduction (**Fig. 20–22**). Radiographic landmarks used to assess the quality of reduction of the anterior column are the iliopectineal line and whether or not the fragment is sufficiently lateralized on the obturator oblique view. If the surgeon is satisfied with the reduction of the anterior column and this is the only component of the fracture, additional screws can be placed into the plate proximal to the iliopectineal eminence, through the lateral window, and into the posterior column to improve fixation, and into the pubic ramus and body through the medial window (**Fig. 20–29A–D**).

Reduction and Fixation of the Posterior Column through the Ilioinguinal Approach (see Video 20–2, Disk 2)

In the setting of an anterior column/posterior hemitransverse or associated both-column acetabular fracture, the anterior column is first reduced as already described. Next, the surgeon can proceed with reduction and fixation of the posterior column. In the setting of a large posterior column fragment that includes the majority of the quadrilateral and retroacetabular surface, fixation can be accomplished with screws only. The reduction maneuver used to reduce the posterior column is to apply a lateralization force through the quadrilateral surface. This can be done with a large angled-jaw reduction forceps: one point is placed through the interspinous notch onto the outer ilium, and the second point of the clamp is inserted through the middle window onto the quadrilateral surface. If needed, a plate or disk can be used to distribute force. If this clamp is placed more posteriorly, it will provide lateralization of the posterior column fragment. A common error is to not have enough length through traction prior to posterior column reduction. If the fracture line on the retroacetabular surface is oblique in orientation, lateralization of the fragment is impossible without sufficient traction. Therefore, traction should be applied to the limb during this step to help reposition the posterior column. Once sufficient lateralization has been achieved, a second, smaller reduction clamp can be placed through the middle window (**Fig. 20–30A–F**). One point of the clamp is placed on the iliopectineal eminence or anterior wall and the other one along the quadrilateral surface, pulling the posterior column in a cephalad direction to reduce the fracture line at the pelvic brim. A bone hook placed into the lesser sciatic notch may help to facilitate this reduction.

Screw fixation into the posterior column is aimed anteriorly and caudally along the posterior column to exit the bone

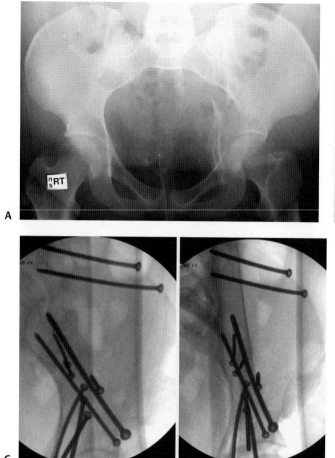

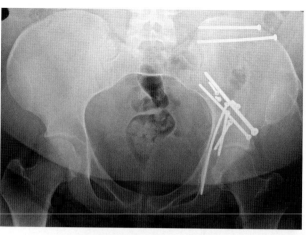

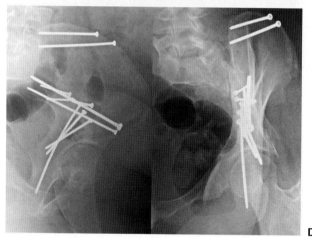

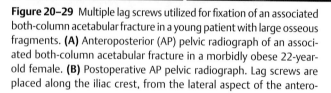

Figure 20–29 Multiple lag screws utilized for fixation of an associated both-column acetabular fracture in a young patient with large osseous fragments. **(A)** Anteroposterior (AP) pelvic radiograph of an associated both-column acetabular fracture in a morbidly obese 22-year-old female. **(B)** Postoperative AP pelvic radiograph. Lag screws are placed along the iliac crest, from the lateral aspect of the antero-

inferior iliac spine back into the posterior iliac crest, from the anterior column into the intact ilium (in anterior to posterior direction), and into the posterior column. **(C)** Intraoperative fluoroscopic views of these screws. Note that the screws heading from the lateral aspect of the anteroinferior iliac spine back into the posterior iliac spine relies on a thick corridor of bone in this area. **(D)** Judet views at 2 years.

distal to the ischial spine. Fixation can be performed either outside or through the plate. A typical starting point is 1 cm lateral to the pelvic brim and about 2 cm anterior to the sacroiliac joint **(Fig. 20–31A,B).** From this starting point, the drill should be directed halfway between the posterior border of the greater sciatic notch and posterior obturator ring. If further compression of the fracture site is indicated or if the surgeon would like the screw to help facilitate the reduction, the screw can be placed in a lag fashion. If the position is to be maintained, lag screw fixation is not recommended. It is very common that these screws are not perpendicular to the fracture line and may further facilitate a malreduction. The second screw is commonly placed either through the plate or outside the plate in a more lateral direction to help close the lateral portion of the posterior column fracture.

Reduction and Fixation of Transverse Fractures from the Ilioinguinal Approach

Reduction of the transverse fractures from the ilioinguinal can be difficult. This is likely due to the rotation of the

fragment through the intact symphysis. In most transverse fractures there is a medialization of the posterior portion of the ischiopubic segment. There is also a sagittal plane rotation of the ischiopubic segment around the displaced femoral head. It is control of this sagittal plane displacement that can be difficult through the ilioinguinal. The reduction can be visualized from the pelvic brim to the anterior rim through the lateral window. The posterior limb of the transverse can be visualized and palpated through the middle window or even better visualized through the Stoppa extension.[19] As already described, reduction forceps placed from near the brim of the ischiopubic segment through the middle window to the outer ilium through the interspinous notch can facilitate lateralization and derotation of the posterior column. The femoral head should be distracted during the rotation maneuver. Fixation can then be accomplished with screws placed from the pelvic brim into the inferior lateral posterior column. This helps to reduce rotation by closing the posterior limb of the fracture more laterally. A screw can also be placed percutaneously into the anterior limb of the transverse fracture. Plate

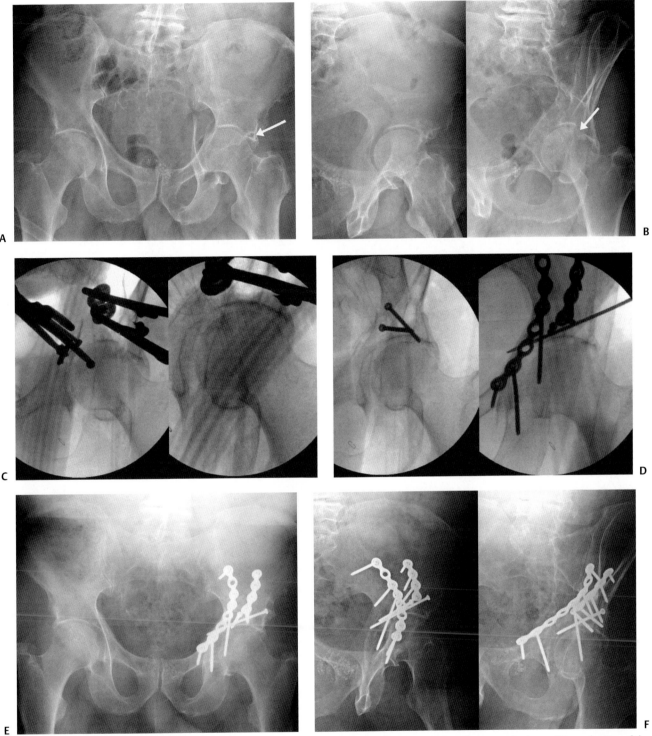

Figure 20–30 Anterior column fracture with significant quadrilateral surface involvement in a 61-year-old male sustained from a low-energy fall. **(A)** There is significant articular impaction and medialization of the femoral head. The intact radiographic acetabular roof is represented by only the most lateral 2 cm (arrow). **(B)** Judet views. The iliac oblique view (left panel) demonstrates no involvement of the posterior column. The ilioischial line was involved on the anteroposterior (AP) radiograph secondary to the significant quadrilateral surface involvement. The obturator oblique view (right panel) demonstrates medialization of the femoral head, displacement of the anterior column, and significant displacement between the intact ilium and the displaced anterior column articular surface (arrow). **(C)** Intraoperative fluoroscopic views of the reduction of the anterior column to the intact ilium via the ilioinguinal approach. The view on the left demonstrates inability to reduce the fracture until a Schanz pin was placed in the proximal femur at the level of the lesser trochanter. A laterally directed force was then applied, which allowed for the anterior column to be clamped to the intact ilium. **(D)** Lag screws were then placed from the anterior column into the intact ilium. Two plates were then placed from the intact ilium onto the anterior column due to the patient's significant osteoporosis. A supra-acetabular lag screw was then placed for fixation of the quadrilateral surface. **(E)** AP pelvic radiograph at 1 year. **(F)** Judet films at 1 year.

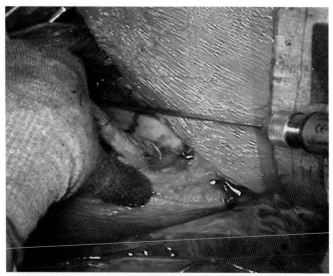

A

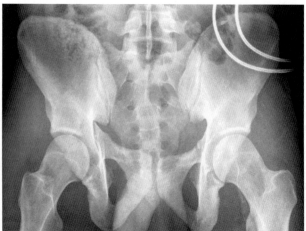

B

Figure 20–31 After reduction of the anterior column in an anterior column/posterior hemitransverse or associated both-column fracture, the posterior column is reduced. A short angled-jaw forceps is placed through the middle window from the pectineal eminence region onto the quadrilateral surface. Lag screws are then placed from the internal iliac fossa into the posterior column. **(A)** Intraoperative photograph. **(B)** Corresponding C-arm view.

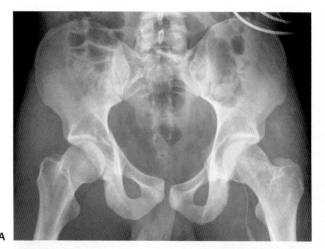

A

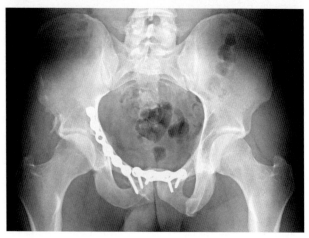

C

B

Figure 20–32 An ilioinguinal approach may be utilized for certain transverse acetabular fractures: a juxtatectal transverse acetabular fracture with associated pubic symphysis disruption. **(A)** Anteroposterior (AP) pelvic radiograph at the time of injury. **(B)** Cephalad (outlet) view of the pelvis. Slight asymmetry of the joint space on the right side was the indication for surgical intervention in this young individual. **(C)** AP radiograph at 1 year.

fixation will help neutralize the rotational forces. The best indication for a transverse fracture to be approached through the ilioinguinal is a fracture that exits in the typical location anteriorly just underneath the anterior-inferior spine, with a very low minimally displaced exit of the fracture line through the posterior column. These fractures will typically have their greatest displacement at the pelvic brim because of sagittal rotation of the ischiopubic segment around the femoral head. Due to the lack of medialization and displacement posteriorly, rotational reduction of the fragment is simplified (**Fig. 20–32A–C).**

Extended Ilioinguinal Approach

Both-column fractures with a fracture line extending from the iliac crest into the sacroiliac joint posteriorly are difficult to reduce with the traditional ilioinguinal approach. Weber and Mast described a lazy lateral position to facilitate an extension of the traditional approach to the outer table of the posterior ilium in these circumstances.[17] This helps to visualize the entirety of the fracture line on the outer aspect of the bone. The fracture line on the internal aspect of the joint, then, is not reduced indirectly, as would be the case when a traditional ilioinguinal approach was used to expose only the internal aspect of the pelvis. Following reduction with screw and superior plate fixation of this fracture line, reduction and fixation of the anterior column and subsequent posterior columns can proceed as already described. This specific fracture pattern is also a good indication for an extended iliofemoral approach.

Reduction and Fixation through the Extended Iliofemoral Approach

After completion of the extended iliofemoral approach, the entire outer aspect of the upper ilium, the supra-acetabular bone to the anterior inferior spine, the posterior column to the subcotyloid groove, and the entire posterior border of the bone are exposed. If needed, further dissection on the internal aspect of the ilium can be performed. If this is done, care must be taken not to detach the entire ilium from its surrounding soft tissues, which will decrease the vascularity of the bone fragments. Therefore, in the circumstance of a fracture extending up into the iliac crest, the soft tissue attachments to the anterior portion of the ilium should be maintained in the region of the anterior-superior and anterior-inferior iliac spines. Visualization of the reduction can be performed on the internal aspect as well as the external aspect of the bone. In the circumstance of a delayed approach to a transverse, T-shaped, or associated transverse-posterior wall acetabular fracture, elevation of the abdominal muscles from the iliac crest and the iliopsoas from the internal aspect of the ilium can also result in a devitalized anterior ilium. Therefore, in this circumstance, dissection along the anterior aspect of the ilium, including release of the rectus femoris and elevation of the iliopsoas from the internal aspect of the ilium from

the psoas gutter posteriorly, is the recommended approach for visualization and clamp access to these fracture lines as they come from the pelvic brim to the anterior rim of the acetabulum.

Reduction through the extended iliofemoral approach for associated both-column fractures or anterior plus posterior hemitransverse fractures begins posteriorly on the iliac crest, moving caudally to the sciatic buttress to reduce the anterior column first, and then reduce this to the posterior column. In the setting of an older fracture, especially with a transverse component, elevation of the superior gluteal neurovascular bundle from the superior-anterior aspect of the greater sciatic notch will be necessary. Soft tissues can then be elevated off the quadrilateral surface and sciatic buttress to help with clamp access and digital evaluation of fracture lines in this region.

Anterior Column Plus Posterior Hemitransverse and Associated Both-Column Fractures

It is common in this circumstance to limit the dissection to the outer aspect of the bone. Smaller areas of detachment of the abdominal muscles from the iliac crest will allow clamp access and digital palpation of the fracture lines in the internal iliac fossa. If a wedge-shaped fracture is included as part of the anterior column, reduction and fixation of this fragment into position is necessary prior to proceeding more anteriorly. Fractures of the anterior or posterior column that enter the sacroiliac joint along the internal aspect are easily visualized along the lateral aspect of the posterior ilium with the extended iliofemoral approach. After the wedge-shaped fragment of the ilium has been reduced, it is common to place a small plate along the lateral surface underneath the iliac crest to neutralize the pull of the abdominal muscles medially. This can then function to neutralize forces that may displace this fragment during subsequent reduction maneuvers. As with the reduction maneuver with the ilioinguinal approach, a Farabeuf clamp placed in the interspinous area or a Shanz pin placed in the anterior-superior iliac spine will help control rotation of the anterior column during reduction. It is also important in the lateral position to be able to control medial displacement of the femoral head. An orthopaedic table can help to facilitate repositioning of the femoral head to indirectly reapproximate some of the fracture lines.

Once this is done, further lateralization of the anterior column fracture fragment can be performed by using a two-screw technique and a Farabeuf clamp in the supra-acetabular bone and also along the iliac crest. This, along with the pointed reduction forceps at the iliac crest, can in most circumstances reduce the anterior column. If further lateralization of the anterior column is necessary, a King Tong clamp with one point placed along the pelvic brim and one point the lateral aspect of the intact ilium can be helpful. A Shanz pin placed in the proximal femur can help to lateralize the medialized femoral head. Once positioned, the preferred vector for interfragmentary fixation is from a region just lateral to the anterior-inferior iliac spine into the sciatic buttress or posterior-superior iliac spine. An interfragmentary screw can also be used along the iliac crest. The rotational force on the anterior column can be neutralized with a small reconstruction plate just above the greater sciatic notch extending across the anterior column fracture line. Placement of the plate within one fingerbreadth above the greater notch ensures good bone opposite the plate. Reduction of the posterior column should be done in similar fashion to that described for the Kocher-Langenbeck approach. A Shanz pin placed in the ischium will help to control rotational alignment.

Depending on the orientation of the fracture line, a two-screw technique with a Farabeuf clamp can be utilized for the reduction along the retroacetabular surface. Also, a pointed reduction clamp is best used along the peripheral rim. This can help to reduce the acetabular rim followed by a placement of a second clamp at or near the greater sciatic notch to complete the reduction of the posterior column. Short interfragmentary screws can be placed just anterior to the greater sciatic notch anchoring into the posterior column along the quadrilateral surface or posterior border of the bone. Longer interfragmentary screws can be placed from the anterior surface of the posterior gluteus medius tubercle directed toward the ischial spine. The posterior column can then be neutralized with a plate from the subcotyloid groove to the supra-acetabular bone near the anterior-inferior spine (**Fig. 20–33A–E**).

Transverse Fractures

For fractures with a transverse component, simultaneous control of the anterior and posterior portions of the fracture can be obtained. The reduction still typically proceeds much like that in the prone position. A Shanz pin placed in the ischium will help to control rotation of the lower ischiopubic segment. The posterior and anterior aspects of the transverse fracture are simultaneously controlled with clamps. Pointed reduction clamps or angled-jaw reduction forceps are placed through the greater notch onto the quadrilateral surface or anterior pelvic brim, and a two-screw technique (with Farabeuf clamp) can be used anteriorly. Alternatively, a two-screw technique can be used on both the anterior and posterior columns. Interfragmentary fixation can then be obtained from the supra-acetabular bone again into the posterior border of the posterior column fracture or along the quadrilateral surface. Screws can also be placed into the anterior column from a position along the posterior border of the gluteus medius tubercle and ~3 to 4 cm above the acetabulum. Similar to the posterior column fixation for the both-column fracture, a screw can be placed from above the greater sciatic notch slightly more anterior and directed into the posterior column. This can then be neutralized with a plate along the peripheral rim from the subcotyloid grove to the supra-acetabular bone.

In the case of a T-shaped fracture, evaluation of the posterior column fracture line is usually much easier through the extended iliofemoral, and therefore reduction is started with this fragment. This is done in a similar fashion as already described. Plate neutralization of the fragment following reduction is indicated along the posterior border of the bone to allow fixation of the posterior column, independent of the anterior column fragment. The anterior portion of the T-shaped fracture can be more difficult to reduce. The fracture can be followed along the internal aspect of the ilium to the pelvic brim. A small Shanz pin can be used as a reduction aid in the anterior column fracture fragment to assist with reduction. Clamps placed from the supra-acetabular bone to the pelvic brim as well as clamps placed from the iliopectineal eminence to the retroacetabular surface can facilitate reduction of the anterior column and thus the vertical stem of the T-shaped fracture. Anterior column fixation can then be placed in a similar manner to that described for the transverse fracture pattern, with screw fixation from the posterior aspect to the gluteus medius tubercle into the anterior column. The entire fracture can then be neutralized with a plate from the ischial tuberosity to the supra-acetabular bone along the peripheral rim. Commonly, screws from the cephalad portion of the plate will go from the intact ilium into the anterior column fracture fragment, further facilitating its fixation (**Figs. 20–33A–E** and **20–34A–D**).

Reduction and Fixation through Sequential Approaches

Although the use of a simultaneous Kocher-Langenbeck and ilioinguinal approach has been described,[26] the authors tend to follow the advice of Letournel[2,4] and Matta[3] to optimize one surgical approach to reduce the fracture. However, there may be indications to perform an ilioinguinal approach followed by a Kocher-Langenbeck approach. One such indication is that of a T-shaped fracture with wide displacement of the anterior column and posterior column without other reasons to perform an extended iliofemoral approach (**Fig. 20–35A–D**).

Rehabilitation

Acetabular fracture patients are kept toe-touch (< 10 kg) weight bearing for 8 to 12 weeks after surgery. Immediate range of motion exercises of the hip are begun and emphasize hip flexion and extension, and internal and external rotation. Continuous passive motion machines are not routinely utilized postoperatively but may be helpful in some cases. Abductor strengthening exercises are emphasized beginning at week 6. Stationary biking and low-resistance weight training are begun at week 6 to 12. Progressive weight bearing is begun at week 8 to 12, with progression from crutch or walker ambulation to a cane in the next 2 to 6 weeks. The patient is informed that muscle strength can

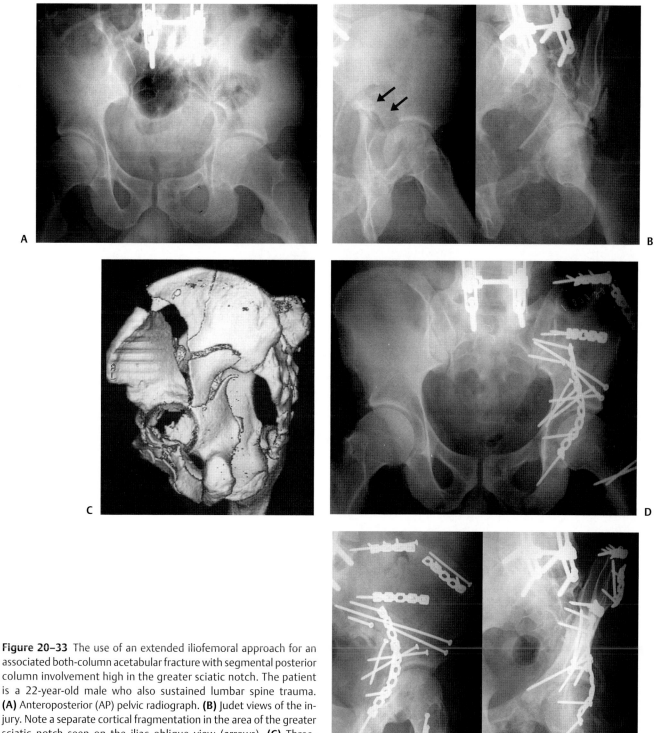

Figure 20–33 The use of an extended iliofemoral approach for an associated both-column acetabular fracture with segmental posterior column involvement high in the greater sciatic notch. The patient is a 22-year-old male who also sustained lumbar spine trauma. **(A)** Anteroposterior (AP) pelvic radiograph. **(B)** Judet views of the injury. Note a separate cortical fragmentation in the area of the greater sciatic notch seen on the iliac oblique view (arrows). **(C)** Three-dimensional computed tomographic reconstruction of the injury. **(D)** AP pelvic radiograph at 1 year. **(E)** Judet views at 1 year.

Tips and Tricks

- The obturator oblique view **(Fig. 23–3C)** is an important film in the evaluation of a patient with a high-energy mechanism, groin pain, and no obvious finding on the AP pelvic radiograph. It nicely depicts subtle fractures of the posterior wall, femoral neck, or femoral head.

- Roof arc measurements must be done with the leg out of traction and are not valid if the hip is subluxed. Roof arc measurements are not utilized with associated both-column or posterior wall acetabular fractures.

- Dynamic stress views can be done in patients whose fractures meet criteria for nonoperative management otherwise.

- Common errors with the Kocher-Langenbeck approach are not making the limb down the leg distal enough, and not dividing the insertion of the gluteus maximus muscle. This does not allow for enough mobilization of the abductor mass for optimal visualization.

- With the Kocher-Langenbeck approach, the sciatic nerve is best found on the posterior aspect of the quadratus femoris. The surgeon should initially not try to find the nerve in the area of the piriformis muscle because this area is generally distorted by the fracture.

- With the Kocher-Langenbeck approach, the quadratus femoris muscle belly should be left undisturbed as the deep branch of the medial femoral circumflex artery lies deep to the muscle belly. It thus protects the major blood supply to the femoral head.

- With the Kocher-Langenbeck approach, transection of the piriformis and obturator internus tendon should be 1.5 cm from their insertion on the proximal femur. Transection closer to the femur places the deep branch of the medial femoral circumflex artery at risk.

- The capsular attachments to a posterior wall acetabular fracture should be maintained.

- The inferior one third to one half of the gluteus minimus is often devitalized by the posterior wall acetabular fracture. It should be debrided at the end of the case to help prevent heterotopic ossification.

- In the ilioinguinal approach, the iliopectineal fascia separates the muscular window (iliopsoas muscle and accompanying femoral nerve) from the vascular window (external iliac artery and vein). The iliopectineal fascia runs from the pectineal eminence to the sacroiliac joint. It is divided or excised.

- The anterior exposure of the extended iliofemoral approach consists of the division of three fascial layers: fascia over the tensor fascia lata muscle, fascia over the rectus femoris, and an aponeurosis over the vastus lateralis. Underneath the last layer are vessels of the lateral femoral circumflex artery, which are ligated.

- Common mistakes of posterior wall acetabular fracture fixation are poor visualization of the cephalad portion of the fracture, inaccurate reduction of marginal impaction, and over-contouring of the posterior wall acetabular plate.

- Certain factors complicate the treatment of a transverse or transverse with posterior wall acetabular fracture from a Kocher-Langenbeck approach. These factors include transtectal fracture, injury to the contralateral sacroiliac joint, injury to the anterior pelvic ring (symphysis disruption or parasymphyseal fracture), and separate osteochondral fragments in the articular dome. Especially in a young patient ($<$ 45 years), if more than one of these factors is present, strong consideration of an extended iliofemoral approach should be entertained.

- It is not uncommon for a transverse fracture reduction to appear "perfect" on the posterior column, but still be malrotated along the quadrilateral surface and pelvic brim. This can best be assessed by digital palpation of the fracture line through the greater sciatic notch. It can be corrected by use of an ischial tuberosity Shanz pin and/or a clamp on the anterior column component of the fracture **(Fig. 20–20).**

- A key concept in treating an associated transverse with posterior wall acetabular fracture is that of first addressing the transverse component of the fracture, and second repairing the posterior wall component of the fracture.

- Anterior column fractures are generally medialized and externally rotated. They are reduced by a pointed reduction clamp along the iliac crest, and a second clamp placed with one tong on the pelvic brim portion of the anterior column, and one tong on the outer aspect of the intact innominate bone. The reduction is facilitated by use of a Farabeuf clamp on the interspinous area for rotational control. The quality of reduction is assessed by visualization of the reduction of the anterior column to the intact ilium through the lateral and medial windows of the ilioinguinal approach, and by palpation of the outer aspect of the innominate bone.

- Reduction of a transtectal transverse acetabular fracture or delayed management of a transverse fracture ($>$ 3 weeks from injury) is facilitated by an extended iliofemoral approach. It allows direct visualization and clamp application on both the anterior and posterior aspects of the transverse fracture. It also allows for direct visualization of the articular surface reduction.

- Reduction and fixation of a pelvic injury (e.g., sacroiliac joint disruption, symphysis injury) generally precedes fixation of the acetabular fracture.

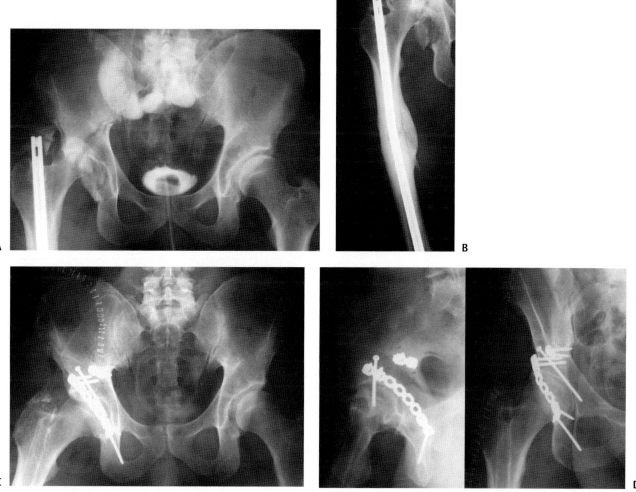

Figure 20–34 An irreducible posterior hip dislocation in a 32-year-old male in the setting of a transtectal transverse with posterior wall acetabular fracture. The patient has heterotopic ossification at the top of his previously placed prominent intramedullary nail. An extended iliofemoral approach was utilized for reduction and fixation.

(A) Injury anteroposterior (AP) pelvic radiograph. **(B)** AP radiograph of the femur at the time of injury. **(C)** AP postoperative radiograph of the pelvis. **(D)** Judet views demonstrating appropriate postoperative alignment of the fracture. The patient developed avascular necrosis and required a total hip arthroplasty at 18 months posttrauma.

improve in the first year after surgery and therefore strengthening is emphasized during this time period. Patients generally are able to return to desk-type work in the first 6 to 12 weeks following surgery but are not able to return to heavy labor until at least 4 to 6 months following surgery.

New Techniques

Trochanteric Flip Osteotomy

Siebenrock et al have described the Ganz trochanteric flip osteotomy.[23] The surgical approach is similar to a Kocher-Langenbeck approach but involves a 1.5 cm osteotomy of the greater trochanter, leaving both proximal and distal muscle attachments to the trochanter in-

tact. This produces a so-called digastric osteotomy. The greater trochanteric fragment remains attached superiorly to the gluteus medius and minimus, and inferiorly to the vastus lateralis. A Z-shaped capsulotomy of the anterior hip capsule can then be performed, which allows for a surgical dislocation of the femoral head with flexion, adduction, and external rotation of the hip. This approach may also be helpful in the setting of a Pipkin IV (femoral head fracture associated with an acetabular fracture) injury **(Fig. 20–36A–D)**. With one surgical approach, a femoral head fracture and a posterior wall acetabular fracture may be addressed. In addition, the osteotomy may be performed without a surgical dislocation of the hip to visualize a more anterior/cranial extension of a posterior wall acetabular fracture without devitalization of the abductors **(Figs. 20–36A–D** and **20–37A–J)**.

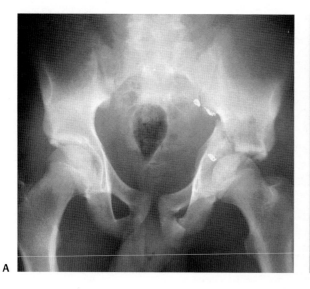

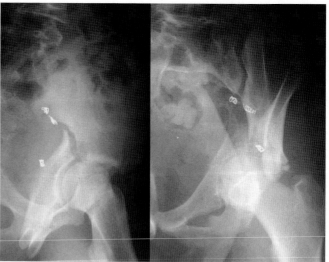

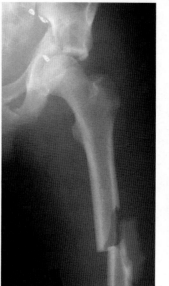

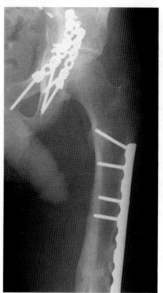

Figure 20–35 The use of planned sequential approaches for a T-type acetabular fracture in a 16-year-old male. The patient has an associated femoral shaft fracture. The patient was hemodynamically unstable and underwent angiographic embolization. **(A)** Injury anteroposterior (AP) film of the pelvis. **(B)** Judet views of the pelvis. The iliac oblique view demonstrates high and significant displacement of the posterior column. The obturator oblique view demonstrates high and significant displacement of the anterior column. **(C)** The associated femoral shaft fracture. **(D)** AP radiograph of the hip taken at 2 years postinjury. The patient has a normal hip.

Acute Total Hip Arthroplasty

Historically, the results of total hip arthroplasty after fracture of the acetabulum were compromised by high rates of loosening of the acetabular component and need for revision.[27] Modern arthroplasty techniques and implants, however, combined with appropriate stabilization of the pelvis, have led to much better results recently.[28,29] The predictable results of acute total hip arthroplasty in the setting of an acetabular fracture may be appealing, particularly in the geriatric patient with significant osteoporosis, fracture comminution, and articular damage or impaction. In general, the technique is that of fixation of the fracture followed by a total hip arthroplasty. For transverse, transverse with posterior wall, and posterior wall acetabular fractures, this may be accomplished through the Kocher-Langenbeck approach **(Figs. 20–38A,B** and **20–39A–C).** For anterior column, anterior column–posterior hemitransverse, and both-column fractures, this may be accomplished through the Levine approach.[29]

Percutaneous Screw Fixation

Closed reduction and percutaneous screw fixation has recently been advocated for the treatment of displaced acetabular fractures in the elderly and for minimally displaced fractures in younger patients.[30,31] The obvious advantage to such a technique is the minimally invasive nature of such an approach. The concerns are the ability to obtain an appropriate reduction. Starr et al had an average of 3 mm of displacement after such treatment.[31] On occasion, there may be extenuating circumstances such as medical instability or severe soft tissue injury that make

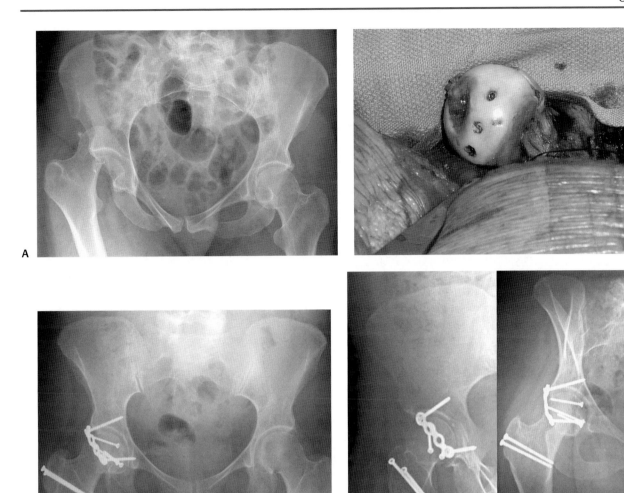

Figure 20–36 The use of a Ganz trochanteric flip osteotomy with surgical dislocation of the hip for treatment of a Pipkin IV fracture of the right hip. **(A)** Injury anteroposterior (AP) radiograph of the pelvis. **(B)** Intraoperative view of the femoral head with fixation of the femoral head. **(C)** AP pelvis at 1 year. **(D)** Judet views at 1 year.

such an approach reasonable. Recently, computer-based surgical navigation has been used for fixation of acetabular fractures.[32] However, these techniques are of limited usefulness because of their reliance on specialized, expensive equipment, and because of the fact that anatomical fracture reduction is necessary to achieve the best outcome in most acetabular fractures, which requires open approaches as described in this chapter.

Outcomes

The outcome of operatively managed acetabular fractures has improved considerably since the 1970s. Professor Emile Letournel is credited for this improvement. He elucidated the interpretation of plain radiographs of the pelvis, presented a classification system for acetabular fractures,

and developed operative approaches and tactics for their surgical management.[2,4] Letournel stressed the importance of understanding the plain radiographs of the acetabular fractures. In addition, he stressed that the appropriate fracture classification allows the surgeon to choose the correct surgical approach and surgical reduction technique for a given fracture displacement. Finally, he stressed that the goal of an open reduction/internal fixation of an acetabular fracture is a perfect reduction. As noted following here, there is a strong correlation between the quality of the reduction and the patient's clinical outcome.

Quality of Fracture Reduction

Letournel and Judet documented the outcome of 569 acetabular fractures treated within 3 weeks after injury.[33]

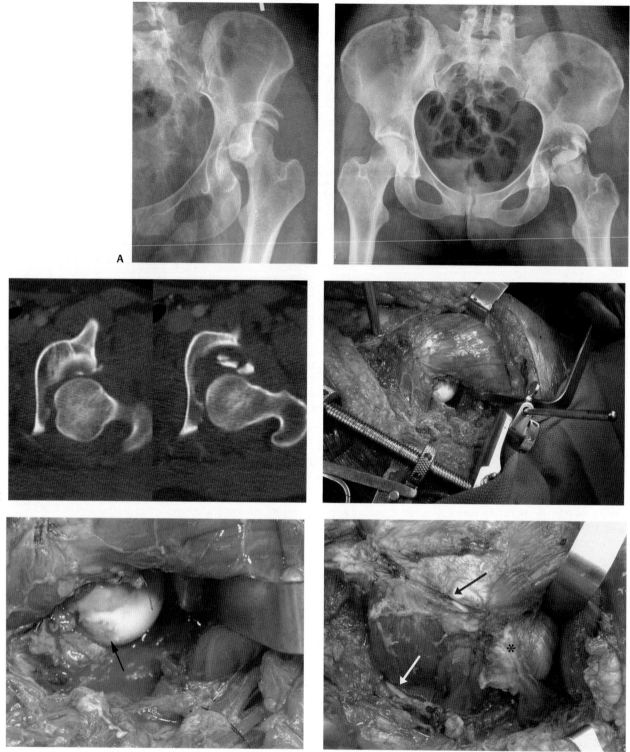

Figure 20–37 The case of a complex superior posterior wall acetabular fracture that necessitated the use of a trochanteric flip osteotomy. **(A)** Anteroposterior (AP) injury radiograph of the hip. **(B)** Attempt at closed reduction of the hip did not result in a concentric reduction. **(C)** Computed tomographic (CT) scan of the left hip demonstrates the large posterior wall acetabular fracture, which extends very anterior. Note extension close to the anterior-inferior iliac spine. Intra-articular fragments are also seen. **(D)** Intraoperative view from the surgeon's perspective standing posteriorly. The gluteus medius and minimus is being retracted anteriorly. A femoral distractor is distracting the hip joint. **(E)** Significant contusion on the posterior aspect of the femoral head is seen (arrow). **(F)** Intraoperative view of the significant cranial displacement of the posterior wall. The sciatic nerve is seen on the posterior border of the quadratus femoris (white arrow), and the piriformis is identified (*). The gluteus is being reflected anteriorly. The trochanteric flip osteotomy is outlined utilizing electrocautery (black arrow) before the osteotomy is performed.

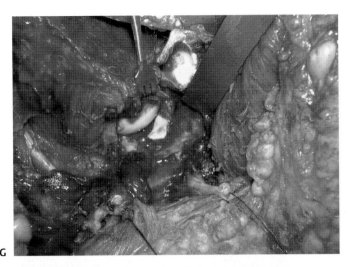

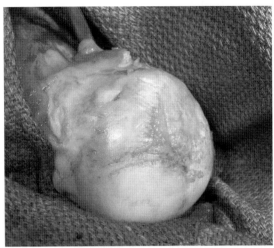

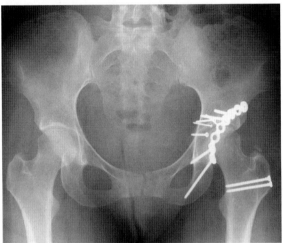

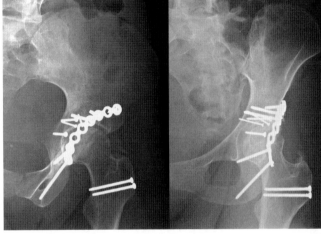

Figure 20–37 *(Continued)* **(G)** After the osteotomy is performed, the entire superior aspect of the femoral head and the superior posterior wall fracture is seen. **(H)** Significant full cartilage damage to the posterior aspect of the femoral head is seen. **(I)** AP radiograph of the pelvis at 2 years postinjury. Although the hip joint appears without significant arthritis, the long-term prognosis is very guarded secondary to the known cartilaginous injury to the femoral head. **(J)** Judet views at 2 years postinjury.

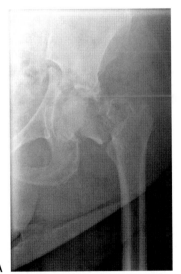

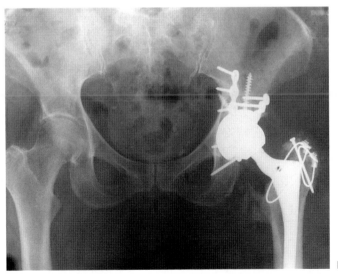

Figure 20–38 Acute total hip arthroplasty after fixation of an acetabular fracture. The patient is a morbidly obese 72-year-old female with insulin-dependent diabetes mellitus. **(A)** Anteroposterior radiograph of the hip. The injury is a transtectal transverse with posterior wall acetabular fracture, vertical shear femoral neck fracture, and comminuted greater trochanteric fracture. The patient underwent open reduction internal fixation of the acetabular fracture and total hip arthroplasty as well as open reduction internal fixation of the greater trochanter. This was all done through a Kocher-Langenbeck approach. **(B)** Six-month pelvic radiograph.

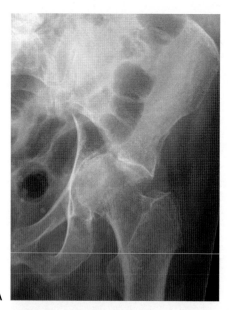

A

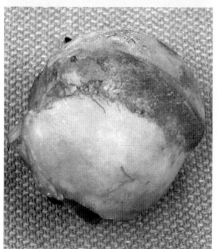

B

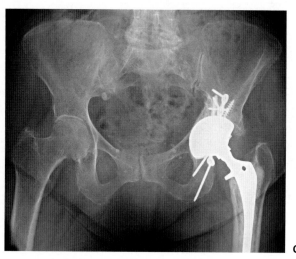

C

Figure 20–39 Case example of immediate total hip arthroplasty in the setting of a displaced transverse with posterior wall acetabular fracture. The patient is an 82-year-old female. She was initially treated nonoperatively for 3 weeks postinjury. **(A)** Significant impaction of the femoral head is seen. **(B)** The femoral head damage is confirmed at the time of total hip arthroplasty. The patient underwent fixation of the transverse component of the fracture and total hip arthroplasty. **(C)** Anteroposterior pelvic radiograph at 2 years.

They classified their quality of reductions into perfect reductions (all radiographic landmarks restored) or imperfect reductions (all radiographic landmarks not restored). They also defined surgical secondary congruence, which generally occurred in both-column fractures. In these cases, the articular surface around the head was internally fixed as perfectly as possible, but there was a recognized malreduction between the innominate bone and the joint. Letournel obtained a perfect reduction in 73.7% of the cases, with 4.8% having secondary surgical congruence. The correlation of the type of fracture and quality of reduction is seen in **Table 20–3.** They noted that the rate of perfect reductions dropped from 75% in the first 2 weeks after injury to 62% in the third week following injury. Furthermore, the quality of the reduction improved with Letournel's experience. In the first 5 years of his operative management of acetabular fractures (1958 to 1962), a per-

fect reduction was achieved in 68% of cases, whereas in the last 6 years documented (1984 to 1990), he achieved a 90% rate of perfect reductions.

Matta reported on a series of 262 operatively treated acetabular fractures.[3] He judged the reduction based on an assessment of the maximal displacement of any of the normal radiographic lines of the acetabulum as seen on any one of the three radiographic views of the acetabulum. An "anatomical" reduction was defined as one with less than 1 mm of displacement, an "imperfect" reduction had 2 to 3 mm of displacement, and a "poor" reduction had more than 3 mm of displacement. He also judged some reductions as having surgical secondary congruence. Overall, the postoperative reduction was anatomical in 71% of cases, imperfect in 20% of cases, and poor in 7% of cases. Surgical secondary congruence was obtained in 3% of cases. He noted that the quality of reduction was related to fracture type, with 96%

Table 20—3 The Correlation of Fracture Type with Quality of Fracture Reduction by Letournel and Judet

Fracture Type	Percentage of Perfect Reductions
Posterior wall	93.7
Posterior column	76.9
Anterior wall	77.7
Anterior column	86.4
Transverse	71.4
T-shaped	70.0
Transverse/posterior wall	67.5
Posterior column/posterior wall	90.0
Anterior column/posterior hemitransverse	68.0
Both column	60.7
Overall percentage of perfect reductions	73.7

Source: Data from Letournel E, Judet R. Fractures of the Acetabulum. 2nd ed. Berlin: Springer-Verlag; 1993:524.

of the simple fracture types reduced anatomically, whereas only 64% of the associated fracture types were reduced anatomically. Age greater than 40 years correlated with worse reduction quality of reduction. Fifty-seven percent of patients older than 40 years had an anatomical reduction compared with 78% of patients less than 40 years old. The initial displacement of the fracture did not correlate with the quality of the reduction.

Moed et al pointed out that the quality of a posterior wall fracture reduction is best assessed with a postoperative CT scan rather than plain film analysis.[34] They reviewed 67 patients, of which 61 had a 4-year average follow-up. The quality of the fracture reduction as measured from plain films of the pelvis was graded as anatomical in 65 of 67 cases. However, CT scans demonstrated a fracture incongruity of $\geq$ 2 mm in 11 patients and a fracture gap > 2 mm in 52 patients. In 24 hips, at least one aspect of the fracture gap was $\geq$ 1 cm in size. Only 15 of the 67 hips were described as anatomical on the basis of postoperative CT analysis. Fracture gaps $\geq$ 10 mm or a total gap area $\geq$ 35 mm^2 were associated with a poor result.

Radiographic and Clinical Results of Operatively Treated Acetabular Fractures

Letournel and Judet demonstrated a strong correlation between the quality of reduction and osteoarthritis.[2,33] With at least 1 year of follow-up, a 10.2% incidence of osteoarthritis was seen after a perfect reduction and a 35.7% incidence of osteoarthritis after an imperfect reduction.

The most commonly utilized clinical grading system is the modified Merle d'Aubigne and Postel scale. It was initially developed for assessing the results of hip arthroplasty,[35] adopted by Letournel and Judet,[36] and modified by Matta.[3] Pain, gait, and range of motion of the hip are each assessed and given a maximal score of 6 points per category. The three individual scores are then summed to derive the final clinical score.

In a study of 262 acetabular fractures followed for at least 2 years, Matta reported an overall clinical result of excellent in 40%, good in 36%, fair in 8%, and poor in 16%.[3] Clinical results paralleled the quality of the reduction (**Table 20–4**). A perfect reduction was associated with an overall good or excellent clinical result in 83% of cases. With an imperfect reduction (2 to 3 mm displacement on any acetabular view), a good or excellent clinical result was obtained in 68% of cases. When the reduction was poor (9 of 18 hips), a good or excellent clinical result was obtained in only 50% of cases. In his series, 6% of patients had a total hip arthroplasty at an average follow-up of 6 years.

Matta identified several factors that were correlated with a worse clinical result:[3]

- An imperfect reduction (2 mm of displacement on any acetabular view)

Table 20—4 Correlation of Quality of Reduction of Acetabular Fracture and Clinical Outcome

Quality of Reduction	Clinical Outcome			
	Excellent	Good	Fair	Poor
Anatomical ($n = 185$)	82 (46%)	68 (37%)	10 (5%)	25 (12%)
Imperfect ($n = 52$)	17 (33%)	18 (35%)	7 (14%)	10 (18%)
Poor ($n = 18$)	3	6	2	7
Surgical secondary congruence	2	3	2	

Source: Data from Matta JM. Fractures of the acetabulum: accuracy of reduction and clinical results in patients operated within three weeks after the injury. J Bone Joint Surg Am 1996;78-A:1632–1645.

Table 20—5 The Correlation of Fracture Type with Percentage of Good–Excellent Clinical Results

Percentage of Good–Excellent Clinical Results		
Fracture Type	Letournel	Matta
Posterior wall	82	68
Posterior column	91	63
Anterior wall	78	67
Anterior column	88	83
Transverse	95	89
T-shaped	88	77
Transverse/posterior wall	74	70
Posterior column/posterior wall	47	90
Anterior column/posterior hemitransverse	85	87
Both columns	82	77
Overall average	81	76

Source: Data from Letournel E, Judet R. Fractures of the Acetabulum. 2nd ed. Berlin: Springer-Verlag; 1993 and Matta JM. Fractures of the acetabulum: accuracy of reduction and clinical results in patients operated within three weeks after the injury. J Bone Joint Surg Am 1996;78-A:1632–1645.

- Traumatic injury to the articular surface or bone of the femoral head
- Age of the patient > 40 years. However, age itself may not be an independent predictor of outcome because age was also correlated with the ability to achieve a perfect reduction.

Clinical results did not correlate with fracture type in either the series of Letournel and Judet or that of Matta **(Table 20–5)**.[3,33]

Results of Operative Fixation of Posterior Wall Acetabular Fractures

Although posterior wall fractures are often thought of as relatively "simple" fractures, the clinical results demonstrate that their overall outcome is not always optimal. Letournel and Judet had overall 83% good to excellent results with posterior wall fractures.[33] Matta had 68% good to excellent results with posterior wall fractures.[3] This was despite the fact that the reduction (as assessed by plain films) was perfect in 93 to 100% of cases. This highlights the issue that Moed et al raised in their paper, noting that plain films are not adequate to document the quality of reduction of a posterior wall fracture.[34] In another paper, Moed et al reported on the clinical results of 100 posterior wall acetabular fractures.[37] These authors emphasize urgent reduction of associated hip dislocations and the goal of anatomical reconstruction of the acetabular articular surface. Eighty-nine percent of the cases had a good or excellent result, and 8%

required a second hip surgery.[37] Factors that contributed to a poor result included older age at the time of injury (> 50 years), a delay in the time to reduction of the hip dislocation, and intra-articular comminution. Other factors that had a trend toward a statistically significant poorer outcome included marginal impaction of the fracture and involvement of the weight-bearing dome by the fracture.

Results Following Delayed or Revision Fixation of Acetabular Fractures

Results following delayed fixation of acetabular fractures are less desirable than those with acute fractures. Letournel and Judet reported 64.4% good to excellent clinical results in fractures treated between 3 weeks and 4 months postinjury.[38] Johnson et al reported on 188 fractures operated on at an average of 43 days postinjury.[39] Good to excellent results were obtained in 65% of patients. Complications in this group were also significant: 20 postoperative sciatic nerve palsies, eight infections, five pulmonary embolisms, and 26 cases of avascular necrosis.

Even worse clinical results are seen with the revision of malreduced acetabular fractures. Mayo et al reported on the clinical results of reoperation of 64 patients with a surgical malreduction or secondary loss of reduction.[40] In 56% of cases, a reduction within 2 mm was achieved. The clinical outcome was 42% good or excellent at an average of 4.2 years follow-up. Furthermore, the time from injury to reoperation also affected the clinical outcome. Fifty-seven percent of patients reoperated on within 3 weeks of injury had a good or excellent result, whereas only 29% of patients reoperated on after 12 weeks of injury had a good or excellent result.

Functional Outcomes

Although the modified Merle d'Aubigne and Postel clinical score[35] is the most commonly used clinical grading system, it is not a true patient-derived functional outcome score. Moed et al have demonstrated that patients with an operatively treated acetabular fracture had high Musculoskeletal Function Assessment (MFA) scores that correlated with the d'Aubigne and Postel scores.[41] The high MFA scores demonstrate that complete return to preinjury functional level is uncommon.

Complications

Fractures of the acetabulum commonly are a result of high-energy trauma. Therefore, it is common that patients may have other associated musculoskeletal or multisystem injuries. Surgical reconstruction can be a labor- and time-intensive endeavor, and medical optimization of the patient prior to surgery is imperative. Despite this, complications of the injury or subsequent surgery occur. Identification of potential problems early in the postinjury course can help to limit subsequent complications. Adequate training and experience in the field of acetabular surgery will have an impact on the surgeon's complication rates.

Injury to the acetabulum and subsequent reconstruction can be associated with complications of deep vein thrombosis, infection, neurological injury, vascular injury, malreduction, intra-articular hardware, and failure of fixation. Following fixation, late complications can include nonunion, malunion, avascular necrosis, heterotopic ossification, and posttraumatic arthritis. Avoidance of early complications has a significant influence on the appearance of late complications and subsequent poor outcomes.

Deep Vein Thrombosis

Deep vein thrombosis following fractures of the pelvis or acetabulum is common.[42–46] Pulmonary embolism is much less common. The potential for significant morbidity or mortality from thromboembolism has led most individuals to use some form of perioperative prophylaxis. This is usually in the form of mechanical devices on the lower extremities along with some form of chemical prophylaxis. The authors utilize low molecular weight heparin (Lovenox 40 mg SQ daily) until the night before surgery, and beginning again on postoperative day 2 for 3 weeks. An alternative is postoperative coumadin.[47] Preoperative screening with ultrasonography is increasingly used, especially in patients that have been transferred from another center for definitive care or in patients in whom there has been a delay of more than 2 days before surgery is performed. If such screening is positive, a vena cava filter is inserted before surgery. Prophylaxis against pulmonary embolism with inferior vena cava filters should be considered in those individuals that are unable to undergo chemical prophylaxis in the perioperative period. These are commonly patients with multiple injuries, including intracerebral or intraparenchymal brain injuries or injuries to the spleen or liver that are being monitored clinically.

Infection

Reported rates of infection following acetabular fracture have ranged from 4 to 12%.[3,11,48] Perioperative antibiotic prophylaxis for infection is recommended in all patients undergoing acetabular fracture surgery. A careful evaluation of the soft tissue envelope for possible abrasions, open injuries, or soft tissue degloving injuries will help to optimize a surgical plan to avoid soft tissue complications. Avoidance of incisions through the degloved areas or possible percutaneous treatment of the degloving injury with incisions remote from the surgical reconstruction can decrease the risk of soft tissue complications following surgery. Meticulous prepping

and draping of the patient as well as careful handling of the soft tissues and attention to the bones' vascularity are important for the prevention of infection. Devitalized muscle should be removed prior to closure, potential spaces should be drained, and antibiotics continued until the drains are removed or serous-type drainage has stopped from the wound. Careful postoperative monitoring of pelvic wounds is very important. Any signs of continued drainage or hematoma should be treated aggressively with early evacuation and debridement.

Large degloving injuries (so-called Morel-Lavallée) lesions represent a separation of the subcutaneous tissue from the underlying muscle fascia.[49] Hak et al reported that bacterial cultures were positive in these degloving injuries in 46% of 24 cases.[49] Furthermore, performing an internal fixation in these cases, even after aggressive debridement, was associated with an infection in three of 24 cases. Tseng and Tornetta reported on the treatment of 19 patients with a Morel-Lavallée lesion in which the patients had early (within 3 days) percutaneous debridement via "brushing" and subsequent lavage and closure over drains through two 2 cm incisions.[50] Fracture fixation occurred on a delayed basis, and no cases of deep infection ensued.

Neurological Injury

A careful examination prior to reconstruction can also define neurological compromise from the injury. It is mandatory that a full and thorough neurological examination is documented prior to surgical reconstruction. Preoperative injury to the sciatic nerve has been reported in up to 30% of injuries.[51]

Sciatic nerve injury secondary to surgery has been reported in up to 16% of patients. Letournel and Judet recommended that the patient be operated in a prone position with the knee flexed and the hip extended to relax the sciatic nerve, as well as use of specific nerve retractors to decrease the potential for iatrogenic nerve injury.[2] Others have recommended the use of intraoperative somatosensory evoked potentials or spontaneous electromyography to assess nerve function during surgery.[52] Middlebrooks et al concluded that intraoperative monitoring was not justified secondary to the low level of postoperative nerve dysfunction seen when appropriate precautions are taken to protect the nerve intraoperatively.[53] Intraoperative monitoring may be indicated for surgeons during their learning curve or for delayed surgeries that may require extensive mobilization of the soft tissues and bone. Prognosis for recovery of the sciatic nerve following traumatic injury is poor compared with that from iatrogenic injury.[54]

Iatrogenic nerve injury or planned transection of the lateral femoral cutaneous nerve of the thigh can occur with the ilioinguinal approach.[55,56] This can result in lateral thigh numbness, or less commonly but more importantly, pain. It is important to discuss this possibility with patients preoperatively. Care of the nerve intraoperatively or sharp incision of the nerve if it is damaged during surgery can result in a decreased risk of postoperative meralgia paresthetica.

Vascular Injury

Injury to vascular structures of the pelvis is less commonly associated with acetabular fractures than with pelvic fractures. Nonetheless, it can occur. Injuries to the superior gluteal artery in association with fractures high into the posterior column occur from the fracture itself or during mobilization and reduction of such a fracture. If injury occurs intraoperatively, the natural reaction of the surgeon is to place a clamp in this area. However, this should be avoided because this will risk injury to the superior gluteal nerve. Rather, packing is successful in most instances. If needed, isolation of the vessel lumen should be established with subsequent suture ligature. In rare occasions, an urgent embolization via angiography must be performed if the vessel cannot be controlled operatively. Angiography

may be performed after packing with a hemostatic biodegradable sponge and superficial wound closure.

Preoperative angiography to assess superior gluteal artery patency prior to an extensile approach has been advocated.[57] In addition, consideration of a change in operative approach was recommended by the same authors if a vascular injury is identified. However, Reilly et al evaluated patency of the superior gluteal artery in 41 patients undergoing extensile approaches. In only one patient was there absence of a Doppler flow signal. They reported no associated flap complications in this series of patients treated with an extended iliofemoral approach.[58]

Injury to the external iliac artery can occur during operative intervention with the ilioinguinal approach. This can occur by laceration with a sharp instrument or from thrombosis. Prolonged retraction through the middle window of the ilioinguinal approach can cause femoral artery thrombosis. Intraoperative digital evaluation of the femoral arterial pulse while working in the middle window is mandatory. In addition, close postoperative moni-

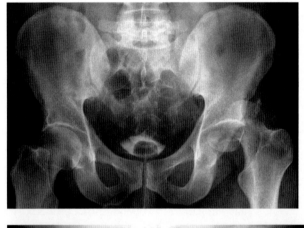
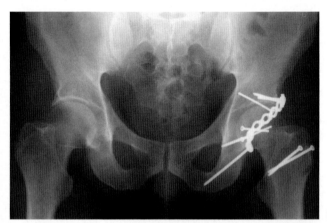
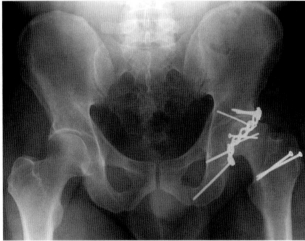
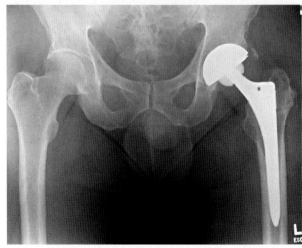

Figure 20–40 Avascular necrosis following an acetabular fracture temporally first involves the femoral head and subsequently demonstrates acetabular involvement. **(A)** Irreducible hip dislocation with a femoral head fracture and small superior-posterior wall acetabular fracture. A closed reduction under sedation was not possible. **(B)** Anteroposterior pelvis radiograph at 1 year status post–open reduction internal fixation of the femoral head and the posterior wall

utilizing a Ganz trochanteric flip osteotomy and a surgical dislocation of the hip. At 1 year postoperatively, the patient was completely asymptomatic. **(C)** Beginning at month 22 postinjury, the patient began to have significant pain in the left hip. Avascular necrosis is seen involving the superolateral aspect of the femoral head; the acetabular side of the hip joint is relatively well maintained. **(D)** The patient underwent a total hip arthroplasty.

toring is advised, with vascular checks every 1 to 2 hours in the first 12 hours postoperatively. If a traumatic laceration occurs during the operation, this should be repaired. Likewise, if a thrombosis occurs in the external iliac artery during the surgery, it may be surgically explored. If altered flow to the lower extremity is noted after closure, an emergent arteriogram is indicated with the thought of possible treatment for a presumed external iliac artery thrombosis.

Posttraumatic Arthritis

The goal of acetabular fixation surgery is a normal hip without arthritis. Clearly, one of the most common long-term complications following acetabular fracture surgery is posttraumatic arthritis, as noted earlier in the Outcomes section.

Avascular Necrosis

Avascular necrosis (AVN) occurs in 1 to 5% of cases.[3,11,59] The diagnosis of AVN should be reserved for those cases with typical radiographic changes noted in the femoral head, including subchondral lucencies, collapse of the femoral head, and eventual destruction of the joint (**Fig. 20–40A–D**). Radiographic changes associated with avascular necrosis first occur in the femoral head and subsequently advance to the hip joint. Progressive loss of joint space associated with deformation or fragmentation of the femoral head is more likely associated with malreduction and femoral head wear than with avascular necrosis. If seen early, it can also be an indication of infection of the hip joint.

Heterotopic Ossification

Heterotopic ossification about the hip is likely secondary to the initial traumatic event as well as any subsequent surgical reconstruction. Certain individuals may be at an increased risk for formation of heterotopic ossification. Significant heterotopic bone formation is more commonly seen in males, patients with associated head injuries, and fractures where there is a delay to surgery.[60–63]

The surgical approach will also influence the incidence of significant postoperative heterotopic ossification, with extensile approaches such as the extended iliofemoral approach having the highest rate, and the ilioinguinal approach having the lowest rate.[3,62] The practice of debriding devitalized skeletal muscle,[64] the use of postoperative oral indomethacin,[65–67] and postoperative radiation[61,63,68–70] have all been recommended. One randomized study showed limited efficacy of 6 weeks of postoperative indomethacin compared with no prophylaxis.[71] In contrast, Moore et al randomized a group patients undergoing acetabular surgery to receive a similar 6-week course of indomethacin or an 800 cGy dose of radiation therapy and found no significant difference between the two treatment arms.[72] Currently, radiation therapy is recommended in a single dose (700 cGy) postoperatively in patients felt to be at high risk. If clinically significant heterotopic ossification does occur, relatively early resection is usually performed at 4 to 12 months postoperatively. Although no published series has documented the efficacy of early intervention, recurrence has not been found to be a problem (**Fig. 20–41A–F**).

Pearls

- The obturator oblique view allows evaluation of the anterior column, posterior wall, and ischial ramus (**Fig. 20–3C**).
- The iliac oblique view (**Fig. 20–3B**) is used to evaluate the posterior column, anterior wall, and iliac wing.
- The classification system of Judet and Letournel consists of five elementary and five associated fracture types (**Fig. 20–4, Table 20–2**).
- Roof arc angles are used to define involvement of the roof of the acetabulum and are described by a vertical line drawn through the center of the femoral head and another from the center of the femoral head to the point where the fracture enters the articular surface on each of the three pelvic radiographs. These must be done with the leg out of traction, and the femoral head must not be subluxed.[6]
- Roof arcs cannot be used to evaluate either the both-column fracture pattern (because the acetabulum medializes along with the subluxated femoral head, referred to as secondary congruency) or posterior wall fractures (because these fractures rarely disrupt the superior articular surface on any view).
- Using a CT scan, fracture lines that violate the subchondral ring within 1 cm of the condensation of the acetabular roof

are considered to involve the weight-bearing roof of the acetabulum.[7]
- Biomechanical studies suggest that the posterior column is more important than the anterior column to stability of the hip during single-leg stance.[8]
- Nonoperative treatment of acetabular fractures should be considered for
  - Fractures that do not involve the weight-bearing articular surface as defined by roof arc angles on plain radiographs or by CT
  - Fractures that are displaced less than 2 mm within the superior articular surface and maintain congruence between the femoral head and acetabulum with the involved leg out of traction
  - Fractures of the posterior wall with less than 20% involvement of the articular surface and no incarcerated fragments
  - Fractures that have secondary congruence following an associated both-column fracture
- Fractures that extend up into the iliac crest including anterior column, anterior column/posterior hemitransverse, and associated both-column fractures

(Continued)

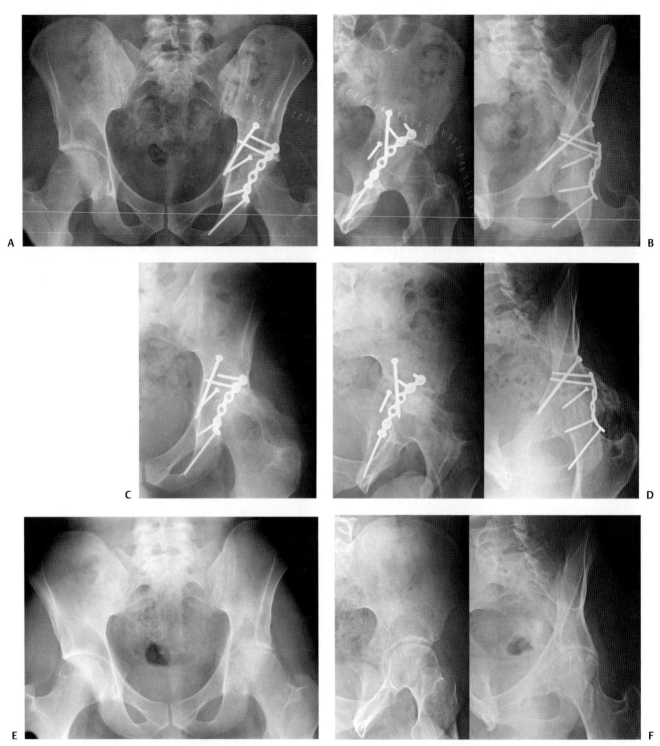

Figure 20–41 Heterotopic ossification following an acetabular fracture. **(A)** Postoperative anteroposterior radiograph of the pelvis following open reduction internal fixation of a transverse with posterior wall acetabular fracture utilizing a Kocher-Langenbeck approach. **(B)** Postoperative Judet views. **(C)** Four months postoperatively, the patient developed Brooker IV heterotopic ossification about the hip. **(D)** Judet views of the hip at 4 months. **(E)** The patient underwent removal of the heterotopic ossification and hardware at 6 months postinjury. He regained nearly normal motion of the left hip. **(F)** Judet views after removal of the heterotopic ossification.

Pearls *(Continued)*

- When an elderly patient sustains an acetabular fracture from a fall, it is usually an anterior column or anterior column/posterior hemitransverse fracture.
- An associated both-column fracture separates all portions of the articular dome from the intact ilium. The inferior lateral edge of the intact portion of the innominate bone represents the "spur sign," which is best seen on the obturator oblique view.
- Surgical indications for the Kocher-Langenbeck approach include posterior wall, posterior column, posterior column/posterior wall, most transverse, most transverse with posterior wall, and most T-type fractures.
- Surgical indications for an ilioinguinal approach include anterior wall, anterior column, anterior column/posterior hemitransverse, and most both-column fractures.
- Surgical indications for an extended iliofemoral approach include a transtectal transverse or transverse with posterior wall, a T-type fracture with wide displacement of both the anterior and posterior columns, and both-column fractures with significant involvement of the sacroiliac joint. It allows for simultaneous control of both the anterior and posterior columns and direct visualization of the articular surface reduction of the hip by distraction of the femoral head outside of the hip.

- The clinical series of Matta closely correlates reduction quality with clinical results.[3] A perfect reduction was associated with an overall good or excellent clinical result in 83% of cases. With an imperfect reduction (2 to 3 mm displacement on any acetabular view), a good or excellent clinical result was obtained in 68% of cases. When the reduction was poor (greater than 3 mm), a good or excellent clinical result was obtained in only 50% of cases. Factors that Matta found were correlated with a worse clinical result included an imperfect reduction (2 mm of displacement on any acetabular view), traumatic injury to the articular surface or bone of the femoral head, and age of the patient > 40 years. The rate of conversion to a total hip arthroplasty was 6%.
- Avascular necrosis following acetabular fracture surgery by experienced surgeons is rare (1 to 3%).[3,11]
- Heterotopic ossification more frequently occurs in those surgical approaches that involve the elevation or injury to the hip abductors. Thus increasing heterotopic ossification occurrence is seen in the following order: ilioinguinal approach, Kocher-Langenbeck approach, extensile approaches (e.g., extended iliofemoral approach). The role of indomethacin remains controversial.

On the DVDs

Video 20–1 (Disk 2) Kocher-Langenbeck Approach for a Transverse Posterior Wall Acetabulum Fracture The detailed steps of the KL approach in the prone position with use of a specialized fracture table are shown. Distraction of the hip joint through use of the table allows for easy retrieval of incarcerated fragments of the posterior wall. Precise anatomic reduction of multiple fragments is seen.

Video 20–2 (Disk 2) Ilioinguinal Approach for Associated Both-Column Acetabulum Fracture The development of the three windows of the ilioinguinal approach is demonstrated. The approach is utilized for a step-wise reconstruction of a complex injury. Clamp application, screw fixation, and assessment of reduction quality are key concepts which are discussed.

References

1. Judet R, Judet J, Letournel E. Fractures of the acetabulum: classification and surgical approaches for open reduction: preliminary report. J Bone Joint Surg Am 1964;46:1615–1636
2. Letournel E. Acetabulum fractures: classification and management. Clin Orthop Relat Res 1980;151:81–106
3. Matta JM. Fractures of the acetabulum: accuracy of reduction and clinical results in patients operated within three weeks after the injury. J Bone Joint Surg Am 1996;78:1632–1645
4. Letournel E, Judet R. Fractures of the Acetabulum. 2nd ed. Berlin: Springer-Verlag; 1993
5. Beaule PE, Dorey FJ, Matta JM. Letournel classification for acetabular fractures: assessment of interobserver and intraobserver reliability. J Bone Joint Surg Am 2003;85-A:1704–1709
6. Matta JM, Anderson LM, Epstein HC, Hendricks P. Fractures of the acetabulum: a retrospective analysis. Clin Orthop Relat Res 1986;205:230–240

7. Olson SA, Matta JM. The computerized tomography subchondral arc: a new method of assessing acetabular articular continuity after fracture (a preliminary report). J Orthop Trauma 1993;7:402–413
8. Vrahas MS, Widding KK, Thomas KA. The effects of simulated transverse, anterior column, and posterior column fractures of the acetabulum on the stability of the hip joint. J Bone Joint Surg Am 1999;81:966–974
9. Hak DJ, Hamel AJ, Bay BK, Sharkey NA, Olson SA. Consequences of transverse acetabular fracture malreduction on load transmission across the hip joint. J Orthop Trauma 1998;12:90–100
10. Tornetta P III. Nonoperative management of acetabular fractures: the use of dynamic stress views. J Bone Joint Surg Br 1999;81:67–70
11. Mayo KA. Open reduction and internal fixation of fractures of the acetabulum: results in 163 fractures. Clin Orthop Relat Res 1994;305:31–37

12. Jimenez ML, Vrahas MS. Surgical approaches to the acetabulum. Orthop Clin North Am 1997;28:419–434

13. Babinski MA, Machado FA, Costa WS. A rare variation in the high division of the sciatic nerve surrounding the superior gemellus muscle. Eur J Morphol 2003;41:41–42

14. Gautier E, Ganz K, Krugel N, Gill T, Ganz R. Anatomy of the medial femoral circumflex artery and its surgical implications. J Bone Joint Surg Br 2000;82:679–683

15. Letournel E. The treatment of acetabular fractures through the ilioinguinal approach. Clin Orthop Relat Res 1993;292:62–76

16. Teague DC, Graney DO, Routt ML. Retropubic vascular hazards of the ilioinguinal exposure: a cadaveric and clinical study. J Orthop Trauma 1996;10:156–159

17. Weber TG, Mast JW. The extended ilioinguinal approach for specific both column fractures. Clin Orthop Relat Res 1994;305:106–111

18. Kloen P, Siebenrock KA, Ganz R. Modification of the ilioinguinal approach. J Orthop Trauma 2002;16:586–593

19. Cole JD, Bolhofner BR. Acetabular fracture fixation via a modified Stoppa limited intrapelvic approach: description of operative technique and preliminary treatment results. Clin Orthop Relat Res 1994;305:112–123

20. Mears DC, MacLeod MD. Acetabular fractures: triradiate and modified triradiate approaches. In: Wiss DA, ed. Master Techniques in Orthopaedic Surgery, Fractures. Philadelphia: Lippincott–Raven; 1998:697–724

21. Reinert CM, Bosse MJ, Poka A, Schacherer T, Brumback RJ, Burgess AR. A modified extensile exposure for the treatment of complex or malunited acetabular fractures. J Bone Joint Surg Am 1988;70:329–337

22. Griffin DB, Beaule PE, Matta JM. Safety and efficacy of the extended iliofemoral approach in the treatment of complex fractures of the acetabulum. J Bone Joint Surg Br 2005;87:1391–1396

23. Siebenrock KA, Gautier E, Ziran BH, et al. Trochanteric flip osteotomy for cranial extension and muscle protection in acetabular fracture fixation using a Kocher-Langenbeck approach. J Orthop Trauma 1998;12:387–391

24. Brumback RJ, Holt ES, McBride MS, et al. Acetabular depression fracture accompanying posterior fracture dislocation of the hip. J Orthop Trauma 1990;4:42–48

25. Norris BL, Hahn DH, Bosse MJ, Kellam JF, Sims SH. Intraoperative fluoroscopy to evaluate fracture reduction and hardware placement during acetabular surgery. J Orthop Trauma 1999;13:414–417

26. Routt ML, Swiontkowski MF. Operative treatment of complex acetabular fractures: combined anterior and posterior exposures during the same procedure. J Bone Joint Surg Am 1990;72:897–904

27. Romness DW, Lewallen DG. Total hip arthroplasty after fracture of the acetabulum: long-term results. J Bone Joint Surg Br 1990;72:761–764

28. Mears DC, Velyvis JH. Acute total hip arthroplasty for selected displaced acetabular fractures: two- to twelve-year results. J Bone Joint Surg Am 2002;84-A:1–9

29. Beaule PE, Griffin DB, Matta JM. The Levine anterior approach for total hip replacement as the treatment for an acute acetabular fracture. J Orthop Trauma 2004;18:623–629

30. Parker PJ, Copeland C. Percutaneous fluoroscopic screw fixation of acetabular fractures. Injury 1997;28:597–600

31. Starr AJ, Jones AL, Reinert CM, et al. Preliminary results and complications following limited open reduction and percutaneous screw fixation of displaced fractures of the acetabulum. Injury 2001;32(Suppl 1):SA45–SA50

32. Crowl AC, Kahler DM. Closed reduction and percutaneous fixation of anterior column acetabular fractures. Comput Aided Surg 2002;7:169–178

33. Letournel E, Judet R. Fractures of the Acetabulum. 2nd ed. Berlin: Springer-Verlag; 1993:521–581

34. Moed BR, Carr SE, Gruson KI, Watson JT, Craig JG. Computed tomographic assessment of fractures of the posterior wall of the acetabulum after operative treatment. J Bone Joint Surg Am 2003;85-A:512–522

35. Merle D'Aubigné RM, Postel M. Functional results of hip arthroplasty with acrylic prosthesis. J Bone Joint Surg Am 1954;36-A:451–475

36. Letournel E, Judet R. Fractures of the Acetabulum. 2nd ed. Berlin: Springer-Verlag; 1993:566

37. Moed BR, Willson Carr SE, Watson JT. Results of operative treatment of fractures of the posterior wall of the acetabulum. J Bone Joint Surg Am 2002;84-A:752–758

38. Letournel E, Judet R. Fractures of the Acetabulum. 2nd ed. Berlin: Springer-Verlag; 1993:591–633

39. Johnson EE, Matta JM, Mast JW, Letournel E. Delayed reconstruction of acetabular fractures 21–120 days following injury. Clin Orthop Relat Res 1994;305:20–30

40. Mayo KA, Letournel E, Matta JM, Mast JW, Johnson EE, Martimbeau CL. Surgical revision of malreduced acetabular fractures. Clin Orthop Relat Res 1994;305:47–52

41. Moed BR, Yu PH, Gruson KI. Functional outcomes of acetabular fractures. J Bone Joint Surg Am 2003;85-A:1879–1883

42. Geerts WH, Code KI, Jay RM, et al. A prospective study of venous thromboembolism after major trauma. N Engl J Med 1994;331:1601–1606

43. Borer DS, Starr AJ, Reinert CM, et al. The effect of screening for deep vein thrombosis on the prevalence of pulmonary embolism in patients with fractures of the pelvis or acetabulum: a review of 973 patients. J Orthop Trauma 2005;19:92–95

44. Gruen GS, McClain EJ, Gruen RJ. The diagnosis of deep vein thrombosis in the multiply injured patient with pelvic ring or acetabular fractures. Orthopedics 1995;18:253–257

45. Montgomery KD, Potter HG, Helfet DL. The detection and management of proximal deep venous thrombosis in patients with acute acetabular fractures: a follow-up report. J Orthop Trauma 1997;11:330–336

46. Stover MD, Morgan SJ, Bosse MJ, et al. Prospective comparison of contrast-enhanced computed tomography versus magnetic resonance venography in the detection of occult deep pelvic vein thrombosis in patients with pelvic and acetabular fractures. J Orthop Trauma 2002;16:613–621

47. Fishmann AJ, Greeno RA, Brooks LR, Matta JM. Prevention of deep vein thrombosis and pulmonary embolism in acetabular and pelvic fracture surgery. Clin Orthop Relat Res 1994;305:133–137

48. Kaempffe FA, Bone LB, Border JR. Open reduction and internal fixation of acetabular fractures: heterotopic ossification and other complications of treatment. J Orthop Trauma 1991;5:439–445

49. Hak DJ, Olson SA, Matta JM. Diagnosis and management of closed internal degloving injuries associated with pelvic and acetabular fractures: the Morel-Lavallée lesion. J Trauma 1997;42:1046–1051

50. Tseng S, Tornetta P. Percutaneous management of Morel-Lavallée lesions. J Bone Joint Surg Am 2006;88:92–96

51. Helfet DL, Schmeling GJ. Management of complex acetabular fractures through single nonextensile exposures. Clin Orthop Relat Res 1994;305:58–68

52. Helfet DL, Anand N, Malkani AL, et al. Intraoperative monitoring of motor pathways during operative fixation of acute acetabular fractures. J Orthop Trauma 1997;11:2–6

53. Middlebrooks ES, Sims SH, Kellam JF, Bosse MJ. Incidence of sciatic nerve injury in operatively treated acetabular fractures without somatosensory evoked potential monitoring. J Orthop Trauma 1997;11:327–329

54. Fassler PR, Swiontkowski MF, Kilroy AW, Routt ML. Injury of the sciatic nerve associated with acetabular fracture. J Bone Joint Surg Am 1993;75:1157–1166

55. Matta JM. Operative treatment of acetabular fractures through the ilioinguinal approach: a 10-year perspective. Clin Orthop Relat Res 1994;305:10–19

56. de Ridder VA, de Lange S, Popta JV. Anatomical variations of the lateral femoral cutaneous nerve and the consequences for surgery. J Orthop Trauma 1999;13:207–211

57. Juliano PJ, Bosse MJ, Edwards KJ. The superior gluteal artery in complex acetabular procedures: a cadaveric angiographic study. J Bone Joint Surg Am 1994;76:244–248

58. Reilly MC, Olson SA, Tornetta P, Matta JM. Superior gluteal artery in the extended iliofemoral approach. J Orthop Trauma 2000;14: 259–263

59. Letournel E, Judet R. Fractures of the Acetabulum. 2nd ed. Berlin: Springer-Verlag; 1993:545–551

60. Ghalambor N, Matta JM, Bernstein L. Heterotopic ossification following operative treatment of acetabular fracture: an analysis of risk factors. Clin Orthop Relat Res 1994;305:96–105

61. Johnson EE, Kay RM, Dorey FJ. Heterotopic ossification prophylaxis following operative treatment of acetabular fracture. Clin Orthop Relat Res 1994;305:88–95

62. Webb LX, Bosse MJ, Mayo KA, Lange RH, Miller ME, Swiontkowski MF. Results in patients with craniocerebral trauma and an operatively managed acetabular fracture. J Orthop Trauma 1990;4: 376–382

63. Bosse MJ, Poka A, Reinert CM, Ellwanger F, Slawson R, McDevitt ER. Heterotopic ossification as a complication of acetabular fracture: prophylaxis with low-dose irradiation. J Bone Joint Surg Am 1988;70:1231–1237

64. Rath EM, Russell GV, Washington WJ, Routt ML. Gluteus minimus necrotic muscle debridement diminishes heterotopic ossification after acetabular fracture fixation. Injury 2002;33: 751–756

65. McLaren AC. Prophylaxis with indomethacin for heterotopic bone: after open reduction of fractures of the acetabulum. J Bone Joint Surg Am 1990;72:245–247

66. Moed BR, Maxey JW. The effect of indomethacin on heterotopic ossification following acetabular fracture surgery. J Orthop Trauma 1993;7:33–38

67. Moed BR, Karges DE. Prophylactic indomethacin for the prevention of heterotopic ossification after acetabular fracture surgery in high-risk patients. J Orthop Trauma 1994;8:34–39

68. Anglen JO, Moore KD. Prevention of heterotopic bone formation after acetabular fracture fixation by single-dose radiation therapy: a preliminary report. J Orthop Trauma 1996;10:258–263

69. Moed BR, Letournel E. Low-dose irradiation and indomethacin prevent heterotopic ossification after acetabular fracture surgery. J Bone Joint Surg Br 1994;76:895–900

70. Burd TA, Lowry KJ, Anglen JO. Indomethacin compared with localized irradiation for the prevention of heterotopic ossification following surgical treatment of acetabular fractures. J Bone Joint Surg Am 2001;83-A:1783–1788

71. Matta JM, Siebenrock KA. Does indomethacin reduce heterotopic bone formation after operations for acetabular fractures? A prospective randomised study. J Bone Joint Surg Br 1997;79:959–963

72. Moore KD, Goss K, Anglen JO. Indomethacin versus radiation therapy for prophylaxis against heterotopic ossification in acetabular fractures: a randomised, prospective study. J Bone Joint Surg Br 1998;80:259–263

21 Hip Dislocations and Femoral Head Fractures

Jeffrey A. Geller and Mark Cameron Reilly

Hip dislocation is a relatively uncommon injury associated with high-energy trauma. The mechanism is an axial force directed through the lower extremity causing the femoral head to extrude out of the hip joint. Dislocations may occur in isolation or in association with fractures of the femoral head or acetabulum. Thirty percent of patients with hip dislocations do not have an acetabular fracture.[1] Forty-two to 84% of hip dislocations are caused by automobile crashes, with the majority of these patients unrestrained by a safety belt. Other traumatic causes include motorcycle crashes, falls, and pedestrian and sports-related injuries.[2,3] Most dislocations of the hip are posterior, although anterior and inferior (obturator) dislocations may also occur.

The evaluation of a patient with a hip dislocation begins with an urgent evaluation in the trauma emergency department. Routine advanced trauma and life support protocols should be followed, including the "ABCs" (Airway/Breathing/Circulation) of the primary survey. One must maintain a high index of suspicion for a posterior hip dislocation when a patient presents with a shortened extremity with the affected hip held in a flexed, adducted, and internally rotated position. After an anterior dislocation, the affected hip usually remains in extension and neutral or slight abduction. Any motion of the dislocated hip will elicit immediate pain in the awake and alert patient. The initial standard radiographic trauma series, including an anteroposterior (AP) pelvis radiograph, will confirm the dislocation; however, the physician must be certain to recognize any concurrent fractures about the hip that might change the treatment protocol, specifically an associated acetabular fracture, femoral head fracture, or femoral neck fracture. Once the full spectrum of the injury is recognized, immediate relocation of the hip should be attempted. A full trauma evaluation must be performed in any patient presenting with a hip dislocation due to the high energy required to cause a hip dislocation and the high rate of associated systemic injuries. In one review of hip dislocations, up to 95% of patients had at least one other organ-system injury. Thirty-three percent of patients had other orthopaedic injuries, 15% had abdominal injuries, 24% had closed-head injuries, 21% had thoracic injuries, and 21% had craniofacial injuries.[1]

Closed reduction of a hip dislocation can usually be done in the trauma suite under directed conscious sedation if the patient is stable for such an intervention. If the reduction attempt is unsuccessful, however, the physician must be prepared to take the patient to the operating room to perform the reduction under general anesthesia. If closed reduction cannot be performed, open reduction must be done. Full radiographic evaluation, including computed tomography (CT), should be performed prior to proceeding to open reduction to identify the structure blocking reduction because a small posterior rim fracture or femoral head fracture may change the surgeon's plan for reduction. Previous investigations have shown that early concentric reduction yields the best long-term results, whereas longer delays uniformly lead to poor results, including avascular necrosis of the femoral head, arthrosis of the hip joint, or neurological injury.[2,4–6] Typically, reduction should be performed in less than 6 hours after the dislocation to reduce the risk of avascular necrosis (AVN). Hougaard and Thomsen reported in 1986 that the rate of AVN increased from 4.8% when reduction of the hip was performed within 6 hours versus 52.9% after greater than 6 hours.[7] After reduction, repeat radiographs should be obtained to confirm reduction and assess congruence of the hip joint. Complete radiographic evaluation should include a repeat AP pelvis off the backboard, Judet views, as well as an AP and lateral view of the hip joint. A CT scan may be of additional benefit to further identify bony fragments in the hip joint or more fully evaluate concurrent acetabular or femoral head or neck fractures.

The hip joint is a ball-and-socket joint that is second only to the shoulder for the magnitude of composite joint motion. The acetabulum is the confluence of the pubis, ischium, and ilium and forms the housing for the femoral head. There is an intimate relationship between the femoral head and the acetabulum. In the uninjured, nondysplastic hip, there is no translational motion between the acetabular and femoral surfaces. The joint is highly constrained by soft tissues, including the stout fibrocartilaginous acetabular labrum, the transverse acetabular ligament, and the hip joint capsule. All of these structures combine to afford the hip with the critical functions of both weight-bearing stability during gait and extraordinary motion. Injury to any of these structures can lead to symptomatic instability or frank dislocation. In a typical posterior hip dislocation without acetabular fracture, the posterior soft tissue capsule is avulsed from its attachment to the labrum, and the femoral head extrudes through the superior gemellus muscle or in

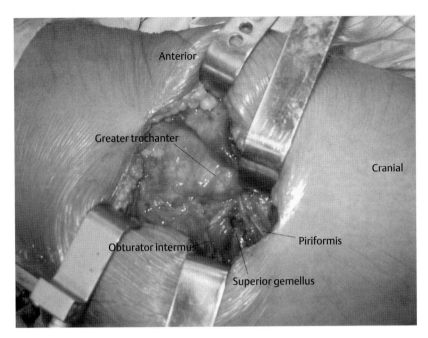

Anterior

Greater trochanter

Cranial

Obturator intermus

Piriformis

Superior gemellus

Figure 21–1 Intraoperative view of open reduction of an irreducible pure dislocation of the left hip. A "dislocation cavity" is usually seen between the piriformis and obturator internus. The femoral head often causes muscle damage to the piriformis, inferior border or gluteus minimus, and superior gemellus muscle belly.

the interval between the piriformis and obturator internus tendons. This can be visualized quite clearly when an open reduction is done **(Fig. 21–1).**

Classification

Hip dislocation can encompass a wide spectrum of injuries with associated fractures. For simplicity's sake, hip dislocation is divided into four categories:

1. Hip dislocation without fractures
2. Hip dislocation with fracture of the acetabulum
3. Hip dislocation with fracture of the femoral head
4. Hip dislocation with fractures of the femoral head and acetabulum

Hip dislocation in association with acetabulum fracture is discussed in Chapter 20; therefore, this chapter focuses on the remaining three entities. Historical classifications of hip dislocations, however, typically include associated acetabular fractures in their classification system. In 1951, Thompson and Epstein classified posterior hip dislocations.[8] This system was devised to incorporate fractures and dislocations based on severity of associated fracture. The types are as follows:

- Dislocation with or without minor fracture
- Dislocation with single large fracture of the posterior rim of the acetabulum
- Dislocation with comminuted fracture of the rim, with/without a large major fragment
- Dislocation with fracture of the acetabular floor
- Dislocation with fracture of the femoral head

Stewart and Milford classified hip dislocations in 1954 as well; however, their system focused on postreduction hip stability.[9] This system is as follows:

- Simple dislocation without fracture
- Dislocation with one or more rim fragments but with sufficient socket to ensure stability after reduction
- Dislocation with fracture of the rim producing gross instability
- Dislocation with fracture of the head or neck of the femur

Despite these attempts to organize these injuries into a single clear-cut system, the most commonly used classification scheme remains an anatomical description based on the location of the femoral head, specifically posterior, anterior or inferior (obturator), and medial. Posterior hip dislocations are by far the most common direction of dislocation, with reported incidences of 89 to 92%.[3,10] Anterior dislocations occur at a rate of ~8 to 11%.[3,10] Inferior or obturator dislocations are rare, and associated femoral neck or shaft fractures have been reported. A medial dislocation by definition involves fracture of the quadrilateral surface of the acetabulum and is more appropriately considered as a displaced acetabular fracture. Other dislocations reported in the literature include bilateral dislocations[11–15] or a totally "floating" pelvis, whereby there is a bilateral hip dislocation with concomitant unstable lumbar spine injury.[16] Bilateral dislocations can occur in opposite directions of dislocation and have a higher association with a motorcycle injury **(Fig. 21–2A,B).**[12–17]

As previously discussed, dislocation may also occur in conjunction with fractures of the femoral head. Femoral head fractures are rare injuries that are due to shear

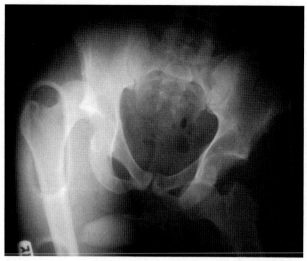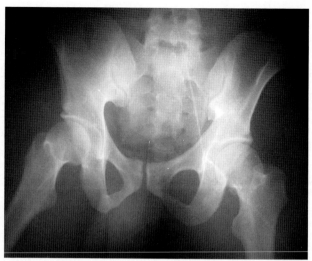

A   B

Figure 21–2 Bilateral hip dislocations. **(A)** The right hip has a posterior hip dislocation. The left hip has an anterior hip dislocation. **(B)** An anteroposterior radiograph of the pelvis after the hips are relocated.

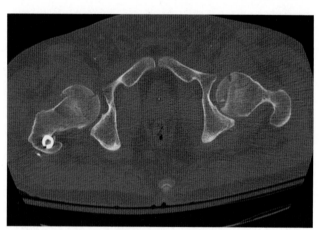

Figure 21–3 Computed tomographic scan demonstrating the typical frontal plane orientation in the anteromedial aspect of the femoral head present in a femoral head fracture.

stresses imparted upon the femoral head while dislocating out of the acetabulum and may occur in up to 16% of hip dislocations.[18] The location of the femoral head fracture is based upon the position of the hip at dislocation. Because most hip dislocations are posterior, the associated femoral head fracture has an anteromedial location caused by the contact between the femoral head and the posterior rim of the acetabulum during dislocation **(Fig. 21–3)**. Although the anterior dislocation of the hip is rare, it is associated with a higher likelihood of femoral head fracture—usually an infrafoveal impaction fracture.[10]

The most widely utilized and well-known classification scheme is that put forth by Pipkin in his original description of femoral head fractures in 1957 **(Fig. 21–4A–D)**.[17] His classification was derived from Thompson and Epstein's classification of posterior hip dislocations with an associated

femoral head fracture and divides femoral head fractures based on location relative to the fovea.

- Pipkin I: infrafoveal
- Pipkin II: suprafoveal
- Pipkin III: type I or II plus femoral neck fracture
- Pipkin IV: type I or II plus acetabular fracture-dislocation

The type I fracture is characterized by a rupture of the ligamentum teres as the majority of the femoral head dislocates. The remaining portion of infrafoveal femoral head remains in the acetabulum and often has a small periosteal or capsular pedicle of soft tissue. In type II fractures, the ligamentum teres remains attached to the femoral head fragment. In type III and IV fractures, associated fractures of the femoral neck or acetabulum are seen. The dislocated portion of the femoral head comes to rest on the posterior rim or retroacetabular surface and may frequently have areas of impaction or fragmentation. Because the typical femoral head fracture involves the anteromedial portion of the femoral head, the radiographic studies that demonstrate the fracture best are the obturator oblique Judet radiograph and the CT scan.

Nonoperative Treatment

Closed Reduction of Posterior Hip Dislocation

After identification of a hip dislocation with or without femoral head or acetabular fracture, a closed reduction should be promptly performed. This should be the case whether or not the injury will be definitely treated nonoperatively. Several methods of closed reduction of a posterior hip dislocation have been described. The most commonly used method is the Bigelow maneuver

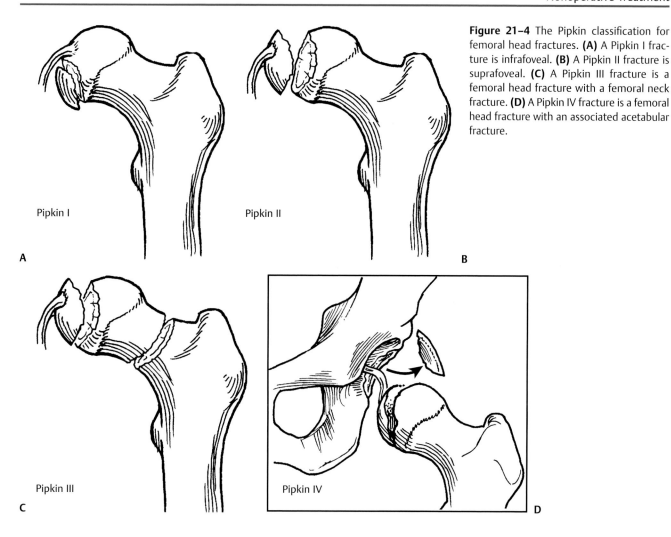

Figure 21–4 The Pipkin classification for femoral head fractures. **(A)** A Pipkin I fracture is infrafoveal. **(B)** A Pipkin II fracture is suprafoveal. **(C)** A Pipkin III fracture is a femoral head fracture with a femoral neck fracture. **(D)** A Pipkin IV fracture is a femoral head fracture with an associated acetabular fracture.

Pipkin I

Pipkin II

Pipkin III

Pipkin IV

(Fig. 21–5A–C).[18] Using this method, the patient lies supine. An assistant provides downward pressure on the anterior-superior iliac spine, while the person performing the reduction pulls in-line traction, flexes the hip to 90 degrees, and applies internal rotation and adduction until reduction is achieved. An alternate technique is the Allis method **(Fig. 21–6).**[19] An assistant stabilizes the pelvis while the reducer pulls in-line traction. The hip is flexed to 90 degrees, and gentle alternating internal and external rotation helps coax the hip back into position. The Stimson method has the patient lying prone with the affected extremity hanging off the end of the exam table **(Fig. 21–7).** The hip and knee are flexed to 90 degrees, and a downward force is applied to the calf.[20] This can often only be tolerated under general anesthesia.

Closed Reduction of Anterior or Inferior Hip Dislocation

Allis also described a method for reduction of anterior hip dislocations using traction and countertraction until re-

duction is obtained.[19] Walker described a method for reducing inferior dislocations. This may be done by applying axial traction combined with an internal rotation force in conjunction with a lateralizing force on the proximal femur.[21]

All reduction maneuvers require sufficient analgesia to allow for muscular relaxation and should be performed with a slow constant force to avoid any further trauma to the hip. Reduction attempted only with conscious sedation should be limited to a single attempt. If unsuccessful, general anesthesia with muscle relaxation should be performed prior to the second attempt to prevent further articular cartilage damage or create an iatrogenic femoral neck or acetabular fracture. A small percentage of hip dislocations will not be able to be reduced closed, even with general anesthesia. Possible etiologies of this include

- Inadequate muscle paralysis
- Reduction of the femoral head being prevented by the hip capsule or short external rotators of the hip **(Fig. 21–8)**
- A femoral fracture that makes control of the proximal femur difficult

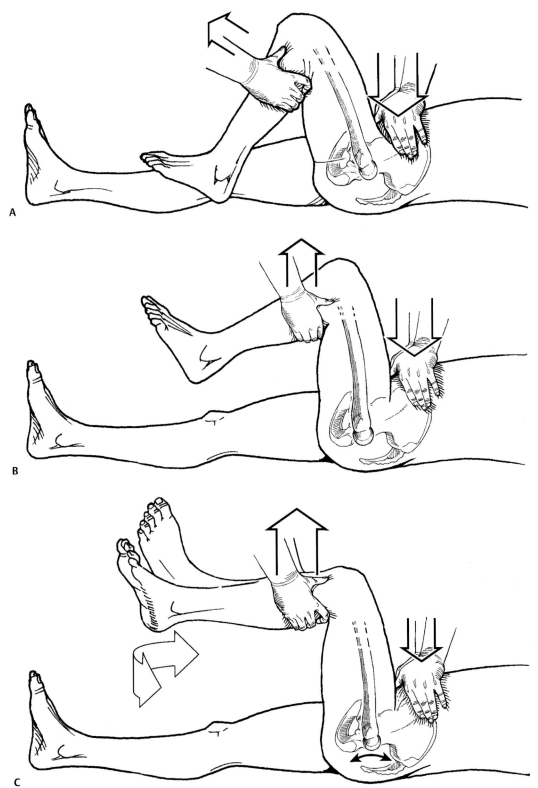

Figure 21–5 The Bigelow method (most common method) for reducing a posterior hip dislocation. The patient lies supine. **(A)** An assistant provides downward pressure on the anterior-superior iliac spines, while the person performing the reduction pulls in-line traction, **(B)** flexes the hip to 90 degrees, and **(C)** applies internal rotation and adduction until reduction is achieved.

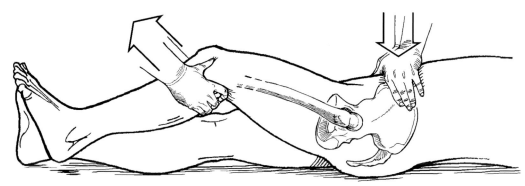

Figure 21–6 The Allis method for reduction of a posterior hip dislocation. An assistant stabilizes the pelvis while the reducer pulls in-line traction. The hip is flexed to 90 degrees, and gentle alternating internal and external rotation helps coax the hip back into position.

In this situation, attempted reduction under general anesthesia may be performed and may be aided by a Schanz pin in the proximal femoral region (at the level of the lesser trochanter) to aid the reduction of the hip dislocation. If a closed reduction is not possible in the operating room, then a decision should be made at that point by the treating surgeon to proceed with an open reduction of the hip dislocation or consider expeditious referral of the patient. In general, if a closed reduction under appropriate sedation with a qualified team is not successful, it is unlikely that a closed reduction under general anesthesia will be successful. This information

may be helpful for the general orthopaedic surgeon who does not wish to openly address the injury.

Once the hip dislocation is successfully reduced, if complete radiographic evaluation fails to reveal an associated acetabular or femoral head fracture, the patient may be treated with a weight bearing as tolerated protocol using an assistive device if necessary. The patient should be educated and counseled to avoid positions that might allow redislocation. *The use of an abduction orthosis is rarely of benefit.* If there is a small fragment of posterior wall fracture, this may be treated similarly to dislocation without fracture (see Chapter 20). If there is

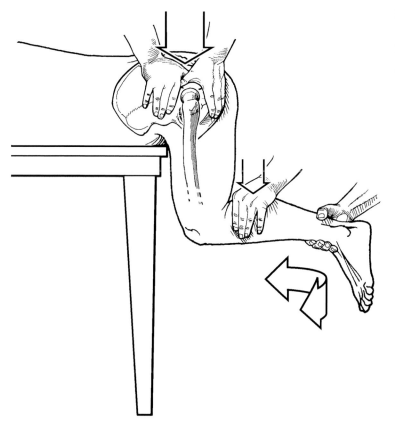

Figure 21–7 The Stimson method for reduction of a posterior hip dislocation The patient is lying prone with the affected extremity hanging off the end of the exam table. The hip and knee are flexed to 90 degrees, and a downward force is applied to the calf.

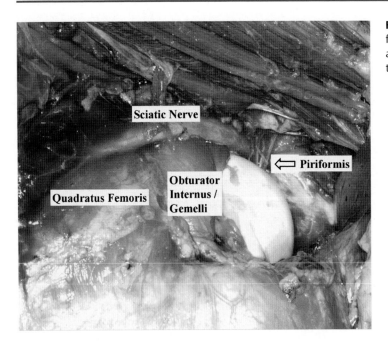

Figure 21–8 The case of an irreducible hip dislocation. The femoral head is seen to be buttonholed through the capsule and between the piriformis and obturator internus muscle/tendon.

any question about the stability of the hip joint, the surgeon should fluoroscopically evaluate the hip stability under anesthesia.[22] If subluxation of the femoral head is noted on any view (AP and Judets) of the hip (while under flexion, axial loading, and internal rotation), operative stabilization of the posterior wall should be performed. Assistive ambulatory aids may be temporarily used until the acute pain has subsided; however, full progression to unassisted ambulation should be implemented as soon as tolerated.

Rarely when a femoral head fracture is present is nonoperative treatment appropriate. Femoral head fractures may be treated nonoperatively when they are small, infrafoveal, displaced less than 1 mm, and not associated with any intra-articular debris. Otherwise, due to the highly disabling nature of this injury and the associated complications, nonoperative treatment is relatively rare.[23]

Indications for Surgical Treatment

Most femoral head fractures will require operative treatment. Small infrafoveal fractures, although not necessarily contributing to hip stability, may unite in a malreduced position and block hip motion. The typical displacement seen in infrafoveal fractures is a caudal and anterior displacement of the fragment. Healing in this position may impinge against the edge of the cotyloid fossa and reduce hip rotation or adduction. Unless a small infrafoveal fracture remains well reduced after reduction of the associated hip dislocation, primary excision of the fragment should be performed.

Surgical Treatment

Surgical Anatomy, Surgical Approaches, and Surgical Technique

A more detailed description of the surgical anatomy and surgical approaches is seen in these respective sections in Chapters 20 and 22.

Pipkin I or II Fracture (see Videos 21–1, 21–2, Disk 3)

The type of surgical treatment of the femoral head fracture is determined by the size and location of the fragment. Small infrafoveal fractures may be appropriate for excision and capsular repair. This is typically performed with the patient in the lateral position through a Kocher-Langenbeck approach. After incision of the fascia lata and splitting the fibers of the gluteus maximus, the gluteus medius and minimus can be carefully retracted anteriorly. The tendon of the piriformis muscle is transected at least 1 cm from the greater trochanter to protect the ascending branch of the medial femoral circumflex and the blood supply to the femoral head from injury. The dislocation usually occurs through the substance of the superior gemellus muscle, and some damaged muscle usually requires debridement. The tendon of the obturator internus muscle together with the remaining gemelli is also transected. The quadratus femoris is not taken down from the femur—also to protect the blood supply to the femoral head. The traumatic capsulotomy will be easily visualized, and the hip should be redislocated under carefully controlled circumstances. If difficult to achieve, the traumatic capsulotomy may be extended along the rim of the acetabulum, with care taken not to damage the acetabular labrum. Once dislocated, the hip is flexed, and the femoral head fragment may be retrieved from the joint by visualizing the interior of the acetabulum anterior to the femoral neck. Illumination of the interior of the joint may be helpful and may be achieved with the use of a headlight or a flexible light source.

Careful preoperative scrutiny of the CT scan will tell the surgeon how many femoral head fragments to expect to retrieve from the interior of the joint, and palpation will confirm that no intra-articular fragments are left behind. Once the fragment is removed and the joint irrigated, the ruptured ligamentum teres is generally debrided to ensure that its remnant does not become interposed between the femoral head and the acetabular articular surface after reduction. The femoral head is then reduced and the capsulotomy repaired. If a direct capsular repair is not possible, suture anchors may be used to reattach the capsule to the rim of the acetabulum. The anchors should be directed away from the joint to ensure that their tips do not inadvertently penetrate the articular surface during insertion. The short external rotators are repaired prior to wound closure.

Large femoral head fragments or those with a suprafoveal location are critical for hip stability, and congruence of the weight-bearing surface of the femoral head and these fragments should be treated with open reduction and internal fixation. Through the Kocher-Langenbeck approach, even with the femoral head dislocated and the hip maximally flexed, internally rotated, and adducted, the anteromedial location of the fracture is impossible to fully visualize. Even if the fragment can be reduced, fixation of the fragment is not possible with anterior to posterior lag screws. For this reason, the surgical approach of choice for fixation of femoral head fractures is the Smith-Petersen approach. The patient is positioned supine on a radiolucent table. Alternately, a traction table designed for use in ac-

etabular surgery may also be used. An incision is made from the anterior-superior iliac spine ~7 cm distally in line with the lateral border of the patella. The tensor fascia is opened over the tensor fascia lata muscle. This helps protect the lateral femoral cutaneous nerve from injury. The tensor fascia lata is retracted laterally, and the fascia overlying the rectus femoris is incised, identifying the reflected and direct heads of the rectus proximally. Typically, both heads of the rectus are transected, and the rectus femoris is retracted medially. The capsular fibers of the lateral border of the iliopsoas muscle are identified and are sharply dissected off the anterior hip capsule as far medially as the iliopsoas bursa. A retractor may be placed under the psoas tendon and used to retract medially. The anterior hip capsule is now exposed, and a T-shaped capsulotomy is performed with one limb paralleling the rim of the acetabulum and the stem of the T parallel to the femoral neck. Care must be taken to avoid damaging the acetabular labrum.

The femoral head is now dislocated anteriorly by external rotation and traction. If the traction table is used, the hip may be extended as well, improving the ease of dislocation. Once dislocated, the leg is placed in the "figure of four" position. The femoral head fragment typically will remain attached to the ligamentum teres and stay within the acetabulum. Generally, the ligamentum teres and any capsular attachments to the fragment should be maintained if possible to prevent the femoral head from becoming completely avascular. Frequently, however, the reduction cannot be obtained without sacrificing one of the two soft tissue attachments because the femoral head fragment will not reach to the remaining head in the dislocated position. Once reduced, the femoral head fragment is fixed with the use of countersunk standard screws or variable-pitch headless screws. Typically, the screws are of small diameter: 2.0, 2.7 or 3.5 mm screws may all be useful **(Fig. 21–9)**. There are frequently areas of impaction and shear injury to

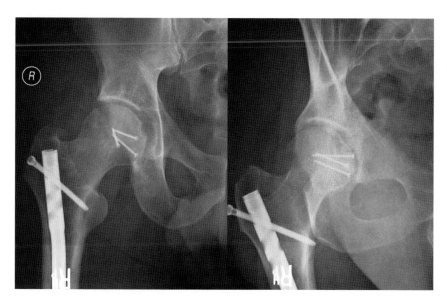

Figure 21–9 For fixation of a femoral head fracture, screws are seen to be oriented from anterior to posterior. The obturator oblique radiograph demonstrates the quality of reduction.

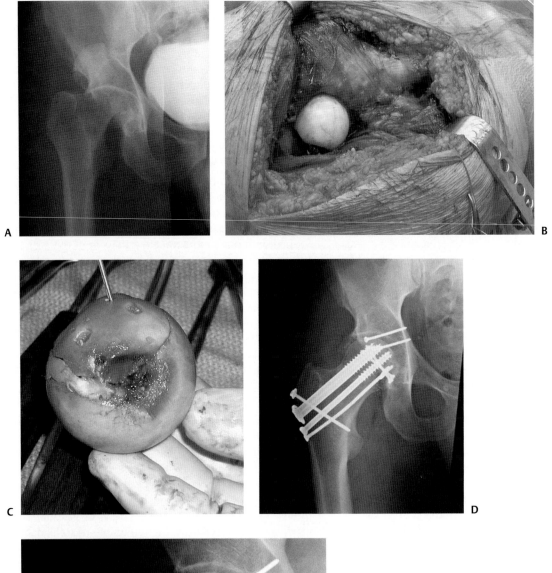

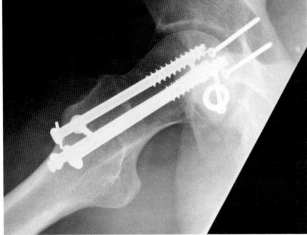

Figure 21–10 The case of a Pipkin III fracture-dislocation of the femoral neck and head in a 32-year-old male. No closed reduction was possible. **(A)** An anteroposterior (AP) radiograph of the hip. **(B)** A Kocher-Langenbeck approach of the hip was performed because the femoral head was dislocated in this direction. This intraoperative photo demonstrates that the femoral head is free-floating. **(C)** The femoral head was a free fragment, which allowed for reduction and fixation of the femoral head. **(D)** The femoral neck following reduction and fixation, which was possible through the posterior approach. AP radiograph of the hip is demonstrated here. Long-term prognosis is guarded. **(E)** The lateral view of the reduction. (Case courtesy of Frank Shuler, MD, PhD.)

the surrounding cartilage at the site of impact, and this may require additional small screw or absorbable pin fixation. Once fixation is achieved, the hip is carefully reduced after irrigation and palpation of the acetabulum have confirmed that there are no remaining intra-articular fragments. The anterior capsulotomy is repaired, and the direct head of the rectus femoris is reattached to the anterior-inferior iliac spine either through a drill hole or with the use of suture anchors.

In rare circumstances, the posterior hip dislocation may be irreducible due to either the femoral head fracture or the intact portion of the head being buttonholed through the posterior traumatic capsulotomy. In this circumstance, the Smith-Petersen approach may not allow the necessary exposure to relocate the head. If this occurs, a posterior approach to perform an open reduction of the dislocation may be followed by an anterior approach for the fixation of the fracture.

Pipkin III Fracture

The Pipkin type III fracture is a fracture of the femoral neck in association with either an infrafoveal or a suprafoveal femoral head fracture (**Fig. 21–10A–E**). The femoral head fracture will generally remain in the acetabulum while the neck–head fragment dislocates posteriorly. The surgical reduction and fixation of these fractures must be performed urgently to minimize the additional disruption of the blood supply to the femoral head. Either a Watson-Jones or a Smith-Petersen approach will allow reduction and fixation of the combined injury. The neck–head fragment must first be reduced into the acetabulum. If the femoral head fragment is small, fixation of the femoral neck first allows manipulation of the leg to assist in the reduction of the femoral head fragment. When the femoral head fragment is large, the fractures must often be reduced simultaneously. If the fragments have no remaining soft tissue attachments or the patient is elderly or has a low functional demand activity level, consideration may be given to primary prosthetic replacement.

Pipkin IV Fracture

Pipkin IV fractures are typically a Pipkin I or II fracture pattern in association with a posterior wall acetabulum fracture (**Fig. 21–11**). Because it is the posterior rim of the acetabulum that impacts against the femoral head and causes the fracture (and vice versa), a large femoral head fracture is often seen in conjunction with a small rim avulsion. Similarly, small femoral head fractures may be seen in conjunction with large posterior wall fragments. The two injuries should be considered independently in determining the appropriate surgical treatment, but it is rare for this injury to require reduction and fixation of both the femoral head and acetabular fractures.

For small femoral head fragments, a Kocher-Langenbeck approach is typically utilized to perform an excision of the

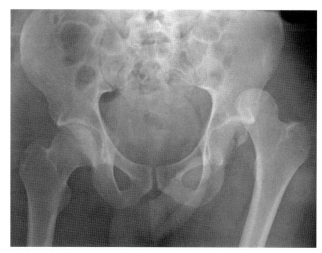

Figure 21–11 Typical radiograph of a Pipkin IV injury. A small peripheral posterior wall fracture is seen.

femoral head fragment and a reduction and internal fixation of the posterior wall fracture. A reduction and fixation of larger femoral head fragments may be attempted, but, as already described, the posterior approach to the hip affords neither the optimal visualization for reduction nor fixation of the femoral head. If reduction and fixation is determined at this point to be desirable but not achievable, a sequential staged Smith-Petersen approach may be utilized for the treatment of the femoral head fracture.

Larger femoral head fragments requiring open reduction and internal fixation are best treated with the Smith-Petersen approach primarily. Following fixation of the femoral head, the hip joint should be stressed to see whether the posterior wall fracture is of sufficient size to compromise the stability of the hip joint. If the hip subluxates posteriorly, a staged Kocher-Langenbeck approach can be utilized for fixation of the posterior wall fracture. If no subluxation is noted, the posterior wall fracture may be appropriate for nonoperative management.

A final option is the use of the trochanteric flip (digastric) osteotomy as described by Siebenrock et al in combination with an anterior capsulotomy and dislocation to provide access to both fractures with a single surgical approach (**Fig. 21–12**).[24] The patient is positioned in the lateral position on a radiolucent table. The Kocher-Langenbeck approach as already described is performed. A trochanteric osteotomy is performed, creating a trochanteric fragment of ~1.5 cm thickness, with the gluteus medius and minimus attached proximally and the vastus lateralis attached distally. The piriformis tendon remains attached to the proximal femur, protecting the blood supply to the femoral head. The traumatic capsulotomy is extended along the rim of the acetabulum. The hip is flexed and externally rotated and the femoral head dislocated anteriorly. The femoral head fragment is reduced and fixed with lag screw fixation and the hip reduced. The posterior wall fracture may then be

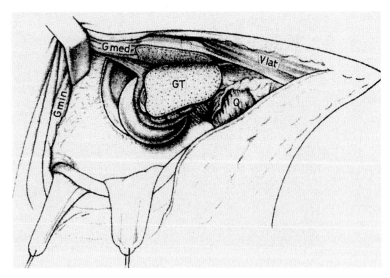

Figure 21–12 A schematic of the Ganz trochanteric flip osteotomy approach for dislocation of the femoral head. This approach may be utilized for treatment of a Pipkin IV injury. Gmin, gloteus maximus muscle; Gmed, gluteus medius muscle; Vlat, vastus lateralis muscle; GT, greater trochanter; Q, quadratus femoris muscle. (With permission from Siebenrock KA, Gautier, E, Ziran BH, et al. Trochanteric flip osteotomy for cranial extension and muscle protection in acetabular fracture fixation using a Kocher-Langenbeck approach. J Orthop Trauma 1998;12:387–391.)

reduced and fixed and the entire capsulotomy, traumatic and surgical, repaired **(Figs. 21–13A–J** and **21–14A–E).**

Rehabilitation

Following internal fixation of a Pipkin (I to IV) injury, the patient will have aggressive range of motion exercises of the hip with quadriceps and abductor strengthening exercises. Toe-touch weight bearing is used for the first

8 weeks, with progressive weight bearing after that point. A stationary bike is helpful to aid in recovery. No braces or hip flexion precautions are utilized.

New Techniques

Fracture tables that allow for leg extension and external rotation may allow for better visualization of the femoral head injury.

Tips and Tricks

- If the patient has an irreducible Pipkin IV injury where both the femoral head and posterior wall should be fixed, the first approach should be a posterior approach. Attempting to reduce the hip dislocation from anterior is not wise because the femoral head is usually buttonholed through the external rotators of the hip.
- The screws utilized for fixation of the femoral head fracture should be countersunk and well below the cartilage layer of the femoral head.
- Occasionally, a small but superior-posterior wall fracture is critical to stability of the hip in a Pipkin IV injury. If the wall fragment is too small for fixation, repair of the capsule with anchor sutures may be advisable.
- If a Smith-Peterson approach is utilized for fixation of a femoral head fracture, devitalization of the tensor fascia

lata muscle should be avoided because this can lead to heterotopic ossification.
- The typical malreduction of a femoral head fracture is to have the femoral head fragment displaced inferiorly. For this reason, visualization of the superior aspect of the femoral head is essential to judge the quality of the reduction.
- If the Smith-Petersen approach is used for fixation of a femoral head fracture, the figure-of-four position is helpful to visualize and internally fix the femoral head. This entails flexion, abduction, and external rotation of the leg, and is aided by a towel bump underneath the involved hip's buttock. Alternatively, a fracture table can be utilized for extension and external rotation of the hip.

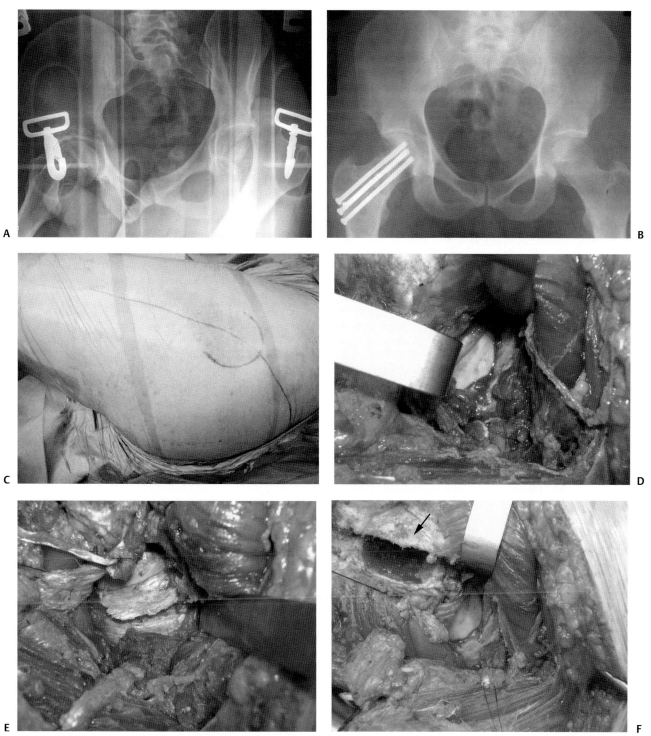

Figure 21–13 A 32-year-old male was involved in a motor vehicle collision and sustained a left fracture-dislocation of the hip. The patient also had a minimally displaced right femoral neck fracture. **(A)** Injury anteroposterior (AP) radiograph of the pelvis. **(B)** AP pelvis radiograph after open reduction and internal fixation of the right femoral neck fracture. The left hip joint space is noted to be wide with an osseous fragment superior to the femoral head. The inferior one third of the femoral head has significant irregularity. **(C)** The patient underwent a Ganz trochanteric flip osteotomy. This was chosen because the surgeon needed complete visualization of the acetabulum and femoral head. The skin incision is seen here. The patient is positioned lateral on a bean bag. **(D)** This intraoperative view demonstrates the "dislocation cavity" with significant devitalization of the inferior aspect of the gluteus minimus and avulsion of the labrum from the posterior wall. **(E)** The superior-posterior wall fracture is seen. **(F)** The trochanteric flip osteotomy is performed. The 1.5 cm osseous fragment (arrow) maintains its attachments to the gluteus medius and minimus.

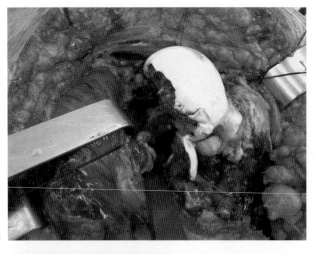

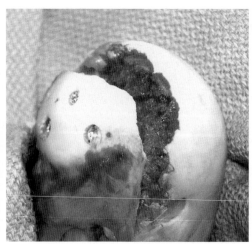

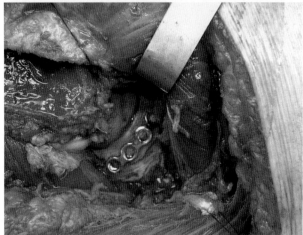

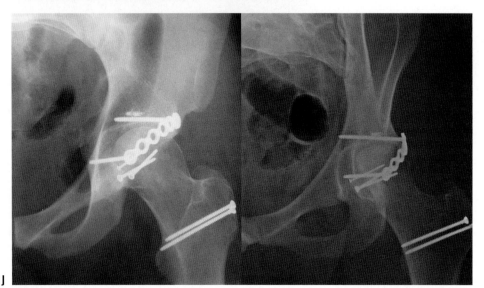

Figure 21–13 *(Continued)* **(G)** The capsulotomy is completed anteriorly, continuing the traumatic capsulotomy. With adduction, flexion, and external rotation of the hip, the entire femoral head is seen. As noted here, the actual osseochondral pathology is often worse than expected from radiographic studies. There are several osseochondral fragments that are not reconstructible. **(H)** Fixation of the femoral head. An attempt was made to maintain the sphericity of the femoral head. **(I)** Fixation of the posterior wall. **(J)** Postoperative films at 1 month. It is recognized that the prognosis long term is guarded. The patient, however, did complete a 100 mile bike ride at 1 year postinjury. (Case courtesy of Philip J. Kregor, MD.)

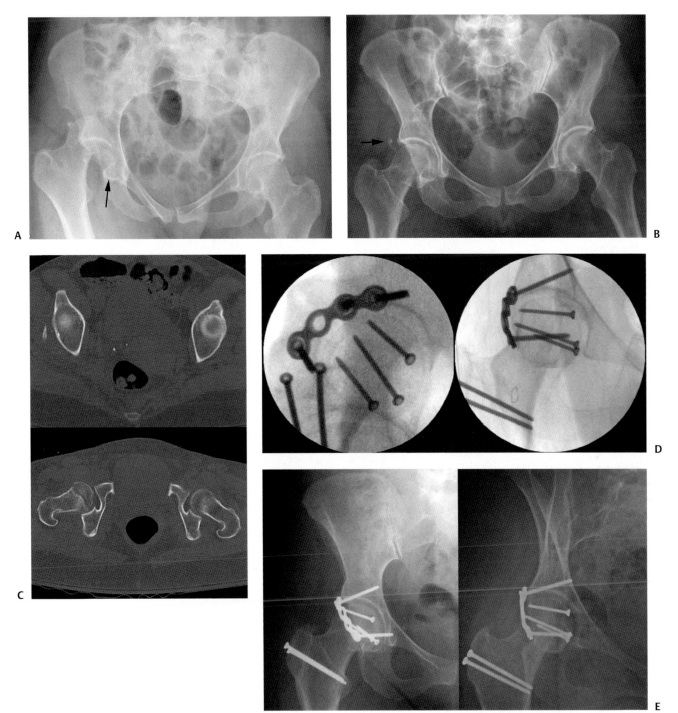

Figure 21–14 This 57-year-old female was involved in a motor vehicle collision and sustained a right hip fracture-dislocation. **(A)** Injury antero-posterior (AP) pelvis radiograph that shows a relatively large fragment of the femoral head in the acetabulum (arrow). **(B)** The patient underwent a closed reduction under conscious sedation in the emergency room. The AP radiograph of the hip is seen here. A subtle irregularity of the sphericity of the femoral head is seen. Additionally, a small superior-posterior wall fracture is seen (arrow). **(C)** Postreduction computed tomographic scan of the right hip. The small posterior wall acetabular fracture is seen. The femoral head fracture is displaced 3 to 4 mm. **(D)** The patient underwent a Ganz trochanteric flip osteotomy for complete visualization and exposure of the injury. Intraoperative views show a peripheral plate on the superior-posterior wall fracture and three anterior to posterior 2.7 mm lag screws utilized for fixation of the femoral head fracture. Two screws are used for fixation of the greater trochanter. **(E)** AP and obturator oblique views of the right hip at 1 year postinjury. The patient has a normal hip. However, it should be noted that this is a short follow-up period. (Case courtesy of Philip J. Kregor, MD.)

Outcomes and Complications

Long-term results following simple traumatic dislocation of the hip are surprisingly poor, even with prompt appropriate reduction. Dreinhofer et al reported on 50 patients followed for an average of 8 years after hip dislocation.[25] Fair and poor results were found in 53% of posterior dislocations and 25% of anterior dislocations. Avascular necrosis, arthrosis, and heterotopic ossification all contributed to poor outcome. Hougaard and Thomsen found that 88% of 100 hip dislocations followed for an average of 14 years had a good or excellent outcome if the hip dislocation was reduced within 6 hours of injury. When the dislocation was reduced after 6 hours, only 42% had a long-term good or excellent result.[7] Upadhyay and Moulton also found that, at an average follow-up of over 12 years, 24% of posterior hip dislocation patients had clinical and radiographic evidence of a poor outcome.[26] All of these studies underscore the severity of the injury and the importance of good patient communication regarding prognosis.

There are few reports documenting long-term outcome after hip dislocation with femoral head fracture. Dreinhofer et al reported on 26 patients and found 15 of them to have fair or poor results when followed for an average of 5 years.[27] Swiontkowski et al reported on 24 patients followed for more than 2 years. Twelve patients were treated with an anterior approach, whereas the other 12 were treated with a posterior approach. The functional outcome in each group was similar. There were no cases of avascular necrosis in the anterior group, but there was an increase in the incidence of heterotopic ossification formation—possibly due to the elevation of the tensor fascia lata muscle from the lateral ilium.[23] Stannard et al also found a 3.2-fold higher incidence of avascular necrosis in those patients operated through the Kocher-Langenbeck approach versus those operated through the Smith-Petersen approach (**Fig. 21–15A–E**).[28]

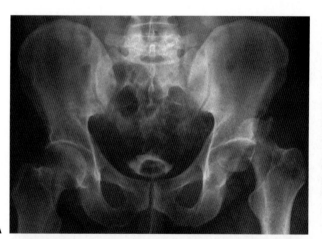

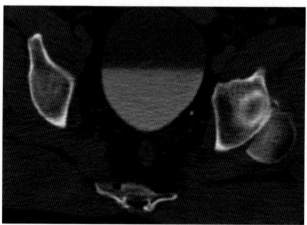

Figure 21–15 A 27-year-old male was involved in a motor vehicle collision and sustained an irreducible Pipkin IV fracture-dislocation of the left hip. **(A)** Anteroposterior (AP) injury radiograph. A closed reduction of the left hip under conscious sedation was not possible. **(B)** Injury computed tomography showing the femoral head wedged on the supra-acetabular surface. **(C)** The patient underwent open reduction and internal fixation of both the femoral head and the posterior wall acetabular fracture at ~12 hours postinjury. **(D)** AP and obturator oblique radiographs at 18 months postinjury. The patient had a normal hip at this point. **(E)** At 2 years postinjury, the patient had severe pain in his left hip. Osteonecrosis of the femoral head was seen. The patient had a total hip arthroplasty at 25 months posttrauma. (Case courtesy of Philip J. Kregor, M.D.)

- With a posterior hip dislocation, the affected hip is held in a flexed, adducted, and internally rotated position. After an anterior dislocation, the affected hip usually remains in extension and neutral or slight abduction.
- Posterior hip dislocations are the most common dislocation, with reported incidences of 89 to 92% of all dislocations.[3,10]
- Femoral head fractures may be treated nonoperatively when they are small, infrafoveal, displaced less than 1 mm, and not associated with any intra-articular debris. Otherwise, due to the highly disabling nature of this injury and the associated complications, nonoperative treatment is relatively rare.[23]
- Through the Kocher-Langenbeck approach, even with the femoral head dislocated and the hip maximally flexed, internally rotated, and adducted, the anteromedial location of the

fracture is impossible to fully visualize. In addition, the posterior approach does not allow internal fixation of the femoral head fragment. For this reason, the Smith-Petersen approach is advisable for most femoral head fracture reduction and fixation.
- The Ganz trochanteric flip osteotomy is a surgical approach option for visualization, reduction, and fixation of both the femoral head and posterior wall fractures of a Pipkin IV injury, if this is desired.
- Hougaard and Thomsen found that 88% of 100 hip dislocations followed for an average of 14 years had a good or excellent outcome if the hip dislocation was reduced within 6 hours of injury. When the dislocation was reduced after 6 hours, only 42% had a long-term good or excellent result.[7]

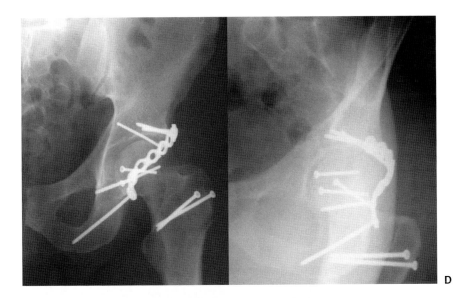

D

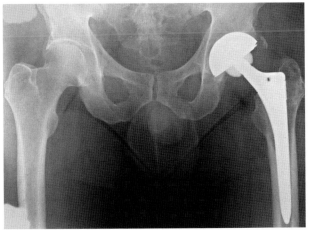

E

On the DVDs

Video 21–1   (Disk 3)   ORIF of Infrafoveal Femoral Head Fracture   This video demonstrates open reduction and internal fixation of a large Pipkin I femoral head fracture using countersunk screws.

Video 21–2   (Disk 3)   ORIF of a Pipkin II Femoral Head Fracture Using the Smith-Petersen Approach   This video shows open reduction of a Pipkin II femoral head fracture using the Smith-Petersen approach. The details of the approach are reviewed.

References

1. Hak DJ, Goulet JA. Severity of injuries associated with traumatic hip dislocation as a result of motor vehicle collisions. J Trauma 1999;47:60–63
2. Yang RS, Tsuang YH, Hang YS, Liu TK. Traumatic dislocation of the hip. Clin Orthop Relat Res 1991;265:218–227
3. Sahin V, Karakas ES, Aksu S, Atlihan D, Turk CY, Halici M. Traumatic dislocation and fracture-dislocation of the hip: a long-term follow-up study. J Trauma 2003;54:520–529
4. Garrett JC, Epstein HC, Harris WH, Harvey JP, Nickel VL. Treatment of unreduced traumatic posterior dislocations of the hip. J Bone Joint Surg Am 1979;61:2–6
5. Epstein HC, Wiss DA, Cozen L. Posterior fracture dislocation of the hip with fractures of the femoral head. Clin Orthop Relat Res 1985;201:9–17
6. Cornwall R, Radomisli TE. Nerve injury in traumatic dislocation of the hip. Clin Orthop Relat Res 2000;377:84–91
7. Hougaard K, Thomsen PB. Traumatic posterior dislocation of the hip: prognostic factors influencing the incidence of avascular necrosis of the femoral head. Arch Orthop Trauma Surg 1986;106:32–35
8. Thompson VP, Epstein HC. Traumatic dislocation of the hip: a survey of two hundred and four cases covering a period of twenty-one years. J Bone Joint Surg Am 1951;33-A:746–778
9. Stewart MJ, Milford LW. Fracture-dislocation of the hip: an end-result study. J Bone Joint Surg Am 1954;36:315–342
10. DeLee JC, Evans JA, Thomas J. Anterior dislocation of the hip and associated femoral-head fractures. J Bone Joint Surg Am 1980;62:960–964
11. Sinha SN. Simultaneous anterior and posterior dislocation of the hip joints. J Trauma 1985;25:269–270
12. Soltanpur A. Bilateral traumatic dislocation of the hip. Injury 1983;14:349–350
13. Sethi TS, Mam MK, Kakroo RK. Bilateral traumatic anterior dislocation of the hip. J Trauma 1987;27:573–574
14. Tezcan R, Erginer R, Babacan M. Bilateral traumatic anterior dislocation of the hip: brief report. J Bone Joint Surg Br 1988;70:148–149
15. Kuhn DA, Frymoyer JW. Bilateral traumatic hip dislocation. J Trauma 1987;27:442–444
16. Levine RG, Kauffman CP, Reilly MC, Behrens FF. "Floating pelvis": a combination of bilateral hip dislocation with a lumbar ligamentous disruption. J Bone Joint Surg Br 1999;81:309–311
17. Pipkin G. Treatment of grade IV fracture-dislocation of the hip. J Bone Joint Surg Am 1957;39-A:1027–1042, passim
18. Bigelow HJ. Luxations of the hip joint. Boston Med Surg J. 1870;5:1–3
19. Allis OH. An Inquiry into the Difficulties Encountered in the Reduction of Dislocations of the Hip. Philadelphia: Dornan Printer; 1896:85
20. Stimson LA. A Treatise on Fractures and Dislocations. Philadelphia: H.C. Leas Son; 1912:797
21. Walker WA. Traumatic dislocations of the hip joint. Am J Surg 1940;50:545–549
22. Tornetta P. Non-operative management of acetabular fractures: the use of dynamic stress views. J Bone Joint Surg Br 1999;81:67–70
23. Swiontkowski MF, Thorpe M, Seiler JG, Hansen ST. Operative management of displaced femoral head fractures: case-matched comparison of anterior versus posterior approaches for Pipkin I and Pipkin II fractures. J Orthop Trauma 1992;6:437–442
24. Siebenrock KA, Gautier E, Ziran BH, Ganz R. Trochanteric flip osteotomy for cranial extension and muscle protection in acetabular fracture fixation using a Kocher-Langenbeck approach. J Orthop Trauma 1998;12:387–391
25. Dreinhofer KE, Schwarzkopf SR, Haas NP, Tscherne H. Isolated traumatic dislocation of the hip: long-term results in 50 patients. J Bone Joint Surg Br 1994;76:6–12
26. Upadhyay SS, Moulton A. The long-term results of traumatic posterior dislocation of the hip. J Bone Joint Surg Br 1981;63B:548–551
27. Dreinhofer KE, Schwarzkopf SR, Haas NP, Tscherne H. Femur head dislocation fractures. Long-term outcome of conservative and surgical therapy [in German]. Unfallchirurg 1996;99:400–409
28. Stannard JP, Harris HW, Volgas DA, Alonso JE. Functional outcome of patients with femoral head fractures associated with hip dislocations. Clin Orthop Relat Res 2000;377:44–56

22 Intracapsular Hip Fractures

George J. Haidukewych

Intracapsular hip fractures remain among the most common, yet potentially devastating, injuries that the orthopedist will encounter. Due to the tenuous blood supply and the high mechanical stresses in this anatomical region, complications such as nonunion and osteonecrosis are not uncommon. The number of intracapsular hip fractures continues to increase proportionately with the ever-growing elderly population. In North America, 220,000 fractures of the hip occur each year, equating to a $9 billion cost to the health care system.[1] These fractures typically occur after low-energy falls in older patients with poor bone quality, but also occur in younger patients as a result of high-energy trauma. The optimal treatment of intracapsular hip fractures remains controversial. Typically, for physiologically older patients with poor bone quality, prosthetic replacement has been favored. Multiple studies have documented excellent prosthesis survivorship, predictable pain relief, and, perhaps most importantly, a low reoperation rate.[2,3] For physiologically younger patients, however, anatomical reduction and internal fixation is recommended, with efforts focused on preserving the femoral head. This chapter reviews the surgical treatment of intracapsular hip fractures and will be stratified based on the physiological age of the patient. Of course, *physiological age* is a relative term, and the appropriate treatment should be individualized to each patient. For purposes of this chapter, *elderly* is defined as a chronological age of 65 years or older.

Most patients with an intracapsular hip fracture are elderly and present with pain in the involved hip, typically in the groin, after a low-energy fall. The limb may be foreshortened and held in external rotation. The diagnosis should also be considered whenever a patient presents with a femoral shaft fracture after high-energy trauma. High-quality radiographs, including an anteroposterior (AP) and lateral view of the femoral neck, should be obtained. Usually such a "trauma AP" radiograph is obtained with the leg in external rotation, which does not give the best view of the femoral neck. A good profile of the femoral neck can be seen either with the leg internally rotated or with an obturator oblique (Judet) view of the pelvis. Often the computed tomographic (CT) scan of the chest, abdomen, and pelvis that is usually obtained in the polytraumatized patient will include some sections through the femoral neck; these should routinely be scrutinized using bone windows **(Fig. 22–1A–C)**. In polytraumatized patients,

other life-threatening injuries should be treated first, then the femoral neck fracture should be treated urgently.[4] Medical optimization is recommended preoperatively, especially in frail elderly patients with multiple comorbidities.[5] In general, patients should be brought to surgery as soon as medical clearance is obtained.

Occasionally a patient will present with groin pain in the absence of any identifiable trauma. Radiographs may be completely normal. In this setting a femoral neck stress fracture or nondisplaced fracture should be suspected, and a magnetic resonance imaging (MRI) scan should be obtained. In this setting, MRI provides rapid fracture diagnosis, avoids ionizing radiation, excludes other potential causes of hip pain, and provides information on fracture verticality and anatomical location (femoral neck or intertrochanteric).[5–7] This information may influence fixation device selection and is superior to a bone scan for diagnosis.[8]

Classification

Multiple classification schemes have been proposed for intracapsular hip fractures.[9] The most commonly utilized is the Garden classification **(Fig. 22–2)**.[10,11] Although there are four subtypes in this classification, most surgeons prefer to simply group these fractures into those that are nondisplaced (Garden I and II) and those that are displaced (Garden III and IV). Generally, the prognostic significance and treatment method chosen follow from the simple consideration of fracture displacement. The Abbeitsgemeinshaft für Osteosynthesefragen/Orthopaedic Trauma Association (AO/OTA) classification is also utilized but is slightly cumbersome. It takes into account other important variables such as fracture verticality and location of the fracture in the femoral neck **(Fig. 22–3A–C)**.[12] It distinguishes subcapital, transcervical, and basicervical fractures. Finally, Pauwels classified fracture patterns into three broad categories depending on the orientation of the fracture: those with < 30 degrees (Pauwels I), 30 to 50 degrees (Pauwels II), and ≥ 50 degrees of verticality measured from the horizontal (Pauwels III) **(Fig. 22–4)**.[13] Fractures with these increasing angles of verticality are thought to behave in fundamentally distinct ways that may influence both fixation device selection and salvage options if fixation fails, as discussed in detail later in the chapter.

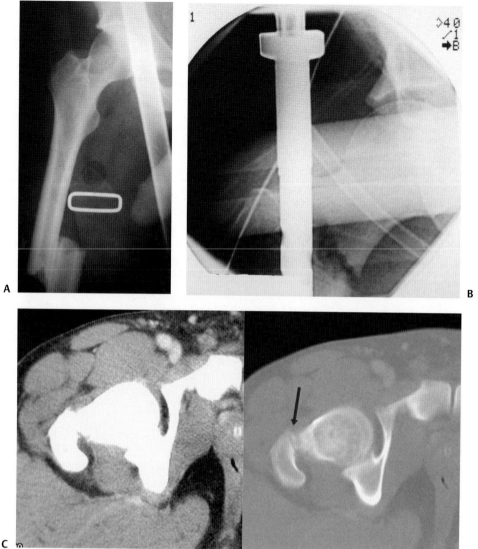

Figure 22–1 Example of a missed femoral neck fracture in a trauma patient. **(A)** Anteroposterior radiograph of the femur in a patient with a femoral shaft fracture. The limb is externally rotated, and the femoral neck appears normal. The patient had a trauma computed tomographic (CT) scan, and the radiologist specifically reported that

there were no fractures in the pelvis or proximal femur. **(B)** Intraoperative imaging during femoral nailing showed a femoral neck fracture. **(C)** Review of the CT scan showed that the fracture was not visible with soft tissue windows (left panel) but was clearly visible when bone windows were used (right panel).

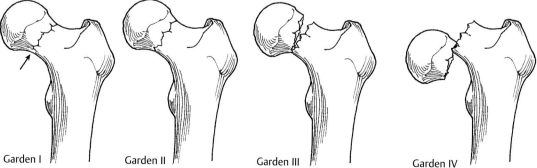

Figure 22–2 Garden classification of femoral neck fractures (from left). Garden I: An incomplete fracture with valgus impaction. Garden II: A complete fracture that is nondisplaced. Garden III: A complete fracture that is partially displaced. Garden IV: A complete fracture that is totally displaced.

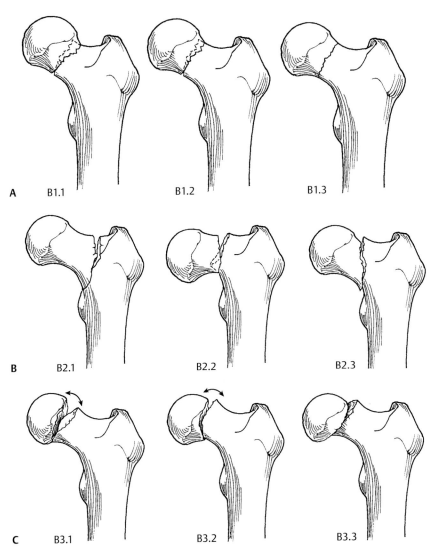

Figure 22–3 Arbeitsgemeinschaft für Osteosynthesefragen/Orthopaedic Trauma Association (AO/OTA) classification of femoral neck fractures. In this alphanumeric scheme, the femoral neck fracture is a type 31-B fracture. **(A)** Illustrates the 31-B1 fractures (subcapital fracture with slight displacement): B1.1 impacted in valgus > 15 degrees; B1.2 impacted in valgus < 15 degrees; B1.3 nondisplaced fracture. **(B)** Illustrates the 31-B2 fractures (transcervical fracture): B2.1 basicervical neck fracture; B2.2 midcervical fracture; B2.3 midcervical shear-type fracture. **(C)** Illustrates the 31-B3 fractures (displaced, subcapital fracture): B3.1 moderate displacement in varus and external rotation; B3.2 moderate displacement with vertical translation and external rotation; B3.3 marked displacement.

Nonoperative Treatment

It is difficult from the literature to define which fractures are nondisplaced and which are minimally displaced. Previous literature often classified the valgus-impacted fracture as nondisplaced. For the purpose of this chapter, fractures that require a reduction maneuver to achieve acceptable alignment will be considered displaced, whereas those that are either pinned in situ due to valgus impaction or truly anatomically nondisplaced will be considered nondisplaced.

Femoral neck fractures are treated operatively in all but the most frail, essentially nonambulatory patients who have prohibitive medical comorbidities and nondisplaced or stable, valgus-impacted fractures. Indications for nonoperative treatment of a displaced femoral neck fracture in an elderly patient are extremely rare. Without some form of operative stabilization (either arthroplasty or internal fixation), the patient may have significant pain and difficulty with mobilization. The prognosis after such treatment is poor due to pulmonary complications, decubi-

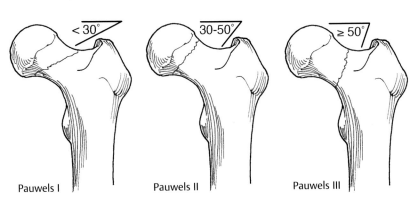

Figure 22–4 Pauwels classification (from left). Pauwels I: Fracture line with < 30 degrees verticality. Pauwels II: Fracture line with 30 to 50 degrees verticality. Pauwels III: Fracture line with ≥ 50 degrees verticality.

tus ulcers, thromboembolism, and further deconditioning and loss of independence. In such cases, nonoperative treatment should be chosen only if the anesthetic risk is truly life threatening. Otherwise, operative management of the displaced femoral neck fracture in the elderly adult should be the norm. Nonoperative treatment of the nondisplaced or valgus-impacted (Garden I or II) femoral neck fracture in the elderly adult can be performed with good results, but not reliably so. In general, nonoperative management would consist of toe-touch weight bearing (if possible) for 8 to 12 weeks with close radiographic monitoring of the fracture site. However, rates of nonunion for nondisplaced or valgus-impacted fractures treated nonoperatively are as high as 39%.[14] Additionally, if late displacement occurs, the fracture reduction may be more difficult, or the fracture may need to be treated with prosthetic replacement. Finally, fracture displacement may increase the rate of osteonecrosis and nonunion. Therefore, even nondisplaced fractures should be treated with some form of internal fixation regardless of patient age, except in the patient with the most severe surgical risk.

There is generally no role for nonoperative treatment for femoral neck fractures in the young adult (physiological age < 65 years), except in situations of life-threatening polytrauma or severe medical problems/anesthetic risk. In such circumstances, there is no later "good" alternative for delayed treatment. Occasionally, a true stable valgus-impacted femoral neck fracture may be encountered in a young adult and treated successfully nonoperatively.

Indications for Surgical Treatment

Displaced fractures are typically treated with open reduction and internal fixation (ORIF) in younger patients (physiological age < 65) and some form of prosthetic replacement in older patients. Factors such as activity, medical comorbidity, and bone quality should be considered when deciding appropriate treatment. Chronological age alone should not be used as a decision-making guide because it does not always reflect physiological age.[5] Nondisplaced or valgus-impacted femoral neck fractures, regardless of age, are treated with screw fixation, except in the situations already noted. It should be recognized, however, that the nondisplaced femoral neck fracture in the young patient is rare.

Surgical Implant Options in the Young Patient

Scores of techniques and devices for internal fixation of femoral neck fractures have been recommended. Although bone quality in the femoral head is often the limiting factor as to whether a successful result is obtained in older patients, in younger patients bone quality is typically normal, and the fracture pattern becomes a very important factor in selecting the appropriate fixation device. Fracture verticality (shear angle) has been recognized by many

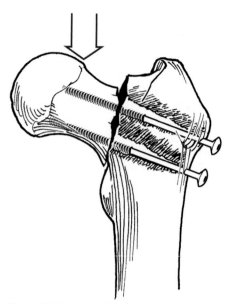

Figure 22–5 A Pauwels III femoral neck fracture will not be adequately addressed with screws alone. The loading vector (arrow) is nearly parallel to the fracture line and cannot be resisted by the supporting bone.

authors to be a contributing factor for potential instability by virtue of increasing shear stresses imparted by forces across the hip with increasing fracture verticality.[13] Fractures with less verticality (e.g., more horizontal) tend to be relatively stable and experience compression with loading. These are typically treated with screw fixation. Fractures that are more vertical, such as the Pauwels III fracture (**Figs. 22–4, 22–5**), result in higher shear stresses challenging the internal fixation device and may be inadequately stabilized with cannulated screws alone.[15–21] The metaphyseal bone in the proximal femur, especially in patients with poor bone quality, may not provide sufficient support to the shafts of the screws to prevent inferior and posterior displacement of the proximal fragment (**Fig. 22–5**). Therefore, some authors have recommended the use of an additional screw that engages the calcar region, placed perpendicular to the primary fracture line (**Fig. 22–6A,B**).[22] When a vertical fracture line is present, a fixed-angle device may also be used to stabilize the fracture. The sliding hip screw device, by virtue of its fixed neck-shaft angle, may minimize shear at the fracture site. Others have recommended the use of a 95 degree dynamic condylar screw (personal communication, Roy Sanders, MD). By virtue of its 95 degree entry into the femoral head, this device theoretically has the ability to lag and compress the fracture perpendicular to the vertical fracture line, a principle critical to the most ideal application of a lag screw. These devices have the disadvantage of requiring more extensive exposure and removal of bone from the femoral head for implantation. Also, care must be taken to avoid rotation of the head and neck fragment during insertion.

Other authors have used an angled blade plate to treat unstable high shear-angle injuries with good results.[20] Well-designed clinical and biomechanical studies that compare fixation constructs for the displaced, unstable

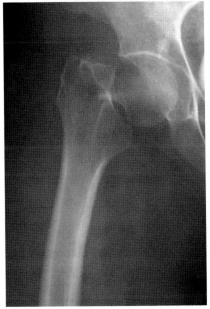
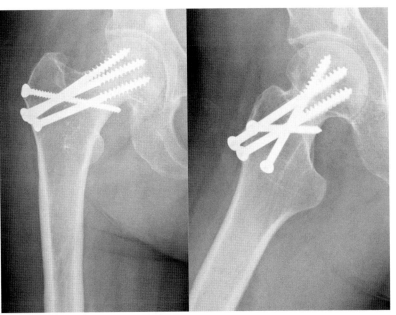

A
B

Figure 22–6 Example of a vertical (Pauwels III) femoral neck fracture in a 53-year-old female who sustained multiple fractures as the result of a motor vehicle collision. **(A)** Injury radiograph of the femoral neck fracture. **(B)** Follow-up films taken 2 years after injury. Note the use of a horizontal screw to counteract the shear forces of this vertical femoral neck fracture. The patient had a normal hip. (Courtesy of Philip J. Kregor, MD)

femoral neck fracture are lacking, but in general, when a fracture is noted to have high fracture verticality and a tendency to shear, fixation with parallel cannulated screws alone is not recommended. It should be noted, however, that the vast majority of femoral neck fractures can be treated successfully with three well-placed, parallel cancellous screws. The use of more than three screws does not appear to offer significant mechanical advantage.[23] The one exception to this may be the case in which there is significant posterior femoral neck comminution, in which case a fourth screw may offer a biomechanical advantage.[24] A recent meta-analysis of fixation methods demonstrated the superiority of screws over pins and showed no clear advantage for an implant with a side plate.[25]

The author prefers to treat valgus-impacted, low shear-angle subcapital and transcervical fractures with three parallel, cannulated, cancellous screws. High shear-angle transcervical and so-called basicervical fractures are treated with a low-angle sliding hip screw device with the addition of a proximal cancellous derotation screw **(Fig. 22–7A–C)**.

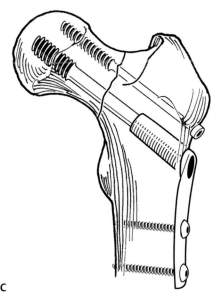
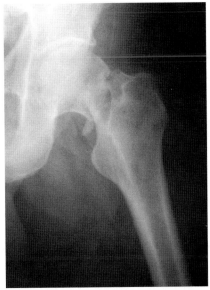
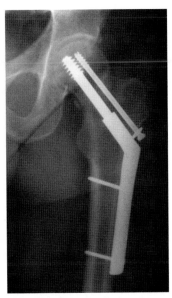

A–C

Figure 22–7 A high shear-angle, vertical femoral neck fracture may be treated with a low-angle (125 to 130 degrees) sliding hip screw device after the addition of a proximal cancellous derotation screw.

(A) Schematic of fixation. **(B)** Case example of a vertical Pauwels III femoral neck fracture. **(C)** Treatment with a sliding hip screw and a derotation screw.

Further research is needed to fully define the optimal internal fixation device for the high shear-angle femoral neck fracture, but in theory, fixed-angle devices will resist shear much more effectively than cancellous screws alone, especially in osteoporotic bone.

Surgical Options in the Elderly Patient

Displaced Fractures in the Physiologically Older Patient: General Principles

Controversy surrounds the optimum management of displaced fractures in the older patient. Few will argue that the best femoral head is the patient's own, if it can be preserved without avascular necrosis or nonunion. For example, a patient in the seventh decade of life who is extremely active, healthy, and has excellent bone quality may benefit from an attempt at ORIF. Recent data have documented, however, that even in such fit patients, arthroplasty may provide a more predictable form of fracture management with a low rate of reoperation.[2,3] Also of concern is the fact that reoperation rates approaching 40% have been reported for such patients following ORIF, even with contemporary techniques and internal fixation devices.[26] Primarily due to the challenges of obtaining excellent fixation of the proximal fragment in osteopenic bone and the high rate of reoperation due to fixation failure, prosthetic replacement is considered by many to be the treatment of choice for displaced fractures in older patients.[2,3] It is critical to individualize the decision making in this patient population, and further data will be necessary to determine which treatment method is best.

Once the decision to perform prosthetic replacement has been made, even more controversy surrounds the choice of prosthesis (unipolar, bipolar, or total hip arthroplasty) and the method of prosthetic fixation, cemented or uncemented. Decision making should be guided by patient activity, estimated life expectancy, and bone quality and is discussed in detail later in the chapter.

Uncemented Hemiarthroplasty

The use of first-generation, one-piece, uncemented, monopolar hemiarthroplasty of the Austin-Moore type should be reserved for minimally ambulatory patients with displaced fractures.[3,5,27] These devices have demonstrated concerning rates of subsidence, thigh pain, and acetabular erosion when these implants are used for ambulatory, active patients.[27–29] The author currently reserves the use of such implants for the most medically infirm, minimally or nonambulatory nursing home residents with displaced fractures, especially those with advanced dementia or severe cardiopulmonary comorbidities. These outdated designs probably function simply as spacers, and it is doubtful that any ever achieve sufficient bony stability to allow unrestricted pain-free ambulation.

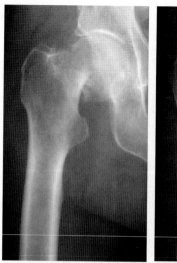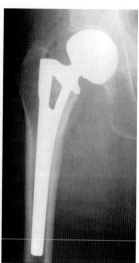

A   B

Figure 22–8 Displaced femoral neck fracture in a minimally ambulatory nursing home resident with multiple cardiopulmonary comorbidities. **(A)** Injury anteroposterior radiograph. **(B)** Treatment with an uncemented modular hemiarthroplasty.

Current second-generation uncemented hip fracture prostheses offer multiple femoral sizes and antirotation fins to allow better fit and fill of the proximal femur, thereby providing improved rotational stability. Additionally, some systems offer modular neck sleeves, allowing more accurate soft tissue balancing and restoration of leg length and femoral offset. If proximal fenestrations are present, they should be filled with cancellous bone from the femoral head in an attempt to improve prosthetic fixation **(Fig. 22–8A,B)**. Newer designs offer improved metaphyseal geometries and roughened surfaces that may facilitate bony ongrowth while avoiding the substantial additional expense of a porous ingrowth surface.

Cemented Hemiarthroplasty

A recent meta-analysis of the literature regarding the treatment of displaced femoral neck fractures in elderly patients suggests that, in general, cemented hemiarthroplasty provides superior clinical results when compared with uncemented hemiarthroplasty.[3] This is not surprising because cement offers the advantages of immediate, secure prosthesis fixation in femoral canals that are often capacious and osteopenic. There is, however, some risk of sudden death when performing cemented hemiarthroplasties for femoral neck fracture. Elderly patients have diminished pulmonary reserve and fatty marrow contents. Parvizi et al recently evaluated risk factors for sudden death after primary hip arthroplasty.[30] The overall risk of sudden death when performing a cemented arthroplasty for acute hip fracture was approximately one in 500. The nonelective nature of the operations and the multiple comorbidities of the elderly cohort likely contributed to the mortality rate. Careful lavage and drying of the femoral canal are recommended to minimize potential embolization debris, and very gentle, if any, cement pressurization is used in the patients that are more medically frail. In one series, this appeared to decrease the rate of intraoperative embolization.[30,31] To summarize, cement offers better results for the vast majority of patients, but it should be used with caution in more frail patients. The role of some form of femoral canal venting with a vent tube or a drill hole remains controversial.

Bipolar versus Unipolar Hemiarthroplasty

Once the decision to perform a hemiarthroplasty has been made, another point of controversy surrounds the use of either a fixed unipolar or a bipolar type of bearing. The bipolar design rationale provides the theoretical benefit of transferring stresses from the articular cartilage to the internal metal-on-polyethylene bearing.[32] Although the preservation of motion at the bipolar bearing over time has been the source of much debate, it is unknown whether any rotation in the sagittal plane occurs at the bipolar interface. Additionally, the amount of bearing motion necessary to decrease stresses in the acetabular cartilage is unknown. Even minuscule amounts of rotation could theoretically cause less stress on the articular cartilage and improve acetabular erosion rates over unipolar designs. Although the amount of motion these bearings allow in vivo is unknown, what is most important is whether patients with these bearings have predictable pain-free ambulation and a low rate of revision for symptomatic acetabular wear. A recent series has documented excellent long-term survivorship of a bipolar hemiarthroplasty for older patients with displaced femoral neck fractures with a very low rate of reoperation for acetabular erosion.[28] The main mode of failure at follow-up was femoral loosening, not acetabular wear. The available literature suggests that the use of a bipolar bearing, at longer follow-up, does appear to favorably decrease acetabular erosion rates over those reported for unipolar designs in ambulatory patients.[3] This fact needs to be weighed against the additional cost of the bipolar bearing and the potential for increased rates of polyethylene wear. The bipolar bearing provides additional interfaces such as locking rings that may potentially cause higher rates of volumetric polyethylene wear and lead to osteolysis in more active patients.

Several prospective randomized and nonrandomized studies exist that compare the results of unipolar and bipolar hemiarthroplasties for displaced fractures of the femoral neck.[3,29,33–37] In general, there appears to be no difference in function, morbidity, or mortality or other complications at short to midterm follow-up. With longer follow-up, however, the bipolar bearing does appear to have some advantage in lower reoperation rates and a very low rate of symptomatic acetabular wear.[3] This is not surprising because patients that live longer are probably more active, and therefore place more stress on the residual acetabular cartilage. Further research is necessary to more definitively determine

whether there is any clear advantage of one choice over the other. The author currently attempts to "demand match" by using cemented stems with bipolar bearings for community ambulators and unipolar bearings for housebound or nursing home ambulators (**Fig. 22–9A–C**).

The Role of Total Hip Arthroplasty

Historically, total hip arthroplasty has been reserved for displaced femoral neck fractures in patients with preexisting symptomatic acetabular degenerative change.[38] This combination of pathology, however, is extremely rare. Most patients with severe arthritis have stiff, thick hip capsules and tend to fracture in the intertrochanteric (extracapsular) region, not the femoral neck. More recently, there has been a trend to expand the indications for total hip arthroplasty to include patients with acute, displaced femoral neck fractures, even in the absence of acetabular pathology. Multiple studies have demonstrated that pain relief, functional improvement, and prosthesis durability are excellent; however, the most problematic complication of total hip arthroplasty for treatment of acute femoral neck fracture is dislocation.[26] Cumulative dislocation rates have averaged 10% across multiple series, even in the hands of experienced arthroplasty surgeons.[38] Multiple reasons have been postulated for this relatively high dislocation rate, including the fact that these patients do not have the typically stiff soft tissues associated with degenerative joint disease and likely regain motion quickly, perhaps allowing impingement and dislocation. There are additional patient variables, including dementia, adduction and flexion contractures, poor soft tissues with advancing age, and inability to follow hip precautions postoperatively. Despite these concerns, in recent studies, including a large prospective, randomized study by Keating et al, total hip arthroplasty demonstrated superior functional outcome when compared with internal fixation or cemented hemiarthroplasty.[26] Additionally, there does not appear to be an increase in morbidity, mortality, or cost in this patient cohort.

The decision on whether to pursue total hip arthroplasty or hemiarthroplasty should be based on patient factors such as activity level, physiological age, expected longevity, and the status of the acetabular articular surface. In general, it should be noted from the available literature that the vast majority of older "community ambulatory" patients treated with cemented hemiarthroplasty will have reasonable function, no or minimal pain, a low reoperation rate, and a dislocation rate of less than 2%.[28] This fact should be weighed against the generally better function but higher dislocation rate associated with total hip arthroplasty.

If total hip arthroplasty is undertaken, consideration should be given to the use of surgical approaches, such as the anterolateral approach, that have been generally associated with a lower dislocation rate.[39] Careful attention to

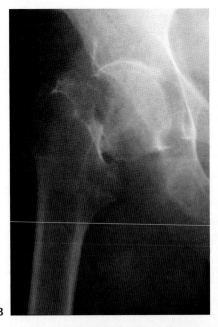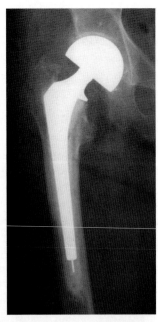

A,B

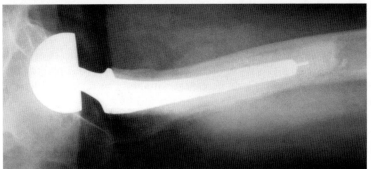

C

Figure 22–9 Displaced femoral neck fracture in a 70-year-old community ambulator. **(A)** Anteroposterior (AP) injury radiograph. **(B)** Postoperative AP radiograph after cemented bipolar hemiarthroplasty. **(C)** Postoperative lateral radiograph.

component positioning, including the selected use of larger-diameter femoral heads or elevated lipped liners, should be considered. It is important to realize that the main reason for dissatisfaction and reoperation for total hip arthroplasty performed in this setting is not aseptic loosening due to polyethylene wear, but recurrent dislocation. The author routinely uses 32 mm heads and an anterolateral approach when performing total hip arthroplasty for acute femoral neck fracture, if the acetabular component size allows for adequate polyethylene liner thickness (**Fig. 22–10A–C**). With recent improvements in the wear characteristics of high molecular weight polyethylene via cross-linking, in vitro data suggest improvement in volumetric polyethylene wear rates with larger-diameter heads when compared with older bearing surfaces. Larger heads confer improved stability by allowing a greater range of motion prior to impingement and dislocation. There are no data, however, to prove that larger head size has any effect on dislocation rate in this patient cohort. Further data are needed to more clearly define the indications for total hip arthroplasty in the setting of the acute displaced femoral neck fracture; however, it may have a role for the more active elderly patient.

Surgical Treatment

Surgical Anatomy

Osseous Anatomy

The mean neck shaft angle of the adult femoral neck is ~130 ± 7 degrees with 10 ± 7 degrees of anteversion.[40-42] These angles are variable, and scrutinizing radiographs of the contralateral hip can assist the surgeon in evaluating accuracy of reduction if internal fixation is planned, or when determining appropriate offset, prosthesis size, and leg lengths if prosthetic replacement is planned.

Vascular Supply to the Femoral Head

An understanding of the blood supply to the femoral head is important to the appropriate treatment of these injuries.[43] Gautier et al investigated the surgical vascular anatomy of the femoral neck by performing a latex injection study that documented perfusion of the femoral head (**Fig. 22–11**).[44] The major blood supply of the femoral head is based posteriorly, arising from the deep branch of the medial

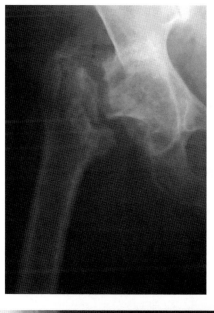
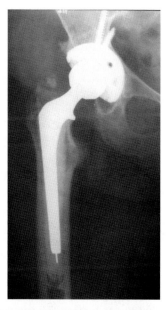

A,B

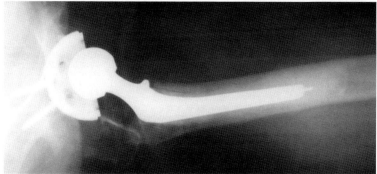

C

Figure 22–10 Femoral neck fracture in a patient with severe preexisting osteoarthritis of the hip. **(A)** Antero-posterior (AP) injury radiograph. **(B)** Postoperative AP radiograph following total hip arthroplasty. **(C)** Post-operative lateral radiograph of total hip arthroplasty.

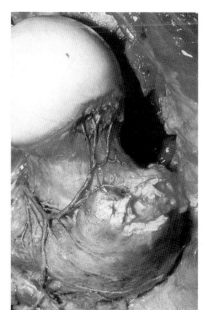
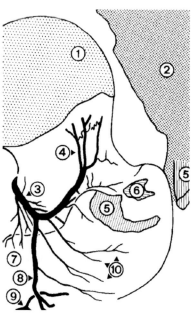

Figure 22–11 Demonstrates the vascularity of the femoral head. Structures demonstrated include the deep branch of the medial femoral circumflex artery (MFCA, 3); the terminal subsynovial branches of the MFCA (4); the insertion of the gluteus medius (5); the insertion of the piriformis (6); the lesser trochanter with nutrient vessels (7); the trochanteric branch (8); the branch of the first perforating artery (9); and the trochanteric branches (10). (Used with permission from Gautier E, Ganz K, Krugel N, et al. Anatomy of the medial femoral circumflex artery and its surgical implications. J Bone Joint Surg Br 2000;82:679–683.)

femoral circumflex artery. This deep branch passes posterior to the obturator externus muscle, anterior to the obturator internus muscle, and finally anterior to the piriformis muscle. It penetrates the synovial fold between the gluteus minimus and the piriformis, and then courses along the posterosuperior aspect of the femoral neck in its intracapsular course. It finally divides into two to four subsynovial retinacular vessels that supply the majority of the femoral head.[44] Other sources of femoral head blood supply include the artery of the ligamentum teres and the inferior metaphyseal artery.[45-50] The artery of the ligamentum teres supplies the small area of the femoral head near the ligamentum teres insertion. The terminal branches of the deep branch of the medial femoral circumflex artery have an anastomosis with the artery of the ligamentum teres. As shown by Sevitt, this anastomosis may be important in the revascularization of the femoral head following a femoral neck fracture.[51] The inferior metaphyseal artery arises from the lateral femoral circumflex artery and supplies a small portion of the inferior femoral head.[45-50] The blood supply to the femoral head can be interrupted by fracture displacement or compression from an intracapsular

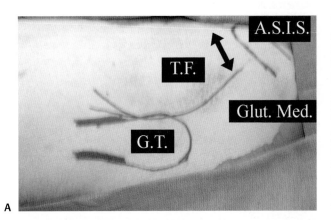

A

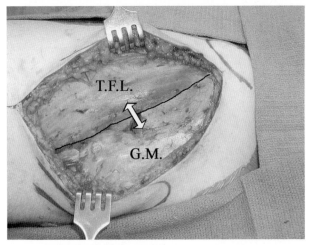

B

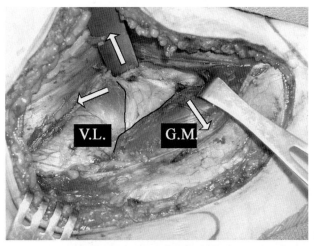

C

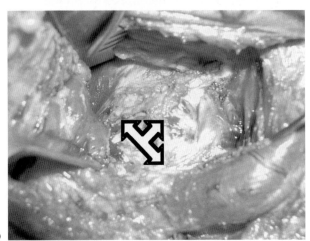

D

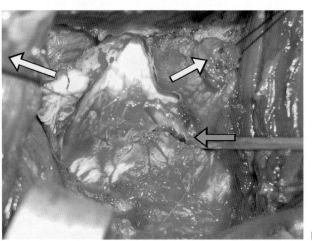

E

Figure 22–12 The Watson-Jones approach for fixation of a femoral neck fracture in a young adult. **(A)** The skin incision is a curvilinear incision centered over the anterior aspect of the greater trochanter that begins 3 to 4 cm posterior to the anterior-superior iliac spine (ASIS). It uses the interval between the fascia tensor (TF) and gluteus medius (GM) muscles. **(B)** Identification of the interval relies upon the fat stripe located between the TFL muscle and the GM muscle (arrow). **(C)** The TFL is retracted anteriorly, and the GM is retracted posteriorly. The origin of the vastus lateralis (VL) often overlies the anterior hip capsule. It is also reflected distally to expose the anterior hip capsule (arrows demonstrate retraction of muscles). **(D)** A T capsulotomy can then be performed in the hip capsule (arrow). **(E)** With the capsulotomy (white arrows) performed, the femoral neck fracture (gray arrow) may be visualized. (Courtesy of Philip J. Kregor, MD)

hematoma. Theoretically, kinking of any vessels not already disrupted by the fracture is possible by fracture displacement; as a result, urgent reduction and capsulotomy may improve perfusion to the femoral head.[52] Additionally, conditions for potential revascularization may be theoretically optimized by stable internal fixation. Claffey demonstrated that these vessels may be intact with displacements of less than one half the diameter of the femoral neck.[49] Therefore, in younger patients it has been recommended that femoral neck fractures should be treated in an urgent fashion. The data are mixed on the efficacy of capsular decompression in an attempt to decrease the rate of osteonecrosis.[4,28,43,52–56] Most traumatologists currently recommend urgent reduction and stable internal fixation with capsulotomy for younger patients because, in this cohort, all efforts are focused on preserving the femoral head. Capsulotomy is relatively simple, adds little operative time, and does not expose the patient to substantial additional risk. Until further clinical data are available, the author recommends capsulotomy for younger patients. The impact of capsulotomy or aspiration of the hip on the final outcome of these injuries, however, has not been clearly elucidated by the available literature and remains controversial. In all likelihood, the fate of the femoral head is determined at the time of injury for the vast majority of patients; however, it may be impossible to predict accurately which patients may benefit from capsulotomy.

The hip capsule has maximum volume with slight flexion and external rotation of the limb. Patients are typically more comfortable in this so-called antalgic position, and attempts to place these patients in traction and internal rotation preoperatively may theoretically decrease capsular volume available for a hematoma and have negative effects on perfusion of the femoral head. In one study, gentle skin traction in the antalgic position was effective in decreasing intracapsular pressures.[57] A supportive pillow under the knee is usually adequate for patient comfort.

Surgical Approaches

Watson-Jones Approach (see Video 22–1, Disk 3)

The patient is placed supine, either on a completely radiolucent table or on a fracture table. Although use of the fracture table facilitates fluoroscopic visualization using the cross-table lateral view and provides rotational control, it may not allow for optimal rotational control of the lower extremity necessary to "fine-tune" the femoral neck reduction. With use of a radiolucent table, a small bump is placed underneath the buttock. The skin incision is a curvilinear one that is centered over the anterior aspect of the greater trochanter and begins 3 to 4 cm posterior to the anterior-superior iliac crest (**Fig. 22–12A**). The location of the avascular interval between the tensor fascia lata muscle and the gluteus medius muscle is identified by the white fat stripe dividing the two muscle bellies (**Fig. 22–12B**). The muscle belly of

the vastus lateralis may be quite large in the young adult and may overlie the hip capsule along the intertrochanteric ridge. It is reflected distally, thus exposing the thick anterior hip capsule (**Fig. 22–12C,D**). A T capsulotomy is then performed. To ensure that the center of the T is along the axis of the femoral neck, fluoroscopy may be utilized. The medial/superior extent of the capsulotomy is developed to the level of the labrum. A Hohman retractor may be placed along the anterior acetabulum to afford appropriate visualization of the femoral neck (**Fig. 22–12E**).

Hardinge Approach

A reasonable and more familiar alternative to the Watson-Jones approach is the lateral approach to the hip described by Hardinge et al.[58] Instead of developing the interval between the tensor fascia lata and gluteus medius, the anterior third of the abductors is released in continuity with a sleeve of the anterior vastus lateralis origin (**Fig. 22–13**). This approach is the author's preference, especially in muscular patients. The capsule is identified and, if not disrupted, incised in an inverted T-shaped fashion. It is helpful to tag the ends of the capsule with sutures to assist with intraoperative retraction. The hematoma is evacuated, and a pointed Hohman retractor placed along the medial calcar region or on the anterior acetabular rim can retract the anterior soft tissue and assist in visualization of the fracture fragments. In larger patients a headlight can help with visualization as well.

Modified Smith-Petersen (modified Heuter) Approach

The modified Smith-Petersen approach can be helpful for ORIF of a subcapital femoral neck fracture, or for placement of a hemiarthroplasty or total hip arthroplasty through a single incision on a specialized fracture table.[59] If this approach is utilized for internal fixation, a separate incision must be made on the lateral aspect of the femur for placement of screws. The patient is placed supine, either on a completely radiolucent table with a bump underneath

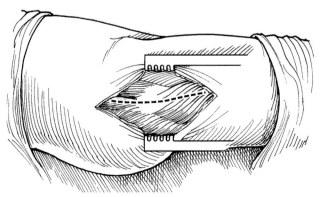

Figure 22–13 The Hardinge approach to the hip. The anterior third of the gluteus medius is released in continuity with the vastus lateralis.

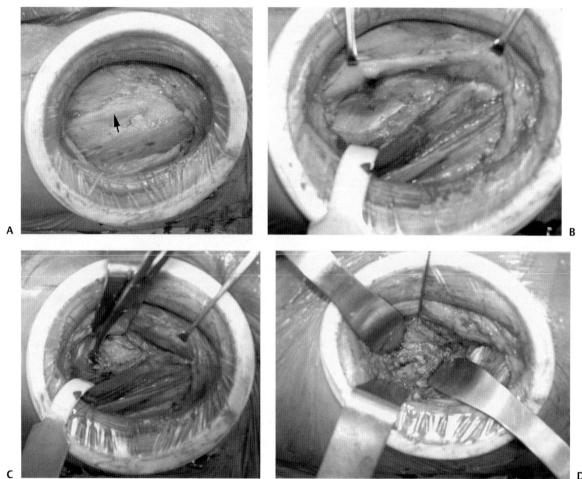

Figure 22–14 **(A)** The modified Hueter approach relies upon the delineation of the fatty stripe between the sartorius and the tensor fascia lata muscle (arrow). **(B)** The fascia of the tensor fascia lata muscle is then incised. Retraction of the fascial layer and lateral retraction of the tensor fascia lata muscle exposes the fatty tissue overlying the hip capsule. The muscle belly of the rectus femoris is also seen.

(C) Branches of the lateral circumflex artery are coagulated. **(D)** A capsulotomy is then performed. In this case retractors are placed around the superior and inferior neck because the patient is undergoing an anterior total hip arthroplasty as described by Matta et al.[59] (Courtesy of Philip J. Kregor, M.D.)

the buttock or on a fracture table. An incision of 10 to 12 cm is made over the muscle belly of the tensor fascia lata muscle (**Fig. 22–14A**). By making the fascial incision over the tensor fascia lata muscle, the surgeon avoids injury to the major branch of the lateral cutaneous nerve of the thigh. However, some smaller branches may be sacrificed. This incision begins ~2 cm posterior and 1 cm distal to the anterior-superior iliac spine, and is directed slightly lateral. The fascia lata is incised over the tensor fascia muscle, and the interval between the sartorius and tensor fascia muscle is developed (**Fig. 22–14B**). Retractors are then utilized to reflect the tensor laterally and the sartorius medially. The straight head of the rectus femoris may then be identified originating from the anterior-inferior iliac spine (AIIS). The reflected head of the rectus femoris is then seen over the superolateral hip capsule. For ORIF, these may then be released, leaving a stump of tissue on the AIIS for later repair. A T capsulotomy can then be made, as already noted for the Watson-Jones approach (**Fig. 22–14C,D**).

Surgical Approaches for Arthroplasty

The surgical approaches (posterior and anterolateral) for arthroplasty are described in the appropriate sections under Surgical Techniques.

Surgical Techniques

Role of Hip Capsulotomy in Open Reduction and Internal Fixation of Femoral Neck Fracture

It is controversial whether capsulotomy prevents osteonecrosis and whether it should be performed during fixation. Multiple clinical series have documented low rates of avascular necrosis and nonunion with in situ fixation in the absence of capsulotomy or other form of hip capsule decompression in the older patient.[15,60–62] In the younger patient with a nondisplaced fracture, however, there is the theoretical concern that the hip capsule may not be disrupted by the injury, and these patients may benefit the most from some form of capsulotomy or hematoma decompression. This may also be the case in the displaced femoral neck fracture. There are no comparative data of series with and without capsulotomy to substantiate this speculation. The two clinical series with the lowest rates of avascular necrosis and nonunion in the treatment of a displaced femoral neck fracture in a young adult both had a formal hip capsulotomy as a prescribed part of the treatment.[63,64] The author currently reserves capsulotomy for younger patients with acute, traumatic, nondisplaced fractures and all patients with displaced fractures that undergo successful closed reduction. Hip capsulotomies are not performed in the treatment of stress fractures or nondisplaced fractures in older patients that are treated with screw fixation because there is no evidence that capsulotomy affects outcome in this setting.

Internal Fixation of a Nondisplaced or Valgus-Impacted Femoral Neck Fracture (see Video 22–2, Disk 3)

The patient is positioned supine on a fracture table. The well leg is gently abducted, avoiding the lithotomy position, which may cause potential increase in well leg compartment pressures. It is critical to ensure that excellent AP and lateral fluoroscopic views that allow imaging of the entire femoral head and neck are possible before preparation and draping. The skin is then prepared and draped, and intravenous prophylactic antibiotics, typically a first-generation cephalosporin, are given. The decision regarding whether to perform the surgery percutaneously or through a small incision is based on surgeon preference and is typically influenced by patient size. The ideal location for the incision can be estimated by placing a guide pin or other metal object along the skin of the anterior thigh and using AP fluoroscopy to estimate the trajectory of the screws. The incision is made where this line intersects the lateral aspect of the femur. It is critical that *the starting point for all screws is above the level of the lesser trochanter* to avoid potential late iatrogenic subtrochanteric fracture (**Fig. 22–15**). Below this level, the cortex of the lateral femur represents the tension side of the subtrochanteric region, an anatomical region that experiences enormous tensile forces with weight bearing. Multiple cortical perforations during guide pin or screw placement in this area are not recommended. Also, screw placement in an inverted V pattern with two screws inferiorly and one screw superiorly is discouraged because of potential stress cracks between the two typically large screw heads on the lateral femoral tension cortex.

The position of the screws in the femoral head and neck is believed to be important to the success of an in situ pinning.[65–72] Placing the first screw "low" along the calcar bone supports the shaft of the screw, thereby minimizing potential inferior displacement of the proximal fragment (**Fig. 22–16A**). Placing the second screw posteriorly along the posterior cortex of the femoral neck is important to

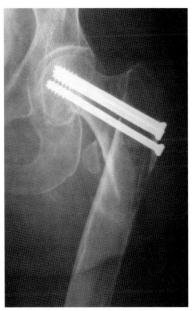

Figure 22–15 A subtrochanteric femur fracture can occur at the site of screw insertion. For this reason, multiple inferior screws should be avoided.

prevent posterior displacement of the proximal fragment (**Fig. 22–16B**). A third screw is typically placed anteriorly, forming a triangular pattern (**Fig. 22–17**). This is especially important for fractures in osteopenic patients because the femoral neck is often "hollow" and lacks adequate cancellous bone to support the shafts of the screws and prevent screw toggle. In general, maximizing the "spread" between screws so that they are as near the femoral neck cortex as possible is encouraged (**Fig. 22–17**). In highly comminuted fractures, some have advocated the use of a fourth screw, thus forming a diamond-shaped pattern; however, the clear advantage of additional screws has not been proven in clinical studies.[16,23,24]

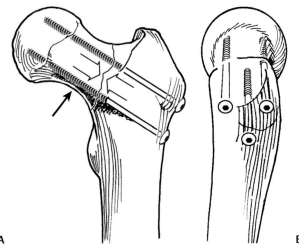

A   B

Figure 22–16 Recommended screw placement. Note the proximity of screw shafts to the cortex of the femoral neck. (**A**) Anteroposterior view. (**B**) Lateral view.

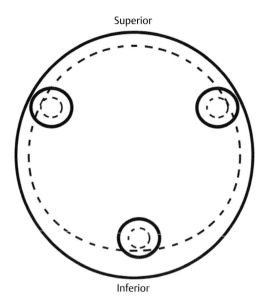

Superior

Inferior

Figure 22–17 Cross-sectional diagram of the femoral neck demonstrating the desired screw "spread" in the femoral neck.

It should be noted that valgus-impacted fractures distort the normal anatomy of the proximal femur. The femoral head is usually impacted into the valgus and somewhat posteriorly relative to the femoral neck. In this situation, screw placement should be guided by the femoral neck. Screws tend to be inserted in the inferior head on the AP view and anterior head on the lateral view in this situation (**Fig. 22–18A–C**).

When appropriate guide pin placement has been confirmed, measurements are taken and the screws are inserted. Screws are placed as parallel as possible and tightened sequentially to allow uniform fracture compression. Multiple commercially available guides are designed to assist parallel guide pin placement. It is important to obtain AP, oblique, and true lateral fluoroscopic views to ensure that all screw threads have crossed the fracture site and that the screw tips have not penetrated the subchondral bone of the femoral head. Most cannulated cancellous screw systems offer short and long thread lengths. Short thread lengths are typically chosen to allow all threads to cross the fracture line and allow compression. Washers are used as indicated for osteopenic patients to prevent overpenetration of the lateral femoral cortex.[73] The wound is closed with interrupted suture for the fascia, subcutaneous tissue, and skin.

Open Reduction and Internal Fixation of Displaced Intracapsular Hip Fractures

The patient is positioned on a fracture table or a radiolucent table, if other injuries dictate. It is the author's preference to use a fracture table when possible due to the improved fluoroscopic visualization of the proximal fragment it offers, when compared with the patient supine on a radiolucent table. Additionally, it allows reduction maneuvers to be

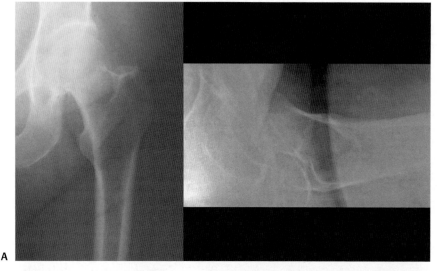

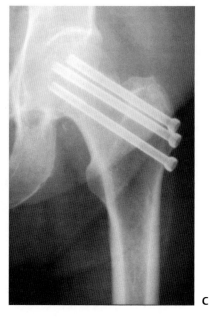

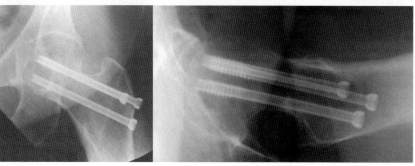

Figure 22–18 Example of a valgus-impacted femoral neck fracture in a 72-year-old female. **(A)** Anteroposterior (AP) and lateral injury radiographic views. **(B)** Postoperative AP and lateral views. **(C)** Follow-up film at 2 years demonstrating uneventful healing.

fine-tuned and held in place. A gentle attempt at closed reduction is performed. This involves good muscle relaxation, axial traction, and internal rotation of the limb. AP and lateral fluoroscopic views are carefully scrutinized to evaluate fracture reduction. If excellent closed reduction is obtained, then the fracture is stabilized as the fracture pattern dictates (as discussed in the section on fixation device selection). Because the quality of reduction is an important determinant of outcome, this step is not rushed, and the radiographs must be carefully scrutinized. Radiographic parameters that are evaluated include assessment of restoration of the normal femoral neck length, restoration of the normal neck-shaft angle, restoration of Shenton's line, and lack of retroversion as viewed on the lateral radiograph. Subtle malreduction and/or malrotation of the femoral neck may lead to lack of stability and failure and may be difficult to discern on fluoroscopic images. The best view in which to scrutinize the reduction is an AP of the hip with the leg internally rotated, combined with a good cross-table radiograph. If there is any concern regarding the quality of reduction as viewed fluoroscopically, a plain film radiograph should be obtained intraoperatively. Capsulotomy is usually performed after the internal fixation is completed. This usually requires extending the wound somewhat proximally because most internal fixation devices used do not routinely require such proximal exposure. The author prefers to pass a Cobb elevator along the anterior capsule and confirm its location with fluoroscopy. A long-handled no. 15 scalpel blade is then used to cut down along the anterior femoral neck as the Cobb retracts and protects the anterior soft tissue.

If imperfect closed reduction is obtained, then open reduction is indicated.[5,52,55] Multiple vigorous attempts at closed reduction may compromise any remaining vascularity to the femoral head or cause bony comminution and are therefore not recommended. The exact amount of angulation or displacement that defines an acceptable reduction has not been well documented. Some authors have recommended a slight valgus reduction because this position is more stable with compression; however, any varus tilt of the proximal fragment should not be accepted.[5,52,55] Anatomical reduction in both AP and lateral planes is recommended.

Any of the three approaches described under Surgical Approaches can be utilized for open reduction. The Watson-Jones approach has been most utilized. The Smith-Petersen approach may be helpful in subcapital fractures, and the Hardinge approach may be helpful in very muscular patients.

Usually the femoral head is located posterior to the femoral shaft. A helpful technical tip to assist with obtaining reduction is to initially distract the entire distal femoral fragment laterally with the help of a large bone hook or Shanz pin in the region just above the lesser trochanter (**Fig. 22–19A,B**). This can disimpact a malaligned fracture and allow free positioning of the fracture fragments with a dental pick or Schanz pin used as a reduction aid in the femoral head fragment. The distal fragment is then allowed to settle back on the proximal fragment, and the reduction is confirmed visibly, by palpation with a finger, and with fluoroscopic imaging. Evaluating the accuracy of reduction can be quite challenging in comminuted fractures, especially when attempting to judge correct rotation (anteversion). Evaluating cortical widths fluoroscopically can assist with determining accuracy of reduction. Having a radiograph of the contralateral side can assist the surgeon in judging the neck-shaft and anteversion angles that are

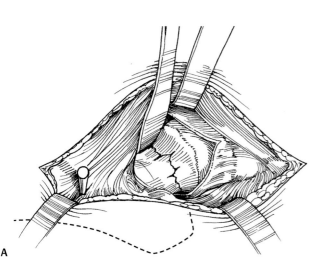

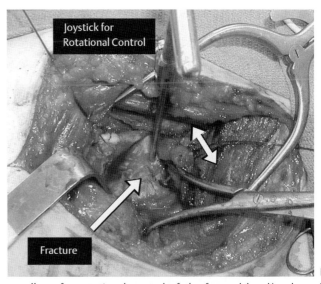

Figure 22–19 Reduction strategy for a femoral neck fracture in a young adult via the Watson-Jones approach. **(A)** Illustration of the femoral neck fracture after it is exposed. With the T capsulotomy performed, the femoral neck fracture is well visualized. **(B)** In this clinical case, a Schanz pin placed in the femoral neck allows for rotational control of the femoral head/neck, and a pointed reduction clamp allows for compression of the femoral neck fracture. The long arrow points to the fracture which is directly seen. The double arrow delineates the interval between the tensor fascia and gluteus medius muscle.

"anatomical" for the particular patient. When reduction is deemed satisfactory, provisional fixation with multiple 2 mm Kirschner wires is recommended to avoid rotation of the proximal fragment during definitive stabilization. In addition, modified clamps may be utilized to help obtain compression across the femoral neck fracture before screw introduction (**Fig. 22–19B**). The choice of fixation device used for definitive stabilization is based on the fracture configuration and surgeon preference and has been discussed previously. After definitive stabilization, the capsule is typically either left completely open or very loosely approximated with a few absorbable sutures to allow adequate drainage of any subsequent hematoma. A deep drain is recommended. If partially released, the abductors are repaired with heavy nonabsorbable suture and a layered closure performed in the usual fashion.

Special Case: Ipsilateral Femoral Neck/Femoral Shaft Combination in the Young Adult (see Video 22–3, Disk 3)

A femoral neck fracture is present in 2 to 6% of patients with femoral shaft fractures.[74–78] The femoral neck fracture is often not initially diagnosed, being missed in up to 33% of cases.[76] This may arise from the fact that the proximal aspect of the femur is often externally rotated in the setting of a femoral shaft fracture (**Fig. 22–1A–C**). An intraoperative plain film AP pelvis at the end of the intramedullary nailing of the femur with the legs internally rotated (putting the femoral neck on profile) lessens the risk of a "missed fracture."[79] The most accurate visualization of the femoral neck occurs with 15 degrees of internal rotation, and therefore may not be optimally seen in an AP pelvis radiograph of a patient with a femoral shaft fracture. If there is a suspicion of a femoral neck fracture before femoral shaft fixation, this may be investigated with use of an obturator oblique Judet view of the pelvis because this puts the femoral neck "on profile." Additionally, a good-quality cross-table lateral of the hip may also indicate the presence of a femoral neck fracture. Finally, abdominal and pelvic CT scans that are often a part of trauma protocols may also detect a minimally displaced femoral neck fracture (**Fig. 22–1A–C**).

The treatment options and algorithms differ according to whether the fracture is recognized *before* treatment of the femoral shaft fracture, or is recognized *during or after* fixation of the femoral shaft fracture. If the femoral neck fracture is recognized before treatment of the femoral shaft fracture, the femoral neck fracture takes "first priority." Treatment options include ORIF of the femoral neck (with placement of screws in the anterior and posterior aspect of the femoral neck) followed by antegrade intramedullary nailing, cephalomedullary nailing (e.g., Russell-Taylor reconstruction femoral nailing), ORIF of the femoral neck followed by retrograde intramedullary nailing of the femur, and ORIF of the femoral neck followed by plate fixation of the femoral shaft fracture. The first two options have a potential disadvantage

of compromising the femoral neck reduction or fixation by the subsequent nailing procedure. However, acceptable results have been reported with both treatments. Wu and Shih utilized antegrade intramedullary nailing followed by screw fixation in 22 patients.[77] No cases of osteonecrosis or nonunions were noted at an average follow-up of 26 months. Wiss et al reviewed their experience with 33 consecutive adult patients with ipsilateral femoral neck and shaft fractures between 1984 and 1987.[80] All but one patient sustained a Pauwels III (vertical shear fracture), with 67% of them being basilar neck fractures and 33% of them being transcervical. Their surgical protocol was a reduction of the femoral neck fracture, followed by intramedullary nailing of the femoral shaft fracture. In nine cases, provisional Kirschner wire fixation of the femoral neck was performed before intramedullary nailing. Initially, standard first-generation intramedullary nails were utilized. With these nails (19 patients), five of 19 cases resulted in a varus nonunion of the femoral neck, with two of these five also developing avascular necrosis. They concluded: "Reamed antegrade femoral nailing and supplemental cancellous screw fixation of the femoral neck fracture has not proven uniformly successful."

Randelli et al reported on a series of 27 ipsilateral femoral neck and shaft fractures treated with the Russell-Taylor reconstruction nail.[81] Fifty-two percent of the fractures were displaced (Garden III or IV fractures). A closed reduction of the femoral neck fracture was then performed, followed by provisional Kirschner wire fixation in the anterior aspect of the femoral neck. A reamed Russell-Taylor reconstruction nail was then placed, utilizing the proximal interlocking screws for definitive fixation of the femoral neck. They reported one case of avascular necrosis, one case of a femoral shaft varus malunion, and four cases of heterotopic ossification about the hip.

Rather than performing fixation of the femoral neck around an antegrade nail, other options include ORIF of the femoral neck followed by either retrograde intramedullary nailing or plate fixation of the femoral shaft. Swiontkowski et al reported a series of 15 patients treated with urgent ORIF utilizing lag screws of the femoral neck, followed by either retrograde intramedullary nailing or plate fixation.[76] Although all fractures healed, two patients did develop avascular necrosis of the femoral head.

Thus the treatment for the high-energy, displaced femoral neck fracture combined with a femoral shaft fracture remains without one single best treatment option. Mandatory for a good result with all treatment modalities, however, is an anatomical reduction and fixation of the displaced femoral neck fracture.

A femoral neck fracture may become evident *during or after* fixation of a femoral shaft fracture. This may be possible because

- The femoral neck fracture was not visible on the injury films of the hip because the proximal femur was externally rotated.

- A nondisplaced fracture of the femoral neck became displaced with intramedullary nail fixation.
- True iatrogenic creation of a femoral neck fracture occurred during nail insertion.

Simonian et al reported on the latter situation. Four apparently iatrogenic femoral neck fractures occurred in a series of 315 intramedullary nailings of the femoral shaft.[82] In these cases, the femoral neck fracture may be reduced and internally fixed with the intramedullary nail left in place. The fracture should be addressed as already discussed regarding femoral neck fixation in the young adult. In rare cases, the nail may need to be removed to obtain an appropriate reduction of the femoral neck.

Arthroplasty for Displaced Femoral Neck Fractures (see Video 22–4, Disk 3)

Femoral Canal Preparation: General Principles

The goal of femoral canal preparation, regardless of stem type chosen, is to align the femoral component with the central aspect of the femoral canal in both coronal and sagittal planes. Achieving rotational stability of the component is critical as well. The appropriate component anteversion varies based on whether the anterior or posterior approach is utilized and the native anteversion of the host femur. There is a strong tendency for varus and flexion malalignment with the use of the anterolateral approach due to the surgeon's desire to protect the remaining abductors during canal preparation (**Fig. 22–20A,B**). It is probably preferable to release slightly more of the abductors initially

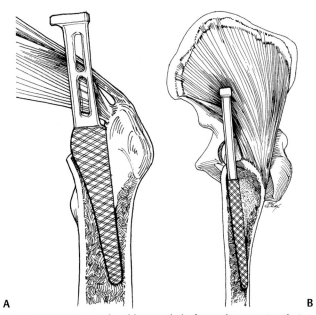

Figure 22–20 Potential problems with the femoral preparation during the Hardinge approach for hip arthroplasty. **(A)** Varus canal preparation due to trochanteric overhang and abductor musculature. **(B)** Flexion canal preparation should be avoided.

and perform a secure repair later than to damage the abductors with reamers or broaches during canal preparation. Scrutiny and templating of the preoperative radiographs can estimate the amount of trochanteric overhang and thereby assist the surgeon in anticipating the amount of trochanteric bone that must be reamed to avoid varus stem alignment. Such malalignments are less problematic with femoral preparation performed through the posterior approach due to easier retraction of the abductor mass and better visualization of the posterolateral portion of the femoral neck. It is important to note that the anteroposterior dimension of the proximal femur will limit the ultimate size of the femoral component in the elderly patient because the femoral isthmus is generally quite capacious with advancing age. The femur should be broached until visible proximal fit and fill are obtained, the broach will not advance with gentle hammer blows, and rotational stability is obtained.

Anterolateral Approach for Arthroplasty

The patient is positioned in the lateral decubitus position with hip rests or some form of positioning device to carefully maintain the patient in a stable lateral position. Evaluation of the horizontality of the gluteal crease can assist in determining whether the pelvis is appropriately aligned. The lateral knee of the down leg should be well padded to protect the peroneal nerve. The skin is then prepared and draped in the usual fashion, and intravenous antibiotics, typically a first-generation cephalosporin, are given. An incision centered on the greater trochanter is made with a slight curve posteriorly. This is deepened through the fascia, and the trochanteric bursa is excised from the lateral aspect of the trochanter. The size of the abductor mass is evaluated, and ~40% of the anterior insertion is released. This can be done either with a pure abductor tendon release or in continuity with a sleeve of the anterior vastus lateralis, depending on the quality of the tissues and surgeon preference. Some authors have recommended the release of a small sliver of bone from the anterior trochanter with the abductor tendons to allow secure reattachment and bone-to-bone healing.[58] The capsule is exposed. It is preferable to preserve the capsule and the labrum for stability reasons if a hemiarthroplasty is being performed. The capsule is incised in an inverted T-shaped fashion, and the edges are tagged with a suture. The hip is then dislocated and placed in a sterile pocket on the anterior aspect of the operating table. The top of the lesser trochanter is palpated, and a femoral neck cut is made based on preoperative templating of the appropriate level of neck resection. With most femoral neck fractures, the definitive neck cut involves simply freshening the proximal femur with a saw blade. Performing the definitive neck cut immediately will allow greater exposure to remove the femoral head fragment, which remains in the acetabulum. The femoral head fragment can be removed either with a corkscrew driven into the center of the head fragment or with a grasping rongeur. Removing the entire head in one piece is preferable if possible to facilitate accurate sizing of the hemiarthroplasty.

The acetabulum is then evaluated for cartilage wear and inspected for free fracture fragments. Fracture fragments can often be found posteriorly along the femoral neck or in the cotyloid fossa. If a hemiarthroplasty is being performed, the diameter of the removed femoral head is measured with a pass-through hole gauge or a caliper. A combination of this measurement and preoperative templating can assist in determining the appropriate size of the hemiarthroplasty component. Acetabular trials are also used to accurately size the hemiarthroplasty component. Ideally there is a solid "suction" type fit into the acetabular cavity. Trials often have slots to allow visual assessment of appropriate seating. It is important not to oversize the component, which can lead to peripheral loading, instability, and pain, nor to undersize the component, which can lead to medial erosion, instability, and pain as well. It is typical to require a hemiarthroplasty the identical size of the resected femoral head or occasionally a millimeter larger. It is unusual to require a hemiarthroplasty component smaller than that of the resected femoral head. Once appropriate acetabular sizing has been determined, attention is turned to the proximal femur. Great care should be taken to protect the remaining abductor insertion while femoral canal preparation is performed. Due to the concern of injuring the remaining abductors during femoral preparation, there is a tendency to prepare the femoral canal in varus and flexion. In very soft osteopenic bone, it is recommended that reaming be performed by hand. Once appropriate reaming and broaching are performed to achieve rotational stability of the trial, a trial reduction is performed. Most systems offer a choice of neck shaft angle. The appropriate neck shaft angle that restores the patient's offset can be estimated by templating the opposite unfractured side preoperatively. The trials are assembled and the hip reduced.

If the capsule has not been released all the way to the labrum and retracted well with tag sutures, reduction can be difficult due to soft tissue interposition. Vigorous attempts at trial reduction can cause the broach to rotate in the proximal femur, leading to proximal femoral fracture. If reduction is difficult, the neck resection level should be reevaluated, and the capsule released further, if necessary. In general, the center of rotation of the femoral head corresponds to the tip of the greater trochanter. Leg lengths are evaluated, and the hip is placed through a full range of motion. It is ideal to be able to flex the hip in neutral to over 90 degrees and internally rotate the hip fully without any tendency for posterior dislocation. When using the anterior approach, it is very important that the hip be stable with full extension and external rotation as well. It is wise to follow the native anteversion of the femoral neck during femoral preparation when performing a hemiarthroplasty

through the anterior approach. Any excessive anteversion can potentially result in impingement and anterior instability. The femoral canal should be irrigated and dried prior to placement of a cement restrictor plug. The restrictor is inserted to a depth of approximately 2 cm distal to the prosthesis tip and centralizer if used. The femoral canal is then prepared with irrigation, suction, and careful drying, and the cement is then introduced under pressurization, unless there is some concern about potential for hemodynamic instability with cementation. The author considers all elderly hip fracture patients as "high risk" for infection and routinely adds antibiotics (gentamicin) to the cement mixture. The cement is allowed to cure with the component held in the desired amount of anteversion and then all extraneous cement is removed.

The acetabulum is then irrigated and evaluated for any bony or cement debris. If repeat trial reduction reveals excellent stability, then the real hemiarthroplasty components are assembled, and the hip is reduced. It is important to check the stability of the hip and leg lengths multiple times during the operation. The capsule is closed with heavy absorbable suture, and the abductors are securely reattached to their bed with heavy no. 5 nonabsorbable suture through bone. A deep drain is placed, and the fascia is closed with absorbable sutures. The subcutaneous tissues and skin are closed in the usual fashion. The patient is placed in a lightly compressive dressing and a hip abduction pillow and transferred to the recovery room.

Posterolateral Approach for Hemiarthroplasty

The patient is positioned in a lateral decubitus position, and intravenous antibiotics are given, typically a first-generation cephalosporin. An incision is centered over the greater trochanter and curved more posteriorly than that typical for an anterior approach. The fascia is opened, and the bursa is excised from the posterior aspect of the trochanter. The leg is internally rotated, putting the posterior structures under tension. The piriformis tendon is located superiorly with blunt dissection, and a blunt retractor can be placed in the interval between the piriformis and the gluteus minimus proximally. The piriformis, short external rotators, and capsule are then released subperiosteally from the posterior aspect of the femur as a single thick musculocapsular sleeve for later reattachment. Secure anatomical repair of this flap at the completion of the procedure may decrease the risk of dislocation. The hip is internally rotated further, and a femoral neck cut is made using preoperative templating and the lesser trochanter as a guide to the appropriate level of neck resection. The femoral head is removed in a similar fashion to that described for the anterolateral approach. Appropriate acetabular sizing and femoral component preparation are performed. It is important when using the posterior approach to ensure that the arthroplasty is stable in flexion and internal rotation to allow stability when seated, and the adducted, flexed, internally rotated so-called position of sleep. Upon completion of the arthroplasty, the posterior capsulotendinous flap is secured in its anatomical location through drill holes in bone with nonabsorbable suture. Deep drains are placed under the fascia. The subcutaneous tissues and skin are closed in the usual fashion.

Total Hip Arthroplasty: Surgical Technique of Acetabular Preparation

If total hip arthroplasty is the therapeutic option chosen for the patient, then the acetabulum is carefully exposed circumferentially, typically removing the capsule and labrum. It is critical to have excellent circumferential visualization of the acetabular rim prior to reaming. Pointed Hohman retractors levering on the outside of the acetabular rim should be used with caution in osteopenic patients. The acetabulum is carefully reamed until a concentric bleeding bed of cancellous bone remains. It is important to realize that in sharp contradistinction to the patient population with degenerative arthritis, the acetabular cartilage in most hip fracture patients is essentially normal; therefore, the dense subchondral bone present in the patient with degenerative arthritis will not be present. These patients will usually not have the medial osteophyte and lateralized hip center that is so common in patients with osteoarthritis; therefore, very careful reaming is recommended to prevent penetration of the medial wall or damage to one of the acetabular columns. Often the final reamer can be used on reverse to impact, rather than remove, bone. The appropriate cup size can be estimated from preoperative templating, from reamer fit, and with trials.

The decision to implant a cemented or uncemented acetabular component is based on surgeon preference and bone quality. The author prefers to use uncemented components in this setting. These components allow intraoperative flexibility by offering various polyethylene liner and head size options that may be advantageous in this patient population, which is plagued by concerning dislocation rates. It is recommended that the difference in the true diameter of the last reamer used and that of the acetabular component should not exceed 2 mm to minimize the risk of fracture. The uncemented acetabular component is then carefully impacted in the appropriate amount of abduction and anteversion. From the anterolateral approach it is important not to place excessive anteversion on the acetabular component. Anterior instability from impingement of the neck of the femoral component on the posterior rim of the cup can be problematic. It is wise in osteopenic patients to augment initial cup stability with screws. If a cemented cup is chosen, cement anchoring holes are typically made with a curet in the ilium, ischium, and pubis, and the component is cemented into this bed. To avoid undesirable inferior cement extravasation, the inferior aspect of the acetabular component is inserted first, then the cup is tipped into the appropriate abduction and

anteversion. This causes the excess cement to extravasate superiorly, facilitating removal of any extraneous cement. It is important to hold the cup securely in the desired position during cementation. Trial reduction and closure are performed in a similar fashion described previously.

Tips and Tricks

- In ORIF of the femoral neck, 4.0 mm Schanz pins in the femoral neck and a 5.0 Schanz pin in the proximal femur (at the level of the lesser trochanter) can be utilized as rotational reduction aids.
- Direct visualization of the femoral neck fracture reduction best determines the quality of the reduction. In general, reliance on fluoroscopic interpretation may lead to malreduction.
- The common deformity in a malreduction of the femoral neck is varus and anterior apex angulation. Restoration of Shenton's line can be used to judge the restoration of the normal neck-shaft angle radiographically. Careful appraisal of the cross-table lateral is helpful to ensure that the normal anteversion for the femoral neck has been re-created.
- In arthroplasty for a femoral neck fracture, "cutout" of the corkscrew is common and problematic when removing an osteoporotic femoral head. This can be minimized by holding the femoral head with the surgeon's thumb during insertion of the corkscrew. The corkscrew should be directed toward the center of the femoral head.
- Careful preoperative templating is mandatory when planning a hemiarthroplasty or arthroplasty for a femoral neck fracture in an elderly adult. Often, the injured patient has poor-quality rotated films that make good preoperative templating difficult. If the surgeon relies on a femoral neck cut 1 cm above the lesser trochanter, this will lead to leg length differences in patients with a valgus or varus neck. Therefore, a good-quality AP pelvis radiograph should be obtained at the time the patient undergoes anesthesia if the films are not adequate. The hips should be internally rotated, with a slight amount of traction on the involved limb, and the pelvis should be flat on the x-ray cassette.

Rehabilitation

One of the major advantages of surgical treatment of femoral neck fractures is the ability to mobilize the patient immediately postoperatively. In general, patients treated with prosthetic replacement can bear weight as tolerated. Hip dislocation precautions should be taught by physical therapy to minimize the risk of dislocation. If ORIF was performed, weight-bearing decisions should be guided by bone quality, fracture pattern, and quality of fixation. Typically, patients will "self-regulate" weight bearing based on pain; thus weight bearing can progress as tolerated, which may also facilitate functional rehabilitation.[83–85]

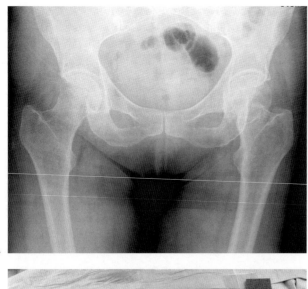

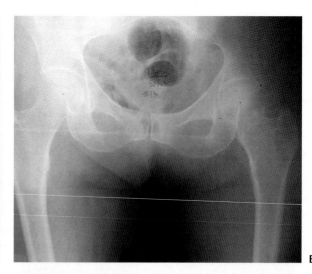

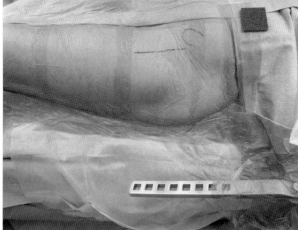

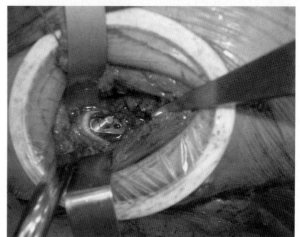

Figure 22–21 The case of a femoral neck in a very active 72-year-old female treated by total hip arthroplasty. The surgical approach was a single anterior modified Hueter approach, as described by Matta et al.[59] **(A)** Anteroposterior (AP) radiograph of the pelvis showing a left femoral neck fracture. **(B)** Templating x-ray. A no. 13 femoral stem and a 52 or 54 mm acetabular cup are planned. A femoral neck cut 19 mm above the top of the lesser trochanter is planned. **(C)** Supine positioning on the fracture table (OSI ProFx table). The Smith-Petersen approach is drawn on the skin. **(D)** With extension, external rotation, and adduction of the leg, the proximal femur may be exposed and broaching performed. Here, the broach is in place before trialing of neck sizes.

New Techniques

Improved Fixation in Osteoporotic Bone

The major limiting factor to achieving stable internal fixation of the proximal fragment is poor bone quality. New techniques and implants will likely focus on some method of improving local screw purchase. Bioactive coatings may improve screw purchase and speed healing, thereby placing less stress on the internal fixation device. Insufflation of cement, calcium phosphates, or other such materials through ports in fixation devices may provide improved screw purchase.[86,87] Perhaps with such innovations the indications for internal fixation will expand, and fixation failure rates will decrease. Prophylactic fixation of the contralateral hip with injectable synthetic bone cements or other "orthobiologics" will be investigated because it is recognized that the risk of a contralateral hip fracture in elderly patients is concerning.

Single-Incision Anterior Approach for Hip Arthroplasty on an Orthopaedic Table (see Video 22–5, Disk 3)

Matta et al have described a modification of the Hueter anterior approach to the hip with utilization of a specialized orthopaedic fracture table (ProFix, Orthopedic Systems Inc., Union City, California).[59] This approach was originally described by Judet and Judet in 1947.[88,89] The use of the fracture table allows placement of the acetabular component and femoral component through a ~10 cm modified Hueter approach, with the patient supine. The table allows hyperextension, adduction, and external rotation of the leg. This, combined with proximal femoral elevation via use of a table hook, allows visualization of the proximal femur through the

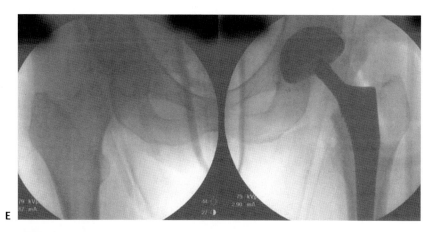

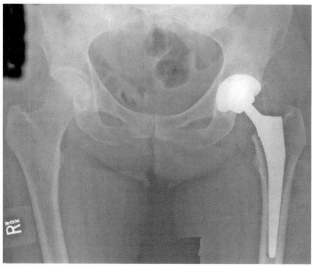

Figure 22–21 *(Continued)* **(E)** Intraoperative fluoroscopic views of both hips. Offset and neck length can be compared "real time" with the opposite side. **(F)** Postoperative AP radiograph. (Courtesy of Philip J. Kregor, MD)

modified Hueter approach. Fluoroscopic control of placement of the implants is possible. Matta et al reported on 494 primary total hip arthroplasty surgeries performed with this technique.[59] The majority of the arthroplasties were uncemented (442 hips); the remaining were hybrid. Ninety-six percent of the acetabular cups were placed in the accepted range of 35 to 50 degrees of abduction; 93% of the acetabular cups were placed in the target range of 10 to 25 degrees of anteversion. Leg length discrepancy averaged 3 mm, with a range of 0 to 26 mm. Three patients had dislocations, with an overall dislocation rate of 0.61%. Overall, there were 17 operative complications, including three greater trochanter fractures and three ankle fractures. These complications are the result of manipulation of the leg by the table to expose the proximal femur for femoral canal broaching and femoral component insertion. This surgical technique may have particular advantages in the elderly, including

- Supine positioning of the patient
- Total preservation of the abductors
- Low rate of dislocation (particularly helpful in bedridden patients)
- Accurate intraoperative assessment of component positioning and leg length restoration

The technique has not been described specifically for femoral neck fractures, but both hemiarthroplasties and arthroplasties may be utilized with this approach **(Fig. 22–21A–F)**.

Outcomes

Internal Fixation in Young Adults

Historically, the displaced femoral neck fracture in a young adult was associated with an 86% incidence of osteonecrosis and a 59% chance of nonunion. Noting these poor results, Swiontkowski and Gerber et al recommended a protocol of emergent open reduction and rigid fixation with cancellous lag screws.[52,63] They also emphasized direct visualization of the fracture via a Watson-Jones approach. Swiontkowski et al reported that 20 patients had a 0% nonunion rate and a 20% incidence of osteonecrosis.[64] Gerber et al reported on a series of 54 patients with an overall 10% rate of osteonecrosis and a 17% rate of delayed union or nonunion.[63] In a retrospective review of a 25-year experience from the Mayo Clinic, 73 femoral neck fractures

(51 displaced, 22 nondisplaced) in patients between the ages of 15 and 50 years were followed until union or conversion to hip arthroplasty, or for at least 2 years.[55] Fifty-two fractures were treated with cannulated screws, and 17 were treated with a sliding hip screw. Thirty-seven of 51 displaced fractures were treated with a closed reduction and internal fixation, and 14 were treated with an ORIF. Overall, 73% of the fractures healed after one operation and had no osteonecrosis at 2 years. Twenty-three percent of the fractures developed osteonecrosis, and 8% developed a nonunion. In considering only the displaced fractures, 10% developed a nonunion and 27% developed osteonecrosis. The overall rate of femoral head retention was 82% at 6.6 years.

Femoral Neck Fractures in Elderly Adults

Outcomes of a femoral neck fracture in an elderly (> 65 years of age) adult should be judged not only by fracture complications but also by mortality rates and functional outcomes. A recent meta-analysis by Bhandari et al provides a relatively concise, though not exhaustive, overview of the key factors related to the outcomes following arthroplasty versus internal fixation in patients 65 years of age or greater.[2] Their meta-analysis included 14 reports published between 1969 and 2002 with valid comparative data regarding internal fixation versus arthroplasty. The pooled sample size from the meta-analysis was 1901 patients. Several key concepts were elucidated:

- Arthroplasty (hemiarthroplasty or total hip arthroplasty) substantially reduces the prevalence of surgical revision, with the revision rates ranging from 0 to 24% in arthroplasty groups and 10 to 49% in the internal fixation group. Compared with internal fixation, arthroplasty reduced the relative risk of revision surgery by 77%. According to these data, for every six patients treated with arthroplasty instead of internal fixation, one revision surgery could be avoided. In looking specifically at internal fixation cases, the risk of reoperation trended toward an increase in cases treated with screws alone versus a compression hip screw.
- Arthroplasty is associated with an increased risk of infection, more surgical blood loss, and a longer operating time.
- There is a trend toward increased mortality at 1 year after arthroplasty compared with internal fixation. One-year mortality rates were 23% (226/981) in arthroplasty patients, and 20% (160/783) in internal fixation patients.
- For internal fixation, the rates of nonunion were 18.5%. Avascular necrosis was seen in 9.7% of cases.
- The overall dislocation rate following all types of arthroplasty was 0.82%. However, when looking at total hip arthroplasty, the mean dislocation rate was 6.9%. There was no statistical evidence that the type of

approach (anterolateral vs posterior) affected dislocation rates. (This is in contrast to the previous meta-analysis by Lu-Yao et al, which reported a trend of higher dislocation rates with a posterior versus an anterolateral approach.[3])
- The overall estimated conclusion was that for every 100 patients treated with arthroplasty instead of internal fixation, 17 revision surgeries can be avoided, but at the expense of four more wound infections, four additional deaths, and one hip dislocation.

Complications

Medical Complications

Associated injuries are common in younger patients, whereas postoperative medical complications are common in elderly patients. All patients with a femoral neck fracture are at high risk of venous thromboembolism, so some form of prophylaxis is indicated, usually involving both mechanical methods and pharmacological agents. Consultation and concomitant medical management with an internist may result in shorter hospital stays and a lower rate of complications in a recent study. Early mobilization and aggressive pulmonary toilet may decrease complication rates. The elderly patient population undergoing surgical treatment for femoral neck fracture has demonstrated a significantly higher mortality than age-matched controls.[5,35,83,90–93] It has been recommended that elderly patients be either referred or evaluated and treated for osteoporosis to potentially decrease the incidence of other fragility fractures.[94]

Nonunion

Fortunately, nonunion of the femoral neck fracture in young patients is relatively uncommon.[5,52,55,95,96] The treatment of nonunion in the younger patient is focused on preservation of the native femoral head.[97] There are two general categories of treatment methods used to salvage femoral neck nonunions in young patients. The first are corrective osteotomies, typically valgus intertrochanteric osteotomies, which convert the deforming shear force of a vertical fracture line to the compressive force of a horizontal fracture line (**Fig. 22–22A–C**). Multiple studies have documented the efficacy of this procedure in achieving bony union even in the face of small patches of avascular necrosis.[98–102] The functional outcomes, however, have been good but not outstanding, probably due to the decreased offset and abductor efficiency with valgus osteotomy.[103] Interestingly, most nonunions in young patients demonstrate high fracture verticality with varus tilt and foreshortening of the femoral neck. Often these have been treated previously with cannulated screws (**Fig. 22–22A–C**). It is extremely unusual to see a nonunion of a low shear angle fracture in a young

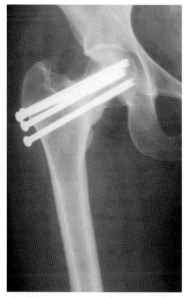
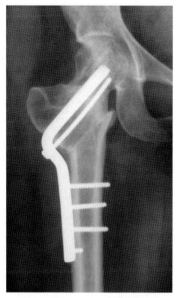

A,C

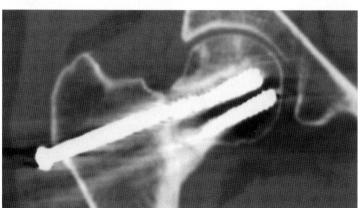

B

Figure 22–22 Nonunion of a vertical femoral neck fracture in a young patient treated with multiple cannulated screws. **(A)** Note varus displacement and inferior shearing of the proximal fragment. **(B)** Computed tomographic scan confirming nonunion. **(C)** Postoperative view after valgus intertrochanteric osteotomy. The patient went on to heal without problems.

patient. The other broad category of salvage options includes some form of bone grafting. This may either be a nonvascularized graft (with or without a muscle pedicle) or a free vascularized osseous graft. The Meyers quadratus pedicle graft has perhaps been the most widely studied.[104,105] The exact indications for each of these bone-grafting techniques, however, have not been well elucidated. A summary of the clinical results of these various bone-grafting options are detailed in **Table 22–1**.[104–111]

In general, nonunion in the older patient is treated with prosthetic replacement. Failure is typically due to poor bone quality and is not amenable to repeat internal fixation attempts. Nonunion rates in elderly patients as high as 40% have been reported.[5,112] The results of hip arthroplasty for salvage of failed treatment of femoral neck fractures have been documented by many authors.[97,113–116] Either hemiarthroplasty or total hip arthroplasty can be successful depending on the status of the articular cartilage and surgeon preference. Pain relief is probably more predictable with total hip arthroplasty, however. These reconstructions typically have certain unique technical challenges and are

also plagued by concerning rates of instability. Limb shortening, bony defects from previous hardware, often broken, deformity, and osteopenic bone all pose challenges to the successful arthroplasty in this setting. Pain relief and functional improvement, however, are predictable.

Osteonecrosis

Osteonecrosis after femoral neck fracture may or may not be symptomatic.[4,52,55,95,117,118] Rates of osteonecrosis of ~25% for displaced fractures have been reported.[5,114] A discussion of all the treatment options for avascular necrosis for the young patient after femoral neck fracture is beyond the scope of this chapter. In general, femoral head salvage operations are considered for symptomatic patients with precollapse osteonecrosis. Many methods for attempts at salvage or delay of total hip arthroplasty have been recommended, with varying results, including bone grafting, either free vascularized or nonvascularized, or some form of proximal femoral osteotomy designed to reposition the necrotic area out of the weight-bearing dome.[117] The

Table 22-1 Summary of Results of Various Bone-Grafting Techniques for Nonunion of the Femoral Neck

Series	No. Patients	Mean F/U	Mean Age	% AVN Preop	Type of Graft	% Fracture Union	% AVN Progression	% Converted to THA
LeCroy et al[106]	22	85 mos	29	All 16/22 stage I and II 6/22 III and up	Free vascularized fibula	20/22 (91%)	13/22 (59%)	2/22 (9%)
Nagi et al[107]	40 neglected fractures	68 mos	35	8/40 (20%)	Free vascularized fibula	37/40 (93%)	7/40 (18%)	3/40 (8%)
Hou et al[108]	5 neglected fractures	2 years	24	None	Iliac crest pedicle (deep circumflex iliac artery)	5/5 (100%)	None	None
Leung et al[109]	15	3.5 years	38	None	Iliac crest pedicle (deep circumflex iliac artery)	15/15 (100%)	1/15 (7%)	1/15 (7%)
Nagi et al[110]	26	29 mos	39	4/26 (15%)	Autograft fibula nonvascularized	25/26 (96%)	0	None
Baksi[105]	56	35 mos	42	34/56 All stage I and II (61%)	Quadratus femoris muscle-pedicle	42/56 (75%)	2/34 (6%)	Not stated
Meyers et al[104]	32	14 followed > 1 year	16–79	Not stated	Quadratus femoris muscle-pedicle	23/32 (72%)	Not stated	Not stated
Henderson[111]	77	69 followed to union	46	Not stated	Autograft fibula or tibia, nonvascularized	46/49 (69%)	Not stated	Not stated

AVN, avascular necrosis; F/U, follow-up; THA, total hip arthroplasty.

amount and location of femoral head involvement are prognostic as well. The treatment of advanced avascular necrosis with femoral head collapse, however, is typically managed with hemiresurfacing arthroplasty, total hip arthroplasty, or hip arthrodesis based on patient age, activity, and the status of the acetabular cartilage.[119] Elderly patients with symptomatic osteonecrosis are typically managed with hip arthroplasty.

Pearls

- The major blood supply to the femoral head is provided by the lateral retinacular branches of the deep branch of the medial femoral circumflex artery.[44]
- Historically, a displaced femoral neck fracture in a young adult was associated with an 86% incidence of osteonecrosis and a 59% chance of nonunion.[119]
- Basic tenets of modern-day fixation of a high-energy femoral neck fracture in a young adult include (1) urgent reduction and stabilization, (2) direct visualization of the fracture, and (3) rigid fixation via cancellous lag screws.
- No randomized, prospective study has investigated the timing of surgery or the role of capsulotomy on the outcome of a femoral neck fracture in a young adult. However, two studies with a low incidence of osteonecrosis and nonunion in young patients both performed a capsulotomy and performed internal fixation in an urgent manner.[63,64]
- Rates of nonunion for a displaced femoral neck fracture in a young adult range from 0 to 17%. Rates of avascular necrosis for the same entity range from 10 to 23%.[54,63,64]
- Posttraumatic osteonecrosis of the femoral head may not be symptomatic.[100]
- The two treatment options for a femoral neck nonunion in a young adult are a valgus intertrochanteric osteotomy and a vascularized fibular graft.[100,106]

- In treatment of a femoral neck fracture, three screws are generally sufficient.[23] Maximal spread of the screws in the neck is important, with one screw inferiorly along the neck and another screw posteriorly in the neck. In cases with extreme osteoporosis or posterior neck comminution, a fourth screw may be advantageous.[24]
- A femoral neck fracture in combination with a femoral shaft fracture is seen in ~2 to 6% of all femoral shaft fractures.[74–78] They are most commonly seen in the proximal one-third transverse diaphyseal fracture. An intraoperative plain film is helpful to avoid missing the femoral neck injury. Treatment of the femoral neck fracture takes first priority. Rates of avascular necrosis in this situation are lower than with an isolated femoral neck fracture.[120]
- Rates of nonunion for nondisplaced or valgus-impacted fractures treated nonoperatively are as high as 39%.[14]
- A recent meta-analysis of comparative trials between internal fixation and arthroplasty for femoral neck fractures in elderly patients demonstrated lower revision rates but higher wound infection rates, higher 1 year mortality, and higher dislocation rates in the arthroplasty cases. One year mortality rates were 23% for arthroplasty patients and 20% for internal fixation patients.[2]

On the DVDs

Video 22–1 (Disk 3) Watson-Jones Approach for ORIF of Femoral Neck The steps of a Watson-Jones approach for optimal visualization of a femoral neck fracture are shown. The approach allows for clamp placement and for use of reduction aids to insure anatomic reduction.

Video 22–2 (Disk 3) Closed Reduction and Pinning of a Femoral Neck Fracture This video demonstrates treatment of a femoral neck fracture using 7.3 mm cannulated screws. Proper placement of the screws to avoid the "stick in a can" phenomenon is emphasized.

Video 22–3 (Disk 3) ORIF of a Femoral Neck and Subtrochanteric Femur Fracture with Locking Proximal Femur Plate This video demonstrates ORIF of a complex femoral neck/subtrochanteric femur fracture using the Watson-Jones approach. A sys-

tematic approach to reduction and fixation of this severe injury is demonstrated, with the use of a locking precontoured proximal femur plate to stabilize the fracture.

Video 22–4 (Disk 3) Hemiarthroplasty of a Displaced Femoral Neck Fracture This video reviews hip hemiarthroplasty using a Kocher-Langenbeck approach. The details of the approach are reviewed.

Video 22–5 (Disk 3) Hemiarthroplasty of a Displaced Femoral Neck Fracture via the Anterior Approach A specialty fracture table allows for hemiarthroplasty through a 10 cm modified Hueter approach. Advantages include: supine positioning, avoidance of abductor devitalization, and real-time fluoroscopic control of component position.

References

1. Ray NF, Chan JK, Thamer M, et al. Medical expenditures for the treatment of osteoporotic fractures in the United States in 1995: report from the National Osteoporosis Foundation. J Bone Miner Res 1997;12:24–35

2. Bhandari M, Devereaux PJ, Swiontkowski MF, et al. Internal fixation compared with arthroplasty for displaced fractures of the femoral neck: a meta-analysis. J Bone Joint Surg Am 2003;85: 1673–1681

3. Lu-Yao GL, Keller RB, Littenberg B, et al. Outcomes after displaced fractures of the femoral neck: a meta-analysis of one hundred and six published reports. J Bone Joint Surg Am 1994;76:15–25

4. Jakob M, Rosso R, Weller K, et al. Avascular necrosis of the femoral head after open reduction and internal fixation of femoral neck fractures: an inevitable complication? Swiss Surg 1999;5: 257–264

5. Kyle RF, Cabanela ME, Russell TA, et al. Fractures of the proximal part of the femur. Instr Course Lect 1995;44:227–253

6. Hirata T, Konishiike T, Kawai A, et al. Dynamic magnetic resonance imaging of femoral head perfusion in femoral neck fracture. Clin Orthop Relat Res 2001;393:294–301

7. Speer KP, Spritzer CE, Harrelson JM, et al. Magnetic resonance imaging of the femoral head after acute intracapsular fracture of the femoral neck. J Bone Joint Surg Am 1990;72:98–103

8. Rizzo PF, Gould ES, Lyden JP, et al. Diagnosis of occult fractures about the hip. Magnetic resonance imaging compared with bone-scanning. J Bone Joint Surg Am 1993;75:395–401

9. Caviglia HA, Osorio PQ, Comando D. Classification and diagnosis of intracapsular fractures of the proximal femur. Clin Orthop Relat Res 2002;399:17–27

10. Garden RS. Malreduction and avascular necrosis in subcapital fractures of the femur. J Bone Joint Surg Br 1971;53:183–197

11. Zlowodzki M, Bhandari M, Keel M, et al. Perception of Garden's classification for femoral neck fractures: an international survey of 298 orthopaedic trauma surgeons. Arch Orthop Trauma Surg 2005;125:503–505

12. Fracture and Dislocation Compendium. Orthopedic Trauma Association. Committee for Coding and Classification. J Orthop Trauma 1996;10(Suppl l):v-ix, 31–35

13. Bartonicek J. Pauwels' classification of femoral neck fractures: correct interpretation of the original. J Orthop Trauma 2001;15: 358–360

14. Tanaka J, Seki N, Tokimura F, et al. Conservative treatment of Garden stage I femoral neck fracture in elderly patients. Arch Orthop Trauma Surg 2002;122:24–28

15. Parker MJ. Prediction of fracture union after internal fixation of intracapsular femoral neck fractures. Injury 1994;25(Suppl 2): B3–B6

16. Weinrobe M, Stankewich CJ, Mueller B, et al. Predicting the mechanical outcome of femoral neck fractures fixed with cancellous screws: an in vivo study. J Orthop Trauma 1998;12:27–37

17. Hammer AJ. Nonunion of subcapital femoral neck fractures. J Orthop Trauma 1992;6:73–77

18. Estrada LS, Volgas DA, Stannard JP, et al. Fixation failure in femoral neck fractures. Clin Orthop Relat Res 2002;399:110–118

19. Deneka DA, Simonian PT, Stankewich CJ, et al. Biomechanical comparison of internal fixation techniques for the treatment of unstable basicervical femoral neck fractures. J Orthop Trauma 1997;11:337–343

20. Broos PL, Vercruysse R, Fourneau I, et al. Unstable femoral neck fractures in young adults: treatment with the AO 130-degree blade plate. J Orthop Trauma 1998;12:235–239 discussion 240

21. Alho A, Benterud JG, Solovieva S. Internally fixed femoral neck fractures: early prediction of failure in 203 elderly patients with displaced fractures. Acta Orthop Scand 1999;70:141–144

22. Parker MJ, Porter KM, Eastwood DM, et al. Intracapsular fractures of the neck of femur: parallel or crossed Garden screws? J Bone Joint Surg Br 1991;73:826–827

23. Swiontkowski MF, Harrington RM, Keller TS, et al. Torsion and bending analysis of internal fixation techniques for femoral neck fractures: the role of implant design and bone density. J Orthop Res 1987;5:433–444

24. Kauffman JI, Simon JA, Kummer FJ, et al. Internal fixation of femoral neck fractures with posterior comminution: a biomechanical study. J Orthop Trauma 1999;13:155–159

25. Parker MJ, Blundell C. Choice of implant for internal fixation of femoral neck fractures: meta-analysis of 25 randomised trials including 4,925 patients. Acta Orthop Scand 1998;69:138–143

26. Keating JF, Grant A, Masson M, et al. Randomized comparison of reduction and fixation, bipolar hemiarthroplasty, and total hip arthroplasty: treatment of displaced intracapsular hip fractures in healthy older patients. J Bone Joint Surg Am 2006;88: 249–260

27. Sharif KM, Parker MJ. Austin Moore hemiarthroplasty: technical aspects and their effects on outcome, in patients with fractures of the neck of femur. Injury 2002;33:419–422

28. Haidukewych GJ, Israel TA, Berry DJ. Long-term survivorship of cemented bipolar hemiarthroplasty for fracture of the femoral neck. Clin Orthop Relat Res 2002;403:118–126

29. Faraj AA, Branfoot T. Cemented versus uncemented Thompson's prostheses: a functional outcome study. Injury 1999;30:671–675

30. Parvizi J, Holiday AD, Ereth MH, et al. The Frank Stinchfield Award: sudden death during primary hip arthroplasty. Clin Orthop Relat Res 1999;369:39–48

31. Pitto RP, Blunk J, Kossler M. Transesophageal echocardiography and clinical features of fat embolism during cemented total hip arthroplasty: a randomized study in patients with a femoral neck fracture. Arch Orthop Trauma Surg 2000;120:53–58

32. Dalldorf PG, Banas MP, Hicks DG, et al. Rate of degeneration of human acetabular cartilage after hemiarthroplasty. J Bone Joint Surg Am 1995;77:877–882

33. Bochner RM, Pellicci PM, Lyden JP. Bipolar hemiarthroplasty for fracture of the femoral neck: clinical review with special emphasis on prosthetic motion. J Bone Joint Surg Am 1988;70:1001–1010

34. Calder SJ, Anderson GH, Jagger C, et al. Unipolar or bipolar prosthesis for displaced intracapsular hip fracture in octogenarians: a randomised prospective study. J Bone Joint Surg Br 1996;78: 391–394

35. Kenzora JE, Magaziner J, Hudson J, et al. Outcome after hemiarthroplasty for femoral neck fractures in the elderly. Clin Orthop Relat Res 1998;348:51–58

36. Lo WH, Chen WM, Huang CK, et al. Bateman bipolar hemiarthroplasty for displaced intracapsular femoral neck fractures: uncemented versus cemented. Clin Orthop Relat Res 1994;302:75–82

37. Ong BC, Maurer SG, Aharonoff GB, et al. Unipolar versus bipolar hemiarthroplasty: functional outcome after femoral neck fracture at a minimum of thirty-six months of follow-up. J Orthop Trauma 2002;16:317–322

38. Lee BP, Berry DJ, Harmsen WS, et al. Total hip arthroplasty for the treatment of an acute fracture of the femoral neck: long-term results. J Bone Joint Surg Am 1998;80:70–75

39. Woo RY, Morrey BF. Dislocations after total hip arthroplasty. J Bone Joint Surg Am 1982;64:1295–1306

40. Reikeras O, Bjerkreim I, Kolbenstvedt A. Anteversion of the acetabulum and femoral neck in normals and in patients with osteoarthritis of the hip. Acta Orthop Scand 1983;54:18–23

41. Reikeras O, Hoiseth A. Femoral neck angles in osteoarthritis of the hip. Acta Orthop Scand 1982;53:781–784

42. Reikeras O, Hoiseth A, Reigstad A, et al. Femoral neck angles: a specimen study with special regard to bilateral differences. Acta Orthop Scand 1982;53:775–779

43. Kregor, PJ. The effect of femoral neck fractures on femoral head blood flow. Orthopedics 1996;19:1031–1036; quiz 1037–1038

44. Gautier E, Ganz K, Krugel N, et al. Anatomy of the medial femoral circumflex artery and its surgical implications. J Bone Joint Surg Br 2000;82:679–683

45. Howe WW, Lacey TI, Schwartz RP. A study of the gross anatomy of the arteries supplying the proximal portion of the femur and the acetabulum. J Bone Joint Surg Am 1950;32A:856–866

46. Trueta J, Harrison HM. The normal vascular anatomy of the femoral head in adult man. J Bone Joint Surg Br 1953;35B:442–461

47. Catto M. A histological study of avascular necrosis of the femoral head after transcervical fracture. J Bone Joint Surg Br 1965;47:749–776

48. Chung SM. The arterial supply of the developing proximal end of the human femur. J Bone Joint Surg Am 1976;58:961–970

49. Claffey TJ. Avascular necrosis of the femoral head: an anatomical study. J Bone Joint Surg Br 1960;42-B:802–809

50. Crock HV. An atlas of the arterial supply of the head and neck of the femur in man. Clin Orthop Relat Res 1980;152:17–27

51. Sevitt S. Avascular necrosis and revascularisation of the femoral head after intracapsular fractures: a combined arteriographic and histological necropsy study. J Bone Joint Surg Br 1964;46:270–296

52. Swiontkowski MF. Intracapsular fractures of the hip. J Bone Joint Surg Am 1994;76:129–138

53. Drake JK, Meyers MH. Intracapsular pressure and hemarthrosis following femoral neck fracture. Clin Orthop Relat Res 1984;182:172–176

54. Gill TJ, Sledge JB, Ekkernkamp A, et al. Intraoperative assessment of femoral head vascularity after femoral neck fracture. J Orthop Trauma 1998;12:474–478

55. Haidukewych GJ, Rothwell WS, Jacofsky DJ, et al. Operative treatment of femoral neck fractures in patients between the ages of fifteen and fifty years. J Bone Joint Surg Am 2004;86-A:1711–1716

56. Maruenda JI, Barrios C, Gomar-Sancho F. Intracapsular hip pressure after femoral neck fracture. Clin Orthop Relat Res 1997;340172–180

57. Harper WM, Barnes MR, Gregg PJ. Femoral head blood flow in femoral neck fractures: an analysis using intra-osseous pressure measurement. J Bone Joint Surg Br 1991;73:73–75

58. Dall D. Exposure of the hip by anterior osteotomy of the greater trochanter: a modified anterolateral approach. J Bone Joint Surg Br 1986;68:382–386

59. Matta JM, Shahrdar C, Ferguson T. Single-incision anterior approach for total hip arthroplasty on an orthopaedic table. Clin Orthop Relat Res 2005;441:115–124

60. Asnis SE, Wanek-Sgaglione L. Intracapsular fractures of the femoral neck: results of cannulated screw fixation. J Bone Joint Surg Am 1994;76:1793–1803

61. Chiu FY, Lo WH. Undisplaced femoral neck fracture in the elderly. Arch Orthop Trauma Surg 1996;115:90–93

62. Robinson CM, Saran D, Annan IH. Intracapsular hip fractures: results of management adopting a treatment protocol. Clin Orthop Relat Res 1994;302:83–91

63. Gerber C, Strehle J, Ganz R. The treatment of fractures of the femoral neck. Clin Orthop Relat Res 1993;292:77–86

64. Swiontkowski MF, Winquist RA, Hansen ST Jr. Fractures of the femoral neck in patients between the ages of twelve and forty-nine years. J Bone Joint Surg Am 1984;66:837–846

65. Booth KC, Donaldson TK, Dai QG. Femoral neck fracture fixation: a biomechanical study of two cannulated screw placement techniques. Orthopedics 1998;21:1173–1176

66. Bout CA, Cannegieter DM, Juttmann JW. Percutaneous cannulated screw fixation of femoral neck fractures: the three point principle. Injury 1997;28:135–139

67. Chua D, Jaglal SB, Schatzker J. Predictors of early failure of fixation in the treatment of displaced subcapital hip fractures. J Orthop Trauma 1998;12:230–234

68. Lindequist S, Tornkvist H. Quality of reduction and cortical screw support in femoral neck fractures: an analysis of 72 fractures with a new computerized measuring method. J Orthop Trauma 1995;9:215–221

69. Saito N, Miyasaka T, Toriumi H. Radiographic factors predicting non-union of displaced intracapsular femoral neck fractures. Arch Orthop Trauma Surg 1995;114:183–187

70. Smyth EH, Shah VM. The significance of good reduction and fixation in displaced subcapital fractures of the femur. Injury 1974;5:197–209

71. Springer ER, Lachiewicz PF, Gilbert JA. Internal fixation of femoral neck fractures: a comparative biomechanical study of Knowles pins and 6.5-mm cancellous screws. Clin Orthop Relat Res 1991;267:85–92

72. Stafford P, Goulet R, Norris B. The effect of screw insertion site and unused drill holes on stability and mode of failure after fixation of basicervical femoral neck fracture. Crit Rev Biomed Eng 2000;28:11–16

73. Zlowodzki M, Weening B, Petrisor B, et al. The value of washers in cannulated screw fixation of femoral neck fractures. J Trauma 2005;59:969–975

74. Bennett FS, Zinar DM, Kilgus DJ. Ipsilateral hip and femoral shaft fractures. Clin Orthop Relat Res 1993;296:168–177

75. Winquist RA, Hansen ST Jr, Clawson DK. Closed intramedullary nailing of femoral fractures: a report of five hundred and twenty cases. J Bone Joint Surg Am 1984;66:529–539

76. Swiontkowski MF, Hansen ST Jr, Kellam J. Ipsilateral fractures of the femoral neck and shaft: a treatment protocol. J Bone Joint Surg Am 1984;66:260–268

77. Wu CC, Shih CH. Ipsilateral femoral neck and shaft fractures: retrospective study of 33 cases. Acta Orthop Scand 1991;62:346–351

78. Zettas JP, Zettas P. Ipsilateral fractures of the femoral neck and shaft. Clin Orthop Relat Res 1981;160:63–73

79. Tornetta P III, Creevy WR, Kain M. Avoiding missed femoral neck fractures: improvement by using a standard protocol in cases of femoral shaft fractures. In: Orthopaedic Trauma Association Annual Meeting, Hollywood, FL, 2004

80. Wiss DA, Sima W, Brien WW. Ipsilateral fractures of the femoral neck and shaft. J Orthop Trauma 1992;6:159–166

81. Randelli P, Landi S, Fanton F, et al. Treatment of ipsilateral femoral neck and shaft fractures with the Russell-Taylor reconstructive nail. Orthopedics 1999;22:673–676

82. Simonian PT, Chapman JR, Selznick HS, et al. Iatrogenic fractures of the femoral neck during closed nailing of the femoral shaft. J Bone Joint Surg Br 1994;76:293–296

83. Koval KJ, Skovron ML, Aharonoff GB, et al. Predictors of functional recovery after hip fracture in the elderly. Clin Orthop Relat Res 1998;348:22–28

84. Koval KJ, Sala DA, Kummer FJ, et al. Postoperative weight-bearing after a fracture of the femoral neck or an intertrochanteric fracture. J Bone Joint Surg Am 1998;80:352–356

85. Koval KJ, Friend KD, Aharonoff GB, et al. Weight bearing after hip fracture: a prospective series of 596 geriatric hip fracture patients. J Orthop Trauma 1996;10:526–530

86. Eriksson F, Mattsson P, Larsson S. The effect of augmentation with resorbable or conventional bone cement on the holding strength for femoral neck fracture devices. J Orthop Trauma 2002;16:302–310

87. Stankewich CJ, Swiontkowski MF, Tencer AF, et al. Augmentation of femoral neck fracture fixation with an injectable calcium-phosphate bone mineral cement. J Orthop Res 1996;14:786–793

88. Judet J, Judet R. The use of an artificial femoral head for arthroplasty of the hip joint. J Bone Joint Surg Br 1950;32:166–173

89. Judet R, Judet J. Technique and results with the acrylic femoral head prosthesis. J Bone Joint Surg Br 1952;34:173–180

90. Eiskjaer S, Ostgard SE. Risk factors influencing mortality after bipolar hemiarthroplasty in the treatment of fracture of the femoral neck. Clin Orthop Relat Res 1991;270:295–300

91. Hudson JI, Kenzora JE, Hebel JR, et al. Eight-year outcome associated with clinical options in the management of femoral neck fractures. Clin Orthop Relat Res 1998;348:59–66

92. Michelson JD, Myers A, Jinnah R, et al. Epidemiology of hip fractures among the elderly: risk factors for fracture type. Clin Orthop Relat Res 1995;311:129–135

93. Nilsson LT, Jalovaara P, Franzen H, et al. Function after primary hemiarthroplasty and secondary total hip arthroplasty in femoral neck fracture. J Arthroplasty 1994;9:369–374

94. Gardner MJ, Flik KR, Mooar P, et al. Improvement in the under-treatment of osteoporosis following hip fracture. J Bone Joint Surg Am 2002;84-A:1342–1348

95. Dedrick DK, Mackenzie JR, Burney RE. Complications of femoral neck fracture in young adults. J Trauma 1986;26:932–937

96. Tooke SM, Favero KJ. Femoral neck fractures in skeletally mature patients, fifty years old or less. J Bone Joint Surg Am 1985;67:1255–1260

97. Jackson M, Learmonth ID. The treatment of nonunion after intracapsular fracture of the proximal femur. Clin Orthop Relat Res 2002;399:119–128

98. Wu CC, Shih CH, Chen WJ, et al. Treatment of femoral neck nonunions with a sliding compression screw: comparison with and without subtrochanteric valgus osteotomy. J Trauma 1999;46:312–317

99. Müller ME. Intertrochanteric osteotomy: indication, preoperative planning, technique. In: Schatzker J, ed. The Intertrochanteric Osteotomy. New York: Springer-Verlag; 1984:25–66

100. Marti RK, Schuller HM, Raaymakers EL. Intertrochanteric osteotomy for non-union of the femoral neck. J Bone Joint Surg Br 1989;71:782–787

101. Ballmer FT, Ballmer PM, Baumgaertel F, et al. Pauwels osteotomy for nonunions of the femoral neck. Orthop Clin North Am 1990;21:759–767

102. Anglen JO. Intertrochanteric osteotomy for failed internal fixation of femoral neck fracture. Clin Orthop Relat Res 1997;341:175–182

103. Mathews V, Berry DJ, Trousdale RT, et al. Clinical and functional results of valgus intertrochanteric osteotomy for femoral neck fracture nonunion. 69th Annual Meeting of the American Academy of Orthopaedic Surgeons, Dallas, TX, 2002

104. Meyers MH, Harvey JP Jr, Moore TM. The muscle pedicle bone graft in the treatment of displaced fractures of the femoral neck: indications, operative technique, and results. Orthop Clin North Am 1974;5:779–792

105. Baksi DP. Internal fixation of ununited femoral neck fractures combined with muscle–pedicle bone grafting. J Bone Joint Surg Br 1986;68:239–245

106. LeCroy CM, Rizzo M, Gunneson EE, et al. Free vascularized fibular bone grafting in the management of femoral neck nonunion in patients younger than fifty years. J Orthop Trauma 2002;16:464–472

107. Nagi ON, Dhillon MS, Goni VG. Open reduction, internal fixation and fibular autografting for neglected fracture of the femoral neck. J Bone Joint Surg Br 1998;80:798–804

108. Hou SM, Hang YS, Liu TK. Ununited femoral neck fractures by open reduction and vascularized iliac bone graft. Clin Orthop Relat Res 1993;294:176–180

109. Leung PC, Shen WY. Fracture of the femoral neck in younger adults: a new method of treatment for delayed and nonunions. Clin Orthop Relat Res 1993;295:156–160

110. Nagi ON, Gautam VK, Marya SK. Treatment of femoral neck fractures with a cancellous screw and fibular graft. J Bone Joint Surg Br 1986;68:387–391

111. Henderson MS. Ununited fracture of the neck of the femur treated by the aid of the bone graft. J Bone Joint Surg Am 1940;22:97–106

112. Rogmark C, Carlsson A, Johnell O, et al. A prospective randomised trial of internal fixation versus arthroplasty for displaced fractures of the neck of the femur: functional outcome for 450 patients at two years. J Bone Joint Surg Br 2002;84:183–188

113. Hagglund G, Nordstrom B, Lidgren L. Total hip replacement after nailing failure in femoral neck fractures. Arch Orthop Trauma Surg 1984;103:125–127

114. Haidukewych GJ, Berry DJ. Hip arthroplasty for salvage of failed treatment of intertrochanteric hip fractures. J Bone Joint Surg Am 2003;85-A:899–904

115. Mabry TM, Prpa B, Haidukewych GJ, et al. Long-term results of total hip arthroplasty for femoral neck fracture nonunion. J Bone Joint Surg Am 2004;86-A:2263–2267

116. McKinley JC, Robinson CM. Treatment of displaced intracapsular hip fractures with total hip arthroplasty: comparison of primary arthroplasty with early salvage arthroplasty after failed internal fixation. J Bone Joint Surg Am 2002;84-A:2010–2015

117. Lavernia CJ, Sierra RJ, Grieco FR. Osteonecrosis of the femoral head. J Am Acad Orthop Surg 1999;7:250–261

118. Protzman RR, Burkhalter WE. Femoral-neck fractures in young adults. J Bone Joint Surg Am 1976;58:689–695

119. Franzen H, Nilsson LT, Stromqvist B, et al. Secondary total hip replacement after fractures of the femoral neck. J Bone Joint Surg Br 1990;72:784–787

120. Alho A. Concurrent ipsilateral fractures of the hip and femoral shaft: a meta-analysis of 659 cases. Acta Orthop Scand 1996;67:19–28

23 Intertrochanteric Femur Fractures

Gregory Tennant and Jorge Alonso

Intertrochanteric hip fractures have an incidence of nearly 200,000 per year in the United States alone; their incidence is expected to increase dramatically as the population ages. The typical patient with an intertrochanteric fracture is older and more osteopenic than patients that sustain femoral neck fractures.[1] Intertrochanteric fractures are managed by surgical stabilization for two reasons. Most importantly, surgery is performed so that the affected patient can be immediately mobilized, thereby avoiding the complications of prolonged recumbency in these typically frail patients. Second, when treated nonoperatively, varus malunion inevitably occurs, so that surviving patients treated nonoperatively have leg shortening and abductor dysfunction. Thus intertrochanteric fractures are nearly universally repaired. The role of the orthopaedic surgeon continues to encompass not only initial management and surgical fixation but also postoperative care and mobilization. Decisions about the timing of surgery and the method of surgical stabilization must consider the patient's overall health, fracture pattern, and postoperative goals and risks.

Complications related to fixation of intertrochanteric hip fractures were once very common due to the combination of poor bone quality and the severe mechanical loads in this region of the femur. Older, fixed-angle devices often failed by screw cut-out in the femoral head, implant breakage, or side plate pull-off from the femoral shaft. The rate of fixation failure dropped dramatically after the introduction of the sliding hip nail/screw.[2] These devices were later modified to the modern sliding hip screw and became the treatment of choice for almost all intertrochanteric fractures. More recently, there has been recognition of specific fracture subtypes for which alternative methods of stabilization are more appropriate. This chapter focuses on the appropriate use and surgical technique of the sliding hip screw and the cephalomedullary device for the treatment of intertrochanteric hip fractures.

Classification

Many classifications of intertrochanteric femur fractures have been proposed; none has gained widespread clinical use. This is due in part to the fact that, for the past several decades, nearly all intertrochanteric fractures were treated surgically with a sliding hip screw, obviating the need for detailed fracture classification. This has now changed with recognition of specific fracture patterns that are too unstable for fixation with a sliding hip screw.

When evaluating an intertrochanteric fracture, it has been useful to divide the injury into stable and unstable patterns. Both Evans[3] and Kyle et al[2] have presented simple classification systems that are based on the degree of fracture stability after reduction. In most intertrochanteric fractures, the primary fracture line parallels the intertrochanteric line, extending from proximal-lateral to inferomedial (**Fig. 23–1**). The most important feature separating a stable from an unstable pattern is the presence of a displaced fragment in the region of the lesser trochanter (**Fig. 23–2**). Reverse obliquity fracture patterns are less common and sometimes occur as part of a fracture with subtrochanteric extension. This pattern begins inferolaterally and extends in a proximal-medial direction, parallel to the axis of the femoral neck (**Fig. 23–3**). Evans noted that medial cortical involvement and/or comminution, failure to obtain medial cortical apposition, and the reverse obliquity pattern are the major components resulting in failure to obtain postanatomical reduction stability.[3] Kyle

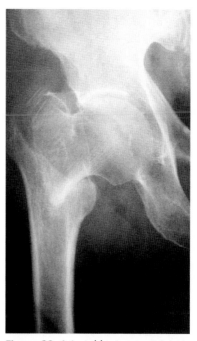

Figure 23–1 A stable, two-part intertrochanteric femur fracture demonstrating the primary fracture line along the intertrochanteric line.

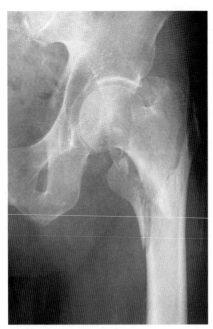

Figure 23–2 An unstable intertrochanteric fracture with loss of the posteromedial buttress.

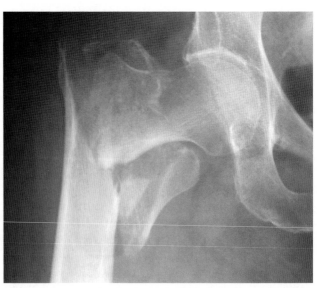

Figure 23–4 Example of a comminuted intertrochanteric fracture with an associated fracture of the femoral neck. This pattern is very unstable and prone to complications.

et al analyzed over 600 intertrochanteric fractures and found that the degree of collapse of the sliding hip screw correlated with increasing instability of the posteromedial buttress.[2] In a more recent paper from the same institution, Kyle and colleagues describe another pattern of fracture in which a fracture at the base of the femoral neck is associated with severe comminution of the trochanteric region **(Fig. 23–4).**[4] This pattern had the most fracture collapse and the greatest risk of hardware failure. Haidukewych et al reported a series of reverse obliquity fractures and documented high failure rates with this use of sliding hip screws in this pattern.[5] Thus, for practical

purposes, one need recognize three patterns of intertrochanteric fracture: stable injuries with an intact or reducible posteromedial buttress, those with loss of the posteromedial buttress, and the reverse obliquity pattern.

The Arbeitsgemeinschaft für Osteosynthesefragen/Orthopaedic Trauma Association (AO/OTA) Comprehensive Classification of Fractures addresses these injuries with the well-known alphanumeric system.[6] Types A1 through A3 are simple fractures. Types B1 through B3 are multifragmentary with involvement of the greater or lesser trochanters. Types C1 through C3 describe the reverse obliquity fracture pattern.

Nonoperative Treatment

Although some authors have described protocols for the nonoperative management of ambulatory patients with intertrochanteric fractures,[7] nonoperative management is rarely appropriate. Currently, there are very few indications for nonoperative management of intertrochanteric hip fractures. Such treatment should only be considered for the rare fracture that is not visible on radiographs (if the patient can be safely and comfortably mobilized) and for bedridden patients that are too ill to undergo surgery **(Fig. 23–5A,B).** If such patients can be made comfortable, can sit, and can be moved for hygiene, then nonoperative treatment may be considered, with the recognition that the patient may not survive long. Lyon and Nevins reported on nonoperative management of nonambulating nursing home patients.[8] They recommend early mobilization to a chair and analgesic pain control. Such a nonoperative approach accepts a trade-off between the typical deformity of varus, external rotation, and shortening of the

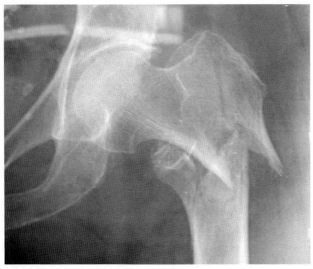

Figure 23–3 A reverse obliquity fracture.

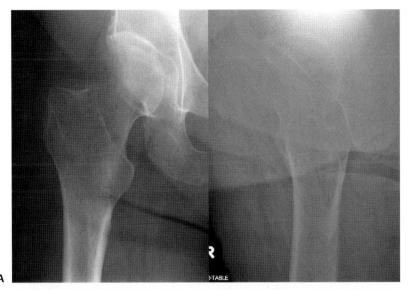

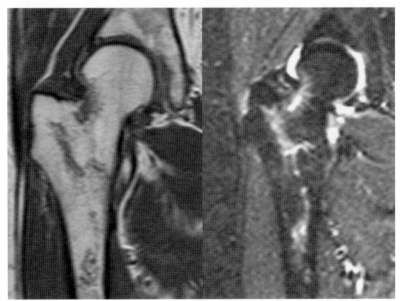

Figure 23–5 An occult intertrochanteric fracture of the upper femur. **(A)** Plain radiographs of an elderly patient with hip pain after a fall appear normal. **(B)** T1-weighted (left panel) and T2-weighted (right panel) magnetic resonance images showing bone marrow edema and a fracture line in the trochanteric region. The patient was treated nonoperatively.

proximal femur that develops without stabilization in favor of early patient mobility.

Occult fractures of the intertrochanteric region of the femur, which by definition are nondisplaced and difficult to see on traditional radiographs, can be readily assessed with the use of magnetic resonance imaging (MRI) **(Fig. 23–5A,B).** MRI offers rapid, dependable detection of these nondisplaced or incomplete fractures that are often seen in the elderly patient with hip pain following minor trauma.[9,10] MRI was found to be more accurate and more effective for the early detection of occult fractures than both computed tomographic (CT) scan and scintigraphy.[11] Pathology needing operative intervention is much more likely to be found in patients older than 70 years.[10] Once they are identified, treatment of these fractures depends on the degree of pain, the patient's health

and comorbidities, as well as functional demands. Those patients who are nonambulators and can be mobilized to a chair comfortably may be treated nonoperatively as long as their fracture does not displace. For most patients, occult fractures should be treated operatively with a sliding hip screw. This simple procedure allows the patient to walk and move about with less pain and no risk of fracture displacement.

Indications for Surgical Treatment

With the exception of medically unstable patients, nearly all intertrochanteric proximal femur fractures will be treated surgically. Surgical stabilization of these fractures offers the optimal means for early mobilization and for early rehabilitation toward regaining a preinjury functional level. Surgical timing seems to be a more controversial topic than the surgical indications themselves. Although Kenzora et al noted an increase in surgical mortality with hip surgery on the same day of admission,[12] others warn of operative delay. Ring stressed that only minimal medical improvement occurs when patients have long-standing chronic ailments, recommending early fixation over delay for medical optimization.[13] McNeill noted when surgical stabilization was delayed more than 48 hours after admission for a nonmedical issue, there was a 10-fold increase in mortality.[14] This would indicate that, although intertrochanteric hip fracture fixation should not be considered an emergent procedure, unnecessary surgical delays should be avoided. Surgical stabilization should be performed in an urgent manner.

Surgical Treatment

Basic Concepts

Kaufer determined that the strength of fixation of an intertrochanteric hip fracture after reduction and stabilization is determined by five distinct variables: bone quality, fragment geometry, fracture reduction, implant design, and implant placement.[15] Two of these variables are not under the surgeon's control: bone quality and fragment geometry, or fracture pattern. These may be considered to be static variables. Three of these factors are related to the surgeon rather than the patient, that is, fracture reduction, implant design, and placement of the implant. These are considered to be dynamic variables because the surgeon has the ability to control the quality of reduction, the implant chosen, and the implant position. Studies have shown that the position of the implant within the femoral head is an important determinant of outcome.[2,16,17] Im et al looked at factors associated with loss of reduction in a series of 66 elderly patients with apparently stable intertrochanteric fractures and found that iatrogenic comminution of the lateral cortex during surgery was statistically associated with excessive displacement after surgery.[18] Thus the surgical technique of open reduction and internal fixation must be done in a way to optimize these dynamic factors and overcome the static variables to create a stable construct.

Surgical Anatomy

The bony anatomy of the proximal femur is made up of four distinct parts: the femoral head and neck, greater trochanter, lesser trochanter, and subtrochanteric region or shaft. Each of these can be involved within the parameters of the intertrochanteric proximal femur fracture. Each

has its own set of deforming forces that must be understood to obtain a suitable reduction.

The intracapsular portion of the femoral head and neck is generally undisturbed, with the extracapsular neck region being occasionally involved in an intertrochanteric fracture. The hip abductors provide a deforming force through their insertion on the greater trochanter, whereas the gluteus minimus and short external rotators will tend to externally rotate the proximal shaft away from the head and neck fragment **(Fig. 23–6).** The hip adductors also provide a strong deforming force to the femoral shaft through their insertion on the medial proximal femoral shaft. The fragment containing the lesser trochanter will tend to be flexed and adducted due to the pull of the iliopsoas tendon. The hamstrings and quadriceps provide an additional

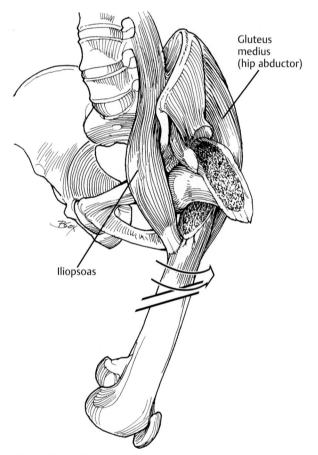

Figure 23–6 Deforming forces about an intertrochanteric fracture. The hip abductors insert on the greater trochanter and cause proximal displacement of this fragment, whereas the gluteus minimus and short external rotators will tend to externally rotate the proximal shaft away from the head and neck fragment. The hip adductors also generate a deforming force to the femoral shaft through their insertion on the medial femoral shaft. The fragment containing the lesser trochanter will tend to be flexed and adducted due to the pull of the iliopsoas tendon. The hamstrings and quadriceps provide an additional axial shortening force across the fracture.

axial shortening force across the fracture. Simple fractures display more predictable displacement patterns that are easily reduced, whereas more complex fractures can have widely separated fragments with multiple displacement planes due to the multiple deforming muscle forces.

Surgical Technique

Reduction

Obtaining optimum reduction of the intertrochanteric femur fracture is the key to successful surgery. This is best achieved through the use of a fracture table. The ability to evaluate the injury pattern and manipulate the fragments indirectly in three dimensions while applying traction to varying degrees is essential. Once the patient is securely positioned on the fracture table, one should first evaluate the injury pattern and displacement using three fluoroscopic views: the anteroposterior (AP) of the hip, lateral, and a true lateral femoral neck view taken with the C-arm angled ~20 degrees from horizontal **(Fig. 23–7A–C)**. The femoral neck view accounts for the anteversion of the proximal femur and is helpful during reduction and during pin or screw placement.

To reduce the fracture, one should first apply gentle traction to the leg (applied through the foot or a traction pin) and then correct any external rotation deformity of the distal fragment, aligning it appropriately with the neck fragment. The leg of the injured side should be aligned with the patella pointing straight up during this correction. Once a provisional reduction of the fracture is obtained with acceptable rotation and length on the AP view of the hip, one should then move the C-arm to obtain lateral and femoral neck views. Using the lateral view of the hip, one may fine-tune the reduction with respect to flexion or extension of the distal fragments by elevating or lowering the foot while maintaining all previous reduction maneuvers. Finally, having corrected all three planes of deformity, one may check the true lateral of the femoral neck using the 20 degree lateral view.

Occasionally, acceptable reduction will not be obtainable with the fracture table alone. Commonly, posterior sagging of the fracture occurs, which can only be seen using the lateral fluoroscopic projection. When present, posterior sag must be corrected and maintained manually **(Fig. 23–8)**. In severe cases the fracture fragments may need to be disimpacted before they can be reduced. In cases of high-energy trauma, incarcerated muscle and significant fracture displacement can all account for inability to achieve an acceptable reduction. In these cases, one can first obtain a provisional correction of alignment, rotation, and length with the fracture table and then use

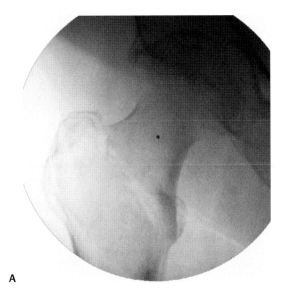

A

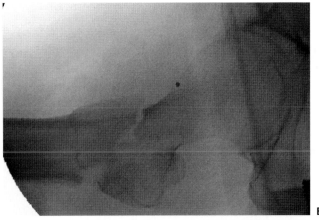

B

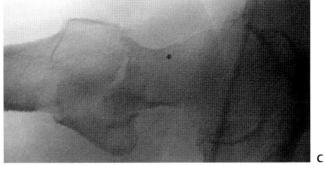

C

Figure 23–7 The three fluoroscopic views typically used during open reduction and internal fixation of intertrochanteric femur fractures. **(A)** Anteroposterior view of the hip. **(B)** Lateral view of the hip. **(C)** A true lateral femoral neck view taken with the C-arm angled ~20 degrees from horizontal.

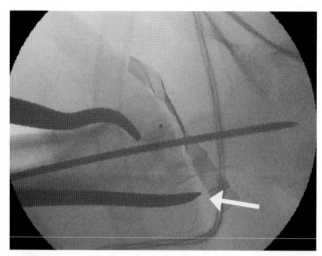

Figure 23–8 A lateral fluoroscopic projection shows a blunt elevator (white arrow) placed below the femur that is used to push upward and correct posterior sag. It is important that this maneuver is maintained throughout the various steps of inserting the implant.

more traditional reduction clamps, pins, or both to obtain and maintain fracture reduction during fixation. Often, a pointed reduction clamp placed from the medial calcar to the shaft will help to maintain reduction during fixation (**Fig. 23–9**). An important point about the technique is that the reduction must be obtained prior to fixation and

maintained during fixation because the recommended implants will not correct a malreduction, nor will they allow for fragment manipulation after insertion.

Surgical Fixation

Implant Choice

There are three general categories of implants used for intertrochanteric fractures: the screw and side plate, the cephalomedullary nail, and the fixed angle plate. Much recent discussion has concerned the relative merits of the sliding hip screw versus the cephalomedullary nail. Although the hip screw and side plate remains the preferred implant for fixation of stable intertrochanteric fractures (**Fig. 23–10A,B**), the cephalomedullary nail has increased stability in unstable fracture patterns, especially the reverse obliquity type (**Fig. 23–11A,B**).[19] The screw and side plate construct, in contrast to the cephalomedullary nail, fails to fully control the reverse obliquity fracture, lending to its higher failure rate when used in this pattern.[20] The cephalomedullary nail, although associated with less initial blood loss, is also associated with a higher rate of periprosthetic fracture when compared with the hip screw and side plate.[21]

The Gamma nail (Stryker Orthopaedics, Mahwah, New Jersey) is the most studied of the trochanteric nails. Ac-

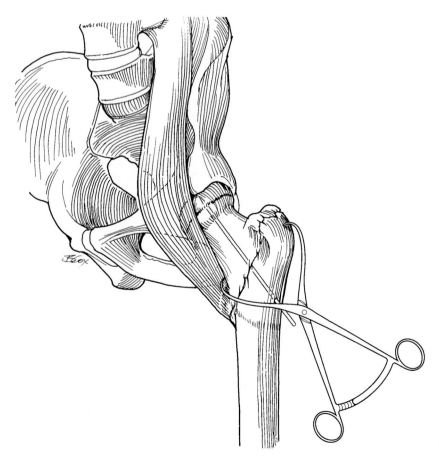

Figure 23–9 Example of a pointed reduction clamp placed from the medial calcar to the shaft to maintain reduction of an unstable fracture during fixation.

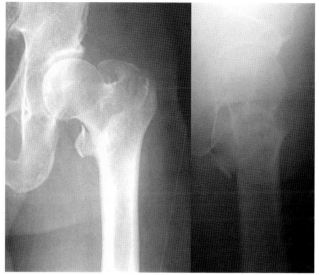

A

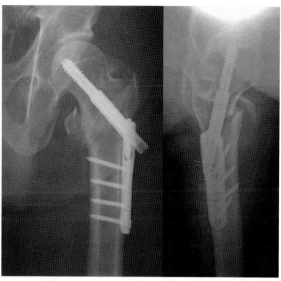

B

Figure 23–10 A "typical" intertrochanteric fracture treated with a sliding hip screw. **(A)** Anteroposterior and lateral radiographs of the hip showing a stable intertrochanteric fracture with a small, mini-

mally displaced lesser trochanter fragment. **(B)** After closed reduction and internal fixation with a sliding hip screw.

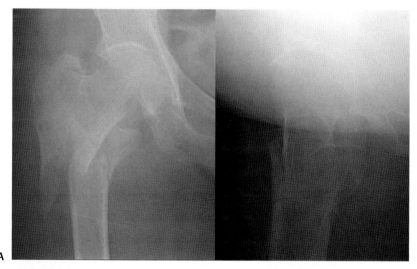

A

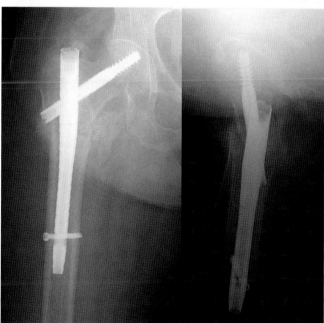

B

Figure 23–11 An unstable reverse obliquity fracture treated with a cephalomedullary nail. **(A)** Anteroposterior and lateral radiographs of the hip showing an unstable reverse obliquity fracture. **(B)** After closed reduction and interlocking nailing with a short cephalomedullary nail. In general, longer nails are preferred because of the risk of a later fracture at the tip of the nail.

cording to both Lindsey et al[22] and Davis et al,[23] benefits of the Gamma nail are as follows.

1. Provides stable fixation of the head and neck
2. Allows for controlled collapse and impaction of the fracture to increase stability
3. Decreases the lever arm on the proximal fragment compared with a lateral plate due to its intramedullary placement
4. Intramedullary reaming provides bone graft.
5. Provides excellent axial and rotational control
6. Allows early weight bearing
7. Requires minimal dissection for insertion
8. Serves as a load-sharing implant

The traditional fixed-angle device, that is, the 120 or 130 degree blade plate, has little place for use during fixation of routine intertrochanteric fractures. Laros and Moore,[24] along with Esser et al,[25] found higher complication rates with the fixed- angled device. These included higher rates of nonunion, joint penetration resulting from fracture collapse, and additional fractures.

In contrast, a 95 degree fixed-angle plate still has some merit for fixation of the more unstable fracture patterns. This may be a 95 degree blade plate or a 95 degree condylar screw **(Fig. 23–12A–C)**. Unstable intertrochanteric fractures, including the reverse obliquity fracture, can be stabilized using this device, but its use requires considerable skill, and there is little margin for error during insertion. The 95 degree blade plate offers excellent proximal fixation that opposes the fracture plane and allows for the possibility of lag screw fixation across the fracture site.

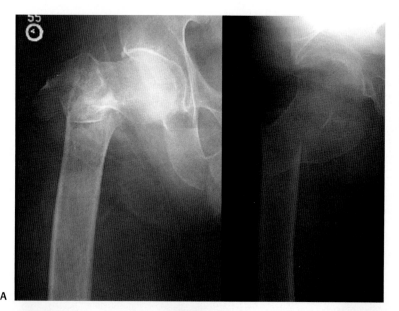

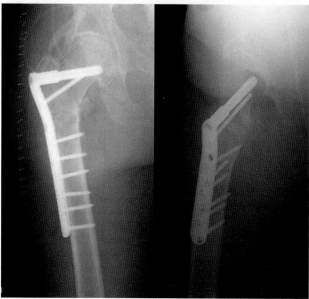

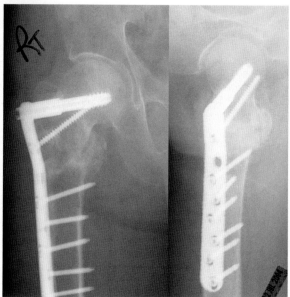

Figure 23–12 An unstable reverse obliquity fracture treated with a fixed-angle, 95 degree condylar screw. **(A)** Anteroposterior and lateral radiographs of the hip showing an unstable reverse obliquity fracture. **(B)** After open reduction and internal fixation with a 95 degree dynamic condylar screw. **(C)** Final views after fracture healing reveal no loss of fixation or collapse of the fracture as would be expected with a sliding hip screw.

A

B

C

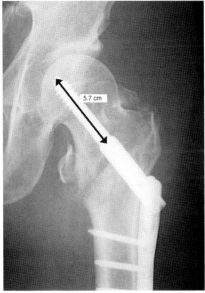
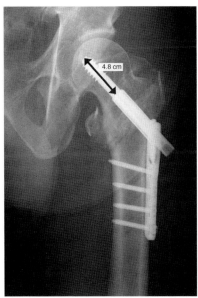
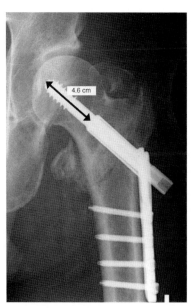

A–C

Figure 23–13 Example of compression occurring along the axis of the hip screw following surgery. **(A)** Postoperative radiograph; note the length of the screw extending beyond the barrel is 5.7 cm, and the end of the screw is barely visible lateral to the side plate. **(B)** Follow-up radiograph taken 1 month later. Much more of the barrel ex- tends lateral to the side plate, and the length of screw extending beyond the barrel is now reduced to 4.8 cm. **(C)** Another radiograph taken 3 months after surgery shows a little further collapse, with the length of the screw extending beyond the barrel now 4.6 cm.

In general, one should consider using the sliding hip screw and side plate with the maximal angle that allows screw placement into the center of the femoral head for fixation of stable intertrochanteric fractures **(Fig. 23–10A,B)**.[26] One should reserve cephalomedullary devices for unstable fractures, especially those with a reverse obliquity component, because the mechanical advantage of intramedullary placement is important for stabilizing these fractures **(Fig. 23–11A,B)**.[27] These implants have the additional advantage of avoiding disruption of the fracture hematoma, and they minimize any additional periosteal stripping at the fracture site. However, because neck-shaft angle options of intramedullary nails are limited to the angle "built in" (typically 130 degrees), it may be more difficult to achieve central positioning of the lag screw within the femoral head with these devices.[28] This is especially true in patients with a neck-shaft angle less than 125 degrees, in whom a sliding hip screw would allow better implant placement within the femoral head.[28]

Sliding Screw and Side Plate (see **Video 23–1, Disk 3**)

Sliding hip screws are excellent devices for fractures that have an intact medial cortical buttress and minimal comminution at the fracture site. The keys to successful use of this device are preoperative planning, understanding the fracture pattern and its anticipated stability following reduction, and understanding the biomechanics of sliding hip screws. The sliding capability of the screw and side plate will allow for compression of the stable fracture during postoperative weight bearing without loss of fixation **(Fig. 23–13A–C)**. Preoperative planning is essential for optimal use, with the best templating source being the opposite hip. Therefore, good radiographs must be obtained prior to entering the surgical suite. Appropriate radiographs include the standard AP pelvis, AP and lateral of the injured hip, and a low pelvis with the legs internally rotated. The internally rotated view is the best for determining implant angle because it gives a true view of the neck-shaft angle and a true depiction of fracture anatomy **(Fig. 23–14A,B)**. Both the implant angle and the anticipated screw length can be templated, ensuring that both the surgeon and the staff are prepared for the case.

Kyle and colleagues have characterized the sliding forces that influence the function of sliding hip screws.[26] Sliding is optimized when the axis of the barrel and screw is close to the angle of the joint reaction force (159 degrees) **(Fig. 23–15)**. This requires a so-called high-angle hip screw. Hip screws with a lower, more anatomical neck-shaft angle (e.g., 135 degrees) are not as well aligned with the joint reaction force, which then has a component vector that acts perpendicular to the axis of the barrel to jam the screw. Thus the forces that initiate sliding of the hip screw are optimum when a valgus reduction is achieved.

Once the patient is positioned on the fracture table and an acceptable reduction has been obtained and carefully scrutinized using fluoroscopy in the AP, lateral, and 20 degree lateral neck view, one should confirm that preoperative antibiotics have been received within 30 minutes of incision. Although there are several choices of skin

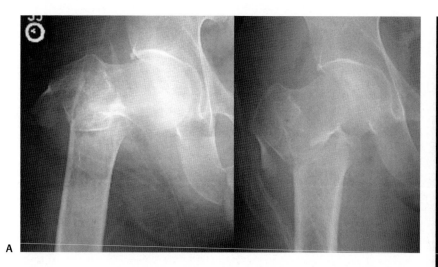

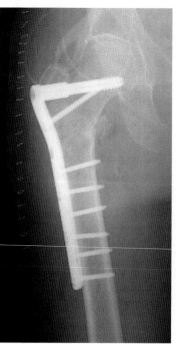

Figure 23–14 Example of the utility of traction x-rays. **(A)** On the left, an angulated, ill-defined fracture is seen. On the right, the traction view clearly establishes that this is a fracture with a reverse oblique component, possibly changing the operative plan from a sliding hip screw to **(B)** a fixed-angle device.

preparation, the authors prefer to use DuraPrep (3M Corporation, St. Paul, Minnesota) on the skin and drape with an adhesive barrier "curtain" drape. Once the patient is positioned, prepped, and draped, one should reconfirm that the fluoroscopy imaging works and position the C-

arm such that it can maneuver through each view without moving the base of the machine.

To place the incision, outline the greater trochanter and the path of the femoral shaft with a marking pen prior to incision. The incision is started along the lateral

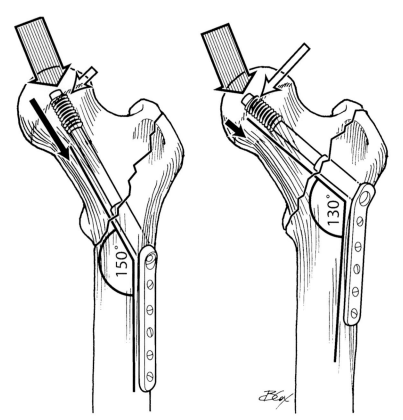

Figure 23–15 The forces acting to initiate sliding of a sliding hip screw. The joint reaction force is shown (large arrow). With a high-angle hip screw (left panel), the axis of the screw is nearly parallel to the joint reaction force, with little force acting to jam the screw. When a lower-angle device is used (right panel), the component of the joint reaction force acting along the barrel is smaller (small arrow), and the corresponding jamming force is greater. Thus greater force is required to initiate sliding, and the implant may be more likely to function as a rigid device.

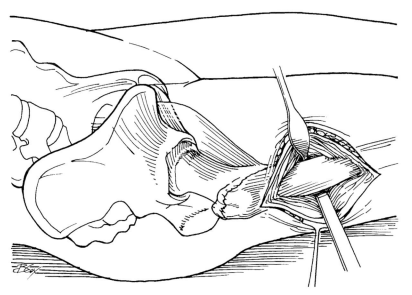

Figure 23–16 The lateral approach to the thigh used for placement of a sliding hip screw.

aspect of the thigh ~10 cm below the tip of the greater trochanter. The incision should be ~1 cm posterior to the midline and is ~15 cm in length with a gentle posterior to anterior orientation, matching the course of the proximal femur **(Fig. 23–16)**. Dissection is carried down to the iliotibial band. Having identified the iliotibial band, this layer should then be incised in line with the skin incision, allowing direct visualization of the vastus lateralis muscle. At this point, the vastus may be split bluntly in line with the proximal femur to gain direct access to the fracture, or it may be elevated by dissecting it from the lateral intramuscular septum. If a vastus split is chosen, it should be performed bluntly and carried proximally and distally along the path of the muscle fibers. If the vastus is elevated from the lateral intramuscular septum down to the linea alba of the femur, the muscle is gently released from the femoral shaft in a submuscular fashion. Both options allow appropriate visualization for use of the sliding screw and side plate. The Hohman retractor is excellent for maintaining good retraction of the vastus muscle during fixation.

Once appropriate exposure has been obtained, fluoroscopy is used to localize the appropriate starting point for the femoral head screw guide pin **(Fig. 23–17A,B)**. This point will vary depending on the implant angle templated preoperatively. For higher-angle (more valgus) implants, the starting point will be more distal on the femur. Using the appropriate implant angle targeting guide, the pin is then driven from the posterolateral cortex into the center of the femoral neck, aiming slightly anteriorly to take into account the anteversion of the femoral neck. This is an excellent point at which to confirm that the implant angle, starting point, and guide pin trajectory are appropriate, using all three fluoroscopic views, before proceeding any further **(Fig. 23–17A,B)**. If any adjustments are made to the guide pin, including a change of starting position or change

of angle used, this step will need to be repeated until the guide pin is centered in the neck, targeting the center of the femoral head in all three views. Once the guide pin is in an appropriate position on all three views, it is advanced to the subchondral bone at the apex of the femoral head.

A common error at this point is to place the starting point of the guide pin too anterior on the shaft of the femur, as seen on the lateral and 20 degree views, or to have a starting point that is too proximal. If either error is made, it is impossible to place the tip of the guide pin at the apex of the femoral head **(Fig. 23–17A,B)**. To ensure appropriate screw placement in the lateral views, the guide should be oriented in a posterolateral position for guide pin placement. This compensates for the normal 20 degrees of femoral anteversion between the neck and shaft. The guide pin is then advanced through the central aspect of the femoral neck directly toward the apex of the head. A proximal start point will place the screw superior in the head, which increases the likelihood of implant failure from cut-out. An angular mismatch between the neck–shaft angle and the implant will also result in poor guide pin placement within the femoral head. Finally, be sure that the guide is perfectly flat on the femoral shaft during wire placement because failure to do so will result in a gap between the lateral cortex and the plate.

An important concept to understand regarding ideal position of the guide pin in the femoral head is the tip–apex distance (TAD) described by Baumgaertner et al.[16,17] The TAD is a measure of the distance from the apex of the femoral head to the tip of the inserted guide pin as measured on both the AP and lateral radiographic views. The TAD is the sum, in millimeters, of the distance on the AP view from the tip of the implant added to that on the lateral view **(Fig. 23–18A,B)**. The risk of cut-out increases dramatically when the TAD exceeds 25 mm.[16,17]

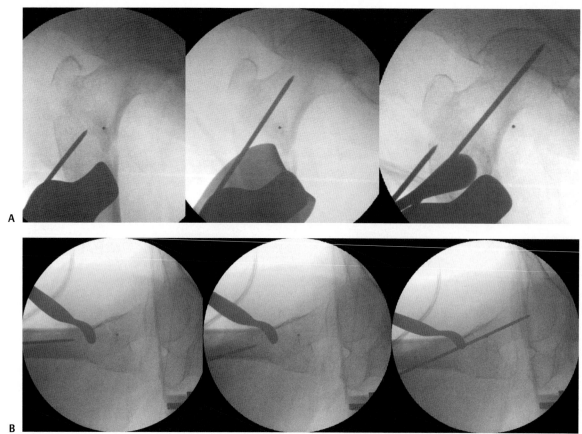

Figure 23–17 Fluoroscopy is used to localize the appropriate starting point for the femoral head screw guide pin. **(A)** These three panels illustrate successive steps in obtaining central positioning of the guide pin using the anteroposterior view. A guide pin is started and advanced a few centimeters into the femoral neck. In the middle panel, it is apparent that the pin is angled too superiorly. The right-panel was taken after the guide pin was redirected into the center of the femoral head. **(B)** These three panels illustrate successive steps in obtaining central positioning of the guide pin using the lateral view. On the left panel, a guide pin is placed on the lateral cortex. In this case it was starting too anterior. In the middle panel, the pin is moved posterior on the femur and then aimed anteriorly to account for the anteversion of the femoral head. On the left, the pin is advanced into the center of the femoral head.

Once the guide pin has been properly inserted, a direct measurement is taken of screw length and reaming depth. Most systems do not include the threaded terminal 10 mm of the guide pin in this measurement, and it is useful to add 5 mm to the measured value. At this point, the triple reamer should be preset for the desired length and slowly advanced over the guide pin **(Fig. 23–19)**. One should use intermittent fluoroscopy to monitor the reamer depth as it advances because serious complications can occur if the guide pin penetrates the pelvis.[29] Visualization during reaming allows the surgeon to make appropriate changes in reaming depth as well as monitor for advancement of the guide pin into the hip joint. In general, it is not necessary to ream to the end of the guide pin; instead, one should stop advancing the reamer 5 mm short of its tip. Once the triple reamer seats to the preset depth, it will no longer advance, so, if more length is needed, adjust the reamer setting in increments of 5 to 10 mm and repeat the reaming process. The guide pin will need to be in its proper position in the head for screw insertion; there-

fore, if it is pulled out with the reamer, replace it prior to inserting the screw.

The cutting tap is then placed over the guide pin and advanced by hand to the reaming depth. This step is not necessary in patients with poor bone density. The cannulated screw, equal in length to the final reaming depth, is then advanced by hand over the guide pin until it is seated in subchondral bone. At this point, the guide pin may be removed, and the surgeon begins application of the side plate.

The side plate barrel is advanced over the previously inserted screw, and the side plate is impacted down to bone, aligning with the femoral shaft. Some systems are "keyed" and require correct rotational orientation of the screw during insertion to align the plate with the bone. Adjustments may be made in screw rotation at this time to obtain proper plate alignment. Once impacted, the plate is then affixed to the proximal femoral shaft with two to six bicortical screws using standard technique. Two screws are sufficient for most stable fractures, but more screws

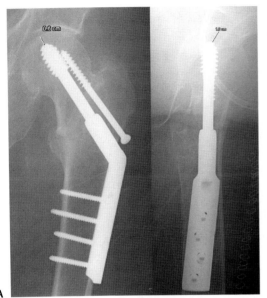

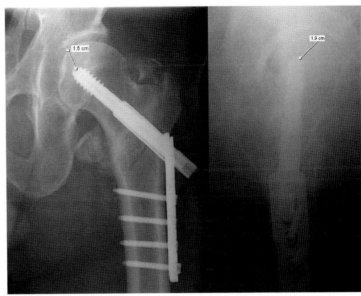

A

B

Figure 23–18 The tip–apex distance (TAD) used to determine positioning of the guide pin within the femoral head. **(A)** An example of ideal screw positioning with less than 1 cm of distance between the tip of the screw and the apex of the femoral head in both views. In this case, the TAD measures 16 mm. **(B)** In this example, the TAD measures 35 mm, exceeding the desired amount by 1 cm. Fortunately, this fracture went on to union in this case.

may be needed in cases of severe osteoporosis to prevent screw pull-out from the femoral shaft **(Fig. 23–20A–D)**.

One should be sure that the shaft of the large femoral head screw has enough engagement within the barrel of the side plate to allow for impaction and compression. If the screw is too short, there is a risk of both disengagement of the screw from the side plate and jamming of the screw, with catastrophic failure. In very small patients, a short barrel may be necessary because the length of the barrel itself can sometimes prevent fracture collapse.

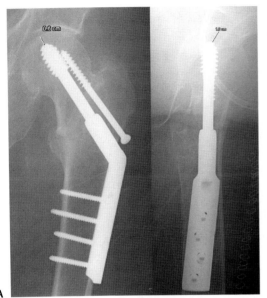

Figure 23–19 The triple reamer is advanced over the guide pin to the preset depth.

Overall, the hip screw and side plate construct has an excellent track record for fixation of intertrochanteric hip fractures, provided that it is not used with reverse obliquity fractures.

Cephalomedullary Nail (see Video 23–2, Disk 3)

In general, antegrade femoral nails are designed for insertion in either the piriformis fossa or the tip of the trochanter. For the purposes of this review, the latter are referred to as trochanteric nails. Trochanteric nails typically have a more pronounced proximal angulation to facilitate their slightly eccentric starting point and have a larger proximal diameter than nails designed for insertion in the piriformis fossa. Because intertrochanteric fractures typically disrupt the region of the piriformis fossa, trochanteric nails are generally considered when intramedullary fixation of trochanteric fractures is desired. The trochanteric starting point is also more accessible than the piriformis fossa in obese patients. There are many variations of the trochanteric nail; some have one large femoral neck screw, whereas others use two smaller-diameter screws. Most are available in both short and long lengths. These devices require the same reduction strategies as with the hip screw and side plate but may be inserted using a percutaneous technique unless fracture clamps are required. These are excellent devices for both simple and complex intertrochanteric fractures, including the reverse oblique pattern **(Fig. 23–11A,B)**. The intramedullary position of these implants yields enhanced mechanical advantage over the hip screw because there is a shorter lever arm from the femoral head to the load-bearing axis of the implant. Fixation of the nail distally is not dependent on

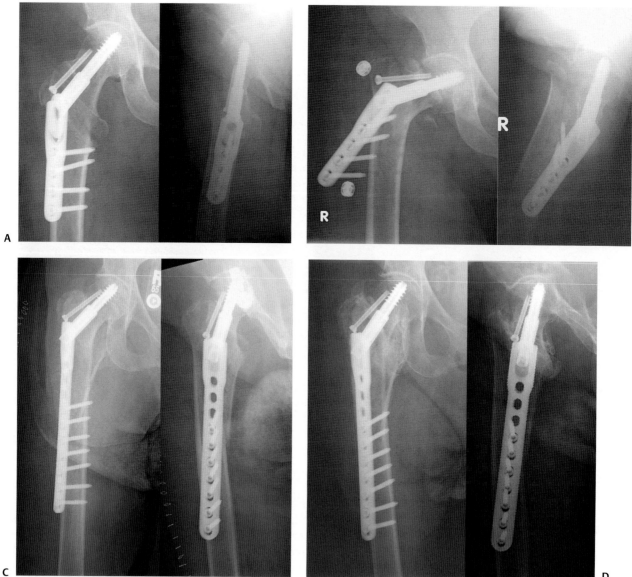

A

B

C

D

Figure 23–20 An example of a side plate that pulled off the femoral shaft due to inadequate fixation. **(A)** Anteroposterior and lateral views after repair of a peritrochanteric fracture with a four-hole slide plate. **(B)** Two views of the hip taken just 10 days later after a minor

fall, showing that the screws had pulled out with a new fracture line propagating through the empty screw holes. **(C)** Anteroposterior and lateral views after revision fixation with a longer side plate. **(D)** Final views after fracture healing.

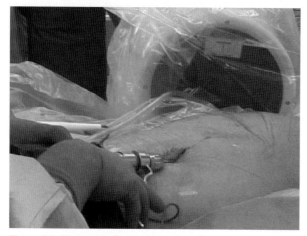

Figure 23–21 Incision for trochanteric nailing.

screw fixation; instead, the nail is surrounded by intact cortical bone. The distally placed screw provides rotational control of the implant. Compression is obtained across the fracture in the same manner as with a hip screw and side plate, but in addition, many cephalomedullary nails also have compression devices that allow for immediate maximal compression intraoperatively.

Patient positioning on the fracture table and initial fracture reduction are performed as described previously. The incision for cephalomedullary nail insertion is made approximately 3 to 5 cm above the greater trochanter and is generally 2 to 4 cm in length. The incision is also angled from posterior to anterior as it moves distally to align with the proximal shaft and anterior bow of the femur (**Fig. 23–21**). In obese patients, the location of the incision may vary

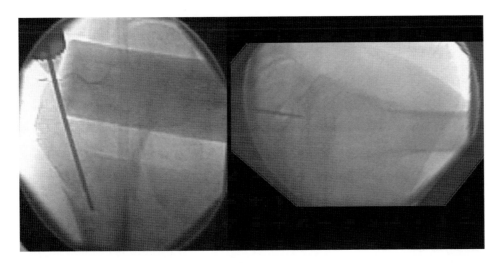

Figure 23–22 Anteroposterior (AP) and lateral images taken during surgery showing the starting point for a trochanteric nail. The guidewire is placed on the medial aspect of the tip of the trochanter on the AP view (left panel) and on the anterior third of the trochanter on the lateral view (right panel).

according to the soft tissues. Blunt dissection is performed down to the gluteus medius fascia. This fascial layer is then split sharply using a knife, but extending distally toward the greater trochanter, thus allowing for appropriate instrument passage toward the trochanteric or piriformis fossa start point. Then, the starter awl or guide pin is now advanced to the greater trochanter or piriformis fossa.

The proper starting point is essential for nail insertion. With a trochanteric nail, the starting point must be in the anterior third of the trochanter on the lateral view and 20 degree neck view, and must also be at the medial aspect of the apex of the trochanter on the AP view **(Fig. 23–22).**

Once the appropriate starting point has been identified, and after ensuring that the fracture remains reduced, the starting pin or awl is advanced into the intertrochanteric region approximately 3 cm. This should be performed in line with the femoral shaft on the lateral view and toward the lesser trochanter on the AP view. If a starting pin is

used, it will need to be overreamed to create an opening sufficient for guidewire and nail placement **(Fig. 23–23).**

The ball-tipped guidewire is now advanced through the starting hole and advanced past the subtrochanteric region within the intramedullary canal. The guidewire should be inserted past the isthmus of the femur to ensure appropriate wire placement and to prevent wire back-out during reaming. The position of the guidewire should be confirmed on both AP and lateral radiographic projections prior to reaming **(Fig. 23–24).**

Once guidewire placement is confirmed, the intertrochanteric region and proximal femoral canal must be prepared for nail placement. Most systems for cephalomedullary nailing recommend a standard proximal and distal reaming diameter for nail placement. Once the distal reaming diameter has been achieved, the surgeon should advance to the recommended proximal opening width by reaming only within the intertrochanteric region with the

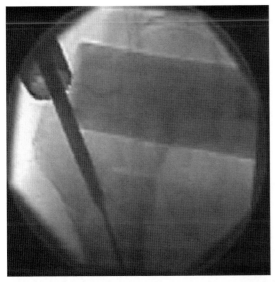

Figure 23–23 The proximal femur is gently opened with a large-diameter cannulated reamer that is inserted over the previously placed guidewire.

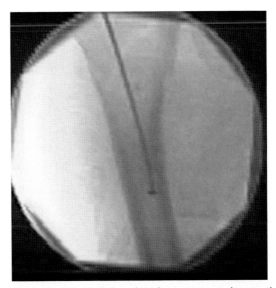

Figure 23–24 A ball-tipped guidewire is inserted across the fracture into the distal femur.

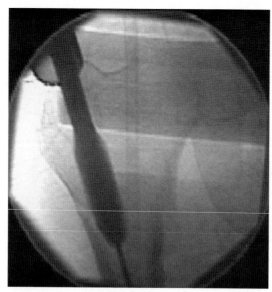

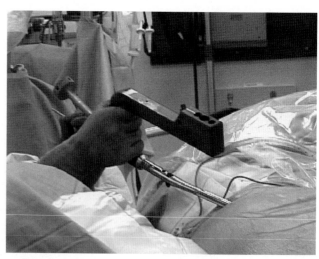

Figure 23–26 The assembled nail with the attached jig for proximal interlocking is inserted by hand over the guidewire.

Figure 23–25 A special large-diameter reamer (typically 17 mm) is used to open the trochanteric region to accommodate the large-diameter proximal portion of the nail.

larger reamers **(Fig. 23–25)**. All reaming should be done by passing a flexible reamer over the guidewire, and care must be taken to ensure that the guidewire remains in place during reamer advancement and removal. The end of the guidewire can be firmly gripped with a Kocher clamp during reamer removal, and guidewire position should be confirmed radiographically between reamer passes if there is any concern of guidewire position change. Another useful tip for reaming is to place a mallet at the lateral aspect of the reamer as it enters the starting hole. By placing a medial force through the mallet, it is easier to prevent lateralization of the starting hole and loss of the lateral cortex of the greater trochanter. The proximal femur is now prepared for nail insertion.

The cephalomedullary nail is assembled with its outrigger targeting device and is now advanced into the proximal

femur by hand over the guidewire **(Fig. 23–26)**. Care must be taken to avoid a varus or valgus stress to the nail during advancement. This can result in loss of reduction, fracture extension involving the femoral neck or greater trochanter, and possibly creation of a subtrochanteric fracture. The nail is gently advanced over the guidewire while using an anterior-posterior rotational force applied through the outrigger. Nail depth and orientation are checked radiographically on the AP view, and once the appropriate seating depth has been achieved, the nail outrigger is placed with approximately 20 degrees of anteversion to target the femoral neck and head. The appropriate depth for the nail will place the lag screw in the center of the femoral neck and head, or slightly inferior to the center on the AP radiographic view. At this point, the ball-tipped guidewire should be removed.

Lag screw/helical blade guide pin placement will require coordinating the guide pin trajectory on the AP, lateral, and femoral neck lateral views **(Fig. 23–27)**. If properly

Figure 23–27 The femoral head lag screw is inserted with biplanar fluoroscopic imaging. The guide pin is inserted into the center of the femoral head on both views.

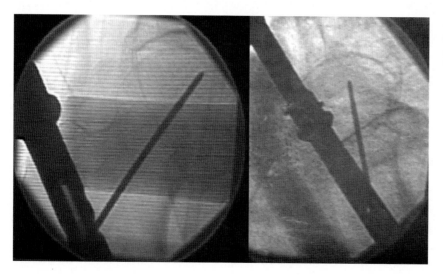

placed, the guide pin will advance into the subchondral bone in the center of the femoral head on all three radiographic views. One should start first with the AP view and advance the guidewire through the targeting device and halfway up the femoral neck using fluoroscopy. If the pin trajectory is inappropriate for the neck-shaft angle, it is recommended that the pin and nail be removed and that the appropriate angled nail be used. If the wire is advancing too high or low within the neck, the wire should be removed, and the nail depth should be gently adjusted.

Once appropriate nail angle and depth are confirmed, with the guide pin advanced to the transcervical level, the guidewire should be viewed in the lateral and femoral neck lateral views. If adjustments are required, the pin must be fully removed prior to correcting the nail anteversion. The wire should be advanced and reevaluated with fluoroscopy after each adjustment of the nail until the proper anteversion of the guide pin is obtained. While still using the lateral view, the pin is advanced into the subchondral bone of the femoral head. Guide pin placement within subchondral bone at the center of the femoral head must be confirmed not only on the femoral neck lateral view but also on the AP view prior to proceeding with lag screw/helical blade placement. One should attempt to place the screws as close to the apex of the femoral head as possible; use of the same TAD criteria described for the sliding hip screw is appropriate (see section Surgical Fixation: Sliding Screw and Side Plate; **Fig. 23–18**). Once optimal guide pin position within the femoral head has been achieved, the lag screw/helical blade length must be determined. Overreaming of the guide pin is recommended, and the lag screw/helical blade is then advanced over the pin to final seating depth and orientation within the femoral head (**Fig. 23–28**). The system-specific slide mechanism

should be tightened to allow for fracture compression. Distal locking of the nail is recommended for unstable patterns where rotational control is indicated.

Fixed-Angle Device (95 Degrees)

Fixed-angle devices such as the blade plate or dynamic condylar screw have limited use in peritrochanteric fractures of the upper femur. Their use is primarily confined to the most unstable fracture patterns, such as reverse obliquity fractures. The indications and techniques for these devices are thoroughly discussed in Chapter 24.

Rehabilitation

Accepted postsurgical protocol for intertrochanteric fractures requires 24 hours of intravenous antibiotics, as well as deep venous thrombosis (DVT) prophylaxis. A first generation cephelasporin is utilized. If the patient is penicillin-allergic, vancomyin is utilized. Both mechanical and chemical DVT prophylaxis is recommended in the postsurgical period. Patients are generally allowed to bear weight as tolerated because cognitively intact patients will generally "autoprotect" the affected extremity.[30] Koval et al showed that patients with unstable patterns placed less weight upon the repaired extremity than did those patients who presented with stable fracture patterns.[30] In a separate study, Koval et al showed that allowing patients to bear weight to tolerance resulted in no increased rate of fixation failure.[31]

Successful rehabilitation with therapy has been shown to be less dependent on factors such as sex, fracture type, and type of operation and most dependent on the level of patient function prior to injury and age.[32] Standardized formal rehabilitation including physical therapy and social services has not been shown to improve patient recovery in the 3 and 6 month interval.[33]

New Techniques

Recently, the use of external fixation had been critically explored for use in definitive treatment of intertrochanteric hip fractures. Moroni et al, in a series of 40 fractures, showed that primary external fixation using hydroxyapatite-coated pins was as effective as the 135 degree hip screw for the treatment of pertrochanteric fractures.[34] This technique required less operative time, minimized blood loss, and showed significantly less overall postsurgical pain. Also, overall reduction was maintained at 6 months. External fixation continues to be explored.

Because of the fact that most intertrochanteric fractures are associated with osteopenia, the use of composite fixation has been of interest. Traditionally, surgeons have used bone cement (PMMA) to fill in areas of severe comminution.[35] Because PMMA is nonresorbable and may interfere with fracture healing, there has been recent interest in the use of resorbable implants that may be

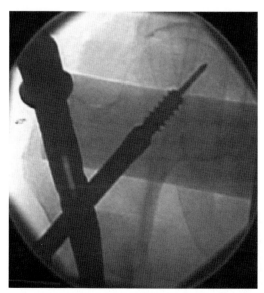

Figure 23–28 The final screw is inserted over the guide pin.

Tips and Tricks

- The internally rotated view is the best radiographic view for preoperative planning to determine implant angle because it gives a true view of the neck-shaft angle and a true depiction of fracture anatomy.
- Fracture reduction must be obtained prior to fixation because the implants will not correct malreduction, nor will they allow for fragment manipulation after insertion.
- Beware of posterior sag, and maintain manual correction of this throughout the procedure.
- A pointed reduction clamp placed from the medial calcar to the lateral femoral shaft will help to maintain reduction during fixation **(Fig. 23–9).**
- A common error during guide pin placement is start the pin too anterior on the shaft of the femur, as seen on the lateral and 20 degree views, or to have a starting point that is too proximal. If either error is made, it is impossible to place the tip of the guide pin into the apex of the femoral head. To ensure appropriate screw placement in the lateral views, the guide should be oriented in a posterolateral position for guide pin placement. This compensates for the normal 20 degrees of femoral anteversion between the neck and shaft.
- When measuring the length of the lag screw, be aware that most systems do not include the threaded terminal 10 mm of the guide pin in this measurement. It is therefore helpful to add 5 mm to the measured value.
- In general, it is not necessary to ream to the end of the guide pin; instead, one should stop advancing the reamer 5 mm short of its tip.
- Tapping is not necessary in many older patients with osteopenic bone.
- Make sure that the shaft of the large femoral head screw has enough engagement within the barrel of the side plate to al-
low for impaction and compression. If the screw is too short, there is a risk of both disengagement of the screw from the side plate or jamming of the screw, with catastrophic failure. In very small patients, a short barrel may be necessary because the length of the barrel itself can sometimes prevent fracture collapse.
- With a trochanteric nail, the start is in the anterior third of the trochanter on the lateral view and 20 degree neck view, and at the medial aspect of the apex of the trochanter on the AP view. When using a piriformis nail, the starting point is on the lateral aspect of the fossa on the AP view, and on the anterior aspect of the fossa on the lateral and 20 degree lateral femoral neck views.
- A useful tip for reaming is to place a mallet at the lateral aspect of the reamer as it enters the starting hole. By placing a medial force through the mallet, it is easier to prevent lateralization of the starting hole and loss of the lateral cortex of the greater trochanter.
- Always insert a trochanteric nail by hand after sufficient reaming to avoid inadvertent fracture of the femoral shaft.
- In general, longer nails are preferred because of the reduced risk of later fracture at the tip of the implant and less risk of fixation failure. However, when inserting a long trochanteric nail, beware of mismatch between the bow of the femur and the nail, leading to possible perforation of the anterior distal femoral by the tip of the nail.
- In patients with severe osteopenia, composite fixation may be necessary. In these circumstances, consider augmenting the surgical fixation with polymethyl methacrylate (PMMA). The authors recommend the use of Palacos (Biomet Orthopedics, Inc., Warsaw, Indiana) because of its favorable handling characteristics.

remodeled into bone. Currently, there are numerous calcium phosphate cements that are commercially available, and which may allow the surgeon to "fill in" areas of comminution or improve the density of the bone, increasing the strength of fixation and preventing collapse of the fracture. Using a biomechanical model, Elder et al found that augmenting fixation with Norian SRS (Synthes, Paoli, Pennsylvania) increased stiffness of the fracture construct and minimized displacement of the sliding hip screw.[36] These researchers also found that medial bone surface strain was closer to the intact state and that side plate strain was lower relative to controls. However, there was no difference in the load to failure between Norian-augmented and control femora.[36] The authors concluded that augmentation of unstable intertrochanteric fractures improved overall fracture stability, facilitated load transfer across the fracture, and decreased shortening of the proximal femur and stress on the sliding hip screw.[36] In another study, Norian cement–augmented specimens had less shortening (1 mm

vs 17 mm) and twice the initial construct stiffness compared with control specimens.[37]

As in other areas of surgery and traumatology, interest in minimally invasive techniques has led to the development of alternative approaches for these injuries as well. DiPaola and colleagues have presented a minimally invasive adaptation of the sliding hip screw technique.[38] However, Gotfried in particular deserves credit for advancing this approach to intertrochanteric fractures with his percutaneous compression plate.[39] This device had a low rate of complications in an independent series of 130 patients.[40]

Outcomes

The outcome after an intertrochanteric fracture is not well described. In the past, the outcome was judged to be successful if the patient survived and the fracture healed. Functional measurements of outcome were not considered in detail. In terms of fracture union, osteoporosis, fracture geometry, and the surgical technique are strong predictors of outcome. Specifically, to optimize the outcome for a given fracture, the surgeon must anatomically reduce the fracture, choose the most appropriate implant, and insert the implant correctly. These issues are thoroughly discussed elsewhere in this chapter.

Recently, the assessment of outcomes has become more sophisticated with the validation of general health outcome assessment tools and specific hip function scores. Interestingly, when such analyses are done, one of the strongest predictors of outcome turns out to be the level of preinjury function.[41] Of all proximal femoral fractures, patients with unstable intertrochanteric fractures have the poorest functional outcome scores, but this group of patients is the most debilitated before injury as well.[41]

Surgeons treating intertrochanteric fractures must choose between two primary methods of treatment: a sliding hip screw or a cephalomedullary nail. The sliding hip screw is certainly the "gold standard" for managing these fractures,[2] but the very feature—sliding—that allows fracture impaction to increase stability and healing also contributes to loss of femoral offset and femoral shortening after healing. Intramedullary nails, by virtue of their greater stability and intramedullary position, may allow for fracture healing with less deformity, and possibly better abductor function.[27,42] One recent comparative study found better walking ability in patients with unstable fractures that were treated with a Gamma nail.[27] There have been many comparative trials published; most have methodological shortcomings that make their interpretation difficult. To keep abreast of this issue, Parker and Handoll have performed a series of comprehensive meta-analyses that are published as part of the Cochrane Library of Systematic Reviews.[43] In their latest biennial report, 32 randomized clinical trials were analyzed. Twenty of these, including a total of 3646 patients, compared the Gamma nail with a sliding hip screw. Patients treated with a Gamma nail had an increased risk of intra- and postoperative fracture of the femur and an increased rate of reoperation. The rate of wound infection, mortality, or medical complications was similar in both sets of patients. It was not possible to analyze other outcomes.

Five other studies, involving 623 people, compared the intramedullary hip screw with the sliding hip screw. Again, fracture fixation complications were more common in the intramedullary hip screw group; in fact, all cases of perioperative femoral fracture occurred in the nailing group. In keeping with the findings for the Gamma nail, postoperative complications, mortality, and functional outcomes were similar in the two groups. A few other trials evaluated the proximal femoral nail, an experimental mini-invasive static intramedullary nail, and the Medoff sliding plate (Medpac, Valencia, California); none provided sufficient evidence to establish that there was any improved outcome with these newer devices. Two studies in-

volving a total of 65 patients with reverse oblique or transverse fractures at the level of the lesser trochanter found intramedullary nails (Gamma nail or proximal femoral nail) to be associated with better intraoperative results and fewer fracture fixation complications than extramedullary implants (a 95 degree blade plate or dynamic condylar plate). The conclusion of the Cochrane reviewers is that, given the lower overall complication rate of the sliding hip screw compared with intramedullary nails, the sliding hip screw appears to be superior for most trochanteric fractures. Intramedullary nails do appear to have advantages for selected fracture types, such as reverse obliquity and subtrochanteric fractures.[43]

A more detailed description of outcome of intertrochanteric fractures was recently provided by Chirodian et al, who reported on 1024 consecutive cases managed with a sliding hip screw.[44] The patients' mean age was 82 years, and 78% were female. Seventy-five percent of the fractures were judged to be unstable. At 1 year follow-up, 69% of patients were alive. The vast majority (95%) had minimal or no pain, 85% had returned to their prefracture living arrangement, and 50% regained their level of mobility. Complications of surgical fixation occurred in 4% of cases, and just fewer than 3% required further surgery as a result. These data confirm that the overall fixation failure and reoperation rates for trochanteric fractures fixed with a sliding hip screw are low. The final outcome in surviving patients is good, and most patients return to their prefracture level of accommodation and mobility.[44]

Complications

Complications after intertrochanteric fracture can be broadly grouped into systemic complications and local complications. Systemic complications include mortality, myocardial infarction, thromboembolism, and pressure ulceration. Because intertrochanteric fractures commonly occur in debilitated, chronically ill patients, there is clearly increased mortality; White et al calculated that the standard mortality ratio is six times higher in patients with hip fractures than the general population matched for age.[45] Mortality is dramatically increased in patients with chronic renal disease (63%),[46] malnourishment (70%),[47] and diabetes (80%).[48] Other factors that are associated with a higher risk of mortality include delay to surgery more than 24 hours,[45] dementia, postoperative pneumonia, malignancy, advanced age, and deep wound infection.[49] Patients with hip fractures are among those at highest risk for thromboembolic complications, and all should be treated with either or both mechanical and pharmacological prophylaxis. Mechanical compression devices, such as sequential pneumatic compression stockings or intermittent plantar compression pumps, have demonstrated effectiveness in reducing deep venous thrombosis in hip fracture patients.[50] A relatively new drug, fondaparinux, is a synthetic factor XA inhibitor, and is the only agent approved by the Food and Drug Administration for prevention of deep vein thrombosis in hip fracture patients. In one large, randomized, clinical trial, fondaparinux was compared with Lovenox and was associated with an incidence of venous thromboembolism by day 11 of 8.3% (52 of 626 patients) compared with 19.1% (119 of 624 patients) in the enoxaparin group ($p < .001$).[51] The risk reduction with fondaparinux was 56.4% (95% confidence interval, 39.0 to 70.3%). Importantly, there were no significant differences between the two groups in the incidence of death or clinically relevant bleeding.[51] Recently, the Seventh American College of Chest Physicians Conference on Antithrombotic and Thrombolytic Therapy: Evidence-Based Guidelines were published.[52] For patients undergoing hip fracture surgery, these guidelines recommend the routine use of fondaparinux, low molecular weight heparins, warfarin (target INR 2.5; range 2.0 to 3.0), or low-dose unfractionated heparin. These guidelines also recommend that patients with hip fractures receive thromboprophylaxis for at least 10 days.[52]

Local complications include wound infection, nonunion, and loss of fixation or hardware failure or both. Wound infection remains common in these debilitated patients. It is clear that hip fracture patients undergoing surgery require prophylactic intravenous antibiotics. Southwell-Keely et al recently reported the results of a meta-analysis of the literature and found 15 randomized controlled trials that addressed this topic. It was shown that antibiotic prophylaxis reduced overall wound infections compared with placebo and was equally effective for deep and superficial infections.[53] One dose of intravenous antibiotics was as effective as multiple doses. Antibiotic use also reduced the incidence of urinary tract infection but had no significant effect on mortality.[53]

Loss of fixation is a common complication in these patients, especially those with osteopenia and severe comminution. Numerous studies have shown that the quality of the bone, fracture stability, quality of reduction, type of implant, and position of the implant influence outcome.[2,4,16] Proper position of the implant in the center of the femoral head, as determined by the so-called TAD, appears to be an important means of reducing loss of fixation.[16] Regardless of the quality of reduction and fixation, failure of fixation occurs more commonly in the unstable fracture patterns when sliding hip screws are used; intramedullary devices perform better in these fractures.[5] However, a peculiar failure phenomenon, called the Z-effect, has recently been observed in some unstable fractures treated with short trochanteric nails with two lag screws. Because of differential loading of the two screws (one in tension and one in compression), this type of construct may fail when one of the screws backs out while the other penetrates into the femoral head (**Fig. 23–29**).

When nonunion occurs, there are essentially two options: hip arthroplasty with a calcar-replacing stem, or repeat reduction and fixation, usually with a valgus osteotomy. Bartonicek et al reported on 15 patients with varus malunion or nonunion following intertrochanteric fractures and who were treated with a valgus intertrochanteric osteotomy.[54] Fourteen patients (93%) healed without complications. One patient underwent successful revision for loss of fixation after a fall 6 weeks after surgery. The average leg lengthening after osteotomy was 2 cm (range 1 to 5 cm). In all patients, hip flexion was greater than 90 degrees, and Harris hip score increased from 73 points to 92 points. Osteoarthritis or avascular necrosis of the femoral head did not develop in any case, and the au-

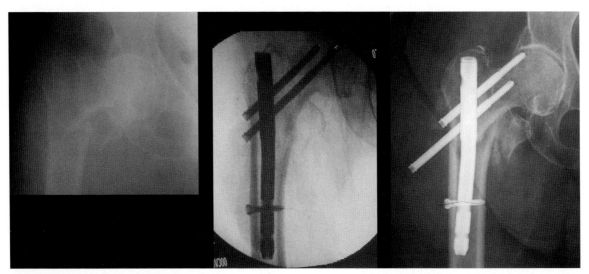

Figure 23–29 Examples of the so-called Z-effect. In the left panel, a three-part intertrochanteric fracture with varus angulation and a displaced posteromedial fragment is shown. The middle panel shows the fracture repaired with a short trochanteric nail with two lag screws in the femoral head. In the right panel, fixation failure is shown with the two lag screws moving in opposite directions. (Courtesy of William Ricci, MD)

thors concluded that valgus intertrochanteric osteotomy is an effective procedure for treating trochanteric malunion or nonunion.[54] When loss of fixation is associated with cut-out or protrusion of the femoral head screw, arthroplasty is necessary. Haidukewych and Berry reported the Mayo Clinic's experience with 60 patients treated with arthroplasty for failed intertrochanteric fractures.[55] Total hip arthroplasty was done in 32 patients; three fourths had a cemented cup, another 27 underwent bipolar hemiarthroplasty, and one had a unipolar hemiarthroplasty. Femoral reconstruction was done in most cases with a calcar-replacement design, extended-neck stem, or long-stem implant. Of 44 patients followed for a mean of 5 years, 39 had no or mild pain, whereas five had moderate or severe pain. In all of the patients with pain, the pain was in the region of the greater trochanter. Forty patients walked, 26 using one-arm support or less. Twelve patients suffered a total of 13 medical complications postoperatively. Survivorship analysis using revision of the implant for any reason as the definition of failure revealed a survival rate of 100% at 7 years and 87.5% at 10 years. These authors consider that hip arthroplasty is an effective salvage procedure for the failed treatment of an intertrochanteric fracture in an older patient, but note

that calcar-replacement and long-stem implants are often required.[55]

Pearls

- The most important feature separating a stable from an unstable intertrochanteric fracture is the presence of a displaced fragment in the region of the lesser trochanter.
- MRI is more accurate and more effective for the early detection of occult intertrochanteric fractures than both CT scan and scintigraphy.[11]
- The sliding hip screw and side plate remains the preferred implant for fixation of stable intertrochanteric fractures, whereas the cephalomedullary nail provides more stability of unstable fracture patterns, especially the reverse obliquity type.[19]
- One of the major biomechanical advantages of an intramedullary device compared with a lateral plate is that the intramedullary implant has a smaller lever arm than a lateral plate due to its intramedullary placement.
- The risk of implant failure increases dramatically when the TAD exceeds 25 mm.

On the DVDs

Video 23–1   (Disk 3)   ORIF of an Intertrochanteric Fracture Using Sliding Screw and Side Plate   This video demonstrates ORIF of a high energy intertrochanteric femur fracture following a skiing injury in a 45-year-old man. We review the proper placement of screws in the femoral head and neck to avoid cutout, as well as the tip-to-apex distance.

Video 23–2   (Disk 3)   Intramedullary Nailing of an Unstable Intertrochanteric Fracture   This video reviews the use of intramedullary nailing to treat intertrochanteric fractures. The correct starting point and indications for intramedullary nailing are discussed.

References

1. Alffram PA. An epidemiologic study of cervical and trochanteric fractures of the femur in the urban population: analysis of 1,664 cases with special reference to etiologic factors. Acta Orthop Scand Suppl 1964;65:1–109

2. Kyle RF, Gustilo RB, Premer RF. Analysis of six hundred and twenty-two intertrochanteric hip fractures. J Bone Joint Surg Am 1979;61:216–221

3. Evans EM. The treatment of trochanteric fractures of the femur. J Bone Joint Surg Br 1949;31B:190–203

4. Kyle RF, Ellis TJ, Templeman DC. Surgical treatment of intertrochanteric hip fractures with associated femoral neck fractures using a sliding hip screw. J Orthop Trauma 2005;19:1–4

5. Haidukewych GJ, Israel TA, Berry DJ. Reverse obliquity fractures of the intertrochanteric region of the femur. J Bone Joint Surg Am 2001;83-A:643–650

6. Fracture and dislocation compendium. Orthopaedic Trauma Association Committee for Coding and Classification. J Orthop Trauma 1996;10(Suppl 1):v–ix, 31–35

7. Clawson DK. Intertrochanteric fractures of the hip. Am J Surg 1957;93:580–587

8. Lyon LJ, Nevins MA. Management of hip fractures in nursing home patients: to treat or not to treat. J Am Geriatr Soc 1984;32:391–395

9. Lim KB, Eng AK, Chng SM, Tan AG, Thoo FL, Low CO. Limited magnetic resonance imaging (MRI) and the occult hip fracture. Ann Acad Med Singapore 2002;31:607–610

10. Chana R, Noorani A, Ashwood N, Chatterji U, Healy J, Baird P. The role of MRI in the diagnosis of proximal femoral fractures in the elderly. Injury 2005;36 (available at http://www.sciencedirect.com/ science/journal/00201383)

11. Lubovsky O, Liebergall M, Mattan Y, Mosheiff R. Early diagnosis of occult hip fractures MRI vs CT scan. Injury 2005;36:788–792

12. Kenzora JE, McCarthy RE, Lowell JD, Sledge CB. Hip fracture mortality: relation to age, treatment, preoperative illness, time of surgery, and complications. Clin Orthop Relat Res 1984;186:45–56

13. Ring PA. Treatment of trochanteric fractures of the femur. Br Med J 1963;53(3):654–656

14. McNeill DH. Hip fractures: influence of delay in surgery on mortality. Wis Med J 1975;74:129–130

15. Kaufer H. Mechanics of the treatment of hip injuries. Clin Orthop Relat Res 1980;146:53–61

16. Baumgaertner M, Curtin S, Lindskog D, Keggi J. The value of the tip–apex distance in predicting failure of fixation of peritrochanteric fractures of the hip. J Bone Joint Surg Am 1995;77:1058–1064

17. Baumgaertner MR, Solberg BD. Awareness of the tip-apex distance reduces failure of fication of trochanteric fractures of the hip. J Bone Joint Surg Br 1997;79:969–971

18. Im G-I, Shin Y-W, Song Y-J. Potentially unstable intertrochanteric fractures. J Orthop Trauma 2005;19:5–9

19. Bridle SH, Patel AD, Bircher M, Calvert PY. Fixation of intertrochanteric fractures of the femur: a randomized prospective comparison of the gamma nail and dynamic hip screw. J Bone Joint Surg Br 1991;73:330–334

20. Watson JT, Moed BR, Cramer KE, Kargas DE. Comparison of the compression hip screw with the Medoff sliding plate for intertrochanteric fractures. Clin Orthop Relat Res 1998;348:79–86

21. Hardy DC, Descamps PY, Krallis P, et al. Use of an intramedullary hip-screw compared with a compression hip-screw with a plate for intertrochanteric femoral fractures: a prospective, randomized study of one hundred patients. J Bone Joint Surg Am 1998;80:618–630

22. Lindsey RW, Teal P, Probe RA, Rhoads D, Davenport S, Schauder K. Early experience with a gamma interlocking nail for peri-trochanteric fractures of the proximal femur. J Trauma 1991;31:1649–1658

23. Davis J, Harris MB, Duvall M, D'Ambrosia R. Peritrochanteric fractures treated with a Gamma nail: technique and report of early results. Orthopedics 1991;14:939–942

24. Laros GS, Moore JF. Complications of fixation in intertrochanteric fractures. Clin Orthop Relat Res 1974;101:110–119

25. Esser MP, Kassab JY, Jones DH. Trochanteric fractures of the femur. J Bone Joint Surg Br 1986;68:557–560

26. Kyle RF, Wright TM, Burstein AH. Biomechanical analysis of the sliding characteristics of compression hip screws. J Bone Joint Surg Am 1980;62:1308–1314

27. Utrilla AL, Reig JS, Muñoz FM, Tufanisco CB. Trochanteric Gamma nail and compression hip screw for trochanteric fractures: a randomized, prospective, comparative study in 210 elderly patients with a new design of the Gamma nail. J Orthop Trauma 2005;19:229–233

28. Walton NP, Wynn-Jones H, Ward MS, Wimhurst JA. Femoral neck-shaft angle in extra-capsular proximal femoral fracture fixation: does it make a TAD of difference? Injury 2005;36:1361–1364

29. Mueller M, Jähnich H, Butler-Manuel A. Inadvertent guide wire advancement in hip fracture fixation with fatal outcome. Injury 2005;36:679–680

30. Koval KJ, Sala DA, Kummer FJ, Zuckerman JD. Postoperative weight bearing after a fracture of the femoral neck or an intertrochanteric fracture. J Bone Joint Surg Am 1998;80:352–356

31. Koval KJ, Friend KD, Aharonoff GB, Zuckerman JD. Weight bearing after hip fractures: a prospective series of 596 geriatric hip fracture patients. J Orthop Trauma 1996;10:526–530

32. Thorngren KG, Norrman PO, Hommel A, Cedervall M, Thorngren J, Wingstrand H. Influence of age, sex fracture type and pre-fracture living on rehabilitation pattern after hip fractures in the elderly. Disabil Rehabil 2005;27:1091–1097

33. Beaupre LA, Cinats JG, Senthilselvan A, Scharfenberger A, Johnston DW, Saunders LD. Does standardized rehabilitation and discharge planning improve functional recovery in elderly patients with hip fracture? Arch Phys Med Rehabil 2005;86:2231–2239

34. Moroni A, Faldini C, Pegreffi F, Hoang-Kim A, Vannini F, Giannini S. Dynamic hip screw compared with external fixation for treatment of osteoporotic pertrochanteric fractures: a prospective, randomized study. J Bone Joint Surg Am 2005;87:753–759

35. Bartucci EJ, Gonzalez MH, Cooperman DR, Freedberg HI, Barmada R, Laros GS. The effect of adjunctive methylmethacrylate on failures of fixation and function in patients with intertrochanteric fractures and osteoporosis. J Bone Joint Surg Am 1985;67:1094–1107

36. Elder S, Frankenburg E, Goulet J, Yetkinler D, Poser R, Goldstein S. Biomechanical evaluation of calcium phosphate cement-augmented fixation of unstable intertrochanteric fractures. J Orthop Trauma 2000;14:386–393

37. Yetkinler DN, Goodman SB, Reindel ES, Carter D, Poser RD, Constantz BR. Mechanical evaluation of a carbonated apatite cement in the fixation of unstable intertrochanteric fractures. Acta Orthop Scand 2002;73:157–164

38. DiPaola M, Rozbruch SR, Helfet DL. Minimal incision technique using a two-hole plate for fixation of stable intertrochanteric hip fractures. Orthopedics 2004;27:270–274

39. Gotfried Y. Percutaneous compression plating for intertrochanteric hip fractures: treatment rationale. Orthopedics 2002;25:647–652

40. Peyser A, Weil Y, Liebergall M, Mosheiff R. Percutaneous compression plating for intertrochanteric fractures: surgical technique, tips for surgery, and results. Oper Orthop Traumatol 2005;17:158–177

41. Cornwall R, Gilbert MS, Koval KJ, Strauss E, Siu AL. Functional outcomes and mortality vary among different types of hip fractures: a function of patient characteristics. Clin Orthop Relat Res 2004;425:64–71

42. Pajarinen J, Lindahl J, Savolainen V, Michelsson O, Hirvensalo E. Femoral shaft medialisation and neck-shaft angle in unstable pertrochanteric femoral fractures. Int Orthop 2004;28:347–353

43. Parker M, Handoll H. Gamma and other cephalocondylic intramedullary nails versus extramedullary implants for extracapsular hip fractures in adults. Cochrane Database Syst Rev 2005; Oct 19(4):CD000093

44. Chirodian N, Arch B, Parker MJ. Sliding hip screw fixation of trochanteric hip fractures: outcome of 1024 procedures. Injury 2005;36:793–800

45. White BL, Fisher WD, Laurin CA. Rate of mortality for elderly patients after fracture of the hip in the 1980's. J Bone Joint Surg Am 1987;69:1335–1340

46. Tierney GS, Goulet JA, Greenfield ML, Port FK. Mortality after fracture of the hip in patients who have end-stage renal disease. J Bone Joint Surg Am 1994;76:709–712

47. Foster MR, Heppenstall RB, Friedenberg ZB, Hozack WJ. A prospective assessment of nutritional status and complications in patients with fractures of the hip. J Orthop Trauma 1990;4:49–57

48. Davidson TI, Bodey WN. Factors influencing survival following fractures of the upper end of the femur. Injury 1986;17:12–14

49. Wood DJ, Ions GK, Quinby JM, Gale DW, Stevens J. Factors which influence mortality after subcapital hip fracture. J Bone Joint Surg Br 1992;74:199–202

50. Westrich GH, Rana AJ, Terry MA, Taveras NA, Kapoor K, Helfet DL. Thromboembolic disease prophylaxis in patients with hip fracture: a multimodal approach. J Orthop Trauma 2005;19:234–240

51. Eriksson BI, Bauer KA, Lassen MR, Turpie AG. Fondaparinux compared with enoxaparin for the prevention of venous thromboembolism after hip-fracture surgery. N Engl J Med 2001;345:1298–1304

52. Geerts WH, Pineo GF, Heit JA, et al. Prevention of venous thromboembolism: the Seventh ACCP Conference on Antithrombotic and Thrombolytic Therapy. Chest 2004;126(Suppl 3):338S–400S

53. Southwell-Keely JP, Russo RR, March L, Cumming R, Cameron I, Brnabic AJ. Antibiotic prophylaxis in hip fracture surgery: a meta-analysis. Clin Orthop Relat Res 2004;419:179–184

54. Bartonicek J, Skala-Rosenbaum J, Dousa P. Valgus intertrochanteric osteotomy for malunion and nonunion of trochanteric fractures. J Orthop Trauma 2003;17:606–612

55. Haidukewych GJ, Berry DJ. Salvage of failed internal fixation of intertrochanteric hip fractures. Clin Orthop Relat Res 2003;412:184–188

24 Subtrochanteric Femur Fractures

Stephen H. Sims

Fractures of the subtrochanteric region of the proximal femur can be especially challenging to manage and warrant special consideration to obtain consistently satisfactory results. The subtrochanteric zone of the femur is generally considered to include the area extending 5 cm distally from the inferior border of the lesser trochanter or the junction of the proximal one third and middle third of the femoral shaft (**Fig. 24–1**). Fractures that have their major displacement in this area are considered subtrochanteric fractures despite the possibility that some of these fractures may extend into the trochanteric area proximally or the distal femoral shaft. Subtrochanteric fractures occur with a bimodal distribution.[1-5] Those fractures seen in young patients tend to occur as a result of high-energy trauma and often have significant comminution, whereas fractures occurring in older patients are often caused by lower-energy injuries.

Features unique to subtrochanteric fractures that complicate treatment include both anatomical and biomechanical characteristics. The subtrochanteric area of the femur is primarily cortical bone that heals more slowly and tends to fracture with comminution. The femoral medullary canal widens in the intertrochanteric area, which makes intramedullary fixation in this region more difficult because of the possibility of less secure fixation and higher risk of malunion. Intramedullary nails do not fill the capacious proximal canal and therefore will not effect a reduction of the fracture as the nail is passed across the fracture site, as may occur in the midshaft area. If the fracture is malaligned as the nail is passed, it will remain in the malaligned position; therefore, the fracture has to be held in a reduced position as the intramedullary fixation is accomplished. In the subtrochanteric region, special reduction techniques may be needed because there are strong deforming forces across these fractures. Biomechanically, the subtrochanteric area of the proximal femur is an area of high stress concentration, which has led to high rates of implant failures in the treatment of these fractures.[6]

There are large muscles that insert on the proximal femur and create strong deforming forces across the fracture that make fracture reduction difficult. The gluteus medius and gluteus minimus insert on the greater trochanter and function as strong hip abductors. The piriformis, gemellus superior, and gemellus inferior also insert in this area and function as external rotators of the hip. The iliopsoas inserts on the lesser trochanter and acts to flex and externally rotate the hip. These muscles account for the deformity typically seen in these fractures (**Fig. 24–2**). The proximal

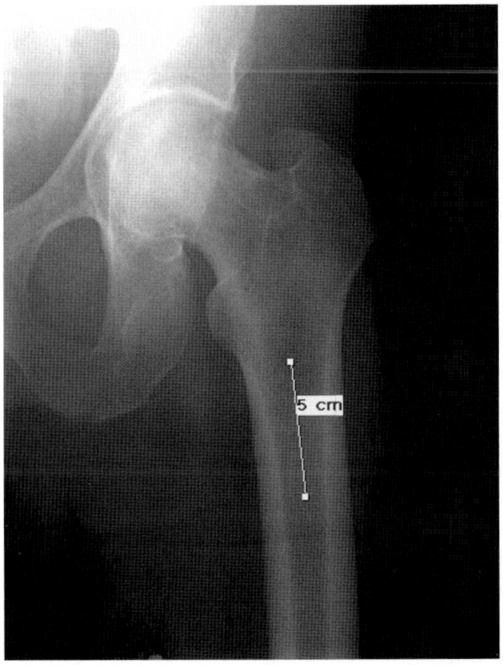

Figure 24–1 Depiction of the subtrochanteric zone of the femur.

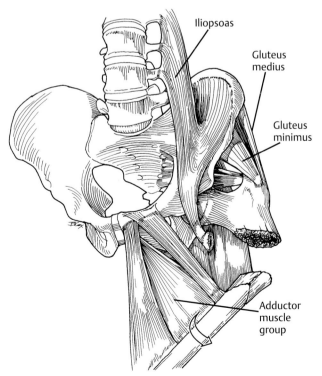

Figure 24–2 Muscle insertions on the proximal femur account for the typical displacements seen in subtrochanteric fractures.

fragment is flexed, abducted, and externally rotated, and the distal segment is adducted and shortened by the action of the adductors and hamstrings. Unlike many fractures where the reduction is accomplished by moving the distal segment into alignment with the stationary proximal fragment, reduction of these fractures requires movement of both segments because it is not possible to move the distal segment alone into satisfactory alignment with the proximal fragment. This understanding is critical to gaining acceptable alignment regardless of the type of fixation selected.

The high mechanical stresses in this area occur as a result of the compressive force of the body's weight as well as additional forces generated by the muscles that insert upon the fracture fragments. These forces have been studied by numerous investigations. Major compressive stresses in the femur are greatest in the medial cortex 1 to 3 in. below the lesser trochanter and can exceed 1200 lb per square inch.[6] This area is the most highly stressed area in the body. Tensile stresses of approximately 25% less are experienced at the lateral cortex slightly more proximal.[6]

Classification

Numerous classification systems for subtrochanteric fractures have been proposed. Most of these classification systems are not currently useful and will not be discussed in deference to those that are more useful. The Russell-Taylor classification is based on the presence or absence of fracture involvement at the lesser trochanter and posteromedial buttress and the presence or absence of extension into the greater trochanter and piriformis fossa (**Fig. 24–3**).[2] This classification is particularly useful in selecting a biomechanically appropriate implant for definitive treatment. In this classification, group I fractures do not have extension into the piriformis fossa and/or greater trochanteric area and thus are considered to be most suitable for treatment with intramedullary nails with standard piriformis fossa starting points. Type IA fractures do not involve the lesser trochanter and/or posteromedial buttress; therefore, standard locking nails can be used for treatment of this fracture pattern. Type IB fractures do involve the area of the lesser trochanter and therefore are not treated with standard locking nails but instead can be treated by nails with cephalomedullary proximal locking. Group II fractures have extension into the piriformis fossa and greater trochanteric area and are therefore less suitable for intramedullary fixation using an implant with a piriformis fossa starting point. These fractures are best treated with either 95 degree fixed-angle implants or trochanteric entry nails. Group IIA fractures do not have involvement of the lesser trochanteric area and thus have an intact posteromedial buttress. Group IIB fractures have significant involvement of the lesser trochanteric area and lack an intact posteromedial buttress, which has implications for treatment and increases the risk of implant failure.

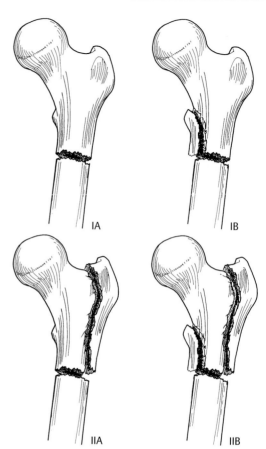

Figure 24–3 Russell-Taylor classification of subtrochanteric fractures.

The Arbeitsgemeinschaft für Osteosynthesefragen/Orthopaedic Trauma Association (AO/OTA) comprehensive classification of fractures considers these fractures as diaphyseal fractures.[7] The femoral shaft is represented as bone 3 and segment 2 (diaphyseal segment). The proximal limit of the diaphyseal segment is a transverse line passing through the inferior edge of the lesser trochanter. Although this classification is not used for the general clinical management of these injuries, it is useful in collecting data for descriptive purposes and research.

Nonoperative Management

There is little role for the nonoperative management of these injuries in the adult. Nonoperative treatment requires prolonged immobilization with associated significant morbidity and mortality to the patient. High rates of local complications also occur with nonoperative treatment, including nonunions, malunions, and soft tissue complications.[8-10] Nonoperative treatment is reserved for the rare case of a nonambulatory patient with a low-energy fracture and minimal pain for whom surgery is felt to be too risky to the patient or unlikely to succeed.

Indications for Surgical Treatment

Treatment for subtrochanteric fractures in adults is primarily operative. Operative options include plates or intramedullary implants. Intramedullary nails are typically placed with closed methods, although open reduction and nailing of displaced or highly unstable fractures is occasionally necessary. In contrast, plating of femur fractures has been traditionally performed with open techniques, but recently less invasive techniques of indirect fracture reduction and plate fixation have been reported.[11–16]

Intramedullary implants include those with standard proximal locking, those with cephalomedullary proximal locking, and intramedullary hip screw implants with a trochanteric entry point. Plate options include 95 degree fixed-angle implants such as condylar blade plates or dynamic condylar screws, 135 degree sliding hip screws, and the Medoff sliding plate[17] (Medpac, Inc., Valencia, California). Fixed-angle plates are preferred; higher rates of complications are noted when sliding plates are used to repair subtrochanteric fractures, especially when the primary fracture line has a reverse obliquity component **(Fig. 24–4A,B)**.[18–20] Indications for each of these implants with advantages, disadvantages, and techniques will be further discussed.

Intramedullary Nails

Standard interlocking intramedullary nails offer the advantage of familiarity to most surgeons, the biomechanical ad-

vantages of an intramedullary implant, the ability to be placed by a closed technique, and good outcomes. Nails with standard proximal interlocking screws are suitable only for subtrochanteric fractures that are completely distal to the lesser trochanter **(Fig. 24–5A–D)** (see **Video 24–1, Disk 3**). Cephalomedullary locking (sometimes called second-generation) intramedullary nails offer the same advantages of intramedullary fixation but are technically more demanding because the proximal interlocking screw must be placed in the appropriate position in the femoral head. These implants are suitable for fractures that extend above the lesser trochanter but do not involve the piriformis fossa or greater trochanter **(Fig. 24–6A,B)**. So-called intramedullary hip screws are newer options for those complex fractures with proximal trochanteric extension. Intramedullary hip screws (also referred to as trochanteric nails) are designed to be inserted through a trochanteric starting point and incorporate a large hip screw or blade device that is inserted into the femoral head **(Fig. 24–7A,B)** (see **Video 24–2, Disk 3**). These implants offer the advantages previously outlined for intramedullary devices and extend the indications for the use of intramedullary implants. However, trochanteric nails have the unique disadvantage of requiring the removal of a significant amount of proximal femoral bone. To accommodate the large femoral head screw and remain biomechanically sound, the proximal portion of the nail must be large, usually on the order of 17 mm. This requires the surgeon to create a large hole in the tip of the greater trochanter, necessitating significant bone removal and loss of a portion of the area of insertion of the

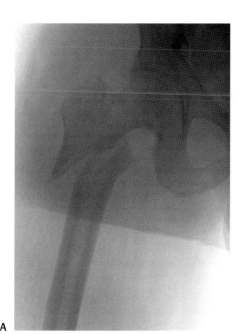
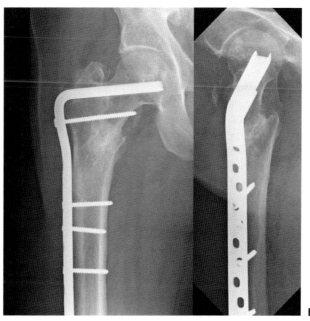

A   B

Figure 24–4 Example of a reverse obliquity fracture. **(A)** Anteroposterior radiograph of the proximal femur showing a fracture with a reverse-oblique orientation. **(B)** Anteroposterior and lateral radiographs after open reduction and internal fixation with a fixed-angle blade plate.

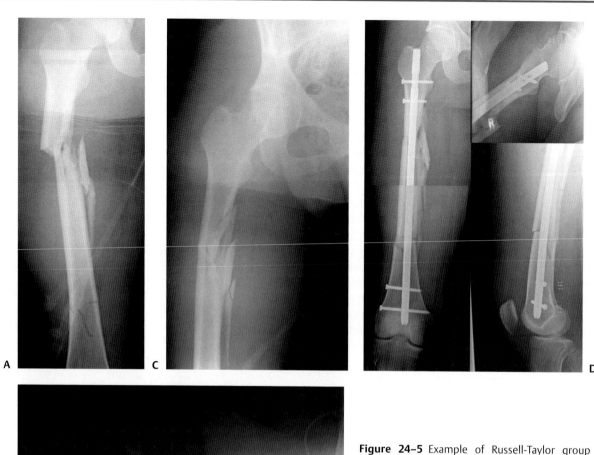

Figure 24–5 Example of Russell-Taylor group IA fracture amenable to treatment with a standard interlocking femoral nail. **(A)** Anteroposterior and **(B)** lateral radiographs of the fracture. **(C)** Example of the so-called obturator outlet view, which is taken more perpendicular to the flexed and externally rotated proximal fragment, thereby giving a more accurate representation of it. Because of its flexed position, the proximal fragment is foreshortened in a standard anteroposterior view. **(D)** Anteroposterior and lateral radiographs after intramedullary nailing with a standard piriformis locking nail.

hip abductors. Insertion of the locking device into the femoral head also requires removal of significant bone from the lateral cortex of the femur as well as removal of bone from the femoral head and neck for its placement. As a result, abductor dysfunction, insertional site pain, and difficulty with later reconstructive options can occur.

Other disadvantages of intramedullary implants include the difficulty with fracture reduction. The fracture has to be reduced prior to passing the guidewire, and the reduction has to be maintained until the nail is fully seated and locked proximally **(Fig. 24–8A–E).** This often requires manipulation of both the proximal and distal fragments. The nail does not aid with the reduction for reasons previously mentioned. Additionally, the starting point can be more difficult to locate due to the abducted position of the proximal fragment.

Plates

Ninety-five degree fixed-angle plate devices can be used for all subtrochanteric fractures but are particularly indicated for those with proximal trochanteric extension where the use of a nail with a piriformis starting point would be contraindicated **(Figs. 24–9A–C** and **24–16A–F).** (see **Video 24–3, Disk 3**) The condylar blade plate offers the unique advantage of needing minimal bone removal and the ability to accomplish an indirect reduction once the blade has been placed in the correct position in the femoral head. Its primary disadvantage is biomechanical; the extramedullary position on the lateral cortex of the femur results in increased stresses in the implant and on the implant–bone interface. An additional disadvantage is that many surgeons are unfamiliar with its use.

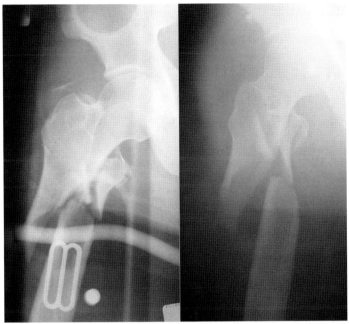
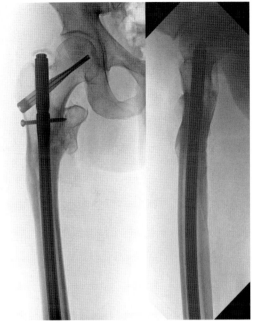

A

B

Figure 24–6 Example of Russell-Taylor group IB fracture amenable to treatment with a cephalomedullary interlocking femoral nail. **(A)** Anteroposterior and lateral radiographs. Note the reverse-oblique pattern of the primary fracture line and the involvement of the lesser trochanter. **(B)** Anteroposterior and lateral radiographs after intramedullary nailing with a second-generation interlocking nail inserted through the piriformis fossa.

This author's algorithm for the treatment of subtrochanteric femur fractures is as follows: For fractures 2 or 3 cm or more distal to the lesser trochanter, a standard locking piriformis fossa entry intramedullary nail is used. Subtrochanteric fractures that extend proximally into the area of the greater trochanter or trochanteric fossa are treated with a 95 degree condylar blade plate in patients with good bone quality. A trochanteric nail is used in older patients with poor bone quality. For those fractures with extension into the area of the lesser trochanter but no involvement of the piriformis fossa or greater trochanter, either a 95 degree condylar blade plate or cephalomedullary nail with a piriformis starting point is used; the choice depends on other factors.

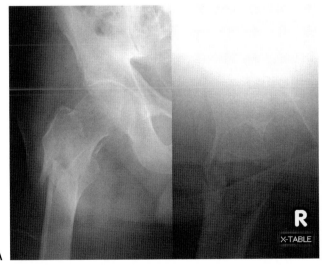
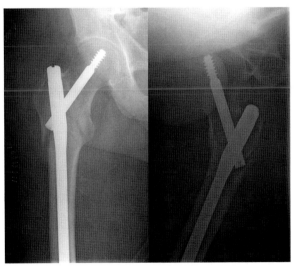

A

B

Figure 24–7 Example of Russell-Taylor group II fracture amenable to treatment with a trochanteric nail. **(A)** Anteroposterior (AP) and lateral radiographs of a proximal femur fracture. The AP view demonstrates a reverse-oblique pattern with what appears to be a splaying apart of the proximal segment, suggesting an additional fracture in the coronal plane. Although it is difficult to see on the lateral, there are secondary fracture lines entering the piriformis fossa. **(B)** Postoperative radiographs after trochanteric nailing.

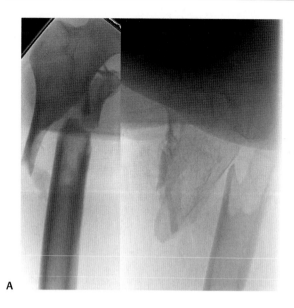

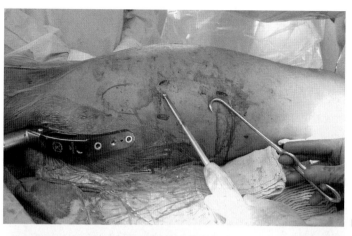

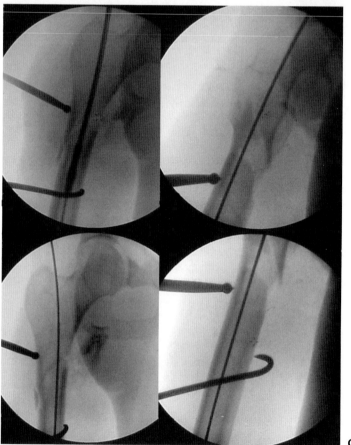

Figure 24–8 Examples of reduction techniques. **(A)** Anteroposterior and lateral views of an unreduced subtrochanteric fracture demonstrating the typical displacement. Note the amount of displacement of the proximal segment on the lateral view. **(B)** Intraoperative photo of a bone hook and ball-tipped pusher, and their respective locations of insertion. **(C)** Intraoperative fluoroscopic image showing these instruments as they are used to reduce the fracture on AP and lateral view.

Surgical Treatment

The operative technique for three common methods of fixation of subtrochanteric fractures including a cephalomedullary locking intramedullary nail with a piriformis fossa starting point, a trochanteric nail, and a 95 degree condylar blade plate will be described in some detail.

Surgical Techniques

Positioning

Patient positioning is the same for all three of these fixation techniques. Either supine or lateral positions may be used depending on the surgeon's preference, the presence of other injuries, and the patient's body habitus.

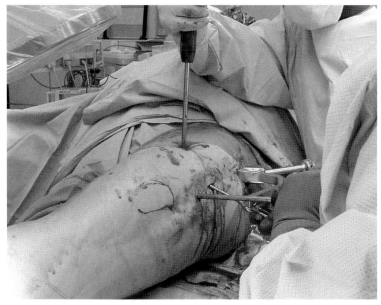

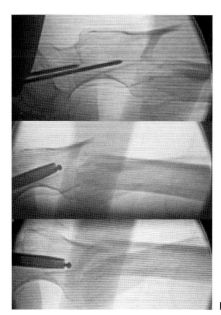

D   E

Figure 24–8 *(Continued)* **(D)** Intraoperative photograph of the instruments being used. **(E)** Intraoperative views of another case in which a reduction rod was used to "steer" the proximal fragment to

the distal femur. In addition, a ball-tipped pusher is used to correct the flexion of the proximal fracture segment.

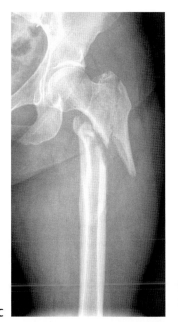

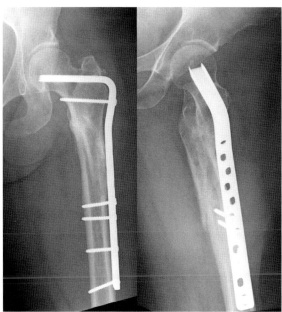

A,C

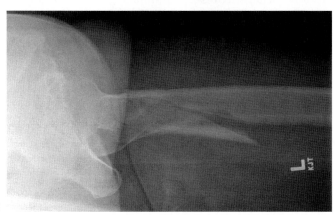

B

Figure 24–9 Example of Russell-Taylor group IIB fracture that is not amenable to nailing and was treated with a fixed-angle plate. **(A)** Anteroposterior radiograph of the proximal femur showing a high subtrochanteric fracture with involvement of the piriformis fossa. **(B)** Lateral radiograph of the injury. **(C)** Postoperative radiographs taken 3 months after injury.

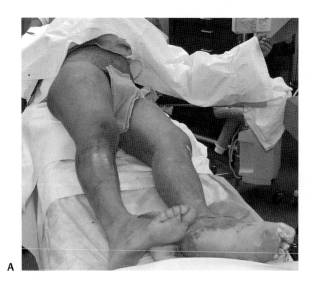

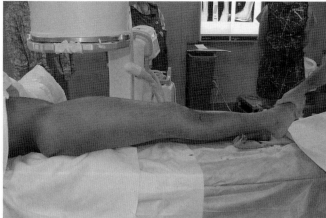

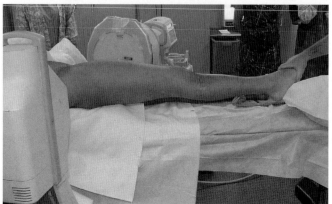

Figure 24–10 The authors preferred patient positioning. **(A)** The patient is on a radiolucent table with a bump under the involved buttock which tilts the pelvis approximately 30–50 degrees. **(B)** The AP projection. Because the pelvis is tilted, this generally gives a good radiograph of the femoral neck profile. **(C)** Fluoroscopic imaging in the lateral plane.

Lateral positioning facilitates exposure of the proximal femur and reduces the posterior sag that can occur with supine positioning. The author prefers to position the patient on a radiolucent table with large bumps located beneath the affected hip and ipsilateral shoulder to maintain the patient somewhere between the supine and lateral position **(Fig. 24–10A–C).** The bump must be large enough to roll the patient sufficiently forward so that when the C-arm is in the full lateral position (i.e., x-ray beam parallel to the floor), an unencumbered lateral view of the hip can be seen. If the soft tissue shadow of the contralateral thigh overlaps the image of the hip, then the patient needs to be rolled more toward the lateral position with a larger bump to raise the affected side even higher. Typically, the patient will be positioned at an angle of approximately 30–50 degrees to the bed. Because the proximal fragment is externally rotated due to the pull of the short external rotators, this position will give a true lateral view of the hip. The lower abdominal area, pelvic area, and entire lower extremity are prepped and draped into the field. Prior to positioning and draping, the opposite extremity measurements of rotation and length of this extremity should be determined. Rotational alignment can be clinically measured with medial and lateral thigh rotation, and length is measured with a

radiographic ruler for comparison with the affected extremity after fixation.

Cephalomedullary Nail (see Video 24–1, Disk 3)

Operative treatment with a cephalomedullary nail requires that the fracture first be reduced. The proximal fragment will be flexed, abducted, and externally rotated due to the pull of the attached muscles. Fracture reduction is accomplished with repositioning of the proximal fragment and the distal fragment. Repositioning of the fragments is accomplished with the use of a ball-spike pusher from a pelvic set or similar device placed through a stab incision anteriorly near the distal end of the proximal fragment **(Fig. 24–8A–C).** This tool is used to push the proximal fragment out of its flexed position. A second ball-spike pusher placed through a stab incision laterally at the distal end of the proximal fragment can be used to push the proximal fragment out of the abducted position. Sometimes a single ball-spike pusher can be placed anterolaterally to create the correct combined vector to push the proximal fragment out of the flexed and abducted position. The distal fragment will usually be medially translated and can be reduced by placing a bone hook through a stab incision at the proximal portion of the distal fragment to pull this portion of the femur laterally and into alignment with the proximal portion. Manual traction on the extremity will need to be maintained throughout all of these maneuvers or the patient could be placed on the fracture table if additional personnel are not available for this function. The starting point in the piriformis fossa will be much more easily accessible with the proximal fragment held in the reduced position; conversely, it will be difficult to locate if the proximal fragment is unreduced in the abducted and flexed position.

An alternative method of fracture reduction that can be used in simple fracture patterns is to use a reduction rod (**Fig. 24–8D**). These are shorter cannulated rods that many femoral nail implant sets contain. To use them, the starting point is obtained in the proximal fragment while it is unreduced to the shaft. The upper segment is reamed, usually to 11 mm, to accommodate the reduction nail. This device is then inserted to the fracture, and then the handle of the reduction nail is used to reduce the upper fragment to the distal fragment. Once reduced, a guidewire is placed across the fracture, and reaming may commence. When the reduction rod is removed, another means of maintaining reduction is needed; this method is best used for Russell-Taylor group IA fractures (simple subtrochanteric fractures below the lesser trochanter).

Nail insertion and locking can be done through small incisions. The location of the incision proximally over the buttock area for nail insertion can be determined using the guidewire from the nail set and fluoroscopy (**Fig. 24–11**). The guidewire is placed on the skin over the thigh in line with the femur. Fluoroscopy ensures that the guidewire is in line with the femoral canal and over the trochanteric fossa. The entry point for the nail is usually significantly proximal to the greater trochanter. A guidewire can be placed overlying the piriformis fossa on an AP radiograph and its position confirmed via fluoroscopy. The proximal aspect of the guidewire allows the surgeon to make a mark which designates the cephalad-caudad position of the skin incision. The location for the incision in the anterior-posterior direction can be determined by palpating the greater trochanter and proximal femur and moving directly proximal from these landmarks.

The guidewire is then pushed through the skin at this point. It should be placed in the piriformis fossa in line with the femoral canal on the anteroposterior (AP) and lateral x-ray views (**Fig. 24–12A–C**). A 2 cm skin incision is made around the guidewire insertion point at the skin. Standard locking first-generation nails are started at a point directly in line with the intramedullary canal. Because the femoral neck is slightly anterior to the femoral shaft, cephalomedullary nails are started more anteriorly in the piriformis fossa to facilitate central screw insertion in the femoral neck on the lateral x-ray. The reduction must be maintained while the guidewire is placed to be sure it traverses the proximal femoral fragment in the correct path. The guidewire should appear absolutely parallel to the proximal femur. If the femur is allowed to return to the flexed and abducted position, the guidewire will likely pass the proximal femur from proximal lateral to distal medial, which will lead to a varus malposition and on the lateral x-ray will cross from proximal anterior to distal posterior, leading to a flexed malposition of the fracture that will be difficult to correct later. After the guidewire is correctly placed in the proximal femur, the proximal canal is opened with the starter reamer drill over the guidewire. The starter guidewire and drill are removed, and a bead-tip guide rod is passed into the proximal fragment, while maintaining the reduction with the use of the ball-spike pushers, traction, and/or a bone hook. The guide rod can then be passed across the fracture into the distal femur. Fluoroscopy can be used to be certain that the guide rod is passed into the center of the distal femur as seen on the AP and lateral x-ray of the knee.

The canal is then sequentially reamed to allow for a canal-filling implant to be placed. The canal should be reamed 1.5 mm larger than the selected nail. The nail length is determined by indirect measurement using a second guide rod of equal length or by use of a calibrated measuring device placed over the guidewire from the manufacturer to provide a direct measurement reading. It is critical to maintain the reduction throughout the reaming process because the nail will follow the path reamed in the proximal femur when it is passed over the guide rod. The proximal femur may require additional overreaming to allow for the nail to be placed because many cephalomedullary nails have a larger diameter in the proximal portion of the nail (15 to 17 mm). While the reduction is maintained, the nail is then passed over the guide rod. It will be important to be mindful of the degree of nail rotation by watching the proximal locking guide. Nail rotation should be maintained to allow placement of the proximal locking guide into the center of the head. Prior to fully seating the nail, a lateral x-ray of the proximal femur can be taken that will show the neck and head of the femur, and the proximal locking guide will also be seen on the x-ray. The nail can be rotated to align the proximal locking guide with the axis of the head and neck, which will appear with the locking guide overlying the neck

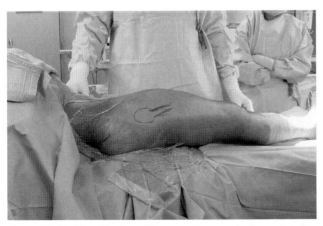

Figure 24–11 Identification of the percutaneous starting point after the patient's limb has been prepped and draped. Note that the bony landmarks are drawn, and the starting point is in line with the femoral canal in both coronal and sagittal planes.

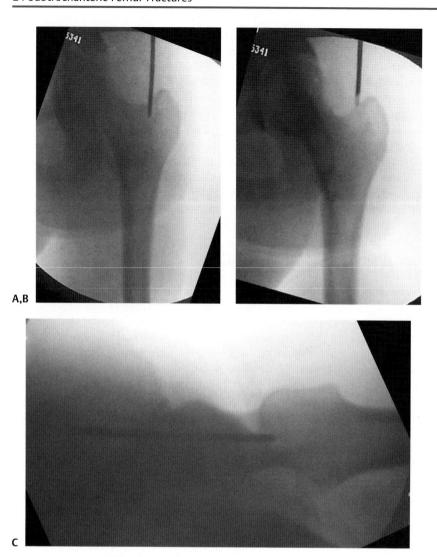

Figure 24–12 Localization of the starting point for femoral nailing. **(A)** When the guidewire is correctly positioned, its tip will be seen in the base of the piriformis fossa on the anteroposterior view. **(B)** When the guide pin appears to be on the top of the femoral neck, it is too anterior. **(C)** Correct positioning on the lateral view.

and head on the lateral x-ray. The nail is fully seated to a point where the proximal locking guide will be in the appropriate location in the femoral head as seen on the AP x-ray.

A guide pin is then inserted into the femoral head and again checked on the AP x-ray to be sure the position is appropriate. On the lateral x-ray, the position of the guide pin can be checked by rotating the locking guide anteriorly and posteriorly to ensure that the pin is centered in the head. Proximal locking is then accomplished. Finally, distal locking is performed by standard freehand technique. Prior to fully seating the nail, it is important to check a lateral x-ray of the distal femur to be sure the nail remains centered in the canal. Because the anterior bow of the nail is less than the bow of the native femur, it is possible during nailing of proximal fractures to have the nail perforate the anterior femoral cortex distally. The axial alignment is restored if the fracture was maintained reduced throughout the nailing process. It is straightforward to assess alignment using AP and lateral x-rays. In contrast, the rotational alignment can be difficult to judge, and there is a tendency to leave the patient's femur externally rotated **(Fig. 24–13A–F).** If a horizontal lateral x-ray of the proximal

femur has been yielding a true lateral picture of the hip, then the knee should be held internally rotated to match the anteversion of the opposite hip (usually 10 to 15 degrees). The rotation should be checked prior to, during, and after nail placement and prior to and after distal locking.

An easy method for reliably measuring rotation is to obtain a perfect lateral view of the knee, which is usually obtained with the C-arm fully rotated to the lateral position. The degree of rotation on the C-arm is then noted (e.g., 90 degrees). The C-arm is then moved to the hip and orbited toward an AP view by 5 degree increments until a perfect lateral view of the hip is obtained and the degrees of rotation on the C-arm are noted (e.g., 75 degrees). The difference between these measurements is the amount of anteversion of the femur (in the example noted, 15 degrees). Several factors can be used to help assess the proper length. Often, assessment of the fracture pattern will allow the length to be determined simply by bone-to-bone contact. In those comminuted fractures where the fracture pattern does not allow determination of length, the injured extremity will have to be matched to the opposite extremity. The length of the opposite femur can be measured preoperatively in the

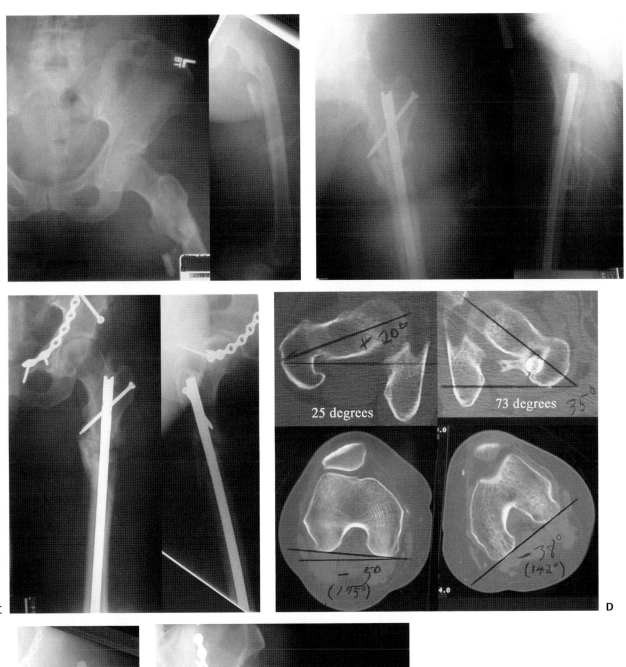

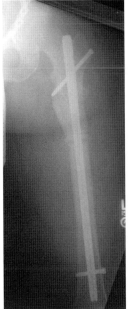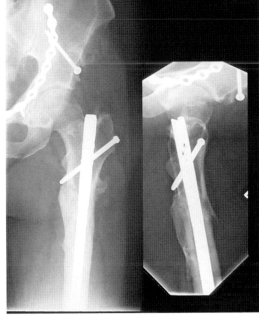

Figure 24–13 Example of rotational deformity following nailing of an open subtrochanteric fracture. **(A)** Poor-quality films of the pelvis and femur showing a both-column acetabular fracture and a subtrochanteric femur fracture. **(B)** Postoperative films after reamed intramedullary nailing done in the lateral position. Note the antibiotic beads in the open wound. **(C)** Films after the fracture had clinically united. The patient complained of her foot turning in differently. **(D)** A limited axial computed tomographic scan was done with cuts through the femoral neck and condyles bilaterally. The relative difference in rotation between the two sides was 48 degrees. **(E)** A percutaneous rotational osteotomy was done just below the original fracture. **(F)** Final follow-up films are shown.

A

B

C

D

E,F

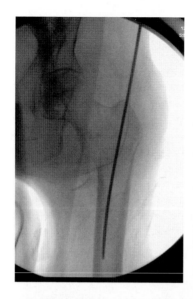

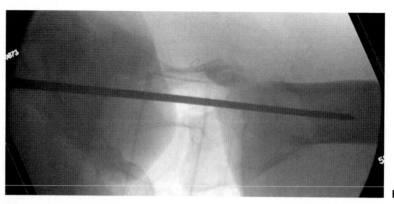

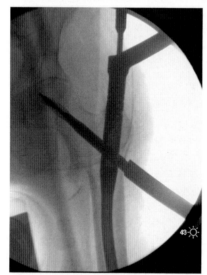

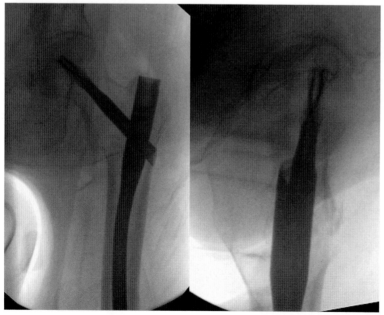

Figure 24–14 Intraoperative C-arm views of the appropriate starting point for trochanteric nailing. **(A,B)** Intraoperative fluoroscopic views of the upper femur showing ideal positioning of the guidewire. **(C)** Intraoperative imaging during proximal interlocking. **(D)** Final anteroposterior and lateral views.

computed tomographic (CT) scan by taking a scout film and using a cursor to measure the length of the femur. Additionally, a point from the top of the piriformis fossa to the physeal scar can be measured as a possible nail length on the opposite extremity. This is often possible because many patients with these fractures will be taken to CT scan preoperatively for other reasons. Finally, the length of the opposite extremity can be measured in the operating room (OR) prior to final positioning for surgery by using a long radiographic ruler that is often provided in most femoral nail implant sets.

Upon completion of the procedure, sterile dressings are applied, the drapes are removed, and the patient is placed flat on the OR table. All instruments should be kept sterile and the C-arm kept in the room in case changes need to be made. The length should be measured by comparison with the opposite extremity, as should rotation of the hips. If these are not symmetric, then it is rather simple to remove the distal locking screws and make the appropriate adjustments and redo the distal locking as long as the instruments have been kept sterile.

Trochanteric Nailing (see Video 24–2, Disk 3)

The operative technique for fixation with a trochanteric femoral nail involves the same patient positioning and reduction maneuvers as described for the cephalomedullary nails with a piriformis starting point. As previously described, the reduction must be maintained while establishing the starting point, inserting the guide rod, reaming, nail placement, and proximal locking. The location of the incision is again determined by placing a guidewire over the anterior thigh at the appropriate angle over the greater trochanter. The guide pin can be pushed through the skin to be centered with the medullary canal on the lateral view and be at the tip of the trochanter on the AP view (**Fig. 24–14A–D**). An incision is made in the skin that is 2 to 3 cm long and in line with

the femur, which usually begins 2 to 4 cm proximal to the tip of the greater trochanter. While the proximal femur is maintained in the correct alignment as previously described, the guide pin is inserted into the greater trochanter. The proper placement of the starting point is critical and must be rechecked prior to opening the canal with the large proximal reamer (17 mm). The starting point should be in line with the medullary canal and centered on the neck as seen on the lateral view and at the tip of the greater trochanter on the AP view (**Fig. 24–14A–D**). If the abducted position of the proximal fragment is not corrected, the starting point will be too far lateral and lead to eventual varus malalignment. Short and long nails are offered, and arguments can be made for the use of either for intertrochanteric fractures, but for subtrochanteric fractures the long nails should be used. Proximal locking is done according to the manufacturer's instructions utilizing all of the steps for imaging and placement of the screw within the femoral neck and head described in the previous section for cephalomedullary nails (**Fig. 24–14A–D**). Distal locking is performed and overall femoral alignment checked, as also described earlier.

Ninety-five Degree Condylar Blade Plate (see Video 24–3, Disk 3)

Open reduction and internal fixation of subtrochanteric femur fractures with a 95 degree condylar blade plate offers the advantages of minimal bone removal, the ability to pretension the construct, and the ability to use the plate to accomplish an indirect reduction. The disadvantage is the unfamiliarity of many surgeons with the use of this implant; thus it is felt to be more technically demanding, and it usually requires an open procedure. The patient is positioned as described for the intramedullary nail techniques, and the C-arm is brought in from the opposite side of the bed. If needed, the patient can be placed on a fracture

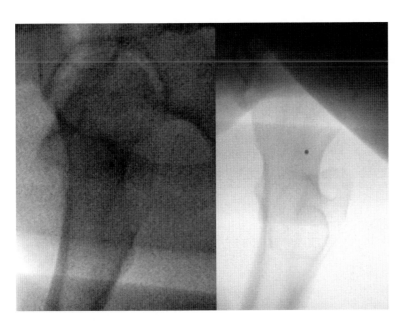

Figure 24–15 Intraoperative C-arm views showing improved femoral neck visualization after tilting the C-arm toward the patient's head, accounting for the neck-shaft angle, and giving a truer view of the length of the femoral neck. The left panel shows a true lateral fluoroscopic image of the hip. The right panel shows the modified lateral image taken with the C-arm canted 20 degrees toward the patient's head and rotated slightly over the top toward the obturator oblique projection of the pelvis. Note that the femoral neck is better visualized.

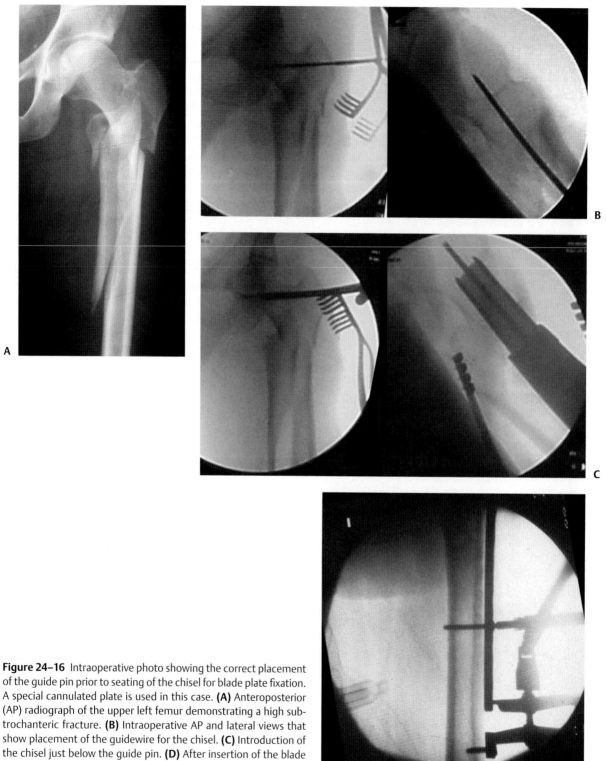

Figure 24–16 Intraoperative photo showing the correct placement of the guide pin prior to seating of the chisel for blade plate fixation. A special cannulated plate is used in this case. **(A)** Anteroposterior (AP) radiograph of the upper left femur demonstrating a high subtrochanteric fracture. **(B)** Intraoperative AP and lateral views that show placement of the guidewire for the chisel. **(C)** Introduction of the chisel just below the guide pin. **(D)** After insertion of the blade plate, compression is achieved using the articulated tensioner.

table; just as for nailing, lateral positioning may facilitate exposure and fixation. Alternatively, a femoral distractor can be used to help regain length in fractures with significant comminution and shortening. Prior to prepping and draping, the surgeon should be certain that good AP and lateral x-ray views of the hip and femur can be obtained. One problem with lateral imaging of the femoral neck is

the foreshortening that occurs because the femoral neck is angled 40 degrees or so to the femoral shaft **(Fig. 24–15)**.

If the patient is in the full lateral position, by tilting the upper portion of the vertically oriented C-arm 20 to 30 degrees toward the patient's head, a true lateral view of the femoral neck can be obtained **(Fig. 24–15)**. For this reason, as well as the fact that the proximal fragment is in a flexed,

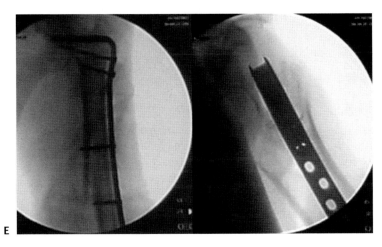

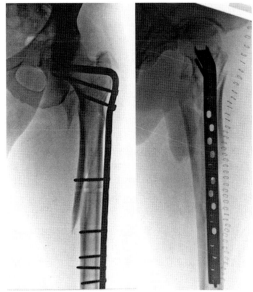

Figure 24–16 *(Continued)* **(E)** Intraoperative fluoroscopic views of the fixation construct. **(F)** Final AP and lateral radiographs.

abducted, and externally rotated position, good AP and lateral views of the proximal fragment require some rehearsal prior to prepping and draping the patient and starting the procedure. Depending on the amount of deformity, the proximal fragment can be reduced to the normal alignment, as previously described, or more commonly left in its abnormal position and the C-arm directed to give the proper x-ray views. As previously described, with the author's preferred positioning technique a large bump beneath the hip and shoulder rolls the patient ~30–50 degrees toward the lateral position; this positioning will correct for the external rotation of the hip so that the image can be directed perpendicular to the floor to obtain an AP view. If the proximal fragment is flexed significantly, then the image can be directed caudally to match the hip flexion to be perpendicular to the proximal fragment. This results in the appearance of an obturator outlet view of the pelvis but a true AP view of the unreduced flexed and externally rotated proximal fragment **(Fig. 24–5A–D).**

For the lateral x-ray of the hip, the C-arm is oriented obliquely to the patient in the proximal to distal direction to account for the abduction and give a true lateral view of the hip and proximal fragment. Once it has been ensured that good x-ray views can be obtained, the entire leg from the toes to above the iliac crest is prepped and draped. An incision is made initially that will only expose the proximal femur for chisel insertion and will later be extended distally for plate insertion. Blood loss may be decreased if the distal part of the incision is not made until after the chisel has been seated. The initial incision is made ~10 cm long beginning 2 to 3 cm proximal to the proximal portion of the greater trochanter and extending distally along the posterior border of the femur. The incision should be kept just distal to the proximal femur to facilitate placement of a K-wire for guidance of the chisel and chisel placement **(Fig. 24–16A–F).** Because the proximal fragment is externally rotated, this will prevent interference from the soft tissues while placing the

K-wire and chisel into the head and neck in the proper orientation. The iliotibial band will be divided, and the gluteus fascia is divided to identify the greater trochanter and the origin of the vastus lateralis at the vastus ridge. The posterior one third to one half of the vastus lateralis origin is released and continued distally with the elevation of the vastus anteriorly when the remainder of the incision is made for exposure for eventual plate placement.

A K-wire of ~ $\frac{7}{64}$ in. diameter is placed from the lateral cortex into the center of the femoral head on the lateral view and at a 95 degree angle into the head on the AP view. It is mandatory that the surgeon pre-operatively plans the direction of this K-wire on a good quality radiograph of the opposite hip. The K-wire is placed just proximal to the location of the chisel placement so it can serve as a guide for its insertion. The starting point on the lateral cortex will be proximal to the vastus ridge from the greater trochanter ending in the inferior portion of the femoral head in the subchondral bone. This K-wire is placed with the proximal fragment in its malaligned position by obtaining good AP and lateral x-ray views of the proximal fragment **(Fig. 24–16A–F).** The 95 degree angle to the proximal fragment can be checked with the 95 degree angle guides. Once the K-wire is placed correctly to serve as a guide, the chisel can be placed just distal to the K-wire. By keeping the chisel parallel to the K-wire in both planes, the chisel can be placed into the center of the head as seen on the lateral view and at a 95 degree angle as seen on the AP view. Some implant systems utilize a cannulated chisel; in such cases the chisel is inserted over the guide pin(s). To correct for the deformity in the sagittal plane as seen on the lateral x-ray, the long face of the chisel must be placed perpendicular to the axis of the proximal fragment as seen on the lateral x-ray.

The seating chisel guide that is slid onto the chisel should lie parallel to the head and neck proximally and the bone on the proximal fragment distal to the neck as seen on the lateral x-ray. Because the proximal fragment is usually flexed, this will require the seating chisel be placed so that the plate would be anterior and appear flexed compared with the distal fragment. This should be checked with alternating AP and lateral C-arm images; careful chisel placement is paramount because this will determine the final alignment of the femur. The lateral cortex of the femur is opened with two or three 4.5 mm drill holes connected together to allow chisel insertion. During insertion, the chisel should be backed out periodically (i.e., every 1 cm of insertion) to disengage to prevent it from becoming so tightly impaled in the bone of the femoral head that it cannot be removed. This is especially important for the last 10 to 15 mm of insertion where the bone is more dense. The chisel should be inserted to a point close to the subchondral bone, which will usually allow for a 70 to 80 mm blade in an adult. If the depth measurement read off the chisel at the lateral cortex is between sizes, then the shorter blade is usually selected to avoid head perforation. The skin incision is now extended distally for its full length to allow placement of the selected plate. The iliotibial band is divided for the length of the incision, and the vastus lateralis is elevated anteriorly.

Great care is taken to preserve the vitality of the fracture zone and maintain soft tissue attachments to all fragments. This means that the use of self-retaining retractors, cerclage wires, and medial stripping is avoided. Only the lateral aspect of the bone need be exposed. With some fractures it is even possible to leave the muscle intact over the fracture area and slide the plate submuscularly past this area. The chisel is removed, and the blade of the 95 degree condylar blade plate is inserted into the path created in the femoral head by the chisel, using the plate holder to maintain the proper orientation. Final seating is done with the impactor after removing the plate holder. The plate will be anterior and flexed relative to the distal fragment of the femur. By rotating the plate and clamping it to the bone with a Verbrugge clamp, the fracture will be reduced. This is an example of using the plate to accomplish an indirect reduction of the fracture. Rotation should be checked clinically and by obtaining lateral x-rays of the knee and hip for comparison, as previously described.

Length can be checked by C-arm images or a radiographic ruler, as previously described. In some instances, especially if length is a concern, a universal distractor can be used by placing a Schanz pin through the proximal hole in the plate and a second Schanz pin in the femur distal to the plate. Distraction can be applied, and if any bone contact can be reestablished, then the universal distractor can be reversed to pretension the construct. If the universal distractor is not used, the articulated tension device should be used to pretension the construct in cases where some bony contact can be reestablished **(Fig. 24–16A–F).** If the muscle was left intact over the fracture zone, blade placement will require abduction of the leg while adducting the hip with the K-wire that had been previously inserted. One or two screws can be added to the proximal fragment for additional fixation, and distal fragment fixation is provided with screws through the plate.

As with the intramedullary nails, the instruments and implants should all be kept sterile until the patient is examined flat on the OR table with all drapes removed to be certain the length and rotation have been restored. If these are not correct, then the patient will need to be reprepped and draped, the distal screws removed, the problem corrected, and the distal screws replaced.

Tips and Tricks

- Reduction of subtrochanteric femur fractures requires movement of both proximal and distal segments because it is not possible to move the distal segment alone into satisfactory alignment with the proximal fragment. This is because of the flexed, abducted, and externally rotated position of the proximal segment. This understanding is critical to gaining acceptable alignment of the fracture no matter what of type of fixation is selected.
- Regardless of the operative method used, lateral positioning facilitates exposure of the proximal femur and reduces the posterior sag that can occur with supine positioning.
- When nailing a subtrochanteric fracture, the nail itself cannot guarantee reduction of the fracture. Instead, fracture reduction must be achieved before insertion of the guidewire and reaming and must be maintained throughout the procedure.
- Because the femoral neck is slightly anterior to the femoral shaft, cephalomedullary nails should be inserted more anteriorly in the piriformis fossa to facilitate central screw insertion in the femoral neck on the lateral x-ray.
- With use of a cephalomedullary nail, the canal should be reamed 1.5 mm larger than the selected nail to allow for some rotation of the nail to obtain optimal position of the screw(s) within the center of the head of the femur.
- Almost all trochanteric nails require additional overreaming to allow for the nail to be placed because many cephalomedullary nails have a larger diameter in the proximal portion of the nail (15 to 17 mm).
- Because the anterior bow of the nail is less than the bow of the native femur, it is possible during nailing of proximal fractures to have the nail perforate the anterior femoral cortex distally.
- External rotation deformity is common.

Rehabilitation

Postoperatively, patients are mobilized as soon as their other injuries allow. On postoperative day 1, ambulation is begun with touch-down weight-of-leg weight bearing to

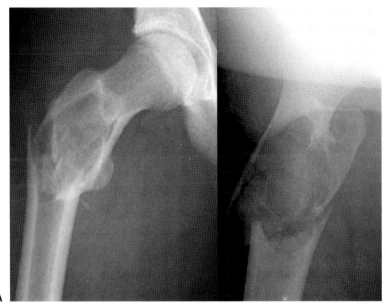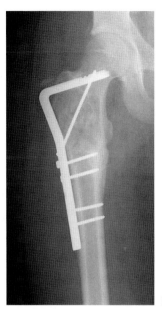

A   B

Figure 24–17 A new locking blade plate by Zimmer (Warsaw, Indiana). **(A)** Radiographs of a 16-year-old with a pathological fracture through a unicameral bone cyst. **(B)** Follow-up radiograph taken after open reduction and internal fixation with a locking blade plate and bone grafting.

neutralize the muscular joint reaction forces. Limited weight bearing is continued for 10 to 12 weeks or until good progression toward healing is demonstrated radiographically. Hip, knee, and ankle range of motion exercises are also begun on the first postoperative day along with leg raising and isometric exercises. Patients are told to expect a limp for at least 6 months and to expect it to be 12 to 18 months before their recovery is complete.

The exception to the preceding protocol is for patients treated with intramedullary fixation for simple fracture patterns that are axially stable with good bony apposition and no proximal trochanteric extension. These patients can be allowed to bear weight as tolerated after surgery.

New Techniques

New techniques to treat these challenging fractures are evolving. The 95 degree angle blade plate as described earlier is a useful treatment modality option for acute peritrochanteric femur fractures. It is also useful in reconstructive cases around the proximal femur, such as malunion and nonunion. However, it does have some disadvantages, including technical execution with its implantation (especially if the surgeon does not perform this routinely); inability to change the path of the seating chisel/blade plate several times; need for a large incision so that the plate may be inserted; and possible loss of bone in the area where the blade should be directed (in reconstructive cases). To improve upon the traditional blade plate, a cannulated locking blade plate has been introduced (Zimmer, Inc., Warsaw, Indiana). The blade has a slot, through which a long, angled screw is placed (**Fig.**

24–17A,B). This construct "locks" the implant to a triangular volume of bone and is very stable.

Even more recently, a locking plate–screw device has recently been released that is anatomically contoured and provides multiple points of fixed-angle screw purchase into the proximal femur (**Fig. 24–18**) (see **Videos**

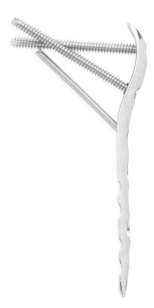

Figure 24–18 The Proximal Femoral Locking Plate by Synthes (Paoli, Pennsylvania). Proximally, the plate has two 7.3 mm screws and a third 5.0 mm screw that is meant to function as a "kickstand" for the first screw. Nonlocking screw may first be placed in the proximal two holes, which may be helpful in the setting of a fracture with an associated basicervical femoral neck fracture or a sagittal plane split in the greater trochanter. Distal screws in the plate may be either locking or nonlocking screws.

24–4, 25–5, Disk 3). It was designed to be user-friendly for the surgeon. Guidewires are placed in the proximal femur, and over these wires, cannulated locked screws are placed. This allows the surgeon to change the placement of these guidewires. Another potential advantage of this locking plate–screw device is that it can be placed using a submuscular approach with minimal stripping of the soft tissues around the fracture. However, the device can also be utilized in a completely open manner, as with a 95 degree angle blade plate. When used openly, the plate is affixed to the proximal femur, based upon a careful preoperative plan and templating of the opposite proximal femur. However, in a slightly different surgical technique, the anatomical contour and nonlocking screw options also allow the plate to be used as an aid in fracture reduction. Nonlocking screws may first be placed through the proximal aspect of the plate, which allows for compression of sagittal plane fractures.

A recent report has utilized the Proximal Femoral Locking Plate (Synthes, Paoli, Pennsylvania) in 31 consecutive patients with peritrochanteric femur fractures, with the plate inserted in a submuscular manner.[21] There was one nonunion reported for a union rate of 97%, with no infections. In all but one case, the neck-shaft angle of the injured side was reduced within 5 degrees of the contralateral side. There was one varus malreduction and one varus collapse, both in patients with ballistic injuries that included significant comminution and bone loss. Both healed uneventfully.

For the submuscular technique, the patient is placed in the supine position on a fracture table. Boot traction is utilized in lower-energy fractures in elderly patients. Distal femoral pin traction is utilized in higher-energy fractures generally sustained in younger patients. Preoperative reduction is performed under fluoroscopy. A lateral incision over the greater trochanter is made extending ~8 to 10 cm. The vastus lateralis fascia is incised off the vastus ridge in an L-shaped fashion, and a limited subvastus approach is created elevating 4 to 5 cm of the vastus off the lateral proximal femur. The plate is slid submuscularly along the lateral border of the femur through this incision using fluoroscopic guidance. Indirect reduction is obtained using table traction and using the plate as a template. A Schanz pin can be placed into the greater trochanter to manipulate the proximal fragment out of either or both external rotation and varus. A wood-handled elevator may be utilized to correct flexion deformity of the proximal segment. Guidewires for the proximal locking screws are then placed and their position verified on fluoroscopy in both AP and lateral planes. A small incision is made over the distal portion of the plate to confirm appropriate alignment of the plate on the lateral cortex of the femur, and the distal plate is held in place with a guidewire. Proximal fixation is then obtained using conical nonlocking screws if sagittal plane compression is

needed. Placement of these nonlocking screws also serves the purpose of bringing the plate down to the bone. The plate is designed for two 7.3 mm and one 5.0 mm locking screws to be placed into the proximal fragment. Distal fixation is then performed through the distal incision and percutaneously along the shaft. Conical screws in the proximal segment are exchanged for locking screws prior to closure unless there is excellent bony purchase (**Figs. 24–19A–F**).

The proximal femoral locking plate has potential advantages over traditional implants for the treatment of comminuted peritrochanteric femur fractures. This plate is applicable to all fractures in the pertrochanteric region, regardless of greater trochanterii or femoral neck involvement. Ninety-five degree blade plates or intramedullary nail devices may displace nondisplaced or sagittal plane fractures of the proximal femur. In contrast, locked and nonlocked screws may be placed in the proximal femur in a nonaggressive manner. The resultant fixed-angle construct prevents shortening and varus collapse as can be seen with traditional implants.

Outcomes

As mentioned earlier in this chapter, obtaining successful outcomes following the treatment of subtrochanteric femur fractures poses a unique set of challenges related to the anatomical and biomechanical characteristics of this area. The use of biomechanically improved implants and surgical techniques emphasizing the preservation of the blood supply to the fracture zone through indirect reduction has led to reports of acceptable results in the more recent literature as opposed to the earlier reports of frequent nonunions and hardware failures.

For the more distal subtrochanteric fractures involving diaphyseal bone that are amenable to a standard locking nail inserted through the piriformis fossa (first-generation nail), the results are similar to those reported for all femoral shaft fractures with high union rates and good return to function.[22–26]

The use of intramedullary nails with a piriformis starting point and cephalomedullary proximal locking, the so-called second-generation intramedullary nail, offers improved biomechanics over standard proximal locking nails and has led to its common use for those fractures at or involving the lesser trochanter but with no proximal extension into the greater trochanter of the piriformis fossa.[27–30] High union rates have been reported for subtrochanteric fractures with the use of this implant with restoration of acceptable alignment and length.[2,31–35] Union rates have averaged 10 to 12 weeks with low complication rates and low incidence of need for additional surgeries.[35] Return of function has been related to patient age and preinjury function. Younger patients have regained full mobility and

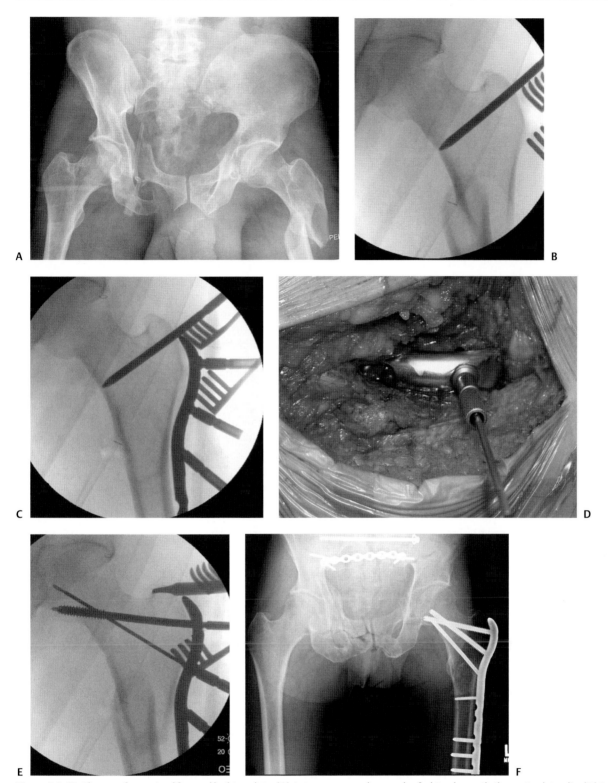

Figure 24–19 The use of a proximal femoral locking plate. **(A)** Antero-posterior pelvic radiograph showing a left proximal femoral fracture as well as a Zone II sacral fracture. Although the femoral fracture itself is amenable to nailing, such management might result in injury to the lumbosacral plexus because of the unstable sacral fracture. Therefore, plate fixation was chosen. **(B)** With distal femoral traction, a Schanz pin is used to correct the varus and external rotation deformity of the proximal segment. **(C)** The proximal femoral locking plate is then slid in a submuscular fashion beneath the vastus lateralis. **(D)** Intraoperative photo after placement of the proximal femoral guidewire. **(E)** A conical (nonlocking) screw is used to bring the plate down to the bone without using devitalizing clamps. It is later changed to a locking screw. Note the medial translation of the femoral shaft. **(F)** Radiograph of the pelvis taken 5 months later. Note the reduction of the distal femur to the plate. This was done with the nonlocking 4.5 mm screw. The patient's pelvic ring injury was also stabilized, as shown.

returned to their prefracture level of activities, whereas those patients over the age of 60 have demonstrated less favorable functional results.[33]

The use of trochanteric entry cephalomedullary nails has allowed expanded use of intramedullary fixation to include its use for proximal fractures with involvement of the piriformis fossa. Additionally, its use has been advocated for all complex proximal femur fractures due to its perceived ease of insertion and improved biomechanics. High union rates and low complication rates have been reported in several large series with the use of this implant to treat subtrochanteric fractures.[1,4,17,36–38] Union rates of 96 to 98% have been reported at 1 year follow-up, with 8 to 12% of patients requiring a second operation to gain the union or treat complications. One large series specifically looked at low-energy subtrochanteric fractures in elderly patients (median age of 78.5 years) treated with a trochanteric entry long cephalomedullary nail and reported functional outcomes with at least 1 year follow-up in 211 patients.[38] Fracture healing was complete in 98% of patients, and 8.9% required a second operation. Functional outcomes were similar to those shown for other proximal femur fractures in elderly patients with high mortality rates during the first year (24%), a trend toward an increased level of social dependency (only 53.1% of those living at home prior to injury able to return to their home), and an increased incidence of patients unable to walk or requiring assistance to walk (only 44.9% of those able to walk without assistance prior to injury were able to walk without assistance at 1 year postinjury).

A concern specific to the trochanteric entry cephalomedullary nails is the insertion site and need for removal of a large amount of bone from the proximal femur. The removal of a significant amount of bone from the greater trochanter at the area of the insertion of the abductors has raised concerns as to the long-term effects on abductor strength and gait. Additionally, insertion site pain may be increased with these large implants. There are no studies that can verify these concerns at present. These implants require a large entry hole due to their proximal diameters (typically 17 mm) and removal of significant bone for the head fixation. This significant bone removal may create some difficulties with future operations and concerns if implant removal is needed.

The use of 95 degree fixed-angle devices can be applied for all subtrochanteric fractures, including those with involvement of the lesser or greater trochanter or piriformis fossa. Early reports with these fixation devices found nonunion rates as high as 16 to 20% and infection rates as high as 20%.[3,5,13] The use of prophylactic antibiotics and the implementation of surgical techniques stressing indirect reductions, preservation of the vitality of the fracture zone, and prestressing of the construct have decreased these complications to nonunion rates of 0 to 7% and corresponding very low infection rates.[4,11,12,14–16,18,39]

Complications

The treatment of subtrochanteric femur fractures continues to evolve, and the complication rates have been decreased to more acceptable rates with improved operative techniques and the use of biomechanically improved implants. A wide range of the rates of the most common complications exist in the literature due to the techniques employed in the operative treatment of these fractures, the spectrum of fracture patterns that are treated, and the preinjury status and associated injuries of the patients treated. Common complications include delayed union and nonunion with resultant failure of fixation or hardware breakage, malunion, infection, persistent pain, and loss of function.[1,3–5,10–16,19,20,33–38,40–47] All of these complications have been addressed earlier in this chapter. Careful operative technique, close patient follow-up, and familiarity with multiple techniques of treatment of these fractures can minimize the incidence and long-term effects of these complications. Most malunions result from improper alignment at the initial surgery and not from loss of alignment. It is critical to carefully check the alignment of the operated extremity, comparing it to the opposite extremity prior to leaving the operating room; if the alignment is not symmetric, revision should be done at this time. The most common malalignment will be varus, flexion, external rotation, of the proximal segment. Shortening may also occur. Nonunions have been treated successfully with high rates of fracture union and clinical and functional improvement with revision of the internal fixation and bone grafting.[48–50]

Pearls

- After a subtrochanteric fracture, the proximal fragment of the femur is flexed, abducted, and externally rotated, while the distal segment is adducted and shortened by the action of the adductors and hamstrings.
- It has been calculated that the compressive stresses in the femur are greatest in the medial cortex 1 to 3 in. below the lesser trochanter and can exceed 1200 pounds per square inch.
- Unlike intertrochanteric fractures, fixed-angle devices are preferred for subtrochanteric fractures because higher rates of complications are noted when sliding plates are used.
- External rotation of the proximal segment is a particular problem after using a nail to repair a subtrochanteric fracture. The arc of rotation of both hips should be checked and compared before the procedure is terminated.

On the DVDs

Video 24–1 (Disk 3) Unreamed Femoral Nailing to Treat Bilateral Femur Fractures in a Multitrauma Patient This video demonstrates a multi-trauma patient with bilateral femur fractures. Unreamed nailing is used to minimize any pulmonary insult to the patient, with an assessment of his function following the first nail to determine if he was able to withstand the second nailing procedure.

Video 24–2 (Disk 3) Trochanteric Nail for Reverse Oblique Subtrochanteric Fracture This video demonstrates the stabilization of a reverse-oblique fracture of the proximal femur with a trochanteric nail (ITST, Zimmer, Warsaw, Indiana). Details of lateral positioning, the nail starting portal, fracture reduction, and nail insertion are covered.

Video 24–3 (Disk 3) Blade Plate Fixation for a Russell-Taylor IA Proximal Femur Fracture A 95-degree-angled blade plate is placed in the appropriate position in the proximal femur, and then the plate is utilized to afford the reduction. The steps in placement of a blade plate and use of the articulating tensioning device are shown.

Video 24–4 (Disk 3) Proximal Femoral Locked Plating for Osteoporotic Subtrochanteric Femur Fracture Advantages of a submuscularly placed locked fixator include: avoidance of abductor devitalization, ability to use the plate to afford the reduction, and appropriate fixation of the osteoporotic proximal segment. Closed reduction techniques and submuscular fixator placement are shown.

Video 24–5 (Same as 22–3, Disk 3) ORIF of Femoral Neck and Subtrochanteric Femur Fracture with Locking Proximal Femur Plate This video demonstrates ORIF of a complex femoral neck/subtrochanteric femur fracture using the Watson Jones approach. A systematic approach to reduction and fixation of this severe injury is demonstrated, with the use of a locking precontoured proximal femur plate to stabilize the fracture.

References

1. Cheng MT, Chiu FY, Chuang TY, Chen CM, Chen TH, Lee PC. Treatment of complex subtrochanteric fracture with the long gamma AP locking nail: a prospective evaluation of 64 cases. J Trauma 2005; 58:304–311

2. Russell TA, Taylor JC. Subtrochanteric fractures of the femur. In: Browner BD, Jupiter JB, Levine AM, Trafton PG, eds. Skeletal Trauma: Fractures, Dislocations, Ligamentous Injuries. 1st ed. Philadelphia: Saunders; 1992:1485–1525

3. Sanders R, Regazzoni P. Treatment of subtrochanteric femur fractures using the dynamic condylar screw. J Orthop Trauma 1989;3: 206–213

4. Vanderschot P, Vanderspeeten K, Verheyen L, Broos P. A review on 161 subtrochanteric fractures: risk factors influencing outcome: age, fracture pattern, and fracture level. Unfallchirurg 1995;98:265–271

5. Waddell JP. Subtrochanteric fractures of the femur: a review of 130 patients. J Trauma 1979;19:582–592

6. Koch JC. The laws of bone architecture. Am J Anat 1917;21:177–298

7. Fracture and dislocation compendium. Orthopaedic Trauma Association. Committee for coding and classification. J Orthop Trauma 1996;10:36–40

8. Hibbs RA. The management of the tendency of the upper fragment to tilt forward in fractures of the upper third of the femur. NY Med J 1902;75:177–179

9. Johnson KD, Johnston DW, Parker B. Comminuted femoral shaft fractures: treatment by roller traction, cerclage wires and an intramedullary nail or an interlocking intramedullary nail. J Bone Joint Surg Am 1984;66:1222–1235

10. Velasco RU, Comfort TH. Analysis of treatment problems in subtrochanteric fractures of the femur. J Trauma 1978;18:513–523

11. Kinast C, Bolhofner BR, Mast JW, Ganz R. Subtrochanteric fractures of the femur: results of treatment with a 95-degree condylar blade plate. Clin Orthop Relat Res 1989;238:122–130

12. Kulkarni SS, Moran CG. Results of dynamic condylar screw for subtrochanteric fractures. Injury 2003;34:117–122

13. Nungu KS, Olerud C, Rehnberg L. Treatment of subtrochanteric fractures with the AO dynamic condylar screw. Injury 1993;24: 90–92

14. Neher C, Ostrum RF. Treatment of subtrochanteric femur fractures using a submuscular fixed low-angle plate. Am J Orthop 2003; 32(Suppl 9):29–33

15. Siebenrock KA, Muller U, Ganz R. Indirect reduction with a condylar blade plate for osteosynthesis of subtrochanteric femoral fractures. Injury 1998;29(Suppl 3):C7–C15

16. Vaidya SV, Dholakia DB, Chatterjee A. The use of a dynamic condylar screw and biological reduction techniques for subtrochanteric femur fracture. Injury 2003;34:123–128

17. Miedel R, Ponzer S, Tornkvist H, Soderqvist A, Tidermark J. The standard gamma nail or the Medoff sliding plate for unstable trochanteric and subtrochanteric fractures: a randomised, controlled trial. J Bone Joint Surg Br 2005;87:68–75

18. Haidukewych GJ, Israel TA, Berry DJ. Reverse obliquity fractures of the intertrochanteric region of the femur. J Bone Joint Surg Am 2001;83-A:643–650

19. Senter B, Kendig R, Savoie FH. Operative stabilization of subtrochanteric fractures of the femur. J Orthop Trauma 1990;4: 399–405

20. Wile PB, Panjabi MM, Southwick WO. Treatment of subtrochanteric fractures with a high angle compression hip screw. Clin Orthop Relat Res 1983;175:72–78

21. Kregor PJ, Corr BR, Zlowodzki MP. Submuscular locked plating of pertrochanteric femur fractures: early experience in a consecutive, one-surgeon series; Presented at Annual Meeting, American Academy of Orthopedic Surgeons, Chicago, IL, March 22–26, 2006

22. Brumback RJ, Uwagie-Ero S, Lakatos RP, Poka A, Bathon GH, Burgess AR. Intramedullary nailing of femoral shaft fractures, II: Fracture-healing with static interlocking fixation. J Bone Joint Surg Am 1988;70A:1453–1462

23. Thoresen BO, Alho A, Ekeland A, Stromsoe K, Folleras G, Haukebo A. Interlocking intramedullary nailing in femoral shaft fractures: a report of forty-eight cases. J Bone Joint Surg Am 1985;67: 1313–1320

24. Wiss DA, Brien WW, Becker V. Interlocking nailing for the treatment of femoral fractures due to gunshot wounds. J Bone Joint Surg Am 1991;75:598–606

25. Wiss DA, Brien WW, Stetson WB. Interlocked nailing for treatment of segmental fractures of the femur. J Bone Joint Surg Am 1990;72:724–728

26. Wiss DA, Fleming CH, Matta JM, Clark D. Comminuted and rotationally unstable fractures of the femur treated with an interlocking nail. Clin Orthop Relat Res 1986;212:35–47

27. Bredbenner TL, Snyder SA, Mazloomi FR, Le T, Wilber RG. Subtrochanteric fixation stability depends on discrete fracture surface points. Clin Orthop Relat Res 2005;432:217–225

28. Kraemer WJ, Hearn TC, Powell JN, Mahomed N. Fixation of segmental subtrochanteric fractures: a biomechanical study. Clin Orthop Relat Res 1996;332:71–79

29. Roberts CS, Nawab A, Wang M, et al. Second generation intramedullary nailing of subtrochanteric femur fractures: a biomechanical study of fracture site motion. J Orthop Trauma 2003; 17(Suppl 8):S57–S64

30. Wheeler DL, Croy TJ, Woll TS, Scott MD, Senft DC, Duwelius PJ. Comparison of reconstruction nails for high subtrochanteric femur fracture fixation. Clin Orthop Relat Res 1997;338:231–239

31. Bose WJ, Corces A, Anderson LD. A preliminary experience with the Russell-Taylor reconstruction nail for complex femoral fractures. J Trauma 1992;32:71–76

32. Broos PL, Reynders P. The use of undreamed AO femoral intramedullary nail with spiral blade in nonpathologic fractures of the femur: experiences with eighty consecutive cases. J Orthop Trauma 2002;16:150–154

33. Garnavos C, Peterman A, Howard PW. The treatment of difficult proximal femoral fractures with the Russell-Taylor reconstruction nail. Injury 1999;30:407–415

34. Kang S, McAndrew MP, Johnson KD. The reconstruction locked nail for complex fractures of the proximal femur. J Orthop Trauma 1995;9:453–463

35. Smith JT, Goodman SB, Tischenko G. Treatment of comminuted femoral subtrochanteric fractures using the Russell-Taylor reconstruction nail. Orthopedics 1991;14:125–129

36. Borens O, Wettstein M, Kombot C, Chevalley F, Mouhsine E, Garofalo R. Long gamma nail in the treatment of subtrochanteric fractures. Arch Orthop Trauma Surg 2004;124:443–447

37. Pakuts AJ. Unstable subtrochanteric fractures: gamma nail versus dynamic condylar screw. Int Orthop 2004;28:21–24

38. Robinson CM, Houshian S, Khan LA. Trochanteric-entry long cephalomedullary nailing of subtrochanteric fractures caused by low-energy trauma. J Bone Joint Surg Am 2005;87:2217–2226

39. Tornetta P. Subtrochanteric femur fracture. J Orthop Trauma 2002; 16:280–283

40. Bedi A, Toan Le T. Subtrochanteric femur fractures. Orthop Clin North Am 2004;35:473–483

41. Craig NJ, Sivaji C, Maffulli N. Subtrochanteric fractures: a review of treatment options. Bull Hosp Jt Dis 2001;60:35–46

42. Di Cicco JD 3rd, Jenkins M, Ostrum RF. Retrograde nailing for subtrochanteric femur fractures. Am J Orthop 2000;29(Suppl 9):4–8

43. Fielding JW, Magliato HJ. Subtrochanteric fractures. Surg Gynecol Obstet 1966;122:555–560

44. Froimson AI. Treatment of comminuted subtrochanteric fractures of the femur. Surg Gynecol Obstet 1970;131:465–472

45. Lechner JD, Rao JP, Stashak G, Adibe SO. Subtrochanteric fractures: a retrospective analysis. Clin Orthop Relat Res 1990;259: 140–145

46. Sims SH. Subtrochanteric femur fractures. Orthop Clin North Am 2002;33:113–126

47. Whitelaw GP, Segal D, Sanzone CF, Ober NS, Hadley N. Unstable intertrochanteric/ subtrochanteric fractures of the femur. Clin Orthop Relat Res 1990;252:238–245

48. Barquet A, Mayora G, Fregeiro J, Lopez L, Rienzi D, Francescoli L. The treatment of subtrochanteric nonunions with the long gamma nail: twenty-six patients with a minimum 2-year follow-up. J Orthop Trauma 2004;18:346–353

49. Haidukewych GJ, Berry DJ. Nonunion of fractures of the subtrochanteric region of the femur. Clin Orthop Relat Res 2004;419: 185–188

50. Pascarella R, Maresca A, Palumbi P, Boriani S. Subtrochanteric nonunion of the femur. Chir Organi Mov 2004;89:1–6

25 Femoral Shaft Fractures

Brent L. Norris and Peter J. Nowotarski

Fractures of the diaphysis of the femur are a result of relatively high-energy trauma. The femur is the strongest and longest bone in our body. Motor vehicle collision is the most common cause of femoral shaft fracture. Secondary causes are pedestrian versus automobile, falls from heights, and gunshot injuries.[1] Although femoral shaft fractures no longer carries the significant mortality previously associated with this injury, mortality following bilateral femoral shaft fractures can approach 30%.[2,3] This is partially attributed to the fact that each femoral shaft fracture can lose two to three units of blood and may substantially impact hemodynamic stability, even in a young healthy patient.[3] However, the predominant risk of mortality is likely related to the associated injuries.[3]

The femoral shaft, or diaphysis, comprises the region extending between 5 cm below the lesser trochanter to 9 cm above the knee joint. The region proximal to this is considered the subtrochanteric femur, and the region distal is considered the supracondylar portion of the femur. Maintenance of mechanical stability to the femoral shaft is crucial for normal ambulation. There are significant axial, bending, and torsional forces on this elongated bone that are essential for normal gait. Furthermore, the femur is surrounded by a large amount of muscle in the diaphysis. These hip and thigh muscle forces allow locomotion to occur and rely heavily on a well-aligned femoral shaft. Because of the significant muscle attachments, fractures of the femoral shaft are often markedly displaced and require significant manipulation to achieve reduction.

The femoral shaft is filled with hemopoietic cells and fatty bone marrow. The fatty marrow is extravasated into the venous and lymphatic system upon fracture and can be further introduced into the vascular tree via instrumentation of the femoral shaft.[4,5] It has been theorized that this fat embolization can potentially lead to a deleterious "second hit" or even fat embolism syndrome in patients who have sustained a femoral shaft fracture undergoing intramedullary instrumentation.[6]

The incidence of femoral shaft fractures in the United States has been estimated around 1 to 1.3 fractures per 10,000 people per year. There is a bimodal distribution, including a peak around the age of 25 and a second peak at around the age of 65. Younger patients sustain femoral shaft fractures usually as a result of high-energy trauma. In contrast the older patient may often sustain a femoral shaft fracture from a lower-energy mechanism secondary to osteoporosis. As would be expected, younger patients with femoral shaft fractures are predominantly high-energy trauma, and the older patient, in contrast, is usually

from pathological changes to the bone and lower-energy mechanisms.

Injuries associated with femoral shaft fractures are frequent and can be divided into two categories, including systemic injury (head, chest, abdominal, and other remote musculoskeletal injury) and regional injuries (skeletal injuries ipsilateral to the limb). Common systemic injuries are significant head or thoracic injuries. Abdominal injuries are less common and associated predominantly with pelvic ring injuries. When femoral shaft fractures are associated with a head or chest injury, treatment can become a quandary, especially as it relates to the timing of fixation.[7,8] Immediate stabilization of femoral shaft fractures, although desirable, may sometimes be deleterious to the other injured systems, and the most appropriate time for definitive treatment remains controversial.[8] The release of inflammatory mediators following intramedullary nailing of a femoral shaft fracture can overwhelm an already injured system, especially the brain or lung.[9,10] This phenomenon is termed the "second hit" and remains central to a continued debate regarding the optimal timing for fixation of femur fractures in multiple trauma.[10] The controversy is further discussed in Chapter 34.

A less common problem that can be encountered is fat embolism syndrome. Gurd has described major and minor criteria to help diagnose this elusive entity, which clinically entails fever, hypoxia, mental status changes, and pathognomonic skin petechiae.[11,12] Fortunately, the incidence of fat embolism syndrome is low; but when it does occur, it can lead to significant pulmonary distress and morbidity. If appropriate ventilatory support is not quickly initiated, mortality may result.

Common regional injuries associated with femoral shaft fractures include a second fracture of the proximal femur, specifically femoral neck fractures.[13] This entity is sometimes missed or may be occult in nature. A relatively high index of suspicion must be maintained to diagnose this relatively common problem (2 to 6% of all femoral shaft fractures). A high-angle Pauwels C-type fracture (a vertical shear fracture pattern) of the femoral neck is a common fracture pattern seen with femoral shaft fractures. If recognized, stabilization of the femoral neck fracture prior to instrumentation of the shaft is recommended.[13] Other associated hip pathology includes posterior hip dislocations; associated acetabular fractures; and, very uncommonly, ipsilateral intertrochanteric, subtrochanteric, and/or supracondylar fractures.[14]

Clinically significant knee ligament injuries have been described in patients with femoral shaft fractures (20 to 30%).[15]

Additionally, patients commonly complain of anterior knee pain following femoral shaft fractures. Patellofemoral injury from a dashboard strike or even occult meniscal tears are often the cause of this pain. The incidence of late meniscal pathology is ~20% and more commonly affects the lateral side.[15] Ipsilateral lower extremity injuries associated with femoral shaft fractures include tibial shaft fracture, ankle fracture/dislocation, and major foot injuries. All these injuries are commonly seen in patients involved in high-speed motor vehicle collisions. Remote skeletal injury, including clavicle and upper extremity injuries, is also common and will limit the patient's ability to mobilize when it occurs.

Associated neurological and vascular injuries are rare. The large muscle envelope surrounding the femur protects the major vascular and neurological structures. When a vascular injury does occur, proper expedient treatment is of paramount importance because it is usually a limb-threatening injury. The vascular integrity should be evaluated whenever there is absent pulse or diminished pulses with an ankle-brachial index (ABI) of less than 0.9.[16] When these are found, an urgent on-table arteriogram should be performed to rule out vascular injury, and definitive treatment should occur simultaneous with stabilization of the femoral shaft fracture.

Classifications

Classification of the femoral shaft fractures is fairly straightforward. There are several systems, although a descriptive classification is probably the most useful. This is commonly what is used when the patient arrives in the emergency room, and includes fracture location, pattern, whether the fracture is open or closed, and associated injuries. This information helps determine treatment, the timing and urgency of such, and the need for involvement of other services. Other classification systems are predominantly for communication, for research protocols, and for evaluating surgical outcomes. In addition to the anatomical classification, the two most commonly used classification systems are the Winquist and the Arbeitsgemunshaft für Osteosynthesefragen/Orthopaedic Trauma Association (AO/OTA) systems.

Winquist and Hansen graded fractures 1 through 4, based on the degree of diaphyseal comminution.[17] The more comminuted the fracture, the more injury the bone and soft tissue sustain and the higher the likelihood for problems with healing. Grade 1 fractures are transverse or short obliques with less than 25% comminution. Grade 2 fractures have 25 to 50% shaft width comminution. Grade 3 fractures have more than 50% but less than 100% comminution. Grade 4 fractures have segmental comminution.

The AO/OTA classification system is predominantly used as a descriptor for research and comparing injuries for publication.[18] The femur is designated by the number 3; the diaphyseal portion of the bone is designated by the number 2. The fractures are then further subdivided into type A, type B, or type C fractures. Type A fractures are simple fracture patterns such as spiral, short oblique, or transverse. Type B fractures are fractures with a small butterfly fragment or bending wedge. Type C fractures are segmentally comminuted injuries (**Fig. 25–1**). This classification system was not necessarily developed for treatment, but more for understanding the personality of the fracture, the time needed for healing, and the complications associated with treatment of this injury.

As previously stated, the most helpful classification system for femoral shaft fractures is a descriptive type. Simply describing the fracture location, either upper middle or lower third of the shaft, the fracture pattern (spiral, short, oblique, transverse, or comminuted), and whether the injury is an open fracture is extremely helpful. Additionally, knowledge of the degree of associated soft tissue injury and other associated injuries, systemic and regional, assists the surgeon in the preoperative decision making.

One final note on open fractures: extrapolating the original Gustilo-Anderson classification for tibia fracture to the femur does not render justice to the magnitude of injury to the soft tissues following a femoral shaft fracture. The tibia is a more subcutaneous bone, and open wounds can be seen with relatively low-energy injuries. This is very uncommon for fractures of the femoral shaft because it is surrounded by muscle, and even a small puncture wound in the anterolateral thigh denotes a very high energy fracture. Furthermore, a significant amount of muscle injury will likely exist below the skin. Therefore, a femoral shaft fracture with any degree of open skin injury denotes a high-energy injury, and usually warrants a type 3 classification from the Gustilo-Anderson system.

Nonoperative Treatment

Nonoperative treatment of an adult femoral shaft fracture in the era of modern medicine is essentially nonexistent. Because of the extreme morbidity and mortality associated with nonoperative care of this injury, surgical management has become the mainstay of treatment. Nonoperative treatment originally consisted of closed manipulation/reduction with skin or skeletal traction. Traction was adjusted periodically as needed to obtain overall gross alignment of the limb. Bed rest was required for upwards of 8 to 10 weeks prior to mobilization. Pins and plaster techniques and cast bracing followed traction treatment but generally showed unfavorable results.[19] Fortunately, in 1940, Gerhard Küntscher introduced intramedullary nailing of the femoral shaft. His pioneering treatment ushered in today's trend of operative management over nonoperative management for this fracture.

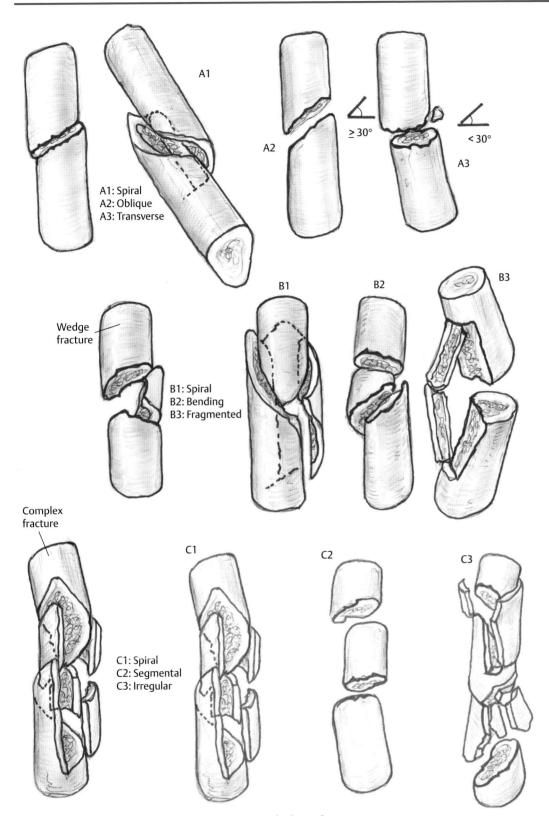

A1

A2

≥ 30°   < 30°

A3

A1: Spiral
A2: Oblique
A3: Transverse

Wedge
fracture

B1   B2   B3

B1: Spiral
B2: Bending
B3: Fragmented

Complex
fracture

C1   C2   C3

C1: Spiral
C2: Segmental
C3: Irregular

Figure 25–1 The AO/OTA fracture classification system for femur fractures.

Indications for Surgical Treatment

Fracture of the femoral shaft in an adult is an indication for surgical management. The type and timing of intervention are the key elements of the decision-making process. There are only a few limited reasons not to pursue surgical stabilization of the femoral shaft, and they include patients that are in extremis (with life-threatening injuries), patients that are medically unfit for anesthesia, and possibly Jehovah's Witnesses who have sustained significant blood loss. All other patients should undergo surgical intervention to repair the femoral shaft in hopes of stabilizing the injury, decreasing pain, and restoring as much function as possible to the limb.

Surgical Treatment

Surgical treatment of femoral shaft fractures can be quite varied, depending on surgical skills and the clinical situation. The type and timing of fixation will depend largely on variables beyond the fracture itself. The associated injuries to the patient are as important as the fracture type and location. Other fractures that affect surgical decision making include the amount of local soft tissue injury and whether the fracture is open or closed. Forms of surgical treatment include external fixation, plate fixation (including compression plating, bridge plating, and percutaneous bridge plating), and intramedullary nailing.

Intramedullary nailing has become the standard by which other treatments are now measured. Although it remains the standard and most common form of treatment, several controversies exist regarding intramedullary nailing of the femoral shaft. These include such things as direction of insertion of the nail (either antegrade or retrograde), how the nail is implanted (either reamed or unreamed), and how the nail is secured to the femur (standard locking, cephalomedullary locking, static locking, or dynamic locking). The position of the patient during instrumentation (supine vs lateral) and the use of a fracture table versus placing the patient free on a radiolucent table are also important variables to be considered. Finally, there are several special situations that influence treatment of the femoral shaft fracture, including the associated femoral neck fracture, the soft tissue injury, open fractures with segmental bone loss, arterial injury, the multiply injured patient, patients with a significant chest injury, and patients with an associated head injury. All of these scenarios will be discussed in detail later in the chapter but are mentioned here to point out the numerous patient and injury conditions that influence the decision-making process.

Surgical Anatomy

Details of the anatomy of the leg will be presented as appropriate with the surgical techniques described in the next section. The quadriceps muscles are located anteriorly, the adductors medially, and the hamstring muscles posteriorly. The preferred approach for plating of the femur is immediately anterior to the lateral intermuscular septum. It is critical to remember the perforating vessels that pierce the septum and control them during the approach. Understanding the anatomy of the hip and knee is critical to the success in intramedullary nailing. The details are discussed in the sections on antegrade and retrograde nailing.

Surgical Techniques

External Fixation

The application of an external fixator to a femoral shaft fracture has been used for several decades. The best indications for placement of an external fixator in a femoral shaft fracture are a patient who is polytraumatized or underresuscitated, a patient with a significant head injury, a patient with a very large contaminated open soft tissue envelope, a patient with an associated ischemic vascular injury, or a patient with other surgical injuries requiring concurrent operating room teams.[20,21] One of the key features to external fixation is the speed with which it can be placed. It should take ~15 to 20 minutes to apply a four-pin fixator to the femoral shaft and gain enough stability to control the limb.

A keen understanding of the relevant anatomy of the hip, thigh, and knee and quality radiographs of the entire femur are required prior to any surgical intervention. Radiographs of the femoral neck region (internal rotation preferred), the entire femoral shaft, and the knee joint are needed to rule out associated skeletal injuries. The fracture level should be identified and measured as it relates to key landmarks about the femur (i.e., the lateral epicondyle and the top of the trochanter). This will assist the surgeon in identifying the level of the fracture by simple palpable landmarks. This is extremely important and facilitates the application of an external fixator when a C-arm is not available, as in the intensive care unit setting.

The patient should be placed on a radiolucent table. The entire limb should be prepped and draped in a sterile fashion, including the hip joint and lateral crest of the ilium. Pins should be placed independently, with two pins fairly close to the fracture and two pins distant to the fracture **(Fig. 25–2A,B)**. The first pin can usually be placed four fingerbreadths below the tip of the trochanter, which should put it at the level of the lesser trochanter. The next pin is based upon the location of the fracture and placed as close to the fracture as possible in the proximal fragment. The next pin would be placed just below the fracture, and the last pin is placed at least two fingerbreadths above the lateral epicondyle. The choice of pin size is usually a 200 × 5 mm Schanz pin to allow for a double-stacked frame laterally. Larger pins (250 to 300 mm × 5 mm) may be needed for obese patients. The pins are placed directly lateral to slightly anterolateral through percutaneous stab wounds.

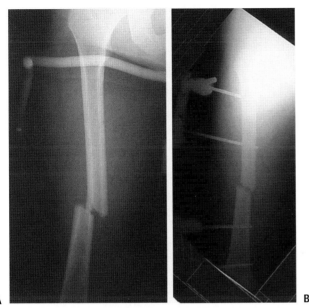

A   **B**

Figure 25–2 (A) Radiograph of a midshaft femur fracture in a hare traction splint. **(B)** External fixator with two pins close to the fracture and two pins distant to the fracture.

The fascia is incised sharply, blunt dissection is carried out down to the level of the femur, and the cortex is palpated. The femur is predrilled with a 3.5 mm drill bit and a triple trocar reaming guide. The pins are then placed bicortically. Each fragment is then independently manipulated with a two-pin bar cluster or multihole pin clamp. A third bar-to-bar clamp is then used to solidify the reduction after longitudinal traction, and correction of the deformity is obtained under fluoroscopic guidance. At this point the frame is locked down, and a second set of bars is applied to strengthen the construct. If the frame is for temporary use only (which is frequently the case), a single-stack frame should be adequate and certainly less expensive. Having said this, carbon fiber or steel bars smaller than 11 mm should be double stacked. The pin sites are then released sharply if there is skin tenting and wrapped with sterile gauze to help with bleeding and drainage at the pin–skin interface. Very few femurs will be treated to union with an external fixator; however, postoperative pin care should begin early on. Half peroxide/half normal saline Q-tip swabs to the pin–skin interface three times a day with rewrapping of the pins will control drainage and decrease risk of pin-tract infection. Range of motion of the hip and knee is usually limited with pins transfixing the quadriceps, but it is allowed and encouraged. Motion problems are one of the more significant disadvantages of management of the femoral shaft fracture with an external fixator.

Plate Fixation

There are two techniques for plate fixation of femoral shaft fractures, compression plating and bridge plating.

Compression plating of fractures is ideal for simple fracture patterns, including spiral fractures, short oblique fractures, and transverse fractures. The more comminution that is present, the more difficult it is to plate the femur with compression techniques. For plating a comminuted fracture, bridge plating is the most useful and desirable technique. Indications for plating include a large associated open wound, surgeon preference for plate fixation; and patients with significant head/chest injury that theoretically could sustain further injury to these organ systems with intramedullary instrumentation.[21] Complex combined femoral neck and shaft fractures or femoral shaft and distal intercondylar femur fractures are also relative indications for plate fixation.[23]

Plate fixation ideally is placed anteriorly and laterally to decrease tensile forces. Plating, unfortunately, has a significant mechanical disadvantage compared with intramedullary nailing because it is off axis to the mechanical load. For this reason, when compression plating is applied, a minimum of 8 cortices above and below the fracture is warranted with a thick 4.5 mm broad plate.

Compression Plating

Patients are placed supine on a radiolucent fracture table. The entire limb is prepped and draped to include the hip and the ilium. A long lateral incision is made centered over the fracture **(Fig. 25–3A,B)**. The fascia lata is incised slightly posteriorly and longitudinally. Surgical dissection requires the entire vastus lateralis muscle to be lifted up and taken off the lateral intermuscular septum **(Fig. 25–4)**. Bleeding from perforating arteries is common and must be controlled. An alternative approach would be through the traumatic wound. Care should be taken to avoid any further injury to the muscle envelope, and using the traumatic wound may facilitate this. Reduction of the fracture is performed directly with reduction clamps. Careful application of a plate-holding clamp is needed to avoid further injury to the bone and its vascularity. If a simple fracture pattern is present, lag screws can be used to provisionally hold the fracture, and a large 4.5 mm broad plate placed laterally can be used as a neutralization plate.

Bridge Plating

In more comminuted fractures where lag screw fixation is precluded, bridge plating should be considered. The plate should be long enough to span the fracture and allow for four bicortical screws proximally and distally. The plate is applied to the proximal fragment and aligned parallel to the bone and secured with two 4.5 mm screws. Reduction of the fracture is usually performed indirectly in a closed fashion. In open fractures, some direct manipulation of fracture fragments is possible but should be minimized to avoid further damage to bone vascularity.

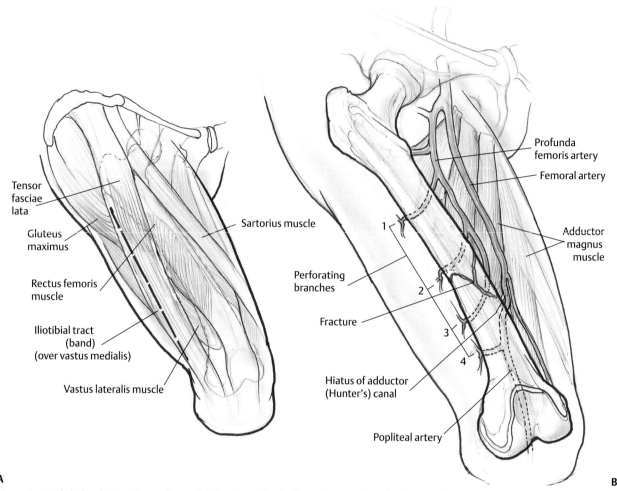

Figure 25–3 **(A)** The skin incision and superficial anatomy for the lateral approach to the femur. **(B)** The vascular anatomy of the femur, depicting the location of the perforating branches encountered during the lateral approach.

Length, axial alignment, and rotational alignment are of significant importance. Comparison radiographs of the opposite limb are sometimes necessary to confirm an acceptable reduction, especially regarding length. See Chapter 4 for details regarding the assessment of alignment (see **Figs. 4–19** through **4–22**). Once the limb and comminuted fracture are aligned appropriately, the plate is secured to the distal fragment with a plate-holding clamp. A third screw is then passed in the distal fragment close to the fracture. Care must be taken to make sure the plate is posterior enough to account for the anterior longitudinal femoral bow. After further review of the length and rotational alignment, the distal fragment is finally secured with the fourth screw at the level of the supracondylar region. If the fracture remains shortened, the distal screws should be removed, and the distal fragment is held to plate with a plate-holding clamp. A push-pull screw with a lamina spreader or the compressor/ distractor (articulating tensioning device) is then used to obtain appropriate length.

Generous use of C-arm fluoroscopy is needed to help confirm adequate alignment and rotation of the fracture. The use of a fracture table may complicate matters, and the authors prefer to operate with the leg draped free on a radiolucent table under appropriate musculoskeletal relaxation. A few of the remaining screw holes are then filled with bicortical 4.5 mm screws totaling a minimum of 8 cortices proximally and distally. The soft tissue envelope is then closed over the plate with suction drainage placed deep to the fascia lata. Bone grafting is applied if the fracture envelope is surgically opened or medial defects are encountered. In open fractures, antibiotic-impregnated bioabsorbable calcium sulfate beads can be used in hopes of stimulating bone formation and eradicating any potential infection that may be present.

Postoperative rehabilitation begins early with range of motion of the hip and knee. This includes use of a continuous passive motion (CPM) machine if necessary. The limb is kept touch-down weight bearing, and isometric quadriceps muscle strengthening is encouraged. Control of the limb, once ob-

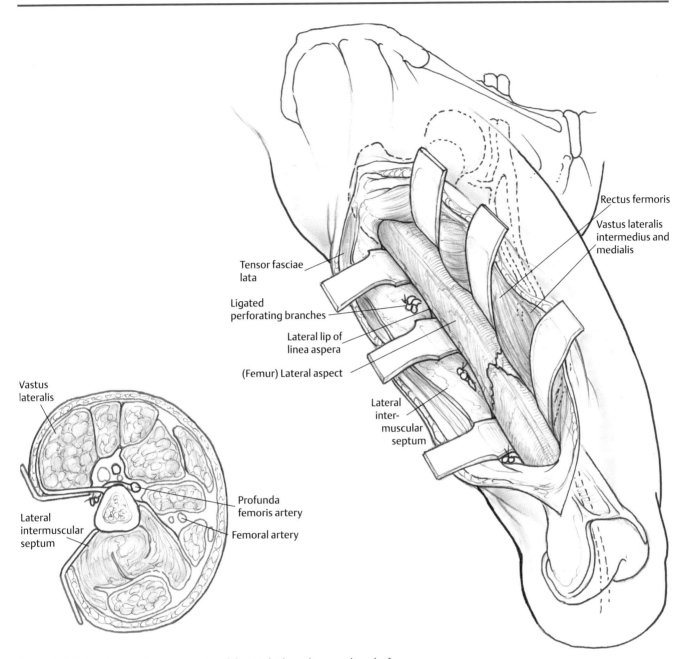

Figure 25–4 The deep anatomy encountered during the lateral approach to the femur.

tained, signifies return of muscle function, and it is reasonable to consider discontinuation of deep venous thrombosis (DVT) prophylaxis at this point (usually anywhere from 3 to 6 weeks). Restricted weight bearing is continued until bridging callus is seen. Restricted weight bearing is used for 12 to 14 weeks in most cases. Weight bearing is advanced slowly, and hopefully patients are full weight bearing by 16 weeks.

Percutaneous Bridge Plating

The patient's limb is prepped and draped sterilely off the fracture table to allow control of the entire limb from the iliac crest to the foot. The hip is placed over a slight bump to allow for elevation of the trochanter. It is important to

remember the impact of the bump when reducing the fracture and establishing the rotational alignment of the lower limb. Fractures amenable to this technique are predominantly comminuted middiaphyseal fractures in patients who cannot undergo intramedullary fixation. The technique is to obtain contralateral limb measurement for length from the tip of the trochanter to the epicondyle region. This length is then equilibrated to a large 4.5 mm broad plate that is slightly prebent to match the lateral aspect of the femur from the vastus ridge to the epicondylar flare.

Two small incisions are made through the fascia lata at the level of the epicondyle laterally as well as over the vastus ridge **(Fig. 25–5A).** The plate is then slid submuscu-

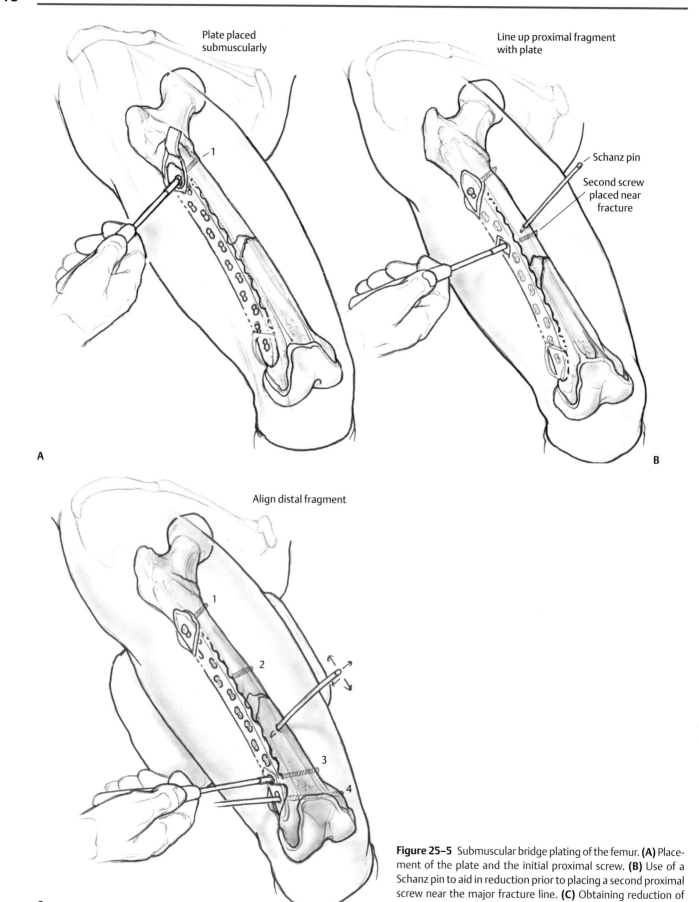

Plate placed
submuscularly

1

A

Line up proximal fragment
with plate

Schanz pin

Second screw
placed near
fracture

B

Align distal fragment

1

2

3

4

C

Figure 25–5 Submuscular bridge plating of the femur. **(A)** Placement of the plate and the initial proximal screw. **(B)** Use of a Schanz pin to aid in reduction prior to placing a second proximal screw near the major fracture line. **(C)** Obtaining reduction of the distal fragment and placing distal screws.

larly beneath the muscle in a retrograde fashion until it is identified coming out of the proximal portion of the wound. A bicortical screw is inserted at the level of the lesser trochanter, securing the plate. At this point surgical manipulation of the fracture is accomplished indirectly with traction, direct pressure, and occasionally with the use of percutaneous Schanz pins (5 mm "joysticks") or long ball-spike pushers. Once the proximal fragment is aligned with the plate, a second screw is applied percutaneously with the use of C-arm guidance (preferably close to the fracture). At this point, with the plate secured with two screws in the proximal fragment, the distal fragment is then manipulated into a reduced position with the use of bumps, traction, percutaneous Schanz pins, or ball-spiked pushers **(Fig. 25–5B)**. Care should be taken to ensure appropriate rotation and length at this point. A third bicortical screw is then applied percutaneously through the plate, securing the bone to the plate. A fourth screw is applied through the plate in the epicondylar region **(Fig. 25–5C)**. Length and rotational alignment are reassessed, and supplemental screw fixation is applied percutaneously for a total of three or four screws proximally and distally.

At this point the patient's wounds are irrigated and closed, and range of motion of the hip and knee is performed. Rotational alignment and length are further scrutinized at this time. Postoperative care includes restrictions in weight bearing and DVT prophylaxis until muscle control of the limb is obtained. Abundant callus formation is usually seen in this situation because the undisturbed muscular envelope helps lead to early periosteal callus formation. Weight bearing is still restricted for a total of 12 to 14 weeks to allow bridging callus to organize and mature. Hip and knee motion, as well as gentle strengthening, is encouraged during the early postoperative period.

Antegrade Intramedullary Nailing (see Videos 25–1, 25–2, 25–3, 25–4, Disk 3)

Intramedullary nailing is currently the best method of fixation for femoral shaft fractures. Although controversy still exists over several aspects of intramedullary nailing, clinical outcomes following intramedullary nailing remain excellent, and complications are minimal.

Antegrade, Piriformis, Reamed, Supine, Fracture Table

The patient is placed supine on a modern fracture table. The fracture table should allow the well leg to be extended at the hip and abducted in reference to the injured leg. The affected limb has a proximal tibial traction pin applied at the level of the tibial tubercle or just below this. A malpositioned tibial traction pin will interfere with reduction maneuvers and should be replaced if this occurs. A tensile K-wire can be applied with a Kirschner bow, or a larger pin can be used for direct traction. A centrally threaded pin is not necessary, although it is preferred when larger-diameter

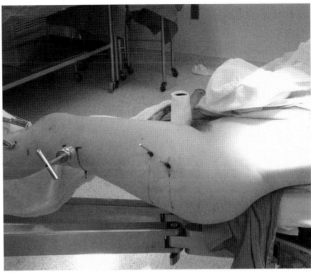

Figure 25–6 Patient in traction on the fracture table with legs in the scissor position.

pins are used. The patient is then placed on the fracture table with the majority of the affected limb prepped and draped in a supine position (iliac crest to the traction pin). Patient positioning is critical to facilitate instrumentation of the proximal femur. Circumferential prepping of the limb is ideal, although not necessary. At least 270 degrees of the lateral aspect of the femur should be exposed. It is not necessary to drape the most medial aspect of the femur into the field. The C-arm is brought in from the opposite side next to the well leg. The well leg is placed in an abducted and down (extended) position (not the lithotomy position) **(Fig. 25–6)**. Patients are often placed in a V position to accentuate the accessibility of the greater trochanter. This position is achieved primarily by moving the patient's head and trunk, with a smaller contribution to the position achieved by adducting the fractured leg **(Fig. 25–7)**.

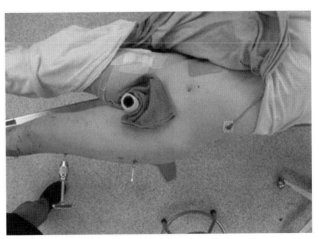

Figure 25–7 Relative adduction of the injured leg is achieved primarily by placement of the patient's trunk and head, with a smaller contribution from adducting the injured leg.

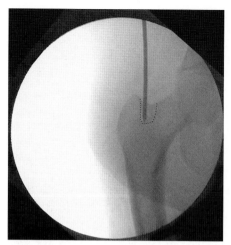

Figure 25–8 Fluoroscopic view of the proximal femur with the dotted line outlining the piriformis fossa.

The reduction maneuvers for more proximal fractures are to place the hip in a more flexed position to help approximate the distal fragment to the proximal fragment. A crutch with a Mayo stand cover or other sterile cover pushing up the distal fragment will help correct the posterior sag of the distal fragment. A significant amount of adduction is also necessary to help overcome some of the forces and help visualize/locate a piriformis starting point on the proximal femur. Rotational alignment should be checked so that the lateral portion of the patella is in line with the anterior-superior iliac spine. With these landmarks in place, the C-arm is brought in to visualize the proximal femur. The proximal femur should show the outline of the femoral neck and the piriformis fossa **(Fig. 25–8)**. We suggest C-arm confirmation of an adequate closed reduction of the femoral shaft fracture prior to prepping, draping, and incision.

After sterile prep and drape, the skin incision is made ~10 to 12 cm above the trochanter. The deep fascia is opened. A 3 mm guide pin is passed down through the musculature in line with the piriformis fossa just medial to the trochanter. A medial or anterior starting point will encroach on the femoral neck and potentially cause either or both femoral neck fracture and damage to the femoral head circulation. Halfway down the piriformis fossa is ideal and confirmed on the lateral view to be aligned with the medullary shaft. This pin is then introduced through the piriformis fossa to just below the lesser trochanter. Anteroposterior (AP) and lateral fluoroscopy should confirm pin placement to be centralized in the canal. A cannulated 13 mm reamer is then passed over the guidewire, opening the proximal femur to the level of the lesser trochanter.

In larger patients, getting a starting point can be quite difficult (especially when the hip remains abducted). A useful tip to help prevent this is to place the patient's pelvis more lateral on the fracture table, adduct the leg, and place a percutaneous spiked pusher or 5 mm unicortical Schanz pin on the proximal fragment, helping adduct this fragment further **(Fig. 25–9A,B)**.

Once the "opening hole" is obtained, a guidewire with a ball tip is passed into the proximal fragment and across the fracture. Surgical manipulation is often necessary to accomplish this task. There are specific techniques to help manipulate fractures into a reduced position. An intramedullary fracture reduction tool (which is also cannulated and has a curved tip) is bulky enough to help effect a reduction from inside the medullary canal **(Fig. 25–10A,B)**. A ball-tipped guidewire is then passed across the fracture once the reduction is obtained. If the "finger" reduction tool is not available, then a Schanz pin to grab the distal fragment can be used to manipulate this fragment into reduction through extramedullary means. The least invasive

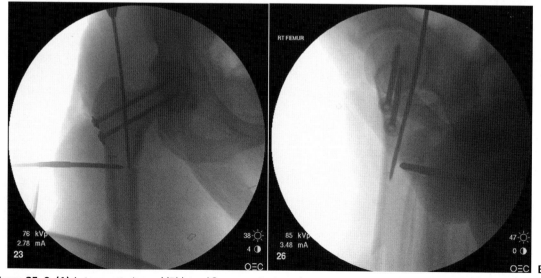

Figure 25–9 (A) Anteroposterior and **(B)** lateral fluoroscopic views demonstrating the use of a Schanz pin to position the proximal fragment for optimal placement of the guidewire.

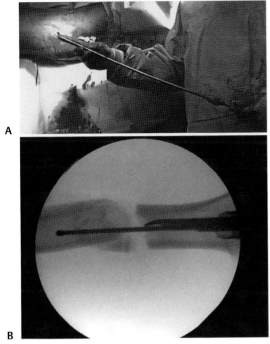

A

B

Figure 25–10 **(A)** Photograph of the intramedullary reduction tool prior to insertion in the femur. **(B)** Fluoroscopic view demonstrating use of the intramedullary reduction tool to assist with passage of the ball-tipped guidewire across the fracture.

techniques include the use of a crutch placed posteriorly beneath the drapes to help correct the flexed or sagging position of the distal fragment. Additional forces can be applied manually to the proximal or distal fragment from the anterior, medial, or lateral aspect to help align the limb.

Once the ball-tipped guidewire is in the distal fragment, the C-arm is brought to the level of the knee, and the guidewire is passed centrally to the level of Blumensaat's line. It is very important to make certain the guidewire is located in the center of the distal femur on both the AP and lateral images. This will help centralize the nail and prevent malalignment in comminuted distal third femur fractures. Lateral images are used to confirm the guidewire is not too anterior so as to eccentrically ream out the anterior cortex. At this point sequential reaming of the femur is performed. The nail diameter should be chosen based on preoperative evaluation of the medullary canal. Intraoperative sizing is commonly done by choosing a nail 1 mm larger than the first reamer that produces endosteal "chatter." However, the nail size should allow for large enough locking bolts to prevent early hardware failure with ambulation (stainless steel 6.4 mm, titanium 5 mm). Once sequential reaming is performed, the ball-tipped guidewire can be replaced with a smooth guidewire via an exchange tube. This step is not necessary with some intramedullary nailing systems, where the ball-tipped guidewire will pass through the tip of the nail.

Measurements for nail length can be performed with a radiolucent ruler or by the subtraction method. The subtraction method uses two guidewires of the same length measured off the tip of the trochanter. The portion of one guidewire inside the femoral canal correlates with the portion of the other guidewire outside the body **(Fig. 25–11)**. When segmental comminution is encountered and the length is in question, the opposite intact femur is measured from the top of the trochanter to the medial epicondyle. If both fractures are comminuted, the same-sized nail should be chosen and placed to the same landmark on each femur. Additionally, some manufacturers have rulers that allow you to measure off the guidewire directly. Once the appropriate length and diameter are chosen, the nail is passed over the smooth guidewire and secured with locking bolts. Again, all reduction forces and maneuvers should be in place, with the fracture reduced during nail passage.

Locking bolts should be placed in a static pattern unless there is a good reason to undergo dynamic locking. This usually means two screws above and two screws below the fracture, preferably 5 cm or more from the site of the fracture. Fractures amenable to dynamic locking are Winquist 1 fractures and possibly some Winquist 2 fractures. These are predominantly at the level of the isthmus where the nail is canal filling and allows for very little toggle of the fracture. Infraisthmal fractures mandate two locking bolts distally, as far away from the fracture as possible.

All proximal insertion jigs for femoral nailing have proximal locking guides. These are generally well targeted. However, they occasionally will miss the locking hole and should be confirmed radiographically. Distal "freehand locking" is still required in antegrade nailing. The freehand technique relies heavily on the use of C-arm fluoroscopy. A "perfect circle" should be obtained of the locking holes and placed in the center of the C-arm screen **(Fig. 25–12)**. The small incision should be made over this circle through the fascia. Blunt tissue dissection to the bone with a hemostat is performed followed by placing a sharp drill bit in the center of the perfect circle **(Fig. 25–13)**. If this is placed eccentrically, when the drill bit is brought perpendicular to the shaft, it will miss the drill hole or cause the screw to be placed eccentrically. Once the drill guide is passed, appropriate depth should be obtained with depth gauges and rechecked by C-arm to confirm it is through the locking hole (on the lateral image) and the appropriate length (on the AP). The wounds are then irrigated and closed, and drains are applied prior to closure of the skin envelope if necessary. Finally, the femoral neck is carefully scrutinized under fluoroscopy to verify absence of femoral neck fracture.

The patient is then removed from the fracture table, and the traction pin is removed from the leg. The knee is examined for ligamentous injury, and femoral length and rotational alignment are confirmed. Postoperatively, the patient is encouraged once again to begin isometric strengthening of the quadriceps. Restricted weight bearing in fracture patterns that are comminuted has been recommended in the past, but stronger biomaterials and new biomechanical

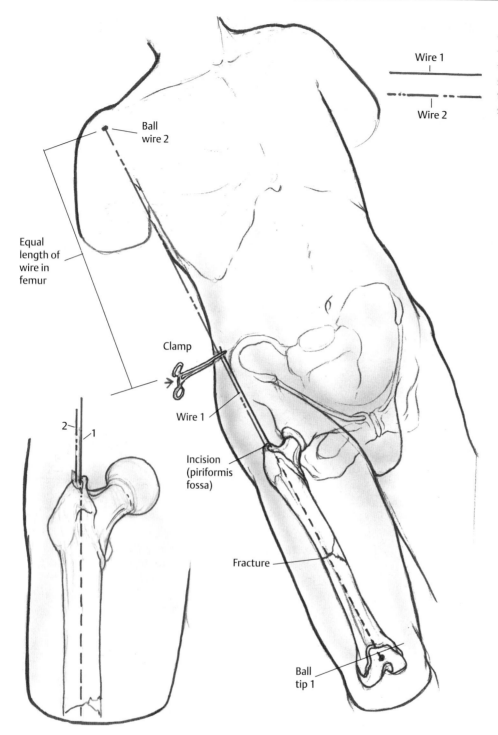

Figure 25–11 The subtraction method for calculating the correct nail size using two ball-tipped guidewires. It is important that both guidewires are of the same length, and that the fracture is at the appropriate length when the measurement is made.

and clinical data suggest early weight bearing as tolerated can be initiated safely. Having said this, most patients will self-limit weight bearing until some healing has occurred. DVT prophylaxis is necessary until muscle control of the limb is regained and the patient is mobile.

Antegrade, Trochanteric, Reamed, Supine

Antegrade intramedullary nailing through a trochanteric starting point supine on a fracture table with a reamed nail

is a relatively new procedure for management of femoral shaft fractures. This requires a new nail with a proximal-lateral bend of ~5 to 8 degrees. Nailing through this starting point with a straight nail will frequently lead to malalignment. The surgical anatomy is essentially the same as the piriformis starting point, with the exception that the starting point of the nail is lateralized to assist in placement of the nail in more obese patients. The piriformis starting point can be quite difficult to obtain in large patients, especially with proximal fractures.

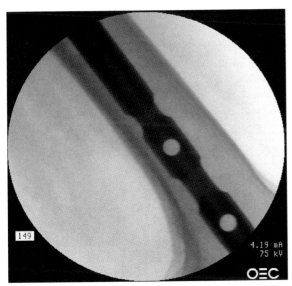

Figure 25–12 A "perfect circle" for interlocking a femoral nail using the freehand technique.

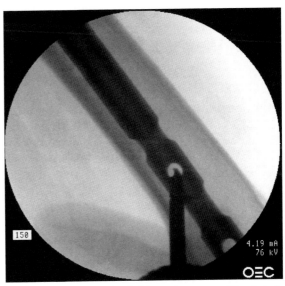

Figure 25–13 Placing the drill bit in the center of the circle for distal interlocking.

The same setup is used as previously described with the C-arm used to visualize the proximal fragment, including the trochanteric ridge, the piriformis fossa, and the femoral head and neck. The guide pin is inserted no more than a couple of millimeters off the tip of the trochanter and down the center of the canal. It is important that the starting point is at the tip of the trochanter and not too far lateral or anterior (**Fig. 25–14**). On the AP image, the guidewire is passed toward the inferior aspect of the lesser trochanter. The cannulated reamer is then taken to the base of the lesser trochanter. Care should be taken to avoid injury to the medial cortex. At this point a similar technique of passing the guidewire, measuring the nail,

and instrumenting of the nail is performed. Entry of the trochanteric nail is somewhat precarious in that it tends to direct the nail toward the lesser trochanter, and care is needed to visualize that a blunt-tipped nail passes around this critical (high stress) region of the femur. Propagation of fracture lines or even bursting of the proximal femur can occur with violation of the medial cortex. Overreaming by 2 mm and inserting the nail with the anterior bow directed laterally (**Fig. 25–15**) followed by rotation of the nail 90 degrees during insertion facilitate nail passage through the subtrochanteric region. Additionally, fractures in the more proximal part of the femur undergoing trochanteric nailing are more prone to varus malalignment, and care should be taken to avoid this complication. This is best facilitated by the use of a fracture table where an acceptable closed reduction can be obtained and maintained during surgery. Fortunately, fractures of the femoral shaft

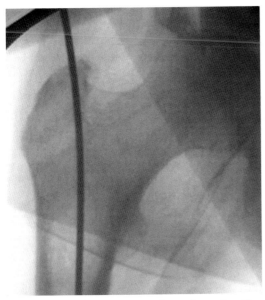

Figure 25–14 The starting point for trochanteric nailing should be at the tip of the trochanter, not farther laterally.

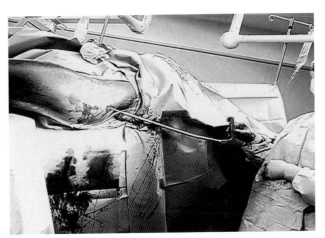

Figure 25–15 Inserting a trochanteric nail with the handle up will direct the anterior bow laterally, easing the passage of the nail through the proximal femur.

will often assist in self-aligning when a canal-filling nail is applied. Rehabilitation is unchanged from previous intramedullary techniques.

Variations of Antegrade Nailing

Significant variations from the foregoing can occur if the surgeon chooses to place the patient in a lateral position for nailing. Advantages of nailing in the lateral position include exposure of the piriformis entry portal. This is much easier because the fatty tissues fall away from the surgeon in this position. The difficulties include visualization of the starting point on the lateral view. This can be overcome with flexion of the leg as well. One of the biggest problems with lateral nailing is the tendency for rotational malalignments. This occurs predominantly from lack of attention to detail in aligning the limb preoperatively and intraoperatively during locking of the nail.[24]

Another variation is nailing fractures off the fracture table in the supine position. There are multiple indications for using a radiolucent table rather than a fracture table when performing a femoral nailing: ipsilateral lower extremity fractures with significant large open wounds that required extensive debridement (especially of the medial aspect of the leg), associated vascular injuries, and finally patients with other surgical injuries requiring simultaneous surgery with other surgical teams.[25] The key point to fracture reduction off the fracture table is the use of appropriate bumps beneath the hip and fracture site to assist in acquisition of a good starting point. Judicious use of percutaneous Schanz pin reduction tools can help align the fracture. A knowledgeable assistant is usually necessary, and attention to detail regarding length and rotation is paramount. The patient should be under full musculoskeletal paralysis to assist in obtaining length of the femur as the large muscle envelope tends to cause shortening and prevent the surgeon from obtaining adequate length.

The final variation is the choice of an unreamed nail. The indications for using an unreamed nail include and are usually restricted to a patient that is extremely unstable and patient with a significant chest injury. Studies promoting unreamed nails from Europe specifically address a second pulmonary injury associated with embolic phenomenon from reaming of the medullary canal. Several North American clinical trials have shown the use of unreamed nails in the femoral shaft to be less effective in achieving union compared with reamed nailing.[26,27] Therefore, the decision to place unreamed nails must be made based on the best information available at the time of surgery. Surgeons must recognize that the use of unreamed nails might jeopardize the outcome of the femoral shaft injury.

Retrograde Intramedullary Nailing (see Videos 25–5 and 25–6)

Surgical anatomy associated with retrograde femoral nailing centers predominantly around visualization of the knee joint and the proximal femur. The nail is inserted through an intercondylar entry portal in the knee joint to just above the notch (Blumensaat's line on lateral fluoroscopic views) and the posterior cruciate ligament fibers. Indications for use of retrograde nailing are multiple and include, but are not limited to, obesity, ipsilateral femoral neck fractures, ipsilateral acetabular fractures, ipsilateral lower extremity fractures, pregnant females, and bilateral injuries.[28]

Retrograde Reamed

The patient is placed on a radiolucent table with exposure of the hip. This may necessitate a small bump under the hip to elevate the trochanter to allow for prepping and draping in this region. The entire limb is prepped and draped from the foot to the iliac crest circumferentially. The use of radiolucent triangles is quite helpful in retrograde nailing, because it bends the knee ~30 degrees, allowing access to the appropriate entry portal for retrograde nailing and clears the patella (**Fig. 25–16**). Once the leg is prepped and draped, the preferred incision is percutaneous over the central portion of the patellar ligament. The ligament is incised through its midline or retracted laterally with a medial peripatellar incision. The opening guide pin is placed percutaneously into the notch just above Blumensaat's line (**Fig. 25–17A**). It should be just anterior to the posterior cruciate ligament and quite low in the notch to avoid patellofemoral articulations. The starting point is slightly lateral to midline to allow central placement up the medullary canal (**Fig. 25–17B**). The guide pin is then advanced into the medullary canal in a center–center position and confirmed on AP and lateral image. The lateral image should confirm pin placement 7 to 8 mm anterior to Blumensaat's line to avoid drilling out the posterior cortex. The opening reamer is then passed through the knee with a tissue protector to avoid injury of the patel-

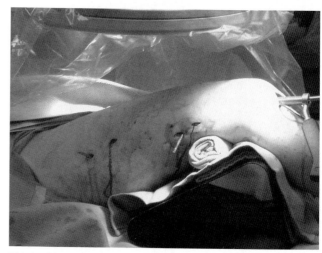

Figure 25–16 Radiolucent triangles help position the knee in approximately 30 degrees of flexion for retrograde nailing.

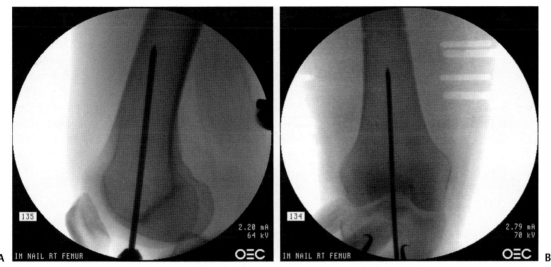

Figure 25–17 **(A)** Lateral view of the start point for retrograde nailing, with the entry just above Blumensaat's line. **(B)** Anteroposterior view with the starting point slightly lateral to midline, allowing the nail to centralize within the canal.

lar ligament, patella, or anterior tibial plateau and the underlying fat pad **(Fig. 25–18).** The opening reamer is advanced 5 to 7 cm into the distal femur. Irrigation of these reamings is then performed to help remove them from the fat pad and potentially the joint itself. The ball-tipped guidewire is then introduced up the medullary canal across the fracture site to the level of the piriformis fossa high in the proximal femur. Reductions are obtained through manual manipulation of the distal fragment or use of Schanz pins in the proximal fragment. The femur is then reamed sequentially, from 9 mm to a maximum of 13 mm. The fracture reduction is maintained during reaming. Larger reamers will encroach on the patellofemoral articulation and should be avoided. A 12 mm or smaller nail is then placed with the nail seated at least 3 to 5 mm deep to the articular surface

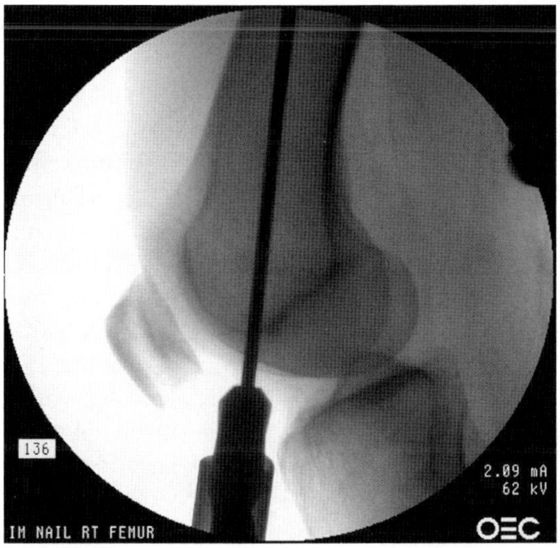

![Figure 25-18 fluoroscopic image]

Figure 25–18 Tissue protector minimizes soft tissue damage during the reaming process.

distally and the tip above the lesser trochanter proximally. Nail depth in the distal fragment is best visualized in the lateral fluoroscopic image. It must be above Blumensaat's line.

The nail is then secured proximally with two locking bolts (anterior-posterior) and distally with two locking bolts (lateral-medial). Proximal interlocking in the AP plane is safest when locking screws are placed proximal to the lesser trochanter to minimize injury to the femoral neurovascular structures.[29] Occasionally, a posteriorly placed blocking screw will be needed in the distal fragment to facilitate a reduction of a fracture and prevent malalignment with apex posterior angulation. This screw guides the nail more anteriorly in the distal segment, securing a more anatomical reduction on the lateral image. Lateral blocking screws are occasionally needed to keep the nail in a more medialized position, securing a better varus–valgus alignment. Once adequate alignment is obtained, the wounds are then irrigated and closed. The knee is ranged to check for stability. The postoperative rehab is similar to antegrade nailing. Weight bearing of the distal fractures should be followed closely to avoid acquired malalignment. DVT prophylaxis, early range of motion, and isometric quadriceps strengthening are encouraged in the early postoperative period.

Special Considerations (see Video 25–7, Disk 3)

Femoral shaft fractures associated with femoral neck injuries are a challenging combination of injuries.[13,23] Most orthopaedic surgeons recognize and appropriately place their attention on the femoral neck fracture for an exacting reduction prior to treatment of the femoral shaft. Use of one implant to treat both fractures is acceptable if anatomical reduction of the femoral neck is obtained and maintained or provisional stabilization is initially performed.

Patients with this injury can either be treated with a cephalomedullary intramedullary nailing after provisional screw fixation of the neck, or with separate fixation techniques for both fractures, including cannulated screws or a fixed-angle hip screw for the femoral neck fracture and a retrograde femoral nail for the femoral shaft fracture. Regardless of the implant chosen, an anatomical reduction of the femoral neck should be performed first and foremost and should take precedence over management of the femoral shaft fracture.[13,23]

Gunshot wounds in today's urban environment are quite common, and treatment of the femoral shaft fracture secondary to a ballistic injury should be performed in a fashion similar to a closed injury.[1] Extensive debridements are no longer needed for low-velocity wounds, and standard traditional nailing can be performed safely with low infection rates. Perioperative antibiotics should be given for 24 hours. However, a shotgun or high-velocity rifle injury is quite different from a low-velocity handgun injury, and aggressive debridement of this wound with provisional stabilization with external fixation would likely be warranted. Once a clean wound is obtained, definitive management with either a plate or an intramedullary nail would be appropriate.

Management of open fractures from blunt trauma, as previously described, can be quite challenging. They are fraught with multiple complications, including infection, segmental bone loss, delayed union, and nonunion. Aggressive management of the soft tissues is of paramount importance if return to maximum function is desired. Devitalized muscle tissue should be debrided but with caution so that extensive muscle loss is avoided. The use of adjunctive treatments such as vacuum-assisted closure (VAC) and/or hyperbaric oxygen for the ischemic wound should be considered in hopes of preserving some muscle in the zone of injury.[30] Sequential debridements are warranted for high-energy injuries.[30,31] Lower-energy injuries, including wounds with small skin envelope injuries, can be treated with aggressive early debridement and closure of the wound. When segmental bone loss is encountered and devitalized fragments are noted in the wound, these fragments should be removed because they increase the risk for infection. When segmental bone loss has occurred, placement of an antibiotic bead spacer is appropriate to help manage the space and to allow for a bone graft to be applied in the future.[31] The authors' current practice is to place calcium sulfate pellets (Osteoset Resorbable Bead Kit, Wright Medical Technology, Inc., Arlington, Tennessee) impregnated with antibiotics (vancomycin 1 g plus tobramycin 1.2 g) or nonresorbable polymethyl methacrylate (PMMA) beads (vancomycin 1 g and tobramycin 3.6 g). PMMA beads are removed at the time of staged bone grafting. Occasionally the soft tissue envelope will facilitate healing and span large segments of bone loss with abundant callus formation. This may obviate the need for bone grafting. Nevertheless, sequential films taken at 6 and 10 weeks should be performed to discern whether bone formation is on schedule. If the gap is large enough and bone formation is not bridging the gap, then intervention with bead removal and bone grafting should be performed.[31] At reoperation, the hardware should be evaluated and assessed if it is to be sufficient to allow bony union. If loose hardware is encountered, the hardware should be revised to a stable construct, and deep cultures should be obtained to rule out possible early infection.[31]

Arterial injury associated with a femoral shaft fracture is a limb-threatening injury. The arterial blood supply should be restored promptly, preferably before 6 hours of ischemia. Ischemia beyond 6 hours will often lead to muscle cell death and a dysfunctional fibrotic limb. Controversy still exists in management of this difficult injury, but suffice it to say arterial blood flow should be restored first. This may be in the form of a temporary shunt to allow the distal tissues to be perfused. With a shunt in place, all three options are open to the surgeon to stabilize the femoral shaft fracture, including external fixation, plate, or intramedullary nailing. In large open wounds, a plate may be chosen because direct visualization is apparent. When fractures are more comminuted, intramedullary nailing is preferred to help maintain alignment and length. In some situations where further debridement will be warranted, external fixation would be the best option. The surgical treatment, once applied, should be followed by direct repair of the arterial injury (rarely) or reverse vein interposition grafting (more common). Additionally, venous structures should be repaired in hopes of improving blood flow out of the limb. Fasciotomies of the leg are necessary when ischemia time reaches 4 to 6 hours. This is prophylactic in nature to prevent any potential adverse effects of reperfusion to the lower limb. If external fixation is applied after the repair, extreme care should be taken at the time of exchange nailing to avoid the dreaded complication of reinjury to the vascular repair.

There remains extreme concern regarding a deleterious "second hit" occurring in the multiply injured patient following surgical management of the femoral shaft fracture (especially with intramedullary nailing).[6] The patient already has a systemic inflammatory response from the initial trauma and a significantly "primed pump." A second stimulus (embolization of fatty contents from the marrow) may be enough to incite further end-organ damage, especially to the lungs and the brain.[10] In these patients, it is important to limit the amount of surgery to the severely injured individual with a less aggressive staged approach of temporary stabilization followed by delayed definitive fixation. Generous use of external fixation is appropriate in this population of patients. Once their systemic inflammatory response has resolved, intramedullary nailing and removal of external fixation has a very low complication rate.[20] This protocol allows the patient to recover from the initial inflammatory response and prevent secondary injury to the vital organs. The term *damage control orthopaedics* has been coined to describe this type of treatment. Definitive surgical treatment is performed when the patient is outside the window of heightened systemic inflammatory response (see Chapter 34).

Conflicting literature exists regarding the most appropriate time for fixation of femoral shaft fractures in head-injured patients.[7,8] Proponents for early stabilization suggest earlier mobilization and the upright head/chest position are favorable. Opponents of this early stabilization feel increasing intracranial pressures with volume expansion are detrimental to the overall outcome. It is the authors' understanding that appropriately resuscitated patients with intracranial pressure monitoring are safe to undergo early intramedullary nailing with the utmost effort to avoid intraoperative hypotension. However, for this to occur, appropriate consultation with neurosurgery is necessary, as well as general surgery trauma personnel to assist in monitoring the patient pre-, intra-, and postoperatively for pressure issues and volume needs.

The optimal timing of intramedullary stabilization of femur fractures in multiple trauma patients and which patients should be treated using damage control orthopaedics remain highly controversial.[4]

New Techniques

Reamer Irrigator Aspirator

The reamer-irrigator-aspirator (RIA) is a new development that allows reaming to be accomplished in a single pass while aspirating the medullary canal and decreasing fat extravasation into the vascular system **(Fig. 25–19).** Early animal data indicate the RIA decreases the exposure of the lungs to fat and marrow contents.[32] Initial clinical testing is promising, allowing the speed of a single-pass

---

Tips and Tricks

- External fixation: the first pin should be placed four finger-breadths below the greater trochanter (at the level of the lesser trochanter).
- External fixation: the last pin is placed at least two finger-breadths above the lateral epicondyle.
- Plating: if the fracture remains shortened, the distal screws should be removed and a push-pull screw with lamina spreader or compressor/distractor (articulated tensioning device) used to obtain length.
- Plating: a bump should be placed under the hip to allow for elevation of the trochanter.
- Percutaneous plating: after obtaining provisional fixation, the length and rotational alignment are reassessed, and supplemental screw fixation is applied percutaneously for a minimum of four cortices proximally and distally.
- Intramedullary nailing: reducing proximal fractures can be difficult. The hip is flexed, and the distal piece is reduced to the proximal fragment. A crutch with a sterile cover can be used to reduce the posterior sag of the distal bone.
- Intramedullary nailing: in large patients getting the piriformis start point is difficult. Place the patient's pelvis more lateral on the fracture table adduct the femur using the post as a fulcrum, and use a percutaneous spiked pusher on the proximal fragment, helping adduct this fragment further. This will help adduct the proximal fragment.
- Intramedullary nailing: intraoperative sizing can be done by choosing a nail that is 1 mm smaller than the diameter where the first reamer encounters significant endosteal chatter.
- Following nailing, carefully scrutinize the femoral neck with an internal rotation view using fluoroscopy.
- Trochanteric nailing: the guide pin should be inserted right at the tip (or a couple of millimeters laterally at the most) of the greater trochanter.
- Trochanteric nailing: insert the nail rotated 90 degrees with the anterior bow directed laterally to ease passage of the nail proximally.
- Retrograde nailing: the use of radiolucent triangles to bend the knee 30 to 40 degrees improves access to the appropriate entry portal.

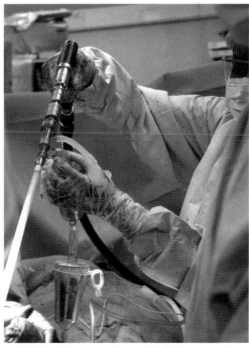

Figure 25–19 The reamer-irrigator-aspirator allows single-pass reaming while minimizing the exposure of the lungs to marrow contents.

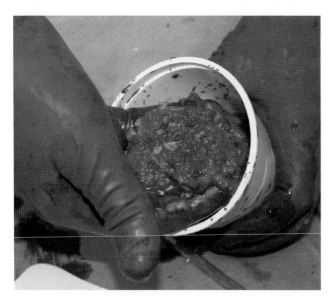

Figure 25–20 The aspirate from the reamer-irrigator-aspirator after reaming of a femur. It may be used for bone graft.

reaming. Research is currently ongoing to evaluate the aspirate that is harvested using the RIA. The fluid and material collected appear to be rich in bioactive substances, and some centers are investigating using it to enhance bone healing **(Fig. 25–20).**

Outcomes

There are several published reports regarding the descriptive outcomes of patients with a femoral shaft fracture.[33,34] Isolated injuries do quite well, and most patients recover fully from their injuries. The limitations in function are largely related to the significance of the soft tissue injury and not necessarily to the fracture pattern. It is paramount to avoid complications, including shortening, malalignment, infection, nerve injury, and arterial injury. In multiple series, isolated femoral shaft fractures treated with intramedullary nailing reveal 98 to 99% union rates, less than 1% infection rate, and less than 5 to 10% incidence of shortening or malalignment.[23,33] Significant nerve and artery injuries are extremely rare in this form of treatment. Published reports of bridged plating (although limited) have been less favorable in that there have been higher rates of malalignment. However, union rates are still relatively high (approaching 90 to 95%). Compression plating in experienced hands yields a 92 to 93% union rate with an infection rate of ~1 to 2%.[22] Either or both delayed union and nonunion with hardware failure approach 3 to 5%. Reports of external fixation for definitive treatment of femoral shaft fractures are rare, and therefore union rates are difficult to determine. A high rate of pin tract problems, delayed union and nonunion, as well as malalignment and knee stiffness are noted following external fixation

of the femur. This is predominantly why this form of treatment has been abandoned and is now mainly used for temporary provisional stabilization.

Published series of femoral shaft fractures in the multiply injured and head injured patients still show high levels of union, and it is only in those fractures that are high-grade open injuries or fractures with segmental loss that union rates drop. Infection risks increase as the amount of soft tissue damage occurs and approaches 7 to 10% in high-grade open injuries (type 3B or higher).[35] Subsequent bone grafting of femoral shaft fractures is occasionally warranted, especially in the setting of an open fracture or segmental loss. Bone grafting should occur early (8 week period) if healing appears to be delayed clinically and radiographically. When intramedullary nails are in place, the surgeon has the luxury of waiting a little longer before deciding if a bone graft is needed.

Complications

Complications of treatment of femoral shaft fractures are numerous and should be treated aggressively. Treatment will often be based on the type of fixation implemented. Infection following intramedullary nailing, although rare, can be quite difficult to diagnose and eradicate when it does occur. Part of the evaluation for infection should include laboratory studies, including complete blood count (CBC), sedimentation rate, and C-reactive protein. These parameters (which can be suggestive of infection) can be monitored during treatment to determine if the treatment is working. Additionally, nuclear medicine imaging studies such as combination technetium and indium-labeled white cell scans may be helpful. However, definitive diagnosis can only be determined with positive tissue cultures.

When infection does occur, debridement of the infected soft tissues is warranted, and occasionally removal of the implant and debridement of the intramedullary canal and local bone segment. Provisional stabilization with external fixation may be needed. Immediate reamed exchange nailing may yield good results when the infection is identified and a susceptible organism is treated with IV antibiotics.[36,37] Treatment of intramedullary infection can be difficult, though, and recent studies have shown antibiotic cement–impregnated intramedullary nails can also help eradicate intramedullary infection.[38] The goal of treatment is to obtain union, and, if infection continues, then hardware removal can be performed following union of the fracture. In cases where plate fixation or external fixation has been used, removal of the devices is warranted if they are loose. A course of parenteral antibiotics followed with subsequent intramedullary nailing and bone grafting can be an effective tool to gain union. Difficulty arises when retrograde intramedullary nailing has been performed and infection ensues. Potential for introducing infection into the knee joint is real and needs to be treated aggressively. Fortunately, this complication has been rare in the published literature to date.

Missed fractures following treatment of femoral shaft fracture has a known incidence of 3 to 7%.[13] Whether these injuries occur at the same time of the femoral shaft fracture or whether they are occult is uncertain. The most dreaded missed fracture is a femoral neck fracture. For this reason, the authors recommend an AP hip with internal rotation radiograph be performed following all intramedullary procedures to confirm that no occult fracture is present. Bony windows of the femoral neck on trauma abdomen/pelvis computed tomographic (CT) scans should be reviewed as well to check for occult femoral neck fractures. If one is identified, aggressive treatment should immediately follow with prompt reduction and stabilization of the femoral neck fracture. Nail removal is not warranted unless wide displacement occurs and reduction cannot be obtained and maintained. Other missed fractures or iatrogenic injuries include propagation of the simple fracture patterns to a more segmental pattern, which can be overcome with the use of static locked nails. When nailing infraisthmal distal fractures, care should be taken to avoid missing the occult spiral fracture into the condyles. When this occurs, it is necessary to provisionally stabilize the condyles with interfragmentary lag screws prior to intramedullary nailing.[39]

Fracture around nails or plates can occur. Fractures with the intramedullary nail in place usually occurs at the proximal portion of the femur around the intertrochanteric/subtrochanteric region, or the distal portion around the supracondylar/intercondylar region. Fractures around plate fixation almost always occur above or below the plate because this is the area of significant stress transfer. Refractures are complicated by the need for a new implant to span the fracture. This will usually necessitate removal of the existing implant prior to definitive stabilization.

Routine removal of implants can also lead to refracture, and for this reason it is suggested that intramedullary nails should remain in place for ~12 to 18 months, and plate fixation probably should not be removed (especially distal femoral blade plates). A period of protective weight bearing following plate and intramedullary nailing for a few weeks is recommended, with restriction from contact sports for a minimum of 2 months.

Delayed and nonunion following treatment with an intramedullary nail can sometimes be overcome by converting load-bearing properties of the statically locked nail to load-sharing properties of the dynamically locked nail (see **Video 25–8, Disk 3**). Removal of the statically locked screw is a simple procedure and will transfer mechanical stress to the fracture site and sometimes promote bone union. When nonunion persists, exchange nailing has shown varying results from 50 to 90% union rates.[36,37] If all options fail, open bone grafting and conversion to compression plating may be the best option, although open bone grafting with exchange nailing is also a consideration.

Fortunately, delayed and nonunions are rare, occurring less than 2% of the time in closed fractures. A higher incidence occurs in open fractures, and infection should be ruled out as the cause of delayed union or nonunion. When complicated by infection, nonunions can be recalcitrant and require multiple procedures to induce union.

When nonunion occurs with plate fixation, hardware failure usually ensues. Therefore, fractures that are slow to heal with plate fixation warrant early aggressive bone grafting prior to hardware failure. If this is not performed, then removal of hardware with refixation and bone grafting is warranted, or conversion to intramedullary nailing with or without bone grafting. As with any nonunion, infection parameters should be obtained and deep cultures should be taken to rule out an occult deep infection as the source of nonunion.

Malunion following intramedullary nailing unfortunately occurs more commonly than previously reported or suspected, with an incidence between 5 and 10%, depending on fracture location and nail direction (antegrade/retrograde).[24] The most common malalignment following intramedullary nailing is rotational malalignment followed by shortening. The more proximal and distal the fracture, the higher the incidence of coronal plane deformity (varus and valgus malalignment). Femoral midshaft malunion is rare with a canal filling nail. When fracture tables are used, shortening is less common, but rotational malalignment can still occur. Attention to detail while placing locking screws will help prevent malrotation deformity. Laterally positioned nailing also increases the risk of rotational malalignment. Malrotation of greater than 20 degrees clinically warrants radiographic evaluation with a rotational CT of the femoral neck and condyles. If malrotation is greater than 20 degrees, derotation is warranted. (It should be noted an external rotation deformity is more common but more easily tolerated compared with an internal rotation deformity.) This can be performed acutely if recognized immediately postoperatively. If healing has occurred, a derotation osteotomy may be necessary. Closed osteotomy can be performed with an intramedullary saw, allowing for correction of the deformity, including length, varus–valgus malalignment, and rotational malalignment.

Intramedullary nailing of the femur, either done antegrade or retrograde, can lead to prominent hardware. Antegrade nail prominence usually manifests itself with abductor irritation and a Trendelenburg-type gait. Trochanteric bursitis has been seen in situations with a starting point over the trochanter or from prominent locking bolts in this region (either transversely or oblique intertrochanteric). The distal locking bolts, especially in retrograde intramedullary nails, can also cause a bursitis affecting either the medial or lateral tissues about the knee. Retrograde nails, if not placed proximal to Blumensaat's line on the lateral radiograph, can be prominent in the notch and can be quite damaging to the patellofemoral articulation. Care should be taken to place the intramedullary device deep enough to avoid this. Most prominent hardware should be managed conservatively until union. Shortly after union, the symptomatic screws can be electively removed. Intramedullary nails should remain in place for 12 to 18 months; however, this may not be possible in very symptomatic individuals.

Prominent plate hardware is, fortunately, very rare. However, when the plate is extended to the distal and proximal region of the femur, symptoms may occur. Occasionally this will warrant treatment, but care should be taken to remove only the symptomatic portion of the plate hardware if possible.

Compartment syndrome of the thigh following femoral shaft fracture is quite rare but in certain situations should prompt vigilance. The risk factors for compartment syndrome include vascular injury, extensive coagulopathy, prolonged external compression (crush injury), persistent hypertension, and use of antishock pneumatic trousers. If compartment syndrome is expected, early release and debridement are mandatory. Because of the extensive muscle injury that can occur with a compartment syndrome of the thigh, massive amounts of myoglobin are released and can be fatal if not recognized early in the course of treatment. Significant morbidity is also associated with a delay in diagnosis and treatment.

Neurological injury, fortunately, is quite rare and related to choice of fixation. With intramedullary nailing, injuries to the sciatic and pudendal nerve have been reported.[39] Pudendal nerve injury results in labial or scrotal loss of sensation and, potentially, impotence. One study reported an incidence of ~10% of antegrade nailings on a fracture table.[40] Traction applied to help obtain the reduction should be released once reduction has been obtained and fixation applied. Studies have shown both the length of time and the magnitude of traction are responsible for these palsies.[39] Nerve injury from plating is rare, although vascular injury with open plating techniques may be slightly increased. During plate fixation, direct fracture manipulation places vasculature structures at a higher risk for injury.

The complication of heterotopic ossification (HO) can and does occur around the hip abductor musculature following antegrade intramedullary nailing. Factors that may effect the formation of HO include magnitude of muscle injury, amount of debris left from the reaming, and other factors related to the physiology of the patient at the time of intramedullary nailing. These other factors are primarily significant head injuries and significant burns, which for reasons unknown stimulate HO. Severe HO may limit hip function, cause significant pain, and induce a limp. These patients need to be evaluated with sequential radiographs and CT scans to clarify the extent/location of heterotopic ossification. Patients with significant HO may necessitate hardware removal and excision of the HO at some point in the course of treatment. If the HO is resected prior to maturation, the use of radiation therapy postoperatively is warranted.

HO can also arise from open fracture wounds and damaged muscle tissue. When this occurs, it predominantly affects quadriceps strength and more importantly knee motion. Knee contractures can occur if the HO is extensive. For this reason, meticulous debridement of damaged muscle is necessary. Use of suction drains to prevent hematoma collection is also recommended. Routine prophylaxis for this form of HO is not recommended; however, if significant HO does occur, excision will likely be needed to restore knee function.

Pearls

- Associated regional injuries include ipsilateral femoral neck fractures, supracondylar extension, and tibial shaft or foot and ankle fractures.
- Mortality following bilateral femoral shaft fractures can approach 30%.
- The incidence of femur fractures is 1 to 1.3 per 10,000 people per year.
- Femoral neck shaft fractures occur in 5% of all femur fractures.
- Knee ligament injuries occur in 20 to 30% of femur fractures and meniscus injuries occur in 20%; meniscus injuries are more frequent on the lateral side.
- At least 8 cortices above and below the fracture should be obtained when plating a femoral shaft.
- Indications for retrograde nails include obesity, ipsilateral neck fracture, ipsilateral acetabular fracture, pregnant females, and bilateral fractures.
- For isolated femurs, union rates are 98 to 99%, infection is less than 1%, and shortening or malrotation is 5 to 10%.
- Bridge plating has union rates of 90 to 95%, but malalignment is a problem.
- Compression plating has 92% union rate, 2% infection, and 3 to 5% hardware failure.
- Infection occurs in 7 to 10% of high grade (type 3B) open fractures.
- Missed fractures occur in 3 to 7% following treatment of femur fractures.

New Horizons

Some new horizons in the treatment of femoral shaft fractures mostly involve treatment with intramedullary nailing. Intramedullary nailing is associated with a high degree of radiation exposure. Certainly, the starting point and distal locking screws require significant use of fluoroscopic imaging. New techniques using computer-assisted surgery will limit the radiation exposure to surgeons. There are several devices on the market that will allow surgeons to place instrumentation and guides from a previous single-shot image. Additionally, several manufacturers have radiolucent drills, which prevent some of the free-hand problems with interlocking screws. Other areas of treatment include the use of the reamer-irrigator-aspirator not only in the treatment of femoral shaft fractures but also in the harvesting of a medullary bone graft. The

intramedullary material harvested has adult stem cells as well as a plethora of growth factors. These exciting new forms of technology are currently being investigated at several institutions and will be at the forefront in treatment of femoral shaft fractures as well as autogenous bone grafting for some time to come.

On the DVDs

Video 25–1 (Disk 3) Tips and Tricks for Femoral Nailing Tips and tricks to allow successful antegrade reaming of the femur are reviewed. Patient positioning, location of the piriformis fossa, and nailing on a conventional table are all presented.

Video 25–2 (Disk 3) Percutaneous Antegrade Femoral Nailing This video demonstrates a unique percutaneous technique for antegrade femoral nailing using the piriformis start portal. The anatomy of the trochanteric region and the technique of determining the appropriate location of the skin incision are reviewed.

Video 25–3 (Disk 3) Trochanteric Antegrade Nailing of the Femur Intramedullary nailing of the femur using a trochanteric starting portal is demonstrated. The correct starting point and techniques of reduction are emphasized.

Video 25–4 (Disk 3) Flexible Elastic Nail for Pediatric Femur Fracture Although not discussed in the text, this video shows the use of stacked titanium elastic nails for stabilization of a transverse femoral shaft fracture in an 8-year-old child. Two nails are inserted retrograde, one each from the medial and lateral femoral condyles.

Video 25–5 (Disk 3) Retrograde Intramedullary Nail for an A Type Supracondylar Femur Fracture A 2.5 cm medial parapetellar approach is utilized for stabilization for an A type supracondylar femur fracture. Emphasis is on correct starting point and fracture reduction.

Video 25–6 (Disk 3) Retrograde Intramedullary Nailing of the Femur This video demonstrates the technique and principles for retrograde nailing of a supracondylar femur fracture using a tendon splitting approach. The importance of the correct starting point is emphasized.

Video 25–7 (Disk 3) ORIF of a Femoral Neck and Shaft Fracture A Watson-Jones approach is used to perform an open reduction and internal fixation of a femoral neck. The shaft fracture is also stabilized with an intramedullary nail.

Video 25–8 (Same as **Video 5–2, Disk 1**) **Compression Plating of a Femur Nonunion** This video demonstrates compression plate fixation of a femur nonunion with a titanium broad LCDCP. The lateral approach to the femur, as well as the importance of debridement of the nonunion and compression of viable bone fragments are stressed.

References

1. Giannoudis PV, Pape HC, Cohen AP, Krettek C, Smith RM. Review: systemic effects of femoral nailing: from Küntscher to the immune reactivity era. Clin Orthop Relat Res 2002;404:378–386
2. Copeland CE, Mitchell KA, Brumback RJ, Gens DR, Burgess AR. Mortality in patients with bilateral femoral fractures. J Orthop Trauma 1998;12:315–319
3. Nork SE, Agel J, Russell GV, Mills WJ, Holt S, Routt ML Jr. Mortality after reamed intramedullary nailing of bilateral femur fractures. Clin Orthop Relat Res 2003;415:272–278
4. Pape HC, Grimme K, Van Griensven M, et al; EPOFF Study Group. Impact of intramedullary instrumentation versus damage control for femoral fractures on immunoinflammatory parameters: prospective randomized analysis by the EPOFF Study Group. J Trauma 2003;55:7–13
5. Giannoudis PV, Pape HC, Cohen AP, Krettek C, Smith RM. Review: systemic effects of femoral nailing: from Küntscher to the immune reactivity era. Clin Orthop Relat Res 2002;404:378–386
6. Pape HC, Hildebrand F, Pertschy S, et al. Changes in the management of femoral shaft fractures in polytrauma patients: from early total care to damage control orthopedic surgery. J Trauma 2002;53:452–462
7. Starr AJ, Hunt JL, Chason DP, Reinert CM, Walker J. Treatment of femur fracture with associated head injury. J Orthop Trauma 1998;12:38–45
8. Starr AJ. Early fracture fixation may be deleterious after head injury. J Trauma 1997;42:981–983
9. Sauaia A, Moore FA, Moore EE, Lezotte DC. Early risk factors for postinjury multiple organ failure. World J Surg 1996;20: 392–400

10. Moore FA, Moore EE. Evolving concepts in the pathogenesis of postinjury multiple organ failure. Surg Clin North Am 1995;75: 257–277
11. Gurd AR, Wilson RI. Fat-embolism syndrome. Lancet 1972;2: 231–232
12. Gurd AR, Connell AM. The origin of fat emboli after injury. Br J Surg 1969;56:614
13. Wolinsky PR, Johnson KD. Ipsilateral femoral neck and shaft fractures. Clin Orthop Relat Res 1995;318:81–90
14. Barei DP, Schildhauer TA, Nork SE. Noncontiguous fractures of the femoral neck, femoral shaft, and distal femur. J Trauma 2003;55: 80–86
15. Blacksin MF, Zurlo JV, Levy AS. Internal derangement of the knee after ipsilateral femoral shaft fracture: MR imaging findings. Skeletal Radiol 1998;27:434–439
16. Mills WJ, Barei DP, McNair P. The value of the ankle-brachial index for diagnosing arterial injury after knee dislocation: a prospective study. J Trauma 2004;56:1261–1265
17. Winquist RA, Hansen ST Jr. Comminuted fractures of the femoral shaft treated by intramedullary nailing. Orthop Clin North Am 1980;11:633–648
18. Orthopaedic Trauma Association Committee for Coding and Classification. Fracture and dislocation compendium. J Orthop Trauma 1996;10(Suppl 1):36–40
19. Crotwell WH III. The thigh-lacer: ambulatory non-operative treatment of femoral shaft fractures. J Bone Joint Surg Am 1978;60: 112–117

20. Scalea TM, Boswell SA, Scott JD, Mitchell KA, Kramer ME, Pollak AN. External fixation as a bridge to intramedullary nailing for patients with multiple injuries and with femur fractures: damage control orthopedics. J Trauma 2000;48:613–623

21. Nowotarski PJ, Turen CH, Brumback RJ, Scarboro JM. Conversion of external fixation to intramedullary nailing for fractures of the shaft of the femur in multiply injured patients. J Bone Joint Surg Am 2000;82:781–788

22. Seligson D, Mulier T, Keirsbilck S, Been J. Plating of femoral shaft fractures: a review of 15 cases. Acta Orthop Belg 2001;67:24–31

23. Watson JT, Moed BR. Ipsilateral femoral neck and shaft fractures: complications and their treatment. Clin Orthop Relat Res 2002; 399:78–86

24. Ricci WM, Bellabarba C, Lewis R, et al. Angular malalignment after intramedullary nailing of femoral shaft fractures. J Orthop Trauma 2001;15:90–95

25. Wolinsky PR, McCarty EC, Shyr Y, Johnson KD. Length of operative procedures: reamed femoral intramedullary nailing performed with and without a fracture table. J Orthop Trauma 1998;12:485–495

26. Shepherd LE, Shean CJ, Gelalis ID, Lee J, Carter VS. Prospective randomized study of reamed versus unreamed femoral intramedullary nailing: an assessment of procedures. J Orthop Trauma 2001;15: 28–33

27. Tornetta P 3rd, Tiburzi D. Reamed versus nonreamed anterograde-femoral nailing. J Orthop Trauma 2000;14:15–19

28. Ostrum RF, DiCicco J, Lakatos R, Poka A. Retrograde intramedullary nailing of femoral diaphyseal fractures. J Orthop Trauma 1998;12: 464–468

29. Riina J, Tornetta P III, Ritter C, Geller J. Neurologic and vascular structures at risk during anterior-posterior locking of retrograde femoral nails. J Orthop Trauma 1998;12:379–381

30. Herscovici D Jr, Sanders RW, Scaduto JM, Infante A, DiPasquale T. Vacuum-assisted wound closure (VAC therapy) for the management of patients with high-energy soft tissue injuries. J Orthop Trauma 2003;17:683–688

31. Christian EP, Bosse MJ, Robb G. Reconstruction of large diaphyseal defects, without free fibular transfer, in Grade-IIIB tibial fractures. J Bone Joint Surg Am 1989;71:994–1004

32. Pape HC, Zelle BA, Hildebrand F, Giannoudis PV, Krettek C, van Griensven M. Reamed femoral nailing in sheep: does irrigation and aspiration of intramedullary contents alter the systemic response? J Bone Joint Surg Am 2005;87:2515–2522

33. Winquist RA, Hansen ST Jr, Clawson DK. Closed intramedullary nailing of femoral fractures: a report of five hundred and twenty cases. J Bone Joint Surg Am 1984;66:529–539

34. Brumback RJ, Reilly JP, Poka A, Lakatos RP, Bathon GH, Burgess AR. Intramedullary nailing of femoral shaft fractures, I: Decision-making errors with interlocking fixation. J Bone Joint Surg Am 1988; 70: 1441–1452

35. Patzakis MJ, Wilkins J. Factors influencing infection rate in open fracture wounds. Clin Orthop Relat Res 1989;243:36–40

36. Hak DJ, Lee SS, Goulet JA. Success of exchange reamed intramedullary nailing for femoral shaft nonunion or delayed union. J Orthop Trauma 2000;14:178–182

37. Weresh MJ, Hakanson R, Stover MD, Sims SH, Kellam JF, Bosse MJ. Failure of exchange reamed intramedullary nails for ununited femoral shaft fractures. J Orthop Trauma 2000;14: 335–338

38. Paley D, Herzenberg JE. Intramedullary infections treated with antibiotic cement rods: preliminary results in nine cases. J Orthop Trauma 2002;16:723–729

39. Butler MS, Brumback RJ, Ellison TS, Poka A, Bathon GH, Burgess AR. Interlocking intramedullary nailing for ipsilateral fractures of the femoral shaft and distal part of the femur. J Bone Joint Surg Am 1991;73:1492–1502

40. Brumback RJ, Ellison TS, Molligan H, Molligan DJ, Mahaffey S, Schmidhauser C. Pudendal nerve palsy complicating intramedullary nailing of the femur. J Bone Joint Surg Am 1992;74: 1450–1455

26 Distal Femur Fractures

Philip J. Kregor and Michael Zlowodzki

The surgical treatment of supracondylar distal femoral fractures with or without intra-articular involvement [Arbeitsgemeinschaft für Osteosynthesefragen/Orthopaedic Trauma Association (AO/OTA) types 33A and 33C] continues to be difficult. Fracture characteristics that make these injuries particularly difficult include osteoporosis, multiplanar articular injury, a short distal femoral block in which to insert fixation, associated open wounds, and possible extensor mechanism injuries. Complications are significant and include infection, knee stiffness, need for bone grafting, malunion, and nonunion.[1-3] There has been an evolution in the treatment of distal femoral fractures in the past 4 decades, with nonoperative methods of treatment being the mainstay of treatment in the 1960s and early 1970s. Although fractures healed without significant difficulty when treated by these methods, there was significant deformity and joint stiffness afterward.[4,5]

With this experience in mind, surgeons began to utilize techniques of open reduction and rigid internal fixation that were popularized by the AO group in the mid-1970s. During this time, Schatzker et al and others began utilizing the 95 degree angled blade plate, the condylar buttress plate, and the dynamic condylar screw (DCS) for rigid fixation of supracondylar and supracondylar/intercondylar femur fractures.[6-9] These devices provided sufficient fixation to allow early range of motion of the knee, decreased knee stiffness, and improved mobility of the patient. These early surgical techniques were associated, however, with a significant risk of infection and need for bone grafting. Both of these complications were attributed to the relatively large surgical exposures utilized in the early experience with open reduction and internal fixation of these fractures. Bone grafting rates with classical open reduction and internal fixation ranged between 0 and 87%.[1] The concept of biological plating was developed by Mast, Jakob, and Ganz.[10,11] The principles of biological plating are:

- Maintenance of soft tissue attachments and vascularity of the cortical bone fragments
- Anatomical restoration of the articular surface
- Restoration of the appropriate length, rotation, and alignment of the metaphyseal/diaphyseal region using indirect methods, without preoccupation with complete anatomical restoration of this region

Bolhofner et al in 1996 demonstrated the efficacy of biological plating for supracondylar femur fractures.[12] In contrast to the early experience with internal fixation, maintenance of the soft tissue viability around the fracture resulted in 100% union. Since then, multiple series have documented the effectiveness of indirect reduction techniques for repair of supracondylar femur fractures.[13-19]

Based on the experience with biological plating, surgeons sought ways that would even further minimize the exposure of the metaphyseal/diaphyseal component of the fracture. This was accomplished by one of two surgical techniques popularized in the 1990s. The first of these was the use of retrograde intramedullary nailing.[20-27] The advantages of intramedullary nailing for long bones are well established. The results of retrograde nailing of the distal femur fracture are associated with lower rates of infection. The second major advance in maintaining the soft tissues around the distal femur fracture was that of submuscular plating.[28-30] With submuscular plating, the articular surface of the distal femur fracture can be maximally visualized and fixed while a plate can be slid along the femoral shaft in a submuscular manner. As with retrograde nailing of the femur, the nonunion and infection rates are quite low with this type of treatment.[13-19,31] However, as expected, whenever the fracture is not directly visualized, malreductions can be problematic (see **Videos 26–1, 26–2, and 26–3**).[14,32]

A recent concept in the evolution of treatment of distal femur fractures is the utilization of locked internal fixators for the distal femur. Previously, maintenance of reduction of the distal femoral block, especially in the setting of significant osteoporosis or a short distal segment, was a significant concern. The locked internal fixators were developed out of the early experience with Schüli nuts in treating patients with significant osteoporosis and revision fixations[33] and also with the utilization of the PC-Fix (Synthes, Paoli, Pennsylvania) for forearm fractures.[34] A biomechanical cadaver study has shown higher axial loads to failure and a lower incidence of loss of distal fixation for a locked internal fixator compared with a blade plate and a retrograde intramedullary nail, especially in osteoporotic bone.[35] Clinically, the use of locked internal fixators in the distal femur has recently been helpful in multiplanar articular injuries, osteoporotic fractures, fractures with short distal segments, and fractures above total knee arthroplasty.[13-19,31,32,36,37] The goals of treatment of a supracondylar/intercondylar femur fracture are:

- Restoration of the articular surface
- Restoration of normal alignment of the limb
- Full or nearly full range of painless motion

- Uneventful healing without need for bone grafting
- Return to former activities and a good functional outcome as assessed by modern-day functional outcome instrument

With these goals in mind, the surgeon should be able to classify the fracture, decide upon operative versus nonoperative treatment, decide upon the mode of surgical treatment (if warranted), and be able to predict certain outcomes given the surgical treatment. This chapter explores in detail each of these aspects of the care of these difficult fractures.

Classification

Müller et al has stated that a good classification scheme allows one to determine the surgical approach and treatment as well as the prognosis for a particular injury.[38] In this realm, the AO/OTA classification for distal femur fractures is quite useful (**Fig. 26–1**). The classification helps to determine the surgical approach, surgical implant, rehabilitation protocol, and outcome. Type A fractures are extra-articular, type B fractures are partial articular fractures, and type C fractures represent a complete intra-articular fracture with dissociation from the diaphysis.

To determine the classification, good quality anteroposterior (AP) and lateral radiographs are essential. If there is any question regarding the characterization of the injury, the surgeon should request and help obtain AP and lateral traction views as well as oblique traction views. A computed tomographic (CT) scan with frontal and sagittal reconstructions may be utilized to characterize the articular injury. Key questions to be asked with these radiographs are:

1. Is there an intercondylar split?
2. If there is an intercondylar split, is it complex or simple?
3. Are there separate osteochondral fragments in the area of the intercondylar notch or between the intercondylar split?
4. Is there an associated Hoffa (frontal plane) fracture? (This can be seen best on the lateral radiograph of the distal femur.)

The answer to the first question differentiates between an A-type and a C-type fracture. The answer to the second question differentiates between a C1/C2 and a C3 fracture. Finally, the answer to the third and fourth questions allows the surgeon to decide if an extensile (lateral parapatellar approach) or less extensile approach (anterolateral approach) is needed. The fourth question is important because Nork et al have demonstrated a 38% incidence of frontal plane (Hoffa) fractures in type C fractures.[39]

In the AO/OTA classification, differentiation between an A1, A2, and A3 fracture simply designates the amount of comminution in the metaphyseal area. As such, this provides little additional information to the surgeon, in terms of both surgical approach and prognosis. That is, a slightly comminuted fracture in the metaphyseal area would be treated in a similar manner and would have no worse outcome than a simple fracture (A1 fracture). It may, however, determine the type of reduction utilized in this area (direct vs indirect reduction).

Classification of a fracture as a type B (partial articular) injury must be accompanied by an accurate description of the condyle fracture, whether it is a medial condyle, lateral condyle, or frontal plane fracture. This has significance in terms of surgical approach and surgical implant used.

Nonoperative Treatment

In 1967, while discussing supracondylar femur fractures, Neer et al stated that "no category of fracture at this level seemed well suited for internal fixation."[4] They evaluated 110 patients with supracondylar femur fractures treated between 1942 and 1966. In those fractures treated with internal fixation, 52% had a satisfactory outcome, whereas in those that received closed treatment, 90% were satisfactory. However, the authors did note a significant varus/internal rotation deformity common with nonoperative treatment with functional cast, bracing, or traction. In 1966, Stewart et al reported on the treatment of 215 supracondylar femur fractures and had a similar conclusion.[5] They noted that 67% of the fractures treated by closed methods had a good or excellent clinical outcome, whereas only 54% of fractures treated by open reduction and internal fixation were rated good or excellent. Twenty of 69 patients treated with open reduction and internal fixation either had a delayed union or a nonunion. These observations, however, must be taken with some perspective. It is clear that with appropriate intervention the clinical results of internal fixation have significantly improved.[12,13,27,40,41] In addition, it should be recognized that the functional expectations for treatment of a supracondylar femur fracture in the 1960s were relatively low and not in keeping with modern-day patient expectations. For example, to have a satisfactory Neer score, the patient could still have pain with fatigue, a restricted function (for example, needing to climb the stairs sideways), have knee motion of only 100 degrees, and have up to 5 degrees of angulation or 0.5 cm of shortening.[4]

With modern-day techniques at the surgeon's disposal, the occasions in which nonoperative treatment is the best treatment option are rare. The situations might include a nonambulatory patient, a patient with significant comorbidities (for example, a recent myocardial infarction in which surgical intervention is not possible), and imminent death. It is quite challenging in the frail and osteoporotic patient to control the distal femoral block/supracondylar fracture in a cast, even if the surgeon accepts the inherent

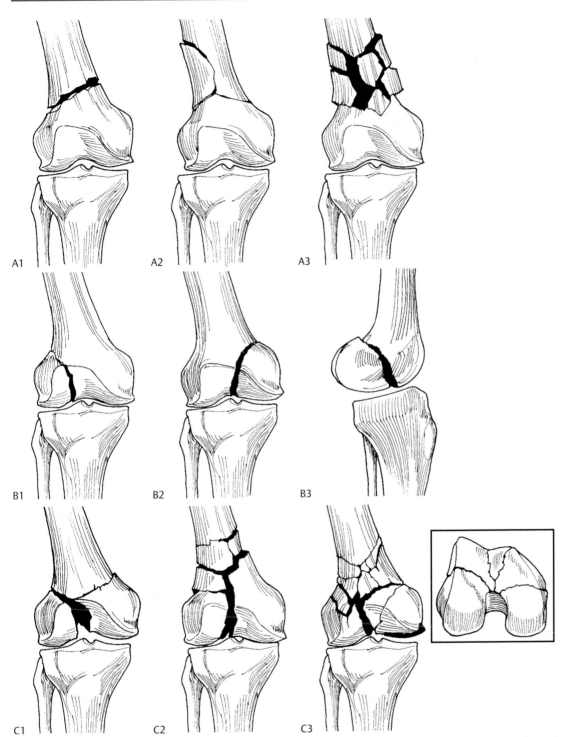

Figure 26–1 The Arbeitsgemeinschaft für Osteosynthesefragen/ Orthopaedic Trauma Association (AO/OTA) classification for distal femurs. From top left: A1: Extra-articular fracture with a simple metaphyseal component. A2: Extra-articular fracture with a wedge fracture in the metaphyseal region. A3: Extra-articular fracture with complex metaphyseal involvement. B1: Partial articular fracture of the lateral condyle in the sagittal plane. B2: Partial articular fracture of the medial condyle in the sagittal plane. B3: Partial articular fracture in the frontal plane (Hoffa fracture); of either medial or lateral femoral condyle or both. C1: Supracondylar/intercondylar femur fracture with a simple metaphyseal component and a simple articular split. C2: Supracondylar/intercondylar femur fracture with a simple articular split and complex metaphyseal involvement. C3: Supracondylar/intercondylar femur fracture with complex articular involvement.

stiffness. Displacement of the fracture in a frail patient may lead to skin pressure sores from the fractured bone ends themselves.

The surgeon may occasionally encounter a nondisplaced supracondylar femur fracture without intra-articular extension. This fracture may be treated in a hinged brace with early range of motion. In an otherwise healthy patient, immobilization in a cast for multiple weeks will result in unacceptable stiffness in a high percentage of cases. In such a case, displacement of the fracture in the hinged brace would represent a surgical indication.

Indications for Surgical Treatment

As noted above, nearly all supracondylar/intercondylar femur fractures should be treated operatively. Particularly in a young person, any attempt to treat such a fracture in a cast, brace, or traction would not reliably accomplish the goals of treatment that were established earlier in the chapter. A nondisplaced supracondylar femur fracture may be treated in a hinged knee brace with immediate motion of the knee. If the fracture displaces with early motion, this is an indication for surgical treatment. Additionally, although the long-term results of articular incongruity and supracondylar femur fractures is not known, the basic tenets of articular reconstruction would warrant operative intervention for any displaced intra-articular fracture, particularly in a young patient.

The foregoing logic also holds for the elderly osteoporotic patient. If medical comorbidities or functional demands warrant nonoperative treatment (for example, in a splint or hinged knee brace), this may still not be possible. For example, excessive pain with nonoperative treatment requiring narcotics, inability to mobilize the patient, potential skin breakdown, or fracture displacement are indications for surgical treatment.

Surgical Treatment

Surgical Anatomy

An understanding of the osseous anatomy of the distal femur is paramount to understanding distal femur fractures and operative intervention. The normal anatomical axis of the distal femur is 6 to 7 degrees of valgus in a male and 8 to 9 degrees of valgus in a female (i.e., a line drawn down the intramedullary canal of the femur bisects a line drawn across the articular surface of the femur by an angle of ~83 to 84 degrees in a male and 81 to 82 degrees in a female). The lateral cortex of the femur slopes ~10 degrees when the end of the femur is viewed head-on, and the medial cortex slopes ~25 degrees **(Fig. 26–2).** Both the medial and lateral femoral condyles are convex and articulate with the corresponding medial and lateral tibial plateau with the

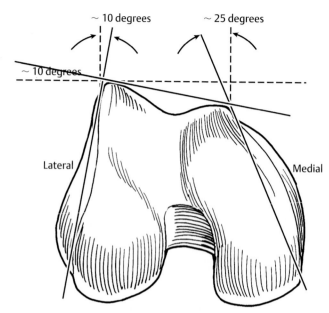

Figure 26–2 End-on view of the distal femoral condyle. The anterior aspect of the femoral condyle slopes ~10 degrees from lateral to medial. The lateral femoral condyle slopes ~10 degrees, and the medial femoral condyle slopes ~25 degrees.

medial and lateral meniscus in between. The intercondylar notch separates the posterior two thirds of the medial femoral condyle from the lateral femoral condyle. The medial and lateral epicondyles are on the posterior portion of the medial and lateral femoral cortex, respectively. The cartilage covering the medial and lateral femoral condyle is ~3 to 4 mm thick. The patella articulates with the femoral trochlea on the anterior-distal aspect of the femoral condyle.

Key surgical points directly relevant to the surgical anatomy relate to the sloping of the medial and lateral femoral condyles and the insertion site for an intramedullary nail placed through the distal articular surface. The lateral femoral cortex slopes ~10 degrees, and therefore a plate must be rotated anteriorly ~10 degrees when it is placed on the lateral cortex of the distal femur. A common surgical error is to have the posterior aspect of the plate (for example, 95 degree angled blade plate) impact upon the posterior aspect of the lateral femoral cortex before the plate is flush with the bone.

The surgeon must also be cognizant of the 25 degree slope of the medial femoral cortex when placing a blade plate, DCS, or any type of screw from lateral to medial. For example, if one is placing a screw from lateral to medial in the anterior aspect of the distal femoral condyle, a screw may perforate the medial femoral cortex but appear to be "in" on the AP radiograph. Similarly, when placing a blade plate or DCS, the surgeon must measure the most anterior aspect of the hole drilled for such a device, so that the screw or side plate will not penetrate the medial femoral cortex. If this is not remembered, prominent hardware in the medial aspect of the femur will become aggravating for the patient.

Surgical Approaches

There are four common approaches that are utilized in the treatment of distal femur fractures. As already noted in the Classification section, the classification scheme is very helpful in determining the surgical approach (**Table 26–1**).

Medial Parapatellar Approach: Retrograde Intramedullary Nailing of the Distal Femur Fracture without Articular Extension (see Videos 26–2, 26–3, 26–4, Disk 3)

The patient is placed supine on a radiolucent table with a bump under the hip on the same side as the injury to tilt the pelvis ~10 to 15 degrees. The knee can be flexed to ~80 to 90 degrees with the use of large towel bumps or a triangular leg support. In the situation of a nonarticular (type A) fracture, an incision ~2 to 2.5 cm long and parallel to the medial aspect of the patellar tendon, inferior to the patella, can be made. No attempt is made to directly visualize the articular surface of the distal femur (**Fig. 26–3A–C**).

Table 26–1 Surgical Approaches for Distal Femur Fractures

Type A fracture
   Medial peripatellar approach (for percutaneous intramedullary nailing)
   Anterolateral approach without exposure of the articular surface (for plate fixation)

Type B fractures
   Anteromedial approach with visualization of the joint surface (for isolated medial femoral condyle fracture)
   Anterolateral approach with visualization of the joint surface (for isolated lateral femoral condyle fracture)
   Posterior approach to the knee joint (for a medial and/or lateral femoral condyle fracture that is too posterior to adequately visualize from an anteromedial or anterolateral approach)

Type C1/C2
   Medial peripatellar approach with visualization of the articular surface (for retrograde intramedullary nailing of the distal femur after reduction and internal fixation of the articular surface)
   Anterolateral approach with visualization of the articular surface (for plate fixation of the distal femur after reduction and internal fixation of the articular surface)

Type C3 fracture
   Lateral peripatellar approach with complete eversion of the patella and visualization of the articular surface (for plate fixation after reduction and internal fixation of the articular surface)

Medial Parapatellar Approach: Retrograde Intramedullary Nailing of Distal Femur Fracture with Articular Extension

In the treatment of a C1/C2 fracture, the articular surface should be visualized to actively reduce the articular surface. Therefore, the medial parapatellar approach is continued cephalad for 2 to 8 cm, depending upon the need for further visualization of the articular surface of the distal femur. The incision described earlier for the small percutaneous medial parapatellar approach is then extended proximally through the skin and subcutaneous tissue and through the medial extensor retinaculum. A division in the extensor mechanism ~8 to 10 mm medial to the patella is made. In general, for visualization of a simple intra-articular split, eversion of the patella is not necessary. Reduction and fixation of the articular surface as described later can then be performed, after which nailing is performed as already noted. The extensor mechanism is then repaired on the medial aspect of the patella with no. 5 nonabsorbable inverted sutures.

Anterolateral Approach to the Distal Femur: Plate Fixation of Fractures without or with Simple Articular Extension (see Video 26–5, Disk 3)

The anterolateral approach of the distal femur is utilized for plate fixation of both type A and type C1/C2 fractures. For type A fractures, no attempt is made to visualize the distal articular surface of the femur. In the C1- and C2-type fractures, such visualization is mandatory. The distal aspect of the anterolateral approach can be utilized for submuscular techniques, whereas a traditional "muscle-sparing" anterolateral approach can be utilized for biological plating of the distal femur.

The skin incision for an anterolateral approach of the distal femur begins at the tibial tubercle and then curves toward the anterior one third of the distal femoral condyle and then up the midlateral aspect of the femoral shaft (**Fig. 26–4A,B**). The distal aspect of the incision is not necessary if the articular surface does not need to be visualized. Dissection is carried down through the skin and subcutaneous tissue sharply to the level of the iliotibial band. The iliotibial band is then divided in line with its fibers. The fibers of the iliotibial band curve anteromedially toward the tibial tubercle. After the iliotibial band is divided, the joint capsule is visualized. Often it is not disrupted even in severely displaced fractures. The joint capsule does not necessarily need to be divided or disrupted in the type A fracture, although doing so may allow the surgeon to accurately assess the plate position on the lateral aspect of the distal femur. For submuscular plating techniques in a C1/C2 fracture, the skin incision is ~10 to 12 cm long, whereas for a type A fracture, it is ~8 to 10 cm long.

The surgeon may wish to perform traditional open plating instead of utilizing a submuscular technique. For a formal open biological plating, an anterolateral approach as described earlier for the submuscular techniques is ex-

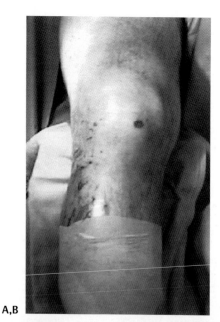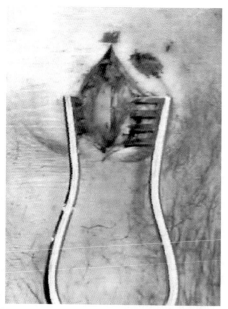

A,B

Figure 26–3 Medial peripatellar approach for retrograde intramedullary nailing of a distal femur fracture without articular extension. **(A)** The knee is on a triangular support. **(B)** A 2 cm incision is made medial to the patellar tendon. **(C)** Guidewire and nail insertion into the distal femur is performed under fluoroscopic control.

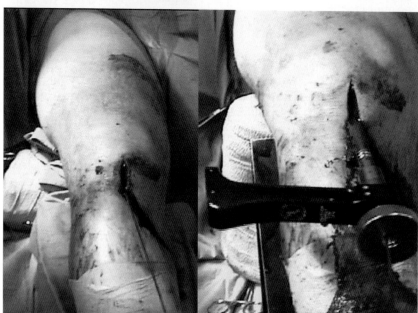

C

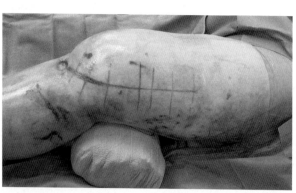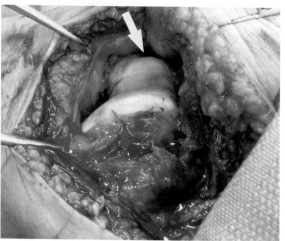

A

B

Figure 26–4 Anterolateral approach to the distal femur with visualization of the articular surface. **(A)** A curvilinear incision is directed from the tibial tubercle over the anterior one third of the distal femoral region. **(B)** A Hohman retractor may be placed over the medial femoral condyle after capsulotomy (arrow) so that the articular surface can be well visualized.

tended proximally up the midlateral aspect of the femur (**Fig. 26–4A,B**). Again, sharp dissection is performed through the subcutaneous tissue, and the iliotibial band is divided. The fascia of the vastus lateralis is then divided roughly between the anterior two thirds and the posterior one third of the vastus lateralis fascia. The muscle belly is then retracted anteriorly with skin rakes while a wood-handled elevator is used to tease the muscle fibers off the posterior aspect of the vastus lateralis fascia and the posterior intramuscular septum, going in a distal to proximal direction. In doing so, multiple perforating arteries are encountered, and these are either ligated or cauterized. No attempt is made to completely strip the lateral aspect of the femur of its periosteum, and certainly no attempt is made to visualize every aspect of the fracture or the anterior/medial aspect of the metaphyseal/diaphyseal component of the fracture. Instead, the muscle fibers are left intact anteriorly over the femoral shaft. Hohman retractors may be placed anterior to the femur within the quadriceps muscle, ~1 cm removed from the anterior surface of the femur, so as not

to have these Hohman retractors strip the muscle belly off the anterior aspect of the femur.

Exposure of the articular surface is performed by dividing the joint capsule from the metaphyseal area down to the level of the lateral meniscus. A Hohman retractor may be carefully placed over the medial aspect of the femoral condyle so as to allow for direct visualization of the articular surface (**Fig. 26–4B**).

Lateral Parapatellar Approach: Plate Fixation of Fractures with Complex Articular Extension (see Video 26–6, Disk 3)

The lateral parapatellar approach of the distal femur was popularized by Krettek et al,[42] and is based on the realization that a medial parapatellar approach (as utilized in total knee arthroplasty) allows for excellent visualization of the articular surface of the femur without devitalization of the metaphyseal and diaphyseal component of the distal femur (**Fig. 26–5A–C**). Its use generally relies on the placement

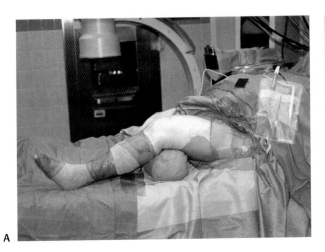

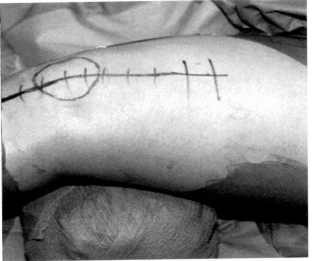

Figure 26–5 The lateral parapatellar approach for a distal femur fracture. **(A)** The patient setup. A bump is placed underneath the left buttock, the entire left hip and left lower extremity are prepped and draped, and supracondylar bumps are placed posterior to the supracondylar region. **(B)** The skin incision is over the lateral half of the patella. **(C)** A division in the quadriceps tendon is performed proximally, and ~8 to 10 mm of the tissue is left on the lateral border of the patella (arrow).

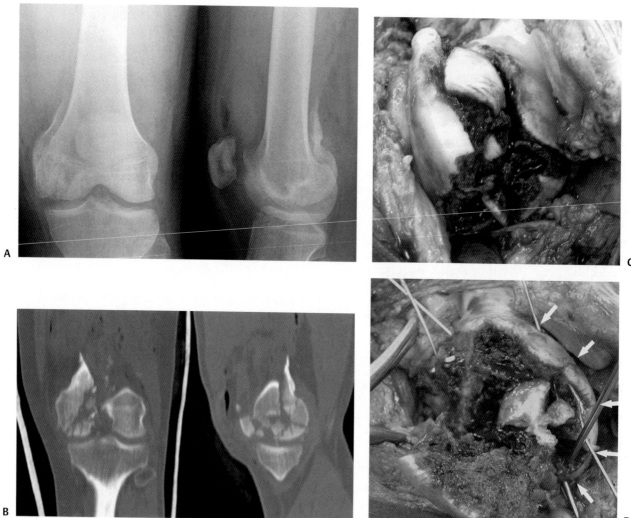

Figure 26–6 A medial femoral condyle fracture in a 32-year-old male highlights the need for appropriate preoperative imaging and techniques for complex articular reconstruction. **(A)** Anteroposterior (AP) and lateral radiographs demonstrate what appears to be a relatively "simple" isolated medial femoral condyle fracture. **(B)** The computed tomographic (CT) scan demonstrates multilevel involvement of the articular surface of the medial femoral condyle. **(C)** A medial peripatellar approach was performed for visualization of the articular surface. Here, the articular surface is seen to be in multiple fragments. **(D)** Provisional K-wire fixation is utilized for reconstruction of the medial femoral condyle near the intercondylar notch. Arrows demonstrate multiple frontal plane fractures (multiple Hoffa fractures).

of a plate in a submuscular manner. The rationale for the incision being made lateral rather than medial is so that this plate can be relatively easily passed from the same incision. The patient is once again positioned supine, with a buttock bump to tilt the pelvis ~15 degrees and a tourniquet utilized as desired. Supracondylar bumps are placed posterior to the distal femur, which aids in neutralizing the hyperextension deformity of the distal femur caused by pull of the gastrocnemius. An incision (~15 cm) is then made just lateral to the midline and based over the lateral aspect of the patella (**Fig. 26–5B**). A full-thickness flap is carried down to the extensor retinaculum. The extensor retinaculum is divided and is later repaired. The quadriceps tendon is divided, separating the lateral 40% from the medial 60%, and this is carried down to the superior pole of the patella. As the arthrotomy is continued around the lateral

aspect of the patella, a cuff of extensor mechanism ~8 to 10 mm thick is left on the lateral aspect of the patella (**Fig. 26–5C**). The incision continues around the distal portion of the patella, finally paralleling the patellar tendon. With the knee in hyperextension, the surgeon can then evert the patella. Care must be taken, especially in osteoporotic individuals, to avoid undue force on the patellar tendon insertion. A common mistake at this juncture is not to release sufficient quadriceps tendon cephalad, which will not allow for appropriate eversion of the patella, thereby placing excess force on the patellar tendon.

With varying degrees of flexion and extension of the knee, often with the knee flexed 70 to 90 degrees and the patella everted, excellent visualization of the articular surface can be obtained. Reduction and fixation as described below are then performed for the complex articular injury.

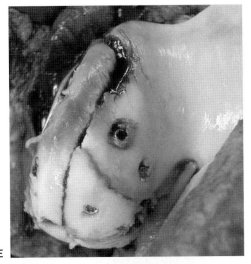

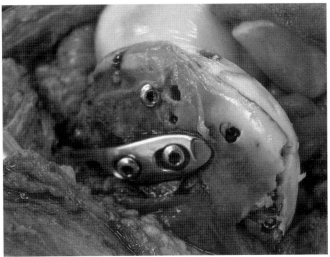

E

F

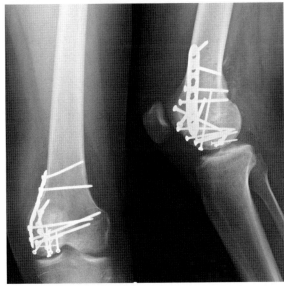

G

Figure 26–6 *(Continued)* **(E)** Reconstruction of the medial femoral condyle and its multiple articular fragments. It is unusual to utilize lag screws directly through the articular surface, but this was felt to be the only surgical option. **(F)** Antiglide medial femoral plate for support of the articular reconstruction. **(G)** AP and lateral radiographs of the knee at 1 year postinjury. The patient's knee range of motion is 0 to 100 degrees. The prognosis is guarded.

Closure of the extensor mechanism is performed with no. 5 nonabsorbable inverted sutures.

In addition to being utilized for these C3 distal femur fracture, the lateral parapatellar approach may be utilized for a complex or very posterior lateral femoral condyle fracture.

Medial Parapatellar Approach: Plate Fixation of Medial Condyle Fractures with Complex Articular Extension

A medial parapatellar approach is performed in an identical way to that described for the lateral parapatellar approach with identical surgical positioning. This approach is quite familiar to most orthopaedic surgeons because it is the approach utilized for a total knee arthroplasty. No significant differences exist from the approach described above other than the incision being made on the medial aspect of the patella. As in the lateral parapatellar ap-

proach, its major use is for that of a complex medial femoral condyle fracture **(Fig. 26–6A–G).** In the setting of a relatively simple medial femoral condyle fracture, one may utilize a standard anteromedial approach.

Medial/Lateral Posterior Approaches: Plate Fixation of Medial/Lateral Condyle Fractures with Complex Articular Extension (Which Cannot Be Visualized Adequately through Anterior Approaches)

Occasionally, a medial and/or lateral condylar frontal plane fracture (Hoffa fracture) may be based so far posterior that there is a concern that the fracture cannot be adequately exposed from an anterior-based approach. In such a case, a posterior-based approach is indicated. The patient is placed in the prone position with the tourniquet high about the thigh with appropriate padding placed underneath the contralateral lower extremity and both upper extremities. A curvilinear midline incision is made over the posterior aspect of popliteal fossa. A full-thickness flap is carried down to the muscle fascia. The sciatic nerve divisions and popliteal artery are identified, and the plane between the medial or lateral gastrocnemius muscle is developed to visualize the femoral condyle. Capsulotomy is then performed with direct visualization of the articular component of the fracture. The necessity for this approach is quite rare but must be kept in mind for the aforementioned surgical indication.

Surgical Techniques

As with the surgical approach, the classification of the fracture will determine the appropriate implant and technique for distal femoral fractures (**Table 26–2**).

Initial Stabilization

Before classifying the injury, the surgeon should perform a preoperative assessment of the injury and the patient. Although a distal femur fracture can be treated in the acute setting (in the first 24 hours after injury), this should only be done with a well-resuscitated patient without life-threatening injuries, a good understanding of the articular injury, confidence in the quality of debridement of open wounds (if applicable), and an appropriate surgical team. If any of these criteria are not met, a spanning external fixator may be placed across the knee joint. Care is taken to keep the pins relatively high on the femur and low on the tibia, so as not to have the pin sites close to the surgical incision site. Stabilization of the sides of the knee joint with a cylinder splint will add stability to this area, and perhaps provide increased patient comfort.

Table 26—2   Possible Implant for Distal Femoral Fractures as Determined by the AO/OTA Classification

Type A or C1/C2 Fractures
1. Dynamic condylar screw[40,43–48]
2. 95 degree angled blade plate[3,12,48–53]
3. Antegrade femoral nail[41,65–67]
4. Retrograde femoral nail[16,20–27,68–74]
5. Locked internal fixator (LISS, lateral condylar buttress plate with locked distal screws)[13–19,31,32,36,37]

Type B fractures
1. Screw fixation[75,76]
2. Screw and plate fixation[75]

Type C3 fractures
1. Standard condylar buttress plate (nonlocked screws)[3,12,40,51,77,78]
2. Locked internal fixator (LISS, lateral condylar buttress plate with locked distal screws)[13–19,31,32,36,37]

AO/OTA, Arbeitsgemeinschaft für Osteosynthesefragen/Orthopaedic Trauma Association; LISS, Less Invasive Stabilization System

Articular Fracture Reduction and Fixation (see Videos 26–5, 26–6, Disk 3)

In simple terms, the treatment of a supracondylar/intercondylar femur fracture can be broken into two steps: (1) articular fracture visualization, reduction, and fixation; and (2) connection of the reconstructed distal femoral articular block to the proximal femur utilizing a plate or retrograde nail. The surgeon must not compromise the first step because of the second step. A common and critical mistake would be to place a retrograde nail or a submuscular plate through a limited approach *without* appropriate visualization and fixation of the articular injury. Although attempts should be made to avoid nonunions and malunions of the supracondylar region, the reality is that they can be relatively easily addressed if they occur. However, poor reduction of the articular surface is catastrophic and cannot be easily dealt with (**Fig. 26–6A–G** and **26–7**). Thus the surgeon should carefully assess the articular injury and ensure that the surgical approach will allow

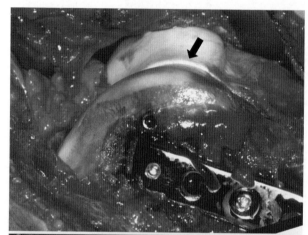

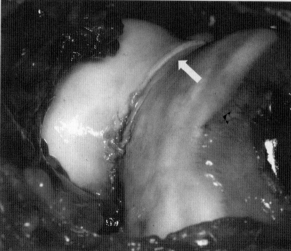

Figure 26–7 Intraoperative photographs of articular surface malreduction (arrows). Although, the metaphyseal component of the fracture was well reduced with a 95 degree angled blade plate, the articular step-off for this simple articular split was 2 to 3 mm. This is not acceptable.

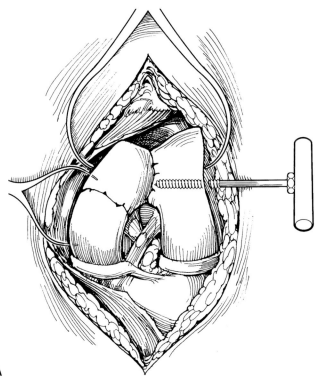

A

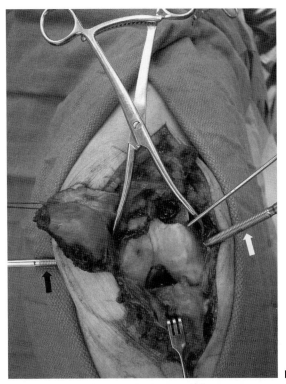

B

Figure 26–8 (A) Multiple reduction tools used for articular reconstruction. A large Weber clamp is utilized to clamp the medial and lateral femoral condyles together. A Schanz pin has been placed in the lateral femoral condyle to act as a reduction aid. A medium Weber clamp is placed through a cortical pilot hole in the medial femoral condyle to reduce the Hoffa fracture. **(B)** Intraoperative view of a similar articular reduction. The patient had an associated patellar tendon disruption. A Schanz pin was placed in the medial (black arrow) and lateral (white arrow) femoral condyles to aid reduction of the articular surface.

appropriate visualization of the articular injury. After the articular injury is exposed, there are several reduction aids and techniques that may be helpful.

Reduction aids for the articular surface that may be helpful include **(Fig. 26–8A,B):**

- Schanz pins utilized as reduction aids in the medial and lateral femoral condyle to assist in reduction of the intercondylar fracture
- Large pointed reduction Weber clamps, or large pelvic reduction clamps, which compress the lateral and medial femoral condyle blocks together
- Provisional K-wires, which can hold reduction of articular blocks until definitive lag screw fixation is achieved
- Dental picks, which are helpful in fine manipulation of articular segments

After reduction is achieved, multiple 3.5 mm cortical lag screws are utilized in a lateral to medial direction for fixation of intercondylar fractures, or in an anterior to posterior direction for fixation of Hoffa fractures. In general, three lag screws are placed from lateral to medial. Lag screws may then be placed in an anterior to posterior direction. A diagonal screw placed from anterolateral to posteromedial may be helpful to "lock in" the entire distal femoral articular

surface in injuries with complex multiplanar involvement **(Fig. 26–9A,B).** Mini-fragment 2.7 mm lag screws may also be utilized, especially for fixation of small osteochondral fragments in the intercondylar notch. Occasionally, screws may need to be placed through the articular cartilage if fragments are exceedingly small. This should be avoided, however, if possible **(Fig. 26–6E).** Meticulous attention to detail and surgical patience must be exercised when dealing with complex articular injuries. When there are multiple fragments, provisional fixation of the entire articular surface is advisable before definitive fixation **(Fig. 26–6D).**

Assessment of the articular surface reduction is conducted through a visual inspection and digital palpation. A common malreduction that can occur is a rotation of one condyle on the other condyle when treating a C1/C2 injury. This can be avoided with a careful inspection of the superior aspect of the intercondylar fracture *as well as* the intercondylar notch area around the fracture. Such malrotation will not be appreciated if only on end view of the distal femur is assessed.

Finally, manipulation of severely osteoporotic osseous fragments is a surgical challenge because clamps or Schanz pins tend to crush the bone (e.g., in a 90-year-old patient). This may be one situation where direct manipulation of the osseous fragments may be advisable, utilizing finger pressure.

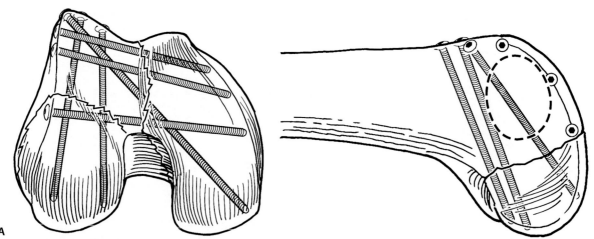

Figure 26–9 Drawings of multiple articular screws utilized for treatment of a type C3 fracture of the distal femur. **(A)** Lag screws may be placed from the lateral to medial femoral condyle, as shown in this end-on view. Anterior to posterior lag screws may be placed for fixation of the Hoffa fracture. Finally, a diagonal screw may be placed from the anterolateral to posteromedial aspect to the articular surface. **(B)** Side view of similar articular screw reconstruction. The dotted line represents the area that can be utilized for placement of the plate.

Blade Plate Fixation of the Distal Femur

The 95 degree angled blade plate is not a commonly used device because it is thought to be a technically difficult device to use. It is utilized for A-type and C1/C2-type fractures. Its use in type C3 fractures is limited because of concern of the disruption of the articular surface fixation with introduction of the blade. Its use has been supplanted by the use of locking distal femoral plates, as well as the use of retrograde nails. It is included here for four reasons:

1. Multiple surgical series have been documented, along with the DCS (with which it has significant similarities).[3,12,40,43–53]

2. The concepts in its use are critical as a foundation for all surgical techniques described following here.

3. It is a device that demonstrates well the concept of indirect reduction of the metaphyseal/diaphyseal component of the fracture. The key concept is that the surgeon must ensure that the blade plate is placed in the distal femur in the appropriate position. If this is properly done, frontal plane (varus/valgus) and sagittal plane (flexion/hyperextension) alignment is ensured.

4. It can be thought of as the first "locked fixator" for the distal femur. The blade component provides excellent frontal and sagittal plane control of the distal femoral block.

The key to understanding the blade plate is to understand which plane of correction is established at each point of the surgical sequence:

1. The varus/valgus angulation of the distal femur is established by the angle with which the blade goes into the distal femoral block with reference to the joint line in the coronal plane.

2. The length and rotation of the femur are determined when the first proximal screw is placed.

3. The flexion/extension (sagittal plane alignment) of the distal segment is determined by the amount of flexion or extension with which the blade goes into the distal segment, and is "locked" into place when a second screw is placed in the proximal femoral fragment.

After the articular surface undergoes reduction and fixation, the blade is placed. The steps in blade plate placement are:

1. Establishment of the varus/valgus angulation of the distal femoral block. A good quality AP radiograph is obtained. A 4.5 mm drill bit is started at a point 1.5 cm from the distal femoral articular surface and at a point between the anterior third and the middle third of the distal femoral condyles (when viewed from the side) (Fig. 26–10A,B). This drill bit (and subsequently the other drill bits, seating chisel, and blade) should be place at a perpendicular orientation to the distal femoral lateral cortex.

2. A second and third 4.5 mm drill bit is placed in the distal femur utilizing the triple hole drill guide, which keeps the drill bits parallel to each other. The positions of the second and third drill bits relative to the first drill hole in the distal femur establish the flexion/extension axis that the blade plate will have on the distal femur. At this point, the most anterior hole is measured because this length determines the maximal length of the blade. If the blade is longer than this distance, the anterior aspect of the blade will protrude out of the medial cortex.

3. A router is used to enlarge the cortical drill holes.

4. A seating chisel is introduced in the same path as the drill bits. The depth of penetration of the blade is used as a second determinant of the length of the blade to

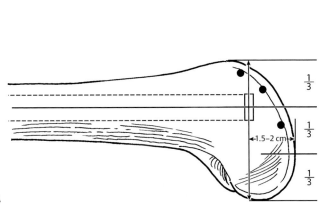

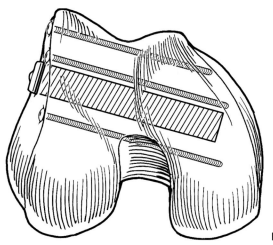

A

B

Figure 26–10 Area for placement of a 95 degree angled blade plate in the distal femur. Note that three lateral to medial lag screws have been placed. **(A)** Side view. The starting point is at the center between the anterior one third and posterior two thirds of the femoral condyles and is ~1.5 cm from the distal femoral articular surface. **(B)** The blade plate is driven in a perpendicular direction to the lateral femoral cortex. Note that the anterior aspect of the blade plate must be short of the medial femoral cortex so that the plate is not prominent.

be chosen. When the seating chisel is driven into the distal femoral block, care must be taken to avoid having the blade become incarcerated in bone. This can particularly be a problem in young hard bone. To avoid this, the seating chisel is "backslapped" after every 10 to 15 mm of forward advancement of the seating chisel into the distal femoral block.

5. The seating chisel is replaced by the blade plate. A large amount of force should not be necessary to introduce the blade plate into the distal femoral block at least for the first half of the blade length because the blade should be following the path already established by the seating chisel.

6. The blade plate is then impacted into the bone with an impactor.

7. The blade plate is then secured to the distal segment by additional screws.

8. The length and rotation of the distal femur are established. This may be aided by use of an external fixator or femoral distractor. The plate is then held on the proximal fragment with an articulating Verbrugge clamp. One screw in the proximal femur will "lock in" length and rotation.

9. The lateral radiograph may then be assessed for flexion/extension at the fracture site. The common deformity is hyperextension of the distal segment. This can be minimized through the use of towel bumps posterior to the supracondylar area. Additional screws may be placed in the proximal segment when this reduction is appropriate.

10. In general, three to four screws in a plate that can accommodate twice that many screws in the proximal segment are utilized for biological plating **(Fig. 26–11A–D).**

Dynamic Condylar Screw Placement for a Distal Femur Fracture

The indications for a DCS in treatment of a distal femur fracture are identical to that of a 95 degree angled blade plate. The advantage of the DCS is that precise sagittal plane alignment (flexion/extension) is not necessary when the DCS is placed in the distal segment. Said another way, the DCS may be placed in the distal femoral block, and the side plate can be rotated on the DCS to ensure that the plate is on the midlateral aspect of the femur proximally. The disadvantage of the device is the relatively large amount of bone that is removed with the DCS and the sagittal plane instability unless screws can be placed in the distal femoral block in addition to the DCS. The point of entry for the DCS is exactly that of the 95 degree angled blade plate, except it is placed at 2.0 (not 1.5) cm from the articular surface.

Retrograde Nailing of the Distal Femur (see Videos 26–2, 26–3, 26–4, Disk 3)

In general, retrograde intramedullary nailing of distal femur fractures is reserved for extra-articular or simple articular fractures. There must be adequate purchase of the nail within the distal femoral block; therefore, at least two points of distal fixation with two distal interlocking screws must be obtained. Typically, a relatively large intramedullary nail (12 to 15 mm) is utilized.

The patient is placed supine on a radiolucent table. Towel bumps or a triangle posterior to the supracondylar region allows for counteraction of the common hyperextension (apex posterior deformity) seen in the distal segment secondary to the unopposed pull of the gastrocnemius.

For a type A fracture, the mini medial parapatellar approach described earlier (2 to 3 cm) is made. A guide pin is then placed under radiographic guidance. The guide pin

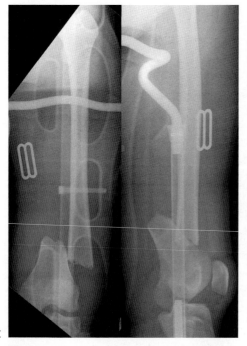
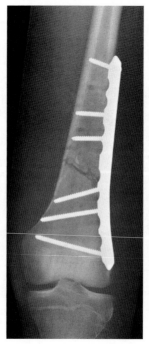
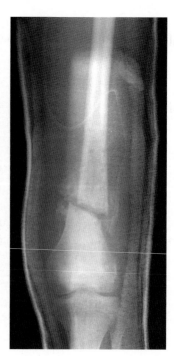

A–C

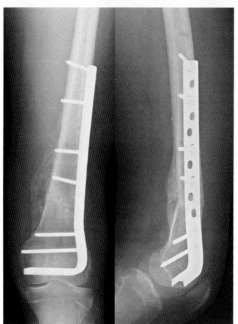

D

Figure 26–11 Utilization of a 95 degree angled blade plate for a distal femur fracture. **(A)** Original injury films. **(B)** The patient was treated with a 4.5 mm broad plate. This construct failed secondary to infection and abscess formation. **(C)** The plate was removed and the infection controlled. **(D)** A 95 degree angled blade plate was placed in the distal femur, and the fracture was compressed utilizing the articulating tension device. Here, complete healing is seen at 4 months.

should appear to be in line with the femoral canal on the AP radiograph. On the lateral view, the guide pin should be visualized at the anterior aspect of Blumensaat's line. The guide pin is then advanced into the distal femur for 8 to 10 cm. A starting hole in the distal femur is then made with a cannulated reamer/drill, usually 12 to 14 mm in diameter. After the starting hole is made, a long guidewire is inserted into the distal femur up to the fracture. The distal femur is then reduced with respect to the femoral shaft in both AP and lateral planes. As with any intramedullary nailing, reaming must take place with the fracture reduced. An external fixator Schanz pin (5 mm diameter in young

bone, 6 mm in elderly bone) can be placed in a lateral to medial direction to control varus/valgus or from an anterior to posterior direction to control the hyperextension deformity, if necessary. The guidewire is then passed up into the proximal femur, depending upon the length required. In general, a retrograde nail is utilized that covers the entire length of the femur. The proximal end of the nail should be above the level of the lesser trochanter. A second guidewire is utilized for an indirect measurement of femoral nail length (as with normal femoral nailing). Preoperative assessment of the width of the intramedullary canal of the femur helps determine the degree of reaming, as does

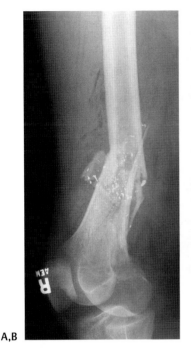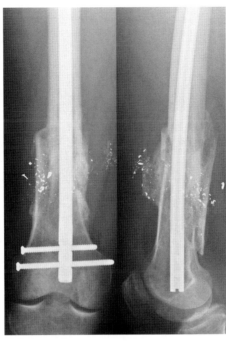

A,B

Figure 26–12 Treatment of a nonarticular distal femur fracture with a retrograde nail. **(A)** Injury radiograph. The mechanism was a ballistic injury. **(B)** Early radiographic healing seen at 3 months. The patient was allowed full weight bearing from the time of initial surgery.

the intraoperative assessment of the "chatter" achieved with such reaming. In general, at least a 12 mm nail is desired, and a 14 to 15 mm nail is utilized in osteoporotic and elderly patients with a more capacious canal. Reaming is usually performed to 1 mm over the desired nail size. The guidewire is left in place while the fracture reduction is confirmed with AP and lateral fluoroscopic views. The assembled nail and interlocking jig are then inserted into the distal femur and across the fracture while the fracture reduction is maintained. The nail should be sunk at least 1 cm below the articular surface of the femur. This should be radiographically and visually confirmed. Two distal interlocking screws are utilized with most nail systems. In some nail systems a special distal "cap" can be used, which allows

for fixed-angle locking of the distal screw. This can be advantageous in osteoporotic bone. Two proximal interlocking screws are then placed; usually these screws go from anterior to posterior and are placed utilizing the freehand method as described for normal routine antegrade femoral nailing in Chapter 25 **(Fig. 26–12A,B).**

For a C1/C2 fracture, the larger medial parapatellar approach is utilized. This allows for reduction and fixation of the articular surface as detailed earlier. The placement of screws must take into account the eventual path of the retrograde nail **(Figs. 26–13A,B** and **26–14A–D).** Screws may be placed anterior and posterior to the nail to lag the lateral condyle to the medial condyle. It is possible to treat a C3 fracture with reduction and fixation of the articular

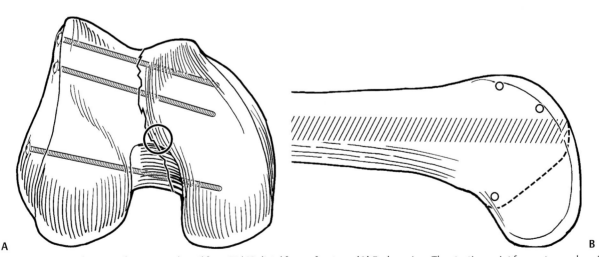

A   **B**

Figure 26–13 Utilization of a retrograde nail for a C1/C2 distal femur fracture. **(A)** End-on view. The starting point for a retrograde nail is anterior to the origin of the posterior cruciate ligament. It is usually just medial in the intercondylar notch. **(B)** On the lateral view, the entry side is in line with the axis of the femur.

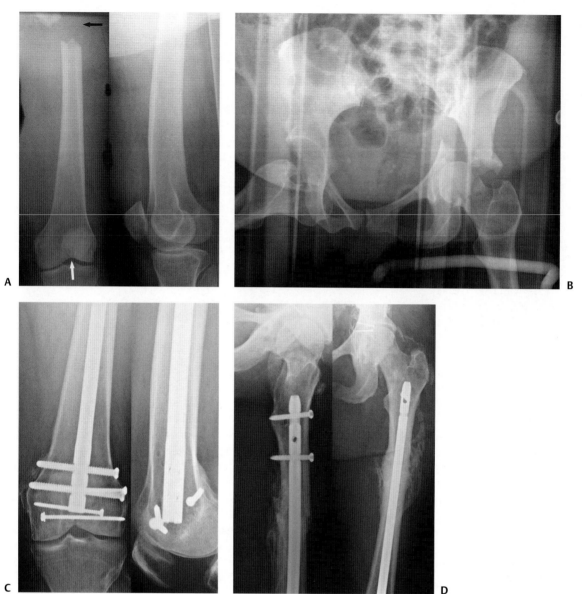

Figure 26–14 Treatment of a C1 distal femur fracture with an associated femoral shaft fracture. Because the patient had an ipsilateral hip fracture-dislocation, retrograde nailing of the femur was chosen instead of antegrade nailing to avoid another incision about the hip. **(A)** Injury radiograph of the femur demonstrates a simple distal articular split. **(B)** Radiograph of the pelvis, showing a left acetabular fracture and complex pelvic ring injury. **(C)** The patient had screw fixation across the articular surface, and then a retrograde nail was placed. Follow-up radiograph at 3 years. **(D)** Follow-up radiographs for the proximal femur at 3 years. The patient developed heterotopic ossification around the acetabular fracture and had plate removal and heterotopic ossification removal at approximately 2 years.

surface followed by retrograde nail placement, but this is probably not advisable. There are other options available, and the introduction of the retrograde nail may disrupt the articular surface reduction and fixation.

Antegrade Nailing of the Distal Femur

Antegrade nailing of a distal femur fracture can be performed, and may be desirable if there is an associated proximal femur fracture. Reduction of the articular surface in a C1 or C2 fracture may be performed as already noted, and antegrade nailing of the femur performed as described in Chapter 25. In most cases, it is advisable to have two interlocking screws distal to the fracture **(Fig. 26–15A–C).**

Locked Plating of the Distal Femur (see Videos 26–5, 26–6, Disk 3)

A variety of locked plating systems have become commercially available in the past 5 years. All have the common feature of multiple fixed-angle locked screws, which provide improved fixation of the distal femoral block. This becomes particularly important when the fracture has a "short" distal

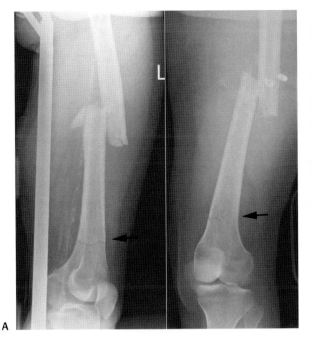

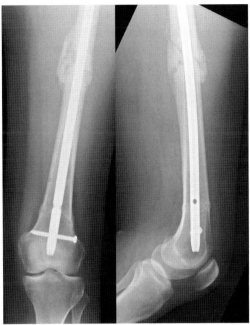

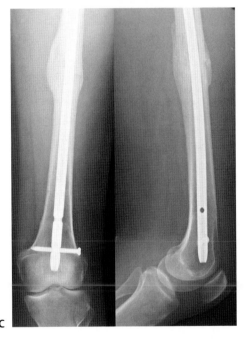

Figure 26–15 Treatment of a nondisplaced supracondylar femur fracture with associated femoral shaft fracture with an antegrade nail. **(A)** Injury radiographs. Note the non-displaced supracondylar fracture (arrow). **(B)** Follow-up radiographs at 2 months. **(C)** Follow-up radiographs at 6 months. In most cases, two distal interlocking screws are utilized.

femoral block, multiplanar articular involvement, or osteoporosis. All of these plating systems were the successors of the condylar buttress plate. Historically, before retrograde nails and locked plates for the distal femur were available, either the 95 degree angled blade plate or the DCS was utilized for simple A and C1/C2 fractures, and the condylar buttress plate was utilized for comminuted C3 injuries. The usual clinical problem with the condylar buttress plate was screw loosening and toggling and subsequent varus collapse.[77]

All of the locked plates provide the mechanical advantages already noted. In addition, they can be passed in a submuscular manner if desired. The Less Invasive Stabilization System (LISS, Synthes, Paoli, Pennsylvania) is a

particular locked plate (fixator), which was the first one available and which has several published series describing its use.[13–19,31,32,36,37] Although the LISS plate is utilized in several of the case examples in this section, the concept of a locked fixator passed in a submuscular manner is more important than specifics of the device itself. The surgical technique that is detailed following here is applicable to any submuscular plating of the distal femur. In addition, each of the implants can be utilized in a completely open fashion, as is detailed in the earlier section on the application of a 95 degree angled blade plate.

The leg lengths and rotational profile of the contralateral extremity, if possible, are examined preoperatively to

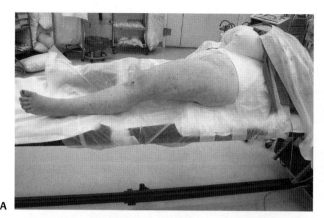

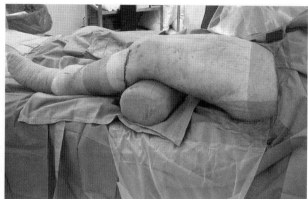

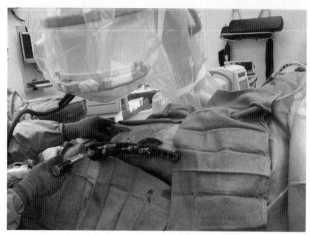

Figure 26–16 Intraoperative patient positioning for submuscular locked plating of the distal femur. **(A)** The patient is positioned on a radiolucent table with a bump underneath the left buttock. The left hip and lower extremity are completely prepped in the surgical field. Appropriate padding is underneath the right lower extremity. **(B)** Supracondylar bumps underneath the left knee. **(C)** Submuscular fixator placement utilizing an outrigger guide.

ascertain the correct rotational profile of the distal femur. A towel bump is then placed under the ipsilateral buttock to counteract the normal external rotation of the lower extremity. If the pelvis is tilted up ∼15 degrees on the involved side, and the rotational profile of the injured femur is correctly reestablished, the foot will usually be 5 to 10 degrees externally rotated at the end of the case. This is a helpful check to avoid serious rotational malalignment. Operative intervention is best performed on a completely radiolucent table, which allows imaging of the entire lower leg. Appropriate padding is placed under the uninvolved extremity, which is secured in place. Prep and drape should allow for complete exposure of the proximal femur and hip region, especially if a longer fixator is to be utilized **(Fig. 26–16A–C).**

The goal of locked submuscular plate fixation of the distal femur is to maintain the soft tissue environment around the metaphyseal/diaphyseal component of the fracture. This is performed utilizing closed reduction techniques. A variety of "aids" facilitate the closed reduction techniques, including:

1. *Early intervention* As mentioned earlier, fractures are addressed as soon as possible. If high-energy, shattered fractures are not stabilized in the first 24 hours, a spanning external fixator is placed to maintain the length of the fractured extremity.

2. *Chemical paralysis* Complete clinical paralysis of the patient is necessary.

3. *Supracondylar towel bumps* Supracondylar towel bumps made of 10, 12, and 15 rolled surgical towels wrapped with an elastic bandage are placed in the area posterior to the supracondylar region. The towel bumps aid in reduction of the common hyperextension of the distal femoral fragment **(Figs. 26–16B** and **26–17).** In addition,

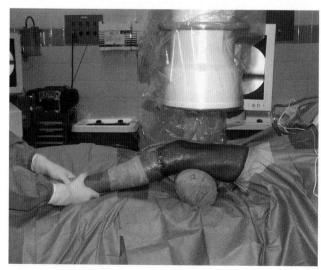

Figure 26–17 Manual intraoperative traction is applied using a supracondylar towel bump as a fulcrum.

the bump acts as a fulcrum for the vector force of the manual traction pull. Relatively small adjustments in the size and location of the towel bumps can make large differences in sagittal plane correction of the fracture.

4. *Manual traction* (**Fig. 26–17**) Hard manual traction is helpful to establish length and rotation, and may facilitate varus/valgus correction. Manual traction is applied to the ankle region, with a force vector that is directed posteriorly. Utilizing the towel bumps as a fulcrum, the manual traction facilitates reduction of the hyperextension deformity of the distal femoral condyle.

5. *Distal femoral condyle Schanz pin* Especially in cases of a very short distal femoral segment, correction of the hyperextension deformity may be difficult. This may be aided by an anterior to posterior Schanz pin, which may act as a reduction aid to derotate the distal fragment into appropriate reduction (**Fig. 26–18**).

6. *Reduction screws* Several of the locked plating systems have the ability to utilize regular nonlocking cortical screws in addition to locked screws in the proximal fragment. These screws may be utilized as reduction aids, especially when the shaft is medialized distally and needs to be brought laterally. It should be emphasized that such a screw should be utilized to "fine tune" the reduction by correcting up to several millimeters of displacement. A screw should not be utilized to correct major displacements. Another type of a reduction screw is that of the so-called whirlybird device, which is essentially a Schanz pin that drills into the bone. The LISS has an outrigger device for introduction of the screws, and

the whirlybird device has a turning nut that turns against the outrigger of the LISS insertion device. It can be utilized to afford small corrections in the frontal plan, or to afford small correction in varus/valgus deformities. Placement of the whirlybird device can also be thought of as a clamp that stabilizes the bone while self-drilling, self-tapping locking screws are placed in the bone. These screws would otherwise push away the bone.

7. *Femoral distractor or external fixator* The femoral distractor or external fixator may be utilized to obtain and maintain the metaphyseal/diaphyseal reduction. However, its use may make fine adjustments in fracture reduction difficult.

8. *Manual pressure* Manual pressure utilizing a large mallet is occasionally necessary to push medially on an adducted or flexed proximal fragment. In addition, it may be utilized on the distal fragment to correct excess valgus (**Fig. 26–19**).

Surgical Sequence of Submuscular Plating (see Videos 26–1, 26–5, 26–6, and 26–7, Disk 3)

Just as with placement of any fixation device for distal femoral fractures, there is a well-defined, stepwise process for locked submuscular plating. Although there may be variations on this sequence, it is helpful to address each step in the surgical sequence. This sequence begins after articular fracture reduction and fixation.

1. *Provisional fracture reduction ("learning the fracture")* Before the plate is inserted, manual traction is applied, the supracondylar bumps are placed, and the fracture reduction is visualized on both AP and lateral fluoroscopy. The surgeon can then note facts such as hyperextension of the distal femoral condyle, flexion or adduction of the proximal femoral shaft, and valgus of the distal femoral condyles. Adjustments in position

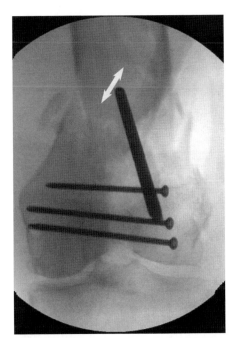

Figure 26–18 An anterior to posterior Schanz pin is placed in the distal femoral block after articular reduction and fixation. This can be utilized to correct a hyperextension deformity in the distal femur.

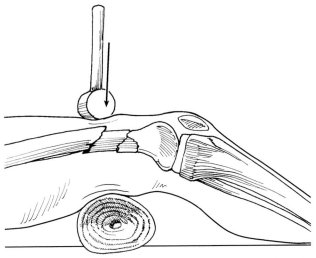

Figure 26–19 Direct pressure from a mallet may be placed on the distal aspect of the proximal segment for reduction of a supracondylar femur fracture.

and size of the supracondylar bumps, vector force direction of manual traction, and correction of deformities utilizing the large mallet can then be made.

2. *Plate insertion* The locked plate is inserted through either the anterolateral incision or a lateral parapatellar approach. Most plates are precontoured to account for the anterior bow of the femur. This step can be done under brief live fluoroscopy and is aided by the tactile sensation of the proximal tip of the plate on the lateral cortex, and the direction of plate insertion compared with the normal anterior bow of the femur. A common tendency is to direct the fixator posteriorly.

3. *Establishment of appropriate placement of the plate on the distal femoral condyle* Several comments are helpful in establishing the correct placement of the distal plate on the lateral femoral condyle:

   - Because the lateral cortex slopes ∼10 degrees, it is necessary to "tilt" the plate to fit the lateral cortex **(Fig. 26–20A)**.
   - The normal position for the given plate should be learned. For example, the LISS fixator normally should be positioned ∼1 to 1.5 cm posterior to the most anterior aspect of the distal femoral condyle and ∼1 to 1.5 cm cephalad to the distal aspect of the femoral condyle **(Fig. 26–20B)**.

After correct placement of the plate on the distal femoral block is established, it is then connected to the distal femoral block. This may be done with a guidewire or one or two screws. If placing locked screws, counterpressure is placed on the medial aspect of the distal femoral condylar region, and the plate is pushed against the bone because locked screws will tend to push away the bone.

4. *Check of reduction–rotation and length with placement of proximal guidewire* A check is made at this point via fluoroscopy in the AP plane to ensure that the proper length of the injured extremity has been reestablished. At this point, the rotational profile of the limb is also assessed using three separate methods: utilizing the knowledge that the foot should be externally rotated 10 to 15 degrees, assessment of the femur with AP fluoroscopy, and evaluation of the skin lines in the distal femoral region. If length and rotation are correct, the proximal end of the plate is affixed to the bone by either a screw or a guidewire, depending upon the system being utilized. A proximal incision may be utilized to ensure that the upper end of the plate is on the midlateral aspect of the bone and that it is in the proper rotation. Additionally, lateral fluoroscopy can be utilized to assess placement of the fixator on the midlateral aspect of the femur, but visualization may be difficult due to the other leg. At this point, corrections in sagittal plane alignment are possible, as noted later. Finally, small corrections of adduction of the proximal fragment, or in varus/valgus alignment of the distal femoral condyle are made.

5. *Placement of screws in the distal femoral block* The common deformities that occur are hyperextension or valgus or both. Hyperextension is corrected by repositioning the supracondylar towel bumps, changing the direction of manual traction, manual pressure, or control of the distal femoral block utilizing a Schanz pin. After the correct placement of the fixator on the distal femoral block is assured *and* after appropriate

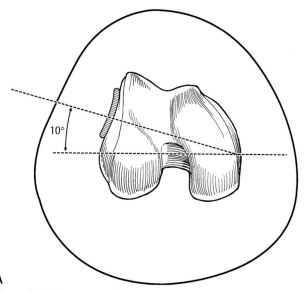

A

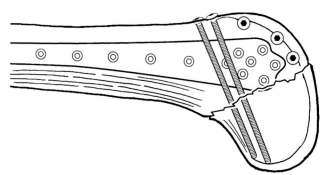

B

Figure 26–20 Drawings of the correct positioning of the Less Invasive Stabilization System (LISS) plate. **(A)** When utilizing the LISS fixator on the distal femur, the hand is raised ∼10 degrees to match the lateral cortical slope. **(B)** When utilizing the LISS fixator, it is brought to an area ∼1.5 cm from the distal articular surface and ∼1 cm from the anterior articular surface. Note anterior to posterior lag screws are placed for fixation of the coronal plane (Hoffa) fracture, and lateral to medial screws are placed for fixation of the intra-articular split.

correction of any deformity is made, several screws may be placed distally.

6. *Appropriate reduction of the proximal femoral shaft, and fixation with additional screws* At this point, any frontal plane (varus/valgus) or sagittal plane (hyperextension/hyperflexion) deformity is corrected,

and additional screws are placed in the proximal femur.

7. *Assessment of fracture reduction and stability* The knee is taken through a full gentle range of motion to ensure fracture fixation adequacy.

8. *Wound irrigation and closure*

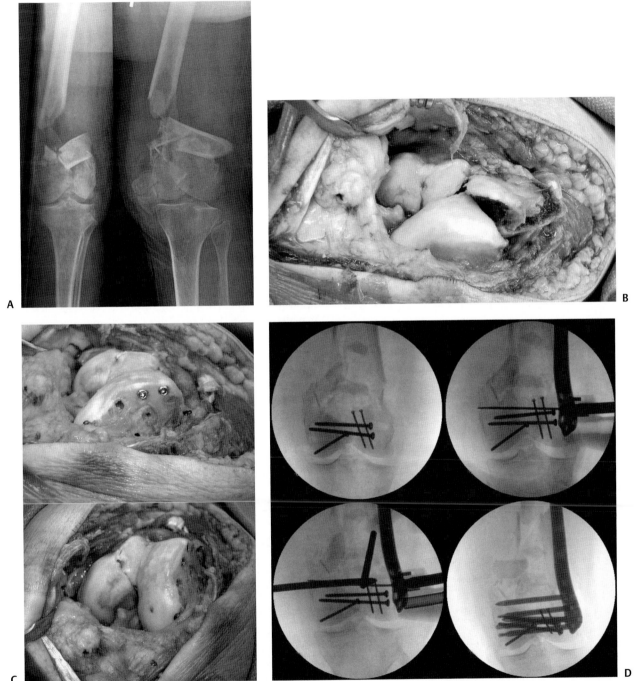

Figure 26–21 Less Invasive Stabilization System (LISS) fixation of a C3 distal femur fracture in a 67-year-old female with preexisting osteoarthritis and insulin-dependent diabetes mellitus. **(A)** Radiograph of injury. **(B)** Intraoperative view of the surface. **(C)** The patient had an associated patellar tendon disruption. A modified lateral peripatellar approach allowed for excellent visualization of the artic-

ular surface. The articular surface is seen here reduced and fixed with multiple lag screws. **(D)** After reduction and fixation of the articular surface, a submuscular plating was then performed. A guidewire is parallel to the joint surface to ensure appropriate reduction to the distal femur. Multiple distal screws were then placed. *(Continued on page 654.)*

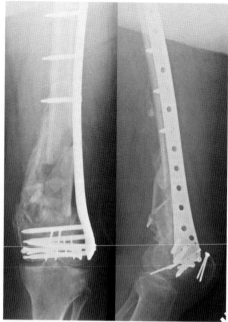

E

Figure 26–21 *(Continued)* Less Invasive Stabilization System (LISS) fixation of a C3 distal femur fracture in a 67-year-old female with pre-existing osteoarthritis and insulin-dependent diabetes mellitus. **(E)** Follow-up radiographs at 4 months demonstrate considerable metaphyseal healing.

Case examples are utilized to demonstrate this sequence (**Figs. 26–21A–E, 26–22A–E,** and **26–23A–D**).

Assessment of Reduction after Fixation of an A- or C-Type Distal Femur Fracture

After fixation of a distal femur fracture, it is important to assess the quality of the reduction in terms of axial alignment, rotation, and length. Specific questions to be asked are:

- How is the valgus/varus alignment?
- Is there hyperextension of the distal femoral condyles?
- Is there any sagittal plane deformity in the diaphysis?
- How is the placement of the fixator or the midlateral aspect of the femur?

The rotation of the limb should be assessed by examining the resting position of the foot, the hip rotational profile, and a radiographic survey of the proximal femur compared with the distal femur/knee joint.[54]

Special Case: Fixation of a Supracondylar Femur Fracture above a Total Knee Arthroplasty (see Video 26–7, Disk 3)

In a setting of a fracture above the femoral component of a total knee arthroplasty, the surgeon must first ensure that there is no loosening of the total knee arthroplasty (**Fig. 26–24A,B** and **26–25A–D**). This is rare, but if it does occur, consideration is given to a total knee revision. Assuming that no loosening is seen, the surgeon may treat the fracture with retrograde nailing or lateral plating.[37,55–59] Retrograde nailing is not applicable to all total knee designs and risks damage to the patellar component and the introduction of particulate debris into the joint. Standard plating utilizing a nonlocking condylar buttress plate or 95 degree angled device has proven efficacious for treatment of these fractures. However, the periprosthetic distal femur fracture is often characterized by a short distal segment in osteoporotic bone. For this reason, locked plating has recently been utilized, and its results are encouraging.[37,56,60] Althausen et al reported low infection rates, no requirement for acute bone grafting, and secure fixation allowing for immediate postoperative immobilization when using the LISS internal

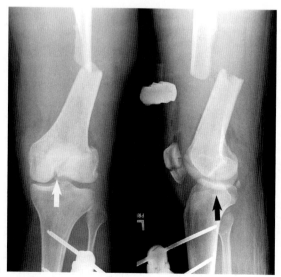

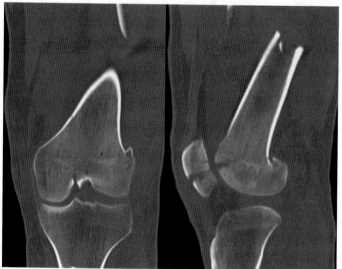

A   B

Figure 26–22 Type III-A open C1 distal femur fracture. **(A)** Radiograph of the injury. The white and black arrows demonstrate the interarticular split. **(B)** The patient had a minimally displaced patellar fracture. The computed tomographic (CT) scan also demonstrates the interarticular split. *(Continued)*

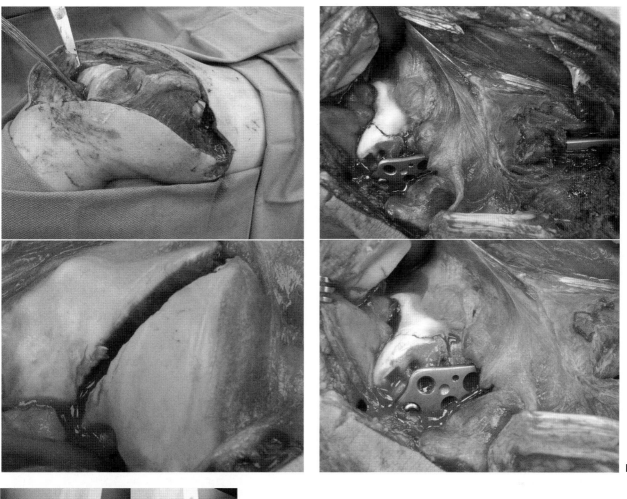

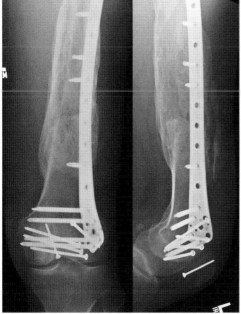

Figure 26–22 *(Continued)* **(C)** A modified lateral peripatellar approach was made utilizing the open wound. Visualization of the articular surface is seen here. **(D)** Fixation of the articular surface was performed, followed by submuscular plating utilizing the Less Invasive Stabilization System (LISS). Note maintenance of the metaphyseal soft tissue around the fracture. **(E)** Complete consolidation of the fracture seen at 1 year. The patient was full weight bearing at 10 weeks. This eventual knee motion was 0 to 130 degrees, symmetrical with the opposite leg.

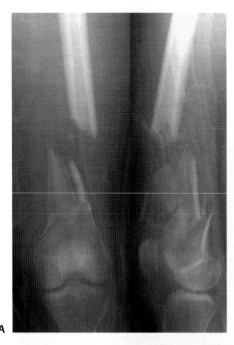

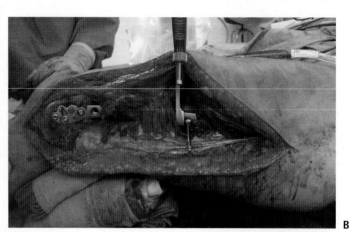

Figure 26–23 Open plating of a C1 distal femur fracture with significant bone loss and 10 cm open wound. **(A)** Injury radiograph. **(B)** The patient underwent irrigation and debridement of the open wound. A lateral approach to the distal femur followed. Note maintenance of the soft tissue environment around the fracture despite an open approach. **(C)** The patient underwent bone grafting at 10 weeks postinjury. **(D)** Complete radiographic healing at 4 months. (Case courtesy of William Ricci, M.D.)

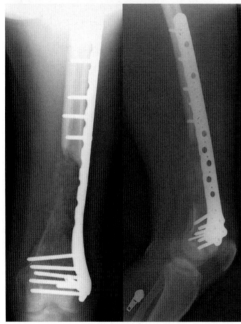

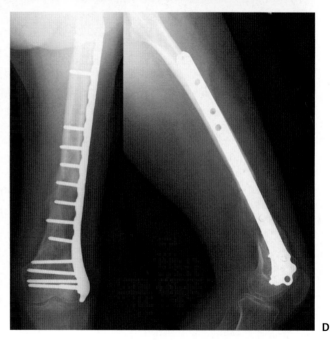

fixator for periprosthetic fractures above the knee.[56] In a case series of 13 fractures, Kregor et al reported no infections, no varus collapse, secondary bone grafting, and one revision total knee arthroplasty for loosening of the femoral component when using the LISS.[37]

Retrograde intramedullary nailing is performed as already described. The old medial peripatellar incision is utilized to expose the femoral component of the total knee arthroplasty. It is important that two distal screws be utilized to obtain adequate purchase in the distal femoral block. It is determined preoperatively if the particular knee arthroplasty will "accept" a retrograde nail. If this is not possible, then plating should be utilized.

The plating technique is the same as noted earlier for the submuscular locked plating of the distal femur. It is helpful to have a good quality lateral radiograph of the distal femur to preoperatively plan placement of the plate and screws.

Reduction and Fixation of a Medial or Lateral Condyle Fracture

A medial or lateral approach is utilized for the respective fracture. If the fracture has a simple articular pattern, an anterolateral or anteromedial approach is utilized. For the more complex fractures, a medial or lateral peripatellar approach

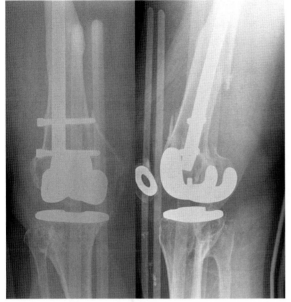

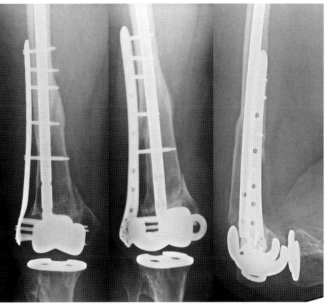

A   B

Figure 26–24 Minimally displaced supracondylar femur fracture at the junction between the tip of an existing antegrade intramedullary nail and a total knee arthroplasty. **(A)** Injury radiographs.

(B) Follow-up radiographs at 3 years posttrauma. The surgical tactic was the placement of the locked fixator posterior to the intramedullary nail to obtain proximal fixation.

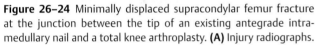

Tips and Tricks

- Significant displacement of a supracondylar femur fracture can lead to similar displacement of fracture fragments, as seen in high-energy tibial plateau fractures or knee dislocations. As such, vascular injury should always be suspected with a displaced, high-energy supracondylar femur fracture. It is prudent in these cases to obtain an ankle-ankle index (AAI) or ankle-brachial index (ABI).[61–63]

- Proper characterization of the articular injury is critical. If the surgeon suspects a supracondylar femur fracture, the question must be asked, Could this be an articular injury? If it is determined that there is an articular injury, the questions are: Are there frontal plane Hoffa fractures? Is this a complex multiplanar articular injury? Are there separate osteochondral fragments? These questions are best assessed by either traction AP/lateral/oblique radiographs of the distal femur or a CT scan with sagittal and frontal reconstructions.

- The surgeon should try to avoid the situation whereby an anterolateral approach is done for a fracture that has a medial Hoffa fracture. In this situation, reduction and fixation of the medial Hoffa fracture may be difficult. However, if this does occur, a separate medial parapatellar approach can be made to visualize and internally fix the medial femoral condyle.

- The common deformity following internal fixation of a supracondylar/intercondylar femur fracture is hyperextension, excess valgus, and excess rotation. Thus the surgeon should understand how to correct these deformities.

- If a "notch" view of the distal femur is seen with an AP radiograph, the distal femur has a hyperextension deformity.

- Screws that are anterior in the distal femoral block and that

appear of appropriate length may be long secondary to the sloped nature of the medial femoral condyle.

- A "one-shot" fluoroscopic view of the distal femur may not give the surgeon a good perception of the overall axial alignment of the distal femur. Scanning with the fluoroscopy unit from proximal to distal allows the surgeon to better determine the presence of any varus or valgus deformities.

- In reducing a complex C3 distal femur articular injury with Hoffa fractures, it is generally advisable to provisionally fix the entire articular surface before definitive fixation. As with any complex articular injury, the ability to determine the exact positioning of separate osteochondral fragments may be difficult until the entire articular surface is reconstructed.

- A 5.0 or 6.0 mm diameter Schanz pin may be placed in the medial femoral condyle from medial to lateral through a percutaneous wound on the medial aspect of the knee. It is then used to reduce the intercondylar fracture. The tip of the screw should not protrude into the fracture site, because it would then prevent reduction.

- A Schanz pin from anterior to posterior in the femoral condylar block will help correct a hyperextension deformity.

- The fixation for a C-type (supracondylar/intercondylar) distal femur fracture should be viewed as two stages: (1) articular block reduction and fixation, and (2) reduction and fixation of the metaphyseal/diaphyseal component of the fracture. The articular block reduction is nearly always by direct reduction (e.g., clamp application). In most cases (except in simple fractures) the metaphyseal/diaphyseal component of the fracture is by indirect reduction.

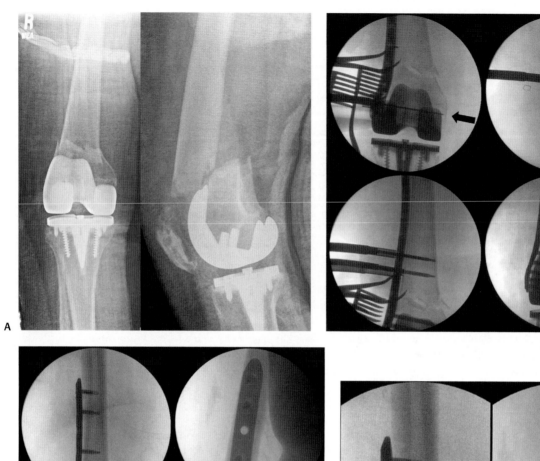

Figure 26–25 The use of a submuscular locked fixator for treatment of a supracondylar femur fracture above total knee arthroplasty. **(A)** Radiograph of the injury. **(B)** Intraoperative fluoroscopic views. A small 8 cm incision is made over the distal femur. The fixator is placed in a submuscular manner. Multiple screws are placed in the distal femur. The guidewire is parallel to the femoral component (arrow). **(C)** Intraoperative fluoroscopic views. **(D)** Fluoroscopic views showing that the upper tip of the plate is centered on the femoral shaft.

may be utilized. Fixation of the articular surface is performed as noted above. In most cases, an antiglide plate is placed on the medial or lateral aspect of the respective femoral condyle. A 4.5 mm narrow plate is routinely used and is undercontoured slightly. The screw just proximal to the fracture prevents shear of the condyle fracture, which might be possible with screw fixation alone **(Fig. 26–26A,B).**

Rehabilitation

Type A fractures: For fractures of the distal femur without articular involvement, the patient is usually partially weight-bearing. Aggressive knee range of motion exercises are immediately begun, as are quadriceps strengthening exercises. After 4 to 6 weeks, progressive weight

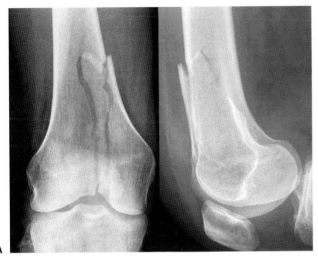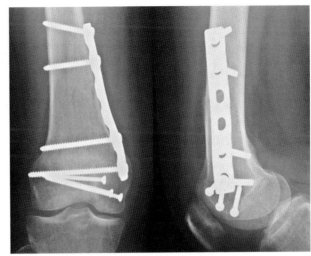

A   B

Figure 26–26 Medial femoral condyle fracture. **(A)** Radiographs of the injury. **(B)** The patient underwent direct visualization of the articular surface, lag screw fixation across the articular surface, and antiglide medial plate placement.

bearing is allowed. This may be modified in patients with severe osteoporosis.

Type B and C fractures: For those patients with an articular injury, progressive weight bearing is not allowed for 10 to 12 weeks. No braces are used.

New Techniques

No significant change in the philosophy or instrumentation in the treatment of distal femur fractures has taken place in the last five years. A greater understanding of the role of locked plating and submuscular techniques is developing. The concept of variable axis locking screws that lock into the plate after being placed at a certain angle has recently been made commercially available.

Outcomes

There is no consensus on the long-term advantages of any type of operative treatment; however, it is clear that operative treatment has considerable advantages over nonoperative treatment. In a relatively recent study (1996), Butt et al compared operative treatment of displaced distal femur fractures in elderly patients using a DCS with nonoperative treatment.[46] The results overwhelmingly favored operative treatment. By the criteria of Schatzker et al,[8] excellent or good results were achieved in 53% of the patients undergoing operative treatment and only 31% of the patients undergoing nonoperative treatment. There were overall fewer complications in the operative group, which also had a shorter average hospital stay. It can be postulated that these results might even be more different with modern-day operative treatment.

Definitive treatment and implant options for supracondylar/ intercondylar femur fractures include plating (blade plate, DCS, condylar buttress plate), antegrade intramedullary nailing, retrograde intramedullary nailing, external fixation, and locked internal fixation (e.g., LISS, locked condylar buttress plate).

Schatzker et al's first experiences with plating (mostly blade plates) in the early 1970s showed greatly improved outcomes compared with nonoperative treatment. In 75% of the patients in which rigid fixation was achieved, good or excellent results were achieved compared with 32% that underwent nonoperative treatment.[8] In 18 of 35 patients, however, rigid fixation could not have been achieved. Of those patients only 21% had a good or excellent result. As seen in Schatzker et al's and other subsequently published case series, functional outcome improved with rigid fixation but did not yield consistently good results.[3,8]

As operative techniques evolved and new implant technologies were developed, the results greatly improved. "Biological" indirect reduction techniques[10] and retrograde intramedullary nailing decreased the need for bone grafting that was used in up to 87% of the cases in earlier series as reviewed by Miclau et al.[1] In a series of 57 fractures (eight A2, 14 A3, 10 C1, 16 C2, and nine C3 fractures; Gustilo type IIIB or IIIC open fractures excluded) treated with blade plates and condylar buttress plates using indirect reduction techniques and no bone grafting, Bolhofner et al reported no nonunions and good or excellent results in 84% of the cases.[12] The advent of retrograde intramedullary nailing also resulted in improved outcomes and decreased infection rates.[20-27] However, the use of retrograde intramedullary nailing is for the most part limited to extraarticular fracture and fractures with simple articular involvement.

Table 26—3   Results of Different Fixation Techniques for Distal Femur Fractures, 1989–2005

Implant/ Technique	Total # of Series	Total *n*	Articular Involvement***	Nonunions (%)	Deep Infection (%)	Secondary Surgical Procedures (%)
AIMN	4	108	22.2% (*n* = 108)	8.3	0.9	23.1
RIMN	15	472	37.1% (*n* = 361)	5.3	0.4	24.2
Internal Fixator (LISS)	8	327	56.9% (*n* = 327)	5.5	2.1	16.2
Compression plate (BP, DCS, CBP, or other)**	16	694	73.0% (*n* = 677)	6.3	4.8	12.7
External fixator	5	69	85.5% (*n* = 69)	7.2	4.3	30.6
Total	48*	1670	58.1% (*n* = 1542)	6.0	2.7	16.8

Source: Data from Zlowodzki M, Bhandari M, Marek DJ, Cole PA, Kregor PJ. Operative treatment of acute distal femur fractures: systematic review of two comparative studies and 45 case series (1989–2005). J Orthop Trauma 2006:366–371.

AIMN, antegrade intramedullary nail; BP, blade plate; CBP, condylar buttress plate; DCS, dynamic condylar screw; LISS, Less Invasive Stabilization System; RIMN, retrograde intramedullary nail. In all treatment options adjunctive screws and/or plates were used to fix the articular surface.

*45 case series, one operative arm of a randomized control trial (RCT) and one comparative study with one LISS and one RIMN arm.

**Primary Implant: BP, 41%; DCS, 33%; CBP, 23%; Other, 3%.

***Some authors did not report on the involvement of the articular surface. The number of patients that articular involvement is reported on is depicted in parentheses and is therefore sometimes lower than total *n*.

The development of locked internal fixators was a further step toward improving outcomes on a more consistent basis, especially by improving distal fixation in osteoporotic bone and facilitating submuscular insertion techniques, which resulted in decreased distal implant "cut-out" rates and decreased infection rates, especially in open fractures.[13–19,31,32,36,37]

Overall, in an evidence-based systematic review, we identified 47 articles with a total of 1670 fractures between 1989 and 2005 reporting on the outcome of operative treatment of acute nonperiprosthetic distal femur fractures.[64] The average nonunion rate was 6.0%, the deep infection rate was 2.7%, and the average secondary surgical procedure rate was 16.8% **(Table 26–3).**

When comparing compression plating techniques (blade plate, DCS, nonlocking condylar buttress plate, and others) with an internal fixator (LISS), there was a statistically nonsignificant trend ($p = .056$) toward lower deep infection rates with the use of an internal fixator (2.1%) compared with compression plating techniques (4.8%) despite a significantly higher percentage of open fractures in the internal fixator group (36 vs 25%).[64]

Complications

Complications in the treatment of distal femur fractures may include nonunion, infection, malunion, and joint stiffness. Extensive soft tissue dissection during the operative procedure destroys the blood supply around the fracture[29,30] and compromises the ability of the body to heal the fracture and to clear pathogens. This may result in higher nonunion and infection rates.

Treatment options for nonunions depend on the primary treatment and may include debridement of the nonunion followed by bone grafting with or without implant exchange. If intramedullary nailing was the primary treatment, exchange nailing is an option with reaming instead of or in addition to bone grafting. Another treatment strategy is to change the fixation technique; for example, from intramedullary nailing to plating or vice versa to change biomechanics at the fracture site and thereby stimulate the biological healing potential of the cells at the fracture site. Infections can be treated with a single or if necessary multiple irrigation and debridements and intravenous antibiotics. Occasionally, plating may lead to local soft tissue irritation, causing pain. In those cases the plate/internal fixator can be removed after the fracture is healed.

Extensive muscle dissection and postoperative rehabilitation restrictions are often due to suboptimal fixation and may also lead to increased knee joint stiffness, especially in articular fractures. On the other hand, minimally invasive techniques can preserve the blood supply and the fracture hematoma and therefore can have a positive effect on fracture healing and infection rates. However, minimally invasive techniques are technically demanding, making bone alignment difficult and therefore potentially increasing the likelihood of malalignment/ malunion. Plating techniques in general have been associated with malreductions. In a series of 57 fractures, Zehnnter et al reported a malalignment of > 5 degrees for varus/valgus in 26%, hyperextension/hyperflexion in 22%, and rotational deformities in 17% of the cases.[53] Functional results appeared to be satisfactory if malalignment was within 5 degrees in any plane. In general, solid fixation with preservation of muscles during the operative procedure also allows for a more aggressive postoperative rehabilitation protocol and can therefore preserve joint motion.

Pearls

- According to the AO/OTA classification of distal femur fractures, type A fractures are extra-articular, type B fractures are partial articular fractures, and type C fractures represent a complete intra-articular fracture with dissociation from the diaphysis.
- To differentiate between C-type injuries, a C1/C2 injury has a simple articular split, and a C3 injury has complex articular involvement.
- Reasonable treatment options for a type A or C1/C2 fracture include antegrade nailing, retrograde nailing, plating with a 95 degree angled device (blade plate or DCS), or plating with an internal fixator. Generally, a C3-type injury should be treated with a locked fixator to allow for placement of multiple screws in the distal femoral block and to avoid varus collapse.
- There is a 38% incidence of frontal plane (Hoffa) fractures in type C supracondylar fractures.[39]
- The common deformity following internal fixation of a supracondylar/intercondylar femur fracture is hyperextension, excess valgus, and excess rotation.
- According to a recent systematic review of the literature,[64] the average nonunion rate was 6.0%, the deep infection rate was 2.7%, and the average secondary surgical procedure rate was 16.8%.
- Historically, the rate of bone grafting for a distal femur fracture has ranged between 0 and 87%.[1]

On the DVDs

Video 26–1 (Same as **Video 4–2, Disk 1**) **Minimally Invasive Percutaneous Plate Osteosynthesis of the Distal Femur** The patient in this video is treated with a DCS plate applied using MIPPO techniques and bridge plating. The surgeon demonstrates tricks for success with MIPPO, including judgment of length and rotation.

Video 26–2 (Same as **Video 25–5, Disk 3**) **Retrograde Intramedullary Nail for A Type Supracondylar Femur Fracture** A 2.5 cm medial parapatellar approach is utilized for stabilization for an A type supracondylar femur fracture. Emphasis is on correct starting point and fracture reduction.

Video 26–3 (Same as **Video 25–6, Disk 3**) **Retrograde Intramedullary Nailing of the Distal Femur** This video demonstrates the technique and principles for retrograde nailing of a supracondylar femur fracture using a tendon splitting approach. The importance of the correct starting point is emphasized.

Video 26–4 (**Disk 3**) **Arthroscopic-Assisted Removal of a Retrograde Nail** Removal of a retrograde intramedullary nail is remarkably facilitated by using an arthroscopic assisted technique. The use of arthroscopy and method of removal are demonstrated.

Video 26–5 (Same as **Video 4–4, Disk 1**) **ORIF of a C2 Distal Femur Fracture with Submuscular Locked Plating** Submuscular locked fixation is performed for a ballistic C2 distal femur fracture in a 34-year-old male. Delayed reconstruction is carried out following placement of a spanning external fixator, originally placed after repair of a vascular injury.

Video 26–6 (**Disk 3**) **Submuscular Locked Fixation of a Combined C3 Distal Femur and C3 Proximal Tibial Fracture** A modified lateral peripatellar approach is utilized for direct visualization of complex articular injuries of both the tibial plateau and distal femur. The steps of submuscular locked fixation are emphasized.

Video 26–7 (Same as **Video 4–3, Disk 1**) **ORIF of a Periprosthetic Distal Femur Fracture with Submuscular Locked Plating** LISS fixation of a distal femur fracture is performed in an osteoporotic distal femur fracture above a total knee arthroplasty. Minimal exposure of the fracture and closed reduction techniques are emphasized.

References

1. Miclau T, Holmes W, Martin RE, Krettek C, Schandelmaier P. Plate osteosynthesis of the distal femur: surgical techniques and results. J South Orthop Assoc 1998;7:161–170
2. Schatzker J. Fractures of the distal femur revisited. Clin Orthop Relat Res 1998;347:43–56
3. Siliski JM, Mahring M, Hofer HP. Supracondylar-intercondylar fractures of the femur: treatment by internal fixation. J Bone Joint Surg Am 1989;71:95–104
4. Neer CS, Grantham SA, Shelton ML. Supracondylar fracture of the adult femur: a study of one hundred and ten cases. J Bone Joint Surg Am 1967;49:591–613
5. Stewart MJ, Sisk TD, Wallace SH Jr. Fractures of the distal third of the femur: a comparison of methods of treatment. J Bone Joint Surg Am 1966;48:784–807
6. Olerud S. Supracondylar, intraarticular fracture of the femur: results of operative reconstruction. Acta Orthop Scand 1971;42:435–437
7. Wenzl H. Results in 112 surgically treated distal femoral fractures [in German]. Hefte Unfallheilkd 1975;120:15–24
8. Schatzker J, Home G, Waddell J. The Toronto experience with the supracondylar fracture of the femur, 1966–72. Injury 1974;6:113–128
9. Schatzker J, Lambert DC. Supracondylar fractures of the femur. Clin Orthop Relat Res 1979;138:77–83
10. Mast JW, Jakob R, Ganz R. In: Planning and Reduction Technique in Fracture Surgery. New York: Springer-Verlag; 1989
11. Gerber C, Mast JW, Ganz R. Biological internal fixation of fractures. Arch Orthop Trauma Surg 1990;109:295–303

12. Bolhofner BR, Carmen B, Clifford P. The results of open reduction and internal fixation of distal femur fractures using a biologic (indirect) reduction technique. J Orthop Trauma 1996;10:372–377

13. Kregor PJ, Stannard JA, Zlowodzki M, Cole PA. Treatment of distal femur fractures using the less invasive stabilization system: surgical experience and early clinical results in 103 fractures. J Orthop Trauma 2004;18:509–520

14. Schütz M, Muller M, Regazzoni P, et al. Use of the less invasive stabilization system (LISS) in patients with distal femoral (AO33) fractures: a prospective multicenter study. Arch Orthop Trauma Surg 2005;125:102–108

15. Fankhauser F, Gruber G, Schippinger G, et al. Minimal-invasive treatment of distal femoral fractures with the LISS (Less Invasive Stabilization System): a prospective study of 30 fractures with a follow-up of 20 months. Acta Orthop Scand 2004;75:56–60

16. Markmiller M, Konrad G, Sudkamp N. Femur-LISS and distal femoral nail for fixation of distal femoral fractures: are there differences in outcome and complications? Clin Orthop Relat Res 2004;426:252–257

17. Weight M, Collinge C. Early results of the less invasive stabilization system for mechanically unstable fractures of the distal femur (AO/OTA types A2, A3, C2, and C3). J Orthop Trauma 2004;18: 503–508

18. Syed AA, Agarwal M, Giannoudis PV, Matthews SJ, Smith RM. Distal femoral fractures: long-term outcome following stabilisation with the LISS. Injury 2004;35:599–607

19. Ricci AR, Yue JJ, Taffet R, Catalano JB, De Falco RA, Wilkens KJ. Less Invasive Stabilization System for treatment of distal femur fractures. Am J Orthop 2004;33:250–255

20. Lucas SE, Seligson D, Henry SL. Intramedullary supracondylar nailing of femoral fractures: a preliminary report of the GSH supracondylar nail. Clin Orthop Relat Res 1993;296:200–206

21. Iannacone WM, Bennett FS, DeLong WG Jr, Born CT, Dalsey RM. Initial experience with the treatment of supracondylar femoral fractures using the supracondylar intramedullary nail: a preliminary report. J Orthop Trauma 1994;8:322–327

22. Gellman RE, Paiement GD, Green HD, Coughlin RR. Treatment of supracondylar femoral fractures with a retrograde intramedullary nail. Clin Orthop Relat Res 1996;332:90–97

23. Janzing HM, Stockman B, Van Damme G, Rommens P, Broos PL. The retrograde intramedullary nail: prospective experience in patients older than sixty-five years. J Orthop Trauma 1998;12:330–333

24. Janzing HM, Stockman B, Van Damme G, Rommens P, Broos PL. The retrograde intramedullary supracondylar nail: an alternative in the treatment of distal femoral fractures in the elderly? Arch Orthop Trauma Surg 1998;118:92–95

25. Danziger MB, Caucci D, Zecher SB, Segal D, Covall DJ. Treatment of intercondylar and supracondylar distal femur fractures using the GSH supracondylar nail. Am J Orthop 1995;24:684–690

26. Gynning JB, Hansen D. Treatment of distal femoral fractures with intramedullary supracondylar nails in elderly patients. Injury 1999;30:43–46

27. Ostermann PA, Hahn MP, Ekkernkamp A, David A, Muhr G. Retrograde interlocking nailing of distal femoral fractures with the intramedullary supracondylar nail [in German]. Chirurg 1996;67: 1135–1140

28. Krettek C, Schandelmaier P, Miclau T, Tscherne H. Minimally invasive percutaneous plate osteosynthesis (MIPPO) using the DCS in proximal and distal femoral fractures. Injury 1997;28(Suppl 1): A20–A30

29. Farouk O, Krettek C, Miclau T, Schandelmaier P, Tscherne H. Effects of percutaneous and conventional plating techniques on the blood supply to the femur. Arch Orthop Trauma Surg 1998;117:438–441

30. Farouk O, Krettek C, Miclau T, Schandelmaier P, Guy P, Tscherne H. Minimally invasive plate osteosynthesis: does percutaneous plating disrupt femoral blood supply less than the traditional technique? J Orthop Trauma 1999;13:401–406

31. Kregor PJ, Stannard J, Zlowodzki M, Cole PA, Alonso J. Distal femoral fracture fixation utilizing the Less Invasive Stabilization System (L.I.S.S.): the technique and early results. Injury 2001;32(Suppl 3): SC32–SC47

32. Schutz M, Muller M, Krettek C, et al. Minimally invasive fracture stabilization of distal femoral fractures with the LISS: a prospective multicenter study. Results of a clinical study with special emphasis on difficult cases. Injury 2001;32:SC48–SC54

33. Kassab SS, Mast JW, Mayo KA. Patients treated for nonunions with plate and screw fixation and adjunctive locking nuts. Clin Orthop Relat Res 1998;347:86–92

34. Haas N, Hauke C, Schutz M, Kaab M, Perren SM. Treatment of diaphyseal fractures of the forearm using the Point Contact Fixator (PC-Fix): results of 387 fractures of a prospective multicentric study (PC-Fix II). Injury 2001;32(Suppl 2):B51–B62

35. Zlowodzki M, Williamson S, Cole PA, Zardiackas LD, Kregor PJ. Biomechanical evaluation of the less invasive stabilization system, angled blade plate, and retrograde intramedullary nail for the internal fixation of distal femur fractures. J Orthop Trauma 2004;18:494–502

36. Wong MK, Leung F, Chow SP. Treatment of distal femoral fractures in the elderly using a less-invasive plating technique. Int Orthop 2005;29:117–120

37. Kregor PJ, Hughes JL, Cole PA. Fixation of distal femoral fractures above total knee arthroplasty utilizing the Less Invasive Stabilization System (L.I.S.S.). Injury 2001;32(Suppl 3):SC64–SC75

38. Müller ME, Allgower M, Schneider R, Willenegger H. Manual of Internal Fixation: Techniques Recommended by the AO-ASIF Group. New York: Springer-Verlag; 1991:750

39. Nork SE, Segina DN, Aflatoon K, et al. The association between supracondylar-intercondylar distal femoral fractures and coronal plane fractures. J Bone Joint Surg Am 2005;87:564–569

40. Ostrum RF, Geel C. Indirect reduction and internal fixation of supracondylar femur fractures without bone graft. J Orthop Trauma 1995;9:278–284

41. Leung KS, Shen WY, So WS, Mui LT, Grosse A. Interlocking intramedullary nailing for supracondylar and intercondylar fractures of the distal part of the femur. J Bone Joint Surg Am 1991;73:332–340

42. Krettek C, Schandelmaier P, Miclau T, Bertram R, Holmes W, Tscherne H. Transarticular joint reconstruction and indirect plate osteosynthesis for complex distal supracondylar femoral fractures. Injury 1997;28(Suppl 1):A31–A41

43. Sanders R, Regazzoni P, Ruedi TP. Treatment of supracondylar-intracondylar fractures of the femur using the dynamic condylar screw. J Orthop Trauma 1989;3:214–222

44. Shewring DJ, Meggitt BF. Fractures of the distal femur treated with the AO dynamic condylar screw. J Bone Joint Surg Br 1992;74: 122–125

45. Ketterl R, Kostler W, Wittwer W, Stubinger B. 5-year results of dia/supracondylar femoral fractures, managed with the dynamic condylar screw [in German]. Zentralbl Chir 1997;122:1033–1039

46. Butt MS, Krikler SJ, Ali MS. Displaced fractures of the distal femur in elderly patients. Operative versus non-operative treatment. J Bone Joint Surg Br 1996;78:110–114

References **663**

47. Jeon IH, Oh CW, Kim SJ, Park BC, Kyung HS, Ihn JC. Minimally invasive percutaneous plating of distal femoral fractures using the dynamic condylar screw. J Trauma 2004;57:1048–1052

48. Huang HT, Huang PJ, Su JY, Lin SY. Indirect reduction and bridge plating of supracondylar fractures of the femur. Injury 2003;34:135–140

49. Sanders R, Swiontkowski M, Rosen H, Helfet D. Double-plating of comminuted, unstable fractures of the distal part of the femur. J Bone Joint Surg Am 1991;73A:341–346

50. Merchan EC, Maestu PR, Blanco RP. Blade-plating of closed displaced supracondylar fractures of the distal femur with the AO system. J Trauma 1992;32:174–178

51. Ziran BH, Rohde RH, Wharton AR. Lateral and anterior plating of intra-articular distal femoral fractures treated via an anterior approach. Int Orthop 2002;26:370–373

52. Yang RS, Liu HC, Liu TK. Supracondylar fractures of the femur. J Trauma 1990;30:315–319

53. Zehntner MK, Marchesi DG, Burch H, Ganz R. Alignment of supracondylar/intercondylar fractures of the femur after internal fixation by AO/ASIF technique. J Orthop Trauma 1992;6:318–326

54. Krettek C, Miclau T, Grun O, Schandelmaier P, Tscherne H. Intraoperative control of axes, rotation and length in femoral and tibial fractures: technical note. Injury 1998;29(Suppl 3):C29–C39

55. Bezwada HP, Neubauer P, Baker J, Israelite CL, Johanson NA. Periprosthetic supracondylar femur fractures following total knee arthroplasty. J Arthroplasty 2004;19:453–458

56. Althausen PL, Lee MA, Finkemeier CG, Meehan JP, Rodrigo JJ. Operative stabilization of supracondylar femur fractures above total knee arthroplasty: a comparison of four treatment methods. J Arthroplasty 2003;18:834–839

57. Chen F, Mont MA, Bachner RS. Management of ipsilateral supracondylar femur fractures following total knee arthroplasty. J Arthroplasty 1994;9:521–526

58. Zehntner MK, Ganz R. Internal fixation of supracondylar fractures after condylar total knee arthroplasty. Clin Orthop Relat Res 1993;293:219–224

59. Gliatis J, Megas P, Panagiotopoulos E, Lambiris E. Midterm results of treatment with a retrograde nail for supracondylar periprosthetic fractures of the femur following total knee arthroplasty. J Orthop Trauma 2005;19:164–170

60. Wick M, Muller EJ, Kutscha-Lissberg F, Hopf F, Muhr G. Periprosthetic supracondylar femoral fractures: LISS or retrograde intramedullary nailing? Problems with the use of minimally invasive technique [in German]. Unfallchirurg 2004;107:181–188

61. Levy BA, Zlowodzki MP, Graves M, Cole PA. Screening for extremity arterial injury with the arterial pressure index. Am J Emerg Med 2005;23:689–695

62. Johansen K, Lynch K, Paun M, Copass M. Non-invasive vascular tests reliably exclude occult arterial trauma in injured extremities. J Trauma 1991;31:515–519

63. Lynch K, Johansen K. Can Doppler pressure measurement replace "exclusion" arteriography in the diagnosis of occult extremity arterial trauma? Ann Surg 1991;214:737–741

64. Zlowodzki M, Bhandari M, Marek DJ, Cole PA, Kregor PJ. Operative treatment of acute distal femur fractures: Systematic review of two comparative studies and 45 case series (1989–2005). J Orthop Trauma 2006:366–371

65. Wu CC, Shih CH. Interlocking nailing of distal femoral fractures: 28 patients followed for 1–2 years. Acta Orthop Scand 1991;62:342–345

66. Dominguez I, Moro Rodriguez E, De Pedro Moro JA, Cebrian Parra JL, Lopez-Duran Stern L. Antegrade nailing for fractures of the distal femur. Clin Orthop Relat Res 1998;350:74–79

67. Butler MS, Brumback RJ, Ellison TS, Poka A, Bathon GH, Burgess AR. Interlocking intramedullary nailing for ipsilateral fractures of the femoral shaft and distal part of the femur. J Bone Joint Surg Am 1991;73:1492–1502

68. Armstrong R, Milliren A, Schrantz W, Zeliger K. Retrograde interlocked intramedullary nailing of supracondylar distal femur fractures in an average 76-year-old patient population. Orthopedics 2003;26:627–629

69. Seifert J, Stengel D, Matthes G, Hinz P, Ekkernkamp A, Ostermann PA. Retrograde fixation of distal femoral fractures: results using a new nail system. J Orthop Trauma 2003;17:488–495

70. Watanabe Y, Takai S, Yamashita F, Kusakabe T, Kim W, Hirasawa Y. Second-generation intramedullary supracondylar nail for distal femoral fractures. Int Orthop 2002;26:85–88

71. Saw A, Lau CP. Supracondylar nailing for difficult distal femur fractures. J Orthop Surg (Hong Kong) 2003;11:141–147

72. Kumar A, Jasani V, Butt MS. Management of distal femoral fractures in elderly patients using retrograde titanium supracondylar nails. Injury 2000;31:169–173

73. Henry SL. Supracondylar femur fractures treated percutaneously. Clin Orthop Relat Res 2000;375:51–59

74. Handolin L, Pajarinen J, Lindahl J, Hirvensalo E. Retrograde intramedullary nailing in distal femoral fractures–results in a series of 46 consecutive operations. Injury 2004;35:517–522

75. Manfredini M, Gildone A, Ferrante R, Bernasconi S, Massari L. Unicondylar femoral fractures: therapeutic strategy and long-term results: a review of 23 patients. Acta Orthop Belg 2001;67:132–138

76. Ostermann PA, Neumann K, Ekkernkamp A, Muhr G. Long-term results of unicondylar fractures of the femur. J Orthop Trauma 1994;8:142–146

77. Davison BL. Varus collapse of comminuted distal femur fractures after open reduction and internal fixation with a lateral condylar buttress plate. Am J Orthop 2003;32:27–30

78. Rademakers MV, Kerkhoffs GM, Sierevelt IN, Raaymakers EL, Marti RK. Intra-articular fractures of the distal femur: a long-term follow-up study of surgically treated patients. J Orthop Trauma 2004;18:213–219

Patella Fractures and Injuries to the Knee Extensor Mechanism

George V. Russell and Robert K. Mehrle

Patella Fractures

The patella is a sesamoid bone connecting the quadriceps tendon and the patellar ligament. As such, the patella is an integral part of the knee extensor mechanism. Anatomically, the fibers of the quadriceps tendon and patellar tendon are in continuity over the dorsal aspect of the patella, whereas medial and lateral expansions of the quadriceps tendon blend with the medial and lateral patellar retinacula.[1] Disruption of both the patella and these lateral expansions is needed to completely disrupt the extensor mechanism (**Fig. 27–1**). Such combined disruption is typical because of the strong tensile loads across the knee; when the patella fails, the soft tissues typically fail as well. The exception occurs when the patella is fractured by a direct blow as the knee is extended; in these injuries the medial and lateral retinacula may be intact, and the extensor mechanism may still function.

Mechanically, the patella increases the extension moment arm of the quadriceps by as much as 50% by displacing its line of action farther away from the center of rotation of the knee.[2] During knee movement, the patella experiences high tensile stresses. Because of its superficial position and its high mechanical loads, the patella is prone to injury by both direct and indirect means. The incidence of patella fractures is 1% of all skeletal injuries.[3] Direct injuries involve trauma to the anterior knee, such as a fall onto the knee or a motor vehicle crash where the dashboard impacts the knee. Less often, the patella fails in tension as a result of indirect extension forces applied through the muscle insertions. Regardless of the mechanism of injury, the resulting fracture and associated retinacular tear lead to partial or complete disruption of the extensor mechanism of the knee (**Fig. 27–1**).

The diagnosis of patella fracture is usually made by the combination of physical examination findings (pain, crepitus, knee effusion, inability to extend the knee actively) and simple anteroposterior, lateral, and tangential (Merchant) radiographs of the knee. Magnetic resonance imaging (MRI) may be useful in cases in which nonoperative treatment is considered to evaluate possible associated retinacular tears or occult osteochondral injury.

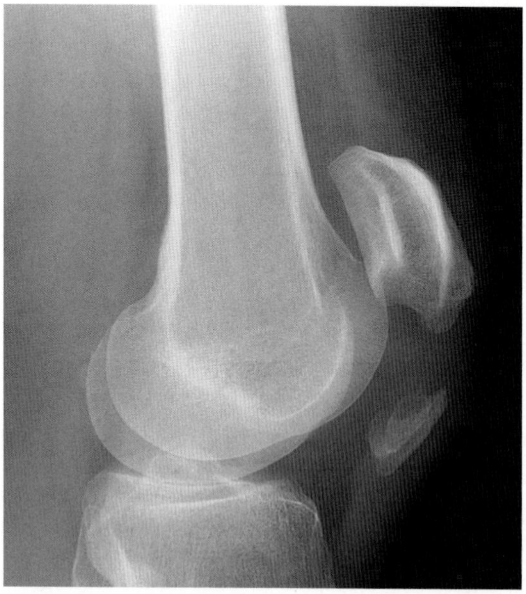

Classification

Patella fractures are typically classified very simply by the orientation of the fracture line(s) as seen on plain radiographs. Transverse patella fractures are the most common and result from direct or indirect mechanisms causing the patella to fail in tension (**Fig. 27–2A,B**). Vertical or stellate fractures usually occur following direct trauma to the anterior knee; in these injuries the primary fracture is oriented about the long axis of the patella (**Fig. 27–3A,B**). Vertical fractures may not result in disruption of the extensor mechanism and may involve the main body of the patella or just the periphery. The surgeon must also distinguish simple fractures, with just two main fragments, from comminuted fractures with many fracture fragments (**Fig. 27–4A–C**). This determination may alter the choice of operative tactic. The tangential view will best show osteochondral fragments. Bipartite patellae exist in 1 to 2% of people and can be confused with a fracture. However, bipartite patellae have a very classic appearance; they occur in the superolateral corner of the patella, are rounded, and have a smooth, sclerotic border (**Fig. 27–5**).

Figure 27–1 Lateral radiograph showing displacement of the inferior pole of the patella.

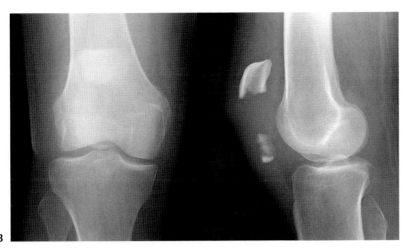

A,B

Figure 27–2 A transverse patellar fracture. **(A)** Anteroposterior (AP) and **(B)** lateral radiographs of the knee reveal a transverse fracture of the patella. On the AP view, the femur obscures the patella, but one can discern an apparent transverse fracture of the patella. The proximal fragment (which is more easily seen) is situated more proximally than where it should be; this is a major clue to the diagnosis if one misses the distal fragment that is overlying the femoral condyles. The diagnosis is obvious on the lateral radiograph.

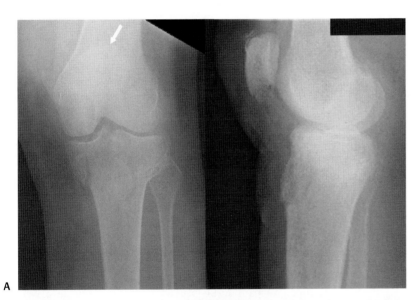

A

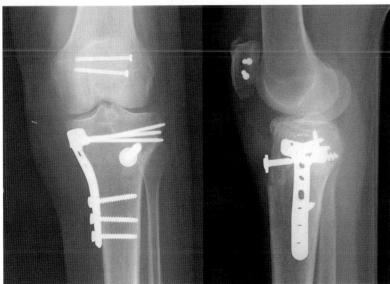

B

Figure 27–3 (A) Anteroposterior (AP) and lateral radiographs of the knee revealing a vertical fracture of the patella (white arrow). On the AP view (left panel), despite the femur, one can see a nondisplaced vertical fracture of the patella. Also seen is a tibial plateau fracture. Unlike a transverse fracture, the plane of a vertical fracture is such that the fracture is not visible on the lateral radiograph (right panel). Nevertheless, the lateral view is still useful because it may demonstrate a joint effusion and can be useful for assessing associated injuries such as exist in this case. **(B)** Postoperative radiographs after open reduction and internal fixation of both the tibial plateau and patellar fractures. Also seen are antibiotic beads placed in the traumatic wounds.

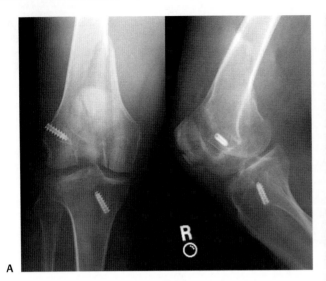

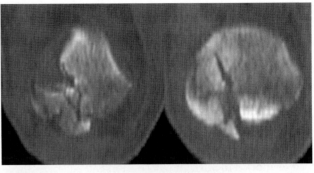

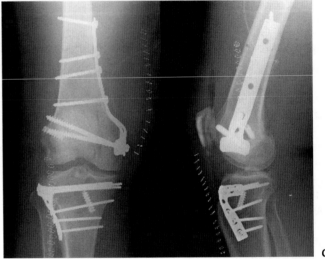

Figure 27–4 A stellate patella fracture. **(A)** Anteroposterior (AP) and lateral radiographs of the knee revealing a supracondylar femur fracture and a poorly defined, minimally displaced, comminuted fracture of the patella. The patient had undergone prior accessory collateral ligament reconstruction with interference screws. **(B)** Computed tomographic images show a stellate fracture pattern, with no fragment being significantly displaced. **(C)** Follow-up radiographs. The patella fracture was treated nonoperatively. The patient was able to perform active knee extension and did not have problems with the patella fracture.

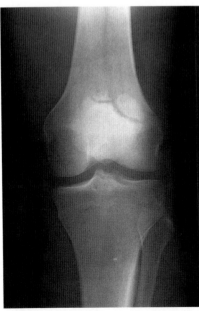

Figure 27–5 Example of a tripartite patella. Radiograph of the knee reveals two sclerotic, rounded fragments involving the superolateral corner of the patella. This is the classic appearance of a tripartite patella with two secondary ossification centers that remain attached to the main patella fragment by a synchondrosis.

Nonoperative Management

Indications for Nonoperative Management

Nondisplaced patella fractures with an intact extensor mechanism may be treated nonoperatively in a cast or brace.[3] When considering nonoperative management, the patient's ability to maintain the knee in extension against gravity should be determined. This distinction can be difficult because of the pain of the injury; intra-articular injection of local anesthetic may help alleviate pain and allow patients to demonstrate motor function. One should be aware of transverse fractures that would be likely to have associated retinacular tears. In contrast, minimally displaced vertical patellar fractures may be more safely treated nonoperatively because the retinacula are likely to be intact. Frequently these fractures involve the lateral portion of the patella with little articular involvement and typically without disruption of the extensor mechanism. Because of this, more latitude is permissible when select-ing patients for nonoperative management. If the fracture is extra-articular and the extensor mechanism is intact, the fracture may be safely treated nonoperatively with early, unrestricted range of motion exercises. For displaced intra-articular fractures or those with an extensor lag, operative management is recommended.

Rehabilitation

Patients are casted with the knee in extension for 4 to 6 weeks, at which time repeat clinical and radiographic examinations are obtained. If the patient is asymptomatic and the radiographs demonstrate evidence of healing, active motion exercises are initiated. The patient begins with knee motion to 30 degrees of flexion and advances by 30 degrees every week until full knee motion is obtained, with a goal of full knee motion by 10 to 12 weeks after injury. Passive motion exercises are to be avoided until one is assured of complete fracture healing to prevent potential fracture displacement.

Severely comminuted patella fractures are generally treated operatively, but those with massive comminution may be better treated with nonoperative management (**Fig. 27–4A–C**).[3] Such fractures are usually the result of a high-energy direct blow to the patella where the extensor mechanism remains intact. These fractures are likened to "candy in a sack" and may be treated with brief immobilization for comfort, followed by progressive range of motion exercises (personal communication, Sigvard T. Hansen, M.D.).

Patella fractures may also be treated nonoperatively in patients who are nonambulatory or in patients who are not surgical candidates or do not desire surgery. Brief immobilization is undertaken for pain control followed by motion as dictated by clinical symptoms. Following nonoperative management, suboptimal knee function can be anticipated.[4] A drop-lock brace can support the knee in extension when needed and may be beneficial in this situation. When the patient is standing, the brace is locked, allowing for ambulation. Two sliding locks on the hinges are released with sitting, allowing for a normal seated posture.[4]

Indications for Surgical Treatment

Because the patella has a large chondral surface, indications for treatment of displaced patella fractures are similar to those of other displaced articular fractures. Fractures that are displaced greater than 2 mm should be operatively reduced and stabilized; however, displacement of 2 mm may be difficult to discern radiographically. All patellar fractures causing disruption of the extensor mechanism of the knee also require operative treatment to restore knee extension, regardless of their apparent amount of displacement. Patellar fractures associated with other fractures about the knee, such as tibial plateau fractures and supracondylar femur fractures, should be surgically treated to allow early knee rehabilitation (**Fig. 27–3A,B**).

The surgeon must choose among three general methods of repair: open reduction and internal fixation, partial patellectomy with tendon reconstruction, and total patellectomy. Total patellectomy is very rarely performed for primary management of patella fractures because at least a portion of the patella can usually be salvaged. Partial patellectomy is usually chosen when the mostly extra-articular distal pole is comminuted; in such cases more secure repair can be obtained by reattaching the patellar tendon to the proximal fragment than by repairing the fracture. This approach spares the need for internal fixation and the patient can be more rapidly rehabilitated without concern of loss of fixation. Occasionally, one might repair a simpler fracture of the upper portion of the patella while excising comminuted fragments of the distal pole, thereby combining both approaches.

Surgical Treatment

Surgical Anatomy

The patella has a somewhat triangular shape, with its apex pointed inferiorly. The proximal three fourths of the articular surface of the patella is covered with articular cartilage, whereas the inferior (distal) pole is extra-articular. The articular surface has a prominent vertical ridge that divides the articular surface into medial and lateral facets. The ridge is located roughly at the junction of the medial and middle thirds of the patella. A second, smaller ridge along the medial patella defines the so-called odd facet. The medial and lateral facets are divided into superior, middle, and inferior portions. Variations in the overall morphology of the patella have been described and classified;[5] the reader is referred to the original source because discussion of this is beyond the scope of this chapter.

The patella has a complex blood supply. A peripatellar vascular plexus receives contributions from six different arteries that form a circular network around the patella. Thus the vascular supply to bone fragments is preserved, even in comminuted fractures. Named vessels include the supreme geniculate artery from the superficial femoral artery and the four geniculate arteries that branch off the popliteal artery. A final anastomosis to the anterior tibial artery is via the recurrent anterior tibial artery.

Surgical Techniques

The patient is simply positioned supine on a radiolucent table with a small positioning pillow placed beneath the ipsilateral hip so that the patella points straight toward the ceiling. A tourniquet may be used, and if so, it is placed proximally on the thigh. The lower extremity is sterilized and surgical drapes are placed. If using a tourniquet, the limb is exsanguinated, and the knee is flexed to advance the patella before the tourniquet is inflated. A vertical midline incision is performed beginning ~6 cm proximal to the patella and extended distally to the tibial tubercle (**Fig. 27–6A**). In the case of an open fracture, the traumatic wound is utilized to the extent possible, with proximal and distal extensions as needed. Surgical incisions to extend

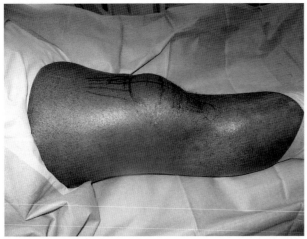
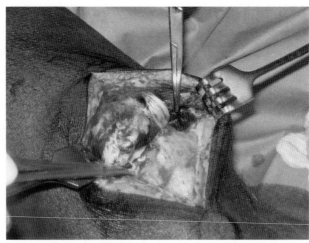

A   B

Figure 27–6 **(A)** Clinical photograph of a patient's leg prepared for surgery. The patella fracture, quadriceps tendon, and patellar tendon are drawn out. The proposed midline incision is marked as well. **(B)** Photograph after exposure of the extensor mechanism.

the traumatic wound should be placed carefully to avoid acute angles that create narrow skin flaps. The incision is carried down to the quadriceps tendon proximally and the patellar tendon distally. The medial and lateral retinacula are exposed to the extent that they are disrupted (**Fig. 27–6B**). At this point, the surgeon must decide on the definitive approach: internal fixation, partial patellectomy, or total patellectomy.

Open Reduction and Internal Fixation (see Video 27–1, Disk 3)

Patella fractures are usually repaired by some combination of a tension-band construct, cerclage wire, and/or interfragmentary screws. The specific construct will depend on the pattern of the fracture and the condition of the soft tissues. For successful repair with a tension band, the primary fracture line must be transverse, and the surgeon must be able to reassemble the fracture well enough so that the fracture fragments can withstand compressive forces. In the case of severe comminution where tension-band fixation is not possible, the surgeon must excise the comminuted segments or choose cerclage fixation.

First, the fracture fragments are identified and the fracture surfaces cleaned of hematoma. The fracture fragments may be gently displaced while maintaining their soft tissue attachments to inspect the underlying articular surface. Typically, the largest fragment is rotated to the side ~90 degrees to accomplish this (**Fig. 27–7A–D**). Associated articular impaction injuries of the distal femur may be observed and can be treated through this surgical exposure. The surgeon must carefully look for any osteochondral fragments from the undersurface of the patella. Free osteochondral fragments are frequently found with patella fractures and must either be stabilized or excised.

After the fracture fragments have been identified, isolated, and cleaned, attention is focused on stabilizing the articular surface. Very small bone fragments may be discarded, whereas attempts are usually made to maintain larger osteochondral fragments. If further exposure of the articular surface of the patella is needed to repair osteochondral fragments, a vertical incision extending from the traumatic tear in the lateral retinaculum may allow the patella to be everted 90 degrees.[6] Alternatively, Berg described the use of tibial tubercle osteotomy to expose comminuted patella fractures.[7] After exposure, the tibial tubercle is predrilled to accept either a 6.5 mm cancellous lag screw or a 4.5 mm bicortical fully threaded screw. An osteotomy of the entire tubercle is made with an oscillating saw; the osteotomized fragment is usually 2 cm wide, 4 cm long, and 1.5 cm thick. The osteotomy can be hinged medially to allow patellar eversion, and repaired securely.[7]

If the osteochondral fragment is stable within the cancellous bed after reduction, no fixation is required because stabilization will be maintained by compression between the main fracture fragments (**Fig. 27–7A–D**). If the osteochondral fragment is unstable, then definitive screw fixation is considered. Using the articular surface of the main fracture fragment as a guide, unstable osteochondral fragments are reduced to the major fragment and stabilized provisionally with small-diameter Kirschner wires as necessary (**Fig. 27–8A–C**). Rigid stabilization of these fragments must be achieved to prevent displacement during postoperative knee motion. To attain such stabilization, the authors have found small-diameter screws to provide the most reliable fixation. Small-fragment 3.0 mm cannulated screws may be placed over the K-wires used for provisional fixation. Mini-fragment 2.0 mm screws may be used for very small fragments. Screws placed directly within the free osteochondral fragment provide the most stable fixation. Bioabsorbable screws may also be used, but the authors prefer metallic screws because of the precision with which they can be placed. Lag screw technique is

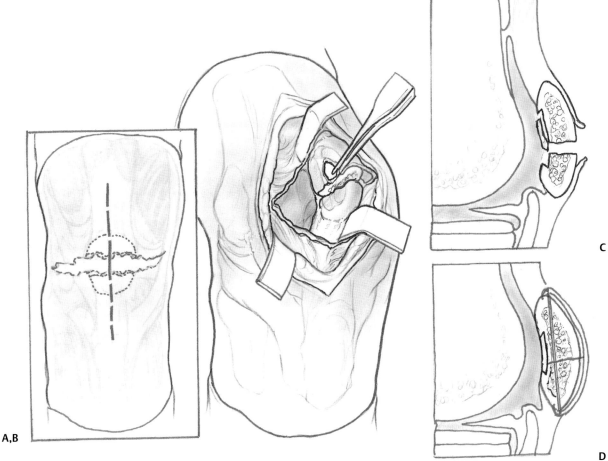

A,B

C

D

Figure 27–7 Drawings of a stable osteochondral fragment. **(A)** The incision is made to expose the knee extensor mechanism. **(B)** The patellar fragments are everted to allow inspection of the articular surface. A separate osseochondral fragment is identified. **(C)** The fragment geometry is such that it keys in place and **(D)** is stabilized by compression between the two main fragments. The Kirchner wires are placed as anterior as possible in the patella.

avoided for fixation of free osteochondral pieces; instead, fully threaded positioning screws should be used **(Fig. 27–8A–C).** For coronally displaced osteoarticular fragments, the screw is placed perpendicular to the articular surface with care to adequately countersink the screw. Sagittally oriented osteochondral fractures are also stabilized with screws, but the screw is placed within the cancellous bone of the fragment roughly parallel to the articular surface. When placing this screw, one must be sure to drill the screw ~2 to 3 mm deep to the articular surface to accommodate the screw head, ensuring the screw head does not impinge along the articular surface.

Attention is next focused on the major fracture fragments, with the goal of creating a simple transverse fracture pattern. The smaller fracture fragments are sequentially reduced and stabilized to the larger ones until a two-part equivalent transverse fracture pattern is achieved. Care must be taken to place the screws sufficiently dorsal in the patella to allow for the more anterior longitudinal Kirschner wires necessary for the tension-band construct. For this type of fixation to be successful, the reconstructed fragments must be fixed well enough that the fracture surfaces can withstand the compression forces generated by the tension band. If such a stable construct cannot be created, it is better to avoid attempting tension-band wiring and instead consider a cerclage wire to hold the comminuted fragments together.

The final step in the reconstruction is to repair the transverse fracture fragments with a tension-band construct. The two fragments of the superior and inferior patella are reduced to one another and held with a Weber or other pointed-reduction clamp **(Fig. 27–9).** Occasionally two reduction clamps are required for adequate control of the fracture reduction. Fracture reduction is verified by palpation or visualization of the articular surface and with fluoroscopy if needed. Using the anterior cortex of the patella as a reduction guide can be misleading. Often, apparently anatomical reduction of the anterior patellar cortex leaves a gap on the articular surface. After assurance of an anatomical reduction, a 2.0 mm Kirschner wire is introduced into the lateral one third of the patella beginning at the inferior pole and exiting proximally through the superior pole **(Fig. 27–10).** Ideally, the Kirschner wire should be

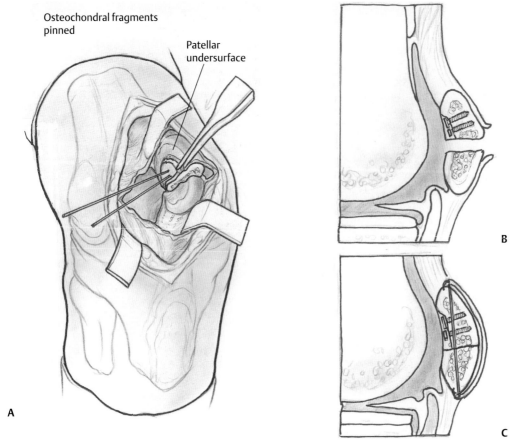

A

Osteochondral fragments pinned

Patellar undersurface

B

C

Figure 27–8 Drawings of an unstable osteochondral fragment. **(A)** Provisional fixation with a K-wire. **(B)** Fixation with a fully threaded positioning screw, and **(C)** final fixation of the primary transverse fracture with a tension band.

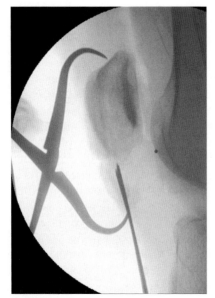

Figure 27–9 Intraoperative fluoroscopic view during repair of a transverse patella fracture, showing that the transverse fracture is reduced and clamped while two K-wires are advanced to the fracture.

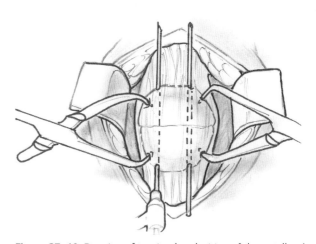

Figure 27–10 Drawing of tension-band wiring of the patella, showing how the primary transverse fracture line is reduced and held with pointed reduction clamps while two K-wires are advanced from distal to proximal across the fracture.

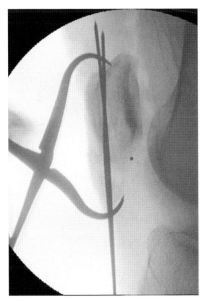

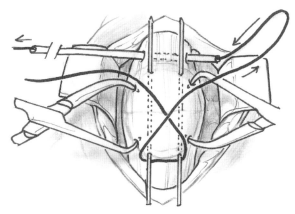

Figure 27–12 Drawing showing placement of an angiocatheter that is inserted transversely into the quadriceps tendon just above, and deep to, the upper end of the K-wires. An 18 gauge surgical wire is then placed around the K-wires in a figure-of-eight fashion.

Figure 27–11 Intraoperative fluoroscopic view showing the position of the K-wires after they are advanced across the fracture.

as close to the dorsal surface (anterior patella) as possible **(Fig. 27–11)**. Depending upon the fracture comminution, this may not always be possible. As the Kirschner wire exits the superior pole of the patella, a small longitudinal incision is made in the quadriceps tendon atop the Kirschner wire. The Kirschner wire is then advanced through the quadriceps tenotomy for ~5 cm. A second Kirschner wire is introduced in a similar fashion in the medial one third of the patella parallel to the initial Kirschner wire **(Fig. 27–11)**. Although the Kirschner wires are typically drilled freehand, Ong and Sherman describe a technique using an anterior cruciate ligament (ACL) drill guide to facilitate drilling the patella and passing sutures.[8]

The tension-band wire is then passed **(Fig. 27–12)**. To facilitate inserting the wire through the quadriceps tendon, a 14 gauge angiocatheter is inserted transversely

into the quadriceps tendon deep to the Kirschner wires, just above the superior pole of the patella. Then, beginning at the inferior pole of the patella, 18 gauge surgical wire is passed deep to the distal ends of the Kirschner wires. The cerclage wire is crossed in a figure-of-eight fashion over the anterior patella, and the end on the same side as the tip of the angiocatheter is inserted through the needle to exit through the hub of the needle on the opposite side. After the wire has been passed through the angiocatheter, the angiocatheter is removed. Two loops are created in the cerclage wire and tightened using heavy needle drivers **(Fig. 27–13A,B)**. The use of two separate twists generates greater compression than a single tightening site. During the tightening process, it is important to ensure that both wires wrap around each other, rather than one wire coiling around the remaining straight wire. If the latter occurs, the twists will simply function as a slip knot, and the construct will loosen. Proper twisting of the wires is facilitated by pulling up on the loops equally as they are simultaneously

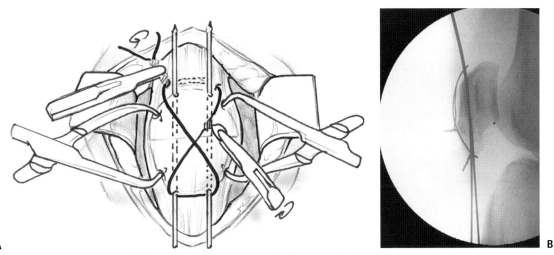

A   B

Figure 27–13 (A) Drawing and **(B)** corresponding intraoperative fluoroscopic view showing the creation of two loops on each vertical segment of the tension-band wire that are twisted, thereby tightening the tension band.

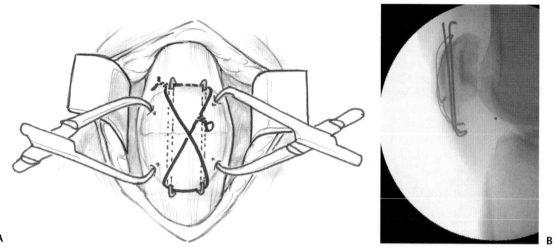

Figure 27–14 (A) Drawing and **(B)** corresponding intraoperative fluoroscopic view demonstrating how the K-wires are cut short and the ends bent, turned, and impacted.

twisted. After tightening, the loops are cut ~1 cm long, bent over, and impacted into the soft tissues. Similarly, the superior ends of the Kirschner wires are cut and curled over using pliers **(Fig. 27–14A,B)**. The Kirschner wires are rotated posteriorly until the curled ends are 10 to 15 degrees posterior to the midcoronal plane and are over the tension-band wire, so that the tension band is captured deep to the Kirschner wires when they are impacted into the superior pole of the patella **(Fig. 27–14A,B)**. The knee is flexed to 90 degrees to ensure fracture stability. The distal ends of the Kirschner wires are cut, leaving ~1 cm. The tourniquet is deflated, and hemostasis is achieved with electrocautery. Retinacular disruptions are repaired with interrupted nonabsorbable suture. The wound is then irrigated and closed over a suction drain.

Biomechanical and clinical studies have proven the tension-band technique as described to be an effective method of stabilizing and treating patella fractures **(Fig. 27–15A,B)**. However, it is technically demanding. The most common error is improper placement of the tension-band wire. Failure to approximate the tension-band wire to bone on the superior and inferior poles of the patella, posterior to the quadriceps and patellar tendons, results in soft tissue interposition. If this happens, gapping of the fracture during knee flexion will occur as the tension band is loaded because sliding is possible along the K-wire until the wire meets the bone.[9,10] The greatest stress is placed on the construct between 30 and 60 degrees of flexion, which is the range when the joint reactive force is greatest. Therefore, the greatest risk of fracture displacement is in this range.[11]

Alternatively, transverse patella fractures may be stabilized with a modified tension-band technique using 4.0 mm cannulated screws (Synthes, Paoli, Pennsylvania) **(Fig. 27–16A,B)**. The transverse fracture is reduced as already described. Using a technique similar to introduc-

ing the Kirschner wires for the tension-band technique, two 1.25 mm guidewires are inserted into the inferior pole of the patella using fluoroscopic imaging. Just before the guidewires exit the superior pole of the patella, the guidewire length is measured using the external sleeve depth gauge. This should correspond to a screw length that is a few millimeters less than the length of the patella, ensuring that the tip of the screw will remain buried in the bone.

The guidewires are then advanced through the superior pole of the patella. A 2 cm longitudinal incision is made through the quadriceps tendon over the guidewires that are then advanced through the quadriceps tendon. The guidewires are overdrilled with the appropriate cannulated drill bit. At this point, a standard depth gauge can be used to determine the length of the screw, which should be 4 to 6 mm less than the measurement determined with the depth gauge. A 4.0 mm partially threaded screw is inserted over each guidewire. It is important to ensure that the screws do not extend beyond the superior pole of the patella because the sharp screw threads may cut the cerclage wire or suture leading to fixation failure and fracture displacement.

After the screws are securely positioned, 18 gauge wire is passed through one screw beginning at the inferior pole. Sufficient wire must be pulled through this screw to allow for passage through the second screw. The wire is then passed through the second screw again, beginning at the inferior pole and exiting through the superior pole. The wire is then secured using the two-loop technique previously described, although in this case the loops are placed superiorly and inferiorly. Alternatively, large-diameter nonabsorbable suture may be used in place of the cerclage wire.

This technique may be particularly helpful in patients with good bone quality in which good screw purchase is assured. Several biomechanical studies have reported

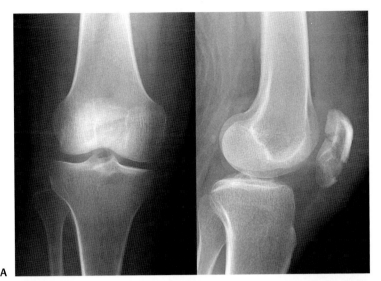

A

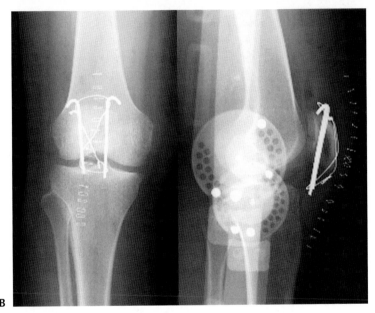

B

Figure 27–15 Tension-band wiring of a transverse patellar fracture. **(A)** Anteroposterior and lateral radiographs of the knee showing a transverse patellar fracture. Although there is not a large gap, the patient could not perform a leg raise, and there was a step-off of the articular surface. **(B)** Follow-up radiographs after fixation using a traditional figure-of-eight tension-band wire technique.

increased strength with the addition of screws, most noticeably in terminal extension.[9,11] This may allow for earlier range of motion in younger patients with good bone quality, whereas the modified tension-band technique is more suitable for elderly patients and fractures with comminution.[12,13]

When the patella is severely comminuted so that two large, stable fragments cannot be constructed, or when there is additional comminution of the periphery of the patella, a cerclage wire or cerclage plating constructs may be utilized for added stability **(Fig. 27–17A–C)**.

Displaced vertical fractures do not require a tension band because they are not subjected to the distraction forces seen with the transverse fractures during knee flexion. For the rare, purely vertical patella fracture, lag screw fixation alone should be sufficient. The patella is exposed through a longitudinal approach over the patella. After ex-

posure of the fracture and removal of fracture hematoma, osteochondral fragments, if present, are stabilized as previously described. The major fracture fragments are then reduced and stabilized with a pointed reduction clamp. Lag screws or positioning screws are utilized to stabilize the fractures.

Partial Patellectomy with Tendon Reconstruction

Partial patellectomy may be considered for severely comminuted patella fractures. Either the superior pole or the inferior pole may be resected, depending on the injury pattern; typically it is the inferior pole that is comminuted **(Fig. 27–18A,B)**. There does not appear to be any correlation between outcome and the size of the remaining patella;[14] therefore, the authors always endeavor to retain at least one large fragment of the patella.

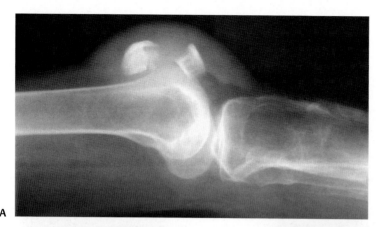

A

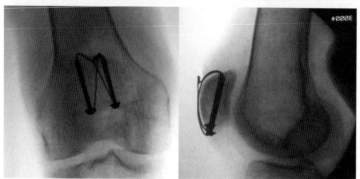

B

Figure 27–16 The modified tension-band technique using cannulated screws. **(A)** Anteroposterior (AP) and lateral radiographs of the knee revealing a displaced transverse fracture of the patella. **(B)** Postoperative views after open reduction and internal fixation with a modified tension-band technique using two cannulated screws. (Case courtesy of Steven Benirschke, M.D.)

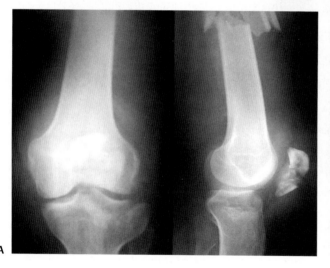

A

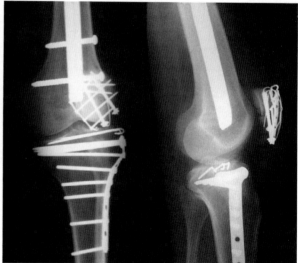

B

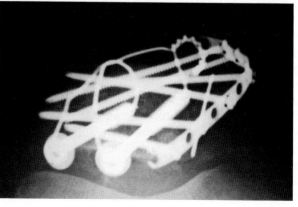

C

Figure 27–17 Peripheral plating of a comminuted patella fracture. **(A)** Anteroposterior (AP) and lateral radiographs of the knee revealing a comminuted fracture of the patella. Fractures of the femoral shaft and tibial plateau are also apparent. **(B)** Corresponding radiographs taken after internal fixation of all fractures. The comminuted patella was repaired with a construct utilizing two cannulated screws placed perpendicular to the primary fracture line, supplemented by a figure-of-eight tension-band wire and a medial peripheral patellar plate. The plate is a mini-fragment semitubular plate, cut off at the ends, which were bent over and impacted into the patella. Multiple 2.0 mm screws were placed across the patella to buttress the articular surface. **(C)** Merchant view of the reconstructed patella. (Case courtesy of Steven Benirschke, M.D.)

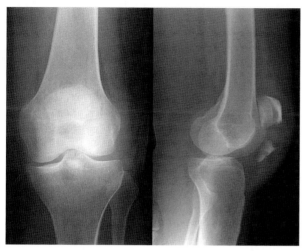
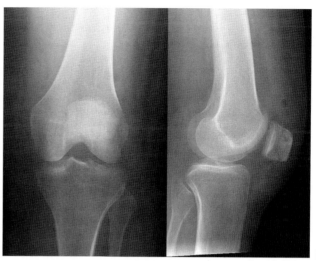

Figure 27–18 A comminuted inferior pole fracture treated with fragment excision and tendon repair. **(A)** Anteroposterior and lateral views of the knee showing a displaced fracture of the distal pole of the patella. **(B)** Radiographic appearance after excision of the distal pole and tendon reconstruction.

The injured pole of the patella is enucleated from the adjacent tendon, preserving as much of the tendon as possible. Anchoring sutures are placed in the corresponding tendon using a tendon-grasping Krakow suture technique (see section on Patellar Ligament Disruption). A 2.0 mm drill bit is used to drill four pilot holes through the long axis of the patella in the midcoronal plane. A suture passer is inserted through the drill holes beginning at the intact portion of the patella to the site where the patella was resected. The suture is passed through the remaining patella and tied over the superior pole of the patella. It is important to maintain the appropriate length of patellar tendon as measured by the Insall-Salvati criteria.[14,15]

Alternatively, the surgeon can remove only the articular cartilage and leave the cortical fragments within the tendon. The advantage of this variation of the technique is that it allows for bone-to-bone healing, which may be stronger, lessening the chance of fixation failure. It is imperative to repair associated retinacular tears, and a cerclage suture can be passed from above the patella to the tibial tubercle to augment the repair. Finally, the vastus medialis obliquus muscle can be advanced to the patellar ligament to improve knee extension.[16]

Total patellectomy has been described for unsalvageable patella fractures, but, while functional, the patient is left with a significant extensor lag and decreased quadriceps muscle power.[17] The key to avoiding extensor lag is to restore appropriate tension of the extensor mechanism; this requires some form of soft tissue imbrication. To effect the repair, multiple tendon-grasping sutures are placed above and below the defect and tied. Although there should be some tension in the extensor mechanism with the knee extended, it is equally important to demonstrate that the repair will allow 90 degrees of flexion without failure.

Rehabilitation

Generally, active range of motion exercises are initiated on the first postoperative day in a supervised setting, allowing up to 90 degrees of flexion depending on the stability of fixation and the condition of the surgical incision. Gentle intraoperative assessment after fixation can help to determine the initial degree of flexion that can be tolerated before excessive tension is put on the repair. In the case of severely comminuted fractures, it is prudent to splint the knee in full extension and only gradually increase flexion. A knee brace with adjustable hinges that locks in extension but can allow increasing degrees of motion is useful. Concurrent straight leg raises are initiated. A continuous passive motion machine may also be beneficial during those periods when the patient is not undergoing supervised physical therapy or walking. Patients are allowed to ambulate full weight bearing with a brace or a knee immobilizer with the leg in full extension. The patient should obtain at least 90 degrees of flexion within the first 4 weeks. Extension exercises must not be forgotten because flexion contractures can be very disabling if allowed to occur.

The patient is seen in the clinic setting 2 to 3 weeks postoperatively for wound examination. Sutures or staples are removed. The patient continues with the postoperative protocol for knee motion exercises and quadriceps strengthening with straight leg raises. Four to 6 weeks postoperatively the patient is again evaluated in the office, and knee radiographs are performed. If the fracture is healing well, active assisted and passive range of motion exercises may be initiated to attain full knee flexion. Resistive exercises using light weights may be initiated 12 weeks postoperatively. The patient is further evaluated in the office every 4 to 6 weeks with advances in strengthening and knee motion until fracture union, and the patient has good strength and is ambulating without an assistive device.

Tips and Tricks

- If one is unsure about whether disruption of the knee extensor mechanism is present, intra-articular injection of local anesthetic may help alleviate pain and allow the patient to demonstrate motor function.
- In the case of an open fracture, the traumatic wound is utilized to the extent possible, with proximal and distal extensions as needed. Surgical incisions to extend the traumatic wound should be placed carefully to avoid acute angles that create narrow skin flaps.
- If further exposure of the articular surface of the patella is needed to repair osteochondral fragments, a vertical incision extending from the traumatic tear in the lateral retinaculum may allow the patella to be everted.
- Rigid stabilization of free osteochondral fragments is needed to prevent displacement during postoperative knee motion. Small-diameter screws provide the most reliable fixation. Small-fragment 3.0 mm cannulated screws may be placed over the K-wires used for provisional fixation. Mini-fragment 2.0 mm screws may be used for very small fragments.
- For successful repair with a tension band, the primary fracture line must be transverse and the surgeon must be able to reassemble the fracture well enough so that the fracture fragments can withstand compressive forces.
- While tightening the tension-band wire, the use of two separate twists generates greater compression than a single tightening site.
- Partial patellectomy is usually chosen when the distal pole is comminuted; in such cases more secure repair can be obtained by reattaching the patellar tendon to the proximal fragment than by repairing the fracture.
- To facilitate inserting the wire through the quadriceps tendon, a 14 gauge angiocatheter is inserted transversely into the quadriceps tendon deep to the Kirschner wires, just above the superior pole of the patella.
- When using cannulated screws and a modified tension band, it is important to ensure that the tips of the screws do not extend beyond the patella because the sharp screw threads may cut the cerclage wire or suture, leading to fixation failure and fracture displacement.
- After total patellectomy, the key to avoiding extensor lag is to restore appropriate tension of the extensor mechanism. Soft tissue imbrication will be necessary.

If the patient is slow to regain motion, a manipulation under anesthesia may be considered after 12 weeks.

For those fractures with marked comminution, tenuous fixation, or problematical wounds, the postoperative protocol should be modified. Generally, these patients are placed in a knee immobilizer or locked hinged knee brace postoperatively, and immediate knee motion is deferred. Straight leg raises are initiated with the knee immobilizer in place. Walking is also permitted with the knee immobilized in extension using crutches or a walker. After discharge, the patients are seen in the clinic setting at 2 weeks for wound examination and radiographs. If the wound is healed, active knee motion is permitted to 30 to 45 degrees with the brace on. A referral is made to a physical therapist, and knee motion and strengthening exercises are sequentially advanced 30 degrees every 2 to 3 weeks until full motion as obtained.

New Techniques

Berg reported the use of tibial tubercle osteotomy in six patients with severely comminuted fractures involving the articular surface.[7] All patients were allowed immediate postoperative continuous knee motion from 0 to 40 degrees of flexion. During walking, the knees were braced in full extension for 4 weeks, and no flexion beyond 70 degrees was allowed during this time. After 4 weeks, progressive range of motion and weight bearing were allowed. All six patients had union of their tibial tubercle osteotomy by 8 weeks without any hardware complications.[7]

Veselko and Kastelec reviewed patients with avulsion of the inferior pole of the patella and compared the results of internal fixation of the distal fragment with a novel basket plate to resection of the distal pole and patellar tendon repair.[18] Their hypothesis was that maintenance of the inferior pole and secure fixation would allow early motion, avoid problems with patella baja, and lead to better outcomes. Ten of 11 patients available for long-term follow-up after internal fixation had a normal patellar height, compared with three of 13 patients following tendon repair. Patella baja was significantly associated with poor function.[18] Although these results suggest that internal fixation may have merit, their protocol may have unfairly biased the patients treated with tendon repair to a poorer result by requiring them to be immobilized. Further study of this approach is necessary.

Fixation failure has been noted in 22% of cases following traditional tension-band wiring of patella fractures.[10] A recent biomechanical analysis found that a horizontally oriented figure-of-eight tension-band construct was more stable than the traditional vertical configuration, with mean fracture displacement during cyclic loading reduced by half (unpublished data, G.A. Brown, M.D., Ph.D.). Clinical confirmation of these findings will be necessary.

Outcomes

Nonoperative treatment yields excellent results in minimally displaced patella fractures with an intact extensor mechanism. Bostrom studied 282 patients with fractures displaced less than 4 mm and/or joint incongruity less than 3 mm; 99% of the patients had good to excellent results after nonoperative treatment.[3]

Patients who have undergone operative stabilization of displaced patella fractures generally have satisfactory results.[3,9,19–22] Although most patients will regain full knee range of motion, several studies have noted worsening results in patients with comminuted fractures due to loss of terminal knee extension and flexion.[21–24] Factors associated with improved outcomes are anatomical reduction and rigid internal fixation.[19,25] Poorer results are associated with fractures with either or both residual displacement and suboptimal fixation. Rigid fixation obtained through optimal surgical technique is important to prevent early failure of fixation. Stable repair allows early knee range of motion, resulting in improved knee motion and quadriceps strength. Residual weakness of the quadriceps muscles may contribute to anterior knee pain; quadriceps rehabilitation should be a primary focus of aftercare. Postoperative physiotherapy must be individually tailored to the specific patient, type of injury, and strength of fixation. Fixation failure can be caused by overly aggressive rehabilitation, including performance of active knee extension in the early postoperative period, as well as patient noncompliance. One might consider a period of cast immobilization in the noncompliant patient to protect the repair, accepting that functional results may be compromised.

Posttraumatic arthrosis may result from nonanatomical reduction causing abnormal patellofemoral alignment and increased joint contact forces. Therefore, care should be taken to ensure that anatomical reduction and rigid fixation are achieved at the time of surgery to optimize patient outcomes. It is important to note that arthrosis may also result from cartilage damage sustained at the time of initial injury and may result in a poor outcome despite anatomical reduction and ideal fixation. Open patella fractures have been associated with compromised results compared with closed fractures.[23,24]

Early reports in the literature of the results of patellectomy were favorable and patellectomy was considered to be a viable treatment for more comminuted fractures.[1,26,27] However, more recent studies have failed to duplicate these results; poor outcomes after patellectomy are related to decreased quadriceps strength and early arthritic changes following patellectomy.[17,28] Clinical studies have demonstrated that quadriceps strength is reduced by one third after patellectomy, and decreased quadriceps mass in patients following patellectomy suggests that these changes are irreversible.[17] Patellectomy is now considered by many to be a treatment of last resort for only the most severe patella fractures.

In contrast, partial patellectomy is a viable alternative in selected patients with comminuted inferior pole fractures. Saltzman et al reported quadriceps strength of 85% of the normal side, and 77% of patients had good to excellent results.[14] Repairing the tendon to the articular edge of the remaining superior fragment improves patellar alignment and reduces posterior tilt of the remaining fragment. This theoretically reduces abnormal contact stress and long-term degenerative changes.[21] Rerupture can compromise the outcome, and a rigid construct obtained through diligent surgical technique is necessary to prevent rerupture.

Complications

Fortunately, perioperative complications associated with operative treatment of patella fractures are relatively infrequent. Potential early complications include wound infection and loss of fixation; later on there may be nonunion and hardware failure, malunion, patellofemoral pain, or stiffness with or without evidence of arthrosis, or hardware prominence.

Loss of motion usually involves the extreme degrees of knee flexion and is mostly asymptomatic. Rarely, if adequate flexion is not achieved by 3 months postinjury, manipulation of the knee under anesthesia and possible arthroscopic debridement can be considered. This complication is best avoided by the institution of early knee motion and careful supervision of the patient following surgery.

Infection may be one of the most devastating complications. Aside from the tenuous skin over the patella and the possibility that hardware could be exposed if the wound breaks down, wound infection could lead to septic arthritis of the knee. Therefore, a high index of suspicion should be maintained for any wound complications. Any increase in pain, wound erythema, or drainage should be promptly and aggressively treated with incision and drainage, with concomitant lavage of the knee because of the high likelihood of associated septic arthritis. Knee inspection and lavage are best done via arthrotomy performed through the associated medial and lateral retinacular tears instead of through the fracture. The implants should remain in place if possible until fracture union. Empirical intravenous antibiotic therapy should be started at the time of initial debridement and then modified based on culture results. Use of antibiotic-impregnated beads can be considered. Suction drains are placed at the completion of the procedure. Knee motion and physical therapy are suspended until the wound is dry, at which point knee motion is reinitiated. Intravenous and/or oral antibiotics are typically continued for 4 to 6 weeks after final wound closure.

Fixation failure is the most common complication after open reduction and internal fixation of patella fractures, occurring in 22% of cases in one recent series, usually as the result of inadequate fixation.[10] Other causes of fixation failure include patient noncompliance and overly aggressive knee motion. Fractures that redisplace, or if the extensor mechanism is disrupted, require repeat open reduction and internal fixation. Similar principles previously described are used, but fracture fixation may be less stable and an extended postoperative immobilization is required.

Knee pain is frequent after a patella fracture. Quadriceps weakness will occur if the patient does not adequately rehabilitate the muscles. Failure to fully rehabilitate the quadriceps muscles may lead to anterior knee pain. Also, tightness of the knee flexor muscles often accompanies quadriceps weakness and may further exacerbate patellofemoral pain. The importance of quadriceps muscle strengthening and knee flexor muscle stretching cannot be overemphasized to patients during postoperative rehabilitation. Patella baja is uncommon but has been reported in the literature and may require tibial tubercle osteotomy to restore proper patella height.[29]

Despite anatomical fracture reduction, isolated patellofemoral arthrosis may occur after patella fractures as a result of chondral injury to the trochlea and the patella. Continued strengthening and stretching exercises with avoidance of high-impact exercises are recommended. Bicycling with low resistance and high cadence strengthens the quadriceps and decreases patellofemoral pain. Nonsteroidal anti-inflammatories are also useful to alleviate symptoms. For extreme, unremitting pain, a patellectomy may be considered. Patellofemoral arthroplasty may also be considered, but it is considered experimental by many. Total joint arthroplasty may be considered for patients in the older age group.

Injuries to the Knee Extensor Mechanism

Injuries to the extensor mechanism of the knee involve either a rupture of the quadriceps tendon or a rupture of the patellar ligament. Quadriceps tendon injuries usually occur in patients older than 40 years of age, whereas patellar ligament injuries typically occur in patients younger than 40.[30] Tendon ruptures about the knee are sometimes related to an underlying systemic disease such as lupus erythematosus or rheumatoid arthritis. Quadriceps tendon and patellar ligament injuries commonly result from a sudden eccentric contraction of the extensor mechanism with the foot planted. Quadriceps tendon ruptures are frequently due to attritional changes in the tendon (tendinopathy) originating in the rectus femoris muscle 2 to 3 cm proximal to the superior pole of the patella. Because of the attritional changes within the quadriceps tendon, patients can sustain a quadriceps tendon disruption as a result of a relatively low-energy eccentric contraction. Patient questioning frequently reveals a prodromal period where the patient had intermittent pain or tendinitis at the insertion of the quadriceps or patellar tendon.[31]

Patellar ligament ruptures typically result during athletic events secondary to a violent eccentric contraction. The most common site of ligament disruption is at the inferior pole of the patella. Midsubstance tears also occur, but much less frequently than those at the patellar insertion site.

The diagnosis of a patellar tendon rupture is readily made by noting the proximal position of the patella (patella alta) that results from loss of its tether to the tibial tubercle and the unopposed pull of the quadriceps muscle (**Fig. 27–19**). The Insall-Salvati ratio divides the length of the patellar tendon by the length of the patella.[15] The normal ratio is 1.02. With rupture of the patellar tendon, the patella can displace as much as 5 cm proximally. Any proximal displacement of the patella increases the distance between the inferior pole of the patella and the

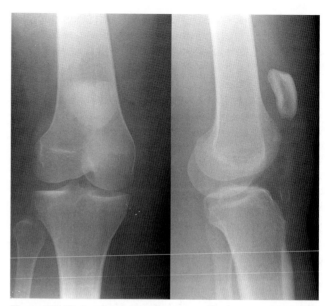

Figure 27–19 A radiograph showing patella alta in a patient with acute patellar tendon rupture.

tibial tubercle, thereby decreasing this ratio. In equivocal cases when patella alta is not present, disruption of the infrapatellar fat pad contour on a lateral knee radiograph was often seen in patients with patellar tendon rupture.[32] Diagnosis of quadriceps tendon rupture can be more difficult. With quadriceps tendon rupture, the patella may appear to be lower than normal or may be in its normal position, and one may have to rely more on clinical suspicion in a patient who can't extend the knee. In a thin patient, a palpable defect in the quadriceps tendon above the patella can confirm the diagnosis. With either tendon rupture, ultrasound or MRI will confirm the diagnosis if there is clinical uncertainty (**Fig. 27–20**).

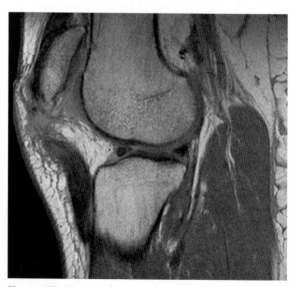

Figure 27–20 Lateral magnetic resonance image of the knee showing a rupture of the patellar tendon.

Nonoperative Treatment

Indications for Nonoperative Treatment

Nonoperative treatment of disruption of the knee extensor mechanism is limited to patients who are not surgical candidates or those patients who are nonambulatory. Patients who are treated nonoperatively can expect significant disability secondary to lack of knee extension, knee extension weakness, and an extensor lag. These patients will require either or both an assistive device for ambulation and a hinged knee brace with a lock. A cylinder cast, knee immobilizer, or locked hinged knee brace may be used to treat these patients.

Rehabilitation

The knee is held in full extension for 6 to 12 weeks. At the completion of immobilization gradual knee flexion exercises are initiated to a maximum of 30 degrees. Knee flexion is then advanced in 30 degree increments every 2 to 3 weeks until 90 degrees of flexion is obtained. Most patients with extensor mechanism disruptions treated nonoperatively will usually require permanent bracing or assistive devices or both.

Indications for Surgical Treatment

Due to the significant morbidity associated with disruption of either the quadriceps mechanism or the patellar ligament, surgery is indicated in most instances.

Surgical Treatment

Surgical Anatomy

The anatomy of the extensor mechanism of the knee is discussed in general terms at the beginning of this chapter (see Patella Fractures). The quadriceps tendon consists of the tendinous fibers of the rectus femoris, vastus medialis, vastus lateralis, and vastus intermedius. The tendon has a laminated structure, with the fibers of the rectus femoris being most superficial.

The patellar tendon is just under 5 cm long and consists mostly of the central fibers of the rectus femoris that cover the patella. The tendon inserts into the tibial tubercle, with some fibers blending with the insertion of the iliotibial tract. Rupture of the patellar tendon usually occurs at the junction of the tendon and the inferior pole of the patella.

Surgical Techniques

Patellar Ligament Disruption

Most surgeons advocate repairing the patellar tendon to the patella using transosseous sutures placed through the long axis of the patella and tied over the top of the patella. The patient is positioned supine on the operative table with a small positioning pillow beneath the ipsilateral hip to rotate the patella until it points upward. A tourniquet is applied to the thigh. Sterile skin preparation and routine draping are performed, the limb is exsanguinated, and the tourniquet is inflated. A midline skin incision is made directly over the patella, extending distally to the tibial tubercle. The exposure is deepened to the patella, patellar ligament, and retinacula. The peritenon over the intact portions of the tendon is opened longitudinally, the patellar ligament disruption is isolated, and the retinacula are exposed and inspected for associated disruptions.

Direct suture repair of patellar ligament injuries is not recommended due to a high rate of rerupture. Instead, these injuries are best repaired to bone with a pull-through suture technique. Fortunately, repair to the patella is facilitated by the fact that most ruptures occur at the osseotendinous junction. Necrotic portions of the tendon are sharply debrided to healthy tissue. Care must be taken to avoid removing too much tendon, which could cause patella baja. A curet or bur is used to debride the superficial cortical bone of the distal patellar pole to bleeding cancellous bone. After this, a pair of locking Krakow sutures are placed in the disrupted patellar ligament using a heavy nonabsorbable suture such as no. 2 or no. 5 Ethibond (Ethicon, Johnson & Johnson, Somerville, New Jersey) (**Fig. 27–21A,B**). The sutures are placed parallel to each other, each grasping ~50% of the width of the tendon, leaving four strands of suture exiting the stump of the tendon. Three parallel, vertical holes are drilled in the patella to receive the pull through sutures. A 2.5 mm drill bit is used to drill a hole from the inferior pole to the superior pole of the patella (**Fig. 27–22**). Care must be taken to ensure the holes are placed in the midsagittal plane of the patella to prevent cut-out of the sutures. When the drill emerges through the superior pole of the patella, it is palpated, a small 1 cm longitudinal incision is placed through the quadriceps tendon, and the drill bit is advanced through the incision. A suture passer is positioned on the end of the drill bit, which is slowly pulled back with the tendon passer following (**Fig. 27–23**). As the tendon passer emerges from the inferior patellar pole, the midline strand of each suture is placed within the loop of the tendon passer. The tendon passer is then pulled proximally, bringing the sutures with it through the patella and out proximally through the quadriceps tendon. The process is repeated with one more drill hole on each side of the central hole. The corresponding suture of that pair is pulled though the patella, and then the paired sutures are tagged with a hemostat. The procedure is repeated until all the sutures are pulled though the patella.

The knee is placed in extension. The paired suture ends are tied to one another with enough tension to approximate the tendon stump to the inferior pole of the patella (**Fig. 27–21A,B** and **27–24**). At this point the knee is flexed to ensure adequate strength of the repair. Generally, the knee is flexed to 90 degrees, but it may be flexed less if

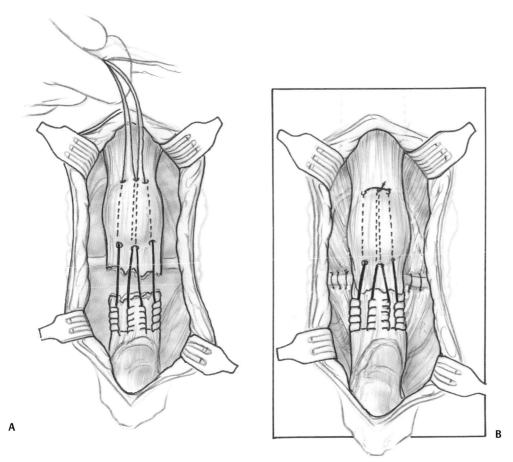

A

B

Figure 27–21 Drawings of a patellar ligament repair. **(A)** Multiple nonabsorbable sutures are placed through drill holes in the patella. Locking suture knots are placed into the patellar tendon. Note that one strand of two separate sutures is placed in the middle tunnel. **(B)** The sutures after they have been tied. The retinacular tear must also be repaired.

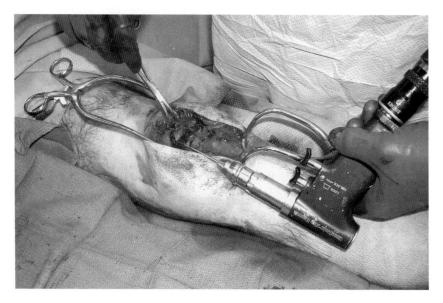

Figure 27–22 Intraoperative photograph showing the first drill hole being made in the patella. A total of three parallel holes are drilled from distal to proximal.

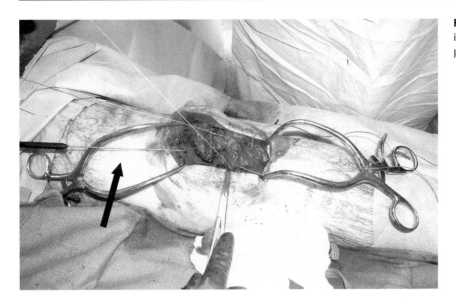

Figure 27–23 Intraoperative photograph showing a suture passer (black arrow) being used to pull sutures through the patella.

there is concern about the repair. If there is a gap at the patella–patellar ligament junction at minimal knee flexion, the pull-through suture technique may have to be repeated. Once assured of firm fixation, the suture knots are buried beneath the quadriceps tendon to avoid prominent suture knots. Defects in the retinacula are then approximated with absorbable suture to reinforce the repair. The wound is then irrigated and closed over a suction drain.

Midsubstance ruptures should also be repaired through bone tunnels. The distally based portions of the tendon are repaired to the patella as described, while the proximal portion of the tendon should be pulled distally and repaired to drill holes placed transversely in the tibial tubercle. The repair is then completed by side-to-side repair

of the tendon fragments with no. 0 absorbable sutures and repair of the retinacular tears as already described.

Quadriceps Tendon Disruption

In contrast to patellar ligament disruptions, many acute midsubstance quadriceps tendon disruptions may be successfully treated with direct suture repair.[30,31] A tourniquet is recommended, and when inflating the tourniquet, the knee must be flexed to prevent retraction of the quadriceps tendon. The surgical exposure is the same as that described for patellar ligament disruptions, except it may require more proximal rather than distal exposure. The quadriceps disruption is identified, and the surrounding retinacula are

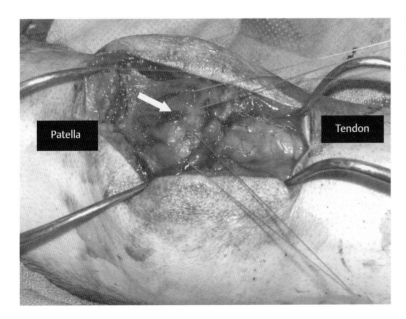

Figure 27–24 Intraoperative photograph showing the sutures being pulled taught, reapproximating the patellar tendon to the patella. Note that the two central sutures exit the same middle drill hole (white arrow).

inspected for associated disruptions. After delineation of the quadriceps tendon disruption, all necrotic portions of the quadriceps tendon are debrided to healthy tissue with a scalpel. Excessive debridement must be avoided to prevent shortening of the tendon that may lead to patella alta or an inability to approximate the tendon disruption. The quadriceps tendon is then repaired using no. 5 Ethibond nonabsorbable suture. The retinacular disruptions are repaired using absorbable suture. After the repair is completed, the knee is flexed to ensure the stability of the repair. Flexion to 90 degrees is ideal but not mandatory.

Quadriceps disruptions at the superior pole of the patella are not suitable for direct suture repair techniques. Although repair to the patella using suture anchors has been reported,[33] there are no long-term results of this technique, and the authors recommend repair using transosseous sutures. After debridement of necrotic tendon, several no. 5 nonabsorbable sutures are placed in the proximal tendon using a locking Krakow stitch. Three to four suture pairs within the disrupted tendon are required for a successful repair. Paired suture strands are marked with a surgical pen to allow for later identification. The superior pole of the patella is roughened with a high-speed bur to bleeding cancellous bone. Marks are made along the superior pole of the patella with a marker or an electrocautery corresponding to the desired positions for suture strands to enter the patella. A 2.5 mm drill bit is then used to drill through the body of the patella in the midsagittal plane beginning at the superior pole. As the drill bit emerges from the inferior patellar pole, a small longitudinal incision is made through the patellar tendon directly over the drill bit. A suture passer is then placed over the drill bit. As the drill bit is retracted, the suture passer is brought through the patella. As the loop of the suture passer emerges from the superior patellar pole, the desired loop of suture is placed within the loop and the suture passer is withdrawn distally, bringing the suture with it through the patella. This is repeated until all suture strands have been passed through the patella (**Fig. 27–25A–D**).

To complete the repair, the knee is positioned in extension. The paired suture ends are tied to one another with care to ensure that the quadriceps tendon is pulled flush against the superior pole of the patella. Ideally, the repair will tolerate flexion to 90 degrees; however, a successful result may be obtained with lesser degrees of flexion. Corresponding retinacular tears are repaired with absorbable sutures.

Scuderi described a popular technique in which a triangular flap (5 cm wide at the base, 7.5 cm long) of the superficial layers of the quadriceps tendon is elevated and turned down to be sewn over the distal tendon.[34] Rarely, if the existing tissue is too necrotic to enable repair as described, a tendon weave as typically used for chronic disruptions may be required to restore the extensor mechanism. Many different techniques have been described using both autograft and allograft weaves to restore knee extension.[31] Despite the

Tips and Tricks

- Ultrasound or MRI will confirm the diagnosis of tendon rupture if there is clinical uncertainty.
- Direct suture repair of patellar ligament injuries is not recommended due to a high rate of rerupture. Instead, these injuries are best repaired to bone with a pull-through suture technique.
- When drilling holes in the patella for suture repair, the holes should be placed in the midsagittal plane of the patella to prevent cut-out of the sutures.
- If the tissue is tenuous during repair of quadriceps tears, the Scuderi technique of turning down a flap of the proximal tendon can be very useful to augment the repair.

technique chosen for reconstruction, the underlying principle is to reestablish independent knee extension.

Rehabilitation

Ideally, after repair of a quadriceps tendon or patellar ligament, motion is initiated within the first few days after surgery; however, the ideal must be balanced with the practical. A recent study of patients not immobilized after repair of traumatic patellar tendon ruptures showed excellent results.[35] For stable repairs where the knee was able to be flexed 90 degrees, early knee motion is recommended. Straight leg raises against gravity are initiated immediately postoperatively. Active knee motion is begun with the assistance of a physical therapist. Passive knee motion should be avoided for the first 4 to 6 weeks to prevent inadvertent rupture of the ligament repair. After 6 weeks, sufficient healing should have occurred to allow for range of motion without restriction. If there is concern about the strength of the repair, knee flexion may be delayed for 4 weeks to allow for initial healing at the repair site. Active assisted knee motion is permissible 4 to 6 weeks postoperatively to assist with knee flexion. Passive knee motion should be avoided during the first 8 weeks postoperatively to prevent inadvertent rupture at the repair site. Full knee motion should be expected in the majority of patients by 12 weeks postoperatively.

Atrophy of the surrounding knee muscles is common after rupture of the extensor mechanism. Muscle strengthening is important for return of normal knee function. A graduated strengthening program is initiated 12 weeks postoperatively. Knee flexion and extension exercises are started with light weights using high repetitions. As strength improves, weight may be added, with a goal of equaling the strength of the contralateral limb. Endurance training is also important in rehabilitation. Stationary bike training is initiated when the patient is allowed unrestricted knee motion. As the patient's strength and endurance improve, resumption of running exercises maybe resumed.

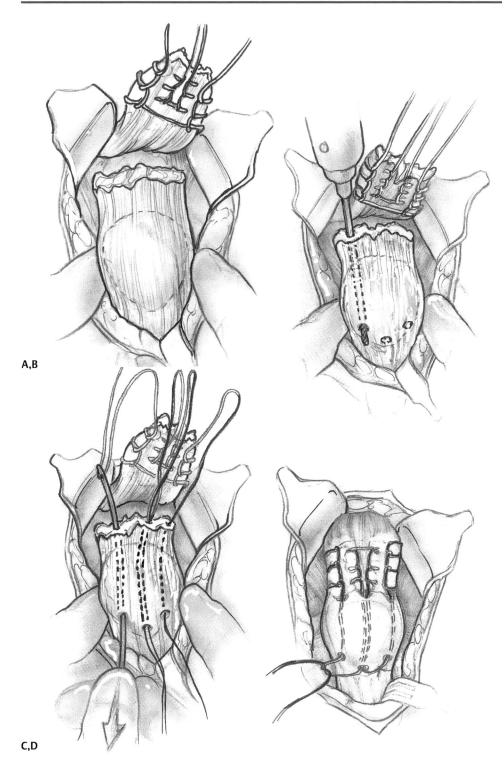

A,B

C,D

Figure 27–25 Drawings of a quadriceps tendon repair. **(A)** Placement of locking sutures in the quadriceps tendon. **(B)** Placement of parallel drill holes in the patella. **(C)** The sutures are brought through the drill holes with a suture passer. **(D)** The sutures are tied over the inferior pole of the patella.

New Techniques

The use of biological material to augment the healing of tendon ruptures is of great interest. Using a rotator cuff tendon model in sheep, Schlegel et al showed that tendon augmentation using swine intestinal submucosa produced a significant increase in stiffness in the augmented tendons.[36] Using a chicken Achilles' tendon model, Kummer and Iesaka tested four different graft biomaterials and found that all of them increased suture fixation strength.[37] Tissue engineering techniques are being used to develop scaffolds that can be seeded with appropriate cells and growth factors.[38] Although all of these techniques are still being evaluated, several such biological patches are clinically available. Although none have been reported for use in tendon ruptures about the knee, their use may be considered on a case-by-case basis. Future work in this area will improve the treatment of tendon ruptures about the knee.

Outcome

Good to excellent results are commonly reported following primary repair of acutely ruptured patella or quadriceps tendon.[30,39,40] Siwek and Rao reported 30 of 30 and 24 of 25 patients had good or excellent results following immediate quadriceps and patellar tendon repair, respectively. Patients undergoing immediate repair of quadriceps and patellar tendon ruptures regained full motion; however, persistent quadriceps atrophy occurred in 75% of patients with quadriceps tendon repair and 35% with patellar tendon rupture.[30] However, in the typically younger patient with patellar tendon rupture, this muscle atrophy did not affect quadriceps strength. Surprisingly, in the typically older patient with quadriceps rupture, the long-term effect on quadriceps strength was not enough to decrease knee function.[30]

Marder and Timmerman reported good results in a series of young patients with primary tendon repair and use of an early, protected physiotherapy program.[40]

Poorer results occur after delayed repair. Wenzl et al found that the outcome after quadriceps tendon rupture was significantly dependent on the time to surgery, with patients repaired within 14 days having much better results.[41] In their paper, the type of repair, kind of postoperative physiotherapy, patient's age, and body mass index had no influence on outcome.[41] For old ruptures, shortening and contraction of the quadriceps as well as degeneration of the tendon tissue make primary repair prone to fail. In such cases, use of preoperative traction, augmentation with allograft tissue, and longer postoperative immobilization may be necessary.[42] Therefore, after delayed repair, more patients experience decreased knee range of motion and increased quadriceps atrophy and strength. Better results were seen after delayed repair of patellar tendon ruptures; however, the results were still not equal to those following immediate repair.[30] Therefore, the most important determinant of patient outcome is timing of repair.

The importance of early postoperative range of motion to patient outcome has been substantiated in several studies in which no postoperative immobilization was used.[40,43,44] In these studies, patients began immediate active flexion and passive extension with hinged brace protection for the first 6 weeks after repair. Patients treated with this protocol experienced no extensor lag and minimal loss of flexion when compared with the opposite knee. In addition, residual quadriceps atrophy and loss of strength were not significant. Thus early range of motion as allowed by the strength of the tendon repair is felt to be important in optimizing patient outcome.

Pearls

- The proximal three fourths of the articular surface of the patella is covered with articular cartilage, whereas the distal pole is extra-articular.
- Bipartite patella exists in 1 to 2% of people and can be easily confused with a fracture. Bipartite patellae have a very classic appearance; they occur in the superolateral corner of the patella, are rounded, and have a smooth, sclerotic border (Fig. 27–5).
- The patella functions biomechanically to increase the extension moment arm of the quadriceps as much as 50% by displacing its line of action farther away from the center of rotation of the knee. The degree of mechanical advantage added by the patella is a function of the amount of knee flexion.
- Vertical fractures of the patella may not result in disruption of the extensor mechanism.

- For displaced intra-articular fractures of the patella and those associated with an extensor lag, operative management is recommended.
- There does not appear to be any correlation between outcome and the size of the remaining patella.
- Quadriceps tendon injuries usually occur in patients older than 40 years of age, whereas patellar ligament injuries typically occur in patients younger than 40.
- Tendon ruptures about the knee are sometimes related to an underlying systemic disease such as lupus erythematosus or rheumatoid arthritis.
- The Insall-Salvati ratio divides the length of the patellar tendon by the length of the patella.[15] The normal ratio is 1.02.

Complications

The knee extensor mechanism is critical to the function of the leg and experiences very high forces during routine activities of daily living. Disability due to pain, decreased motion, and weakness can occur after injury to the patella. Fortunately, complications are infrequent after surgical repair of the knee extensor mechanism. The most common complications are loss of full knee flexion and decreased quadriceps muscle strength. Persistent quadriceps atrophy has been noted, but muscle strength recovery is usually sufficient.[30] Rerupture of the repair is also an infrequent complication. Rerupture rates are typically less than 5% and commonly occur in patients who return to vigorous activities too quickly.[45] Wound complications may occur, and when they happen, repeat surgical debridement and aggressive wound management may be necessary.

On the DVDs

Video 27–1 (Disk 3) Tension Band Wire and ORIF of a Patella Fracture with Minifragment Screws A multifragmentary patella fracture is stabilized through use of both interfragmentary lag screws and tension band fixation. Emphasis is placed on attention to detail in placement of the tension band construct.

Video 27–2 (Disk 3) Patella Nonunion This video is of an elderly gentleman who failed tension band wiring of his patella when he fell during the postoperative period leading to a hardware failure. A revision tension band wiring after debridement of the nonunion is demonstrated.

References

1. Hey Groves EW. A note on the extension apparatus of the knee-joint. Br J Surg 1937;24:747–748
2. Kaufer H. Patellar biomechanics. Clin Orthop Relat Res 1979;144:51–54
3. Bostrom A. Fracture of the patella: a study of 422 cases. Acta Orthop Scand Suppl 1972;143:1–80
4. Pritchett JW. Nonoperative treatment of widely displaced patella fractures. Am J Knee Surg 1997;10:145–147
5. Wiberg G. Roentgenographic and anatomic studies on the patellofemoral joint. Acta Orthop Scand 1941;12:319–329
6. Gardner MJ, Griffith MH, Lawrence BD, Lorich DG. Complete exposure of the articular surface for fixation of patella fractures. J Orthop Trauma 2005;19:118–123
7. Berg EE. Extensile exposure of comminuted patella fractures using a tibial tubercle osteotomy: results of a new technique. J Orthop Trauma 1998;12:351–355
8. Ong BC, Sherman O. Acute patellar tendon rupture: a new surgical technique. Arthroscopy 2000;16:869–870
9. Carpenter JE, Kasman R, Matthews LS. Fractures of the patella. Instr Course Lect 1994;43:97–108
10. Smith ST, Cramer KE, Karges DE, Watson JT, Moed BR. Early complications in the operative treatment of patella fractures. J Orthop Trauma 1997;11:183–187
11. Burvant JG, Thomas KA, Alexander R, Harris MB. Evaluation of methods of internal fixation of transverse patella fractures: a biomechanical study. J Orthop Trauma 1994;8:147–153
12. Benjamin J, Bried J, Dohm M, McMurty M. Biomechanical evaluation of various forms of fixation of transverse patellar fractures. J Orthop Trauma 1987;1:219–222
13. Berg EE. Open reduction internal fixation of displaced transverse patella fractures with figure-eight wiring through parallel cannulated compression screws. J Orthop Trauma 1997;11:573–576
14. Saltzman CL, Goulet JA, McClellan RT, Schneider LA, Matthews LS. Results of treatment of displaced patellar fractures by partial patellectomy. J Bone Joint Surg Am 1990;72:1279–1285
15. Insall J, Goldberg V, Salvati E. Recurrent dislocation of the high riding patella. Clin Orthop Relat Res 1972;88:67–69
16. Gunal I, Taymaz A, Kose N, Gokturk E, Seber S. Patellectomy with vastus medialis obliquus advancement for comminuted patellar fractures: a prospective randomized trial. J Bone Joint Surg Br 1997;79:13–16
17. Lennox IA, Cobb AG, Knowles J, Bentley G. Knee function after patellectomy: a 12- to 48-year follow-up. J Bone Joint Surg Br 1994;76:485–487
18. Veselko M, Kastelec M. Inferior patellar pole avulsion fractures: osteosynthesis compared with pole resection. J Bone Joint Surg Am 2005;87:113–121
19. Levack B, Flannagan JP, Hobbs S. Results of surgical treatment of patella fractures. J Bone Joint Surg Br 1985;67:416–419
20. Curtis MJ. Internal fixation for fractures of the patella: a comparison of two methods. J Bone Joint Surg Br 1990;72:280–282
21. Hung LK, Chan KM, Chow YN, Leung PC. Fractured patella: operative treatment using the tension band principle. Injury 1985;16:343–347
22. Bostman O, Kiviluoto O, Nirhamo J. Comminuted displaced fractures of the patella. Injury 1981;13:196–202
23. Catalano JB, Iiannacone WM, Marczyk S, et al. Open fractures of the patella: long-term functional outcome. J Trauma 1995;39:439–444
24. Torchia ME, Lewallen DG. Open fractures of the patella. J Orthop Trauma 1996;10:403–409
25. Edwards B, Johnell O, Redlund-Johnell I. Patellar fractures: a 30-year follow-up. Acta Orthop Scand 1989;60:712–714
26. Brooke J. The treatment of fractured patella by excision: a study of morphology and function. Br J Surg 1937;24:733–747
27. Mishra US. Late results of patellectomy in fractured patella. Acta Orthop Scand 1972;43:256–263
28. Einola S, Aho AJ, Kallio P. Patellectomy after fracture: long-term follow-up results with special reference to functional disability. Acta Orthop Scand 1976;47:441–447
29. Morshed S, Ries MD. Patella infera after nonoperative management of a patella fracture: a case report. J Bone Joint Surg Am 2002;84:1018–1021
30. Siwek CW, Rao JP. Ruptures of the extensor mechanism of the knee joint. J Bone Joint Surg Am 1981;63:932–937

31. Ilan DI, Tejwani N, Keschner M, Leibman M. Quadriceps tendon rupture. J Am Acad Orthop Surg 2003;11:192–200

32. Chin KR, Sodl JF. Infrapatellar fat pad disruption: a radiographic sign of patellar tendon rupture. Clin Orthop Relat Res 2005; 440:222–225

33. Richards DP, Barber FA. Repair of quadriceps tendon ruptures using suture anchors. Arthroscopy 2002;18:556–559

34. Scuderi C. Ruptures of the quadriceps tendon: study of twenty tendon ruptures. Am J Surg 1958;95:626–635

35. Bhargava SP, Hynes MC, Dowell JK. Traumatic patella tendon rupture: early mobilization following surgical repair. Injury 2004;35:76–79

36. Schlegel TF, Hawkins RJ, Lewis CW, Motta T, Turner AS. The effects of augmentation with swine small intestine submucosa on tendon healing under tension: histologic and mechanical evaluations in sheep. Am J Sports Med 2006;34:275–280

37. Kummer FJ, Iesaka K. The role of graft materials in suture augmentation for tendon repairs and reattachment. J Biomed Mater Res B Appl Biomater 2005;74:789–791

38. DeFranco MJ, Derwin K, Iannotti JP. New therapies in tendon reconstruction. J Am Acad Orthop Surg 2004;12:298–304

39. O'Shea K, Kenny P, Donovan J, Condon F, McElwain JP. Outcomes following quadriceps tendon ruptures. Injury 2002;33:257–260

40. Marder RA, Timmerman LA. Primary repair of patellar tendon rupture without augmentation. Am J Sports Med 1999;27:304–307

41. Wenzl ME, Kirchner R, Seide K, Strametz S, Jurgens C. Quadriceps tendon ruptures: is there a complete functional restitution? Injury 2004;35:922–926

42. Burks RT, Edelson RH. Allograft reconstruction of the patellar ligament: a case report. J Bone Joint Surg Am 1994;76: 1077–1079

43. Levy M, Goldstein J, Rosner M. A method of repair for quadriceps tendon or patellar ligament (tendon) ruptures without cast immobilization: preliminary report. Clin Orthop Relat Res 1987;218: 297–301

44. Lindy PB, Boynton MD, Fadale PD. Repair of patellar tendon disruptions without hardware. J Orthop Trauma 1995;9:238–243

45. Konrath GA, Chen D, Lock T, et al. Outcomes following repair of quadriceps tendon ruptures. J Orthop Trauma 1998; 12:273–279

28 Knee Dislocations and Ligamentous Injuries

James P. Stannard and Robert C. Schenck Jr.

Knee dislocations can be devastating orthopaedic injuries. Knee dislocation is frequently classified as a sports medicine injury. However, it is very rare to see a knee dislocation occur as a result of an athletic injury **(Fig. 28–1)**. The mechanism of injury is usually high-energy trauma such as a motor vehicle accident. Although the incidence has historically been considered low, the true occurrence of knee dislocations is probably higher than originally thought.[1,2] Numerous explanations for this increase include a true increase in high-velocity trauma, a better recognition of the injury itself, and the understanding of "spontaneously" reduced bicruciate knee injuries in trauma. Regardless of the reason for this phenomenon, orthopaedic management of knee dislocations is still a complex, multifactorial treatment dilemma for the orthopaedic surgeon.[3–6] Associated injuries, especially to the popliteal artery, can put the limb at risk and complicate treatment of these injuries. A variety of different treatment methods have been advocated[7] for knee dislocations, and the final outcome can be disappointing despite the most aggressive treatment. Knee dislocations can ultimately result in stiffness, instability, or amputation, and even if salvaged, often function at a level one grade lower than preinjury status.[8]

Numerous methods for treatment have been utilized for dislocations ranging from cast immobilization or external fixation,[9,10] splinting,[11] acute repair of ligamentous structures,[12,13] and staged posterior cruciate ligament and anterior cruciate ligament (PCL/ACL) reconstructions to delayed simultaneous bicruciate reconstruction of the knee.[5,14–16] Selection of the specific treatment plan should be highly patient dependent. Patients with open knee injuries, neurovascular compromise, multiple trauma, or a closed head injury are those patients where cruciate reconstruction has a higher risk of complications, especially that of heterotopic ossification (HO) and stiffness.[17,18] One important consideration is that the patient must be treated as a whole; evaluation must focus not only on the ligamentous injury but also on the potential associated injuries. Knee dislocations frequently traverse a continuum that ranges from low- to high-energy trauma and with varying associated injuries.[2,18–25] Thus, treatment decisions must be based on the specifics of the entire traumatic event.

There are multiple decisions to be made regarding the ligamentous reconstruction of the dislocated knee. The need for a reliable reconstruction of the posteromedial complex (PMC) and posterolateral complex (PLC) are critical for the successful management of the bicruciate knee ligament injury. Furthermore, operative reconstruction of the complete bicruciate revolves around the management of the PCL. The scientific and clinical experience with reconstruction of this critical knee cornerstone is variable at best, but technical advancements continue to improve our treatment options for this ligamentous injury. Various controversies in the management of the PCL include standard transtibial tunnels compared with the tibial inlay method, which avoids the "killer curve" of the graft traversing the back of the tibia, as well as single-bundle versus a two-tailed femoral-sided ligamentous reconstruction are current treatment options. The surgeon caring for a patient with a dislocated knee must have experience and success with one of these treatment options to create a stable knee reconstruction.

Classification

Knee dislocations should be classified by the structures that are torn. The position classification system is based on the direction of the tibia relative to the femur. This system is useful for reduction purposes, but often it is not applicable

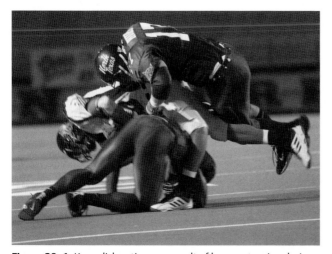

Figure 28–1 Knee dislocating as a result of hyperextension during a football game.

because of the frequency of spontaneous reductions.[20,26,27] An anatomical classification system is useful in determining appropriate treatment and will be discussed in detail later. Finally, the difference between a complete versus incomplete bicruciate knee injury is a useful consideration. The incomplete bicruciate injury involves a more straightforward treatment, usually with early range of motion followed by single cruciate reconstruction.[2,28]

It is now well accepted that a knee can physically dislocate without tearing of both cruciate ligaments. As early as 1975, Meyers et al referred to the knee dislocation with an intact PCL.[29] Shelbourne et al and Cooper et al in separate reports presented patients with a radiographically defined knee dislocation that, upon reduction or operative exploration, demonstrated a functioning PCL.[5,14] In a similar type of an incomplete bicruciate injury, an ACL intact knee dislocation can occur with posterior position of the tibia on the femur with complete tearing of the PCL. Thus describing a knee injury as a dislocation does not clearly define what is torn and gives very little information as to how to treat the injury. Although knee dislocations have been classified historically on the position of the tibia on the femur, a more clinically germane system is to classify dislocations based on what is torn.

In various series of knee dislocations, 20 to 50% of dislocations were reduced at the time of medical evaluation and were considered spontaneously reduced, hence unclassifiable by the position system. The knee ligamentous anatomy is complex, with many combinations of cruciate and collateral disruptions possible with a knee dislocation. Thus it is useful to classify knee dislocations in terms of ligaments involved, and this is best performed at the time of injury (if tolerated) and always during examination under anesthesia (EUA).[2,6]

One should be able to identify one of at least five possible injury patterns based upon an anatomical classification **(Table 28–1)**. This classification system is termed the anatomical system and is based upon ligament function (that is, what is torn) and is very useful in deciding upon treatment and operative incision. The higher the number, the greater the injury to the knee, and in most scenarios, the greater the velocity. Additional designations of C and N

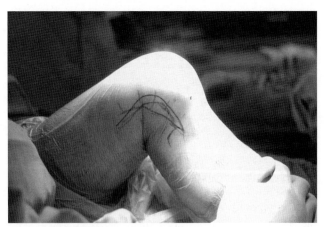

Figure 28–2 Examination under anesthesia demonstrating obvious sag consistent with a complete posterior cruciate ligament injury.

are utilized for associated arterial and neural injuries, respectively. Thus a KDIIILCN implies a complete bicruciate injury with the LCL and posterolateral corner torn with an injury of the popliteal artery and most commonly the peroneal nerve. The anatomical system is useful because it requires the clinician to focus on what is torn, especially directing reconstruction of the corner and collateral ligament involved. It also allows for accurate discussion of injuries between clinicians and allows for comparisons of like injuries in the wide spectrum of knee dislocations. KDV is an injury involving a large condylar fracture about the knee in addition to a multiligament knee injury and identifies as a fracture-dislocation of the knee.

The anatomical classification of knee dislocations considers the functional integrity of the remaining ligaments about the knee and emphasizes the importance of the EUA.[30] Due to the severity of injury and associated pain, an EUA is required to accurately identify what is torn. Lonner and colleagues[2] compared the accuracy of EUA with that of magnetic resonance imaging (MRI) in identifying ligament function. MRI was found to "overcall" ligamentous injuries and was not as accurate as EUA in making the diagnosis of functional ligament injury. MRI does have use in determining types of ligamentous injuries, presence of hyaline cartilage, and meniscal injuries and complements what is found at the time of EUA **(Fig. 28–2)**.[2,19,31–33] MRI is useful preoperatively to gauge an injury prior to EUA and surgical exploration. In our experience, MRI is very important as an adjunct in preoperative decision making but does not substitute for the EUA.[9,19,21,34] Both EUA and MRI are critical to decision making with these complex injuries.

Nonoperative Treatment

Most series that advocated completely nonoperative treatment of knee dislocations were published 15 or more years

Table 28–1 Anatomical Classification

Class	Description
KDI	Cruciate intact knee dislocation
KDII	Both cruciates torn, collaterals intact
KDIII	Both cruciates torn, one collateral torn
	Subset KDIIIM or KDIIIL
KDIV	All four ligaments torn
KDV	Periarticular fracture-dislocation

ago.[3,31,35] Although isolated cases of good function and stability have been reported using nonoperative treatment, many other authors have noted unacceptable rates of stiffness, pain, and instability.[1,8,30,36–42] Nonreconstructive surgery using a spanning external fixator (as opposed to completely nonoperative treatment) may provide more effective treatment to knee dislocation patients who are not good candidates for major ligament reconstructions.[37,38,41,42] All of the nonoperative or nonreconstructive methods rely on indirect healing of ligaments and capsule combined with scar tissue formation to yield a stable knee.[38] In this section, we will review the options and indications for both nonoperative treatment of patients with knee dislocations and surgical treatment that does not involve ligament reconstruction.

Indications

Although many authors strongly support aggressive surgical treatment for patients with acute knee dislocations, as already noted, there are indications to consider nonoperative or nonreconstructive treatment. Patients who should be considered for less aggressive treatment include (1) poor surgical candidates, (2) open dislocations **(Fig. 28–3)**, and (3) patients with a severely damaged closed soft tissue envelope.

Techniques

Cast Immobilization

This technique was commonly utilized to treat knee dislocations prior to the development of modern reconstructive techniques. Problems with casting are numer-

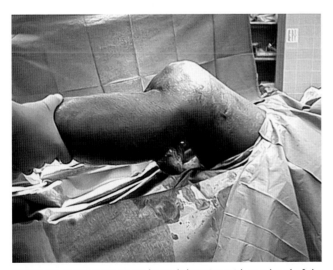

Figure 28–3 Open posterior knee dislocation with one head of the gastrocnemius muscle extruded from the wound.

ous, including lack of access to the soft tissues to monitor wounds or compartments, arthrofibrosis and loss of motion, pain, and instability.[3,31,35,38–40,42] When this technique is selected, it is critical to monitor the patient radiographically for the first 6 weeks to ensure that the knee does not sublux or dislocate within the cast.[38,42] Another important principle is to limit immobilization to a maximum of 6 weeks and then begin aggressive range of motion of the knee.[3,8,36,37,40,42] Immobilization for longer periods of time can contribute to severe arthrofibrosis and pain. Cast immobilization is only appropriate in patients who are unable to undergo surgical treatment.

Hinged Brace with Early Motion

Treatment of knee dislocations with bracing and early motion usually restores motion within a few weeks. However, severe ligamentous laxity is also a frequent result of this technique. Several authors have noted problems with residual laxity despite ligament reconstruction.[1,3,31,41,42] The functional disability due to instability can be quite severe.

External Fixation

External fixation can be used as a temporizing treatment prior to reconstructions in occasional patients who have severe soft tissue injuries, or as definitive care for patients who are not good candidates for reconstruction. External fixation can be an effective method of maintaining reduction without the use of hardware traversing the joint. Major indications for this procedure are high-energy knee dislocations without associated local injuries (such as fracture dislocations), open knee dislocations, severe soft tissue injuries, and patients who have poor rehabilitation potential. Advantages of the technique are good access to open wounds and maintenance of a good reduction. Disadvantages include the potential for loss of motion and scar tissue formation (quadriceps adhesions). The details of this technique are included in the surgical techniques section of this chapter.

Rehabilitation

The duration of immobilization when nonreconstructive surgery or nonoperative treatment is selected is controversial. Many authors agree that a period of immobilization is necessary if early reconstruction is not utilized, with many authors proposing between 4 and 8 weeks.[3,8,36–38,42] Taylor et al[3] noted that immobilization for a period of longer than 6 weeks was associated with severe stiffness and pain. When motion is initiated, rehabilitation should initially consist of active assisted range of motion exercises.

Approximately 3 months following injury, an assessment can be made regarding motion and ligament stability. Subsequent treatment with knee reconstruction, manipulation under anesthesia or lysis of adhesions, or continued functional rehabilitation will depend on the results of that assessment.

Indications for Surgical Treatment and Treatment Algorithm

The vast majority of patients who have sustained knee dislocations should undergo surgical treatment. With the exception of patients who are nonambulators or are critically ill with a chronic medical disease, surgical treatment will benefit nearly all patients following knee dislocations. This section presents an algorithm for the treatment of patients following knee dislocations (**Fig. 28–4**).

Contemporary treatment can be divided into two major categories: treatments that depend on immobilization,and treatments that allow early mobilization of the knee.[38] As already described in the Techniques section of this chapter, the primary treatment method that involves immobilization involves placement of an external fixator spanning the knee joint for 6 to 8 weeks.[37]

Methods that allow early mobilization of the knee involve various repairs and reconstructions of ligaments. The key to all of these methods is early mobilization of the knee joint. The definition of early mobilization varies from 1 day to approximately 4 weeks following surgery. The major theoretical benefit of early mobilization is a reduction of intra-articular scar tissue with a subsequent decrease in pain and improved motion. The risk of early motion is increased wound healing problems and ligamentous laxity. We believe that most patients should be treated by a method that allows early mobilization of the knee joint to improve final range of motion and limit pain and intra-articular scar tissue formation.

Patients who sustain a multiligament knee injury should be evaluated in the emergency department with a careful neurological and vascular exam, with special attention to the vascular supply below the knee and the neurological function of the peroneal and tibial nerves. The patient's skin should be carefully scrutinized to rule out an open dislocation, and a careful exam of the ipsilateral lower extremity should be conducted to detect any associated fractures. If the knee is still dislocated, a reduction should be performed. If the knee is irreducible and the patient has a normal vascular exam, the patient should be taken to the operating room for an open reduction. A splint

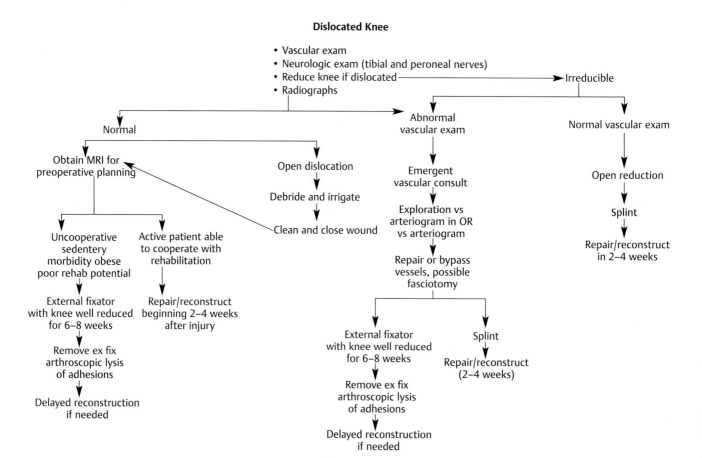

Figure 28–4 Treatment algorithm for patients with knee dislocations. MRI, magnetic resonance imaging; OR, operating room; Ex fix, external fixator.

should be applied and formal repair or reconstruction delayed for approximately 2 to 4 weeks to allow soft tissue recovery. If the vascular exam is abnormal, an emergent consultation with vascular surgeons and open exploration of the popliteal artery should be pursued. Ligament reconstruction is delayed for at least 2 to 4 weeks to allow soft tissue and vascular recovery prior to embarking on extensive reconstructive procedures.

The majority of knee dislocations present with the knee reduced. In this case, a careful vascular exam should be performed to allow the selective use of angiography (see Complications section). Patients with an abnormal vascular exam in terms of pulses, color, and temperature should have an emergent vascular consultation and revascularization with fasciotomy as indicated. Patients with a normal exam and an open dislocation should have an emergent irrigation and debridement. Depending on the severity of the wound, patients with an open dislocation may benefit from placement of a spanning external fixator across the knee. When a clean and closed wound has been achieved, the patient can be considered for ligament reconstruction. Regardless of the initial presentation, an MRI should be obtained prior to ligamentous repair to assist in preoperative planning.

Most patients who are active and cooperative should undergo repair or reconstruction of the torn ligaments in their knee. We recommend initiating repair or reconstruction within 2 to 4 weeks to allow early mobilization of the knee. The ideal timing (if there is an ideal) for ligament repair or reconstruction is not clear based on the literature. Controversy exists regarding repair/reconstruction of all ligaments at one surgery compared with delayed reconstruction of the ACL after early rehabilitation of the PCL, PLC, and PMC. Authors report success with both methods, and each has its advantages. One of the authors of this chapter takes care of all the ligaments at the index surgery, whereas the other does everything except the ACL initially, followed 6 weeks later by ACL reconstruction.

Surgical Treatment

Anatomy

Conceptually, the anatomy of the knee is divided into four defined structures: two cruciates and two collaterals (including the corners). Anatomical arrangement of the popliteus and biceps femoris posterolaterally and the semimembranosus posteromedially allows for musculoskeletal injury of those structures in conjunction with ligamentous trauma.

Important palpable landmarks about the knee include the medial and lateral femoral epicondyles (collateral ligament origins), the tibial (patellar tendon insertion) and Gerdy's (iliotibial band insertion) tubercles, the posteromedial border of the proximal tibia, and the fibular head later-

ally. The frequent need to explore the posteromedial or posterolateral corners in the surgical management of the dislocated knee makes knowledge of these approaches critical. Any approach to the ligamentous corners is based on the femoral epicondyle, posterior tibial border medially, and fibula laterally. With respect to the posterolateral approach, the peroneal nerve must be explored, with neurolysis a critical first step prior to any ligamentous or tendon reconstructive work on the lateral side of the knee. Medially, the tibial tubercle and the insertion of the pes tendons distal to this are noted. These landmarks, along with the medial collateral ligament (MCL) inserting just underneath the pes and along the posterior border of the medial tibia, are important for medial sided approaches to the knee.

The vascular supply about the knee is a complex anastomosis of two separate systems: the intrinsic and extrinsic networks. The intrinsic supply is an anastomotic ring made up of the articular, muscular branches and five geniculates. The geniculates are the superomedial and lateral geniculates, the middle geniculate, and the inferior medial and lateral geniculates. The anastomotic network provides for a rich blood supply to the skin overlying the knee and patella and allows for vascularity even with subcutaneous dissection. When parallel incisions are utilized (such as parallel medial and lateral patellar incisions), the skin flaps are dependent upon the width of the superior and inferior vascular pedicles of the extrinsic system. Planning of such incisions to avoid skin bridge necrosis should have appropriate width of at least 7 to 10 cm between incisions. With proper planning, skin loss is rare, but it can occur and is covered most frequently with a rotationplasty of the medial gastrocnemius muscle. Although the intrinsic/extrinsic vascular system provides adequate vascularity for superficial knee dissections, the anastomotic ring provides inadequate collateral flow to the lower leg with popliteal flow disruption.

The knee joint has a complex anatomical arrangement of muscular and ligamentous attachments. A layer system has been described that is useful to understand the complex and varied anatomy of the posterolateral and posteromedial corners of the knee. The layer system is divided into three sections labeled Roman numerals I, II, and III (**Fig. 28–5**). Layer I is the most superficial fascial layer, with the deeper layers sequentially numbered II and III. Layer I is described as the arciform or Marshall's layer anteriorly, sartorius fascia medially, and ilotibial band and biceps femoris fascia laterally. Layer II includes the patellar tendon, superficial MCL, and the fibular collateral ligament. Layer III is defined as all joint capsular structures, including the functional capsular thickenings of the posterior oblique and arcuate ligaments, the deep MCL, and the mid-one-third lateral joint capsule (responsible for the Segond fracture). Simplistically, but accurately, layer III includes all joint capsular structures but has multiple anatomical variations in thickness, creating distinct ligaments about the posteromedial and posterolateral corners.

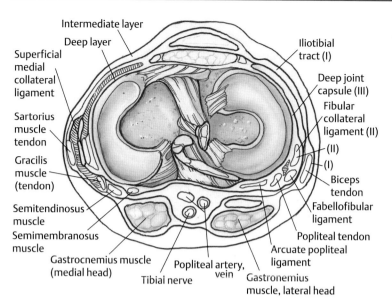

Figure 28–5 Axial view of the structures of the knee using the layer system.

Anteriorly, the joint capsule, or layer III, is thin and adherent to the posterior aspect of the patellar tendon. Posterolaterally, the capsule thickening is named the arcuate ligament (posterior one-third capsule, laterally) and is thickened posteromedially as the posterior oblique ligament (posterior one-third capsule medially). The posterolateral corner and ligaments have great variability and confusing nomenclature when reviewing the anatomical literature.[43] With any posterolateral reconstruction, both the popliteofibular and fibular collateral ligament should be reconstructed.

Posteromedial Approach to the Knee

The posteromedial approach is very useful for access to the vascular structures of the popliteal fossa and is the utilitarian approach to the vessels in a dislocated knee.[26] Variations of this approach have been utilized by Burks and Berg to approach the tibial attachment of the PCL.[16] Open treatment of knee dislocations for reconstruction of the PCL and the posteromedial corner can be accessed via this approach,[44] as well as using it for simultaneous repair of vascular and ligament injuries.[16,26,44] The approaches to the PCL described by Burks and Berg in separate reports utilize a posterior incision into the flexion crease of the knee but utilize a similar deep plane as described following here.

The patient is positioned supine, and the incision is placed along a line from the medial epicondyle to the insertion of the tibial collateral ligament along the posteromedial border of the tibia. With the knee flexed and the hip externally rotated in the "figure-of-four" position, the posteromedial approach can be performed in a supine position and is our preferred approach. The saphenous vein and nerve are identified and should be protected

(Fig. 28–6). The tendons of the pes anserinus can simply be retracted distally. The semimembranosus is variable in its insertion and in our experience usually requires release at its insertion but is tagged for later repair. The medial head of the gastrocnemius muscle is then identified. The remainder of the surgical approach remains anterior to the gastrocnemius, hugging the proximal tibial condyle and medial femoral condyle. The surgeon must continue to isolate the joint line in order not to stray too far distally on the posteromedial tibia. In this approach to the PCL, all retractors must remain anterior to the medial gastrocnemius to avoid injury to the popliteal vessels, and the medial head is routinely *not* released **(Fig. 28–7).** This approach is complex and ideally should be performed on a cadaveric specimen before the first attempt or with an experienced surgeon to clearly understand this anatomical approach and avoid complications. Keeping the knee flexed to 70 degrees relaxes the posterior neurovascular bundle, creating added safety with an approach anterior to the gastrocnemius. In the presence of a knee dislocation and evidence of MCL insufficiency, capsular structures are usually completely disrupted, allowing exposure of the knee joint itself. Access to the lateral side of the knee is limited from this approach.

Posterolateral Approach to the Knee

This approach is useful for reconstruction of posterolateral ligamentous injuries, mobilization of the lateral gastrocnemius muscle for soft tissue coverage procedures, and exploration and repair of the common peroneal nerve. It is frequently useful in knee dislocations and is critical in reconstruction of the posterolateral corner. The peroneal nerve is always isolated prior to deep joint exposure to prevent inadvertent injury to the nerve. In dislocations

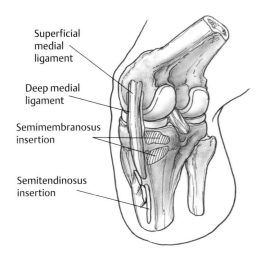

Figure 28–6 Superficial anatomy of the posteromedial approach to the knee.

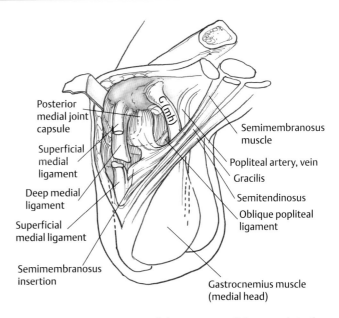

Figure 28–7 Deep anatomy of the posteromedial approach to the knee.

with complete tears of both cruciates, the ligaments are frequently disrupted circumferentially. With dislocations, exposure of the tibiofemoral joint is facilitated by following tissue planes created by the injury.

The patient is placed in the supine position with a tourniquet on the thigh and a small bump under the ipsilateral buttock. The knee joint is best exposed with the knee flexed to 90 degrees, allowing relaxation and protection of the peroneal nerve. The surgeon sits during the procedure, with the skin incision at eye level. The patient's foot is on the table, with the knee flexed to 90 degrees. The skin incision is placed in line with the fibular head and carried in a straight line proximally, then curving onto the lateral thigh. With proximal extension, the incision should curve between the iliotibial band (ITB) and biceps femoris tendon. The incision is carried down to the deep fascia, which is then opened carefully with scissors. At this point the peroneal nerve must be identified and can usually be palpated subfascially as it courses from the biceps femoris through its perineural fat to the fibular neck. The posterolateral approach should always include exposure of the peroneal nerve prior to deep dissection and ligamentous reconstruction **(Fig. 28–8).** The peroneal nerve is best isolated proximally and then released distally, where it wraps around the fibular neck. Once identified, the nerve is protected with a small vessel loop. Once the nerve is identified and protected, exposure of the posterolateral corner and lateral gastrocnemius is relatively straightforward.

Blunt dissection is used to define the plane anterior to the lateral gastrocnemius head **(Fig. 28–9A,B).** In the exposure of combined ligament injuries of the posterolateral knee, the dissection planes are usually already formed secondary to the translation that occurred with the knee injury. The surgeon should not dissect posterior to the gastrocnemius because it places the popliteal neurovascular structures at risk. If the lateral collateral liga-

ments are intact, the PCL cannot be identified from this approach. Furthermore, if the approach is performed for a complete injury of the PCL and posterolateral corner, an intact ACL will prevent access medially to the PCL insertion on the tibia for trough formation. In such a scenario, a posteromedial incision will be necessary to access the PCL insertion site. However, if the ACL, PCL, and LCL are completely torn, with careful dissection, the tibial insertion of the PCL (i.e., inlay) can be exposed and performed from this lateral approach.

Posterior Cruciate Ligament Reconstruction

Much like ACL reconstruction in the 1980s, PCL reconstruction techniques have evolved over the past 10 years. Three distinct approaches to PCL reconstruction now exist. The transtibial reconstruction fixes the PCL graft proximally in a femoral tunnel and distally in a tunnel through the proximal tibia. The tibial inlay technique utilizes a similar femoral tunnel for proximal fixation, but distal fixation is obtained by securing a bone plug into a trough positioned at the anatomical insertion of the PCL. The tibial inlay approach places the bone tendon junction of the distal graft at or near the joint line. Finally, the two-tailed femoral technique is now frequently used in combination with a tibial inlay approach.

Transtibial PCL reconstructions have often resulted in grade I or II laxity. It has been suggested that two major factors may explain late loosening and low-grade laxity following transtibial PCL reconstruction. The first factor is the acute angle the graft must make to round the posterior lip of the tibia when exiting the transtibial tunnel. This has been described as "the killer turn," which may lead to abrasion

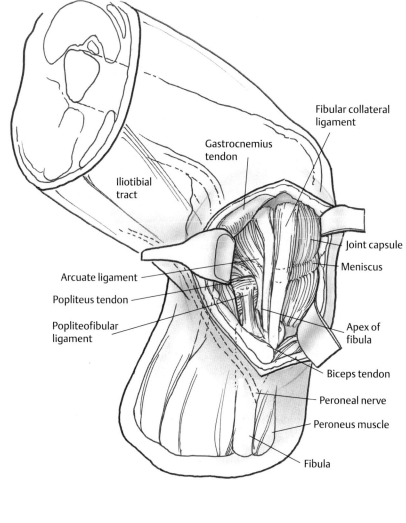

Fibular collateral ligament

Gastrocnemius tendon

Iliotibial tract

Joint capsule

Meniscus

Arcuate ligament

Popliteus tendon

Popliteofibular ligament

Apex of fibula

Biceps tendon

Peroneal nerve

Peroneus muscle

Fibula

and subsequent laxity and failure[16] **(Fig. 28–10).** This first factor is supported by biomechanical studies that show the inlay technique had zero failures compared with 32% in the transtibial technique using a cadaver model with an mechanical testing system (MTS [MTS Systems, Minneapolis, Minnesota]) machine ranging the knee for 2000 cycles. There were also significant differences in graft thinning and elongation between the two techniques. The inlay grafts developed 13% thinning and 5.9 mm of graft elongation over 2000 cycles, compared with 41% thinning and 9.8 mm of graft elongation with the transtibial technique.[45] The second factor is that, although the PCL has at least two distinct bundles functionally, which tighten at different degrees of knee flexion,[46–49] the transtibial endoscopic technique reproduces only the anterolateral bundle. Some contemporary surgical techniques attempt to address these shortcomings of the transtibial method. The tibial inlay technique addresses the potential problems associated with the killer turn by placing a bone block in a trough on the posterior tibia at the site of insertion of the PCL.[16,50–52] The two femoral tunnel technique allows reconstruction of both the anterolateral and posteromedial bundles of the PCL.[53,54]

Tibial inlay techniques at first glance may appear cumbersome but have become more simplified in recent years. Miller and colleagues performed an anatomical study showing that the popliteal artery remains an average of 21 mm posterior to the inlay site when the medial head of the gastroc is left intact.[55] An approach to PCL reconstruction that further simplifies the tibial inlay technique maintains the patient in a supine position throughout the procedure and preserves the origin of the medial head of the gastrocnemius.

Single-Bundle Posterior Cruciate Ligament Reconstruction

This approach can be divided into several steps:

1. Patient positioning, EUA, confirmatory arthroscopy, and notch preparation
2. Femoral tunnel preparation
3. Posteromedial approach and tibial inlay site preparation
4. Graft preparation
5. Tibial-sided graft fixation
6. Femoral-sided graft fixation

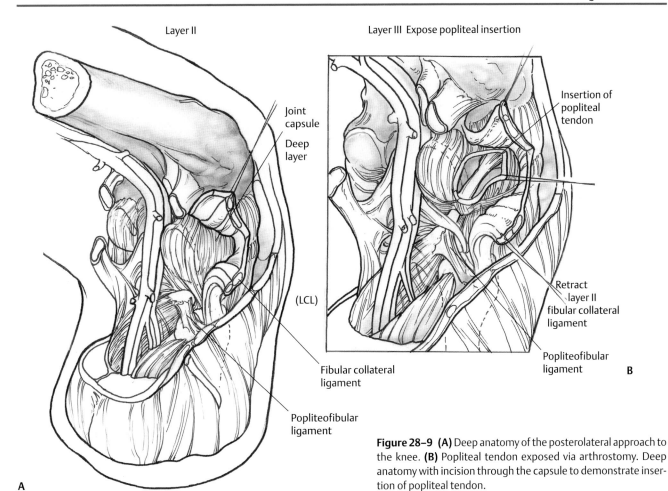

Layer II

Layer III Expose popliteal insertion

Joint
capsule

Deep
layer

(LCL)

Fibular collateral
ligament

Popliteofibular
ligament

A

Insertion of
popliteal
tendon

Retract
layer II
fibular collateral
ligament

Popliteofibular
ligament

B

Figure 28–9 (A) Deep anatomy of the posterolateral approach to
the knee. **(B)** Popliteal tendon exposed via arthrostomy. Deep
anatomy with incision through the capsule to demonstrate insertion of popliteal tendon.

The patient is positioned supine on a standard operating table with the foot of the table up. A careful EUA is
performed determining the ligaments torn. Standard anteromedial and anterolateral arthroscopy portals are

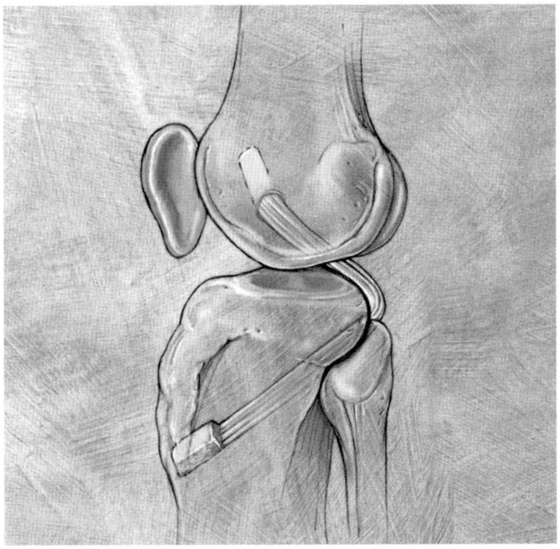

Figure 28–10 The "killer turn" that occurs following transtibial
posterior cruciate ligament reconstruction.

established, and a 30 degree arthroscope is inserted into
the anteromedial portal. A diagnostic arthroscopy is performed, and PCL tear is confirmed. The PCL remnant is
debrided, and the anatomical origin is identified.

Femoral Tunnel Preparation

A long drill-tip guidewire is used for the femoral tunnel
and is inserted into the knee through the anterolateral
portal. The knee is flexed to allow optimal placement of
the guide tip. Under arthroscopic visualization, the tip of
the guidewire is positioned in the center of the anatomical
origin of the anterolateral bundle of the PCL (typically at
the 10:30 position with regard to the notch of a left knee
and 8 mm posterior to the articular surface). The tip of the
guidewire is started inferior and lateral and drilled into
the medial femoral condyle and out through the skin overlying the distal medial thigh. The distal, slotted end of the
guidewire is left outside the anterolateral portal. The drill
is removed, and a 10 mm tunnel reamer is placed over
the guidewire, a 30 × 10 mm femoral tunnel is created in
the medial femoral condyle. The reamer is removed, and the
guidewire is left in place but pulled up into the medial side
with a heavy suture in the guidewire slotted end.

Posteromedial Approach and Tibial-Inlay Site Preparation

All arthroscopic instruments are removed from the knee, and the affected limb is placed in the figure-of-four position. The primary surgeon stands on the contralateral side of the table from the surgical limb. An assistant remains on the ipsilateral side of the table for retraction purposes. The leg is exsanguinated, and the tourniquet is inflated. A 6 to 10 cm skin incision is made over the posteromedial aspect of the knee. The incision overlies the posteromedial border of the tibia and is centered about the posterior joint line. The sartorius fascia is exposed and incised in line with the posteromedial tibia, and the pes tendons are retracted distally **(Fig. 28–7)**. The fascia between the medial head of the gastrocnemius and the posterior border of the semi-membranosus is divided in line with the incision. The semimembranosus is released but tagged for nonabsorbable suture repair at the end of the procedure. The dissection is carried anterior to the gastrocnemius but remains positioned directly on the back of the tibia, knee joint line, and posteromedial femoral condyle. Blunt dissection is performed medially to elevate the popliteus muscle. A blunt Hohman retractor is placed just lateral to the PCL tibial insertion and creates excellent visualization of the back of the tibia to create the trough. Occasionally, positioning the trough in the center of the posterior tibia is difficult. However, with careful observation of the tibial remnant of the PCL, the posterolateral edge of the medial femoral condyle, the joint surface, and lateral meniscus, an anatomical placement can be made. A bur is used to create a trough for the tibial inlay graft. The trough dimensions should be roughly 10 mm wide × 25 mm long × 10 mm deep, extending from the posterior joint line and centered over the midline posterior tibia made in a fashion mimicking the shape of the allograft bone plug. Care is taken not to excessively deepen the trough or place it distally, which may create a killer curve at the tendon–bone junction. A posterior capsulotomy is made at the mid joint line and spread with a Kelly clamp. At this point the tourniquet is released for hemostasis and to minimize tourniquet time.

Graft Preparation

One of the authors' preferred choice of graft is a patellar tendon allograft, whereas the other prefers an Achilles tendon allograft. The Achilles' tendon allows for a two-tailed femoral graft if so desired. A standard triangular bone plug 10 mm in width and 10 mm in depth is fashioned with an oscillating saw from the allograft patella. Two 2.0 mm drill holes are placed in the patellar bone plug, and two no. 5 Ethibond (Ethicon, Johnson & Johnson, Somerville, New Jersey) sutures are placed through the holes to facilitate graft passage. Cancellous bone is removed from the tibial portion of the allograft to create a 25 × 10 × 10 mm rectangular inlay graft mimicking the trough geometry.

Tibia-Sided Graft Fixation

With the affected limb still in the figure-of-four position, a curved Kelly clamp is placed through the inferolateral portal, passed medial to the ACL, and the tip is brought out through the posterior midline capsulotomy. The ends of the no. 5 Ethibond suture are grasped with the Kelly clamp and pulled through the knee and out the anterolateral portal. Traction is placed on the sutures, and the patella bone plug and proximal end of the bone–patella tendon–bone graft are pulled into the intercondylar notch. The slotted guide pin is pulled back through the anterolateral portal with its attached suture. The ends of the Ethibond sutures (attached to the graft) are then threaded through the slot in the distal end of the guidewire in the femoral tunnel. A handheld drill chuck is attached to the drill tip end of the guidewire and used to pull the guidewire and suture ends into the knee, through the femoral tunnel, and out the skin over the medial distal knee. Traction is placed on the sutures, and an arthroscopic grasper is used under arthroscopic visualization to guide the patella bone plug into the femoral tunnel. The tibial inlay graft is then positioned in the posterior tibial trough with the tendon–bone junction at the posterior joint line. Passing the graft into the femoral tunnel requires both patience and care. Once the graft is placed, the surgeon must check graft position, range the knee multiple times, and check the correction of the posterior drawer at 90 degree knee flexion. Graft fixation is delayed until the surgeon is satisfied with graft position, tension, and posterior drawer correction. The authors prefer to fix the tibial side first, keeping the graft at the tibiofemoral joint line to avoid creation of a tibial inlay killer curve. Two 4 mm cannulated screw guide pins are used to secure the inlay graft in the trough. The trajectories for the guide pins are directed anterior to posterior, parallel to the joint line, and at least 1 cm apart. In multiple-ligament injuries, the guide pins can be directed obliquely and lateral to avoid the tibial tunnel for the ACL reconstruction. The guide pins are then overdrilled, and 4 mm cannulated screws are placed in series across the inlay graft to obtain secure tibial fixation **(Fig. 28–11)**.

Femur-Sided Graft Fixation

With the tibial side of the allograft secured, the knee is brought out of the figure-of-four position and flexed over the side of the operating table. The arthroscope is placed back into the anteromedial portal to confirm proper graft placement and alignment. Tension is placed on the Ethibond sutures and patella bone plug, and the knee is taken through multiple knee ranges to minimize graft laxity. An appropriately sized interference screw is placed posterior to the plug through the anterolateral portal. The interference screw is then advanced into the femoral tunnel while performing an anterior drawer maneuver with the knee in 90 degrees of flexion to obtain secure femoral fixation.

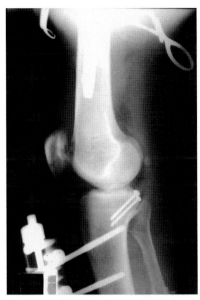

Figure 28–11 Cannulated screws provide secure fixation of inlay graft.

Radiographs are taken in the operating room to verify graft and screw placement, as well as an anatomical position of the knee.

Double-Bundle Inlay Posterior Cruciate Ligament Reconstruction (see Video 28–1, Disk 4)

The anatomical PCL reconstruction is a combination of the tibial inlay[16,50–52] and two femoral tunnel[53,54] techniques. There are many similarities to the single-bundle reconstruction described earlier, especially regarding creation and placement of the tibial inlay trough. The patient should be placed in a supine position to allow arthroscopy using a bump under the knee and allowing the leg to hang off the table. An Achilles' tendon allograft is divided into a larger anterolateral and a smaller posteromedial bundle. The bone block is trimmed, and permanent no. 2 suture is placed into each bundle using Krakow stitches to assist passage into the

appropriate femoral tunnel. The notch is debrided arthroscopically, and any meniscus pathology is addressed simultaneously. When that is complete, a guidewire is drilled ~6 to 8 mm from the articular surface within the footprint of the PCL at the top of the notch. A second guidewire is placed inferior to the first guidewire, making certain to space them so that there will be approximately a 4 mm bone bridge between the two tunnels (**Fig. 28–12**). The tunnel size is selected based on the size of the Achilles' tendon allografts, with a 9 mm anterolateral tunnel and a 7 mm posteromedial tunnel being the most common sizes (**Fig. 28–13**). The arthroscope is then removed from the knee and a posterolateral or posteromedial approach to the knee is performed, depending on associated ligament pathology.

A trough is created in the bone at the site of insertion of the PCL into the posterior tibia utilizing a combination of osteotomes, curets, and occasionally a rongeur. The 0.5 in. curved osteotome is the ideal size for this task. A key tip is that a blunt Hohman or similar retractor must be placed anterior to the gastrocnemius muscle, retracting the muscles and vascular structures posteriorly. Another important point is to keep the knee flexed any time the surgeon is working in the back of the knee. Fixation is obtained with a single 4.5 mm cannulated screw and washer placed utilizing a lag technique by drilling a 4.5 mm hole through the bone block. It is critical not to make the bone block too thin (**Fig. 28–13**), or the allograft may crack when tightened. If this occurs, it can be salvaged with staples. The two bundles are then advanced into the notch and into their respective femoral tunnels. The anterolateral bundle is tensioned at ~80 degrees of flexion, with the posteromedial bundle tensioned at ~15 degrees. Both bundles are secured with absorbable interference screws that are either the same size or 1 mm larger than the size of the tunnel, depending on bone quality. If all four ligament groups in the knee are torn, fluoroscopy may be necessary to confirm that the knee is reduced and that the graft is not overtightened. The initial results utilizing this technique have been very good, with little if any loosening over time and

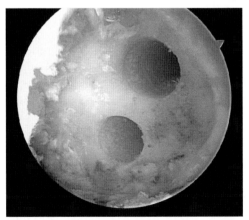

Figure 28–12 The anterolateral and posteromedial tunnels drilled through the medial femoral condyle.

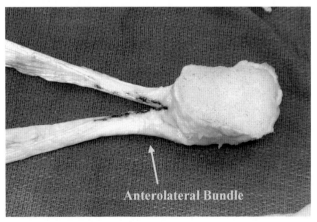

Figure 28–13 Achilles' tendon allograft being prepared for use in posterior cruciate ligament reconstruction.

only a single failure in our first 30 cases. KT-2000 data demonstrated the reconstructed PCL was at least as tight as the uninjured side. Lysholm knee scores and clinical laxity exams were also quite encouraging.[56]

Hamstring Anterior Cruciate Ligament Reconstruction (see Video 28–2, Disk 4)

This technique has gained recent popularity in orthopaedic sports medicine. Cosmetic incisions and relatively easier rehabilitation have made this technique an attractive option. especially for the recreational athlete. It is also useful in competitive volleyball players where patellar tendinitis is frequently debilitating after bone-tendon-bone reconstruction. However, recent studies have shown better long-term stability with a patellar tendon graft on KT-1000 testing; thus a bone-tendon-bone graft remains the gold standard for competitive professional and collegiate athletes. Caution against the use of a hamstring ACL autograft should also be made in a combined ACL/MCL injury or in a bicruciate injury where the tendons may be needed for collateral reconstruction. The technique for hamstring harvest and reconstructions is as follows.

The pes insertion is palpated medial and slightly distal to the tibial tubercle. A 3 cm incision is made in line with the tendons. The sartorius fascia is incised, and each tendon is sequentially hooked with a right-angle clamp. The tendons are detached distally and split into separate tendons, and a Krackow stitch is placed in each end. Harvest is simplified by short-term chemical paralysis of the patient during the procedure. Release of the hamstring from fascial attachments in the thigh must be performed before stripping the tendon from its muscle belly. Once harvested, the remaining muscle is cleaned from the tendon. Krakow sutures are placed in each end, and sizing of the graft is performed. Standard arthroscopic preparation of a tibial tunnel is performed through the harvest incision. Femoral fixation is performed through a variety of techniques and requires accurate placement to promote ideal soft tissue fixation of the graft to the bone tunnels. Femoral tunnel drilling and preparation are determined by the type of fixation utilized.

Modified Two-Tailed Reconstruction of the Posterolateral Corner (see Video 28–3, Disk 4)

The modified two-tailed technique reconstructs three critical components of the deep layers of the posterolateral corner (PLC): the popliteus, the popliteofibular ligament, and the fibulocollateral collateral ligament. The technique involves drilling a 5 mm hole from anterior to posterior through the lateral tibia, exiting where the popliteus tendon traverses the back of the tibia. A retractor or the surgeon's finger should be placed on the posterior tibia while drilling, to prevent damage to the popliteal vessels.

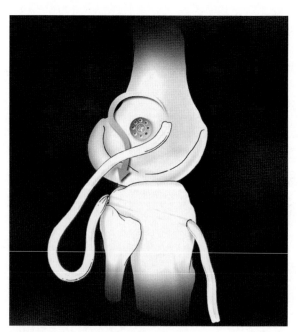

Figure 28–14 Initial graft passage using modified two-tailed posterior cruciate ligament reconstruction.

The tibial tunnel is tapped with a 7 mm tap to allow fixation with a bioabsorbable screw. A tibialis posterior allograft is trimmed to a size of approximately 5 mm and passed into the tunnel from posterior to anterior. It is important to use an allograft that is at least 24 cm in length to be able to reconstruct all three components of the PLC. The graft is secured with a 7 mm bioabsorbable ligament screw that is placed from anterior to posterior **(Fig. 28–14).** A second 5 mm drill hole is made through the proximal fibula, aimed from anterolateral to posteromedial. This tunnel does not need to be tapped. The isometric point on the lateral femoral condyle is then located. The isometric point lies just superior to the point where the FCL and popliteus cross one another on the lateral femoral condyle. A 3.2 mm drill bit is used to drill a hole for a long 4.5 mm bicortical screw going from lateral to medial. An important tip when drilling the screw for a PLC reconstruction in a patient with a multiligamentous knee injury is to remember the location of the femoral tunnel if an ACL reconstruction is necessary. If the PLC screw is not angled from posterior to anterior, it may block reaming of the femoral tunnel for an ACL reconstruction. A spiked ligament washer is used with the screw. An osteotome facilitates decorticating the bone posteriorly and anteriorly around the screw, allowing the allograft to heal to bone in the anatomical locations of the fibular collateral ligament (FCL) and popliteus, respectively. The graft is then taken from the posterior tibia up and around the screw in the lateral femoral condyle **(Fig. 28–14),** back down to the fibular tunnel (the popliteofibular portion should be tucked under the popliteus portion of the graft), through the tunnel, and back to the screw and washer. The graft is tensioned with the foot internally

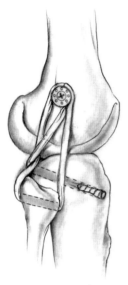

Figure 28–15 Final reconstruction of posterior cruciate ligament using modified two-tailed PLC reconstruction.

rotated and the knee flexed 40 to 60 degrees. The graft reconstructs the popliteus, popliteofibular ligament, and FCL **(Fig. 28–15).**

Posteromedial Complex Reconstruction (Simple Loop)

One posteromedial reconstruction is a simple loop with staple fixation. An incision is made from the medial femoral epicondyle and then distally over the intersection of the tibial collateral ligament where it travels under the pes anserinus tendons. A subretinacular (layer I) tunnel is made from distal to proximal, and then graft harvest is performed **(Fig. 28–16).** The authors prefer to have the semitendinosus left attached distally, but a free semitendinosus graft can be used as well. The graft is harvested from its proximal muscle belly after release of its fascial attachments to the medial gastrocnemius. Remaining muscle is cleared from the tendon, and a Krakow suture is placed in its end. Using a high-speed bur, a tight U-shaped trough is made around the isometric part of the medial epicondyle. The semitendinosus is brought up through its tunnel, placed into the trough, and stapled into place. The graft is brought back down through its tunnel, the knee is ranged multiple times, and the tendon is then stapled to the insertion of the tibial collateral ligament. The knee is placed in a bulky Jones dressing with medial and lateral plaster slabs for 7 to 10 days. Gentle range of motion is begun thereafter in a hinged knee brace. An alternative technique that also reconstructs the posterior oblique ligament also utilizes a semitendinosus autograft, routed around a screw and washer placed at the isometric point, then under the semimembranosus and back to the origin of the autograft **(Fig. 28–17)** (see **Videos 28–4, 28–5, Disk 4**).

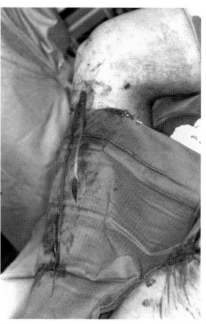

Figure 28–16 Harvest of hamstring tendons for use leaving them attached distally in knee reconstruction leaving them attached distally.

External Fixation-Immobilization

Nonoperative treatment without specific focus on prescribed immobilization creates a ligamentously lax, incompetent knee. However, Taylor and coauthors described very successful results with closed treatment of the simple dislocated knee.[3] In their study, immobilization was utilized for a period of 6 to 8 weeks with good functional results in closed uncomplicated knee dislocations. Interestingly, if immobilization was utilized for less than 6 weeks, the authors found knees to be very mobile but relatively unstable, whereas immobilization longer than 8 weeks produced a stable but stiff knee. Thus the authors recommended a 6 to 8 week period of immobilization for optimal functional results in the simple knee dislocation.[3] The difficulty with external fixation is the process of regaining range of motion after immobilization. Several authors have noted successful treatment of arthrofibrosis using a combination of manipulation under anesthesia (MUA), arthroscopic lysis of adhesions,[25] and postoperative epidural anesthesia (48 to 72 hours) in combination with a continuous passive motion (CPM) machine. External fixation can be utilized in patients with complex injuries that are poor reconstruction candidates. This technique involves immobilization with external fixation for 6 to 8 weeks, followed by removal and MUA with lysis of adhesions as already described.

The fixator is routinely removed in the operating room to allow for EUA, a careful knee manipulation, and arthroscopic lysis of adhesions. The pin sites should be sealed from the operative field prior to arthroscopy. If an active purulent pin tract infection is present, then arthroscopy

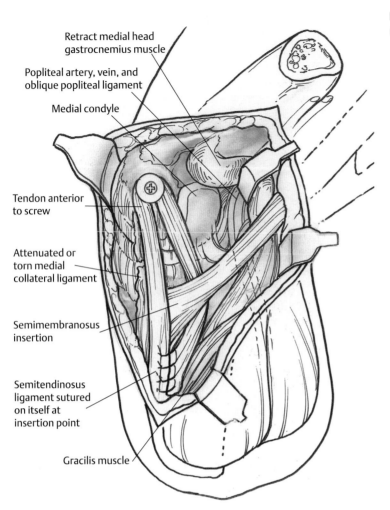

Retract medial head
gastrocnemius muscle

Popliteal artery, vein, and
oblique popliteal ligament

Medial condyle

Tendon anterior
to screw

Attenuated or
torn medial
collateral ligament

Semimembranosus
insertion

Semitendinosus
ligament sutured
on itself at
insertion point

Gracilis muscle

Figure 28–17 Posteromedial corner reconstruction. MCL, medial collateral ligament.

should not be performed. Perioperative epidural anesthesia is recommended to allow pain-free CPM and physical therapy–assisted range of motion exercises for the first 72 hours. Intraoperative postmanipulation radiographs are key to rule out fracture or extensive mechanism disruption. The patient is discharged to home physical therapy and use of a CPM machine. Clinic-based physical therapy should focus the patient on gait training, passive extension (hanging weights in extension, if necessary), and knee flexion exercises. If ligamentous laxity persists after fixator removal and the patient has regained adequate motion, delayed ligament reconstruction may be indicated. A functional early weight-bearing program is tailored to the specific reconstruction. Early motion and protected weight bearing are generally utilized following bicruciate reconstruction. At 6 to 8 weeks the patient should be weight bearing with a well-fitted brace, and functional strengthening can advance. With surgical reconstruction of a dislocated knee, the surgeon should warn the patient of the risk of stiffness. The authors generally counsel patients they have at least a one in five chance of a need for manipulation and postmanipulative epidural and CPM. We usually allow a patient 6 to 8 weeks before recommending MUA

and look for flexion past 90 degrees by 4 weeks postreconstruction.

Rehabilitation

The surgeon must become comfortable with rehabilitation techniques to obtain postreconstructive functional range of motion. Having a patient sit on an elevated table using the contralateral leg to push the knee into flexion is very useful for obtaining knee flexion **(Fig. 28–18).** If available, a stationary bike is very useful to obtain flexion with the seat adjusted to a lower position as flexion gains are made. Flexion contractures are common and easily overlooked. The patient should be evaluated in a prone position, checking heel heights **(Fig. 28–19).** Every centimeter of difference in height is equivalent to approximately 1 degree of a flexion contracture. When treating a flexion contracture, a supine position allows the patient better leverage to obtain a good stretch of the posterior capsule. Hanging weights with the knee in extension in a supine position for 20 minutes twice per day is advisable. Having the patient recline while stretching the knee relaxes the hamstrings and improves patient comfort during this exercise. Use of pain medica-

Tips and Tricks

- Always keep retractors and instruments anterior to the head (medial or lateral) of the gastrocnemius muscle to avoid damage to vascular structures using the inlay technique.
- Flex the knee 90 degrees for a posteromedial or lateral approach to relax the peroneal nerve and move the popliteal vessels out of the way.
- The posterior tibia can be approached medially or laterally for creating the inlay trough if both cruciates are torn. Visualization is easier with the posteromedial approach.
- Use the supine position in the operating room for knee dislocations. Internal and external rotation of the hip will allow posterolateral and posteromedial approaches, including exposure of the posterior tibia for the tibial inlay technique.
- Do not make allograft bone blocks too thin ($<$ 10 mm) for the inlay graft. This will protect against graft cracking and fixation failure when the screw is tightened.
- Tibialis posterior allograft should be at least 24 cm long for reconstruction of the PLC using the modified two-tailed technique. Shorter grafts won't allow FCL reconstruction.
- Plan the direction of the 4.5 mm screw used in PLC reconstruction, keeping in mind the location of the tunnels used for ACL and PCL reconstruction.
- Make allograft bone blocks cylindrical for ACL reconstruction with bioabsorbable pins. It speeds incorporation of the graft and improves fixation.
- Calculate the length of bone/tendon/bone ACL allograft and the femoral tunnel/intra-articular graft to determine appropriate tibial tunnel length.

tions prior to stretching is critical for optimal compliance and resolution of the flexion contracture. The use of ice is a critical component in the resolution of soft tissue swelling and very useful in pain control. Icing is utilized three times per day for 20 minutes at a time and once

prior to bedtime. The use of ice before sleep helps with pain and aids the patient in gaining a better night's rest.

As in any surgical procedure, part of the difficulty is patient anxiety and compliance. Patient education helps decrease anxiety and creates an environment of empathy that improves the overall surgical result. In addition to drawing out the surgical reconstruction for the patient on a large piece of paper (Sharpie pen for this and for extremity identification), the rehabilitation time course is discussed in detail. Three concepts are stressed for patient education:

1. Knee extension ("You need to get your knee to lock straight.")
2. Knee flexion (elevated seated flexion and a stationary bike)
3. Walk normally (The patient should be educated on the difference between a limp and a heel–toe gait. The patient is given the verbal cue to "push off with your toes" to return to a normal walking pattern.)

Patient education is extremely important for successful treatment of knee dislocations.

New Techniques

Placement of a Compass Hinge External Fixator (see Video 28–6, Disk 4)

The Compass Knee Hinge (Smith & Nephew Richards, Memphis, Tennessee) is a hinged external fixator that provides multiplanar fixation across the knee joint while allowing sagittal plane motion. This combination allows remarkable stabilization of the knee joint following dislocations and fracture dislocations. The technique is relatively simple. The patient is placed in a supine position with a roll of sterile sheets under the knee. A fluoroscope is employed to obtain a good lateral view of the knee. A threaded 2.5 mm wire is placed at the isometric point on the lateral femoral condyle and used as a reference wire.

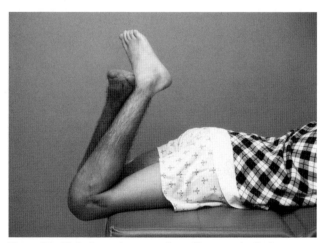

Figure 28–18 Patient using contralateral leg to assist flexion.

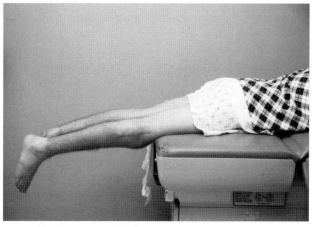

Figure 28–19 Assessing for flexion contracture.

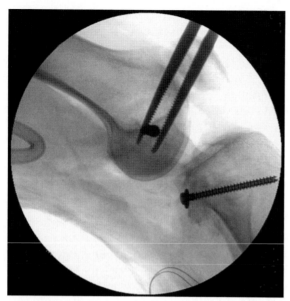

Figure 28–20 Radiographic identification of the isometric point using a line extending from the posterior femoral cortex to Blumensaat's line.

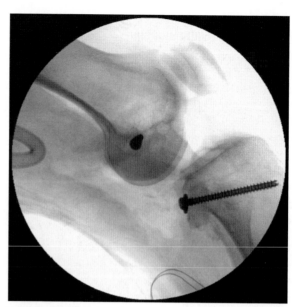

Figure 28–21 Bringing the reference wire into a parallel alignment so that it appears like a dot on a lateral fluoroscopic view.

The isometric point is identified radiographically as the point at which a line drawn from the posterior cortex of the femur intersects with Blumensaat's line (**Fig. 28–20**). The tip of the threaded wire is placed at the isometric point, and the tail end of the wire is brought parallel to the fluoroscope so that it appears as a single dot (**Fig. 28–21**). A mallet is used to tap the end of the wire, seating it in the bone. Again, fluoroscopy is used to check that the wire is parallel with the beam, appearing as a dot rather than a line. When the wire is well seated and parallel, it is drilled all the way across the knee. An anterior-posterior view of the knee is now checked. If the technique has been done correctly, the wire should be parallel with the knee joint

(**Fig. 28–22**). If the wire is not parallel, it should be removed and the procedure repeated.

Once the reference wire has been placed satisfactorily, the hinge is placed over the wire. The femoral pins should both be drilled after placing Rancho cubes (Smith & Nephew, Memphis, Tennessee) (identical to those used with Ilizarov external fixators) facing proximally from the proximal 5/8's ring. The cubes should be placed in the most posterior hole on both the medial and lateral sides. A one-hole cube is used medially, and a three-hole cube is used laterally. A trocar system is included for drilling the half pins. A no. 10 blade should be used to make a skin incision, and then a Kelly clamp or another similar instrument should be used to bluntly dissect down to the bone. Pins (6 mm) are used in the femur, with one placed posteromedially and the other posterolaterally (**Fig. 28–23**).

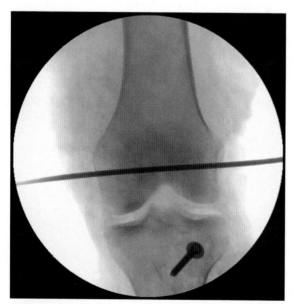

Figure 28–22 Reference wire parallel with the knee joint on an anteroposterior view.

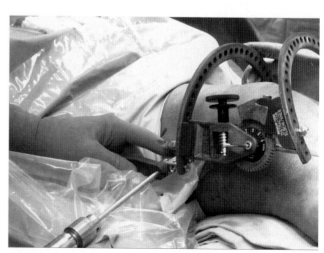

Figure 28–23 Drilling the posteromedial pin for the Compass Knee Hinge.

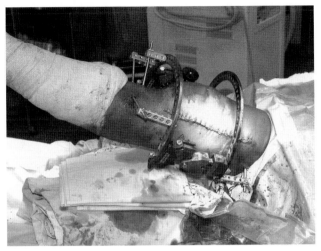

Figure 28–24 Compass Knee Hinge viewed from the lateral side with three tibial pins.

This placement minimizes pain with range of motion of the knee. The thread length on the pin can be read from the drill bit as the second cortex is perforated. Three 5 mm pins are placed in a similar manner in the tibia, using three-, four-, and five-hole Rancho cubes. The pins are placed anterior, anteromedial, and lateral in the tibia (**Fig. 28–24**). Both 5/8's rings are held perpendicular to the shaft of the long bone while the pins are drilled. Care should be taken to evaluate the pin sites with the knee flexed 90 or more degrees (**Fig. 28–25**). If the skin is binding against the pins, it should be released. Finally, all the bolts are tightened, and the range of motion is checked.

The Compass Knee Hinge is worn for approximately 6 weeks. Patients are allowed to bear weight immediately with the hinge locked in extension. Patients are asked to lock the hinge in full extension and maximum flexion for at least 1 hour each per day, with range of motion during

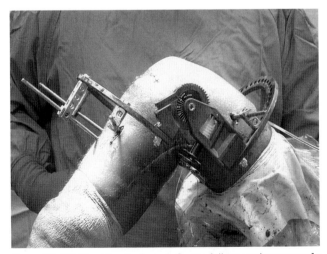

Figure 28–25 Checking the knee in flexion following placement of a Compass Knee Hinge.

the remainder of the day. Pin site care is similar to that provided for any external fixator.

Bone–Patellar Tendon–Bone Anterior Cruciate Ligament Reconstruction with Bioabsorbable Pins (see Video 28–7, Disk 4)

Bone-tendon-bone remains the gold standard for ACL reconstruction. Allograft reconstruction is often advantageous following knee dislocation due to the severity of the soft tissue injury. As documented in the Outcomes section of this chapter, failure is far more common following knee dislocation than following an isolated ACL reconstruction. A relatively new technique for ACL reconstruction involves using bioabsorbable pins to transfix the bone blocks in both the tibia and the femur (RigidFix, DePuy Mitek, Inc., Raynham, Massachusetts). Advantages with this technique include perpendicular fixation and bioabsorbable pins that do not require removal for revision.

The patient is positioned supine with the use of a leg holder or lateral post. Standard arthroscopic portals are utilized, and a systematic examination of the knee is performed. The next step is tibial and femoral tunnel preparation using standard techniques. Our preference is to create 10 or 11 mm bone blocks, with the femoral block ~25 mm in length. It is important to make the bone blocks cylindrical to obtain the best fit possible in the tunnels. A small drill hole is created in the proximal portion of the femoral bone block, and a no. 2 suture is passed through the hole. Two holes are drilled in the tibial bone block with no. 2 suture passed through the holes.

A critical planning step involves factoring the length of the allograft prior to drilling the tibial tunnel. The femoral tunnel is drilled to a depth of 30 to 35 mm. Most patients require an intra-articular distance of roughly 25 mm of graft for an ACL reconstruction. Sixty millimeters (femoral tunnel plus intra-articular portion) should be subtracted from the length of the entire graft to yield the ideal tibial tunnel length. For example, if the entire graft is 105 mm, the tibial tunnel should be at least 45 mm in length to ensure that the bone plug is within the tibial tunnel rather that hanging out distal to the tunnel. Failure to pay attention to this point will make it difficult to achieve adequate tibial fixation.

The RigidFix femoral guide is placed in the femoral tunnel. Two hollow cannulas are drilled into the lateral femoral condyle, oriented so that they will intersect the femoral tunnel (**Fig. 28–26**). The guide is removed, leaving the cannulas in place. The tibial guide is then placed into the femoral tunnel over the guidewire that was placed prior to drilling the femoral tunnel. A measurement is then read from the guide at the articular end of the tibial tunnel (**Fig. 28–27**). The external tibial guide is then calibrated based on this measurement. To gain fixation with both pins through the tibial bone block, 6 to 8 mm is added to the measurement to yield the appropriate setting for the exter-

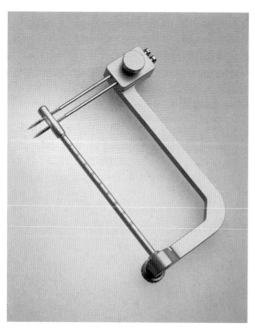

Figure 28–26 Femoral guide with hollow cannulas and bioabsorbable pins. (Courtesy of DePuy Mitek, Inc.)

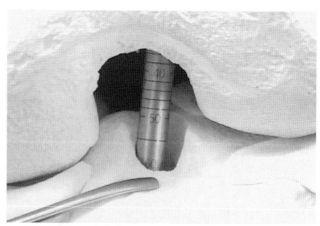

Figure 28–27 Measuring from the tibial guide at the articular surface. (Courtesy of DePuy Mitek, Inc.)

nal guide. For example, if the tibial tunnel measurement is 55 mm, a setting of 61 to 63 mm will yield ideal fixation of the bone block. The guidewire is then pulled into the knee, and two tibial cannulas are drilled from anteromedial to posterolateral **(Fig. 28–28)**. The no. 2 suture from the femoral bone block is then threaded through the guidewire and pulled into the femoral tunnel and out the anterior thigh, pulling the allograft into the femoral tunnel. After seating the graft completely in the femoral tunnel, the bone block is drilled through the previously placed femoral cannulas. A RigidFix absorbable pin is then pushed though the cannula and across the bone block, securely pinning it in

place **(Fig. 28–29)**. A second pin is placed in the same fashion through the other femoral cannula. Traction is then pulled on the tibial bone block, confirming rigid fixation of the femoral bone block. Following this step, the knee is ranged 15 to 20 times with traction to completely seat the graft and pretension it. While maintaining tension, the tibial bone block is pinned with one drill bit through the proximal cannula, and then drilled through the distal cannula. A bioabsorbable pin is then placed through the distal cannula, transfixing the bone block. Finally, the drill bit is removed from the proximal tibial cannula and replaced with a second bioabsorbable pin.

Double Bundle ACL Reconstruction. (see **Video 28–8, Disk 4**) The anterior cruciate ligament has been noted to contain two separate functional bundles, the anteromedial and posterolateral bundles.[56a] It has been proposed that reconstructing both bundles may improve functional outcomes, particularly regarding rotational stability. Reconstruction techniques are being develped for the double bundle ACL reconstruction,[56b] but well designed peer reviewed studies with adequate follow-up will be needed to validate the advantages and disadvantages of the technique.

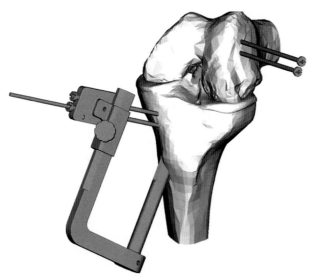

Figure 28–28 Femoral cannulas drilled in place for reconstruction using the RigidFix system. (Courtesy of DePuy Mitek, Inc.)

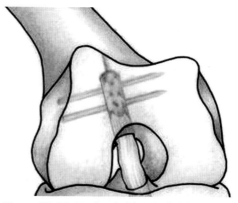

Figure 28–29 Bioabsorbable pins holding femoral bone block in place. (Courtesy of DePuy Mitek, Inc.)

Outcomes (see Videos 28–8, 28–9, Disk 4)

Knee dislocations cover a broad spectrum of injuries, from open high-energy KD-IV patients with a popliteal artery disruption to a chronic, multiligamentous injury with an intact soft tissue envelope and a normal neurological and vascular examination. Many articles regarding knee dislocation are retrospective and have small numbers. There have been no published prospective, randomized studies on knee dislocations. There has been no uniformity in terms of outcome scoring systems used in the literature on knee dislocations. As a result of the above factors, a discussion of the outcomes of knee dislocations can be confusing. This section reviews the published outcome literature on knee dislocations with respect to the following: reconstruction versus nonreconstruction, range of motion, pain, instability, return to work, return to recreational activities or sports, and reported outcome scores. Almekinders and Dedmond have provided an excellent review of the outcomes of knee dislocations.[57]

Reconstruction versus Nonoperative Treatment

There has been a strong trend away from nonoperative treatment of knee dislocations as surgical techniques have improved. At least seven studies have been published that specifically compare nonoperative and operative treatment of knee dislocations.[18,19,24,25,29,31,36] All of the studies are retrospective reviews with a variety of surgical techniques and rehabilitation protocols. When the studies are considered cumulatively, 136 patients treated surgically are compared with 68 patients that are treated conservatively. All seven authors favor surgical treatment, although Roman et al[31] noted motion problems with the patients they treated surgically. The other authors found surgical treatment superior in terms of both motion and stability. Richter et al[36] published the most recent and largest series with 77 patients. They found patients treated surgically had better motion, stability, return to work, and return to recreational activities when compared with patients treated conservatively. They also found patients had better Lysholm (78 vs 65) and International Knee Document Committee (IKDC) scores (41% severely abnormal in the nonoperative group) following surgical treatment. Outcome studies clearly favor surgical treatment for patients following knee dislocations.

Range of Motion

There have been numerous outcome studies published that report on knee motion following dislocations.[1,4,5,7,8,18,19,23–25,28,31,36,56,58–61] When comparing articles published before 1994[4,5,18,19,24,31] with those published since,[1,7,8,25,28,56,60,61] there has been a trend toward an improving total arc of motion. The earlier studies report a mean arc of motion of 106 degrees compared with 121 degrees in the more contemporary studies. Many authors have adopted a rehabilitation program emphasizing immediate motion rather than a period of immobilization. The mean arc of motion achieved in these outcome studies utilizing immediate motion was 124 degrees.[1,7,8,56,60,61] The use of CPM is common.[1,8,56,60,61] The remarkable improvements in knee range of motion following surgical treatment of knee dislocations have frequently required surgical treatment in the form of either manipulation under anesthesia or arthroscopic lysis of adhesions. Reports of the need for surgical intervention to improve knee motion have varied from a low of 13%[8] to a high of 71%[28] for acute dislocations. The mean reported incidence of surgical intervention to augment motion is 38% of the patients in nine different outcome studies.[1,4,7,8,28,56,59–61] The bottom line of the outcome studies cited in this section is that remarkable improvements in motion have been achieved using contemporary surgical techniques, but approximately one third of patients require surgical intervention to improve their motion.

Pain

Pain and motion limitations are more frequent problems than instability following the surgical treatment of knee dislocations. Pain can vary from occasional pain that has minimal impact on daily activities to severe disabling pain. Factors that contribute to pain include articular cartilage injury, chronic instability, arthrofibrosis, and posttraumatic arthritis. Severe pain may yield a nonfunctional knee despite good stability and range of motion. Patients with significant motion limitations frequently experience disabling pain.

The incidence of pain following surgically treated knee dislocations varies in studies.[4,8,19,23,28,36,58,59] Yeh et al[8] and Martinek et al[59] both reported pain in 25% or less of their patients. Sisto and Warren (46%), Mariani et al (56%), Almekinders and Logan (66%), and Richter et al (68%) all reported much more frequent problems with pain following knee dislocations.[4,19,23,36] Noyes and Barber-Westin reported all seven of their acute knee dislocations experienced pain but only one with activities of daily living. On the other hand, 75% of their chronic knee dislocation patients treated with surgery experienced pain with activities of daily living.[28]

Significant pain is clearly an important outcome measure but is frequently not separately reported. It lowers outcome scores. The studies by Almekinders and Logan[19] and Noyes and Barber-Westin[28] both suggest that outcomes may be more favorable in patients treated acutely when compared with patients treated on a delayed basis. This may be a result of chronic instability and subsequent osteoarthritis.[57] Additional outcome studies that specifically address the issue of pain are needed to confirm the relationship of the timing of surgery and chronic pain. Patients who sustain knee dislocations must be prepared for the possibility of significant long-term pain.

Instability

Many authors believe that pain and loss of motion rather than instability are the major problems following knee dislocation. Although the published outcome studies support the severity of the problem with pain and loss of motion, instability is also a major problem. There is a clear trend toward improving stability in more recent studies. One problem in interpreting the literature regarding stability is the wide variety of methods of reporting the results of knee stability examinations. For the purposes of this chapter, instability has been defined as grade 2 or 3 on a scale of 0 to 3, KT1000 or 2000 Ligament Arthrometer (MEDmetric Corporation, San Diego, California) data that are greater than 3 mm side to side difference for either anterior or posterior translation, or greater than 5 mm for total anteroposterior translation, or groups C or D on the IKDC score.

Five outcome studies reported stability data following nonoperative treatment. All five noted instability in virtually all of their patients.[18,19,24,31,36] Using the criteria already defined, virtually every patient treated nonoperatively experienced instability as a final result.

Fifteen outcome studies have been reviewed that report on ligament stability following surgical treatment of knee dislocations.[1,4,5,7,8,18,19,23,24,28,36,56,59-61] Based on the criteria already listed, all of the studies that report on all ligaments involved in the knee dislocation list at least an 18% failure rate. The incidence of instability varies from 18 to 61%, with a mean of 37%. In many cases, more than one ligament meets the criteria for instability. Either or both anterior and posterior instability are reported more frequently than medial or lateral instability. Two papers have reported exclusively on PCL reconstructions and had

failure rates of 0[5] to 3%.[56] One of these papers was focused exclusively on low-energy knee dislocations,[5] and the other reported on the use of a combination tibial inlay and two-bundle PCL reconstruction.[56] Interestingly, both of these papers utilized early motion rehabilitation protocols. Another paper reported on a group of patients treated with a hinged external fixator and had a failure rate of only 7% for all ligament groups.[61] **Table 28–2** provides a summary of the reported outcome results in papers published since 1994.

Return to Work

Knee dislocation is a serious injury that is often associated with other injuries. As a result, patients may have problems returning to their prior level of employment. Several authors have begun reporting on their results, with most able to resume some work.[1,7,8,28,36,56,60] Many are able to resume high-intensity occupations following contemporary reconstruction techniques and extended rehabilitation. The combined results of seven outcome studies demonstrate that 93% of the patients have returned to some type of work, but 31% of the patients have returned to light duty or a less demanding job. Richter et al[36] reported that only 10 of 18 patients who had reconstruction of chronic dislocations returned to work (56%), compared with 50 of 59 (85%) acute dislocations. It is clear from the majority of the outcome studies that it is possible to have patients return to employment, including demanding jobs, following surgical treatment of knee dislocations.

Return to Sports or Recreation

One problem in the literature is differing definitions of return to activity. Many knee dislocation patients are not involved in competitive athletics but are involved in recreational activities such as hunting, fishing, or gardening. Below is a review of the literature and an attempt to quantify

Table 28–2   Instability Outcome Results Reported in Post-1994 Publications

Study (Year)	Clinical Instability (2 or 3)				Ligament Arthrometer			IKDC
	Anterior	Posterior	Medial	Lateral	>3 mm Anterior	>3 mm Posterior	>5 mm Anterior-Posterior	Group C or D
Richter et al[36]	–	–	8 of 72	14 of 72	Mean 5.1	Mean 4.0		
Mariani et al[23]	3 of 23	10 of 23	9 of 23	7 of 23				
Martinek[59]	–	–	–	–				13 of 28
Noyes[28]	1 of 11	2 of 11	–	1 of 6				
Shapiro et al[60]	–	1 of 7	–	–	4 of 7			
Stannard et al[56]	–	1 of 31	–	–			1 of 26	
Stannard et al[65]	8 of 32	1 of 27	–	20 of 56				
Walker et al[64]	–	–	–	–			4 of 13	
Wascher et al[58]	–	2 of 13	–	1 of 13			7 of 12	
Yeh et al[8]	–	–	–	–	25 of 25	9 of 25		

the number of patients that returned to their preinjury level of activity, a lower level of activity, or became sedentary.

Nine outcome studies have been reviewed that report on recreational activities following knee dislocations.[1,4,5,7,19,28,36,56,59] The reported range of patients returning to some activity varies from 0[19] to 97%,[56] with a mean of 65%. Richter at al[36] reported that 56% of their patients who were treated surgically returned to athletic activity, compared with only 17% of their patients treated conservatively. They reported that 49% returned to the same level, with 40% decreased by one level and 10% decreased by two levels using the IKDC score.

The seven studies that reported only on patients who were treated surgically reported 76% of their patients returned to some recreational or athletic activities. However, only 39% were able to return to their preinjury level of competition.[1,4,5,7,28,56,59] Clearly, major improvements have been made in the ability for a patient with a knee dislocation to return to athletic or recreational activities.

Outcome Scores

The major scores utilized to report results following knee dislocations include the Meyers,[29] Lysholm, and IKDC scores. Three outcome studies combined report 36% excellent, 50% good, 10% fair, and 5% poor results following surgical treatment using Meyers criteria.[1,18,29] Meyers reported 0% excellent, 8% good, 15% fair, and 77% poor outcomes following nonoperative treatment.[29]

Eight studies report outcome results using the Lysholm knee score following knee dislocations.[1,7,8,23,25,36,56,60] The mean score for all of the studies was 82.6, with a range of 75 to 89. Two studies reported outcomes of nonoperatively treated knee dislocations using the Lysholm score.[25,36] The mean Lysholm score in these two studies was 65.5. The reported results using the Lysholm knee score clearly favor surgical treatment.

Four outcome studies have used the IKDC scoring system to report their results.[1,23,36,59] This system designates the outcome as group A for a normal knee, group B for a nearly normal knee, group C for an abnormal knee, and group D for a severely abnormal knee. Combining the four studies, the results are as follows: group A—1%; group B—35%; group C—49%; and group D—16%. Richter et al also reported IKDC results on nonoperatively treated patients. They reported group A—0%; group B—6%; group C—53%; and group D—41%.[36] Again, surgical treatment results in notably better results than nonoperative treatment.

Summary

The number of published papers reporting outcome scores has increased dramatically in the recent literature. Several trends are clear from the data. Surgical treatment using contemporary reconstruction techniques clearly yields superior results when compared with nonoperative techniques. Motion and pain remain major problems, but both

appear to be improving with aggressive rehabilitation programs and surgical intervention in the form of manipulation under anesthesia or arthroscopic lysis of adhesions or both. Instability is more of a problem following surgery than many authors acknowledge. Stability to perform activities of daily living is readily achieved, but stability to allow athletics and aggressive rehabilitation is much more elusive. Most authors agree they would rather address instability with secondary operations than have to address arthrofibrosis. The outcomes reported regarding return to work and recreational activities are generally encouraging, although many athletes cannot perform at their previous level of competition. The results with the Lysholm knee score are generally good, with a mean score of 82.6 for all studies utilizing surgical treatment. The IKDC scores have been less encouraging in the published outcome literature, probably due to the final score being the lowest score from all of the components that make up the IKDC. Other scores average the component scores.

Complications

Complications and adverse outcomes are very common following knee dislocations. Pain, loss of motion, and recurrent instability frequently occur after these injuries. Additional complications can be divided into two major categories: injury related and treatment related.[62] This section focuses on several complications related to multiligament knee injuries.

Vascular injuries to the popliteal artery and vein can occur as a result of the injury or the treatment but are certainly more common as a result of the injury. The popliteal artery is at risk for injury due to the anatomy of the region. It is tethered both proximally at the adductor (Hunter's) canal and distally at the soleal arch.[63] Rupture of the artery can lead to disastrous results and amputation because the collateral circulation around the knee is inadequate for lower extremity survival in most individuals.[11,63-65]

The incidence of significant popliteal artery injury varies widely in the literature, with a range of 7 to

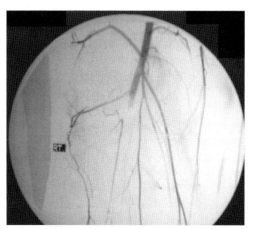

Figure 28–30 Arteriogram demonstrating disruption of the popliteal artery following a knee dislocation.

Table 28—3   Published Cases Using Physical Examination to Determine Need for Arteriography

Study (Year)	No. of Knee Dislocations	No. of Patients with Abnormal Vascular Exam (%)	No. of Patients with Arterial Injury Requiring Surgery (%)	No. of Patients with Normal Vascular Exam (%)	No. of Patients with Arterial Injury Requiring Surgery
Abou-Sayed et al[81]	53	17 (32%)	8 (47%)	36 (68%)	0
Martinez et al[82]	21	9 (43%)	2 (22%)	12 (57%)	0
Dennis et al[80]	38	2 (5%)	2 (100%)	36 (95%)	0
Kendall et al[67]	37	6 (16%)	6 (100%)	31 (84%)	0
Kaufman (1977)[66]	19	4 (21%)	4 (100%)	15 (79%)	0
Treiman (1992)[68]	115	29 (25%)	22 (75%)	86 (75%)	0
Prospective Studies					
Miranda et al[83]	32	8 (25%)	6 (75%)	24 (75%)	0
Stannard (2003)[65]	134	10 (7%)	9 (90%)	124 (93%)	0
TOTAL	**449**	**85 (19%)**	**59 (69%)**	**364 (81%)**	**0**

40%.[12,.20,65–70] The wide range is a result of variability between the studies in terms of method of detection of arterial injury, definition of significant arterial injury, and method of detection of knee dislocations. Many authors have advocated routine arteriography for all patients identified with a knee dislocation[11,20,71–78] (**Fig. 28–30**). Recent articles have questioned the routine use of arteriography and made a strong case for selective arteriography based on the results of physical examination.[12,64,65,67–70,79,80] The term *selective arteriography* is defined as the use of physical examination as the primary screening tool for vascular injuries in patients following knee dislocations. Arteriograms are selectively obtained only on patients who demonstrate abnormal vascular findings on physical exam.[65] **Table 28–3** summarizes the findings of six retrospective[66–68,80–82] and two prospective[65,83] studies employing selective arteriography. The eight studies have evaluated 449 patients with no reported cases in which physical examination failed to detect significant vascular injuries.

Our protocol regarding vascular injury is based upon the use of selective arteriography. Careful physical examination of the dorsalis pedis and posterior tibial arteries, combined with a gross evaluation of the extremity color and temperature, constitutes the primary diagnostic tools used to determine the need for arteriography. If the exam is normal, the patient has a repeat vascular exam approximately 4 to 6 hours later, and again at 24 and 48 hours but does not undergo arteriogram. If there is any asymmetry or abnormality between the two lower extremities, or any history of an abnormal vascular exam by emergency personnel while transporting the patient to the hospital, an arteriogram should be obtained. If there is any doubt, it is clearly wise to err on the side of getting an arteriogram or obtaining a Doppler ankle brachial index.

Nerve injury can occur to either the peroneal or the tibial nerves as a result of either the injury or the treatment. Peroneal nerve injury reportedly occurs in 10 to 42% of knee dislocations. Complete injury is associated with a poor prognosis, with only 37 to 50% of patients obtaining functional recovery with nonoperative treatment.[63,84,85] The indications for neurolysis or nerve grafting are controversial. Some authors are recommending aggressive treatment protocols that include exploration with neurolysis or cable grafting or both. Success varies with the length of the nerve injury, with 14 to 89% improving to grade 3 or 4 strength.[84] Patients who have a peroneal nerve injury and are undergoing posterolateral corner repair or reconstruction should probably be treated with at least a neurolysis.[63,84] Tibial nerve injuries are less frequent than peroneal nerve injuries and often occur in association with popliteal artery and peroneal nerve injuries. Injury to the tibial nerve carries an even worse prognosis than injury to the peroneal nerve.[12,63] Posterior tibial tendon transfer and Achilles' tendon lengthening are surgical treatment options for permanent nerve injuries that may remarkably improve function.

Infection and wound healing problems can occur as a result of either the injury (open dislocations) or the surgical treatment. Open reconstruction following knee dislocations has a reported infection rate of up to 12.5%.[62] Open dislocations have been reported to have wound sepsis in up to 42% of patients.[63,85] Wound healing problems may be more frequent with early surgery and aggressive postoperative motion rehabilitation protocols. A careful evaluation of the degree of soft tissue injury is critical to determining the timing for surgery. Allowing a few weeks for the soft tissue to recover may decrease the incidence of wound problems and infection. Another problem that can occur is the formation of fistulas between the knee joint and the skin. This problem also appears to be more frequent fol-

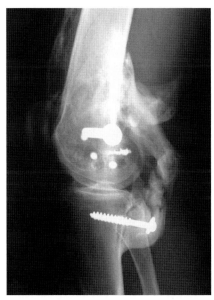

Figure 28–31 Grade IV heterotopic ossification following a knee dislocation.

lowing aggressive early motion rehabilitation. Once established, fistulas may be difficult to eliminate with simple exploration and repair due to the severe soft tissue damage. Flap coverage or capsular repair with tissue substitutes such as xenograft can successfully eliminate a recalcitrant fistula.

HO occurs frequently following high-energy knee dislocations, but there is little data in the literature on this topic. Stannard et al[17] reported on 57 knee dislocations following high-energy blunt trauma. The incidence of HO was 26%, with 12% developing grade 3 (more than 50% of joint space) or 4 (ankylosis of the joint) ossification **(Fig. 28–31)**. The most common location of the ectopic bone was medial, with a posterior location being the second most common. There were significantly more patients who developed arthrofibrosis with HO than patients without HO. There was also a significant association between the development of HO around the knee and developing HO in other anatomical locations. There was a clear trend toward developing HO in patients with open knee dislocations and following infections.[17] There are no clear data regarding what role (if any) early motion or acute surgical treatment may have in the development of HO. Consideration should be given to prophylaxis against HO in patients who have a history of HO or who sustained an open knee dislocation.

Osteonecrosis of the medial femoral condyle is a complication of surgical treatment. It has been reported following PCL reconstruction.[86] Patients complain of pain over the medial femoral condyle. Radiographic findings include flattening of the articular surface and a radiolucency around the condyle. Etiologic factors include drilling the femoral tunnel too close to the articular surface and extensive soft tissue dissection over the condyle during surgery.

Posttraumatic osteoarthritis is another complication of the injury that has been underreported in the literature. Almekinders and Logan[19] have reported degenerative changes in all of their patients at a mean follow-up of 40 months. In contrast, three other papers have noted minimal degenerative changes following surgery.[5,8,60] Most authors agree that surgical stabilization of the knee probably decreases the incidence and severity of posttraumatic osteoarthritis.

Inaccurate or delayed diagnosis occurs frequently following blunt trauma. Knee dislocation is one of the most frequently missed injuries.[62,85] The most common cause of missed dislocations is spontaneous relocation. One solution to this problem is increased awareness and careful examination of the knee of blunt trauma patients. Another solution is increased utilization of MRI, especially in patients with ipsilateral fractures and a knee effusion. Failure to diagnose knee dislocation will frequently result in pain, instability, and loss of motion. More importantly, failure to recognize a spontaneously reduced knee dislocation can lead to amputation of the extremity if a significant popliteal artery injury is not recognized promptly.

Dislocation of the knee is associated with a high incidence of complications, both due to the injury and as a result of surgical treatment. Adverse outcomes also occur frequently. The high energy necessary to cause most knee dislocations will probably ensure that this injury will always be associated with a high risk of complications. However, awareness has improved outcomes by early recognition and treatment as well as strategies to avoid complications.

Pearls

- Outcomes are far more favorable following surgical reconstruction than following nonoperative treatment.
- Range of motion is a mean arc of 121 degrees using contemporary surgical techniques.
- Thirty-eight percent of patients require surgical intervention (manipulation under anesthesia or arthroscopic lysis of adhesions) to improve range of motion following ligament reconstruction.
- Virtually all patients treated nonoperatively have ligamentous instability.
- A mean of 37% of patients have some ligamentous instability following surgical reconstruction.
- Ninety-three percent of patients return to some work, although 31% require light duty or a less demanding job.
- The incidence of significant popliteal artery injury varies from 7 to 40% in the literature. Larger contemporary studies are on the low end of that range.
- Ten to 42% of knee dislocations have peroneal nerve injuries, with less than half of complete injuries making a functional recovery.
- Some HO develops in ~25% of knee dislocations.

On the DVDs

Video 28–1 (Disk 4) Double-Bundle Inlay PCL Reconstruction
This video demonstrates the "Anatomical PCL Reconstruction" technique using an Achilles tendon allograft with two femoral tunnels. We also show the tibial inlay technique through a posteromedial approach.

Video 28–2 (Disk 4) Hamstring ACL Reconstruction This video demonstrates a case using hamstring autograft to reconstruct the ACL over a bioabsorbable pin in the femur.

Video 28–3 (Disk 4) Posterolateral Corner Reconstruction
This video presents the modified two-tailed technique for posterolateral corner reconstruction using either tibialis anterior or tibialis posterior allograft. Methods of determining the isometric point on the lateral femoral condyle are demonstrated.

Video 28–4 (Disk 4) Posteromedial Corner Reconstruction with Autograft This video demonstrates reconstruction of the posteromedial corner using a semitendinosis autograft. The technique reconstructs both the deep MCL and the posterior oblique-ligament.

Video 28–5 (Disk 4) Posteromedial Corner Reconstruction with Allograft This video shows PMC reconstruction using tibialis anterior or posterior allograft using screws and washers at the isometric point on the medial femoral condyle and near the pes anserinus on the tibia.

Video 28–6 (Disk 4) Placement of Compass Knee Hinge External Fixator This video presents step-by-step instuctions on how to place a Compass Knee Hinge external fixator. The technique for determining the isometric point on the femoral condyles is demonstrated.

Video 28–7 (Disk 4) BTB ACL Reconstruction with Bioabsorbable Pins This video demonstrates ACL reconstruction using a bone-patellar tendon-bone graft and bioabsorbable pin fixation. Advantages of this technique include perpendicular fixation of the graft and bioabsorbable pin fixation which allow easy revision if needed.

Video 28–8 (Disk 4) Double-Bundle Anatomical ACL Reconstruction This video reviews the concept of double bundle ACL reconstruction, including the anatomical basis for using the double bundle technique. We then demonstrate one double-bundle ACL reconstruction technique using tibialis anterior allografts with Endobutton (Smith & Nephew Endoscopy, Memphis, Tennessee) femoral fixation and bioabsorbable screw tibial fixation.

Video 28–9 (Disk 4) Posterolateral Bundle of the ACL Reconstruction The posterolateral (PL) bundle of the ACL can be torn with an intact anteromedial bundle. This video shows reconstruction of an isolated PL bundle reconstruction using tibialis anterior allograft.

References

1. Schenck RC. Knee dislocations. American Academy of Orthopaedic Surgeons. Instructional Course Lecture 1994;43:127–136
2. Lonner JH, Dupuy DE, Siliski JM. Comparison of magnetic resonance imaging with operative findings in acute traumatic dislocations of the adult knee. J Orthop Trauma 2000;14:183–186
3. Taylor AR, Arden GP, Rainey HA. Traumatic dislocation of the knee: a report of forty-three cases with special references to conservative treatment. J Bone Joint Surg Br 1972;54:96–109
4. Sisto DJ, Warren RF. Complete knee dislocation: a follow-up study of operative treatment. Clin Orthop Relat Res 1985;198: 94–101
5. Shelbourne KD, Porter DA, Clingman JA, McCarrol JR, Rettig AC. Low velocity knee dislocations. Orthop Rev 1991;20:995–1004
6. Schenck RC, Decoster T, Wascher D. MRI and knee dislocations. In Diduch DR, ed. Sports Medicine Report 2000:89–96
7. Walker DN, Hardison R, Schenck RC. A baker's dozen of knee dislocations. Am J Knee Surg 1994;7:117–124
8. Yeh WL, Tu YK, Su JY, Hsu RW. Knee dislocation: treatment of high-velocity knee dislocation. J Trauma 1999;46:693–701
9. Schenck RC, Hunter R, Ostrum R, Perry CP. Knee dislocations. Instructional Course Lecture American Academy of Orthopaedic Surgeons 1999;48:515–522
10. Schenck RC. Management of PCL injuries in knee dislocations. In: Techniques in Sportsmedicine. Raven Press 1993:143–147
11. Kennedy JC. Complete dislocation of the knee joint. J Bone Joint Surg Am 1963;45:889–904
12. Wascher DC, Dvirnak PC, Decoster TA. Knee dislocation: Initial assessment and implications for treatment. J Orthop Trauma 1997;11:525–529
13. Eastlack RK, Schenck RC Jr., Guarducci C. The dislocated knee: classification, treatment, and outcome. U.S. Army Medical Department Journal 1997;11:2–9
14. Cooper DE, Speer KP, Wickiewicz TL, Warren RF. Complete knee dislocation without posterior cruciate ligament disruption: a report of four cases and review of the literature. Clin Orthop Relat Res 1992;284:228–233
15. Fanelli GC, Gianotti BF, Edson CJ. Arthroscopy assisted combined anterior and posterior cruciate ligament reconstruction. Arthroscopy 1996;12:5–14
16. Berg EE. Positive cruciate ligament tibial inlay reconstruction. Arthroscopy 1995;11:69–76
17. Stannard JP, Wilson TC, Sheils TM, McGwin G Jr, Volgas DA, Alonso JE. Heterotopic ossification associated with knee dislocation. Arthroscopy 2002;18:835–839
18. Frassica FJ, Sim FH, Staeheli JW, Pairolero PC. Dislocation of the knee. Clin Orthop Relat Res 1991;263:200–205
19. Almekinders L, Logan T. Results following treatment of traumatic dislocations of the knee joint. Clin Orthop Relat Res 1992;284:203–207
20. Green NE, Allen BL. Vascular injuries associated with dislocation of the knee. J Bone Joint Surg Am 1977;59:236–239
21. Honton JL, Le Rebeller A, Legroux P, Ragni R, Tramond P. Traumatic dislocation of the knee treated by early surgical repair. Rev Chir Orthop Reparatrice Appar Mot 1978;64:213–219
22. Klein W, Shah N, Gassen A. Arthroscopic management of postoperative arthrofibrosis of the knee joint: indication, technique and results. Arthroscopy 1994;10:591–597
23. Mariani P, Santoriello, Iannone S, Condello V, Adriani. Comparison of surgical treatments for knee dislocations. Am J Knee Surg 1999;12:214–221
24. Meyers M, Harvey JP. Traumatic dislocation of the knee joint. J Bone Joint Surg Am 1971;53:16–29
25. Montgomery T, Savioe F, White J, Roberts T, Hughes J. Orthopedic management of knee dislocations: comparison of surgical recon-

struction of surgical reconstruction and immobilization. Am J Knee Surg 1995;8:97–103

26. Muscat JO, Rogers W, Cruz AB, Schenck RC Jr. Arterial injuries in orthopaedics: the posteromedial approach for vascular control about the knee. J Orthop Trauma 1996;10:476–480

27. Niedzwiedzki T, Hladki W, Mierniczek W. Knee dislocation treatment with temporary tibio-patellar fixation (patellar olecranization). Chir Narzadow Ruchu Ortop Pol 1999;64:209–213

28. Noyes F, Barber-Westin S. Reconstruction of the anterior and posterior cruciate ligaments after knee dislocation: use of early protected post-operative motion to decrease arthrofibrosis. Am J Sports Med 1997;25:769–778

29. Meyers M, Moore T, Harvey JP. Follow-up notes on articles previously published in the journal: traumatic dislocation of the knee joint. J Bone Joint Surg Am 1975;57:430–433

30. Wascher DC. High-velocity knee dislocation with vascular injury: treatment principles. Clin Sports Med 2000;19:457–477

31. Roman PD, Hopson CN, Zenni EJ Jr. Traumatic dislocation of the knee: a report of 30 cases and literature review. Orthop Rev 1987;16:917–924

32. Twaddle BC, Hunter JC, Chapman JR, Simonian PT, Escobedo EM. MRI in acute knee dislocations: a prospective study of clinical, MRI, and surgical findings. J Bone Joint Surg Br 1996;78:573–579

33. Wascher D, DeCoster TA, Schenck RC. 10 Commandments of knee dislocations. Orthopaedic Special Edition 2001;7:28–31

34. Shelbourne KD, Pritchard J, Rettig AC, McCarroll JR, Vanmeter CD. Knee dislocations with intact PCL. Orthop Rev 1992;21: 607–611

35. Reckling FW, Peltier LF. Acute knee dislocations and their complications. J Trauma 1969;9:181–191

36. Richter M, Bosch U, Wippermann B, Hofman A, Krettek C. Comparison of surgical repair of the cruciate ligaments versus nonsurgical treatment in patients with traumatic knee dislocations. Am J Sports Med 2002;30:718–727

37. DeCoster TA. High-energy dislocations. In: Schenck RC Jr., ed. Multiple Ligamentous Injuries of the Knee in the Athlete. Rosemont, IL: American Academy of Orthopaedic Surgeons; 2002:23–29

38. Marder RA, Ertl JP. Dislocations and multiple ligamentous injuries of the knee. In: Chapman's Orthopaedic Surgery. 3rd ed. Philadelphia: Lippincott, Williams & Wilkins; 2001:2417–2434

39. Meyers MH, Moore TM, Harvey JP Jr. Traumatic dislocation of the knee joint. J Bone Joint Surg Am 1975;57:430–433

40. Montgomery JB. Dislocation of the knee. Orthop Clin North Am 1987;18:149–156

41. Sekiya JK, Giffin JR, Harner CD. Posterior cruciate ligament injuries: isolated and combined patterns. In: Schenck RC, Jr., ed. Multiple Ligamentous Injuries of the Knee in the Athlete. Rosemont, IL: American Academy of Orthopaedic Surgeons; 2002:73–90

42. Wascher DC. Bicruciate injuries. In: Schenck RC Jr., ed. Multiple Ligamentous Injuries of the Knee in the Athlete. Rosemont, IL: American Academy of Orthopaedic Surgeons; 2002:91–99

43. Schenck RC. Injuries of the knee. In: Heckman JD, ed. Rockwood and Green: Fractures in Adults. 4th ed. Philadelphia: Lippincott, Williams & Wilkins; 2001:1843–1937

44. Walker D, Rogers W, Schenck RC. Immediate vascular and ligamentous repair in a closed knee dislocation: a case report. J Trauma 1994;36:898–900

45. Markolf KL, Zemanovic JR, McAllister DR. Cyclic loading of posterior cruciate ligament replacements fixed with tibial tunnel and tibial inlay methods. J Bone Joint Surg Am 2002;84:518–524

46. Cross MJ, Powell JF. Long-term followup of posterior cruciate ligament rupture: a study of 116 cases. Am J Sports Med 1984;12: 292–297

47. Fanelli GC, Giannotti BF, Edson CJ. The posterior cruciate ligament arthroscopic evaluation and treatment. Arthroscopy 1994;10: 673–688

48. Hughston JC, Bowden JA, Andrews JR, et al. Acute tears of the posterior cruciate ligament: results of operative treatment. J Bone Joint Surg Am 1980;62:438–450

49. Schulte KR, Chu ET, Fu FH. Arthroscopic posterior cruciate ligament reconstruction. Clin Sports Med 1997;16:145–156

50. Cooper DE. Treatment of combined posterior cruciate ligament and posterolateral injuries of the knee. Oper Tech Sports Med 1999;7:135–142

51. Miller MD, Gordon WT. Posterior cruciate ligament reconstruction: tibial inlay technique—principles and procedure. Oper Tech Sports Med 1999;7:127–133

52. St. Pierre P, Miller MD. Posterior cruciate ligament injuries. Clin Sports Med 1999;18:199–221

53. Clancy WG Jr, Bisson LJ. Double tunnel technique for reconstruction of the posterior cruciate ligament. Oper Tech Sports Med 1999;7:110–117

54. Petrie RS, Harner CD. Double bundle posterior cruciate ligament reconstruction technique: University of Pittsburgh approach. Oper Tech Sports Med 1999;7:118–126

55. Miller MD, Kline AJ, Gonzales J, Beach WR. Vascular risk associated with a posterior approach for posterior cruciate ligament reconstruction using the tibial inlay technique. J Knee Surg 2002;15:137–140

56. Stannard JP, Riley RS, Sheils TM, McGwin G Jr, Volgas DA. Anatomic reconstruction of the posterior cruciate ligament after multiligament knee injuries: a combination of the tibial-inlay and two-femoral-tunnel techniques. Am J Sports Med 2003;31: 196–202

56a. Zantop T, Petersen W, Fu FH. Anatomy of the anterior cruciate ligament. Operative Techniques in Orthopaedics. 2004;15:20–28

56b. Vidal AF, Brucker PU, Fu FH. Anatomic double-bundle anterior cruciate ligament reconstruction using tibialis anterior tendon allografts. Operative Techniques in Orthopaedics. 2005;15:140–145.

57. Almekinders LC, Dedmond BT. Outcomes of the operatively treated knee dislocation. Clin Sports Med 2000;19:503–518

58. Wascher DC, Becker JR, Dexer JG, Blevins FT. Reconstruction of the anterior and posterior cruciate ligaments after knee dislocation: results using fresh-frozen nonirradiated allografts. Am J Sports Med 1999;27:189–196

59. Martinek V, Steinbacher G, Friederich NF, Müeller WE. Operative treatment of combined anterior and posterior cruciate ligament injuries in complex knee trauma. Am J Knee Surg 2000;13:74–82

60. Shapiro MS, Freedman EL. Allograft reconstruction of the anterior and posterior cruciate ligaments after traumatic knee dislocation. Am J Sports Med 1995;23:580–587

61. Stannard JP, Sheils TM, McGwin G, Volgas DA, Alonso JE. Use of a hinged external knee fixator after surgery for knee dislocation. Arthroscopy 2003;19:626–631

62. Fanelli GC. Complications of multiple ligamentous injuries. In: Schenck RC Jr., ed. Multiple Ligamentous Injuries of the Knee in the Athlete. Rosemont, IL: American Academy of Orthopaedic Surgeons; 2002:101–107

63. Ferrari JD. Associated Injuries. In: Schenck RC Jr., ed. Multiple Ligamentous Injuries of the Knee in the Athlete. Rosemont, IL: American Academy of Orthopaedic Surgeons; 2002:31–41

64. Good L, Johnson RJ. The dislocated knee. J Am Acad Orthop Surg 1995;3:284–292

65. Stannard JP, Sheils TM, Lopez-Ben RR, McGwin G Jr, Robinson JT, Volgas DA. Vascular injuries in knee dislocations following blunt trauma: evaluating the role of physical examination to determine the need for arteriography. J Bone Joint Surg. 2003

66. Kaufman SL, Martin LG. Arterial injuries associated with complete dislocation of the knee. Radiology 1977;59-A:236–239

67. Kendall RW, Taylor DC, Salvian AJ, O'Brien PJ. The role of arteriography in assessing vascular injuries associated with dislocations of the knee. J Trauma 1993;35:875–878

68. Treiman GS, Yellin AF, Weaver FA, et al. Examination of the patient with a knee dislocation: the case for selective arteriography. Arch Surg 1992;127:1056–1063

69. Varnell RM, Coldwell DM, Sangeorzan BJ, Johansen KH. Arterial injury complicating knee disruption. Am Surg 1989;55:699–704

70. Wascher DC. High-velocity knee dislocation with vascular injury: treatment principles. Clin Sports Med 2000;19:457–477

71. Alberty RE, Goodfried G, Boyden AM. Popliteal artery injury with fractural dislocation of the knee. Am J Surg 1981;142:36–40

72. Dart CH Jr, Braitman HE. Popliteal artery injury following fracture or dislocation at the knee: diagnosis and management. Arch Surg 1977;112:969–973

73. Gable DR, Allen JW, Richardson JD. Blunt popliteal artery injury: is physical examination alone enough for evaluation? J Trauma 1997;43:541–544

74. Jones RE, Smith EC, Bone GE. Vascular and orthopedic complications of knee dislocation. Surg Gynecol Obstet 1979;149:554–558

75. Lefrak EA. Knee dislocation: an illusive cause of critical arterial occlusion. Arch Surg 1976;111:1021–1024

76. McCoy GF, Hannon DG, Barr RJ, Templeton J. Vascular injury associated with low-velocity dislocations of the knee. J Bone Joint Surg Br 1987;69:285–287

77. McCutchan JD, Gillham NR. Injury to the popliteal artery associated with dislocation of the knee: palpable distal pulses do not negate the requirement for arteriography. Injury 1989;20:307–310

78. Welling RE, Kakkasseril J, Cranley JJ. Complete dislocations of the knee with popliteal vascular injury. J Trauma 1981;21:450–453

79. Applebaum R, Yellin AE, Weaver FA, Oberg J, Pentecost M. Role of routine arteriography in blunt lower-extremity trauma. Am J Surg 1990;160:221–225

80. Dennis JW, Jagger C, Butcher JL, Menawat SS, Neel M, Frykberg ER. Reassessing the role of arteriograms in the management of posterior knee dislocations. J Trauma 1993;35:692–697

81. Abou-Sayed H, Berger DL. Blunt lower-extremity trauma and popliteal artery injuries. Arch Surg 2002;137:585–589

82. Martinez D, Sweatman K, Thompson EC. Popliteal artery injury associated with knee dislocations. Am Surg 2001;67:165–167

83. Miranda FE, Dennis JW, Veldenz HC, Dovgan PS, Frykberg ER. Confirmation of the safety and accuracy of physical examination in the evaluation of knee dislocation for injury of the popliteal artery: a prospective study. J Trauma 2002;52:247–252

84. Goitz RJ, Tomaino MM. Management of peroneal nerve injuries associated with knee dislocations. Am J Orthop 2003;32:14–16

85. Hegyes MS, Richardson MW, Miller MD. Knee dislocation: complications of nonoperative and operative management. Clin Sports Med 2000;19:519–543

86. Athanasian EA, Wickiewicz TL, Warren RF. Osteonecrosis of the femoral condyle after arthroscopic reconstruction of a cruciate ligament: report of two cases. J Bone Joint Surg Am. 1995;77:1418–1422

29 Tibial Plateau Fractures

James P. Stannard and Steven L. Martin

Fractures of the tibial plateau are challenging injuries that are difficult to treat effectively. They may result from relatively low-energy falls in elderly patients with osteoporotic bone, yielding fracture patterns and associated soft tissue injuries that frequently result in good outcomes.[1–7] Alternatively, tibial plateau fractures may occur following high-energy injuries with severe associated injuries to the soft tissues around the knee **(Fig. 29–1).** The outcomes following these injuries are often less favorable.[8–14] Functional outcome following tibial plateau fractures is commonly related to the nature and type of soft tissue injuries. The condition of the surrounding soft tissues is the most critical factor to be considered when surgical treatment of these injuries is being contemplated.[15] Associated injuries to the skin, knee ligaments and menisci, vascular structures, and nerves are all at least as important as the severity of the bone injury in determining functional outcome and the likelihood of the occurrence of complications. Compartment syndrome is another soft tissue complication that may adversely impact results following these injuries.[10,13,15,16] High-energy fractures with severe associated soft tissue injuries treated with open reduction and internal fixation (ORIF) using extensive surgical approaches have yielded poor results and a high incidence of complications.[4,8,9,14,17–19] Contemporary surgeons demonstrating increased vigilance regarding the condition of the soft tissues combined with indirect reduction and limited surgical approaches have achieved remarkable decreases in the occurrence of complications and improvements in outcome following tibial plateau injuries.[10,12,15,20–22]

Simultaneously with the increased recognition of the importance of associated soft tissue injuries with tibial plateau fractures, numerous advances in fixation systems and techniques have been developed. These advances have yielded changes in approach, technique, complications, and outcomes following these injuries. Examples of recent advances have included the use of small-fragment raft screws;[23,24] limited surgical approaches combined with locked plating;[20,25–28] the use of small wire fixators;[21,29–39] arthroscopic assistance in tibial plateau fractures;[15,40] and the use of injectable calcium phosphate bone cement to augment fixation of depressed tibial plateau fractures.[41–43] This chapter focuses on surgical techniques including the incorporation of the recent advances just listed.

Classification

Classification systems should provide either data regarding severity and prognosis of the injury or guidance regarding appropriate treatment. It is very helpful to group tibial plateau fractures into high- and low-energy patterns, which dictate many issues, ranging from type of fixation employed to likelihood of complications. There are two major classification systems frequently employed by orthopaedic surgeons. The first is the system proposed by Joseph Schatzker[7] that divides tibial plateau fractures into six distinct patterns **(Fig. 29–2),** and the second is the system developed by the Arbeitsgemeinschaft für Osteosynthesefragen (AO) and adopted by the Orthopaedic Trauma Association (OTA)[44] **(Table 29–1).** One weakness of both of these classification systems is that they do not relay any information regarding associated soft tissue injuries. Fracture-dislocations can be classified using a modification of the anatomical knee dislocation classification system described in the last chapter.

The Schatzker classification system is the most useful and frequently employed system for tibial plateau fractures.[3,10,15] Type I through III fractures involve the lateral tibial plateau and are often associated with low-energy injuries. Type I is a split or wedge fracture that may occur in young patients. Lateral meniscus tears are associated with this pattern and may prevent reduction of the fracture. Type II is a split depression pattern. This pattern often occurs in patients in their fifth decade of life or later.

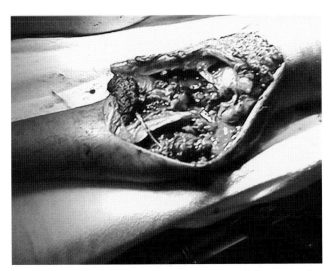

Figure 29–1 Type IIIC open tibial plateau fracture following crush injury.

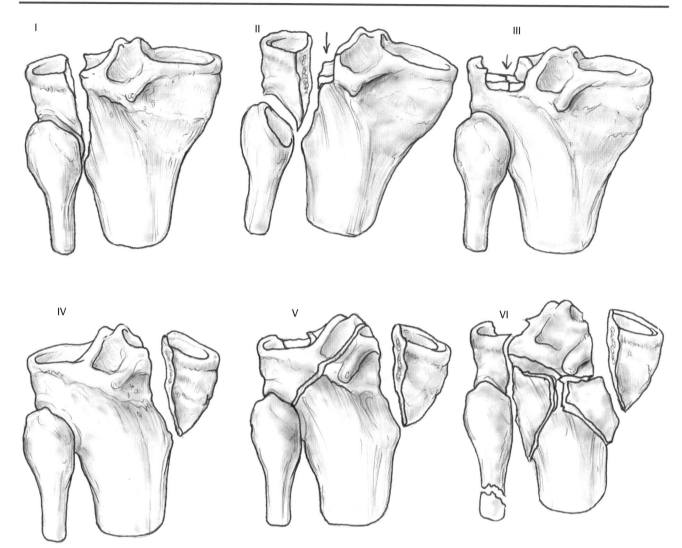

Figure 29–2 Drawings depicting the Schatzker classification of tibial plateau fractures.

Type III is a pure central depression as originally described. This pattern occurs in older patients as a result of lower-energy injuries. Types IV through VI represent high-energy injury patterns that are often associated with additional soft tissue injuries. Type IV is a medial condyle injury. These injuries are less frequent than lateral fractures and may be associated with vascular, neurological, or ligament injuries, including knee dislocations. Type V is a bicondylar tibial plateau fracture that often has the appearance of an inverted Y. The metaphysis and diaphysis remain in continuity in type V fractures. Type VI is a fracture with dissociation of the metaphysis and diaphysis. This pattern

Table 29—1 Arbeitsgemeinschaft für Osteosynthesefragen/Orthopaedic Trauma Association (AO/OTA) Fracture Classification for Tibia/Fibula

Bone	Location		
Tibia/fibula (4)	Proximal segment (41)		
Types	**41A (extra-articular)**	**41B (partial articular)**	**41C (complete articular)**
Groups	41A1. Avulsion	41B1. Pure split	41C1. Articular simple; metaphyseal simple
	41A2. Simple metaphyseal	41B2. Pure depression	41C2. Articular simple; metaphyseal multifragmentary
	41A3. Multifragmentary metaphyseal	41B3. Split depression	41C3. Articular multifragmentary

frequently results from high-energy injuries, is remarkably comminuted and bicondylar, and may have associated ligament and vascular injuries.[3] The skin may be severely damaged with this pattern and requires careful evaluation. All patterns except type I may have depressed articular segments that require disimpaction and possible bone grafting.

The AO/OTA classification employs the designation of number 4 for the tibia and number 1 for the proximal portion of the bone. Consequently, tibial plateau fractures all have the designation of 41. A letter is then added to classify the fractures. The letter *A* indicates a proximal fracture that does not enter the knee joint. A B-type fracture is a unicondylar injury and correlates to Schatzker type I through IV patterns. Although many fractures in the 41B group are low-energy injuries, medial plateau fractures are an important exception. A 41C fracture is a bicondylar injury and correlates to Schatzker type V and type VI injuries. These are normally high-energy injuries. Each of the major patterns (41A, 41B, and 41C) is further subdivided into nine additional patterns. A major advantage of the AO/OTA classification is precision and detail, with 27 subclassifications. This provides a major advantage for research and clinical outcome studies, allowing a comparison of identical fracture types. The classification is cumbersome and difficult to use clinically if taken beyond the major patterns.

Tibial plateau fractures that have associated major ligament injuries are remarkably different injuries than fractures with intact ligaments. Fracture-dislocations can be classified using the anatomical classification for knee dislocations as described in Chapter 28, with a modification to designate the specific ligaments injured. The KD–V injuries are the fracture-dislocations in the anatomical classification. The modification[45] we have proposed uses a decimal point and a number to designate the ligaments injured **(Table 29–2).** A type 1 fracture is a fracture-dislocation that does not involve a bicruciate injury (KD–V.1). A KD–V.2 is a fracture-dislocation that includes a bicruciate injury but has intact medial and lateral ligaments. KD–V.3 is a fracture-dislocation that includes a bicruciate injury and a tear of either the medial or the lateral ligaments, but

not both. Finally, a KD–V.4 injury is a tibial plateau fracture-dislocation that includes tears of all four major ligament groups supporting the knee.

Nonoperative Treatment

The determination of whether a tibial plateau fracture can be treated with closed management as compared with surgical stabilization is a multifactorial decision. Important factors include knee stability, condition of the soft tissue envelope, other skeletal injuries, fracture pattern, the patient's medical condition, and patient expectations. Prior to determining the ideal treatment protocol for a patient with a tibial plateau fracture, a thorough examination of the knee should be performed, and appropriate diagnostic studies should be obtained. The surgeon should pay special attention to the neurovascular status, degree of swelling, condition of the compartments of the lower leg, and condition of the skin. If the fracture is closed, it should be classified using Tscherne's system for grading closed fractures.[12] The condition of the soft tissue is critical, and developing the habit of classifying the soft tissue status will ensure a careful examination. Grade 0 implies soft tissue damage is absent or negligible. Grade 1 correlates with superficial abrasions or contusions. Grade 2 is either deep contaminated abrasions/contusions or impending compartment syndrome. These injuries are due to direct trauma. Grade 3 injuries include extensive contusion or crush with severe muscle damage, degloving injuries, compartment syndrome, or major blood vessel injury associated with the fracture. Severe soft tissue injuries should be allowed to recover for 1 to 3 weeks prior to placing extensive surgical incisions through the damaged soft tissue.

Appropriate imaging studies are important in determining the treatment plan for a patient with a tibial plateau fracture. Initial radiographs should include a good quality anteroposterior and lateral view of the knee and proximal tibia. If the fracture demonstrates substantial distal extension, the same views of the tibia should be obtained. Additional views that can be very helpful include two obliques and a 10 degree caudal radiograph.[3,10,12] Stress radiographs or traction views are also potentially helpful but may not be well tolerated by the patient without anesthesia. In many cases of complex fractures, we wait and obtain these views under general anesthesia using either fluoroscopy or plain radiographs. In most trauma centers, computed tomography (CT) with sagittal and coronal reconstructions has replaced trispiral tomography to evaluate the degree of articular depression and detailed anatomy of the fracture.[46] The CT scan can be very helpful in preoperative planning of reduction and fixation of the fracture. It becomes even more important if minimally invasive techniques of fracture stabilization are planned.

The role of magnetic resonance imaging (MRI) in patients with tibial plateau fractures has been controversial

Table 29–2 Modified Schenck Classification of Fracture-Dislocations

Type	Ligament Injury
V.1	Fracture-dislocation with either ACL or PCL intact
V.2	Fracture-dislocation with ACL and PCL torn
V.3M	Fracture-dislocation with ACL, PCL, and PMC torn
V.3L	Fracture-dislocation with ACL, PCL, and PLC torn
V.4	Fracture-dislocation with ACL, PCL, PMC, and PLC torn

ACL, anterior cruciate ligament; PCL, posterior cruciate ligament; PLC, posterolateral corner; PMC, posteromedial complex.

and somewhat unclear.[3,10] However, numerous manuscripts have been published in the last 10 years or so that clarify the role and benefits of MRI following fractures of the tibial plateau.[47–52] Yacoubian et al[52] found that adding MRI to plain radiographs and CT scanning in 52 patients led to a change in the fracture classification in 21% and a change in the treatment plan in 23% of cases. MRI also improved the interobserver agreement regarding fracture classification and treatment plan. Holt et al[49] reported that MRI led to a change in fracture classification in 48% and a change in the treatment plan in 19% of their patients. They also reported a 48% incidence of previously unrecognized soft tissue injuries in the knee, including two spontaneously reduced knee dislocations. Bennett and Browner[53] confirmed the issue of associated soft tissue injuries of the knee. They detected a 56% incidence using a combination of arthroscopy and examination under anesthesia. Our protocol over the past 3 years for tibial plateau fractures that occur as a result of a high-energy mechanism of injury has included obtaining MRI scans as part of the patient's diagnostic evaluation **(Fig. 29–3A–D)**. We have evaluated

103 patients with MRI following tibial plateau fractures. Numerous soft tissue injuries of the knee have been detected, including 25 medial meniscus tears, 35 lateral meniscus tears, 45 anterior cruciate ligament tears, 41 posterior cruciate ligament tears, 16 posteromedial corner or medial collateral ligament tears, and 46 posterolateral corner (PLC) tears. Most of these injuries are very difficult to detect reliably with physical examination alone in patients with severe tibial plateau fractures. **Table 29–3** summarizes the occurrence of soft tissue injuries of the knee in four published studies[47,49–51] combined with the data we have generated. Published data demonstrate that between 48 and 90% of patients with tibial plateau fractures have significant associated soft tissue injuries of the knee. Our data on 103 patients are similar, with an incidence of 71% soft tissue injuries involving the knee following tibial plateau fracture. Obtaining MRI scans frequently leads to a change in the treatment plan for patients following tibial plateau fractures.[47–53] Published data strongly support routinely obtaining MRI scans in patients following high-energy fractures of the tibial

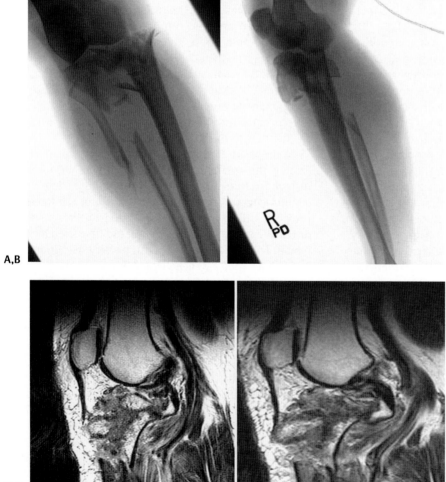

Figure 29–3 (A) Anteroposterior and **(B)** lateral radiographs of a bicondylar tibial plateau fracture. **(C)** Magnetic resonance imaging demonstrates a torn anterior cruciate ligament and **(D)** a posterior cruciate ligament avulsion.

Table 29–3   Soft Tissue Injuries Demonstrated by Magnetic Resonance Imaging following Tibial Plateau Fractures

Author	Fracture	Medial Meniscus Tear	Lateral Meniscus Tear	ACL	PCL	PMC	PLC
Barrow et al[47]	31	10	17	7	0	3	3
Holt et al[48]	21	5	1	3	3	0	4
Kode et al[50]	22	3	9	6	1	5	0
Shepherd et al[51]	20	11	12	2	0	6	1
Stannard et al[27]	103	25	35	45	41	16	46
Total	197	54 (27%)	74 (38%)	63 (32%)	45 (23%)	30 (15%)	54 (27%)

ACL, anterior cruciate ligament; PCL, posterior cruciate ligament; PLC, posterolateral corner; PMC, posteromedial complex.

plateau. Most patients with significant soft tissue injuries of the knee will benefit from surgical management of their fractures.

Nonoperative management utilizing a hinged cast brace is appropriate for some fractures of the tibial plateau. Indications for closed management may include the following fractures: (1) nondisplaced or minimally displaced (< 3 mm),[10,54,55] (2) stable to varus and valgus stress, (3) peripheral submeniscal fractures, (4) low-energy fractures with minimal comminution, and (5) low demand patients with medical contraindications to surgery. The choice of surgical versus nonoperative management must be individualized considering the foregoing indications and other factors such as associated injuries.

Outcome results reported with cast bracing have been variable and often depend on the pattern and stability of the injury.[56–60] A key to obtaining a successful outcome is adequate stability to allow early motion.[58,59] Bicondylar and split depression fractures have both been noted to be associated with less favorable outcome when treated with closed reduction and cast bracing compared with ORIF.[56,60] Poor results have been reported in 10 to 32% of fractures.[56–58,60] Patients with significant knee instability are not good candidates for cast bracing. Therefore, careful physical examination is important in patients who may be candidates for definitive treatment with cast bracing. If there is any concern regarding ligamentous instability, MRI of the knee should be obtained. Early functional motion with limited weight bearing should be employed in patients who are treated with reduction and cast bracing.

Indications for Surgical Treatment

The decision to treat a tibial plateau fracture with surgery is multifactorial, involving patient, fracture, and surgeon factors. Issues to consider regarding the patient include their age, activity, type of employment, associated injuries, and medical problems. Important factors associated with the fracture include the pattern, degree of comminution,

displacement, joint impaction, mechanism of injury or energy imparted to the tissues at the time of injury, condition of the soft tissue around the fracture, and stability of the knee. Surgeon factors to consider include the surgical team's experience and the operating room environment and equipment.

The most important factor to consider prior to embarking on surgical management of tibial plateau fractures is the condition of the local soft tissues. Severe damage to the soft tissue envelope is the most common contraindication to early surgical treatment of tibial plateau fractures.[15] It is important to grade the soft tissue condition and carefully consider this factor following both open and closed fractures. Delaying definitive surgical treatment until optimal soft tissue conditions exist minimizes complications.[10]

Absolute indications for surgery include open fractures, fractures associated with a compartment syndrome, and fractures associated with a vascular injury.[15] Relative indications for surgical stabilization include most displaced bicondylar and medial condyle fractures, lateral plateau fractures that result in joint instability, condylar widening that exceeds 5 mm, fracture-dislocations of the knee, and fractures in the polytraumatized patient that will prevent early mobilization of the patient if the knee is treated nonoperatively.[2,3,10,12,15] **Fig. 29–4** delineates our treatment algorithm for tibia plateau fractures.

Surgical Treatment

Surgical Anatomy

The medial plateau is larger and stronger than the lateral plateau and is concave compared with the convex lateral side. It is important to remember this anatomy when placing subchondral or rafting screws from the lateral side, to avoid intra-articular screws. The lateral meniscus covers a much larger portion of the articular surface than the medial meniscus.[44] Meniscotibial ligaments attach the menisci to the periphery of the tibial plateaus and must be repaired

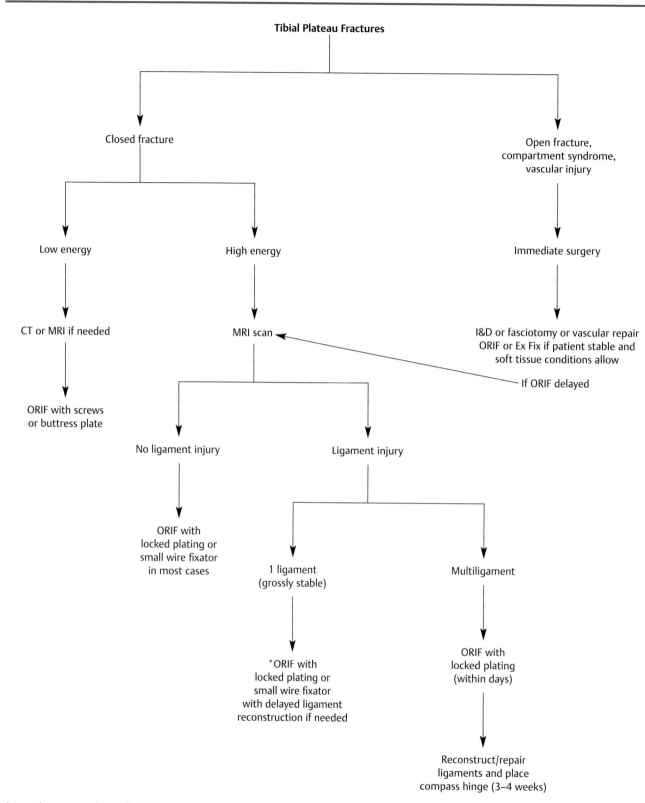

*Consider compass hinge if ORIF does not yield adequate stability for early motion.

Figure 29–4 Treatment algorithm for tibial plateau fractures. CT, computed tomography; MRI, magnetic resonance imaging; I&D, irrigation and debridement; ORIF, open reduction and internal fixation; Ex fix, external fixator.

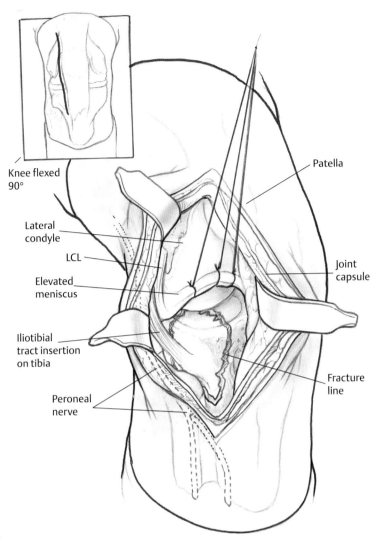

Knee flexed
90°

Lateral
condyle

LCL

Elevated
meniscus

Iliotibial
tract insertion
on tibia

Peroneal
nerve

Patella

Joint
capsule

Fracture
line

Figure 29–5 Meniscus with stay sutures to aid in repair of peripheral meniscus following open reduction and internal fixation of the tibial plateau using a submeniscal arthrotomy.

following either peripheral meniscal tears or submeniscal arthrotomies. It is wise to place stay sutures to repair the peripheral meniscus prior to reduction of the fracture because they are much more difficult to place following reduction (**Fig. 29–5**).

Important landmarks around the proximal tibia include the tibial tubercle, Gerdy's tubercle, the pes anserinus, and the proximal tibiofibular joint. The tibial tubercle is the site of attachment of the patellar tendon. It is important to assess whether the tibial tubercle is involved as a separate fragment in the fracture, to allow stabilization of this critical fragment and early motion of the knee. Gerdy's tubercle is the site of attachment of the iliotibial band, whereas the pes anserinus is the site of attachment of the sartorius, semitendinosus, and gracilis tendons. These landmarks are important for planning surgical incisions and stabilization. The fibular head provides a site of attachment for numerous ligaments and tendons of the PLC, and also acts as a buttress for the proximal lateral portion of the tibial plateau.

Surgical Approaches

The primary surgical approaches employed while stabilizing fractures of the tibial plateau include midline, lateral parapatellar, hockey stick or extended hockey stick, and the posteromedial approach to the knee. A submeniscal arthrotomy can be added to improve articular visualization. Additional approaches that have been described include detachment of the anterior horn of the lateral meniscus[61] and osteotomy of the tibial tubercle for bicondylar fractures.[62] It is critical to achieve stable repair of structures that are detached or osteotomized to improve visualization of the fracture. The surgeon must balance the benefits of improved visualization with the disadvantages of more invasive surgical approaches. We rarely detach the meniscus or osteotomize the tibial tubercle.

The midline and lateral parapatellar incisions are very similar, with the lateral parapatellar simply moved laterally 1 or 2 cm (**Fig. 29–6**). Both incisions allow good visualization of the anterior aspect of the tibial plateau. A submeniscal

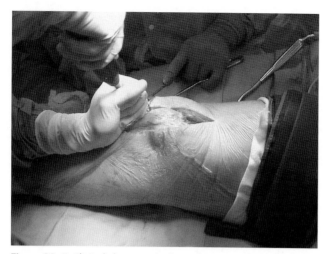

Figure 29–6 Clinical photograph of a midline approach to stabilize a tibial plateau fracture.

arthrotomy can be added to this approach to allow direct visualization of the lateral plateau. Great care must be taken to avoid excessive stripping of the deep tissue, which can be associated with infection and wound dehiscence. The incision should be a sufficient length to allow adequate exposure and placement of a lateral plate without excessive retraction of the soft tissues. It is preferable to have a longer incision and limit aggressive retraction.

The hockey stick approach allows a shorter incision when placing laterally based plates. It also can be extended proximally to allow exposure of the PLC if needed **(Fig. 29–7A,B)**. Distally, the incision starts at a similar location to the lateral parapatellar. The incision should be curved posteriorly just distal to the joint line. The origin of the anterior compartment muscles is then released to allow submuscular plating or elevation of an impacted fragment.

Significant medial fractures (either type IV or those associated with bicondylar fractures) are best approached through a separate posteromedial incision. We do not recommend attempting to place a medial plate through a midline approach because of the excessive stripping necessary to address the posteromedial fragment. A posteromedial approach can be made that allows a large skin bridge if two approaches are being used. The patient is positioned supine, and the incision is placed along a line from the medial epicondyle to the insertion of the medial collateral ligament along the posteromedial border of the tibia **(Fig. 29–8)**. The tendons of the pes anserinus can simply be retracted distally. The semimembranosus is variable in its insertion and in our experience may require release at its insertion but is tagged for later repair. The medial head of the gastrocnemius muscle is then identified. The remainder of the surgical approach remains anterior to the gastrocnemius hugging the proximal tibial condyle and medial femoral condyle. The surgeon must continue to isolate the joint line in order not to stray too far distally on the posteromedial tibia. In this approach all retractors must remain anterior to the medial gastrocnemius to avoid injury to the popliteal vessels, and the medial head is routinely *not* released. Keeping the knee flexed to 70 degrees relaxes the posterior neurovascular bundle, creating added safety with an approach anterior to the gastrocnemius.

A variety of surgical techniques are available for surgeons to stabilize fractures of the tibial plateau and proximal tibia. To have success in addressing the wide variety of fracture and soft tissue conditions associated with trauma in this region, the surgeon should become comfortable with most, if not all, of these techniques. Methods of treating tibial plateau fractures range from relatively simple procedures involving percutaneous subchondral

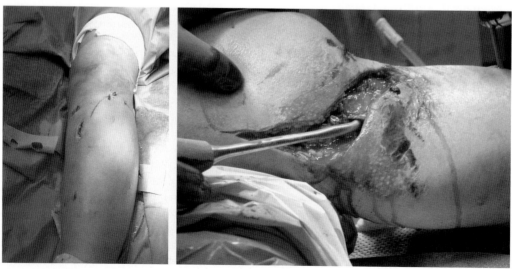

A   B

Figure 29–7 (A) The hockey stick approach drawn on a patient's skin prior to making the surgical incision. **(B)** Extension of the hockey stick approach to allow reconstruction of the posterolateral corner.

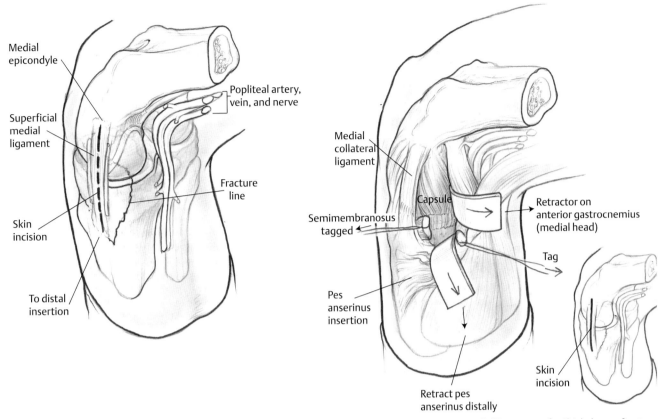

Figure 29–8 The posteromedial approach used for open reduction and internal fixation of a posteromedial fragment of a tibial plateau fracture.

screw fixation to complex locked plate or external fixation constructs. The primary factors we consider when choosing a surgical method are soft tissue condition, energy/comminution of the fracture, and degree of osteoporosis. Low-energy fracture patterns (Schatzker types I through III) generally can be treated with screws alone, conventional plates and screws, or low-profile "anatomical" plates with or without locking screws. Medial condyle fractures (Schatzker type IV) often have a large block of bone that can be stabilized with conventional plates and screws as well. Frequently, associated injuries to skin, neurological, vascular, or ligamentous structures will play a role in our selection of techniques for these fractures. Severe associated soft tissue injuries may require external fixation with either a temporary spanning external fixator, a small wire fixator, or a hinged external fixator. Bicondylar fractures (Schatzker types V and VI) and severely osteopenic bone benefit from either locked plating or small wire external fixation. Finally, fracture-dislocations are an ideal indication for a combination of ORIF combined with a hinged external fixator and ligament repair or reconstruction.

We will discuss in detail several techniques that are helpful in treating fractures of the tibial plateau. The ensuing techniques are not a comprehensive group of the methods that can be used with these fractures but are the methods we most commonly employ.

Surgical Technique

Percutaneous Reduction and Fixation of Low-Energy Fractures

There are three common scenarios encountered by surgeons caring for patients with low-energy (Schatzker types I through III) fractures of the lateral tibial plateau. Type I or split fractures may be treated with either percutaneous ORIF using screws, arthroscopically assisted techniques (discussed later in this chapter), or a lateral buttress plate using open techniques. To accomplish percutaneous fixation, the patient should be positioned supine with a roll of surgical sheets under the knee. A radiolucent table and high-quality fluoroscopy are critical components. Preoperatively, an MRI scan should be obtained to assess for meniscal and ligamentous injuries as well as to assess the fracture pattern. Reduction is achieved either by applying manual traction with a varus force manually or by using a laterally based femoral distractor. If an anatomical reduction is achieved, compression should be obtained with a percutaneously placed, large, pointed fracture reduction clamp. The fracture can then be stabilized with two or three large cannulated screws. Alternatively, the reduction can be temporarily stabilized with several 0.625 Kirschner wires, followed by placing several 3.5 mm "rafting" screws just below the articular surface (**Fig. 29–9**). If an anatomical

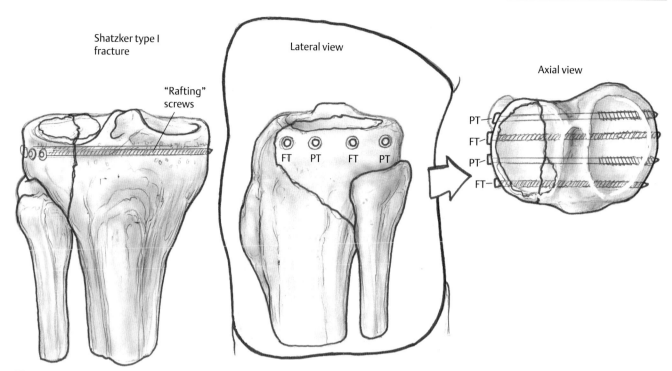

Figure 29–9 Anteroposterior, lateral, and axial drawings of a Schatzker type I tibial plateau fracture treated using percutaneous placement of "rafting" screws. PT, Partially threaded screw; FT, Fully threaded screw

reduction is not achieved, the percutaneous technique should be abandoned for either open or arthroscopic techniques; displacement of as little as 1.5 mm at the joint is associated with significantly increased contact pressure.[54] We rarely use this technique in the setting of severe osteoporosis because screws alone in this bone are insufficient.

Open Reduction and Internal Fixation of Low-Energy Fractures

ORIF is necessary for most type II and III fractures that require surgical stabilization **(Fig. 29–10A–C)**, as well as type I fractures that cannot be anatomically reduced using closed techniques. Surgical approaches that can be used with this technique include the midline, lateral parapatellar, or hockey stick approaches. We generally prefer the lateral parapatellar approach. The exception is the case where the patient has significant injury to the PLC of the knee requiring stabilization. The hockey stick approach is our preferred incision in this instance, allowing extension to repair or reconstruct the PLC either immediately or on a delayed basis. Transverse incision of the lateral meniscal tibial ligament allows a submeniscal arthrotomy. Keeping the knee flexed ~90 degrees aids visualization of the articular surface. Additional tricks that can improve visualization include placing several small traction

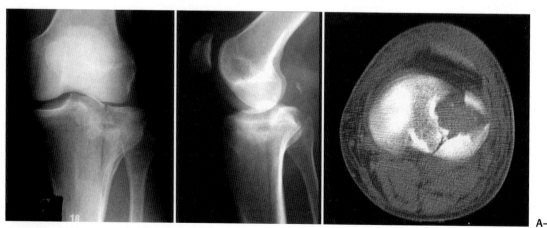

A–C

Figure 29–10 **(A)** Anteroposterior and **(B)** lateral radiographs and **(C)** a computed tomographic scan demonstrating a Schatzker type III tibial plateau fracture with significant impaction.

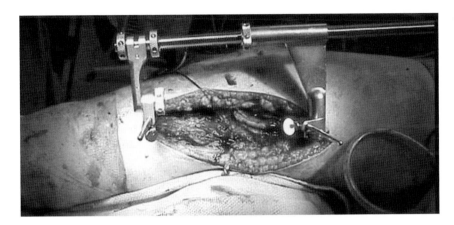

Figure 29–11 Femoral distractor used to improve visualization of the joint and aid in reduction of the tibial plateau.

sutures in the meniscus, or use of the large femoral distractor **(Fig. 29–11)**. The location of the articular impaction can be directly visualized in most cases. Reduction of the joint surface can be accomplished by either "opening the book" by retracting the lateral fragment or creating a cortical window in the metaphyseal flare. If the lateral fracture line ends within the surgical exposure, it is easier to wedge open the fracture like opening a book. The articular depression is then elevated directly using an impactor. It is important to elevate the entire articular depression as a single fragment by placing graft material beneath it if needed, to avoid additional comminution and fragmentation. The impactor should be used to gently tap the articular fragment back into an anatomical reduction under direct vision using the submeniscal arthrotomy. If the condylar fracture line extends beyond the surgical exposure, a cortical window should be created at the metaphyseal flare

(Fig. 29–12). The window can be created using a small (2 mm) drill to make four holes in the shape of a 1 cm square. A small osteotome is then used to connect the dots and create a window. The window can be impacted into the metaphysis and used to elevate the articular surface using an impactor as already described. Once reduced, pointed fracture reduction clamps or Kirschner wires or both should be used to maintain the reduction.

The final stage of surgical stabilization using ORIF involves fixation with a plate **(Fig. 29–13A,B)**. Options include a standard buttress plate, preshaped anatomical plates, and plates that feature threaded holes that allow some or all of the screws to be locked into the plate. All of these implants have advantages and disadvantages. Standard buttress plates are less expensive and have been proven to work well in simple fracture patterns. Anatomical plates save time contouring the plate, and are generally thin in their proximal portion where the soft tissue coverage is often poor. This may decrease patient discomfort or soft tissue complications. Locked plates can be helpful to stabilize the

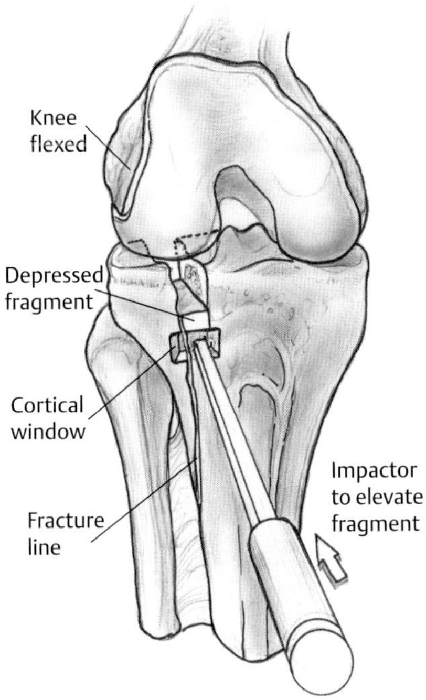

Knee
flexed

Depressed
fragment

Cortical
window

Fracture
line

Impactor
to elevate
fragment

Figure 29–12 Reduction of an impacted fragment through a cortical window.

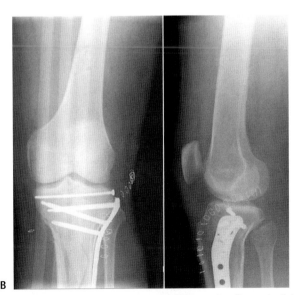

A,B

Figure 29–13 (A) Anteroposterior and **(B)** lateral radiographs following open reduction and internal fixation of a bicondylar tibial plateau fracture with extension into the diaphysis.

medial tibial plateau in Schatzker V and VI fractures where a separate incision does not need to be made medially. In addition, they may be helpful in the setting of severe comminution or severe osteoporosis.

Open Reduction and Internal Fixation with Locked Plating (see Video 29–1, Disk 4)

Locked plating that incorporates threaded screws and threaded holes in plates is a recent development in the surgical treatment of patients with tibial plateau fractures. The absolute indications for using locked plating have not been completely defined. The major advantage of these plates is they exhibit a better potential to withstand applied loads with a gap model (such as is seen with severe comminution or osteopenia) when compared with conventional plates. Each locking screw forms a fixed angle as it locks into place, decreasing the risk of hardware failure in poor quality bone.[20,63–66] Many locked plating systems have some holes that accommodate conventional screws and others that incorporate locking screws. The surgeon must remember the primary advantage of each

type: conventional screws allow compression and can reduce the fracture to the plate, whereas locking screws are less likely to pull out of bone and will not displace the fracture as they are placed. Most low-energy fractures, with the exception of elderly patients with very poor quality bone, do not require locked plating. In addition, most Schatzker types I through IV fractures do not benefit from locked plating, except perhaps in cases of severe osteoporosis. In fact, the locked screws do not compress the medial or lateral tibial plateau to the intact tibia, which is a disadvantage of locked plating. In some cases with a large medial fragment, bicondylar fractures can be adequately stabilized with a single locked plate. If the laterally based plate does not provide adequate fixation of the medial fragment, a medial plate should be added through a separate incision (**Fig. 29–14**).

The technique for most locked plating systems is identical to standard ORIF with buttress plates except for the drilling of the screws. The Less Invasive Stabilization System (LISS, Synthes USA, Paoli, Pennsylvania), which is detailed later in the chapter, is an exception to this rule because it combines minimally invasive and locked plating

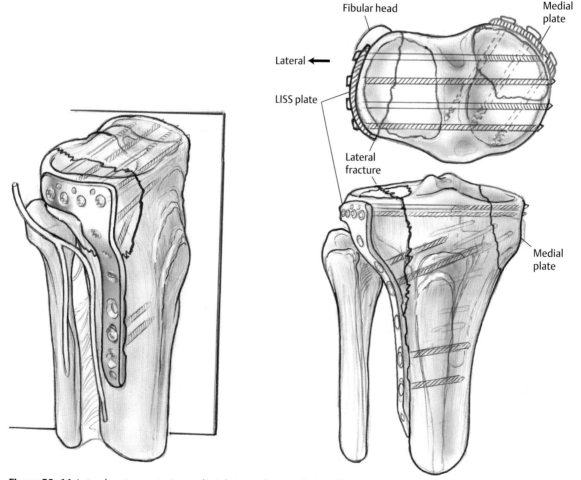

Figure 29–14 Lateral, anteroposterior, and axial views of a laterally based locked plate with a posteromedial plate stabilizing a bicondylar tibial plateau fracture. LISS, Less Invasive Stabilization System.

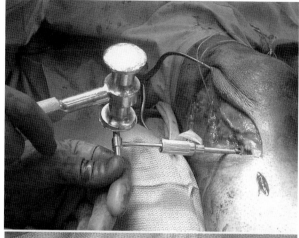

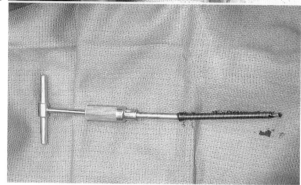

Figure 29–15 (A) Using the broken screw removal set and a mallet to attempt to remove a "cold welded" screw. If the screw can be removed at all, it frequently requires a great deal of force, which **(B)** may deform or break the screw or the screw removal instruments.

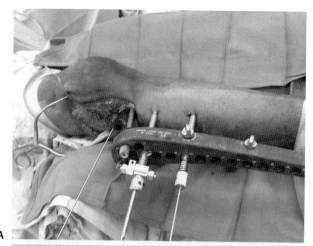

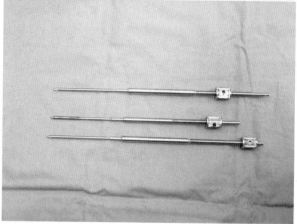

Figure 29–16 (A) Clinical photograph using the "whirlybird" through the Less Invasive Stabilization System (LISS) handle to aid reduction of a bicondylar tibial plateau fracture. **(B)** Photograph demonstrating both the long and short whirlybirds.

techniques. Following reduction and temporary fixation with clamps or K-wires, the locked plate is placed over the proximal tibia. A drill guide should then be screwed into the threaded hole. The hole should be drilled and measured based on the manufacturer's system, and the locking screw should then be drilled into place. It is important to use the guide because drilling from as little as 5 degrees off of the perpendicular can lead to a "cold welding" of the screw head threads with the plate hole threads, or suboptimal "locking" of the screw in the plate. When cold welding occurs, removal of the screw can be extremely difficult **(Fig. 29–15A,B)**. Conventional screws and locked screws should be combined based upon the needs of the individual fracture. Both the locking plates and the screws are more expensive than their conventional counterparts and should only be used where they provide a clear advantage.

Less Invasive Stabilization System (see Videos 29–2, 29–3, Disk 4)

The LISS internal fixation system combines locked plating with a minimally invasive surgical approach. The primary indication for LISS osteosynthesis is high-energy bicondylar fractures. Secondary indications may include periprosthetic fractures, open fractures,[28] and proximal one-quarter tibial shaft fractures.[66] Use of the LISS internal fixator requires a different technique than conventional plate osteosynthesis. It is critical to remember that the screws will not pull the bone to the implant, and therefore the fixator cannot normally be used as a reduction tool. The only exceptions to this occur when using the pull reduction instrument (commonly referred to as the whirlybird) or if conventional screws are used **(Fig. 29–16A,B)**. An important principle to remember is that no screws should be placed through the fixator until the correct length and rotation of the tibia have been restored and the fracture is reduced in both the sagittal and coronal planes **(Fig. 29–17)**. Once the surgeon has begun placing fixed-angle screws, additional reduction will not be possible.

The patient should be placed in a supine position with a roll of towels placed under the knee to assist in the reduction. Generally, a roll that places the knee in 25 to 30 degrees of flexion provides the maximum benefit. However, varying the size and location of the roll can remarkably change the reduction. This process of "learning" the fracture by analyzing the effect of ligamentotaxis on reduction using

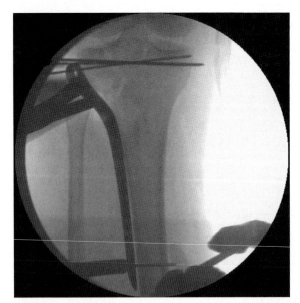

Figure 29–17 Anteroposterior fluoroscopic view demonstrating reduction of the fracture and placement of threaded wires prior to placing any screws.

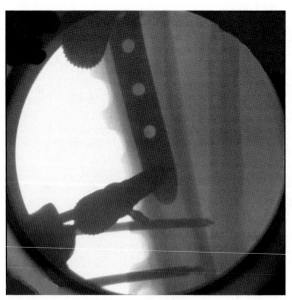

Figure 29–18 It is critical that locked plates are located in the mid-lateral plane so that screws obtain adequate fixation.

longitudinal traction, combined with changing the size and location of the roll, will improve the final reduction and save significant time once the implant has been placed in the submuscular plane. Often manual traction is used to obtain and maintain length, and to "fine-tune" angulation and rotation.

The surgical approach can be accomplished with either a lateral peripatellar or a hockey stick incision. For placement of the LISS fixator itself, a small incision (~5 to 8 cm) is needed. However, the articular component of the fracture requires reduction and stabilization using techniques that are no different than those used with conventional plating. It is important to plan the location of any screws utilized to stabilize the articular reduction, keeping in mind the location of the LISS fixator and screws. We usually stabilize the articular component with a few 3.5 mm screws utilizing a rafting technique. Once a satisfactory reduction of the articular surface has been achieved, a Bovie is utilized to release part of the origin of the anterior compartment muscles to expose the submuscular plane. The LISS fixator should then be attached to the aiming handle.

The LISS fixator is then slid into place using the aiming handle. The surgeon should keep a finger along the anterior crest of the tibia and feel the tip of the fixator pass distally. It is best to keep the tip of the fixator pointing anteriorly because this can avoid injury to the anterior tibial artery and vein and accompanying deep peroneal nerve, which are located on the posteromedial border of the tibia. This also allows a clear understanding of the position of the plate on the tibia in the sagittal plane. It is critical that the implant is located in the middle of the diaphysis of the tibia distally, or the unicortical screws will not have sufficient pull-out strength (**Fig. 29–18**). It should be slid slightly further dis-

tally than the anticipated final position, and then slid back proximally to achieve the best fit to the osseous contour of the proximal tibia. Once placement has been confirmed using fluoroscopy, a 2 mm threaded wire is utilized to stabilize the internal fixator to the proximal tibia. Longitudinal traction is then utilized to obtain length and reduction in the sagittal plane. An incision of the skin corresponding with the location of the most distal hole is made, followed by blunt spreading, placement of the insertion sleeve and trocar, and then connection of the handle to the distal plate with a threaded stabilization bolt. Another 2 mm threaded

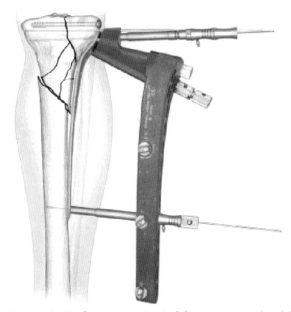

Figure 29–19 The Less Invasive Stabilization System (LISS) fixator pinned to the tibia with slight displacement in the coronal plane.

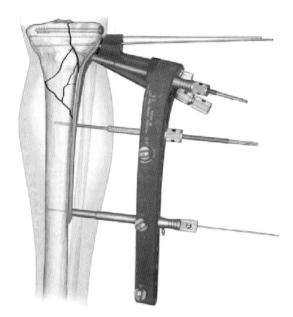

Figure 29–20 The ideal Less Invasive Stabilization System (LISS) configuration with proximal and distal threaded wires as well as whirlybirds just proximal and just distal to the metaphyseal fracture.

wire is utilized to pin the LISS fixator to the midlateral portion of the tibial diaphysis **(Fig. 29–19)**. A lateral view of the tibia using fluoroscopy should be obtained to confirm placement in the midlateral plane. If the fixator is not located in the middle of the tibial diaphysis, the 2 mm wire should be removed and the location adjusted appropriately. An ideal LISS construct involves placing two bicortical whirlybirds, one just proximal and one distal to the fracture **(Fig. 29–20)**. The whirlybird is placed through a stab incision corresponding to the desired hole on the internal fixator. This hole is made by bluntly spreading, placing the drill guide/trocar in

the hole, removing the trocar, and finally drilling the whirlybird into the tibia with irrigation. The whirlybird is then tightened to stabilize and reduce any malalignment of the fracture. No screws should be placed into the LISS fixator until a reduction is obtained and it is stabilized with 2 mm threaded wires proximally and distally in the tibia, and near the fracture with whirlybirds as needed. The LISS fixator does not have an exact fit with the proximal tibia in some individuals due to anatomical variability between patients. Because the locked screws do not pull the fixator snugly against the bone, this can lead to a prominent plate and associated hardware-related pain. An important tip to reduce this possibility can be employed at this point in the case. Prior to placing the proximal screws, a large reduction forceps should be placed through a stab incision medially and also attached to the small wire hole in the proximal anterior portion of the plate.

Tightening the forceps to snug the plate against the tibia prior to placing the proximal screws minimizes the problem of prominent hardware. Care must be taken not to use too much force with this, however, because excessive force may deform the fixator. As soon as one or two screws have been placed, the forceps should be removed **(Fig. 29–21)**. A whirlybird in the proximal segment can also be utilized to accomplish the same purpose.

The final stage of osteosynthesis with a LISS internal fixator involves placing the locked screws. The C, D, and E holes should be utilized with the vast majority of fracture patterns. These screws provide excellent fixation with divergence from one another in three dimensions **(Fig. 29–22)**. A drill guide and cannulated trocar are placed in the E hole. A 2 mm guidewire is then drilled through the trocar, with the position confirmed using fluoroscopy. The length of the screw is measured using the depth gauge provided, and the 2 mm wire and cannulated

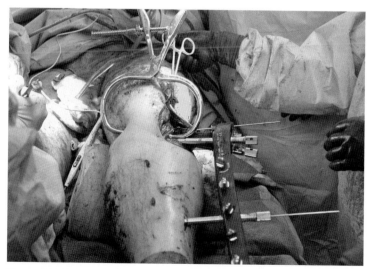

Figure 29–21 Large reduction forceps clamping fixator to the proximal tibia to prevent pain due to prominent hardware.

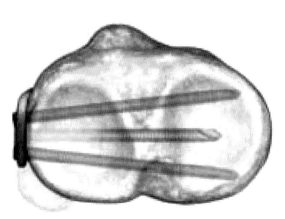

Figure 29–22 Axial view of the tibial plateau with the C, D, and E screws implanted in the plate.

trocar are then removed. A LISS screw is then drilled into the proximal tibia while irrigating. Power drilling should be discontinued just prior to the screw head locking into the holes of the internal fixator. If the screw is powered in the entire way, this may lead to cold welding or an excessive torque force on the surgeon's wrist from the drill. The screw should be locked into the LISS fixator using the torque screwdriver, tightening it until two clicks are heard. This procedure is repeated for the D and C screws. It is important to be aware that the D screw diverges posteriorly. Because the screws are powered in and are threaded, it may be difficult to feel if the posterior cortex is perforated. It is important to place this screw with the knee flexed (to keep the popliteal vessels away from the posterior cortex) after making sure the fixator is not located posteriorly on the tibia. The length of this screw should be adjusted if necessary after obtaining a lateral fluoroscopic view and scrutinizing the location of the D screw. The posterior divergence of this screw is easily remembered if the surgeon realizes that D is for *danger* (to the popliteal vessels). Paying attention to this small technique point allows consistent safe placement of this important screw. If the LISS fixator is placed slightly posterior or is rotated to face posteriorly, this danger can be accentuated. A fourth screw proximally usually replaces the proximal whirlybird. Additional screws should be placed based on the fracture pattern and surgeon's judgment. A minimum of four screws should generally be placed proximally and distally.

The remainder of the case involves placement of the distal screws. The technique includes making a small incision through the skin, bluntly spreading down to bone, placing the drill sleeve/trocar system through the appropriate hole in the aiming handle, attaching the irrigation system, and placing an 18 or 26 mm screw under power. Important points include using irrigation, using a torque-limiting screwdriver at the end of the screw placement, and placing at least four screws distally. The plate also must be in the midlateral plane of the bone to avoid transcortical screw placement. We recommend placing two screws near the fracture site and two screws near the distal end of the plate for maximum stability. The principles involved in screw placement are similar to those involved with placing pins for external fixators. Another important point is that the risk of damage to neurovascular structures rises with more distally placed screws **(Fig. 29–23)**. If the 13-hole plate is being used, great care should be used to bluntly spread down to bone and place the trocar system for holes 10 through 13. Alternatively, a small incision may be used to directly expose the distal three holes on the long LISS plate.

Open Reduction of Medial Tibial Plateau (see Video 29–4, Disk 4)

Fractures of the medial tibial plateau frequently involve high-energy trauma and have associated neurovascular or soft tissue injuries. Careful vascular examination and MRI evaluation are highly recommended to avoid missed diagnoses. Surgical approaches that can be used for this fracture include a medial peripatellar approach or a posteromedial approach to the knee (see detailed description and anatomy in Chapter 28). The posteromedial approach is strongly recommended. Advantages of this approach are that it allows treatment of any posteromedial corner ligament injuries, it is located right over the posteromedial fragment, and it leaves a large skin bridge if the patient has a bicondylar fracture (type V or VI) that requires medial and lateral plating. This approach also makes it easy to place the plate behind and beneath the tendons of the pes anserinus. Fixation of the fracture can be accomplished either with two or three rafting screws or a small buttress plate. Care must be taken to preoperatively plan the position and direction of screws, keeping in mind the location of tunnels and screws that will be necessary for ligament reconstruction in fracture-dislocation patients.

Arthroscopically Assisted Reduction and Internal Fixation of a Schatzker Type III Split Depressed Tibial Plateau Fracture (see Video 29–5, Disk 4)

The arthroscope has become a very useful adjunctive tool in the treatment of lower-energy Schatzker type I through III tibial plateau fractures. As contemporary surgeons improve in arthroscopically assisted fracture surgery, the arthroscope is evolving into a visualization tool, allowing the surgeon to avoid a formal arthrotomy. In this role, arthroscopy may also be useful in select high-energy tibial plateau fractures. In tibial plateau fracture surgery, the arthroscope has two distinct roles. The first is diagnostic, allowing accurate visualization of the articular fracture component and any concomitant intra-articular soft tissue injury. The second is therapeutic, allowing removal of osteochondral debris and assisting in fracture reduction and soft tissue injury repair.

1. *Preoperative planning* This step is critical, and the surgeon should not enter the operating theater without a thorough understanding of the fracture and any potential soft tissue element injuries. Data from the history, exam, plain radiographs, and imaging studies must be mentally collated into an accurate three-dimensional image of the fracture. The surgeon should specifically identify any posterior bone injury that would require a separate posterior corner approach either medially or laterally. The fracture plane orientation relative to the coronal and sagittal planes should be determined as well as the size and location of the central depression fragment. The square area dimension of the depression (i.e., size of the depressed fragment) and adequacy of the rim are more important to the mechanical stability and loading of the lateral compartment than is the distance of

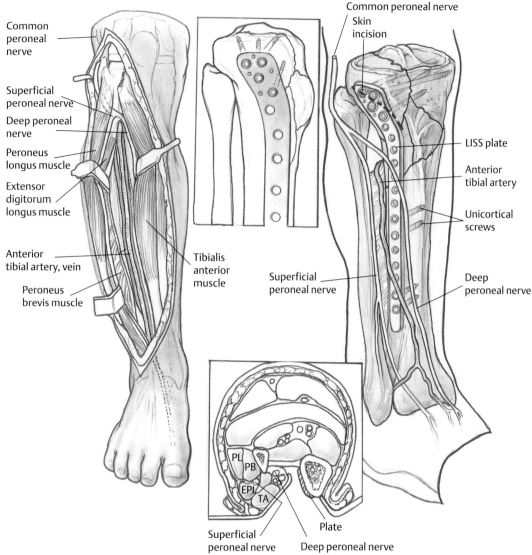

Figure 29–23 The vascular and neurological structures in the anterior and lateral compartments of the leg. There is increased risk for damage of neurovascular structures with percutaneous screw insertion in the distal tibia.

depression. A large area of depression not covered by the lateral meniscus and fractures involving the cortical rim are more unstable and should be treated with ORIF. In contrast, a small central depression fracture with overlying meniscus and a stable rim can be treated nonoperatively with a good functional outcome. Fractures in the gray area between these two extremes require significant surgical decision making.

2. *Patient positioning and operating room setup* The patient is positioned supine on a radiolucent table with a high thigh tourniquet. A leg holder is optional, but I find it most helpful because it stabilizes the femur (proximal segment) in space. In this regard, the extremity is oriented with the patella straight anteriorly. A bump may be required underneath the ipsilateral buttocks. This accurate patient positioning allows a marriage between the preoperative mental fracture

image and the spatial orientation of the knee and proximal tibia in the operating room. The surgeon is then oriented to the sagittal plane perpendicular to the floor and the coronal plane parallel to the floor. The contralateral extremity is positioned out of the way, allowing equal access to the medial and lateral aspect of the operative knee. The foot of the bed can be lowered to allow increased knee flexion if needed. The C-arm is brought in from the contralateral side (**Fig. 29–24A**). The arthroscope video screen is at the ipsilateral head of the bed and the C-arm screen is at the contralateral head of the bed, allowing the surgeon to see both screens without having to turn (**Fig. 29–24B**). Biplanar fluoroscopic views are an absolute necessity.

3. *Diagnostic knee arthroscopy* This is a thorough but expedient process, identifying all intra-articular soft tissue and bone injuries. It is helpful to start with a

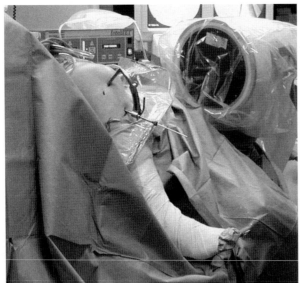

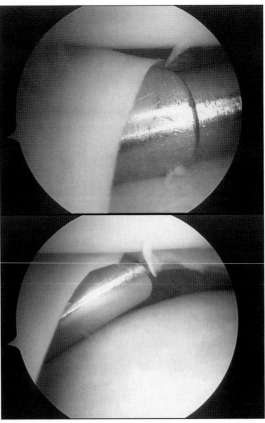

Figure 29–25 Placing a working cannula under the anterior horn of the lateral meniscus remarkably improves visualization of the fracture.

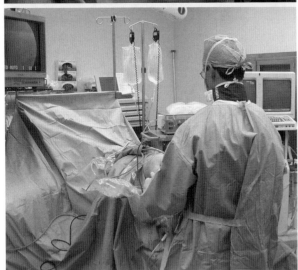

Figure 29–24 (A) Recommended room setup with the C-arm coming in from the contralateral side, compared with **(B)** the tibial plateau fracture and the video screen being on the ipsilateral side near the patient's head.

gentle exam under anesthesia to assess the overall stability of the knee. All landmarks should be marked, including the patella, patellar tendon, joint line, fibular head, and peroneal nerve. Because of swelling, this exercise is helpful even for experienced surgeons. Place a superomedial outflow portal and start with a lateral peripatellar scope portal with inflow through the scope cannula. It is important to always have good outflow to allow unimpeded fluid egress out of the knee. Flow into the leg compartments should always be watched for with frequent evaluation of the compartment soft tissue tension. It is preferable to use gravity inflow. A short period of joint lavage is required to remove blood clots, cartilage, and bone debris. A medial peripatellar portal is then established using arthroscopic and spinal needle guidance. For Schatzker

type I through III fractures of the lateral compartment, the scope is switched over to the medial portal viewing lateral. A lateral inframeniscal portal is then created. The previously made anterolateral skin portal is used, placing a spinal needle under the meniscus. This is confirmed using the arthroscope from the anteromedial portal. Then, using a no. 11 blade knife, a portal under the anterior horn of the lateral meniscus is created in a horizontal fashion. Placement of a working cannula in this location lifts the meniscus up, markedly improving the fracture visualization (**Fig. 29–25**).

4. *Fracture reduction* The organized hematoma and small loose cartilaginous fragments along the fracture are debrided. The major depressed area and the plane of the major split fracture can then be identified. Accurate elevation of the depressed segment requires pushing the fragment from below en masse. This necessitates consistent tunnel placement from below. Use of a knee ligament guide improves the reliability of this step. The tip of the guide pin is then placed in the center of the depression and is drilled from the tibial metaphysis up to 1.5 to 2 cm below the fragment (**Fig. 29–26A,B**). A relatively vertical tunnel allows more uniform elevation with a bone tamp. Pin placement is confirmed with biplanar fluoroscopy. The guidewire is then overdrilled with a cannulated reamer that allows the bone tamp to

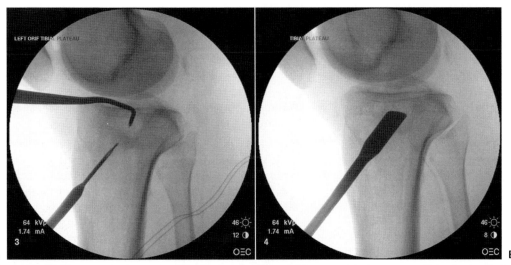

Figure 29–26 Fluoroscopic views using **(A)** a ligament guide and **(B)** a cannulated reamer or dilator to elevate the depressed fragment during arthroscopically assisted open reduction and fixation of a tibial plateau fracture.

pass freely. A coring reamer allows salvage of bone graft from the tunnel for later use. Then the depressed fragment is elevated en masse up to a 1 mm overreduction with the plateau. The reduction is confirmed with the arthroscope, viewing from the anteromedial portal **(Fig. 29–27A,B)**. Generally, light taps with a small hammer allow more controlled reduction than manual pushing for this critical step. An assistant is helpful for this portion of the case. A large bone fracture clamp is then used to compress the major split fracture. The clamp should be placed perpendicular to the fracture plane. The true fracture plane is identified on preoperative images and is confirmed via intraoperative arthroscopy and fluoroscopy. An intra-articular spinal needle can be placed perpendicular to the fracture plane and confirmed with the arthroscope.

5. *Fracture fixation* Fixation is fracture-pattern specific as defined in the ORIF section of this chapter. Screws can first be placed in a raft under the elevated fragment. It is helpful to use a cannulated screw system and place

an initial guide pin under the fragment. The position of the guide pin can then be confirmed via fluoroscopy and by placing the arthroscope up the reamed tunnel from below. If the guide pin is in the correct position, it can be visualized in the tunnel directly beneath the cancellous bone of the elevated fragment. The guide pin is replaced with a cancellous screw. It must be recalled that the medial cortex of the tibia slopes. If this fact is not remembered, screws placed in this location are too long and cause pain on the medial aspect of the knee. Ideally, two screws are placed directly under the fragment. This forms a mechanical buttress against inferior displacement. The biomechanics of fixation of the split portion of the fracture follows the principle of a "fixation ladder." The more comminuted the fracture pattern and the poorer the bone quality, the higher up the fixation ladder the surgeon must go to achieve a stable reduction allowing for early range of motion. Two well-placed screws may be adequate for a stable split-type lateral plateau fracture

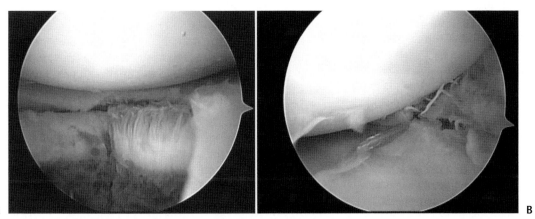

Figure 29–27 Arthroscopic views **(A)** before and **(B)** after reduction of a depressed tibial plateau fracture.

in a compliant patient with good bone quality. Several screws and a small fragment antiglide plate may be necessary for a split depression fracture with metaphyseal comminution in a patient with good bone quality. In contrast, this same fracture in a patient with poor bone quality may require a buttress plate with fixation into the more cortical proximal metadiaphyseal region. The surgeon must match the fixation to the fracture pattern, bone quality, and patient. One must not start at the bottom of the ladder and climb upward intraoperatively. The proper rung on the ladder can be chosen with good preoperative planning. Furthermore, biomechanical stability should not be compromised because the surgeon is attempting to do the case in a percutaneous manner.

Incisions for this step must follow logical planning. It is more soft tissue friendly and cosmetically pleasing to use a 3 to 4 cm longitudinal anterolateral incision midway between the lateral edge of the patella and the fibular head. This one incision can be used for the placement of multiple percutaneous screws, bone clamp placement, percutaneous plating, and outside to inside repairs of the anterior horn portion of a peripheral lateral meniscal tear. A limited lateral peripatellar arthrotomy can be performed through a proximal extension of this incision as well. This is preferable to multiple vertical or horizontal stab incisions. The window of the 3 cm incision can be moved proximally and distally with flexion and extension of the knee and anteriorly and posteriorly with retractors during the different phases of the bone and soft tissue repair.

6. *Grafting of any bone voids or defects* The goals of bone grafting are usually structural and to act as an osteoconductive substance. Bone graft for osteoinduction and as a source of osteoprogenitor cells is generally not a requirement in plateau fractures. If structural support is needed, the surgeon can choose between autograft, allograft, or injectable calcium phosphate cement (see New Techniques section). An osteoconductive scaffold can be achieved with any number of synthetic bone graft substitutes. An injectable bone graft substitute works well in minimally invasive cases and is injected up the tibial tunnel from below. The injection process can be monitored with fluoroscopy. The joint can be visualized via arthroscopy to insure that the material does not extravasate into the joint.

7. *Soft tissue repair* Ligamentous injuries are addressed in the fracture-dislocation section. It is important to perform meniscal repair after the major split fracture is compressed and the osseous architecture is restored. Longitudinal peripheral meniscal tears generally reduce back into place after the fracture gap is closed. All longitudinal tears that are in the peripheral vascular zone should be repaired. Load transfer of the involved plateau is greatly improved if the meniscus is retained. The surgeon should be proficient in a variety of techniques that may be required with low-profile, all-inside anchoring devices for posterior horn tears, inside-out or all-inside suturing techniques for mid-zone injuries, and outside-in suturing reserved for anterior horn tears. Meniscal repair equipment should be readily available for all cases.

8. *Quick knee and leg inspection* Arthroscopically inspect the joint, confirming fracture reduction and soft tissue repair and looking for any retained loose bodies. The leg and thigh compartments should be assessed for the possibility of compartment syndrome at the end of each case. If there is any concern, compartment pressures should be measured as detailed in Chapter 3.

9. *Postoperative care* This is covered later in the chapter. By avoiding a formal arthrotomy, the patient and treating surgeon are generally rewarded with a rapid return of knee motion. Weight bearing is still restricted for 6 to 8 weeks. Most low-energy fractures treated percutaneously can be performed as an outpatient or with a single overnight stay.

Small Wire or Hybrid External Fixation (see Video 29–6, Disk 4)

All the knowledge, skills, and tools for minimally invasive fracture surgery must be available to the surgeon for successful small wire fixation of tibial plateau fractures. The surgeon must become the conductor of the minimally invasive orchestra, bringing together all these tools and techniques in the operative concert. When only one step in the orchestrated sequence is not performed well, the end result can be disharmonious chaos. The patient will perceive this unrecognizable melody as pain and a poor clinical and functional outcome. When each step is performed correctly, and is conducted together with other steps properly, the results can be spectacular.

The primary indication for small wire fixation in proximal tibial fractures is a periarticular fracture with a soft tissue envelope that is not conducive to the formal open operative techniques described earlier in this chapter. The main zone of injury is metaphyseal with a relatively small proximal fragment that does not allow intramedullary nailing or standard half-pin unilateral external fixation as viable treatment options. Additional challenges are often present with articular and diaphyseal fracture extensions. When all these elements are present, as seen in some high-energy proximal tibial fractures, the small wire fixator becomes a powerful and, by default, necessary fracture tool.

The surgeon must always look critically at the status of the soft tissues and weigh the risk:benefit ratio of operative intervention. The timing of surgery is critical. Local swelling and soft tissue injury can temporarily alter local tissue perfusion and oxygenation. Surgery using incisions through these poorly vascularized areas can lead to the disastrous complications of wound necrosis and deep infection. For those fractures with intra-articular extension, traction radiographs either with manual distraction or after placement of a temporary spanning external fixator are extremely helpful in deciding the timing of surgery. If the joint portion of the fracture is nondisplaced, or reduces well with ligamentotaxis, then percutaneous small wire external fixation can generally be performed within the first 3 to 5 days. If there are displaced intra-articular fractures that do not reduce with ligamentotaxis, then surgery must be delayed until the soft tissues will allow at least limited open reduction of the articular fracture portion.

1. *Preoperative planning* This is arguably the most critical step. For this reason, small wire fixation is not the treatment of choice for the emergent treatment of tibial plateau fractures in the middle of the night regardless of surgeon experience. As discussed earlier, a temporary spanning external fixator is placed if the joint and fracture are unstable and length and/or angulation cannot be maintained with a knee immobilizer or cylinder cast. This allows for soft tissue observation, traction films, CT scanning, and, most importantly, preoperative planning. The small wire frame can be completely assembled preoperatively using full-length radiographs of the tibia. Select a ring size, using the contralateral leg, that allows for a minimum of two fingerbreadths' clearance posteriorly and one fingerbreadth anteriorly. In the trauma setting when in between ring sizes, it is preferable to err on the larger size to allow for extremity swelling. Draw the ring levels provisionally on the anteroposterior (AP) radiograph. Two levels of fixation in each major fragment are biomechanically desirable with as close to a 90 degree spread of wire and half-pin fixation as possible. The proximal tibial segment generally has one ring with a drop wire. The distal segment has a ring 2 cm below the major metaphyseal fracture and a second ring just above the ankle. A joint-spanning frame is generally not required as long as two levels of fixation can be achieved in the proximal segment. Select threaded rods of appropriate length and preassemble the small wire frame.

2. *Patient positioning and operating room setup* The temporary spanning external fixator, if present, is removed prior to prepping. This provisional fixator has been exposed to hospital bacterial flora over a period of time. A high thigh tourniquet is used for the limited open reduction portion of the case. The authors have found it useful to use a leg holder on the proximal to midthigh with the patella straight anteriorly. Stabilizing the proximal knee spatially is important, as discussed in the arthroscopic section. A fracture table

is optional, but one must have the capability for intermittent traction/distraction for ligamentotaxis purposes. A femoral distractor can be used for the articular reduction phase but generally gets in the way of the ring fixator. Alternatively, a sterile ankle arthroscopy traction device may be used (Smith & Nephew Dyonics, Memphis, Tennessee). This allows 360 degree access to the leg by placing it off the operating room table and above the contralateral leg and provides axial alignment to the fracture. Traction can be taken on and off as needed throughout the case. The C-arm is placed perpendicular to the extremity from the contralateral side.

3. *Reduction and internal fixation of the articular fracture component* It is important to think of this as a separate step. This emphasizes the importance of anatomical reduction of the joint. The soft tissue injury may be severe, but direct longitudinal incisions without soft tissue undermining or periosteal stripping are generally tolerated. Accurate placement of reduction clamps and cannulated screws orthogonal to the major fracture plane in the first 15 mm of the proximal tibia compresses the joint fracture. Fixation wires should not be placed in the first 15 mm of the proximal tibia unless absolutely necessary. This prevents penetration of the joint capsular reflection on the proximal tibia, reducing the risk of pin tract sepsis with joint sepsis postoperatively. Step 4 should not be performed until the surgeon is satisfied with the articular reduction. Once the frame is placed on the lower extremity, the ability to get good radiographic images of the joint diminishes dramatically.

4. *Application of the small wire fixator and the reduction of the metaphyseal diaphyseal components of the fracture* Once the joint and the major proximal plateau segment have been reconstructed, this is then attached to the distal shaft segment using the small wire frame restoring the mechanical axis. The frame becomes a neutralization device spanning the metadiaphyseal comminution percutaneously without soft tissue disruption. Accurate alignment in the sagittal, coronal, and rotational planes is demanding. Frequent use of alignment rods to assist in fluoroscopic imagery is important. The first and most critical step is the placement of reference wires 1 and 2. The first wire is placed parallel to the knee joint 15 to 18 mm below the joint line. The preassembled frame is then clam-shelled open, placed over the extremity, and attached to this proximal reference wire. The second reference wire is placed parallel to the ankle and attached to the distal ring. These wires are tensioned and attached with the appropriate wire fixation bolts and nuts. This imparts an initial reduction to the fracture. Wires number 3 and 4 are placed in the proximal and distal fragments just above and below the major metadiaphyseal fracture. These reduction olive wires are placed

directionally to allow fracture manipulation. The wires are attached to their respective ring or drop post and fixation bolts and nuts are applied but not tightened. Sagittal (lateral) plane angulation or translation can be corrected by attaching the bolts to the rings one and two holes away from the direction of angulation or translation. This creates an arch in the wire in the direction of the sagittal plane angulation or translation. Coronal plane angulation is then corrected first by attaching wire tensioners to wires 3 and 4 and in an opposing, dueling fashion.

The tensioners are attached on the side opposite to the olive bead on the wire. These wires are then pulled in opposite directions by the tensioners while the reduction is viewed with AP fluoroscopy. Once satisfactory fracture reduction is achieved in the coronal (AP) plane, the trailing wire fixation bolt and nut are tightened on each wire. Both wires are subsequently tensioned. As the wire straightens with tensioning, a reduction is achieved in the sagittal plane. The bone is pulled in the direction of the concavity of the arched wire. Reduction is confirmed with lateral fluoroscopy, and the leading wire fixation bolts and nuts are then tightened. These reduction wires should be replaced and removed at the end of the case because there will be soft tissue compression and necrosis locally around the wire, which can lead to pin tract sepsis. Rotational alignment is confirmed clinically, matching the rotational alignment of the well leg. Generally, the patella is aligned with the second toe.

The difficult portion of the operation is now completed. The surgeon should be completely satisfied with the mechanical axis reduction at this point. Reduction after this point with a standard type of ring fixator is not possible. For subacute fractures and for multilevel segmental fractures where initial accurate reduction is difficult, a Taylor Spatial Frame (Smith & Nephew) can be used. This type of frame will allow computer-assisted correction of the reduction in the postoperative period. The rest of the case consists of completing the frame construct with at least three wire or half-pins in each major weight bearing segment. Due to the small proximal segment of bone, wires are generally used proximally, and half-pins distally. Hybrid wire and half-pin combinations can be used to achieve this 90 degree fixation spread. Wires can be placed through safe transfixation zones in a relatively transverse fashion and half-pins can be placed in the sagittal plane. This forms an inverted T configuration achieving a 90-degree spread. A book that describes safe zones for transfixation is helpful.

5. *Postoperative care* This step is also critical. These patients must be seen frequently in follow-up. Compressive dressings are placed around wires and pins close to the joints to limit soft tissue motion.

Partial weight bearing is allowed (joint reduction permitting). Dry, well-healed pin sites are generally treated with daily soap and water cleansing with a shower. Knee range of motion is encouraged as tolerated. Flexion in the frame is limited to ~90 degrees due to the proximal ring. Frame removal is dictated by radiographs but generally can be done by 3 to 4 months. Exceptions are for open fractures with diaphyseal extension where longer frame times are the rule.

Rehabilitation

Loss of knee motion is the most common problem following fractures of the tibial plateau. Surgical fixation with sufficient stability to allow early motion is critical. Many surgeons have advocated continuous passive motion (CPM) in the early post-operative period. We use early motion with CPM following high-energy fractures of the tibial plateau. It is important to begin slowly (we start with a zero to 30° range of motion) and consider the soft tissue injury when determining how quickly to advance motion. Overly aggressive use of CPM can lead to wound healing problems over the proximal tibia.

The timing for initiating weight bearing will vary considerably, depending on the injury pattern and stability of fixation achieved. We have initiated weight bearing as soon as the patient wishes when a Compass Knee Hinge (Smith & Nephew) is used, and by 4 to 6 weeks (as soon as any callus is visible) when locked plating with the LISS system is used. Conventional ORIF with unstable fracture types or severe articular fractures may require 10 to 12 weeks prior to weight bearing.

Fracture-Dislocation of the Knee

The combination of a fracture extending into the knee joint with multiple ligament injuries represents a severe injury that can be very difficult to diagnose. The most common articular fracture associated with knee ligament injuries is a tibial plateau fracture. Performing a good physical examination of the knee following a tibial plateau fracture is often quite difficult for several reasons: pain, associated soft tissue injuries, other injuries, and the problem of trying to discern if instability is the result of the fracture or a ligamentous injury. An important diagnostic aid is a good physical examination under anesthesia following stabilization of the tibial plateau fracture. An adequate exam requires obtaining enough stability to stress the knee in varus and valgus. Although locked plating techniques have improved stability immediately following osteosynthesis, many surgeons are hesitant to aggressively stress the knee following stabilization of markedly comminuted fractures. The diagnostic challenge described here yields a high incidence of missed ligamentous injuries.

Tips and Tricks

- The axial CT scan at the level of the tibial plateau joint surface is most helpful to understand the sagittal and coronal fracture planes of the tibial plateau fracture, and thus to plan eventual plate and screw placement.
- If a fasciotomy is needed for a tibial plateau fracture with associated compartment syndrome, it is important to draw out all incisions to be used in the future for treatment of the fracture itself. Often the fracture has an initial spanning external fixator placed across it. However, placement of the lateral fasciotomy incision slightly more posterior and distal than usual will help avoid potential conflicts with future incisions.
- A laterally placed large femoral distractor or longitudinal traction with varus stress helps reduce type I fractures to allow percutaneous fixation.
- Use a cortical window to help disimpact depressed articular segments and elevate the whole segment as a unit in type II and III fractures.
- Rafting screws provide significantly better local depression stiffness when compared with large fragment buttress constructs in type II and III (articular depression) fractures.[23]
- The extended hockey stick approach allows both ORIF with a lateral plate and repair or reconstruction of the PLC on either an immediate or delayed basis in cases with PLC ligament damage.
- Keep the knee flexed 90 degrees and place traction sutures in the meniscus to improve visualization for a submeniscal arthrotomy.
- The femoral distractor can be utilized for a consistent varus stress to open up the lateral joint line and visualize the lateral tibial plateau via a submeniscal arthrotomy. However, care must be taken in order not to collapse the medial column in cases of Schatzker V and VI tibial plateau fractures. In these cases, it may be necessary to first fix the medial column. Alternatively, a medial femoral distractor or external fixator can be used as a neutralizing force to prevent medial column collapse.
- Locked plates should be used with marked comminution or severe osteopenia in low-energy fracture types, but they are unnecessary in most cases.
- Laterally based locked plates may be helpful in the treatment of bicondylar tibial plateau fractures when the medial tibial plateau is one segment and does not need to be addressed by a separate posteromedial approach. In such cases, the locked screws will provide sufficient resistance to varus collapse.

- Laterally based locked plates are generally not helpful in bicondylar tibial plateau fractures in which a separate approach needs to be made posteromedially because of articular involvement or displacement of the medial tibial plateau. In these cases, standard plates can be used posteromedially and laterally.
- Locked screws do not reduce the fracture to the implant.
- Drill locked screws perpendicular to the threaded hole to avoid problems with cold welding the screw.
- With the LISS, use the whirlybird to reduce the fractures to the implant in the coronal plane.
- Do not place any locked screws until an acceptable temporary reduction has been achieved. Because the screws form a fixed angle, additional reduction will not be possible after locked screws have been placed.
- When using minimally invasive techniques, "learn" the fracture by experimenting with varying longitudinal traction and the placement and size of a "bump" under the fracture prior to sliding the implant into the submuscular plane. This can remarkably ease and improve the reduction.
- The LISS implant must be centered in the midlateral plane of the tibia for the unicortical screws to have sufficient purchase.
- Always use bicortical whirlybirds with LISS.
- Use a percutaneous clamp on the proximal portion of the plate to reduce the plateau to the LISS implant and minimize pain/soft tissue irritation due to a prominent implant.
- Use the irrigation system when drilling diaphyseal LISS screws to avoid osteonecrosis as a result of high temperatures.
- Use the C, D, and E screws on the LISS in most if not all cases.
- *D* is for *danger*—it diverges posteriorly on the LISS. Flex the knee and be careful of plate location to protect the popliteal vessels.
- Place at least four unicortical screws proximally and distally with the LISS.
- When using the 13-hole LISS, use great care to avoid damage to neurovascular structures when approaching holes 10 through 13.
- The posteromedial approach is ideal for type IV fractures or bicondylar fractures with a large posteromedial fragment.
- High-energy bicondylar fractures are best treated with either minimally invasive submuscular locked plating or a small wire fixator.

MRI is a critical diagnostic tool for recognizing fracture-dislocations of the knee. It is critical to obtain the MRI scan prior to surgical stabilization of the fracture because both internal and external fixators cause severe artifact that remarkably limits the usefulness of the scan. Several studies, as noted in the nonoperative treatment section of this chapter, have documented a high incidence of patients with tibial plateau fractures who also have concomitant ligament or meniscus injuries. Weigel and Marsh reported on long-term outcomes following high-energy fractures of the tibial plateau. They examined the knee ligaments on 20 patients and found

12 (60%) had more than 5 mm of laxity in at least one direction after a mean follow-up of 98 months. The knee score for patients with ligament injuries was a mean of 89 compared with a mean of 93 for patients with no ligament injury. More significantly, only 58% of patients with unstable knees were working compared with 88% of the patients with stable knee examinations.[22] Unrecognized and therefore untreated fracture-dislocations frequently have poor results despite well-aligned and united fractures. The outcome most frequently involves pain and loss of motion, although instability may also be reported. Delamarter and Hohl reported 40% of their patients had poor clinical outcomes with conservative treatment of knee injuries associated with fractures compared with 16% poor results with surgical treatment of the knee injury.[1]

Treatment of patients with combined articular fractures and ligament injuries is complex. Many contemporary authors advocate early repair or reconstruction of ligaments. It is critical to obtain adequate stability of both the osseous and ligamentous injuries to allow early motion following surgery. We have found the Compass Knee Hinge (CKH) (Smith & Nephew) combined with minimally invasive locked plating using the LISS very helpful with fracture-dislocations. The CKH allows early motion following multiligament knee injuries with no rotational or varus/valgus stress on reconstructions **(Fig. 29–28)**. Our early results using the hinge have demonstrated only a 7% ligament failure rate with the hinge compared with a 29% failure rate without the CKH. The difference was significant, with a p value of $< .05$.[67] Our current protocol involves use of the hinge combined with reconstructions and osteosynthesis in virtually all patients with a combination fracture-dislocation of the knee.

New Techniques

Compass Knee Hinge (see Video 29–7, Disk 4)

The detailed technique for placing a CKH appears in Chapter 28. There are no solid data regarding the appropriate surgical timing for patients with fracture-dislocations. The condition of the soft tissues will dictate how aggressively surgical stabilization can be safely pursued. If soft tissue conditions allow, we recommend ORIF of the fracture within a few days of the injury, using minimally invasive locked plating techniques. We allow the soft tissues to recover for approximately 2 or 3 weeks, and then commence repair or reconstruction of ligamentous injuries and placement of a CKH. Sagittal plane range of motion is initiated on the first day following surgery, with a gradual increase to flexion of 90 degrees over the first few weeks. PLC and anterior cruciate ligament (ACL) reconstruction may have to be delayed due to fracture comminution in the area of drilling of fibular head and tibial tunnels, respectively. We have been able to reconstruct the PLC early in most cases.

Fracture-dislocations represent a severe injury with instability of both the osseous and soft tissue envelopes. Aggressive treatment using contemporary techniques and early rehabilitation will be necessary to obtain good functional outcomes. When evaluating our patients with PCL reconstructions who had associated ipsilateral fractures, we found a significant decrease in Lysholm knee scores, return to work, and return to athletic participation when compared with patients who did not have a fracture. The first key to successful treatment of these patients is recognizing the entire spectrum of the injury. We recommend MRI prior to osteosynthesis or ligament reconstruction. After this

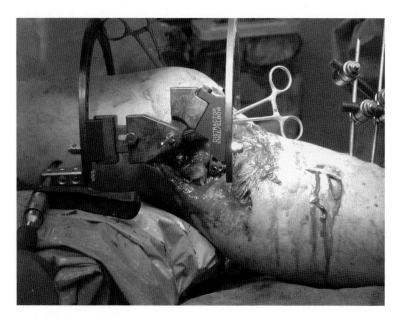

Figure 29–28 Placing the lateral femoral pin of a Compass Knee Hinge in a patient following a fracture-dislocation of the knee.

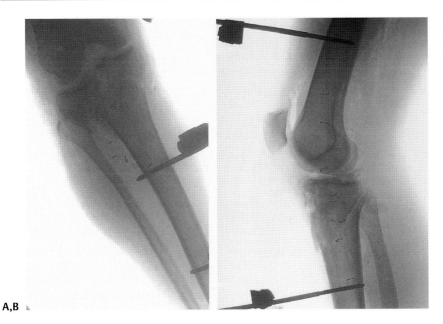

Figure 29–29 (A) Anteroposterior and **(B)** lateral radiographs demonstrating the use of a spanning external fixator to temporarily reduce a bicondylar tibial plateau fracture and provide a relatively stable environment to allow early recovery of the surrounding soft tissues.

A,B

critical diagnostic test, appropriate preoperative planning can be conducted and a successful outcome is obtainable.

Spanning External Fixator

A recent trend in many trauma centers has involved the use of temporary fixation spanning the knee joint **(Fig. 29–29A,B)**. Advantages of this technique are that it stabilizes the soft tissues and allows recovery prior to initiating large surgical exposures. There are two major disadvantages, however. The first is the expense of external fixation that is only used for a few days or weeks. If data were developed that demonstrated improved outcomes or decreased complications, the expense would certainly be justified. The second major disadvantage is that external fixators cause severe artifact during MRI. If spanning fixators are placed prior to obtaining an MRI, significant injuries may be missed and may have an adverse impact on outcome. Our policy at this time is to use spanning fixators if the fracture and knee are so unstable that the knee will not remain reduced in a knee immobilizer or there is significant (e.g., 2 to 3 cm) shortening at the fracture site. This is a rare experience in our practice. We most frequently use a knee immobilizer and delay surgery for 3 days to 2 weeks to allow recovery of the soft tissues. If spanning external fixation is employed, the pin sites should be carefully planned to be out of the planned surgical incisions for the final ORIF of the tibial plateau.

Injectable Calcium Phosphate Bone Cement

Injectable calcium phosphate cements have been developed for use with fractures. Depressed tibial plateau fractures are one of the potential indications of this cement. Studies suggest a reduced time to full weight bearing when cement augmentation is used.[41] A goat study has been published by Welch et al[43] that evaluated the use of calcium phosphate cement compared with cancellous autograft in 10 mm impacted lateral defects. Results demonstrated that the prevalence and degree of fracture subsidence were significantly reduced with the calcium phosphate cement. They also noted that the cement was rapidly resorbed, with the volume fraction of the cement decreased to only 4% after 6 months. Their conclusion was that cancellous autograft did not maintain anatomical reduction, but that calcium phosphate cement did maintain reduction. A clinical study by Lobenhoffer et al[42] documented 26 cases of complex tibial plateau fractures augmented with calcium phosphate bone cement. They allowed early weight bearing, at a mean of 4.5 weeks (range 1 to 6 weeks). Two cases (8%) had a partial loss of reduction, with one (4%) requiring revision. Lysholm knee scores in their patients demonstrated excellent outcomes in 15 (58%), good in six (23%), and fair in five (19%). The early data are encouraging regarding clinical outcome and early return of function in patients with impacted tibial plateau fractures. All of the studies noted here used Norion (Synthes, Paoli, Pennsylvania). Additional studies are needed to confirm the early encouraging results and to further define the role of calcium phosphate cement in tibial plateau fractures.

Outcomes

Assessing outcomes reported in the literature following tibial plateau fractures is very difficult for several reasons. There is no universally accepted outcome score, and many papers have combinations of low-energy isolated fractures mixed with high-energy fractures in patients following trauma. Additionally, techniques for treating fractures of the tibial plateau have changed remarkably with the advent of minimally invasive osteosynthesis, small wire fixators, and locked plating. To overcome some of these obstacles, we will be reporting three separate categories: ORIF more than 10 years ago, ORIF in the past 10 years, and small wire external fixators.

Five different papers reported outcome scores on tibial plateau fractures treated with ORIF at least 10 years ago. Seventy-five percent of the patients were reported to have outcome scores that qualify as either good or excellent, whereas 25% had scores that were fair or poor.[6,7,17,22,55] Contemporary studies that have been published in the past 10 years report outcomes that are good or excellent in 84% of patients compared with fair or poor results in 16%.[20,22,40,68] Patients treated with small wire external fixators (either circular or hybrid) had 70% good or excellent compared with 30% fair or poor outcomes.[21,29,30,34,36,37,39,69] The studies use a variety of outcome measures, but there is a trend toward improved results with more contemporary techniques of ORIF.

Reported rates of union are good in all three categories, with 100% union reported with contemporary ORIF,[27,30,40] compared with 99% for older studies using ORIF[1,9,17,55] and for small wire external fixators.[21,29–34,36,37,39,69] On the other hand, there are notable differences reported in the incidence of malunion. Contemporary ORIF was associated with a 5% incidence of malunion in the only study that reported malunion,[20] compared with 19% with ORIF reported a decade or more ago.[1,9,55] Small wire fixator studies also reported a high incidence of malunion, with 14% noted in six different studies.[31–33,37,39,69]

Loss of knee motion is a frequent complication. Many studies do not give details of exact motion, but only note that many patients do not achieve a full range of knee motion. Eight studies reported motion following the use of small wire fixators, with a mean range of motion of 1 to 105 degrees.[21,29,31,32,36,37,39,69] Four studies reported motion following ORIF in the past 10 years, with a mean range of motion of 2 to 124 degrees achieved.[20,22,27,40] Although regaining knee motion following fractures of the tibial plateau remains a critical problem, recent advances using ORIF with locked plating and minimally invasive techniques have yielded remarkable improvements.

There is limited long-term outcome data available on patients following tibial plateau fractures. Many surgeons have assumed that a result of posttraumatic osteoarthritis was inevitable over time. However, a 20 year follow-up is reported in a study out of Sweden, which documented no degeneration in results between 7 and 20 years postoperatively.[5] Less than 20% of the fractures in this study were bicondylar. A recent study published by Weigel and Marsh from the University of Iowa has documented long-term results following high-energy bicondylar fractures. Their findings are similar to the Swedish study, with no deterioration in the results between 2 and 8 years following injury.[22] Both studies strongly suggest that severe arthritis is not an inevitable consequence of fracture of the tibial plateau, and that good long-term functional outcomes can be achieved.

Complications

Surgical treatment of tibial plateau fractures, particularly ORIF of bicondylar fractures, has been associated with reported complication rates ranging from 23 to 55%.[4,13,29] Complications associated with tibial plateau fractures include loss of knee motion, deep infection, skin slough or soft tissue dehiscence, knee sepsis, peroneal nerve palsy, failure of fixation, malunion, and compartment syndrome. The most frequent (other than loss of knee motion) and severe complications have related to infection and wound dehiscence. Many authors have advocated respect for the soft tissue injury and delayed ORIF in cases of severe injury, with a resultant decrease in complications.[10,15]

Deep infection following internal fixation of fractures of the tibial plateau ranges from 5 to 80% following ORIF in the published literature that is more than 1 decade old. The mean incidence when six studies are combined is 27%.[3,9,14,17,18,55] Four recent studies that use contemporary stabilization techniques stressing soft tissue handling, locked plating, and minimally invasive techniques have all reported a zero incidence of deep infection. One multicenter study using the LISS reported on 52 patients with open fractures of the proximal tibia and tibial plateau following high-energy trauma. They documented an incidence of only 5.8% deep infections despite the high-energy open fractures.[28] Small wire fixators have been associated with a variable incidence of deep infection, with a range of 0 to 13% and a mean of 6.6%.[21,30,32,34,37] Small wire fixators have also been associated with the occurrence of septic knees as a result of intra-articular wire placement. Four studies have reported a mean of 9.5% (range 4 to 20%).[33,34,36,39] This complication can be minimized by keeping all wires at least 10 to 15 mm below the joint line. Skin slough or soft tissue breakdown has also been reported as a frequent problem, especially in older literature reporting on ORIF of the tibial plateau.[3,10]

Peroneal nerve palsy can occur either as a result of the injury or as an iatrogenic injury. It has been reported as the most frequent complication in some series.[7] There has also been a published report of iatrogenic injury to the peroneal nerve with a small wire due to nerve displacement as a result of the injury.[70] Compartment syndrome also occurs following both open and closed tibial plateau fractures.[16] Careful surveillance and rapid fasciotomies if compartment syndrome develops are indicated.

Failure of fixation has been reported as a frequent complication, with a range of 3 to 31% and a mean occurrence of 16%.[1,40,55,69] Locked plating has been reported to minimize this problem as a result of the improved stability in severely comminuted bone.[20,27] As noted earlier, the reported incidence of malunion varies from 5 to 19%, with the lowest incidence associated with the use of locked plates.[1,9,20,31–33,37,39,55,69]

Tibial plateau fractures are associated with a wide variety of complications. The incidence of complications has decreased over the past 10 years with the increased use of small wire fixators and minimally invasive techniques of ORIF. There has also been increased emphasis on a careful

evaluation of the soft tissues[12] and allowing some recovery of the soft tissue injury prior to extensive open procedures. Although the decreases in complication rates are encouraging, the incidence and variety of complications still remain high. Surgeons must exercise great caution when caring for patients with tibial plateau fractures, especially following high-energy trauma.

Pearls

- Type I fractures occur in young patients and are associated with lateral meniscus tears.
- Type IV fractures are associated with knee dislocations and vascular and neurological injuries.
- Type VI fractures are associated with ligament and vascular injuries as well as skin and soft tissue injury.
- MRI studies demonstrate between 48 and 90% of patients with tibial plateau fractures have either ligament or meniscus injury.
- Indications for nonoperative treatment of tibial plateau fractures:
  - Non- or minimally displaced (< 3 mm)
  - Stable to varus and valgus stress
  - Peripheral submeniscal fractures that are stable
  - Low-energy fractures with minimal comminution
  - Low-demand patients with medical contraindications to surgery
- The medial plateau is larger and stronger than the lateral plateau and is concave compared with the convex lateral side.

- Outcome scores have improved in the past 10 years to yield 84% good or excellent results and 16% fair or poor results with modern techniques of ORIF.
- Nonunion occurs in no more than 1% of fractures regardless of whether ORIF or small wire fixators are used.
- Malunion occurs in 5 to 19% of cases depending on the treatment technique.
- Contemporary ORIF techniques yield an improved arc of motion (122 vs 104 degrees) when compared with small wire fixators.
- Long-term studies indicate that results do not routinely degenerate over extended follow-up.
- Deep infection remains a problem, with an incidence of 27% following ORIF in older literature and 6.6% following the use of small wire fixators. Locked plating with minimally invasive techniques may decrease this complication, with some studies reporting very low infection rates.
- Small wire fixators have an incidence of 9.5% septic knees.
- Failure of fixation occurs in 16% of cases when conventional plates and screws are used.

On the DVDs

Video 29–1 (Same as Video 4–1, Disk 1) Rules of Locked Plating This presentation reviews the "rules" that should be applied by surgeons employing locked plating. Included in this presentation are unicortical locked plating systems designed for minimally invasive submuscular application, as well as hybrid plating that includes mixing locked and unlocked screws. The appropriate order of application of screws is stressed.

Video 29–2 (Same as Video 4–5, Disk 1) ORIF of a Bicondylar Tibial Plateau Fracture with the LISS Internal Fixator The patient in this case sustained a comminuted bicondylar tibial plateau fracture. Minimally invasive fixation using the Less Invasive Stabilization System is demonstrated. The importance of obtaining a reduction prior to placing any locked screws is emphasized.

Video 29–3 (Same as Video 26–6, Disk 3) Submuscular Locked Fixation of a Combined C3 Distal Femur and C3 Proximal Tibial Fracture A modified lateral peripatellar approach is utilized for direct visualization of complex articular injuries of both the tibial plateau and distal femur. The steps of submuscular locked fixation are emphasized.

Video 29–4 (Disk 4) ORIF of a Medial Tibial Plateau Fracture Dislocation with Locked Plating This video demonstrates a Shatzker IV tibial plateau fracture combined with a multi-ligament knee injury. Arthroscopy is combined with locked plating to treat remarkably proximal medial tibial plateau fracture.

Video 29–5 (Disk 4) Arthroscopic-Assisted ORIF of a Tibial Plateau Fracture This video lecture on arthroscopic assisted ORIF of tibial plateau fractures emphasizes room setup, portal placement, and the use of ACL guides and impactors to reduce displaced tibial plateau fractures.

Video 29–6 (Same as Video 2–2, Disk 1) ORIF with a Small Wire Circular External Fixator This video reviews the principles of ORIF of tibial plateau fractures using small wire external fixation.

Video 29–7 (Same as Video 28–6, Disk 4) Placement of Compass Knee Hinge External Fixator This video presents step-by-step instuctions on how to place a Compass Knee Hinge external fixator. The technique for determining the isometric point on the femoral condyles is demonstrated.

References

1. Delamarter R, Hohl M. The cast brace and tibial plateau fractures. Clin Orthop Relat Res 1989;242:26–31

2. Honkonen SE. Indications for surgical treatment of tibial condyle fractures. Clin Orthop Relat Res 1994;302:199–205

3. Koval KJ, Helfet DL. Tibial plateau fractures: evaluation and treatment. J Am Acad Orthop Surg 1995;3:86–94

4. Lachiewicz PF, Funcik T. Factors influencing the results of open reduction and internal fixation of tibial plateau fractures. Clin Orthop Relat Res 1990;259:210–215

5. Lansinger O, Bergman B, Korner L, Andersson GBJ. Tibial condylar fractures: a twenty-year follow-up. J Bone Joint Surg Am 1986;68: 13–19

6. Savoie FH, Griend RAV, Ward EF, Hughes JL. Tibial plateau fractures: a review of operative treatment using AO technique. Orthopedics 1987;10:745–747

7. Schatzker J, McBroom R, Bruce D. The tibial plateau fracture: the Toronto experience 1968–1975. Clin Orthop Relat Res 1979;138: 94–104

8. Honkonen SE. Degenerative arthritis after tibial plateau fractures. J Orthop Trauma 1995;9:273–277

9. Mallik AR, Covall DJ, Whitelaw GP. Internal versus external fixation of bicondylar tibial plateau fractures. Orthop Rev 1992;21:1433–1436

10. Mills WJ, Nork SE. Open reduction and internal fixation of high-energy tibial plateau fractures. Orthop Clin North Am 2002;33:177–198

11. Moore TM. Fracture-dislocation of the knee. Clin Orthop Relat Res 1981;156:128–140

12. Tscherne H, Lobenhoffer P. Tibial plateau fractures: management and expected results. Clin Orthop Relat Res 1993;292:87–100

13. Watson JT. High-energy fractures of the tibial plateau. Orthop Clin North Am 1994;25:723–752

14. Young MJ, Barrack RL. Complications of internal fixation of tibial plateau fractures. Orthop Rev 1994;23:149–154

15. Wiss DA. Tibial Plateau Fractures: Master Techniques in Orthopaedic Surgery on CD-ROM in Fractures [electronic resource]. Philadelphia: Lippincott Williams & Wilkins; 2000

16. Andrews JR, Tedder JL, Godbout BP. Bicondylar tibial plateau fracture complicated by compartment syndrome. Orthop Rev 1992; 21:317–319

17. Blokker CP, Rorabeck CH, Bourne RB. Tibial plateau fractures: an analysis of the results of treatment in 60 patients. Clin Orthop Relat Res 1984;182:193–199

18. Burri C, Bartzke G, Coldewey J, Muggler E. Fractures of the tibial plateau. Clin Orthop Relat Res 1979;138:84–93

19. Waddell JP, Johnston DWC, Neidre A. Fractures of the tibial plateau: a review of ninety-five patients and comparison of treatment methods. J Trauma 1981;21:376–381

20. Stannard JP, Wilson TC, Volgas DA, Alonso JE. The less invasive stabilization system in the treatment of complex fractures of the tibial plateau: short-term results. J Orthop Trauma 2004;18:552–558

21. Watson JT, Coufal C. Treatment of complex lateral plateau fractures using Ilazarov techniques. Clin Orthop Relat Res 1998;353:97–106

22. Weigel DP, Marsh JL. High-energy fractures of the tibial plateau: knee function after longer follow-up. J Bone Joint Surg Am 2002;84-A:1541–1551

23. Karunakar MA, Egol KA, Peindl R, Harrow ME, Bosse MJ, Kellam JF. Split depression tibial plateau fractures: a biomechanical study. J Orthop Trauma 2002;16:172–177

24. Westmoreland GL, McLaurin TM, Hutton WC. Screw pullout strength: a biomechanical comparison large-fragment and small-fragment fixation in the tibial plateau. J Orthop Trauma 2002; 16:178–181

25. Cole PA, Zlowodzki M, Kregor PJ. Less Invasive Stabilization System (LISS) for fractures of the proximal tibia: indications, surgical technique and preliminary results of the UMC Clinical Trial. Injury 2003;34(Suppl 1):A16–A29

26. Lee MA, Althausen P, Finkeheier C. Operative treatment of complex tibial plateau fractures: a comparison of hybrid external fixation, dual plating, and less invasive surgical stabilization (LISS) fixation. Podium Presentation, 70th Annual Meeting of the American Academy of Orthopaedic Surgeons, New Orleans, LA, February 2003

27. Stannard JP, Wilson TC, Volgas DA, Alonso JE. Fracture stabilization of proximal tibial fractures with the proximal tibial LISS: early experience in Birmingham, Alabama (USA). Injury 2003;34(Suppl 1): A36–A42

28. Stannard JP, Finkemeier CG, Lee J, Kregor PJ. Utilization of the Less Invasive Stabilization System (LISS) internal fixator for open fractures of the proximal tibia: a multi-center evaluation. Podium Presentation, 70th Annual Meeting of the American Academy of Orthopaedic Surgeons, New Orleans, LA, February 2003

29. Ali AM, Burton M, Hashmi M, Saleh M. Outcome of complex fractures of the tibial plateau treated with a beam-loading ring fixation system. J Bone Joint Surg Br 2003;85:691–699

30. Dendrinos GK, Kontos S, Katsenis D, Dalas A. Treatment of high-energy tibial plateau fractures by the Ilizarov circular fixator. J Bone Joint Surg Br 1996;78:710–717

31. Gaudinez RF, Mallik AR, Szporn M. Hybrid external fixation of comminuted tibial plateau fractures. Clin Orthop Relat Res 1996; 328:203–210

32. Kumar A, Whittle AP. Treatment of complex (Schatzker Type VI) fractures of the tibial plateau with circular wire external fixation: retrospective case review. J Orthop Trauma 2000;14:339–344

33. Marsh JL, Smith ST, Do TT. External fixation and limited internal fixation for complex fractures of the tibial plateau. J Bone Joint Surg Am 1995;77:661–673

34. Mikulak SA, Gold SM, Zinar DM. Small wire external fixation of high-energy tibial plateau fractures. Clin Orthop Relat Res 1998; 356:230–238

35. Morandi MM, Landi S, Kilaghbian V, Randelli P. Schatzker type VI tibial plateau fractures and the Ilizarov circular external fixator. Bull Hosp Jt Dis 1997;56:46–48

36. Murphy CP, D'Ambrosia R, Dabezies EJ. The small pin circular fixator for proximal tibial fractures with soft tissue compromise. Orthopedics 1991;14:283–290

37. Stamer DT, Schenk R, Staggers B, Aurori K, Aurori B, Behrens FF. Bicondylar tibial plateau fractures treated with a hybrid ring external fixator: a preliminary study. J Orthop Trauma 1994; 8:455–461

38. Watson JT, Ripple S, Hoshaw SJ, Fyhrie D. Hybrid external fixation for tibial plateau fractures: clinical and biomechanical correlation. Orthop Clin North Am 2002;33:199–209

39. Weiner LS, Kelley M, Yang E, et al. The use of combination internal fixation and hybrid external fixation in severe proximal tibia fractures. J Orthop Trauma 1995;9:244–250

40. Hung SS, Chao E-K, Chan Y-S, et al. Arthroscopically assisted osteosynthesis for tibial plateau fractures. J Trauma 2003; 54: 356–363

41. Larsson S, Bauer TW. Use of injectable calcium phosphate cement for fracture fixation: a review. Clin Orthop Relat Res 2002;395: 23–32

42. Lobenhoffer P, Gerich T, Witte F, Tscherne H. Use of an injectable calcium phosphate bone cement in the treatment of tibial plateau

fractures: a prospective study of twenty-six cases with twenty-month mean follow-up. J Orthop Trauma 2002;16:143–149

43. Welch RD, Zhang H, Bronson DG. Experimental tibial plateau fractures augmented with calcium phosphate cement or autologous bone graft. J Bone Joint Surg Am. 2003;85:222–231

44. AO Principles of Fracture Management. Rüedi TP, Murphy WM, eds. New York, Stuttgart: Arbeitsgemeinschaft für Osteosynthesefragen; 2000:45–58

45. Stannard JP, Sheils TM, Lopez-Ben RR, McGwin G, Robinson JT, Volgas DA. Vascular injuries in knee dislocations: the role of physical examination in determining the need for arteriography. J Bone Joint Surg Am 2004;86:910–915

46. Chan PSH, Klimkiewicz JJ, Luchetti WT, et al. Impact of CT scan on treatment plan and fracture classification of tibial plateau fractures. J Orthop Trauma 1997;11:484–489

47. Barrow BA, Fajman WA, Parker LM, Albert MJ, Drvaric DM, Hudson TM. Tibial plateau fractures: evaluation with MR imaging. Radiographics 1994;14:553–559

48. Brophy DP, O'Malley M, Lui D, Denison B, Eustace S. MR imaging of tibial plateau fractures. Clin Radiol 1996;51:873–878

49. Holt MD, Williams LA, Dent CM. MRI in the management of tibial plateau fractures. Injury 1995;26:595–599

50. Kode L, Lieberman JM, Motta AO, Wilber JH, Vasen A, Yagan R. Evaluation of tibial plateau fractures: efficacy of MR imaging compared with CT. AJR Am J Roentgenol 1994;163:141–147

51. Shepherd L, Abdollahi K, Lee J, Vangsness CT Jr. The prevalence of soft tissue injuries in nonoperative tibial plateau fractures as determined by magnetic resonance imaging. J Orthop Trauma 2002;16:628–631

52. Yacoubian SV, Nevins RT, Sallis JG, Potter HG, Lorich DG. Impact of MRI on treatment plan and fracture classification of tibial plateau fractures. J Orthop Trauma 2002;16:632–637

53. Bennett WF, Browner B. Tibial plateau fractures: a study of associated soft tissue injuries. J Orthop Trauma 1994;8:183–188

54. Brown TD, Anderson DD, Nepola JV, Singerman RJ, Pedersen DR, Brand RA. Contact stress aberrations following imprecise reduction of simple tibial plateau fractures. J Orthop Res 1988;6: 851–862

55. Stokel EA, Sadasivan KK. Tibial plateau fractures: standardized evaluation of operative results. Orthopedics 1991;14:263–270

56. DeCoster TA, Nepola JV, El-Khoury GY. Cast brace treatment of proximal tibia fractures: a ten-year follow-up study. Clin Orthop Relat Res 1988;231:196–204

57. Drennan DB, Locher FG, Maylahn DJ. Fractures of the tibial plateau: treatment by closed reduction and spica cast. J Bone Joint Surg Am 1979;61:989–995

58. Duwelius PJ, Connolly JF. Closed reduction of tibial plateau fractures: a comparison of functional and roentgenographic end results. Clin Orthop Relat Res 1988;230:116–126

59. Scotland T, Wardlaw D. The use of cast-bracing as treatment for fractures of the tibial plateau. J Bone Joint Surg Br 1981; 63B:575–578

60. Segal D, Mallik AR, Wetzler MJ, Franchi AV, Whitelaw GP. Early weight bearing of lateral tibial plateau fractures. Clin Orthop Relat Res 1993;294:232–237

61. Perry CR, Evans LG, Rice S, Fogarty J, Burdge RE. A new surgical approach to fractures of the lateral tibial plateau. J Bone Joint Surg Am 1984;66:1236–1240

62. Fernandez DL. Anterior approach to the knee with osteotomy of the tibial tubercle for bicondylar tibial fractures. J Bone Joint Surg Am 1988;70:208–219

63. Frigg R, Appenzeller A, Christensen R, Frenk A, Gilbert S, Schavan R. The development of the distal femur Less Invasive Stabilization System (LISS). Injury 2001;32(Suppl 3):SC24–SC31

64. Koval KJ, Hoehl JJ, Kummer FJ, Simon JA. Distal femoral fixation: a biomechanical comparison of the standard condylar buttress plate, a locked buttress plate, and the 95-degree blade plate. J Orthop Trauma 1997;11:521–524

65. Zlowodzki M, Williamson S, Cole PA, Zardiackas LD, Kregor PJ. Biomechanical evaluation of the less invasive stabilization system, angled blade plate, and retrograde intramedullary nail for the internal fixation of distal femur fractures. J Orthop Trauma 2004;18:494–502

66. Cole PA, Zlowodzki M, Kregor PJ. Treatment of proximal tibia fractures using the less invasive stabilization system: surgical experience and early clinical results in 77 fractures. J Orthop Trauma 2004;18: 528–535

67. Stannard JP, Sheils TM, McGwin G, Volgas DA. The use of a hinged knee fixator after surgery for knee dislocation. Arthroscopy 2003; 19:626–631

68. Biyani A, Reddy NS, Chaudhury J, Simison AJM, Klenerman L. The results of surgical management of displaced tibial plateau fractures in the elderly. Injury 1995;26:291–297

69. Ali AM, Burton M, Hashmi M, Saleh M. Treatment of displaced bicondylar tibial plateau fractures (OTA-41C2&3) in patients older than 60 years of age. J Orthop Trauma 2003;17:346–352

70. El-Shazly M, Saleh M. Displacement of the common peroneal nerve associated with upper tibial fracture: implications for fine wire fixation. J Orthop Trauma 2002;16:204–207

30 Tibial Shaft Fractures

Franklin D. Shuler and William T. Obremskey

Fractures of the tibial shaft range from injuries with simple fractures and minimal damage to the surrounding soft tissue to severe limb-threatening injuries associated with neurological, vascular, muscular, and skin damage. Tibia fractures are the most common long bone fracture. The risk of having a tibial shaft fracture is 1 to 2 per 125,000 population,[1] with a reported annual occurrence of 492,000 in the United States.[2] Twenty-five percent of these injuries present as open fractures.[1] National statistics from 2002 indicate the following for tibia fractures: hospital discharges (69,559), mean length of stay (5.1 days), and mean charges ($25,107.00).[2] The aggregate cost of this injury is therefore over 1.7 billion dollars.

Tibial shaft fractures can be treated with multiple methods, including casting, plating, intramedullary rod fixation (reamed or nonreamed), and external fixation. This chapter highlights recommended treatment options for tibial shaft fractures and focuses on surgical options and techniques. Although a strong foundation in principles of surgical technique is discussed, individual patient scenarios dictate the ultimate treatment plan, and nonoperative treatment remains a very viable option for some patients with fractures of the tibial shaft.

Classification

In clinical practice, tibial shaft fractures are still commonly classified by simple descriptions of the fracture pattern (transverse, spiral, oblique, etc.), displacement, and location.

More formal classification schemes include the Arbeitsgemeinschaft für Osteosynthesefragen (AO/Muller)[3] classification, which was based on earlier work by Johner and Wruhs **(Fig. 30–1).**[4] The AO/Orthopaedic Trauma Association (AO/OTA) classification[5] was created to help standardize the literature by using an alphanumeric classification indicating increasing energy and complexity of the fracture. Tibia fractures are also classified according to the amount of soft tissue damage. For closed fractures, the Tscherne classification system is used.[6] Tscherne grade 0 injuries have negligible soft tissue injury. Grade 1 has superficial abrasions or contusions. Grade 2 has deep contaminated skin abrasion and significant muscle contusion. Grade 3 has severe soft tissue injury including crush, degloving, compartment syndrome, and other soft tissue injuries. The Gustilo and Anderson classification system[7,8] (types I, II, and III) is used to grade open fractures, and is covered in Chapter 1, Care of the Soft Tissue Envelope. As the type of open fracture increases, so does the risk of deep infection.

Nonoperative Treatment

The treatment of any tibial shaft fracture is designed to restore the length and alignment of the limb and regain function as quickly as possible. Closed treatment of tibial shaft fractures with casting and functional bracing has a long history of effective treatment, particularly in stable tibial shaft fractures.[9,10] Indications for closed management are somewhat arbitrary. A general consensus is that

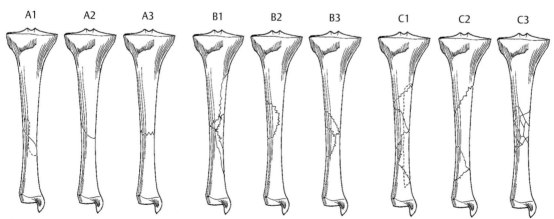

Figure 30–1 The Arbeitsgemeinschaft für Osteosynthesefragen/ Orthopaedic Trauma Association (AO/OTA) classification of tibial shaft fractures assigns a letter (A through C) depending on fracture pattern. Type A fractures are simpler fracture patterns. Type C fractures are associated with fracture comminution, and are higher-energy fractures. These drawings highlight fracture patterns and mechanisms to produce the injuries discussed in this chapter. (From Orthopedic Trauma Association Committee for Coding and Classification. Fracture and dislocation compendium. J Orthop Trauma 1996;10(suppl):1–154)

nonoperative treatment is appropriate for a fracture at least 5 cm away from the distal or proximal tibia, with at least 50% cortical overlap, with initial shortening of < 12 mm, with alignment of less than or equal to 5 degrees varus/valgus or anterior/posterior angulation (after casting), with < 20 degrees of external rotation, and with < 10 degrees internal rotation.[9] An intact fibula is considered to be a relative contraindication to proceed with closed fracture management because of the tendency for tibia varus malalignment.

Sarmiento et al reported on the closed treatment of over 1000 tibial shaft fractures.[9,10] Ninety-nine percent of the fractures with available follow-up healed in 17 to 19 weeks. Ninety-five percent of fractures healed with less than 12 mm of shortening, and 90% healed with ≤ 6 degrees of angular deformity in any plane. Such reliable treatment of stable tibia fractures presents minimal risks and continues to be the standard of care for fractures that meet the criteria for nonoperative management.[9] Although stable tibia fractures can also be treated with intramedullary fixation to promote early mobilization and possibly faster healing, it comes at a risk of operative complications (infection, anterior knee pain, and hardware pain).

Technique for Nonoperative Treatment of a Tibial Shaft Fracture

If a patient and surgeon decide to pursue nonoperative treatment for a stable tibial shaft fracture, a reduction and long-leg cast are often required **(Fig. 30–2A,B)**. The patient should have adequate analgesia for the reduction and casting. This can be done with conscious sedation in the clinic or emergency room setting, but may be performed with fewer problems in an operating room under general anesthesia because immediate imaging is more readily

available and a second reduction and cast application can be performed if needed. As the patient is sedated, the affected limb is placed over the edge or side of the bed. Casting usually requires a surgeon and two assistants. Prior to reduction, one should use an image intensifier to "learn" the exact reduction maneuver. Often, some fracture translation is seen on the anteroposterior (AP) image and is difficult to correct. This translation can usually be improved by external rotation of the fracture, *not* translation of the tibial shaft. We recommend one assistant to hold the thigh and the toes with a 15 to 30 degree bend in the knee **(Fig. 30–2A,B)**. Adequate padding is placed on the pretibial area as well as the calcaneal tuberosity and malleoli. Excessive padding is not desirable because this may contribute to loss of reduction. A short leg plaster cast is applied with the fracture reduced, and a mold is applied to the cast. As the short leg plaster cast is setting, the most experienced surgeon should continue the reduction maneuver and hold the reduction until the plaster sets. An AP and lateral fluoroscopic image or plain x-rays including the entire tibia should be obtained to ensure that an acceptable reduction is obtained. If the reduction is not adequate, the short leg cast should be removed and repeat reduction and casting performed. The reduction is considered acceptable if there is less than 5 degrees of angulation, less than 12 mm of shortening, and less than 50% translation. The leg is extended to ~15 degrees of flexion at the knee using appropriate patella padding, and the cast is extended to an above-the-knee cast. Use of fiberglass decreases the weight and improves the mobility of the patient. A supracondylar femoral mold should be applied as the fiberglass sets to decrease pistoning of the cast.

The patient is allowed to begin ambulation immediately with crutches and touch-down weight bearing. As

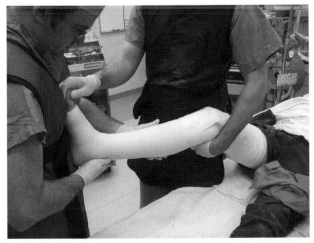
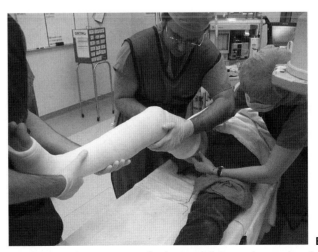

Figure 30–2 Tibial cast application with manipulation under anesthesia. This cast is preferably applied in the operating room with two to three assistants. **(A)** A short leg cast with foot incorporation is applied maintaining the reduction, which was assisted by gravity. Plaster cast application can afford more time for fracture reduction, molding, and maintenance of reduction. **(B)** Conversion to a long leg cast with ~15 degrees of knee flexion with a supracondylar mold applied. Fluoroscopy or formal tibial radiographs are used to confirm acceptable fracture reduction.

the comfort level increases, the patient may progress to weight bearing as tolerated in the long leg cast. Sarmiento et al found that patients who began full weight bearing more than 6 weeks after injury had longer times to union.[10] The patient should follow up at 1 and 2 weeks after cast application to ensure that there has been no change in fracture alignment. If the fracture does not fall into acceptable parameters, the patient and surgeon need to strongly consider operative intervention. A slight degree of angulation of 5 to 10 degrees in the initial cast or at follow-up could be overcome with wedging of the cast.

Cast wedging can be done using open or closed wedging techniques and is best done within 1 to 2 weeks from cast application and fracture. We advocate the use of an opening wedge on the concave side of the deformity. Use

of a closing wedge can result in unacceptable skin compromise. Cast wedging is performed by cutting the cast on the opposite side of the apex of the deformity (concave side). A circumferential cast cut can be made, with deformity correction performed. A solid spacer is placed in the defect left by wedging the cast open, avoiding skin compromise and pinching. A piece of wood, cork, or stacked tongue depressors are often used. Repeat radiographs indicate if correction is sufficient. The reduction is maintained and cast material reapplied.

Between 4 and 6 weeks, patients become significantly more comfortable, and they can be changed to a short leg cast, a functional brace, or a patellar tendon bearing (PTB) cast or brace (**Figs. 30–3A–C** and **30–4A,B**). Classically, Sarmiento et al changed patients to a functional brace be-

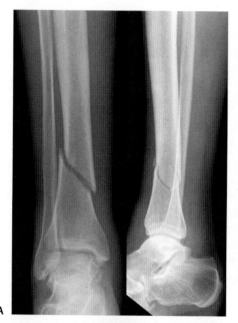
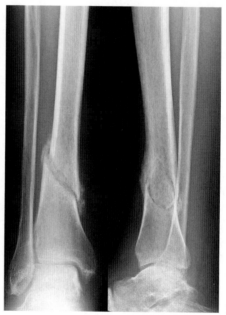
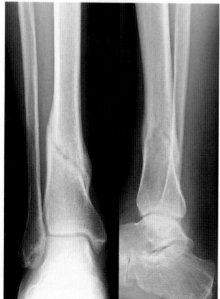

A

B

C

Figure 30–3 Nonoperative treatment of a distal tibial fracture. **(A)** The initial radiographs demonstrate a distal tibial shaft fracture with acceptable alignment and minimal shortening. The patient is permitted to be weight bearing as tolerated by 6 weeks in a fracture brace. Follow-up radiographs are obtained at 2 week intervals until callus formation is noted. **(B)** Radiographs taken at 3 months and **(C)** 6 months demonstrate a healed fracture with acceptable alignment.

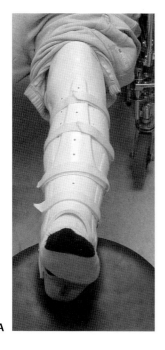

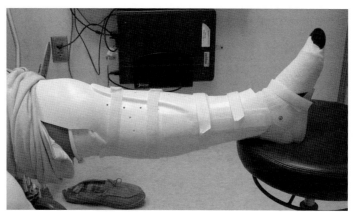

Figure 30–4 A patellar tendon bearing a tibial fracture brace. Clinical photographs of a patient with a nondisplaced middle-third tibia fracture wearing a patellar tendon bearing brace with a foot extension. The foot extension contributes to axial and rotational stability of the brace. **(A)** Frontal view of tibial fracture brace. **(B)** Side view of tibial fracture brace.

tween 4 and 6 weeks after injury.[9,10] This allowed muscle activity of the gastrocsoleus complex and anterior compartment to provide dynamic compression of the fracture and thus in theory increase fracture healing and stability. No prospective randomized study has ever been done to indicate that a functional brace is more efficacious than a cast or a PTB cast. Radiographs are taken at 4 week intervals to ensure maintenance of reduction and alignment and assess healing. When the fracture site has minimal pain and tenderness to palpation or the patient is walking with full weight bearing without much discomfort, the patient can then usually be transitioned to a removable brace. The total period of immobilization varies between 3 and 5 months. There is no reported decrease in range of motion of the knee or ankle, but up to 72% may have limited subtalar motion.[11]

The time to union for tibia fractures treated in a cast may be decreased by up to 4 weeks by the use of ultrasound or electrical stimulation.[12–14] This difference has been particularly notable in patients treated nonoperatively who smoke,[12,13] but the beneficial effect of bone stimulation appears to disappear if an intramedullary nail is placed.[14]

Indications for Surgical Treatment

Studies from the 1980s rarely justified open reduction and internal fixation in closed adult tibial shaft fractures.[11] However, critical analysis of the data presented revealed a 34% malunion rate with significant loss of ankle motion (43%). Documentation that displaced unstable fractures

are not suitable for closed treatment was provided by Hooper et al.[15] In a prospective randomized study comparing tibial shaft fractures with at least 50% displacement and > 10 degree angulation in any direction, Hooper et al compared closed treatment to closed intramedullary nailing. Intramedullary nailing provided a more rapid union rate (15.7 vs 18.3 weeks) with less malunion and shortening. Overall, 24% of the patients failed closed management and were converted to intramedullary nailing. The nonoperative group also had a 10-fold greater chance of malunion. Bone et al[16] reported on 99 patients with unilateral, displaced, isolated, closed fractures of the tibial shaft. Patients were treated with either closed management or reamed intramedullary fixation. An improved time to union (18 vs 26 weeks) was achieved in the intramedullary stabilization group along with an improved functional outcome. Changes in patient expectations have produced a decreased tolerance for malunion, nonunion, and resultant functional loss. It is clear that *unstable* tibial shaft fractures have a decreased rate of malunion, decreased time to union, and improved functional outcome with treatment with intramedullary fixation.

The decision for operative fixation should be made on a case-by-case basis. Indications for surgical treatment of tibial shaft fractures can include the following:

- Open fractures
- Fractures associated with polytrauma or multiple fractures
- Significantly displaced fractures, including shortening > 12 mm
- Fractures associated with compartment syndrome or requiring vascular repair

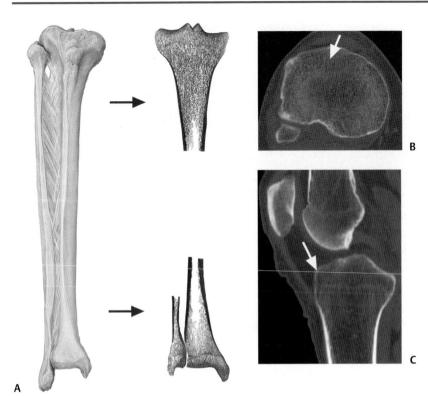

A

B

C

Figure 30–5 **(A)** The cross-sectional anatomy of the tibia. At both proximal and distal segments, the tibia cortex thins, and the tibial medullary canal expands. These metadiaphyseal segments are more difficult to control intramedullary fixation. **(B)** Starting point from axial cut of tibia. **(C)** Starting point on lateral view of tibia. The white arrow highlights an appropriate start point for intramedullary fixation for a diaphyseal fracture.

- Unstable fracture patterns, including distal and proximal shaft fractures
- Fractures that have unacceptable alignment following attempts at closed management

Surgical Treatment

Surgical and Radiographic Anatomy

The tibia has unique topographical and cross-sectional anatomy (**Fig. 30–5**). The medullary cavity of the tibial shaft is relatively straight in longitudinal dimension and relatively triangular in cross section. The straight longitudinal dimension is accessed through an anteriorly based starting point for intramedullary fixation. The posteriorly angulated proximal bend seen on tibial intramedullary implants (Herzog bend, **Fig. 30–6**) is present to help with insertion and avoid posterior tibial cortical penetration during nail insertion.

The proximal and distal tibial metadiaphyseal areas are associated with cortical thinning and medullary cavity expansion. The thinner cortex in these areas causes external fixation pins to have less purchase than in the diaphyseal bone. The decrease in purchase increases the risk of loosening of an external fixator pin. The medullary cavity expansion seen proximally and distally prevents adequate canal filling with intramedullary implants, and malalignment is more common with proximal or distal fractures

(**Fig. 30–7A–C**). Manufacturers of tibial intramedullary implants have recently added obliquely oriented screw patterns and more proximal or distal interlocking options

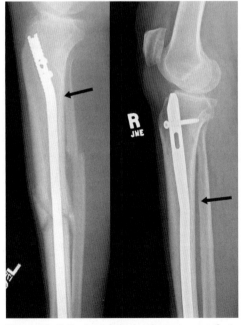

Figure 30–6 Design of tibial nails. A common feature of tibial nails is the proximal apex-posterior bend (Herzog curve, arrows), which facilitates nail insertion from an eccentric anterior starting point and helps prevent posterior cortical penetration during nail insertion.

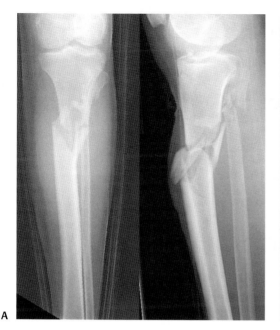 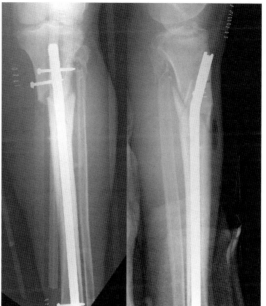

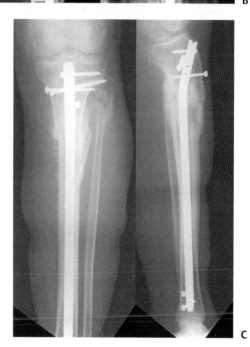

Figure 30–7 Proximal tibial fracture malalignment. **(A)** Anteroposterior and lateral radiographs of an unstable proximal third tibial fracture. **(B)** Radiographs after nailing show persistent medial translation and valgus angulation of the proximal fragment. The starting point is too distal, too anterior and too medial. **(C)** Follow-up radiographs after revision nailing with blocking screws and a new starting point show better alignment.

to provide a surgeon with an increased ability to improve construct stability in the proximal and distal metadiaphyseal areas.

A detailed understanding of cross-sectional anatomy is needed to address tibial shaft fractures and their complications. Placement of external fixation requires an understanding of "safe zones" for hardware placement. The atlas by Lehman et al[17] is an excellent reference for the placement of hardware so that iatrogenic damage to neurological and vascular structures is minimized.

The blood supply to the tibia is derived from intramedullary and periosteal sources. The intramedullary source is important in normal anatomy. The intramedullary supply is derived from a nutrient artery, a branch of the posterior tibial artery. This nutrient artery enters in the proximal aspect of the tibia in a nutrient foramina located in the posterolateral cortex at the origin of the soleus.[18] Upon entering the medullary cavity, it splits into three ascending branches and one descending branch providing endosteal branches. Although the medullary blood supply is important in normal anatomy, following skeletal trauma with fracture, the periosteal blood supply becomes the predominant vascular supply fueling the healing process.[18] The periosteal blood supply is derived from the anterior tibial

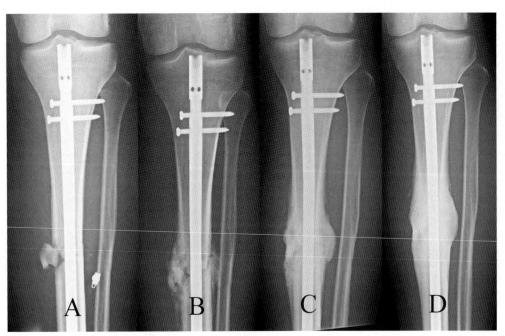

Figure 30–8 Indirect bone healing following tibial nailing. This radiographic series shows progressive tibial callus formation after intramedullary fixation. From left: 1, 2, 4, and 8 months postoperative.

artery. Normally, the periosteal blood supplies ~25% of the normal vascularity to bone. Following skeletal trauma with fracture, this contribution can increase to 100%. Thus soft tissue or periosteal stripping produced by the injury or created surgically can theoretically alter the normal healing process by producing a zone of avascular bone.

The radiographic signs of healing will vary depending on treatment methods used. External fixation, intramedullary fixation, and locked plating techniques ("internal external fixation") heal by a mechanism of indirect bone healing that favors callus formation **(Fig. 30–8)**. In hypertrophic nonunions **(Fig. 30–9)**, callus formation is abundant, with mechanical stability lacking. In contrast, traditional compression plating with anatomical reduction of the fracture fragments results in direct bone healing without motion at the fracture site, and no callus formation is seen on radiographs. "Bridge" plating provides only relative stability and will result in callus formation. If callus is seen following traditional plating, one should be concerned that there is too much fracture motion and that failure of the fracture construct may occur.

Surgical Techniques

The primary objective of this chapter is to highlight surgical techniques used to address tibial shaft fractures. A discussion of intramedullary fixation (with added emphasis on management of proximal and distal fracture patterns), plate fixation, and external fixation is provided.

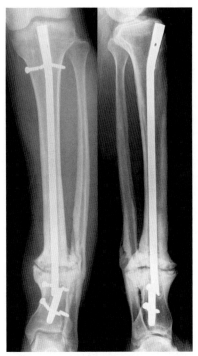

Figure 30–9 A hypertrophic tibial nonunion. This characteristic appearance signifies an appropriate fracture biological healing response with a need for increased mechanical stability. A laboratory evaluation should also be performed (including C-reactive protein and erythrocyte sedimentation rate) to assess for possible infection.

Intramedullary Fixation

Interlocking intramedullary fixation of the tibia has become the dominant treatment for all displaced, unstable and many stable tibial shaft fractures, whether open or closed. Recent controversy has centered on the merits of nailing with large-diameter nails that require reaming, or the use of small-diameter nails that can be placed without reaming.[19,20] Current implants have multiple locking options allowing for improved construct stability as well as improved designs to resist the forces generated during patient mobilization and fracture healing. The indications for nailing have been spreading from the traditional indication of midshaft fractures, to metaphyseal fractures, and even to some fractures of the proximal or distal tibia with simple intra-articular extension.

Currently, a statically locked intramedullary nail is the standard of care for a displaced tibial shaft fracture.[15,16,20,21] It provides a reliable treatment to obtain union and early functional recovery.

Surgical Techniques of Intramedullary Fixation of Diaphyseal Tibial Shaft Fractures (see Videos 30–1, Disk 4)

Patients undergoing intramedullary nailing for a tibial shaft fracture should be placed on a radiolucent table with a bump under the ipsilateral hip. An alternative method uses a traction table with calcaneal pin traction. If patients are placed on a table with calcaneal pin traction, the surgeon should be careful to apply traction only during the reduction phase and locking of the implant. It has been shown that compartment pressures increase significantly during traction, and return to normal after traction is released.[22] One should be concerned about the risk of compartment syndrome if the intracompartmental pressure is raised for a significant period of time during the intramedullary nailing process.

A bump or radiolucent triangle may also be placed under the patient's knee to allow knee flexion (**Fig. 30–10**). This assists with fracture alignment, reduction, and nail insertion. If a surgeon does not have a surgical assistant, a femoral distractor can be placed with two points of fixation, one in the distal tibia or calcaneus and the other at the proximal medial posterior tibia. The femoral or universal distractor can be utilized to help maintain reduction during intramedullary reaming and nail placement (**Fig. 30–11A,B**).

Anterior knee pain has been identified as a common problem after tibial nailing,[23,24] and its incidence may be influenced by the choice of approach that is used to enter the starting point, as well as the location of the starting hole. The appropriate starting point for an intramedullary nail to minimize risk of intra-articular injury has been identified by Tornetta et al (**Fig. 30–12A,B**).[25] This "safe zone" is just anterior to the intermeniscal ligament and on a radiograph is just to the medial side of the lateral tibial spine. On the lateral x-ray it is located just at the anterosuperior margin of the articular

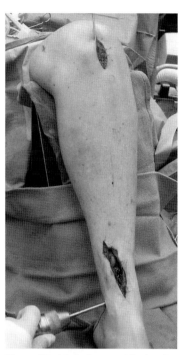

Figure 30–10 Patient positioning for tibial nailing, showing the use of a radiolucent triangle to assist with fracture reduction and nail insertion. With the knee in the flexed position, the proximal tibial starting point is entered.

surface on a slight flat spot that can be seen on a perfect lateral radiograph (**Fig. 30–13A–C**). This ideal starting point may be approached via a medial or lateral peripatellar incision as well as through a patellar tendon–splitting incision. The starting point for the tibial nail should be identified fluoroscopically with the aforementioned bony landmarks with a handheld awl or with a guide pin. When utilizing a guide pin, one must be extremely careful not to have the guidewire aimed too posteriorly. The curved awl design assists with appropriate placement. Both the guidewire and the awl should follow the anterior crest of the tibia (**Fig. 30–13A–C**). Increasing knee flexion over a bump or a radiolucent triangle helps to find the starting tract down the anterior aspect of the tibia. The surgeon must be careful during the insertion, which is initially viewed on the lateral, so that the starting hole does not track too laterally in the anterior plane (**Fig. 30–10**). After the nail insertion site has been ensured to be down the center of the intramedullary canal on the AP image and following the anterior cortex on the lateral image, the starting point is enlarged using the awl or overreaming the tibial guide pin.

The guide pin and awl are removed. Provisional fracture reduction is established (either manually, with traction, or assisted by a distractor) and a ball-tipped guidewire is inserted into the medullary cavity. The guidewire is advanced past the reduced fracture site into a position that is centered in the distal tibia in both planes. For unreamed nail insertion, a T-handled awl can be used for final medullary canal opening. If a tourniquet was used during

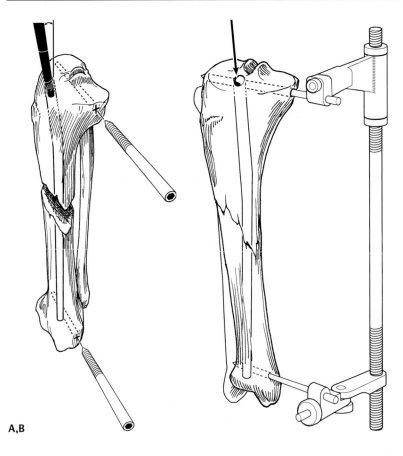

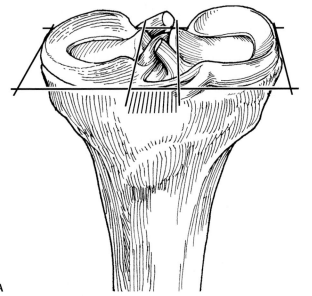

A,B

Figure 30–11 Use of a femoral or universal distractor. The universal femoral or distractor can be placed on the medial side of the tibia to facilitate fracture reduction. This is a tool that can be used for both proximal and distal fracture patterns. Uniplanar external fixation is an appropriate substitution. **(A)** Pins shuld be placed posterior proximally and anterior distally. **(B)** Femoral distractor holding reduction for intramedullary nail placement.

the establishment of the starting site, it is deflated prior to reaming to avoid possible thermal injury.

Initial reaming is performed using an end-cutting reamer with the soft tissues of the extensor mechanism protected. Fracture reduction must be maintained during this initial pass of the reamer because the nail will follow the path that is generated. Reaming is continued with

incremental increases in diameter (0.5 to 1.0 mm) until cortical chatter is obtained. The implant is sized 1 mm smaller than the diameter of the last reamer used to avoid nail incarceration. The nail is inserted over the guidewire into the final position with nail rotation controlled during insertion. Changes in nail rotation are not done without nail advancement to avoid fracture rotation. Final position

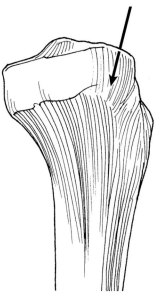

A

B

Figure 30–12 Tibial nail start point. **(A)** The proper starting point for tibial nailing is anterior to the meniscus and shown in the highlighted area. **(B)** On the lateral perspective, one can see that there is enough room anterior to the articular cartilage to allow insertion of the nail at the top of the tibia rather than on the anterior surface.

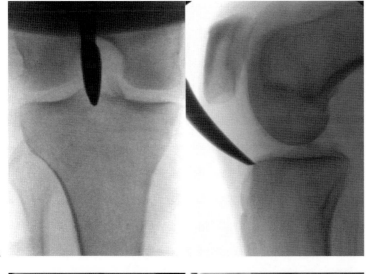

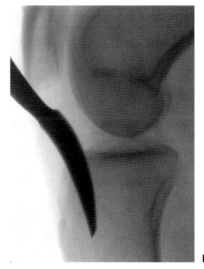

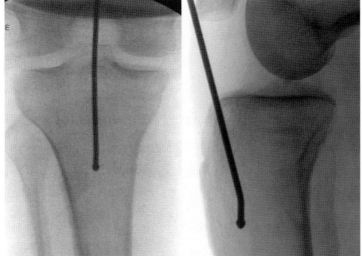

Figure 30–13 Tibial nail radiographic starting point. The sweet spot that was shown schematically in **Fig. 30–12** is shown here radiographically. **(A)** On the anteroposterior image the standard starting point is generally placed overlying the medial aspect of the lateral tibial spine. On the lateral image the awl is placed at the flat point at the anterosuperior margin of the proximal tibial surface. **(B)** The awl is then advanced into the medullary canal of the proximal tibia parallel to the anterior cortex. Increasing knee flexion can assist with this desired anterior pin/awl placement (shown in **Fig. 30–10**). **(C)** The ball-tipped guidewire is advanced into the tibial diaphysis with assistance of biplanar fluoroscopy.

is confirmed using AP and lateral fluoroscopic images, and the guidewire is removed. Larger nails can be placed by reaming an additional 1 to 2 mm greater than the initial reamer size that first produced chatter. This may be most important when nailing metaphyseal fractures. In general, the authors prefer to limit excessive reaming.

The addition of interlocking screws also increases fracture stability. Distal medial to lateral interlocking screws are applied using a freehand technique, with the fracture pattern dictating the appropriate number and position of interlocking screws. More distal fractures or unstable patterns have greater stability following the addition of oblique or multiplanar interlocking screws. Fracture compression is achieved with gentle backslapping after the release of traction or by application of manufacturer-specific compression techniques. Fracture reduction is confirmed with direct visualization of leg alignment and with either or both radiographic and fluoroscopic images. Proximal interlocking is performed using the external alignment guide, with interlocking screws placed in the static or dynamic position with additional construct stability realized by using obliquely oriented screws. In

comminuted fractures, anatomical tibial length and alignment are assessed by comparing to the opposite tibia.

The patient's wounds are closed and sterile dressings applied. Leg muscle compartments are reassessed clinically for elevated pressure; fasciotomy should be performed if there is concern about the development of compartment syndrome. Anatomical leg length and rotation are confirmed with an assessment of knee ligament stability. Alterations in this technique are employed to address the special situation of distal and proximal fracture patterns discussed in the next two sections.

Technique of Open Tibial Shaft Fractures

Intramedullary stabilization has been controversial in open fractures because of concerns that an intramedullary nail would increase the risk of infection. However, comparative studies have found that intramedullary nails had no significant increase in risk of deep infection over external fixation in open fractures.[26,27] The intramedullary nails had equivalent time to union but a significantly decreased incidence of malunion, and required fewer operations to achieve union. Intramedullary nail fixation of open tibial shaft fractures, including type IIIB fractures, has been shown to be safe and effective and is an accepted method of treatment **(Fig. 30–14A–C).** If devitalized segments of bone are encountered during debridement, the surgeon should remove these segments of bone, obtain adequate soft tissue coverage, and plan on early bone grafting of the bony defect 4 to 6 weeks after injury. Biological adjuncts to standard treatments are now available. The use of recombinant bone morphogenic protein-2 (BMP-2) (INFUSE, Medronic, Memphis, Tennessee) in open tibia fractures has recently shown decreased infection rates, decreased time to union, and decreased pain compared with standard intramedullary nailing alone.[28]

Immediate versus delayed closure of soft tissue wounds of open tibia fractures has also been controversial. Standard treatment for many years had included delayed closure after secondary debridement in 48 to 72 hours. Many trauma centers currently obtain adequate debridement at

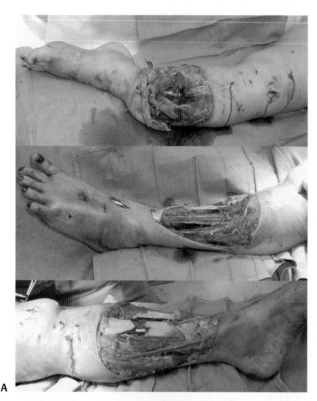
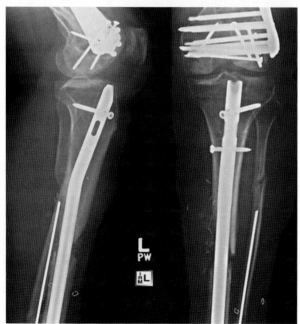

A

B

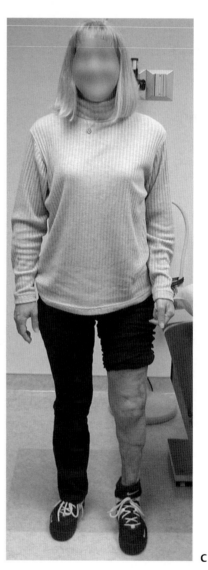

C

Figure 30–14 Open tibia fracture management. **(A)** These intraoperative photos show an open type IIIB tibia fracture with 3 cm of bone loss (upper panel). The foot was viable, and surgical stabilization of the tibia was done with an intramedullary nail, restoring leg length and rotation. Significant periosteal stripping is noted with bone loss and exposed hardware. Soft tissue coverage was obtained, and the patient returned to the operating room at 6 weeks for iliac crest bone grafting. **(B)** Radiographs following bone grafting of the tibial shaft defect. **(C)** Clinical photograph at radiographic union.

the initial operation and if possible perform immediate closure of the wound without subsequent surgical debridement. This early closure technique has not resulted in an increased incidence of superficial or deep infections.[29] A prospective randomized trial is under way with the Orthopaedic Trauma Association to determine the optimum method of care. If an open wound is unable to be closed or felt to need a secondary open debridement, wound coverage can be obtained with moist dressings, a "bead pouch,"[30,31] or a wound vacuum-assisted closure (VAC).[32,33] It is our opinion that the wound should be sealed from the hospital environment to help reduce the risk of exposing the underlying tissues to nosocomial contamination.

Surgical Techniques of Intramedullary Fixation of Proximal Tibial Shaft Fractures

Proximal tibia fractures have a high risk of malalignment when treated by intramedullary nailing **(Fig. 30–7A–C).** When one encounters a proximal tibia fracture, additional techniques are frequently employed to reduce the risk of malalignment when nailing is performed.

When intramedullary fixation is chosen for a proximal tibia fracture, obtaining a proper starting point is absolutely critical. There are several reasons for this. First, because there is no medullary canal in the proximal segment, the implant does not effect any fracture reduction. The lack of any canal-filling effect of the implant is akin to

having a broom handle in a garbage pail. The second reason relates to the three-dimensional anatomy of the upper tibia. The medial cortex of the proximal tibia slopes posteriorly from the anterior apex, whereas the lateral tibia has an anterior "pouch" behind the tibial tubercle. Therefore, when a nail is started medially, the medial cortex rapidly pushes the nail posterolaterally, which causes the valgus and flexion deformity that is so often seen as the nail then engages the midshaft of the tibia **(Fig. 30–7A–C).** By moving the starting point laterally, the guide pin and nail can be directed straight down the canal and still be kept along the anterior cortex of the tibia. This starting point can be facilitated with a lateral peripatellar approach. Additionally, the starting point should be directly parallel to the anterior cortex to avoid the apex anterior deformity that is commonly seen **(Fig. 30–13A–C).** A curet can be used to assist with removal of cancellous bone from the starting point along the anterior crest. Reduction is maintained during guidewire insertion, reaming, and nail insertion. If malalignment is noted, several techniques are suggested.

When malalignment is noted, reduction assistance is required. Tools to assist with fracture reduction include plating with unicortical screws, the use of blocking or "Poller" screws, use of a so-called universal distractor **(Fig. 30–11A,B),** and/or use of pointed reduction clamps. Unicortical plates can be placed on the anteromedial tibia providing temporary reduction of the fracture during reaming and nail placement **(Fig. 30–15A,B).** These plates

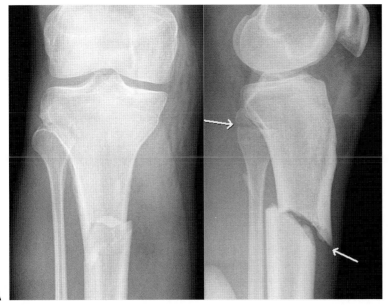

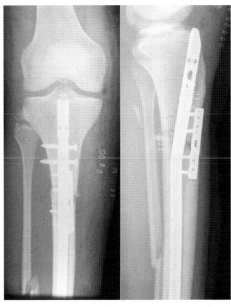

A   **B**

Figure 30–15 Proximal tibia reduction tools—example of plating with unicortical screws. **(A)** This tibia fracture required additional reduction assistance during intramedullary fixation (note the anterior displacement of the proximal fragment; right arrow). (Another arrow demonstrates a fibular head fracture.) **(B)** Postoperative radiographs showing how a short plate was used to maintain reduction of the fracture during nailing. Upon critical assessment, the tibial nail starting point was too medial, contributing to deformity during nail inser-

tion. Unicortical fixation through small-fragment plates (a five-hole, 3.5 mm compression plate was used in this example) allows for passage of the guidewire, reamers, and intramedullary implant while maintaining reduction. The plate can be removed or retained following nail interlocking. It is our preference to limit the use of this technique because of the concern over disruption of the fracture hematoma. A correct (more lateral) starting point would have avoided the problem.

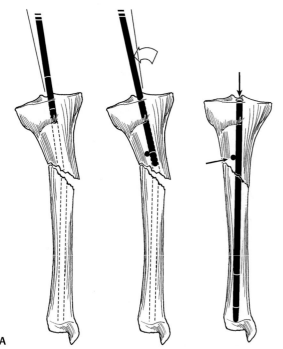

A

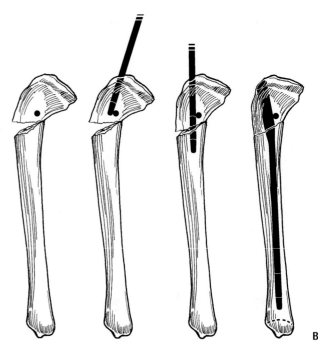

B

Figure 30–16 The use of blocking or "Poller" screws. A blocking screw assists with correcting the apex anterior and valgus angulation. In general, the screw is placed on the concave side of the deformity such that direct contact is made with the intramedullary implant. **(A)** In the coronal plane, the screw is typically placed lateral to the nail. **(B)** In the sagittal plane, the screw is placed posterior to the nail. No discussion of fracture healing inhibition due to galvanic effect (stainless steel contacting titanium) has been noted in the literature.

are particularly useful in addressing segmental tibia fractures (**Fig. 30–7A–C**). Plate choices can vary from one-third tubular plates to dynamic compression plates; locking plates represent a newer option. Reduction and plating should be performed with the knee in an extended position. As the knee is flexed, the plate resists the varus angulation and apex anterior angulation of the proximal fragment. These plates are left in place until nail interlocking is completed. There is debate whether these plates should be removed following interlocking screw application.

Another option to prevent malalignment is by using blocking or Poller screws (**Fig. 30–16A,B**). A blocking screw is a small-fragment cortical screw that is placed to guide the nail; by functionally narrowing the intramedullary canal, such screws can provide additional stability and help to address the primary deformities of the proximal tibia: apex anterior angulation and varus. To prevent the nail from tracking posteriorly, a blocking screw is placed just posterior to the desired nail position; another anterior-posterior blocking screw placed lateral to the nail's ideal tract can keep the nail medial and provide "three-point fixation." This screw serves as a guide rail, steering the nail and fracture to an anatomical fracture reduction. This technique has been well described by several authors[34,35] with good results in proximal third tibial shaft fractures.

Once the proximal deformity has been addressed—if needed—intramedullary reaming or placement of the intramedullary nail may then proceed as usual. Again, the surgeon should ensure that reduction is maintained during this process prior to performing proximal and distal interlocking. Interlocking screw placement should be done in transverse and oblique proximal orientations to provide increased stability.

Surgical Techniques of Intramedullary Fixation of Distal Tibial Shaft Fractures

As with proximal tibia fractures, intramedullary fixation of distal tibia fractures can present challenges. Newer implant designs allow placement of multiple distal interlocking screws in various orientations. Although such implant design modifications can assist with improving fracture stability,[36,37] fracture reduction is paramount. The intramedullary implant does not itself assist with reduction of distal fracture patterns. This is because of the metaphyseal bone expansion that prevents canal filling and can result in malreduction. Malalignment poses a risk of decreased functional and subjective outcomes in distal third tibia fractures treated with intramedullary implants (**Fig. 30–17A–D**).[38] Because the ankle joint has more varus malalignment, ankle scores worsen.[39] Reduction strategies are therefore needed to assist in appropriate alignment and rotation prior

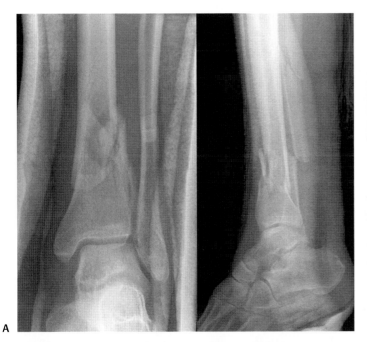
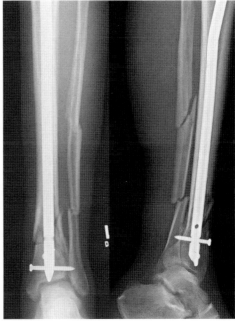

A

B

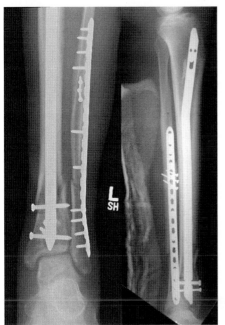
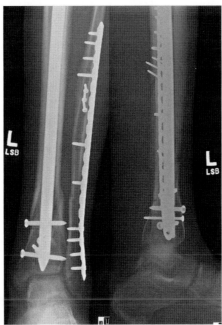

C

D

Figure 30–17 Malreduction of a distal tibia fracture after malreduction. **(A)** Anteroposterior and lateral radiographs of a distal tibia fracture. **(B)** Postoperative x-rays reveal unacceptable valgus and apex-anterior angulation of the distal tibia. **(C)** Revision was performed by plating the fibula to establish lateral column length, and by inserting blocking screws to add stability to the distal tibia. **(D)** Final x-rays after healing.

to intramedullary device placement. Reduction tools include universal distractor placement **(Fig. 30–11A,B),** fibular plating, Steinmann pin placement, distal tibia unicortical plating, and pointed reduction clamping.

A Steinmann pin or Schanz screw can be used to facilitate reduction of distal tibia fractures **(Fig. 30–18A,B).** A smooth pin of sufficient diameter to afford fracture manipulation (at least 2 mm) is placed in the distal tibia. This may be placed anterior to the distal fibula and parallel to the plafond. Placement of the pin parallel to the tibial plafond is critical to assess anatomical fracture reduction and provides a guide to ensure that the final nail placement is perpendicular to the ankle joint. The pin affixed in the distal fracture segment is used as a reduction aid ("joystick") to control fracture translation and rotation, and assist reduction for guidewire placement. It is critical

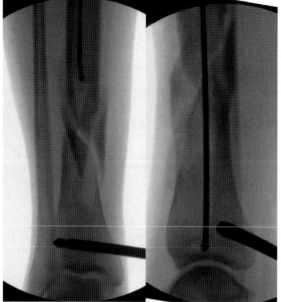
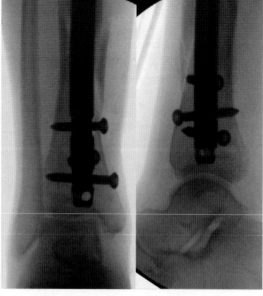

A

B

Figure 30–18 The use of a Steinmann pin to reduce a distal tibia fracture. **(A)** A Schanz screw is placed from medial to lateral in the distal tibia just above and parallel to the plafond. This is used as a joystick to assist with reduction, and as a reference to the alignment of the ankle. The guidewire is placed perpendicular to the

Schanz screw after a reduction is applied. This lateral image confirms that the nail passage will not be blocked by the screw placement. **(B)** Acceptable fracture reduction and stability are achieved using multiple interlocking screws placed in orthogonal and oblique orientations.

to obtain central placement of the guidewire on both AP and lateral images. Central position is confirmed and maintained during reaming. The reduction is maintained during nail placement and interlocking, and the Steinmann pin or Schanz screw is removed.

Distal fibular plating can provide an indirect reduction tool for the distal tibia. Plating of the fibula should be done only if anatomical restoration of fibular length and rotation can be achieved **(Fig. 30–19A,B)**. Additional reduction tools may be required for an anatomical restoration of the

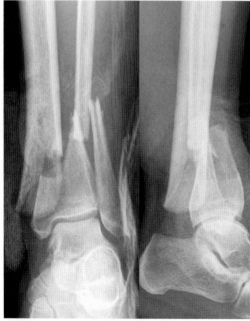
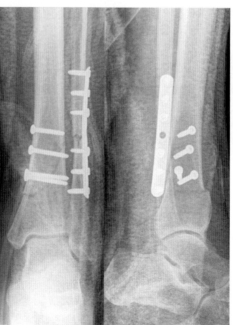

A

B

Figure 30–19 Indirect distal tibia reduction with fibular plating. **(A)** Injury films demonstrate a jagged, oblique, extra-articular fracture of the distal tibial metaphysis. Anatomical restoration of fibular length and rotation is required. **(B)** This case example demonstrates use of

fibular plating with compression lag screw fixation of the distal tibial shaft due to soft tissue envelope concerns. We would typically recommend intramedullary fixation of this fracture pattern with three distal interlocking screws obtainable with newer implant designs.

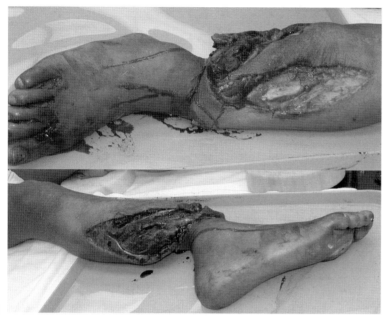
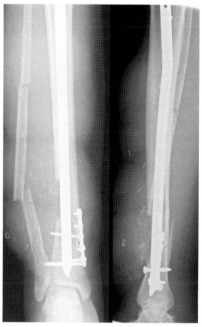

A   B

Figure 30–20 Provisional distal tibia reduction with a tibial plate and unicortical screws. **(A)** Clinical photos of a type III open distal tibial fracture. **(B)** In this case, the fibula has a segmental fracture, and distal fibular plating would not provide adequate indirect reduction of the tibia. Therefore, provisional distal tibia fracture stabilization was performed with a 3.5 mm reconstruction plate placed through the open wound using unicortical screws. Distal interlocking screws were placed at 90 degree orientations to improve fracture stability. Additionally, one screw was placed through the plate and through the intramedullary implant to improve construct stability.

distal tibia. Intramedullary stabilization proceeds after the reduction is maintained. The fibular plate is left in place following intramedullary stabilization. The use of distal tibia unicortical plating is presented **(Fig. 30–20A,B)**. This procedure is analogous to plating used for the proximal tibia **(Fig. 30–15A,B)**.

If intramedullary nailing is to be performed on fractures with intra-articular extension, the articular portion needs to be reduced and stabilized with percutaneously placed lag screws prior to beginning the nailing procedure. Data from multiple authors indicate that intramedullary nailing of distal tibia fractures, even with intra-articular extension, is biomechanically and clinically feasible without significant rates of complications or malalignment.[40–43]

Plate Fixation of Tibial Shaft Fractures (see Video 30–2, Disk 4)

The periosteal blood supply becomes the major source of vascularity after a tibia fracture. A primary concern with plating a tibial shaft fracture is that additional stripping of the periosteal tissues would lead to an avascular bony segment. In an effort to help maintain the fracture environment with minimal disruption, percutaneous plating techniques are gaining popularity to address periarticular fractures with tibial shaft components.

Plate fixation of the tibia is primarily restricted to the proximal and distal fractures. Plate fixation can be performed in the setting of an open tibial shaft fracture where complete periosteal stripping has occurred and anatomical reduction is feasible. If one slides a plate along the bone proximally and distally without further disruption of the blood supply, and anatomical alignment and fixation are feasible, the plate is a reasonable choice. Plate fixation of a tibial shaft fracture may also be necessary if intramedullary nailing is not possible due to a knee arthroplasty or due to a severe proximal or distal tibial periarticular fracture. A prior tibial malalignment may also prevent intramedullary nailing. Plate fixation is also a possible option in children with open epiphyses. In all cases, precontoured percutaneously placed tibial plates are an option. This will decrease the soft tissue insult to maintain the periosteal blood supply to the fracture and decrease the incidence of wound breakdown and deep infection, which has been reported as high as 30% in tibia fracture plating.[44]

Plate fixation employs standard techniques for the tibial shaft and is not specifically covered in this chapter. The development of compression plating techniques by the A.O. group produced some good functional results.[45] A better understanding of the limitations of plating was provided by Johner and Wruhs.[4] They described a series of 212 closed and 79 open fractures that were addressed by plating and discussed a classification scheme that served as the basis for the AO and OTA classifications for tibia fractures. As comminution increased, the rate of complications increased. Complications were reported in 1.5% of simple fractures, in 18.1% of fractures with butterfly fragments, and in 48.3% of comminuted fractures with a 10.3% infection rate in this final group. The recent introduction of percutaneous skeletal fixation is an attempt to help preserve the fracture environment. Initial reports of this fixation technique focused on periarticular injuries. In a series of 14 patients, Collinge et al[46] reported on the use of percutaneous skeletal fixation in complex periarticular tibial shaft fractures. Results demonstrated no malunions with no infections or skin complications in the five patients with closed fractures. One case of osteomyelitis and three superficial infections were reported in nine patients with open fractures. This technique is dependent upon achieving fracture reduction with closed means prior to application of the percutaneous plate construct.

Surgical Techniques of Lateral Submuscular Plate Fixation of Proximal Tibial Shaft Fractures

The results of proximal tibia intramedullary nailing have had an unacceptably high incidence of malunion of up to 30% in the hands of experienced trauma surgeons.[47] Malunion can occur even when the patients use the foregoing techniques to obtain improved reduction during intramedullary reaming and placement of the intramedullary nail. Due to the technical difficulty with intramedullary nailing of proximal tibia fractures, many surgeons now favor percutaneous or submuscular plating of proximal tibia fractures.[48,49] These fixed-angle, locked, precontoured, proximal tibial plates help decrease the risk of malunion and malalignment and require fracture reduction prior to plate application. We prefer to use lateral submuscular techniques for fractures involving the proximal one fifth of the tibial shaft (**Fig. 30–21**). We also use these techniques in fractures involving the articular surface with shaft extension, with discussion in this chapter limited to tibial shaft fractures.

The patient is placed supine on a radiolucent operating room table. A bump is placed under the patient's ipsilateral hip. A tourniquet is placed on the proximal thigh and is often not inflated. An incision is made from Gerdy's tubercle obliquely toward the fibular head. The skin incision is extended down to expose the anterior compartment fascia. The anterior compartment fascia is incised 1 cm lateral to the tibial ridge to facilitate wound closure. A Cobb elevator is used to begin a submuscular dissection on the anterolateral aspect of the tibia. Fracture reduction is achieved and the fixed-angle locking plate can then be attached to an attachment jig or slid by hand down the anterolateral compartment until the proximal aspect of the plate aligns on the anterolateral aspect of the tibia. Multiple views are obtained in the anterior and lateral planes to ensure that the apex ante-

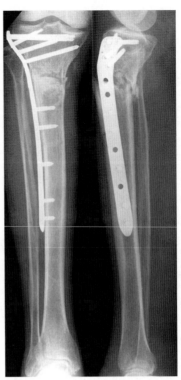

Figure 30–21 Plating of a proximal tibial shaft fracture. We prefer to use lateral locked submuscular plating in proximal one-fifth tibial shaft fractures. This case demonstrates placement of a Less Invasive Stabilization System (LISS) plate. Fracture reduction is achieved prior to plate placement, and the distal extent of the plate should be at least four to six cortical diameters. The length of the plate should generally extend four to six cortical diameters past the fracture.

rior and proximal tibia varus deformities do not occur. The proximal aspect of the plate is ~1 cm distal to the articular surface and is placed for optimal fit on the proximal tibia. After the plate is aligned, it is held with reduction clamps or pull-reduction clamps that are placed through the attachment jig. Once the fracture is anatomically aligned axially and rotationally, any segmental fragmentation in the metadiaphyseal or diaphyseal region can be left undisturbed. Distal plate extension is four to six cortical diameters beyond the fracture site. Plates are often initially fixed to bone with standard nonlocking screws to draw the plate to bone. This technique of submuscular locked plating of proximal tibia fractures has excellent results with ~3% delayed unions or nonunions that require bone grafting.[48,49]

External Fixation of Tibial Shaft Fractures (see Video 30–3, Disk 4)

External fixation can be used to provide either temporizing or definitive stabilization of tibial shaft fractures. Open fractures and fractures in skeletally immature patients are the most common indications for this method. All constructs (pin and bar, tension wire, and hybrid systems) adhere to the same principles of fracture stabilization with minimal soft tissue damage. The initial construct design and rigidity will be altered depending upon patient presentation and expected duration of treatment. External fixation is associated with pin tract infections and higher rates of malunions. A determination of expected patient compliance should also be assessed prior to selection of this treatment method.

Surgical Technique of External Fixation

If external fixator pins are to be placed for temporizing stabilization, fluoroscopy is not necessarily needed, but the pins need to be bridging the fracture site attempting to stay out of the zone of injury. Schanz pins (5 mm) are best used for the tibial shaft, and if necessary external fixator pins can be placed across the ankle into the calcaneus or above the knee to maintain pins away from the zone of injury. If definitive external fixation is to be utilized, external fixator pins should be initially placed close to and far from the fracture site to stay within the two main fragments of bone. Depending on the external fixator system, a thin wire, monolateral, or double-stacked external frame may be utilized to maintain adequate stability.

Increased stability can be obtained with a hybrid fixator with thin wires at the metadiaphysis proximally or distally and combined with tibial shaft Schanz pins. If one utilizes a hybrid fixator proximally, the thin wires should be placed out of the reflected anterior capsule approximately *1.4 cm from the joint to decrease the risk of intra-articular infection.*[50] As a general rule, one may place pins below the level of the fibular head to be sure that they are placed extra-articularly. The surgeon should be cautious about placing thin wires through the fibular head because ~10% of proximal tibia and fibular joints have communication to the knee joint. If a pin tract becomes infected through this portal, it can lead to septic arthritis of the knee. Approximately a 10% incidence of septic arthritis has been reported in the utilization of hybrid fixators about the knee in experienced trauma centers.[51] Neurovascular structures are at risk with thin wire utilization proximally and distally. The surgeon should be well acquainted with cross-sectional anatomy to avoid neurovascular injury. If external fixation is to be utilized distally until union, there appears to be no advantage to bridging versus nonbridging external fixation in terms of late ankle motion. An Ilizarov external fixator frame may also be utilized with highly comminuted fractures, with fractures with severe bone loss, or severe soft tissue injury. Ilizarov frames are extremely helpful with severe fractures or with infected nonunions or for bone transport. Their use is rarely indicated in treatment of acute tibia fractures. A case that highlights multiple treatment methods discussed is shown in **Fig. 30–22A–D.**

Tips and Tricks

Intramedullary Fixation

- The starting point is critical. Change to a more lateral start point at the lateral tibial eminence for proximal fracture patterns.
- To avoid posterior cortical penetration, always focus on a starting point parallel to the anterior tibial cortex on lateral fluoroscopic images. This position is facilitated by increasing knee flexion.
- Maintain acceptable fracture reduction during guidewire placement and reaming. The intramedullary device can only follow the path you create.
- The intramedullary nail does not assist with fracture reduction for proximal and distal fractures due to the loss of canal filling effect resulting from medullary cavity expansion. Additional techniques are frequently required to assist and maintain reduction in these fracture patterns.
- One can increase construct stability by increasing the number of interlocking screws and by changing the orientation of the screws. We recommend for unstable fracture patterns at least two proximal and two distal interlocking screws.
- Completion of intramedullary fixation always has the surgeon reassessing compartment pressures, assessing knee ligament stability, and confirming anatomical fracture reduction with equal leg lengths and rotations.
- For distal and proximal fracture patterns, a plain long cassette radiograph is obtained to better assess alignment.

Plate Fixation

- For percutaneous and submuscular techniques, fracture reduction occurs prior to plate application.

External Fixation

- Place pins outside the zone of injury and outside the knee capsule.
- The most important factor for fracture stability following external fixator application is fracture apposition followed by pin diameter.

New Techniques

Fracture healing always involves a dynamic contest between biomechanical stability and fracture biology (**Figs. 30–8 and 30–9**). Newer intramedullary implant designs offer additional options for distal and proximal interlocking screws. These obliquely oriented screw holes provide a surgeon with an increased ability to improve construct stability for unstable fracture patterns. Any biomechanical construct has biological consequences. One should attempt to minimize the disruption to the soft tissues using all techniques. Augmentation of fracture biology is an exciting new development in

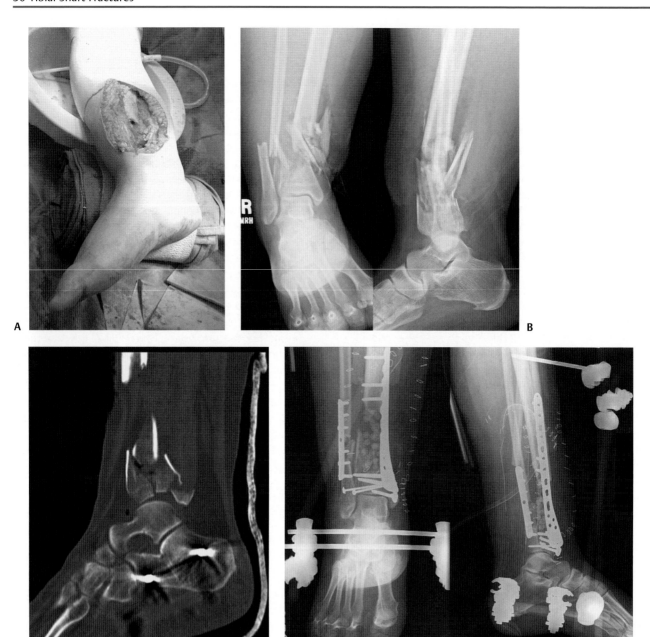

Figure 30–22 The use of multiple treatment methods to treat an unstable, open tibia fracture. **(A)** Photograph following debridement of an open type IIIB tibia fracture with 6 cm of bone loss. **(B)** Preoperative radiographs and **(C)** computed tomographic scan demonstrate the comminuted distal tibial shaft fracture. Alignment was initially achieved with external fixator placement. A repeat wound irrigation and debridement with fracture fixation and soft tissue coverage was performed. **(D)** The mortise radiograph shows fracture fixation using fibular and tibial plating with anatomical restoration of the articular surface. Antibiotic beads were used for 6 weeks. The beads were removed with the membranes left in place with iliac crest bone grafting performed.

the treatment of tibia fractures with growth factors and BMPs currently approved for specific uses.

The use of recombinant BMP-2 (INFUSE) in open tibia fractures has recently shown to decrease infection rates, decrease time to union, and decrease pain compared with standard treatments.[28] One should always review and understand the indications for application of a biologically active product. In particular, recombinant BMP-2 should be applied to an open tibia fracture in a skeletally mature patient following intramedullary fixation if appropriate soft tissue coverage is obtained. Application should occur only if soft tissue stabilization occurs prior to 14 days. As mentioned in the introduction, tibial nonunions are very common, with over 100,000 North Americans having a tibial nonunion per annum (over 10%). Recombinant BMP-7 (OP-1, Stryker Biotech, West Lebanon, New Hampshire) is approved for use as an alternative to autograft in recalcitrant long bone nonunions where autograph is unfeasible and alternative treatments have failed.[52]

Outcomes

The long-term outcome of patients with tibial shaft fractures has been difficult to predict. Sarmiento and Latta found that fracture union and time to fracture union correlated primarily with fracture comminution and open versus closed fractures.[9] No patient-oriented functional outcome measures were done on their patient populations. The patients who are treated in a cast for long periods of time are known to have limited subtalar motion and a low incidence of anterior knee pain. The optimal treatment for closed, displaced tibial shaft fractures is also unclear, as are long-term predictors of outcomes.[53]

Aside from the recent resurgence of periarticular plating, plate fixation of tibia shaft fractures has been uncommonly performed, primarily due to concerns about the risk of infection. In 1976 Gustilo and Anderson[7] reported on open tibial shaft fractures treated with either plate fixation or external fixation. Patients treated with plates were analyzed retrospectively, with a 44% infection rate found among 111 fractures. External fixation results were reported prospectively, with a 9.9% infection rate in 111 fractures. In 1989, Bach and Hansen[44] performed a prospective, randomized study on plate fixation versus external fixation in 59 patients with type II or III tibia shaft fractures. They concluded that the rate and extent of complications were lower with external fixation. Although all tibial shaft fractures healed, there were five plate fixations complicated by osteomyelitis, with three plate fixation failures. One patient developed osteomyelitis after external fixation with three pin tract infections. Malunion was reported in three patients following external fixation (two with 10 degrees AP angulation, one with 25 degrees external rotation). Plating of tibial shaft fracture is currently limited to shaft fractures that have juxta-articular fracture extension.

Displaced tibial shaft fractures have improved outcomes with operative treatment. Hooper et al proved that patients with displaced tibial shaft fractures who are treated with an intramedullary nail have a faster time to union and a faster return to work.[15] If a displaced tibia fracture is to be treated with an intramedullary nail, reaming of the intramedullary canal is controversial. A meta-analysis has been done on nine prospective randomized studies of reamed versus unreamed intramedullary nail placement. It was not conclusive that reaming increases risks of compartment syndrome or infection or decreased time to union.[54] Due to the lack of definitive surgical trials and variation in surgeon opinions, a multicenter international prospective randomized trial is ongoing to determine the optimal treatment of open and closed tibial shaft fractures using either reamed or unreamed tibial nails.

Treatment of open tibial shaft fractures has evolved from external fixation to intramedullary nailing based on data in 1998 from Henley et al,[27] who reported a prospective randomized trial of unreamed interlocking intramedullary fixation versus half-pin external fixation of open tibial fractures (types II, IIIA, and IIIB). There were 104 fractures in the intramedullary fixation group and 70 fractures in the external fixation group. There was a statistically significant difference in malalignment between both groups. The intramedullary fixation group had 92% satisfactory alignment, whereas the external fixation group had 69% satisfactory alignment. There was no statistical difference in infections at the fracture site and time to healing, with 50% of the external fixation patients having at least one pin tract infection. On average the external fixation group also required an additional procedure following the index procedure (2.7 vs 1.7). Results were similar in both groups with equal risk of infection, but fewer secondary procedures were needed in the intramedullary nailing group.

Functional outcomes of patients with intramedullary nailing of displaced tibial shaft fractures have been reported by Dogra et al.[24] In this study, patients are given a disease-specific outcome measure such as the Iowa Knee Score and Iowa Ankle Score. Mean scores for patients with long-term follow-up with these instruments were ~90 of 100 points. The physical component score of the SF-36 (Short Form–36) questionnaires as a measure of overall health and quality of life were significantly lower as compared with general population norms. These data indicate that even after uneventful healing and union of a tibial shaft fracture with a nail, the patient still may have significant disability. Alignment of distal tibial shaft, in particular, may be important for overall patient function because patients with malalignment of distal tibial shaft fractures have been noted to have SF-36 pain scores higher than those patients who have normal anatomical alignment after a distal tibial shaft fracture and internal fixation with an intramedullary nail.[55]

Limb Salvage versus Amputation

Limb salvage versus amputation is one of the most difficult decisions faced by an orthopaedic surgeon. If the patient's life is at risk due to severe hypoperfusion and ongoing active bleeding, this decision may need to be made emergently and in consultation with the trauma service or surgeon. At times, the limb is nearly completely severed with no hopes of reconstruction, and acute amputation decision is easily made. Salvage of extremities is feasible if attempted before 6 hours of warm ischemia. In most cases, the limb is potentially viable and the decision of reconstruction versus amputation can be put off until further information is available. In an unconscious patient with a

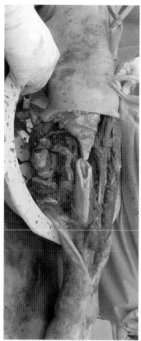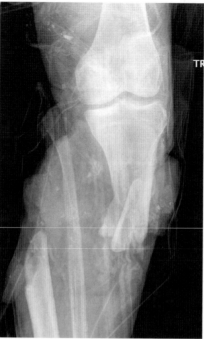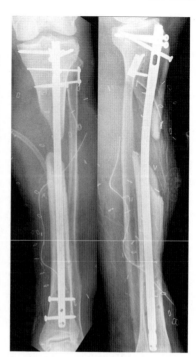

A–C

Figure 30–23 A case where limb salvage decisions were necessary. **(A)** This case is a type IIIB open tibial shaft fracture with segmental bone loss. The patient had a viable foot with posterior tibial artery flow and continuity of the posterior tibial nerve. **(B)** The initial radiographs show a significant bony and soft tissue injury with a dislocated proximal tibia/fibula joint. Correct tibial length and rotation were assisted with fixation of the proximal tibia/fibula joint. **(C)** Intramedullary stabilization performed with three proximal interlocking screws to increase construct stability. The patient decided that he did not want to proceed with soft tissue coverage and later had an uneventful elective below knee amputation.

severe bony injury, the orthopaedic surgeon can place a bridging external fixator across the zone of the injury. If revascularization is required, this can be attempted by the vascular surgeons. If revascularization is not feasible, then amputation should be completed. If the limb is viable, in the next several days the orthopaedic surgeon can have an in-depth discussion with the patient and family about the expectations of limb salvage versus amputation **(Fig. 30–23A–C).** If limb salvage is attempted, the soft tissue can be addressed to obtain debridement and closure as early as possible. The lowest infection rates in severe open tibia fractures have been reported, with definitive closure within 72 hours.[56,57]

The mangled extremity severity score (MESS) was developed in an attempt to predict which limbs were viable **(Table 30–1).**[58] Several other extremity scores have also been developed to assist in decision making. No scoring system has been 100% predictive of amputation. In the largest series of severe lower extremity limbs to date, a MESS score of greater than or equal to 7 (the proposed cutoff for limb salvage vs amputation) was only predictive of amputation in 60% of injuries. In discussing limb salvage versus amputation with patients and families, the orthopaedic surgeon can inform them that both pathways carry significant risks with approximately only

a 50% incidence of return to work with limb salvage or amputation at 2 years. Both treatment groups have significant disability. The amputation group will require fewer operations but appear to have some increase in disability over the course of 5 to 7 years. Georgiadis et al[59] studied the cost of salvage versus amputation; salvage patients averaged seven surgeries compiling a cost of almost $110,000. There were 3 months (89 days) of hospitalization and three complications per patient. Amputation cases had 1.6 operations, 24 hospital days, and one third the cost of salvage.[60] With salvage or amputation, if patients have not returned to work after 2 years they will not return to work. Final outcome of amputation versus limb salvage appears to be more dependent on patient factors such as substance abuse, smoking, education, and social support systems than on medical/surgical factors.[61,62]

Complications

Infection

Infection after tibial shaft fracture is also a challenging problem. Closed tibial shaft fractures have an infection

Table 30—1 The Mangled Extremity Severity Score (MESS)

Variable	Points
Skeletal or soft tissue Injury	
Low-energy (simple fracture, stab, handgun)	1
Medium energy (open fracture, multiple fractures, dislocation)	2
High-energy (shotgun or rifle, crush injury)	3
Very high energy (above + gross contamination, soft tissue avulsion	4
*Limb Ischemia**	
Reduced or absent pulse but perfused	1
Pulseless, paresthesias, diminished capillary refill	2
Cool, paralyzed, insensate, numb	3
[*score doubled if ischemia time > 6 hours]	
Shock	
Systolic blood pressure always > 90 mm Hg	0
Transient hypotension	1
Persistent hypotension	2
Age	
< 30	0
30–50	1
> 50	2

Source: Adapted with permission from Helfet DL, Howey T, Sanders R, Johansen K. Limb salvage versus amputation: preliminary results of the Mangled Extremity Severity Score. Clin Orthop 1990;256:83.

rate of ~1%, open type I fractures have an infection rate of ~5%, type II of 10%, and type III of 15%. Acute infections, defined as less than 4 weeks, can be managed with initial debridement, wound closure, and suppressive antibiotics, with an expected union rate of 90%.[63] In delayed infections, the surgeon needs to assess whether the implants are stable **(Fig. 30–9)**. Stable implants can be retained and infection controlled with debridement and local or systemic antibiotic administration if adequate soft tissue coverage is present. Implants will need to be removed after union occurs if any signs of deep infection persist. If the implants are loose, implants will need to be removed and the infected area debrided until cultures of the infected area are normal and adequate antibiotic treatment has been given. When signs and symptoms of systemic infection and local infection are controlled, reimplantation and grafting can then occur. The critical principle is that all infected and dead tissue must be debrided at the fracture or infection site. If adequate debridement is obtained, good results have also been shown with immediate reimplantation of hardware, antibiotic administration, and adequate soft tissue coverage with 90 to 95% union and cure.[64]

Anterior Knee Pain Following Intramedullary Fixation

The most common complication following intramedullary nailing of the tibia is anterior knee pain. The etiology of this knee pain is not known. In a prospective, randomized study assessing whether a transpatellar approach versus a peritendinous approach for nail insertion can reduce the incidence of knee pain, Toivanen et al[23] demonstrated no significant difference in anterior knee pain or functional testing following these two approaches, with the reported incidence of knee pain ~70%. Participants in this study had planned staged removal of implants. A late outcome study following treatment of isolated tibial shaft fractures with reamed intramedullary nailing demonstrated a 35% incidence of resting anterior knee pain almost 3 years following fracture fixation.[65] Seventy-one percent of these patients also had difficulty with kneeling. There are no current recommendations on how to prevent this complication. Knee pain does not seem to be related to a prominent nail. Pain is relieved in 50% of patients with nail removal, but 3% of patients felt that their pain was worse after nail removal.[65]

Nonunion

Tibial shaft nonunions occur in ~3% of closed fractures and 5 to 15% of open fractures, depending on the severity of the soft tissue injury.[66] A thorough discussion of treatment and evaluation of nonunions is beyond the scope of this text, but some general principles should be adhered to. The surgeon should decide if the nonunion is due to biological or mechanical difficulties. If a hypertrophic nonunion is present, it is most likely a mechanical issue. Hypertrophic nonunion has approximately an 85 to 90% incidence of union with a closed exchanged intramedullary reaming. A nonunion that has bone loss or appears atrophic will probably need an increase in mechanical stability as well as biological stimulation. An increase in mechanical stability can be obtained with enlarged intramedullary nail or plate fixation, or with Ilizarov thin wire frames. Biological stimulation has classically been performed with iliac crest bone graft. Due to the significant morbidity and potential for complications or long-term pain with iliac crest bone graft, several alternatives have been proposed. Good results have been reported with iliac crest aspirate and demineralized bone matrix as well as with equivalent results of iliac crest autograft with recombinant BMP in nonunions.[52,67–69] If a nonunion is present with bony defect, the surgeon has to decide if a large iliac crest or other bone graft will span the defect. Usually defects up to 5 to 6 cm can obtain a union with bone grafting. Defects greater than that may require bone transport or free fibula vascularized graft placement.

Pearls

- Cast treatment is indicated for closed, transverse, oblique, spiral, or comminuted fractures that are 5 cm away from the proximal or distal joint surface and in fractures that have angulation of less than 5 degrees, translation of less than 50%, shortening of less than 1.2 cm, and rotation within 20 degrees of contralateral side.
- Limited subtalar motion is the most common complication after cast treatment of tibia fracture.
- Weight bearing following cast treatment of a tibial shaft fracture should be immediate. A delay of 6 weeks is associated with delayed union.
- An intact fibula is a relative contraindication to nonoperative treatment of a tibial shaft fracture due to the risk of varus malalignment **(Fig. 30–3A–C).**
- Displaced tibial shaft fractures treated with an intramedullary nail will have a decreased time until union and decreased incidence of malunion compared with cast treatment.
- An open tibia fracture treated with an intramedullary nail has no increased risk of infection rate compared with treatment with an external fixator.
- An open tibia fracture treated with an external fixator is more likely to need more operations and a bone graft to get the fracture to heal and has an increased incidence of malunion.
- Thin wire external fixator wires should be placed below the level of the fibular head to decrease risk of septic arthritis.
- Open tibia fracture infection rates are approximately type I—5%, type II—10%, type III—15%.

- Reamed and unreamed tibial nails have equivalent union rates.
- Blocking screws are placed "where you do not want the nail to go."
- Proximal tibial shaft fractures should have the insertion point for nailing anterior and lateral (lateral tibial eminence landmark).
- Proximal tibial shaft fractures addressed with intramedullary nailing can require the use of reduction tools such as unicortical plating, blocking screws, or pointed reduction clamps.
- Distal tibial shaft fractures addressed with intramedullary nailing can require the use of reduction tools such as fibular plating, pointed reduction clamps, or anteromedial (or anterolateral) Schanz pin placement as a reduction tool.
- A universal distractor or external fixator can assist with fracture reductions in proximal and distal patterns.
- Intramedullary fixation of proximal tibia fractures may have malalignment of 30%.
- Anterior knee pain is the most common complication of nailing tibia fractures.
- Nonunion principles are debridement of nonviable tissue, control infection, fracture stability, bone graft, and durable soft tissue coverage.
- Limb salvage versus amputation is multifactorial and requires input from patient, family, and providers.

On the DVDs

Video 30–1   (Disk 4)   Intramedullary Nailing of a Tibia Fracture   Intramedullary nailing of the tibia is shown using a nail that allows nailing in extension. Placement of the starting point is emphasized.

Video 30–2   (Disk 4)   Anterolateral Percutaneous Plating of a Spiral Distal Tibial Shaft Fracture   This video shows reduction and percutaneous plate fixation of a displaced spiral fracture of the distal

tibial metaphysis. The video emphasizes the use of imaging and percutaneous reduction techniques.

Video 30–3   (Disk 4)   External Fixation of the Tibia   This video shows the application of a uniplanar external fixator to the tibia of a 12-year-old child with an unstable tibia fracture and a compartment syndrome. The fixator was applied after fasciotomies and wound VAC application. The stepwise construction of the frame is shown.

References

1. Court-Brown CM, McBirnie J. The epidemiology of tibial fractures. J Bone Joint Surg Br 1995;77:417–421
2. National Center for Health Statistics. Vital and Health Statistics, Detailed Diagnoses and Procedure, National Hospital Discharge Survey, Series 13, No. 122. Healthcare Cost and Utilization Project, http://www.ahrq.gov/hcupnet/, 2002 data base search for ICD-9-CM codes 823.00–823.92
3. Muller ME, Nazarian S, Koch P, Schatzker J. The Comprehensive Classification of Fractures of Long Bones. New York: Springer-Verlag; 1990
4. Johner R, Wruhs O. Classification of tibial shaft fractures and correlation with results of rigid internal fixation. Clin Orthop Relat Res 1983;178:7–25
5. Orthopedic Trauma Association Committee for Coding and Classification. Fracture and dislocation compendium. J Orthop Trauma 1996;10(suppl):1–154
6. Tscherne H, Rojczyk M. Treatment of closed fractures with soft tissue lesions. Hefte Unfallheilkd 1983;162:39–45
7. Gustilo RB, Anderson JT. Prevention of infection in the treatment of 1025 open fractures of long bones. J Bone Joint Surg Am 1976;58:453–458
8. Gustilo RB, Mendoza RM, Williams DN. Problems in the management of type III (severe) open fractures: a new classification of type III open fractures. J Trauma 1984;24:742–746
9. Sarmiento A, Latta LL. Functional fracture bracing. J Am Acad Orthop Surg 1999;7:66–75

10. Sarmiento A, Gersten LM, Sobol PA, Shankwiler JA, Vangsness CT. Tibial shaft fractures treated with functional braces: experience with 780 fractures. J Bone Joint Surg Br 1989;71:602–609

11. Horne G, Iceton J, Twist J, Malony R. Disability following fractures of the tibial shaft. Orthopedics 1990;13:423–426

12. Heckman JD, Ryaby JP, McCabe J, Frey JJ, Kilcoyne RF. Acceleration of tibial fracture-healing by non-invasive, low-intensity pulsed ultrasound. J Bone Joint Surg Am 1994;76:26–34

13. Kristiansen TK, Ryaby JP, McCabe J, Frey JJ, Roe LR. Accelerated healing of distal radial fractures with the use of specific, low-intensity ultrasound: a multicenter, prospective, randomized, double-blind, placebo-controlled study. J Bone Joint Surg Am 1997; 79:961–973

14. Emami A, Petren-Mallmin M, Larsson S. No effect of low-intensity ultrasound on healing time of intramedullary fixed tibial fractures. J Orthop Trauma 1999;13:252–257

15. Hooper GJ, Keddell RG, Penny ID. Conservative management or closed nailing for tibial shaft fractures. J Bone Joint Surg Br 1991;73:83–85

16. Bone LB, Sucato D, Stegemann PM, Rohrbacher BJ. Displaced isolated fractures of the tibial shaft treated with either a cast or intramedullary nailing: an outcome analysis of matched pairs of patients. J Bone Joint Surg Am 1997;79:1336–1341

17. Lehman WB, Paly D, Atar D. Operating Room Guide to Cross Sectional Anatomy of the Extremities and Pelvis. New York: Raven Press 1989

18. Macnab I, de Haas WG. The role of periosteal blood supply in the healing of fractures of the tibia. Clin Orthop Relat Res 1974;105: 27–34

19. Finkemeier CG, Schmidt AH, Kyle RF, Templeman DC, Varecka TF. A prospective, randomized study of intramedullary nails inserted with and without reaming for the treatment of open and closed fractures of the tibial shaft. J Orthop Trauma 2000;14:187–193

20. Keating JF, O'Brien PJ, Blachut PA, Meek RN, Broekhyse HM. Locking intramedullary nailing with and without reaming for open fracture of the tibial shaft: a prospective, randomized study. J Bone Joint Surg Am 1997;79:334–341

21. Bone LB, Kassman S, Stegemann P, France J. Prospective study of union rate of open tibial fractures treated with locked, unreamed intramedullary nails. J Orthop Trauma 1994;8:45–49

22. Tornetta P III, French BG. Compartment pressures during non-reamed tibial nailing without traction. J Orthop Trauma 1997; 11:24–27

23. Toivanen JA, Vaisto O, Kannus P, Latvala K, Honkonen SE, Jarvinen MJ. Anterior knee pain after intramedullary nailing of fractures of the tibial shaft: a prospective, randomized study comparing two different nail-insertion techniques. J Bone Joint Surg Am 2002; 84:580–585

24. Dogra AS, Ruiz AL, Marsh DR. Late outcome of isolated tibial fractures treated by intramedullary nailing: the correlation between disease-specific and generic outcome measures. J Orthop Trauma 2002;16:245–249

25. Tornetta P III, Riina J, Geller J, Purban W. Intraarticular anatomic risks of tibial nailing. J Orthop Trauma 1999;13:247–251

26. Tornetta P III, Bergman M, Watnik N, Berkowitz G, Steuer J. Treatment of grade-IIIB open tibial fracture: a prospective randomized comparison of external fixation and non-reamed locked nailing. J Bone Joint Surg Br 1994;76:13–19

27. Henley MB, Chapman JR, Agel J, Harvey EJ, Whorton AM, Swiontkowski MF. Treatment of type II, IIIA, and IIIB open fractures of the tibial shaft: a prospective comparison of unreamed interlocking intramedullary nails and half-pin external fixators. J Orthop Trauma 1998;12:1–7

28. Govender S, Csimma C, Genant HK, et al. Recombinant human bone morphogenetic protein-2 for treatment of open tibial fractures: a prospective, controlled, randomized study of four hundred and fifty patients. J Bone Joint Surg Am 2002;84:2123–2134

29. DeLong WG Jr, Born CT, Wei SY, Petrik ME, Ponzio R, Schwab CW. Aggressive treatment of 119 open fracture wounds. J Trauma 1999;46:1049–1054

30. Henry SL, Ostermann PA, Seligson D. The antibiotic bead pouch technique: the management of severe compound fracture. Clin Orthop Relat Res 1993;295:54–62

31. Keating JF, Blachut PA, O'Brien PJ, Meek RN, Broekhuyse H. Reamed nailing of open tibial fractures: does the antibiotic bead pouch reduce the deep infection rate? J Orthop Trauma 1996;10:298–303

32. Steiert AE, Partenheimer A, Schreiber T, et al. The V.A.C. system (vacuum assisted closure) as bridging between primary osteosynthesis in conjunction with functional reconstruction of soft tissue—open fractures type 2 and 3. Zentralbl Chir 2004;129(Suppl 1): S98–S100

33. Bihariesingh VJ, Stolarczyk EM, Karim RB, van Kooten EO. Plastic solutions for orthopaedic problems. Arch Orthop Trauma Surg 2004;124:73–76

34. Krettek C, Miclau T, Schandelmaier P, Stephan C, Mohlmann U, Tscherne H. The mechanical effect of blocking screws ("Poller screws") in stabilizing tibia fractures with short proximal or distal fragments after insertion of small-diameter intramedullary nails. J Orthop Trauma 1999;13:550–553

35. Ricci WM, O'Boyle M, Borrelli J, Bellabarba C, Sanders R. Fractures of the proximal third of the tibial shaft treated with intramedullary nails and blocking screws. J Orthop Trauma 2001;15:264–270

36. Bonnevialle P, Savorit L, Combes JM, Rongieres M, Bellumore Y, Mansat M. Value of intramedullary locked nailing in distal fractures of the tibia. Rev Chir Orthop Reparatrice Appar Mot 1996; 82:428–436

37. Gorczyca JT, McKale J, Pugh K, Pienkowski D. Modified tibial nails for treating distal tibia fractures. J Orthop Trauma 2002;16:18–22

38. Kyro A. Malunion after intramedullary nailing of tibial shaft fractures. Ann Chir Gynaecol 1997;86:56–64

39. Puno RM, Teynor JT, Nagano J, Gustilo RB. Critical analysis of results of treatment of 201 tibial shaft fractures. Clin Orthop Relat Res 1986;212:113–121

40. Richter D, Hahn MP, Laun RA, Ekkernkamp A, Muhr G, Ostermann PA. Ankle para-articular tibial fracture: is osteosynthesis with the unreamed intramedullary nail adequate? [in German] Chirurg 1998;69:563–570

41. Richter D, Ostermann PA, Ekkernkamp A, Hahn MP, Muhr G. Distal tibial fracture: an indication for osteosynthesis with the unreamed intramedullary nail? [in German] Langenbecks Arch Chir Suppl Kongressbd 1997;114:1259–1261

42. Hahn D, Bradbury N, Hartley R, Radford PJ. Intramedullary nail breakage in distal fractures of the tibia. Injury 1996;27:323–327

43. Konrath G, Moed BR, Watson JT, Kaneshiro S, Karges DE, Cramer KE. Intramedullary nailing of unstable diaphyseal fractures of the tibia with distal intraarticular involvement. J Orthop Trauma 1997;11: 200–205

44. Bach AW, Hansen ST Jr. Plates versus external fixation in severe open tibial shaft fractures: a randomized trial. Clin Orthop Relat Res 1989;241:89–94

45. Ruedi T, Webb JK, Allgower M. Experience with the dynamic compression plate (DCP) in 418 recent fractures of the tibial shaft. Injury 1976;7:252–257

46. Collinge C, Sanders RW, DiPasquale T. Treatment of complex tibial periarticular fractures using percutaneous techniques. Clin Orthop Relat Res 2000;375:69–77

47. Lang GJ, Cohen BE, Bosse MJ, Kellam JF. Proximal third tibial shaft fractures: should they be nailed? Clin Orthop Relat Res 1995; 315:64–74

48. Cole PA, Zlowodzki M, Kregor PJ. Treatment of proximal tibia fractures using the less invasive stabilization system: surgical experience and early clinical results in 77 fractures. J Orthop Trauma 2004;18:528–535

49. Cole PA, Zlowodzki M, Kregor PJ. Less Invasive Stabilization System (LISS) for fractures of the proximal tibia: indications, surgical technique and preliminary results of the UMC Clinical Trial. Injury 2003;34(Suppl 1):A16–A29

50. DeCoster TA, Crawford MK, Kraut MA. Safe extracapsular placement of proximal tibia transfixation pins. J Orthop Trauma 2004; 18(Suppl 8):S43–S47

51. Marsh JL, Smith ST, Do TT. External fixation and limited internal fixation for complex fractures of the tibial plateau. J Bone Joint Surg Am 1995;77:661–673

52. Friedlaender GE. Osteogenic protein-1 in treatment of tibial nonunions: current status. Surg Technol Int 2004;13:249–252

53. Gaston P, Will E, Elton RA, McQueen MM, Court-Brown CM. Fractures of the tibia: can their outcome be predicted? J Bone Joint Surg Br 1999;81:71–76

54. Bhandari M, Guyatt GH, Tong D, Adili A, Shaughnessy SG. Reamed versus nonreamed intramedullary nailing of lower extremity long bone fracture: a systematic overview and meta-analysis. J Orthop Trauma 2000;14:2–9

55. Obremskey WT, Medina M. Comparison of intramedullary nailing of distal third tibial shaft fractures: before and after traumatologists. Orthopedics 2004;27:1180–1184

56. Godina M. Early microsurgical reconstruction of complex trauma of the extremities. Plast Reconstr Surg 1986;78:285–292

57. Gopal S, Majumder S, Batchelor AB, Knight SL, DeBoer P, Smith RM. Fix and flap: the radical orthopaedic and plastic treatment of severe open fractures of the tibia. J Bone Joint Surg Br 2000; 82:959–966

58. Helfet DL, Howey T, Sanders R, Johansen K. Limb salvage versus amputation: preliminary results of the Mangled Extremity Severity Score. Clin Orthop Relat Res 1990;256:80–86

59. Georgiadis GM, Behrens FF, Joyce MJ, Earle AS, Simmons AL. Open tibial fracture with severe soft-tissue loss: limb salvage compared with below-the-knee amputation. J Bone Joint Surg Am 1993; 75:1431–1441

60. Bondurant FJ, Cotler HB, Buckle R, Miller-Crotchett P, Browner BD. The medical and economic impact of severely injured lower extremities. J Trauma 1988;28:1270–1273

61. MacKenzie EJ, Bosse MJ, Castillo RC, et al. Functional outcomes following trauma-related lower-extremity amputation. J Bone Joint Surg Am 2004;86:1636–1645

62. Haider AH, Edwin DH, MacKenzie EJ, Bosse MJ, Castillo RC, Travison TG. Lower Extremity Assessment Project Study Group. The use of the NEO-five factor inventory to assess personality in trauma patients: a two-year prospective study. J Orthop Trauma 2002; 16:660–667

63. Court-Brown CM, Keating JF, McQueen MM. Infection after intramedullary nailing of the tibia. Incidence and protocol for management. J Bone Joint Surg Br 1992;74:770–774

64. Swiontkowski MF, Hanel DP, Vedder NB, Schwappach JR. A comparison of short- and long-term intravenous antibiotic therapy in the postoperative management of adult osteomyelitis. J Bone Joint Surg Br 1999;81:1046–1050

65. Keating JF, Orfaly R, O'Brien PJ. Knee pain after tibial nailing. J Orthop Trauma 1997;11:10–13

66. Moore ST, Storts RA, Spencer JD. Fractures of the tibia shaft in adults: a ten year survey of such fractures. South Med J 1962; 55:1178–1183

67. Ziran BH, Smith WR, Zlotolow DA, et al. Clinical evaluation of a true percutaneous technique for antegrade femoral nailing. Orthopedics 2005;28:1182–1186

68. Wang L, Li WS, Zhang QS. Autogenous bone marrow graft for the management of nonunion of tibia. Zhongguo Xiu Fu Chong Jian Wai Ke Za Zhi [Chinese Journal of Reparative & Reconstructive Surgery] 2001;15:24–25

69. Hernigou P, Poignard A, Beaujean F, Rouard H. Percutaneous autologous bone-marrow grafting for nonunions: influence of the number and concentration of progenitor cells. J Bone Joint Surg Am 2005;87:1430–1437

31 Distal Tibia Fractures

Sean E. Nork

Fractures of the distal tibia are among the most difficult injuries facing the orthopaedic traumatologist. Although both extra-articular and intra-articular patterns occur with varying severity, the common concern in all of these injuries is the associated soft tissue injury. Their cause is frequently violent, and associated injuries occur commonly. Multiple approaches have been suggested, but there is no consensus regarding the optimal treatment for these injuries and no long-term outcome measures that define the results of either the injury or the treatment.

Most articular fractures of the distal tibial weight-bearing surface are the result of motor vehicle accidents, falls from heights, motorcycle accidents, and industrial injuries. Ankle fractures are usually the result of indirect mechanisms, whereas the majority of pilon fractures are the result of an axial loading mechanism where the talus is forced cranially and into the distal tibia, thus producing the "explosion" fracture of the articular surface. The position of the foot at the time of impact combined with the direction of the applied force will determine the resultant fracture pattern and articular impaction.

The associated soft tissue injury that occurs is frequently more important than the fracture pattern. These injuries are frequently open, especially on the medial side where the distal tibia is in a subcutaneous location. Swelling occurs rapidly and may be exacerbated by the shortening that occurs. The initial and ultimate treatment decisions should be based more on these associated soft tissue concerns than on the osseous injury. Physical examination of the injured lower extremity should include a careful assessment of the local swelling, perfusion, and neurological deficits. Fracture blisters, local skin necrosis, and impaired distal perfusion are commonly observed. Early limb realignment to relieve skin pressure from the osseous deformity should be performed. In addition, gross or micromotion at the fracture site should be minimized to allow the soft tissue swelling to resolve.

The initial radiographic evaluation consists of standard ankle and tibial radiographs. Computed tomographic (CT) scans should be delayed until limb length has been restored. The value of CT scans in assisting with preoperative planning and fracture understanding has been well demonstrated.[1] Similarly, contralateral ankle radiographs are frequently helpful in understanding the unique morphological variations in the distal tibial anatomy and assist with preoperative planning.

Classification

The classification of Rüedi and Allgower is moderately useful and is divided into three types:[2] type I fractures are nondisplaced, type II fractures are characterized by articular displacement, and type III fractures have associated articular comminution and impaction **(Fig. 31–1).** The Arbeitsgemeinschaft für Osteosynthesefragen/ Orthopaedic Trauma Association (AO/OTA) classification incorporates all fractures of the distal tibia, including extra-articular injuries of the distal tibial metaphysis **(Fig. 31–2).**[3] This classification system is much more detailed, describes comminution at multiple levels, and differentiates between partial and complete articular injuries. Similar to other periarticular fractures described by the AO/ OTA classification system, an A-type fracture is extra-articular, a B-type fracture has partial articular involvement, and a C-type fracture has complete (or severe) involvement of the articular surface. However, the reproducibility and usefulness of this classification system have been questioned. Martin et al found better interobserver reliability when classifying fractures into major types with the AO/OTA system (kappa = 0.60) than with that of Rüedi and Allgower (kappa = 0.46).[4] Agreement at the group level with the AO system remained poor (kappa = 0.38).[4] Similar trends were noted when evaluating intraobserver reliability.[4] Swiontkowski et al demonstrated that only moderate agreement (kappa = 0.41 to 0.60) existed with the AO/OTA system, and that determination of the fracture type alone (type A, B, or C) was probably adequate for clinical research.[5] However, for the purposes of describing these injuries and formulating a surgical plan, the fracture group (e.g., C1, C2, or C3) can be helpful.

Nonoperative Treatment

Nonoperative management of distal tibial fractures is recommended only for truly nondisplaced fractures or fractures in patients that have an absolute contraindication for surgical management. Such injuries can be effectively managed with closed reduction and cast immobilization followed by progressive weight bearing and ankle range of motion as radiographic healing progresses. The indications for nonoperative management of displaced, articular tibial pilon fractures are extremely limited. Casting is ineffective in reducing any displaced articular segments, and distraction across a shortened ankle joint is not feasible with this treatment method.

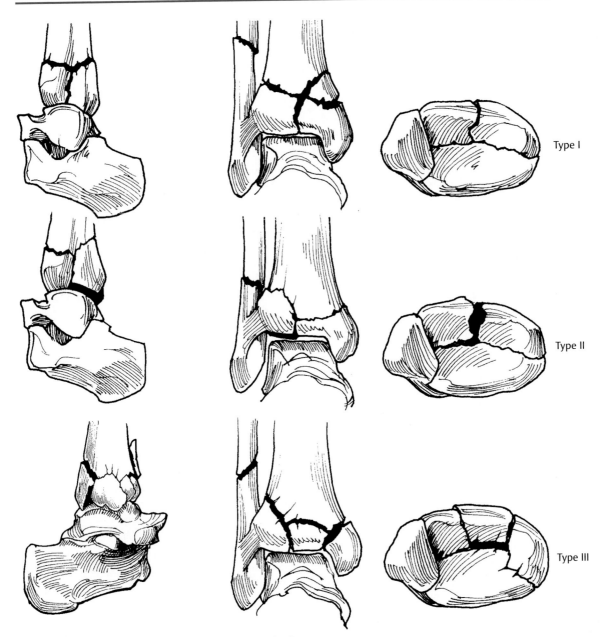

Type I

Type II

Type III

Figure 31–1 The Rüedi and Allgower classification of pilon fractures.

For example, in displaced partial articular injuries (type 43B) of the distal tibia, nonoperative management is ineffective in reducing the displaced fragment in the majority of these injuries. The articular impaction that is frequently associated with these injuries does not respond to ligamentotaxis and will therefore not be reduced with closed methods. Similarly, in displaced complete articular fractures (type 43C), closed methods are ineffective in accurately reducing the articular segments. In the case of an intact fibula associated with a complete articular distal tibial fracture, varus angulation commonly occurs, and closed methods must counteract this tendency. In similar complete articular distal tibial fractures *with* an associated fibular fracture, shortening is expected with associated widening of the joint.

Bedridden patients, paraplegics, and patients with significant medical comorbidities precluding a prolonged anesthetic are all candidates for nonoperative treatment. Casting of pilon fractures has the distinct disadvantage of inhibiting the necessary and ongoing soft tissue evaluations required in management. Other closed methods such as calcaneal traction may allow serial soft tissue evaluations and provide some joint distraction and ligamentotaxis, but patient compliance and prolonged bed rest are required. Alternatively, an ankle joint spanning external fixator (described later) may be used to provide some stability to the fracture.

Significant joint stiffness is expected after the closed treatment of pilon fractures because healing in an acceptable position requires prolonged joint immobilization.

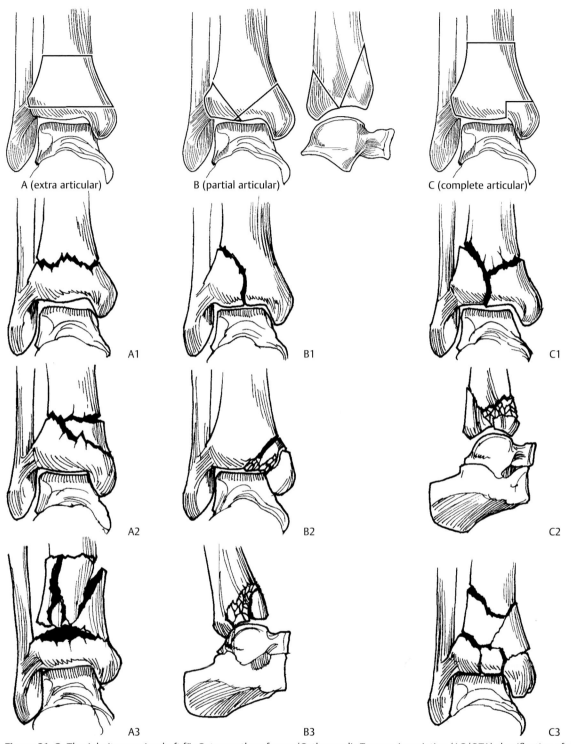

A (extra articular)   B (partial articular)   C (complete articular)

A1   B1   C1

A2   B2   C2

A3   B3   C3

Figure 31–2 The Arbeitsgemeinschaft für Osteosynthesefragen/Orthopaedic Trauma Association (AO/OTA) classification of pilon fractures. The distal tibial fracture would be designated at "4.3" (e.g., 43–C2) injury, followed by the type and group classification above.

Weight bearing and ankle range of motion exercises should be delayed until there is radiographic evidence of healing, frequently requiring at least 12 weeks. Thereafter, progressive weight bearing and mobilization can proceed based upon the patient's comfort in applicable cases.

Indications for Surgical Treatment

The indications for surgical treatment are based on the combination of fracture location, fracture pattern, and the associated soft tissue injury. The presence of open wounds, a failure to obtain or maintain adequate alignment, and other extremity injuries are among the indications for operative fixation. Displaced or unstable extra-articular distal metaphyseal fractures can be effectively treated with several surgical techniques, including external fixation, open reduction and plate fixation, percutaneous reduction and minimally invasive plate fixation, medullary nailing, or combinations thereof. The condition of the surrounding soft tissues should help direct the choice of treatment, each of which has its own certain advantages.

Articular incongruity and talar subluxation are poorly tolerated at the tibiotalar joint. Although there are no strict guidelines for determining how much articular step-off or gap can be tolerated, a visible incongruity at the tibial plafond that is demonstrated on plain radiographs should be considered an indication for operative reduction and fixation in properly selected patients. Nondisplaced fractures may similarly require operative fixation if early motion of the ankle is desired.

Surgical Treatment (see Videos 31–1, 31–2, 31–3, 31–4, 31–5, Disk 4)

General Approach to Open Reduction and Internal Fixation

After evaluating the patient, fracture characteristics, and the integrity of the soft tissue envelope, operative fixation of a pilon fracture can proceed. The overall treatment approach typically consists of a staged protocol with primary restoration of tibial length followed by a delayed reconstruction of the articular surface.[6,7] The basic principles outlined by Rüedi and Allgower over 20 years ago continue to direct our treatment of these injuries.[8] These four sequential principles as originally described consisted of reconstruction of the correct fibular length, anatomical reconstruction of the tibial articular surface, bone grafting of defects, and stable fixation of the fragments by medial buttress plating. Although some flexibility in treatment is important in these injuries, these tenets remain a good starting point during the formulation of an operative strategy. A combination of newer surgical techniques emphasizing meticulous soft tissue handling, limited approaches, and low-profile periarticular implants have allowed for avoidance of the common soft tissue problems that followed medial plating historically.

Surgical Anatomy

The relevant surgical anatomy for the fixation of tibial pilon fractures includes osseous, ligamentous, muscular, and neurovascular structures. Because of the complexity of these injuries, multiple surgical approaches are frequently required. Therefore, a thorough understanding of each approach and the associated anatomical structures is necessary to properly care for these injuries. The most frequent approaches

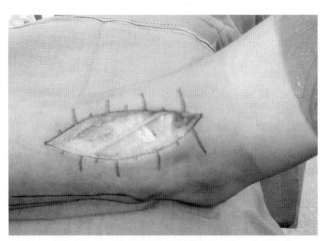

Figure 31–3 Clinical photograph of the superficial peroneal nerve over the fascia in the anterolateral approach.

used include the anterolateral, anterior, anteromedial, posteromedial, and posterolateral. Direct medial approaches to the distal tibia, because of the subcutaneous nature of the bone in that location, are associated with an unacceptably high rate of soft tissue complications, should be avoided, and will not be discussed in this chapter.

An understanding of the basic muscular and tendinous anatomy about the distal tibia and ankle joint is necessary to allow for uncomplicated approaches and dissections in safe planes. The anterior tibial compartment contains, from medial to lateral, the tibialis anterior, the extensor hallucis longus (EHL), the extensor digitorum communis (EDC), and the peroneus tertius. These muscles are all innervated by branches from the peroneal nerve proximally in the leg, enabling distal approaches that are medial, lateral, and between these muscles. The deep peroneal nerve and the anterior tibial vessels are located between the EHL and EDC distally, requiring direct identification and protection in the direct anterior approach. The superficial peroneal nerve is purely sensory and travels from posterior to anterior, crossing the anterolateral surgical incision (**Fig. 31–3**). The peroneal muscles (longus and brevis) occupy the lateral compartment of the leg, have a distal muscle belly posteriorly, and are firmly attached at the distal fibula by the peroneal sheath. The deep posterior compartment muscles are largely tendinous at the level of the ankle joint and include the posterior tibial, the flexor digitorum communis, and the flexor hallucis longus (FHL). The FHL has a very distal muscle belly, and its identification is especially useful in the posterolateral approach to the distal tibia. The gastrocnemius and soleus muscles have a common tendinous insertion at the level of the ankle joint, and their tendon sheath requires protection in any posterior approaches. The tibial nerve and the associated vascular supply posteriorly require protection and identification during posteromedial surgical exposures (**Fig. 31–4**).

An understanding of the ligamentous attachments at the ankle joint is particularly useful when considering

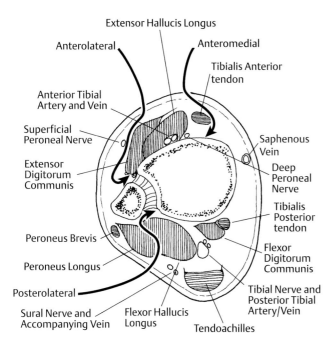

Figure 31–4 The cross-sectional anatomy of the distal tibia demonstrating the relevant neurovascular structures and their relationship to the surgical approaches.

displacement patterns and planes of safe surgical dissection. Frequently, the important ligaments of the ankle remain largely intact after a pilon fracture, producing the commonly observed major fracture segments consisting of the posterolateral (Volkmann's) fragment, the anterolateral (Chaput) fragment, and the medial fragment. As the complexity increases, the number of fragments and the associated comminution increase. However, these three major fragments are observed as a component of most C-type tibial pilon fractures. These fragments typically retain connections with portions of the deltoid (medial fragment or malleolar segment), anterior tibiofibular (Chaput segment), and posterior tibiofibular ligaments (Volkmann's segment). Any surgical approach chosen should respect any remaining ligamentous attachments to these structures.

The relevant osseous anatomy of the tibial pilon includes the distal tibia, the distal fibula, and the talus. The fibula extends distally relative to the tibia, and is firmly attached by the anterior and posterior tibiofibular ligaments. This becomes most relevant when considering a treatment strategy for accurately reducing the tibial articular surface. Any change in either the length or the rotation of the distal fibula will be reflected in the anterolateral and posterolateral segments of the distal tibia. Similarly, because of the intimate articulation between the tibia and fibula at the distal tibiofibular joint, angular deformity of the distal fibula in any plane will have implications on the tibial reduction. The distal tibial articular surface is centrally concave with associated posterior and anterior extensions.

The posterior tibial articular surface extends more distally, making a posterior arthrotomy for joint inspection impractical. Although the anterior tibia extends over the dome of the talus, the entire articular surface of the tibia can be viewed from any of the anteriorly based approaches. The relevant anatomy of the talus includes an understanding of the nonarticular portions because these can be used for placement of Schanz pins that are useful in distraction across the ankle joint. Laterally, there is significantly more room available at the talar neck than on the medial side.

The combination of fracture pattern, associated soft tissue condition, open wounds, patient comorbidities, and surgeon comfort determines the surgical approach(es) to be used. Open wounds may or may not be extended as a component of the surgical approach. Frequently, the soft tissues are the most traumatized over the distal tibia and avoidance of incisions in this region may prove prudent. One of the most important factors in choosing the appropriate surgical approach for a given injury is the location of the fracture lines and the associated comminution.[9,10] The most frequently used approaches for articular injuries are the anterolateral and the anteromedial.

Surgical Approaches and Techniques

Urgent Management Including Open Fracture Treatment

The initial surgical management of tibial pilon fractures requires planning for subsequent procedures based on the injury pattern, associated open wounds, and soft tissue swelling. If open reduction is anticipated, reestablishment of the length of the tibia and fibula is necessary. This assists with resolution of soft tissue swelling, and it also ensures that the definitive open reduction will not require an acute intraoperative limb lengthening.

Fibular fixation (if fractured) is a necessary component of the initial surgical management for three reasons. First, an accurate reestablishment of the proper fibular length and rotation indirectly reduces the tibia due to the strong ligamentous attachments, as already noted. Second, this provides a stable lateral column that a medially based external fixator can be tensioned against to correct any persistent shortening and angulation of the tibia. Third, and most importantly, an accurate fibular reduction maximally reduces the posterolateral tibial articular segment through the posterior tibiofibular ligaments, facilitating later open reduction. The surgical approach for fixation of the fibula should be in a posterolateral location, posterior to the palpable back border of the fibula. This allows for the use of this same incision if a posterolateral approach to the tibia is later chosen, and increases the soft tissue bridge if an anterolateral exposure is required for tibial fixation. Additionally, a posterolateral incision is not located directly over the subcutaneous fibula, helping to minimize wound complications in this location. Fibular fixation is dependent on the location and the mode of failure. Transverse fractures at the ankle joint line are the result of tension forces on the fibula. Conversely, comminuted or wedge fractures proximal to the ankle joint line are typical of valgus overload compressive fractures. The majority of fibular fractures can be treated with a direct open reduction. In some highly comminuted fibular fracture patterns that are not amenable to direct reduction techniques, indirect reduction of the fibula is accomplished. In these instances, no attempt is made to reduce every small cortical fragment, but simply to correct length, rotation, and angulation of the distal fibula. The importance of an accurate reduction of the fibula cannot be overemphasized. Indirect techniques to regain length may be necessary, especially in high-energy pilon fractures with significant shortening and soft tissue swelling. Useful techniques in difficult or comminuted cases include preliminary application of a medial (tibia to calcaneus) external fixator or femoral distractor to regain length, distal fibular plate fixation with application of a proximal push screw to regain length, and application of a small distractor directly to the fibula (**Fig. 31–5A,B**). Precontoured plates may be helpful in a minority of extremely difficult cases because the distal rotation of the fibula can make straight plate applications difficult.

A variety of configurations for ankle-spanning temporary external fixation have been described and work effectively (see **Video 31–1, Disk 4**). Some important principles include placement of all pins remote from any anticipated surgical incisions, avoidance of pin placements into the talus if any anterior exposure is planned, and pin placement into subcutaneous locations to minimize pin site irritation and drainage. Additionally, the external fixator should maintain the foot out of plantar flexion in a neutral position (**Fig. 31–5A,B**). One successful strategy involves construction of a medial triangular external fixator that relies on an intact or plated fibula, against which tension can be applied. The anticipated pin locations are at the medial tuberosity of the calcaneus, transversely in the midfoot into the cuneiforms, and at the anteromedial face of the tibia (two pins) proximal to any subsequent plate applications. After placement of the proximal 5 mm bicortical tibial pin (perpendicular to the anteromedial face of the tibia) and the 5 mm calcaneal tuberosity pin (parallel to the distal tibial coronal plane articular surface), length and coronal alignment can be obtained. Often, even when the fibula is "out to length," the medial column is still short. This can be corrected via

- Manual traction, distracting between the proximal tibial and distal calcaneal pin
- Use of the articulating distractor-compressor clamp, which can aid in gaining length in a controlled manner (**Fig. 31–6**)

During provisional external fixation, the sagittal plane translational and angulatory deformities of the lower leg can also be improved with strategically placed bumps (beneath either the foot or the leg). A 4 mm pin placed transversely across the midfoot from medial to lateral in the cuneiforms is attached to the proximal tibial pin and maintains the foot in a neutral position. Finally, an additional pin is placed into the anteromedial face of the tibia to prevent rotation around the proximal pin. The talus should be accurately reduced and centered in line with the central axis of the tibia (**Fig. 31–7A–C**).

An alternative external fixation scheme involves the use of a centrally threaded 5 mm pin at the calcaneus.

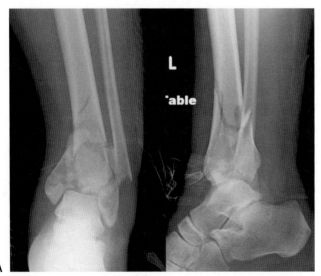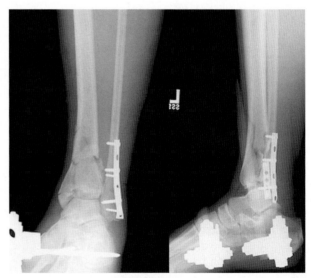

A   B

Figure 31–5 External fixation combined with open reduction and internal fixation (ORIF) of a fibular fracture. **(A)** Injury films. **(B)** Radiographs after fibular plating and spanning external fixation. Note the critical location of the pins for the external fixator. If ORIF of the tibial articular surface is anticipated, pins should be placed away from any planned surgical incisions and plate locations (the proximal tibial pins are so high they are not seen in this x-ray). Pins into the talus should similarly be avoided because all anterior approaches involve some exposure of the talar neck. In this example the distal pins were inserted into the calcaneus and first metatarsal.

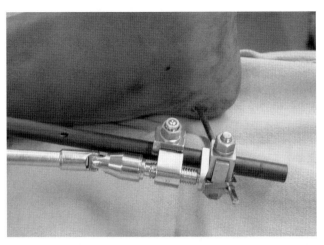

Figure 31–6 The articulating distractor-compressor clamp can be used to regain length with a standard external fixator.

Excellent control of the alignment of the foot in all planes can be obtained by attaching rods to both sides of the foot using a long pin placed through the calcaneal tuberosity. This frame configuration is especially useful in patients who are treated late (and require bilateral distraction to regain length) and in those injuries where the fibula cannot be fixed at the initial operative procedure. Stabilization of either or both the midfoot and the forefoot is still required to maintain the foot in neutral dorsiflexion.

Open fractures require careful preoperative planning about the placement of incisions for the surgical extension of open wounds to allow an adequate debridement. Most commonly, associated open wounds are located medially. If the open wound is small, an anticipated surgical approach, even if completely remote from the open wound, can be used for the initial irrigation and debridement. If

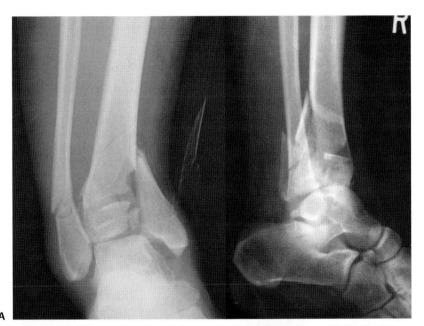

A

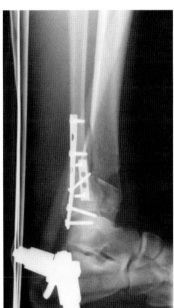

B

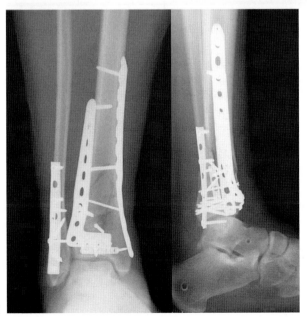

C

Figure 31–7 A closed 43-C3 pilon fracture. **(A)** Injury radiographs demonstrate comminution, varus deformity, and anterior translation of the talus relative to the tibia. **(B)** Following fibular fixation and placement of an ankle-spanning external fixator, the talus is well centered under the tibia on the lateral view. **(C)** An anterolateral approach was used to reduce this fracture. Given the varus and anterior comminution, an anterior plate with screw fixation from anterior to posterior was combined with a medial buttressing plate.

the open wound is large, proximal and distal extensions over the anteromedial face of the distal tibia should be avoided whenever possible. Consistent with the traditional principles of open fracture management, completely devitalized cortical (diaphyseal) fragments require removal. However, every effort should be made to retain all articular segments, irrespective of the soft tissue attachments. If a defect exists after debridement, consideration should be given to placement of antibiotic beads until the time of definitive fixation.

There are situations in which primary definitive fixation of an open pilon fracture may be performed **(Fig. 31–8A–C).** In these cases, clamp application, fracture reduction, articular lag screw fixation, and plate application are all accomplished through the open wound without additional soft tissue stripping. However, the prerequisites of such an approach include

- A complete understanding of the injury, the fracture pattern, and the associated articular involvement
- Confidence that a thorough debridement of the open injury has been done in a timely manner
- An understanding of the techniques through which the surgeon can reduce and internally fix portions of the injury with "minimally invasive" methods
- A well-rested and appropriate surgical team

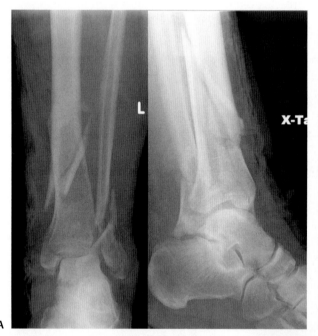

A

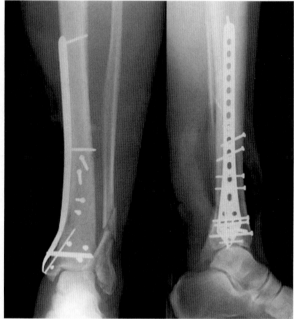

B

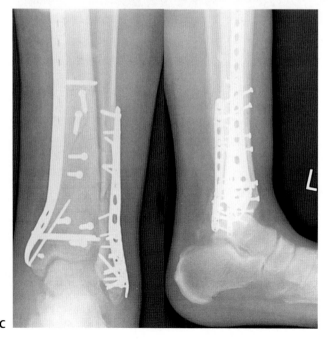

C

Figure 31–8 An open distal tibia fracture with a relatively simple articular injury but with a complex distal fibular fracture. **(A)** Anteroposterior and lateral radiographs of the injury. **(B)** There was a large medial wound that gave direct exposure of the distal tibia as well as the articular surface. The open wound was exploited on the day of injury, allowing fixation of the extra-articular and intra-articular fractures of the tibia. **(C)** The fibula was fixed at a later date when a longer operative procedure could be performed.

If any of these prerequisites for this approach are not met, then a staged protocol consisting of primary fibular plating and external fixation across the ankle joint combined with further debridement and wound closure at a secondary procedure is indicated.

Preoperative Planning

The formulation of a cogent preoperative surgical plan begins with the evaluation of the injury films. Several factors contribute to increasing complexity in these injuries and include proximal fracture extensions, multiple articular fragments, impacted segments, bone loss, and osteopenia. The injury radiographs should be evaluated to determine the primary deformity pattern because this determines the final fixation construct and hence the surgical approach(es) necessary. For example, if the original injury film demonstrates significant varus angulation of the distal tibia, a medial buttressing implant is likely indicated to counteract the inherent tendency for this injury to fail back into varus. Review of the fibular fracture characteristics, combined with the coronal plane angulation of the tibia, provides visual clues regarding the areas of compression and tension failure. Occasionally, the injury radiographs demonstrate a purely axial failure of the tibia with or without fibular failure. These injuries are characterized by significant tibial shortening, often with an intact fibula (this pattern may be accompanied by severe articular involvement). The more commonly observed fracture combinations are varus angulation of the tibia combined with tension failure of the fibula, and valgus angulation of the tibia combined with compressive failure of the fibula. Consideration of tension versus compression failure has implications from a biomechanical standpoint when fixation is considered. Buttress plating is frequently required on the compression failure side, especially if bone contact after reduction is compromised due to cortical impaction. Conversely, large implants are rarely needed to support cortical bone that has failed in tension if the compression failure side has been supported.

CT is essential for the evaluation of the injuries. However, if a staged protocol for fixation is planned (immediate fibular stabilization and ankle spanning external fixation followed by definitive internal fixation as the soft tissue swelling permits), these scans should be delayed until after spanning external fixation has been applied to regain limb length. An exception to this is the situation where the surgeon wishes to internally fix the "simple" articular injury through the traumatic open wound as already noted. CT scans obtained with the extremity in its initial shortened position are frequently of low value due to significant displacement of the fracture fragments and talar shortening. If scans are inadvertently obtained prior to reestablishment of tibial length, they frequently need to be repeated because the overall position of the fragments changes significantly. The axial images are the most useful and provide identification of the major articular fragments,

Table 31—1   Equipment Used for Open Reduction and Internal Fixation of Pilon Fractures

Medium femoral distractor (used to distract between the talus and midshaft of the tibia to allow visualization of the distal tibial articular surface)

Dental picks

Large pointed reduction clamps

Medium pointed reduction clamps

Small pointed reduction clamps

Kirschner wires of varying sizes

2.5 mm terminally threaded pins as joysticks

Small-fragment screws (2.7 and 3.5 mm; with long lengths, e.g., 60–80 mm)

Mini-fragment screws (2.0 and 2.4 mm; with long lengths, e.g., 40 mm)

Headlight to visualize the articular surface

Multiple plates consistent with the screws and preoperative plan

Bone tamps

Allograft bone chips (as necessary) versus a bone graft substitute

cephalad articular impaction, and regions of comminution and fragmentation. The sagittal and coronal reformations provide additional data, especially for identifying impacted segments that are rotated relative to the axial images.

After identification of all the fracture fragments on the CT scan, the findings can be correlated with the findings of the plain radiographs obtained after length has been reestablished. The surgical incisions and implants can then be planned based on the data obtained from the CT scan(s) and the injury radiographs. This should include consideration of the primary failure mode and the translational and angular deformities of the distal tibia (e.g., varus or valgus; anterior translation of the talus relative to the tibial plafond). Locking plates are of minimal use in most distal tibial pilon fractures. However, in cases of severe metaphyseal impact, metaphyseal bone loss, or osteopenia, there may be a role for these implants. Regardless of whether locked plates are used, compression of the articular surface with lag screws (either independently or through a plate) should be performed. For the vast majority of articular fractures unlocked plates combined with screws provide adequate support. A variety of instruments are helpful for reduction and fixation of pilon fractures (**Table 31–1**).

Tourniquet Use

The use of a tourniquet in articular fractures of the distal tibia is not optional but preferred in most circumstances. Limb exsanguination and tourniquet application assist with visualization within a bloodless field. Following the articular reduction, use of the tourniquet can be discontinued. Typically, a low pressure (200 mm Hg) is used to minimize tissue ischemia.

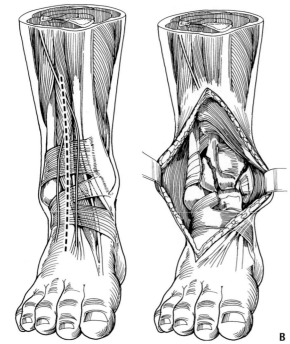

A   **B**

Figure 31–9 (A) The anterolateral approach is useful for fixation of many tibial pilon fractures. The incision is a modification of Bohler's approach and is in line with the fourth metatarsal, extending proximally between the tibia and the fibula. **(B)** The superficial peroneal nerve invariably crosses the surgical incision. The entire anterior compartment musculature can be dissected and retracted from lateral to medial. The exposure of the talar neck allows intraoperative placement of a femoral distractor to improve joint visualization.

Anterolateral Approach for Reduction of Tibial Pilon Fractures

The anterolateral approach **(Fig. 31–9A,B)** is useful in the majority of complete articular (type 43C) pilon fractures, anterior and anterolateral partial articular (type 43B) pilon fractures, and some extra-articular distal tibial fractures that can be stabilized with a plate slid beneath the anterior compartment **(Fig. 31–10A–D)**. The anterolateral approach has the advantage of excellent visualization of the articular surface to the medial shoulder of the ankle while avoiding dissection of the anteromedial tibial face. Impaction at the medial shoulder is difficult to reduce with this exposure. Proximal extension of the incision is limited as well. The approach facilitates accurate articular reduction combined with submuscular and subcutaneous plate applications spanning the metaphyseal comminution.

The patient is positioned supine on a radiolucent operating table extension with the foot brought to the end of the table. A bump consisting of a single rolled blanket placed beneath the ipsilateral hip will assist with positioning the leg in neutral rotation. After the administration of the appropriate antibiotics, the osseous anatomy of the ankle joint is marked with a pen to identify the surgical approach. This incision is centered at the ankle joint, parallel to the fourth metatarsal distally, and parallel to and be-

tween the tibia and fibula proximally **(Fig. 31–11)**. Because of the origin of the anterior compartment muscles from the anterior fibula, proximal extension more than 7 cm from the ankle joint is usually not performed. Distally, the incision terminates slightly distal to the predicted location of the talonavicular joint.

Dissection through the skin and subcutaneous tissues should proceed sharply, with maintenance of full-thickness skin flaps. The superficial peroneal nerve invariably crosses the surgical incision proximal to the ankle joint and should be identified, mobilized, and protected throughout the surgical procedure **(Fig. 31–3)**. The fascia over the anterior compartment of the distal tibia is then incised sharply, beneath the superficial peroneal nerve. Distally, the extensor retinaculum is incised, and the anterior compartment tendons are all retracted medially. The entire anterior compartment musculature, including the peroneus tertius, can then be mobilized and retracted medially. These muscles and tendons are usually easy to mobilize from the underlying anterior tibiofibular ligament, the periosteum of the distal tibia, and the joint capsule. Exposure to the level of the medial shoulder of the distal tibia is possible **(Fig. 31–12)**. Proximally, the dissection is limited to the origin of the anterior compartment muscles from the fibula and the interosseous membrane. Distally, the tendons are retracted medially. The fascia of the extensor digitorum brevis can be incised, with the muscle carefully dissected and retracted medially. This allows exposure of the talar neck for pin placement and femoral distractor application. An arthrotomy can then be performed. The identification (consistent with the preoperative plan) of the proper location for the arthrotomy is critical to avoid unnecessary and damaging devascularization of the distal tibia. The location of the arthrotomy should be at or close to the fracture line separating the anterolateral fracture fragment. Under no circumstances should the anterior tibiofibular ligament be surgically incised. The arthrotomy can be extended distally onto the talar neck. Elevation of the capsule from the anterior distal tibia will allow inspection of the articular segments(s).

Application of a femoral distractor intraoperatively greatly assists with the articular visualization **(Fig. 31–12)**. The previously placed pins for an ankle-spanning external fixator are typically located medially and are of no use for intraoperative distraction. A 4 mm Schanz pin can be placed transversely at the talar neck through the surgical incision. A second 4 mm Schanz pin can then be placed laterally at the tibia, proximal to the anticipated plate application. The location of the anterior compartment neurovascular bundle and the superficial peroneal nerve should be considered during this pin placement, and thus the pin should be placed in the anterior 50% of the tibia. A small distractor can then be applied with the threaded rod located posterolaterally. This will produce distraction across the ankle joint (and not the subtalar joint) combined with plantar flexion because the talar neck is anterior to the axis of rotation of the talus.

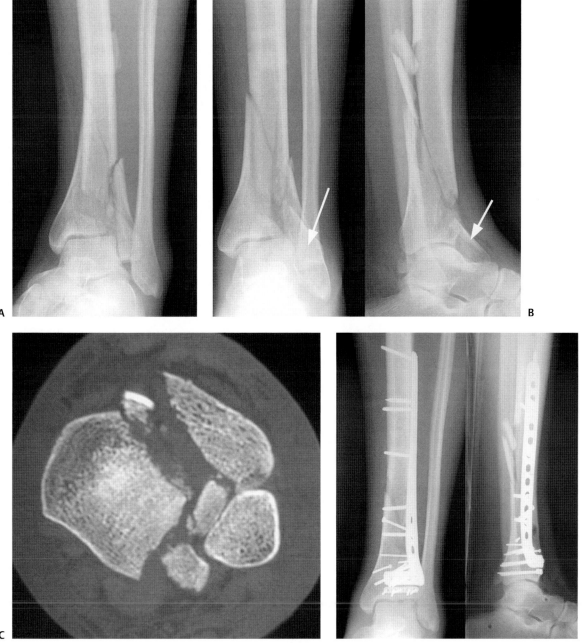

Figure 31–10 Example of a high-energy pilon fracture. **(A)** On initial inspection of the radiographs, the relationship between the talus and the majority of the distal tibial articular surface is relatively normal. **(B)** However, the significant shortening of the talus relative to the intact fibula confirms that the talus should be located distal to the an-

terolateral fragment (arrows). **(C)** The computed tomographic (CT) scan demonstrates the anterolateral fragment and the lateral comminution. **(D)** This fracture pattern is ideally suited for an anterolateral approach with direct visualization of the articular surface and submuscular placement of an anterolateral plate.

Reduction typically proceeds from posterolateral to posteromedial to central to anterior to anterolateral **(Fig. 31–13A–F)**. Because the rotation of the entire articular segment in the sagittal plane will not be known until the final reduction maneuver (i.e., reduction of the anterolateral segment to the remaining reduced articular segments), it is not uncommon for a second (or third) reduction attempt to be required. Typically, an increase in the plantar flexion of the posterior segments is required to correct the commonly observed dorsiflexion deformity of the posterolateral

segment. To proceed with the articular reduction, removal of all hematoma, debris, and early callus is required. The anterolateral segment can be externally rotated on its ligamentous attachment, facilitating exposure into the joint and cancellous surfaces of the metaphysis. Any intercalary anterior cortical fragments and central osteochondral fragments should be retained. The cancellous surface of the medial and posterolateral fragments should be cleaned. This includes cleaning proximally into the interface between the posterolateral segment and the intact tibia to allow mo-

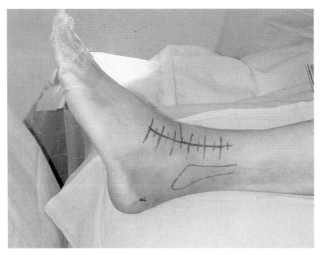

Figure 31–11 Clinical photograph showing the anterolateral approach outlined on the patient with an operative marking pin. The distal fibula is outlined as is the level of ankle joint line. The incision is parallel to the fourth ray of the foot and extends proximally between the tibia and fibula.

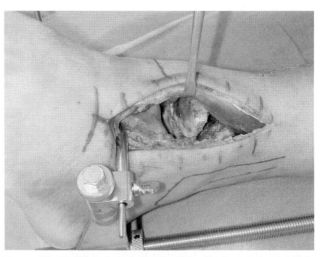

Figure 31–12 Clinical photograph of the final exposure possible through the anterolateral approach. Note the femoral distractor that has been used in this case with a pin in the talus to distract the ankle and facilitate reduction of the articular surface.

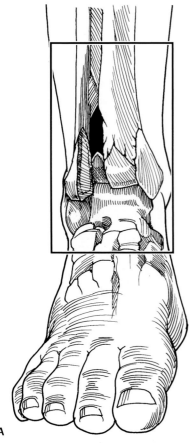

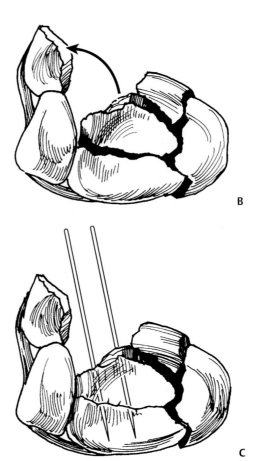

Figure 31–13 (A–F) The joint reduction typically proceeds from posterolateral to medial to anterolateral. The AP schematic shows the major fragment fragments **(A)**. By externally rotating the anterolateral on its ligamentous attachment (laterally), the posterolateral fragment can be viewed, as can any central impaction **(B)**. In this example, the centrally impacted segment is first reduced to the posterolateral segment and held with multiple wires **(C)**. The posterolateral fragment is reduced to the medial segment and held with additional wires. The original wires placed from anterior to posterior are replaced with medial to lateral wires to allow the reduction of the anterior and anterolateral segments **(D)**. The anterior and anterolateral segments are then reduced and stabilized with wires, allowing removal of some of the previously placed wires **(E)**. Finally, plates and screws can be used to fix the pilon fracture, allowing removal of the temporary wires **(F)**.

bilization of this fragment. If a large posterior spike is present, the posterolateral articular segment can be reduced to the intact tibia and held with K-wires placed percutaneously and obliquely from the anterior tibia. Control of the posterolateral segment can be difficult yet facilitated with a joystick placed directly into the anteriorly facing cancellous surface. Additionally, a large, pointed reduction clamp (Weber clamp) can be placed behind the fibula but anterior to the peroneal tendons. This can be placed either through a small posterolateral incision or though a small opening in the posterolateral approach used for plating the fibula (if applicable). One tine of the clamp is applied to the posterolateral tibial articular segment, and the other tine is applied to the anterior tibia.

Reduction then proceeds to the medial segment, which can be reduced using the sagittally oriented articular fracture line located posteromedially. After K-wire stabilization of this reduction, the centrally impacted segments and osteochondral fragments can then be reduced. Dental picks and K-wires (as joysticks) are helpful during this portion of the reduction. These fragments can be temporarily stabilized with K-wires strategically placed (from lateral or medial) to allow for reduction of the anterior articular segments. If an anatomical reduction between these fragments and the posterior pilon is confidently obtained, intraosseous

lag screws can be placed from anterior to posterior. Small screws (2.0 to 2.7 mm) are recommended to allow adequate space for other screws in the distal articular segment. Finally, the anterolateral segment is reduced to the remaining distal tibia. There is frequently a bony spike extending proximally from the anterolateral segment that can be reduced to its corresponding defect in the tibial shaft, ensuring that the rotation and length of this segment are correct. The outer cortex of the anterolateral segment should accurately match the cortical contour of the medial segment, and all intra-articular fracture lines should be reduced anatomically. Any inaccuracies should be corrected at this time. Any anterior distal tibial cortical fragments (whether vascularized or not) should be replaced to ensure an accurate overall reconstruction of the anterior tibial length. The anterolateral segment can frequently be clamped to the medial segment for added stability. The overall reduction can then be confirmed both visually and fluoroscopically if desired.

An alternative reduction strategy includes leaving all impacted central chondral and osteochondral fragments in their native (albeit malreduced) position while the remaining reductions are accomplished (posterolateral to medial to anterolateral). A small cortical window proximally can then be used to reduce the centrally impacted segments while the joint is viewed from below.

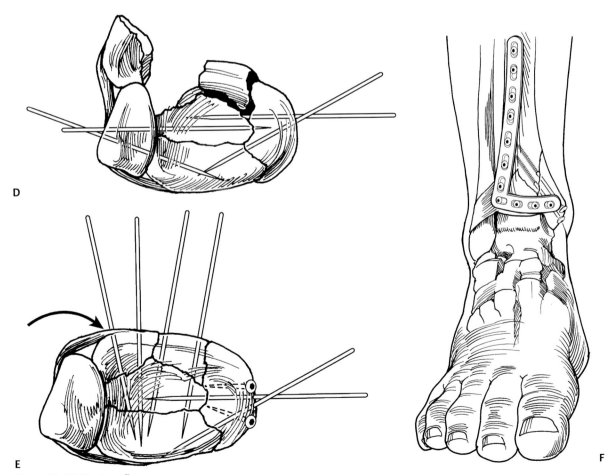

D

E

F

Figure 31–13 (Continued)

A fixation strategy should follow a carefully constructed preoperative plan (**Fig. 31–14A–D**). The goals of fixation should include interfragmentary compression of any articular components combined with stabilization of the articular segment to the tibial diaphysis. The required rigidity of these implants is dependent on the amount of cortical contact, the bone quality, the direction of the initial failure of the distal tibia (varus vs valgus), the presence of any associated bone loss or open wounds, the length of metaphyseal comminution, and the size of the distal articular segment. Small articular segments with extensive meta-

physeal comminution are particularly problematic. Plates can be placed either submuscularly along the anterolateral tibia through the anterolateral incision or subcutaneously along the anteromedial tibia though a small distal incision. Prior to placing a plate along the lateral cortex of the tibia, the femoral distractor frequently must be removed. Either the leading edge of the plate or a small elevator can be used to dissect the anterior compartment muscles from the lateral tibia. Final sagittal plane translational corrections can be accomplished prior to fixation through the plate. Distal fixation requires strategic placement to avoid

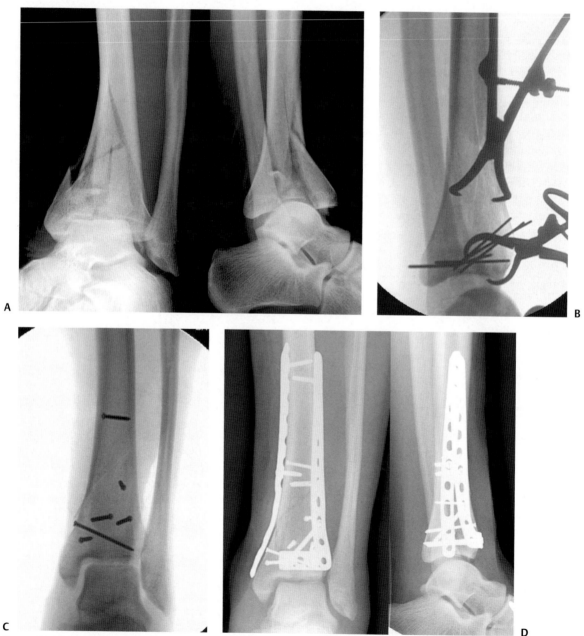

Figure 31–14 A technique for reduction is demonstrated in this simple pilon fracture pattern. **(A)** The anteroposterior and lateral injury radiographs demonstrate the three major articular segments as well as the cephalad location of the talus. **(B)** The articular surface is initially reduced and held with K-wires and clamps. **(C)** In this particular case, multiple lag screws were initially placed, followed by **(D)** submuscular and subcutaneous placement of anterolateral and medial plates.

previously placed hardware or K-wires used in maintaining the articular reduction. Multiple points of fixation in the distal segment are required given the multiple articular fragments. In the setting of a short distal articular segment or in patients with significant osteoporosis, locked distal screws may be advantageous. Proximal screws can be placed either percutaneously (although neurovascular structures are at risk) or through a separate, proximal incision exposing the lateral tibial surface.

Placement of an additional medial plate is possible with only a small distal incision (2 cm in length) placed slightly proximal to the palpable tip of the medial malleolus. This plate may be especially important if the original injury films show a significant varus angulation. The medial plate can be manually advanced in a subcutaneous fashion along the anteromedial face of the tibia. The intended function of the medial implant determines the necessary plate thickness. Implants ranging in rigidity from one-third tubular implants to small-fragment compression plates all have a role. However, flexible implants have been found to be most useful in these applications when considering the balance between maintaining the reduction and minimizing implant prominence. The primary working screw is the one just proximal to the medial fracture exit point. Because the plate is being slid subcutaneously and without any additional surgical exposure, a longer implant can be chosen to increase the torsional rigidity of the construct. A second screw can then be placed through a small stab incision at the top of the plate. The fracture pattern and injury deformities determine the necessary function(s) of the medial implant. In cases where the primary coronal plane deformity is varus, indicating a compressive failure of the medial distal tibia, the plate functions primarily as a buttressing implant, and no fixation into the distal segment is necessary. In instances where the primary coronal plane deformity is valgus, indicating a tension failure of the medial distal tibia, screw fixation into the distal segment may be necessary. Alternatively, a medial plate can be forgone, relying primarily on screw fixations from the medial malleolus into the proximal segment lateral tibial cortex, effectively resisting medial-sided tension failure.

Anteromedial Approach for Reduction of Tibial Pilon Fractures

The anteromedial approach **(Fig. 31–15A,B)** is the most extensile exposure, allowing visualization of the entire distal tibial articular surface. It can be used in virtually all complete articular (type 43C) fractures **(Fig. 31–16A,B)**, and it is especially useful in medial-sided partial articular fractures (type 43B). Subcutaneous plating of extra-articular distal tibial fractures can be approached with this incision as well. The approach provides excellent visualization of the anterior, anterolateral, and medial aspects of the distal tibial articular surface, as well as simultaneous access to the medial malleolus if a fracture exists in that location. Additionally, the approach can be extended prox-

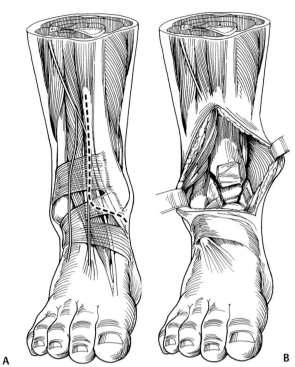

A **B**

Figure 31–15 The anteromedial approach for fixation of tibial pilon fractures. The incision is located over the anterior compartment, lateral to the palpable crest of the tibia. **(A)** The incision curves acutely and medially at the ankle joint. A flap is created over the anteromedial face of the distal tibia, leaving the periosteum attached to the tibial segment. **(B)** A femoral distractor can similarly be placed from the talar neck to the midtibia.

imally to assist with the management of proximal extensions and noncontiguous tibial diaphyseal fractures. The main disadvantage to this approach is its reliance on the survival of a large, full-thickness, anteromedial skin flap in a traumatized and unforgiving soft tissue envelope. As a result, this approach should only be performed through a pristine soft tissue envelope by someone experienced with the approach.

The patient is positioned supine on a radiolucent operating table extension with the foot brought to the end of the table. A bump consisting of a single rolled blanket placed beneath the ipsilateral hip will assist with positioning the leg in neutral rotation. After the administration of the appropriate antibiotics (generally 1 g of cefazolin), the osseous anatomy of the ankle joint is marked with a pen to identify the surgical approach. The surgical incision is curvilinear distally and longitudinal proximally. The incision parallels the long axis of the tibia, 1 to 2 cm lateral to the tibial crest and over the anterior compartment. At the ankle joint, the incision curves relatively acutely (~70 to 80 degrees) in a medial direction and terminates at a point 1 cm distal to the tip of the medial malleolus.

A full-thickness flap must be created. The skin and subcutaneous tissues are carefully dissected from lateral to medial from the underlying anterior compartment fascia

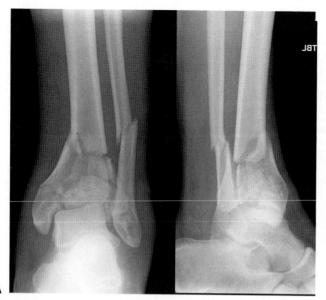

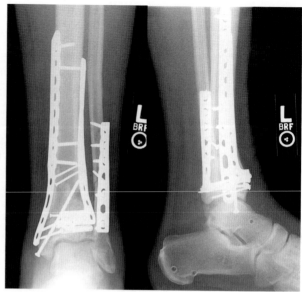

Figure 31–16 The anteromedial approach used to treat an intra-articular distal tibia fracture. **(A)** Anteroposterior and lateral radiographs demonstrating significant comminution extending medially as well as a small medial malleolar segment. These features of the injury make an anteromedial approach appropriate in this fracture. **(B)** A supplemental anterolateral plate can still be placed submuscularly with this approach.

and the periosteum overlying the anteromedial face of the tibia. It is not necessary to expose medially over a large distance. At the distal extent of the incision, the saphenous vein is identified and limits the exposure. The fascia is then incised lateral to the crest of the tibia but medial to the tibialis anterior tendon sheath. Care must to taken to avoid entering this tendon sheath. A single incision into the joint capsule is placed in a location consistent with the preoperative plan and the location of the anterior exit line of the fracture. The arthrotomy is extended distally onto the anteromedial talar neck, which is exposed subperiosteally.

A femoral distractor can then be placed across the ankle joint. To accomplish this, a 4 mm Schanz pin can be placed transversely at the medial neck of the talus in an extra-articular location. This pin is placed through the surgical incision and at the talar neck distal to the medial malleolus. An additional pin can be placed medially at the tibial diaphysis in a location remote from any proposed plate applications. This provides excellent joint exposure through a combination of longitudinal distraction and plantar flexion, allowing visualization to the posterior tibial plafond. Because the deltoid ligament is seldom disrupted, overdistraction and distal displacement of the medial segment(s) occur frequently and may require adjustment (minimization) of the distractive force at the critical point for the medial reduction.

The overall sequence of reduction through this surgical exposure follows a similar strategy as described for the anterolateral approach. The anterior tibiofibular and deltoid ligaments must be maintained and respected during reduction. Access to the posterior articular segments is through whichever anterior fracture exit points are pro-

vided by the injury pattern. The anterolateral fragment can usually be externally rotated on the anterior tibiofibular ligament; the medial fragment can be rotated on the deltoid. The reduction proceeds (typically) from posterolateral to medial to central to anterolateral. This exposure allows optimal visualization for reduction of any separate medial malleolar fractures and medial impaction injuries. The placement of temporary K-wires should be strategic in anticipation of plate applications.

The fixation strategy is dependent on the injury pattern, comminution, and primary deformities. Because this approach is typically used for tibial pilon fractures that fail in varus or for fractures with associated medial impaction or malleolar injuries, medial buttress plating is frequently necessary. This plate can be placed directly on the exposed periosteum of the anteromedial face of the tibia. The proximal extent of the plate can certainly be slid subcutaneously, enabling the proximal surgical exposure to be limited to that necessary for the articular reduction. Additional lateral articular fixations can be easily placed through this incision and frequently consist of small implants compressing the anterolateral fragment to the posterolateral fragment.

Posterolateral Approach for Reduction of Tibial Pilon Fractures

The posterolateral approach is useful in posterior partial articular (type 43B) pilon injuries and as an additional exposure in some complete articular (type 43C) fractures. Because the posterior malleolus extends so far distally, articular visualization is virtually impossible from the posterior approach. Reduction through the posterolateral exposure is therefore limited to cortical reductions of the posterolateral segment(s) to the tibial metaphysis and diaphysis, thereby indirectly reducing the articular surface. As a result, purely posterior pilon fractures (with an intact anterior tibial cortex) can be reduced in an extra-articular fashion only. In some complete articular (type 43C) fracture patterns, it is advantageous to proceed with a posterolateral exposure prior to an anteriorly based exposure, allowing for creation of an accurately reduced posterolateral pillar. Although the exposure is extensile, it is usually limited to the distal tibial metaphyseal and articular segments.

Patient positioning is either prone or lateral. A lateral position has the advantage of allowing a subsequent anterior exposure without having to move the patient to the supine position. This can be accomplished by simply externally rotating the leg in a patient with adequate hip motion. The prone position is more advantageous for the posterolateral exposure but eliminates the possibility of an additional exposure without repositioning the patient.

The location of the incision depends on the integrity of the fibula. If the fibula is intact (no prior fibular incision), the incision is centered between the Achilles' tendon and the peroneal tendons, along the posterolateral aspect of the leg. If a fibular fracture requires stabilization in association with an anticipated posterolateral exposure, this incision should be placed posteriorly. The posterolateral exposure has been well described in texts and numerous publications.[11,12] The sural nerve is protected. The posterolateral border of the peroneal tendons and muscles is developed, with the deep exposure continuing on the lateral side of the flexor hallucis longus muscle. The tibia is then exposed from lateral to medial. Distally, the exposure is di-

rectly from the fibula to the tibia; proximally the muscles are dissected off the interosseous membrane. The posterior tibiofibular ligaments should be respected, as should the posterior joint capsule. This allows exposure medially to the medially malleolus and proximally as far as necessary. The periosteal attachments to the tibia should be respected and maintained except at the fracture line itself. This is especially important if an additional anterior exposure is planned, with additional anterior disruption of the distal tibial osseous blood supply.

The reduction of a large posterolateral fragment relies upon an extra-articular cortical reduction (**Fig. 31–17A,B**). This fragment can be rotated on the posterior tibiofibular ligament to allow removal of hematoma or other debris from within the fracture. To regain length posteriorly, foot dorsiflexion is necessary. If this fails to reestablish the necessary posterior tension, a femoral distractor can be applied from the posterior tibia (with the Schanz pin placed through the incision and directed from posterior to anterior) to the posterior calcaneus (with the Schanz pin place into the calcaneal tuberosity through a midline stab incision). Strategic clamp applications between the posterolateral segment and the intact anterior distal tibia can greatly assist with maintenance of the reduction. Both lag screws directed from posterior to anterior and antiglide plates positioned posteriorly on the tibia allow stable fixation. A plate positioned vertically with a screw placed slightly proximal to the apex of the fracture will provide adequate fixation in most cases. In injuries where an additional anterior exposure is planned and required, strategic placement of the posteriorly based implants will ensure that the anterior reduction maneuvers will not be blocked. Unicortical screws placed through the plate and proximal to the fracture are usually adequate for maintaining the distal reduction.

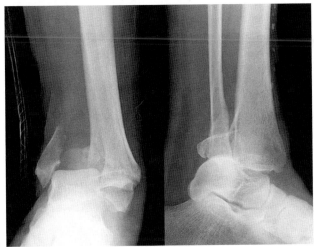
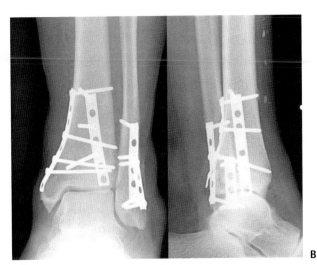

A   B

Figure 31–17 A posteriorly displaced tibial pilon fracture. **(A)** Anteroposterior and lateral radiographs that show the combination of a large posterior articular segment and the fibula fracture. These features of the injury make a posterolateral approach desirable in this trimalleolar variant of a tibial pilon fracture. **(B)** The patient was positioned laterally, allowing reduction and fixation of the posterior tibial articular surface and the fibula. This was followed by a separate medial approach.

Posteromedial Approach for Reduction of Tibial Pilon Fractures

The posteromedial approach is rarely required for fixation of tibial pilon fractures but may be used as an adjunct to an anterior approach in certain circumstances **(Fig. 31–18A–E)**. Because this exposure does not allow direct visualization of the articular surface, reduction is dependent on evaluating the extra-articular cortical reduction, intraoperative imaging, or another method of joint visualization.

The patient is positioned supine on a radiolucent operating table extension with the foot brought to the end of the table. An ipsilateral bump is not needed because external rotation of the limb actually facilitates the exposure. If adequate external rotation of the leg is not obtained, a bump can be placed beneath the contralateral hip to roll the patient toward the injured side. The incision is centered at the ankle joint, between the Achilles' tendon and the posteromedial border of the distal tibia. The interval used for deep dissection is dependent on the location of the major fracture fragments and may be between the tibia and the posterior tibial tendon, between the posterior tibial tendon and the flexor digitorum communis, or between the flexor digitorum communis and the FHL. The latter of these three intervals requires direct exposure and protection of the neurovascular bundle along its length.

The posteromedial exposure allows a direct reduction of the posterolateral and medial fracture fragments. A posteromedial plate can be placed, effectively buttressing the medial fragment. A full-thickness flap can be created dis-tally to allow exposure and fixation of the medial malleolus if necessary.

Treatment of Extra-articular Distal Tibial Metaphyseal Fractures with Plates

Plate fixation of extra-articular distal metaphyseal tibial fractures can be accomplished safely in both closed and open injuries. The treatment approach in high-energy injuries is frequently similar to that in articular tibial pilon fractures, with delayed fixation of the tibia if the soft tissue envelope is such that open procedures are felt to be unacceptably risky. Low-energy closed distal tibial fractures can frequently be treated primarily with plate applications without the need for resolution of soft tissue swelling.

The decision to fix an associated fibular fracture is controversial. However, fibular fixation has several advantages, including indirect reduction of the tibial fracture and establishment of a lateral column to distract against from the medial side. If the fibular fracture appears to be associated with an injury to the ankle itself, this should be stabilized as well.

Plates can be applied to either the anteromedial face of the tibia or the lateral tibial surface. Both locking and non-locking plates have indications depending on the injury characteristics, the quality of bone, and the age of the patient. Surgical approaches include an extended anteromedial approach (as described for an articular pilon fracture), a limited anterolateral approach with submuscular proximal plate application (as described for an articular pilon

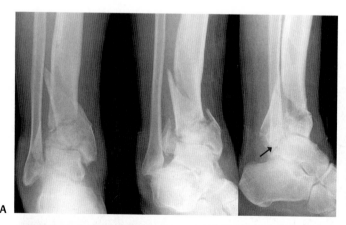

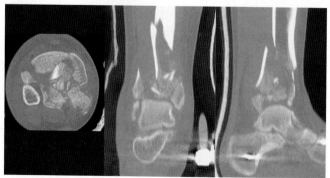

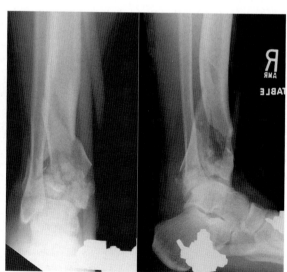

Figure 31–18 A posteromedial approach for internal fixation of a pilon fracture. **(A)** Anteroposterior (left), mortise (middle), and lateral (right) radiographs of a comminuted pilon fracture resulting from a motorcycle accident. The lateral radiograph demonstrates the small posterolateral segment (arrow). **(B)** Following spanning external fixation, the reduction is hardly improved. **(C)** The computed tomographic scan demonstrates the severity of articular comminution.

fracture), and minimally invasive approaches with antero-medial subcutaneous plate applications.

A minimally invasive approach to the anteromedial distal tibia requires an indirect reduction and hence maximal maintenance of the periosteal attachments. A small (2 cm) incision just proximal to the medial malleolus is usually adequate to allow an implant to be passed subcutaneously along the tibial face. A large implant is unnecessary in low-energy injuries. However, high-energy distal tibial fractures with significant comminution or open fractures with bone loss may require implants with significantly more stability and durability. In general, a 3.5 mm plate will suffice, the contouring of which is critical. The surgeon must remember not only the medial concavity of the plate (which can be checked via fluoroscopy), but also that the distal end of the plate is ~20 degrees internally rotated.[13] The sagittal plane deformity can usually be corrected primarily with strategic bump placements beneath either the leg or the heel. However, the coronal plane deformity can be more difficult to manage. In most cases, the plate can be used to reduce the coronal plane angulation and translation, assuming adequate tibial length. If the tibia remains short, a medially applied femoral distractor can greatly assist with regaining length. Distal pin placement for the distractor can be either in the distal tibial segment (providing maximal control) or into the calcaneus. The primary translational deformity of the distal tibial segment determines the order of screw fixations after the plate is placed. If the distal segment remains medially translated (and in varus), placement of a screw just proximal to the fracture in an anatomically contoured or slightly undercontoured plate should complete the reduction. If the distal segment remains laterally translated, placement of a screw into the

distal segment to draw it to the medial implant is usually successful. The use of locked plates in the vast majority of distal tibial fractures is unnecessary. However, in patients with severe osteopenia, open fractures with anticipated delayed healing, and/or open fractures with bone loss, these implants may be of some use. However, the initial reduction maneuvers and screw fixations require unlocked screws to reduce the tibia to the implant. This can be followed by placement of locked implants.

The anteromedial approach, as previously described for intra-articular distal tibial fractures, is mainly reserved for low-energy distal tibial fractures only. Because of the need for the creation of a large medial flap, high-energy injuries should only rarely be treated with this approach. Regardless, the approach requires maintenance of the periosteal envelope and atraumatic plate application. Although the plate can be applied directly within the open wound, indirect reduction of the main fracture components should be performed. The only exception to this may be in the case of a spiral fracture that can be anatomically reduced in an atraumatic fashion. In this case, lag screw fixation and application of a neutralization plate can be accomplished.

The anterolateral approach is limited to exposure of the distal 5 to 7 cm of the tibia, enabling application of a plate combined with a submuscular placement proximally. This approach is the same as that described for articular fractures of the distal tibia. However, the distal exposure can be more limited and no joint arthrotomy is required. This approach frequently requires an additional medial plate placement to resist the tendency for late varus deformity in distal tibial fractures. It is most useful in extremely distal tibial metaphyseal fractures that cannot be adequately stabilized solely from the medial side.

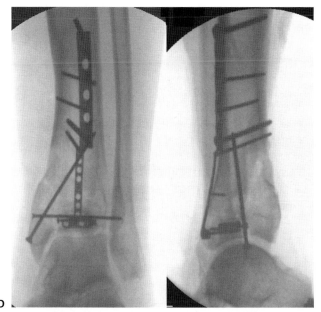

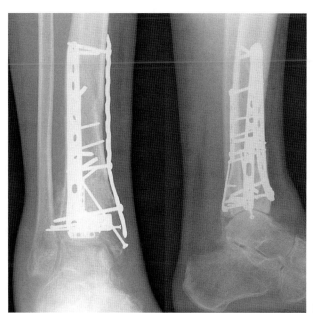

Figure 31–18 *(Continued)* **(D)** Because of the small posterolateral articular segment as well as the separate posteromedial articular fragment, a posteromedial approach was performed. The fixation was limited to

the posterior fragments. The patient then underwent fixation of the remaining pilon through an anterolateral approach. **(E)** There was excellent healing and mild ankle arthrosis visible on 1 year radiographs.

Treatment of Extra-articular Distal Tibial Metaphyseal Fractures with Medullary Nails

Depending on their proximity to the ankle joint articular surface, some distal tibial fractures involving the metaphyseal region are technically pilon fractures. Newer nail designs with multiplanar locking screws positioned close to the distal tip of the implant have expanded the fracture patterns that are amenable to this treatment. As always, a careful preoperative plan as well as an understanding of the geometry of the available medullary implants is important for success. Important in nailing of distal fractures is the understanding that the implant will not assist in reducing the fracture due to the small size of the nail relative to the voluminous anatomy of the distal tibial metaphysis. Additionally, the stability of the ultimate construct is dependent on the interference between the interlocking bolts and the nail, and the interface between the nail and the cancellous bone of the distal tibial segment. Because of the short distance between the proximal interlocking bolt and the fracture, bending stresses are concentrated unabated.

Frequently, associated distal tibial articular or malleolar injuries coexist and should be stabilized prior to nail placement. Strategic screw placement ensures adequate room for nail placement according to the preoperative plan. Medial malleolar injuries can be stabilized with horizontally or vertically oriented screws, depending on the fracture pattern. Medial or anterolateral plates can be used as well, as long as the predicted nail corridor is respected.

Several techniques are useful to ensure placement of the nail across a reduced fracture. These include fibular plating, medial femoral distraction, temporary unicortical plating, percutaneous clamp applications, and joystick manipulations with Schanz pins. In general, reaming of the distal fragment is unnecessary except in young patients with dense metaphyseal cancellous bone. If reaming of the distal segment is anticipated, the fracture should be adequately reduced prior to reamer passage to ensure that a proper path is cut for the nail. The surgeon should maintain tibial alignment and reduction during all aspects of the procedure, including reaming, nailing, and interlocking screw placement. This last point cannot be overemphasized.

As in other techniques for fixation of distal tibial fractures, fibular stabilization is frequently a useful adjuvant. Although most tibial fractures with associated fibular fractures represent an injury that spares the distal ligaments and makes fibular fixation unnecessary for normal ankle function, these same ligamentous attachments assist in tibial fracture reduction. Another useful adjuvant is the femoral distractor, which can easily be placed medially to allow for reestablishment of tibial length and alignment.[14] One pin may be placed from medial to lateral in the proximal posterior tibia, and the other pin is placed either in the distal tibia or the calcaneus. Better control of the fracture can be obtained with placement of the distal Schanz pin into the tibia itself, but it must be placed remote from the anticipated nail location. (Usually this involves placing it somewhat posteriorly in the distal tibia.) For direct manipulation of the distal segment, additional Schanz pins of varying sizes can be placed as joysticks. Similarly, percutaneous clamp applications can assist with reduction. Minimal additional soft tissue dissection should be performed in this already tenuous region of the leg.

If reaming of the distal segment is performed, it is important to ensure that the guidewire is centrally placed in the distal segment of both orthogonal fluoroscopic views. Similarly, the fracture reduction should be maintained by whatever means until nail passage and interlocking are performed. Interlocking with screws at 90 degrees to each other may assist with control of the distal segment. At least two screws (and preferably three) should be placed through the nail in the distal segment. Fracture stability should be confirmed after interlocking. In rare cases where instability exists after interlocking, consideration should be given to either using blocking screws or leaving a two-pin medial external fixator in place for 4 to 6 weeks.

Rehabilitation and Postoperative Management

Postoperatively the drains are left in place for 48 hours or until the output falls to below 10 mL over 8 hours. The wound should remain covered for at least 48 to 72 hours, over which period the patient's leg should be kept elevated except for physical therapy and bathroom visits. The sutures can be removed at 10 to 14 days, depending on healing.

Active ankle and subtalar joint range of motion exercises should begin as soon as the wound is dry, usually between 2 and 5 days after surgery. In articular fractures, non–weight bearing should continue for 12 weeks. A removable posterior splint should remain in place to prevent an equinus contracture. A supervised physical therapy program encouraging active ankle range of motion exercises can be instituted during the first 6 weeks. This can be progressed to include passive exercises between 6 and 12 weeks.

Alternative or "Newer" Techniques

There is no single treatment method that is applicable for all distal tibia fractures. Similarly, multiple treatment approaches have been used with success. Although this chapter has focused primarily on techniques of open reduction, other methods include ankle-spanning unilateral external fixation, articulated external fixation, hybrid frame stabilization, and circular frame (Ilizarov) stabilization. Additionally, each of these methods can be combined with limited open reduction techniques for reduction of articular components of the fracture.

The combination of external fixation and limited internal fixation techniques has been successful in multiple published reports. The important primary goal of these approaches, similar to that in open plating techniques, is to gain an anatomical reduction of the articular surface (when possible) and span from the articular segment to the diaphyseal tibial segment. Whether this is accomplished with plates placed

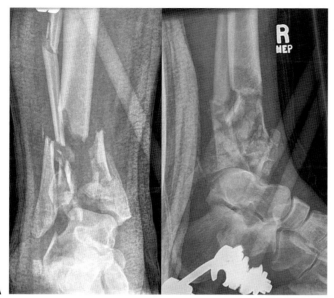

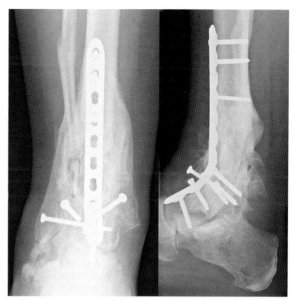

A   B

Figure 31–19 A 60-year-old female polytrauma patient with insulin-dependent diabetes mellitus. **(A)** Radiographs of a right type II open pilon fracture. At the time of initial open fracture irrigation and debridement, significant articular damage was seen. On postinjury day 18, she underwent immediate ankle arthrodesis utilizing an anterior approach and placement of a locked plate. **(B)** Anteroposterior and lateral radiographs of the right ankle at 13 months postinjury. The patient was fully ambulatory and with very minimal pain at the ankle. (Case courtesy of Philip J. Kregor, MD.)

with minimally invasive techniques (as described in this chapter) or with external fixation, the theoretical overall treatment approaches are actually quite similar. The approaches used in these limited techniques are similar to those in open techniques of fixation for the distal tibia. For fine wire fixators, safe corridors have been well described,[15] and a thorough knowledge of the local axial anatomy is necessary. Pin tract infections remain problematic and deep infections occur with these techniques as well. Early weight bearing is possible and encouraged with circular frames applied to the lower extremity, even in articular injuries.

Ankle spanning external fixators have the advantage of avoiding pin tracts that communicate with the fracture lines (and hence with the ankle joint) but do not allow early weight bearing or mobility of the ankle and subtalar joints.

Because these injuries are frequently open and/or associated with some delay in healing, the ideal time for fixator removal (and hence ankle joint motion) is difficult to predict.

There may be a role for primary ankle fusion in some extremely limited and unusual circumstances. This may include open fractures with loss of a significant segment of the articular surface and severe comminution in combination with other patient- or injury-related factors that make open reduction impossible (**Fig. 31–19A,B**).

The use of autogenous bone from the iliac crest to fill in metaphyseal defects following open reduction remains an option. However, allograft bone and bone graft substitutes are being used with increasing frequency to fill these defects. This trend is largely attributed to the relatively common morbidities associated with harvesting iliac crest

Tips and Tricks

- A thoughtful surgical plan should precede even the initial stabilization to assist with the location of surgical incisions as well as the placement of provisional fixation.
- In open pilon fractures, all potential surgical incisions should be marked prior to extending the open wounds at the initial debridement.
- A posteriorly placed fibular incision allows for a wider skin bridge between this incision and a future anterolateral incision.
- If limited approaches are used at the level of the ankle joint, the "7 cm rule" is not applicable. An anterolateral approach can be combined with a posterolateral approach for fibular

(or distal tibial) fixation. Additionally, even a percutaneous medial plate can be placed in combination with these incisions.
- If open reduction and plate fixation of the distal tibia is ultimately planned, the initial spanning external fixation pins should be completely remote from any planned surgical incisions and planned plate applications (even if placed subcutaneously or submuscularly).
- Temporary spanning external fixation should not include pins placed into the talus because the future surgical exposure for the articular reduction will likely include some exposure of the talar neck.

(Continued)

Tips and Tricks (Continued)

- Intraoperative femoral distraction from the talar neck to the tibial diaphysis allows simultaneous joint distraction and plantar flexion, maximizing articular visualization.
- No self-retaining retractors should be used because they produce unrelenting pressure on the soft tissues.
- Sharp dissection should be performed whenever possible.
- Stripping of the periosteum and soft tissue attachments of the distal tibia should be avoided.
- Pilon fractures with associated open posterior wounds are of a particular concern because fixation is usually performed from the anterior aspect of the leg, thereby affecting additional blood supply. Union may be delayed secondary to the traumatic soft tissue injury located posteriorly.
- An accurate articular reduction should be combined with indirect reduction techniques for metaphyseal comminution, if present.
- The anteromedial surface of the distal tibia, irrespective of the surgical approach used, should be maintained with its periosteal attachments.
- The direction of angulation visible on the injury film combined with the pattern of the fibular fracture helps to predict the areas of comminution and articular fragmentation.
- Pilon fractures with valgus angulation and shortening of the fibula usually have lateral distal tibial comminution and compression combined with a tension failure of the medial distal tibia.
- Pilon fractures with varus angulation and associated tension fibular fractures (transverse fractures at the joint level) usually have medial distal tibial articular comminution and tension failure of the lateral distal tibia.
- The tension failure side of the distal tibia typically does not require buttress plating.
- The compressive failure side of the distal tibia typically does require buttress plating. That is, a pilon fracture in significant varus will generally benefit from medial plate application.
- Posterior pilon fractures occur rarely, are difficult to treat, and frequently require a posterior exposure with an associated extra-articular cortical reduction.
- The anterolateral exposure can be used to view the entire articular surface to the apex at the medial shoulder of the ankle. Significant medial malleolar involvement or comminution at the medial shoulder may require a different approach (either entirely or in addition).
- The usual order of reduction in anterior exposures is proper sagittal plane rotation of the posterolateral articular fragment, reduction of the posterolateral and medial fragments, reduction of any intercalary osteochondral fragments to the posterolateral fragment, and reduction of the anterolateral fragment to the medial fragment (and thus to the remaining

distal tibia). Finally, the distal articular block is reduced to the intact tibia.
- Intraosseous small- or mini-fragment screws can be placed to maintain the reduction of separate articular segments. This is most relevant in stabilizing intercalary comminuted fragments to the posterolateral fragment, prior to reduction of the anterolateral segment.
- Rotation of the posterolateral segment can be facilitated by using a large Weber clamp placed either through a lateral stab incision or in the previous posterolateral exposure of the fibula. The one tine of the clamp is placed between the peroneal tendons and the posterior border of the fibula, and onto the posterolateral fragment. The other tine will be on the anterior aspect of the tibia.
- Joysticks placed into intercalary or major fragments (Kirschner wires or 2.5 mm terminally threaded pins) can greatly assist with manipulations and reductions.
- The anterolateral fragment can be externally rotated on the anterior tibiofibular ligament to allow improved joint visualization and reduction. The anterior tibiofibular ligament should not be incised to improve exposure.
- Failure to adequately plantar flex the posterior (or posterolateral) segment occurs commonly, produces a dorsiflexion reduction of the entire articular surface, and should be corrected prior to placing definitive fixation.
- Temporary reduction of the entire articular surface with multiple strategically placed Kirschner wires prior to placement of permanent hardware allows for an initial intraoperative determination of the reduction with adjustments as necessary.
- Retention of all anterior cortical fragments, even those devoid of soft tissue attachments, greatly assists with determining the anterior length (and hence the rotation) of the articular segment.
- Occasionally, simple fractures extending into the tibial diaphysis can be stabilized with multiple lag screws at the time of the fibular fixation and external fixation, effectively turning some complete articular (type 43C) type fractures into partial articular (type 43B) fractures (i.e., stabilization of an entire column of the distal tibia).
- External fixation spanning across the ankle joint will not reduce articular impaction—ever!
- Beware of articular impaction at the seemingly "intact" articular segment in partial articular (type 43B) pilon fractures. There is frequently a ramp of impaction that requires elevation and reduction.
- If a posterior exposure is combined with an anterior exposure, strict maintenance of the periosteum is imperative to minimize the risks of infection and nonunion.

bone graft. As yet, there are no published studies documenting the results of bone-graft substitutes in patients with distal tibial fractures.

Outcomes

The outcomes after surgical treatment of pilon fractures may be more dependent on the associated soft tissue injury than on the osseous injury, the articular reduction, or the treatment method chosen.[16] However, the reported results of operative fixation have changed over time and have influenced the relative popularity of various operative approaches. The initial enthusiasm for open reduction and internal fixation (ORIF) largely stemmed from the good results reported by Rüedi and Allgower.[8,17] Unfortunately, the North American experience with ORIF that followed was disastrous, with frequent complications, particularly with regard to the incidence of deep infection in comminuted fractures.[18,19] Although it has been frequently suggested that the lower-energy, primarily torsional, skiing injuries seen in the former study are not comparable with the higher-energy fractures in the latter, the end result was a recognition of an unacceptably high rate of complications following ORIF of some pilon fractures. As a result, authors sought alternative methods to simultaneously treat the more severe osseous and soft tissue injuries.

Various techniques of external fixation have been recommended to balance the treatment of the soft tissue injury with the underlying articular fracture.[16,20–26] These techniques are associated with a substantial decrease in the wound complications previously reported.[16,20–26] Ankle-bridging external fixation, though potentially associated with significant ankle stiffness, has been associated with low wound complication rates.[21–23,25] Infrequent soft tissue complications, good alignment, and union were all observed after limited internal fixation and application of a hybrid external fixator in one study.[26] Circular external fixation (e.g., Ilizarov technique) has been recommended by several authors, primarily to avoid the cantilever bending forces observed in hybrid fixators.[16,24] Improved results compared with ORIF have been reported in a subset of patients with an associated severe soft tissue injury.[16]

In response to the high rate of soft tissue complications previously reported, a two-staged protocol for ORIF was implemented by several authors.[6,7] This consisted of primary fibular fixation and application of a temporary ankle spanning external fixator followed by definitive ORIF of the articular surface and distal tibia following resolution of the associated soft tissue swelling. This was found to be successful in both open and closed injuries.[6,7] In a more recent retrospective review of several open treatment methods, patients treated with a staged protocol were similarly found to have an acceptable complication rate, improved pain, and better ankle function.[27]

Several studies attempt to review the actual outcomes of surgically treated tibial pilon fractures. Rüedi followed their 9 year results of lower-energy pilon fractures and found frequent degenerative changes despite good initial reductions.[17] More recently, Pollak et al evaluated patients treated with either external fixation or ORIF at a minimum of 2 years after their injuries.[28] Significant disability, pain, swelling, and stiffness were reported. Interestingly, the only injury or treatment characteristic that was found to be related to the outcomes was treatment with external fixation (as opposed to ORIF). Marsh et al looked at their minimum 5 year results after external fixation and percutaneous screw fixation of 35 tibial plafond fractures.[29] Although their follow-up cohort did not include five patients who had already undergone an ankle arthrodesis, they found significant impairment and arthrosis in the majority of the remaining ankles.

Overall, significant improvements in the short-term complications have been observed due to a better understanding and appreciation of the severe associated soft tissue injury in these particular fractures. A staged protocol for open reduction, limited internal fixation combined with external fixation, and circular external fixation have all contributed to a decreased incidence of wound complications and deep infection previously observed with the treatment of pilon fractures. However, the long-term outcomes associated with these injuries remain suboptimal. Ankle stiffness, arthritis, pain, and secondary surgical procedures occur commonly. Despite these delayed complications, a comprehensive surgical approach that optimizes the articular reduction, provides stable fixation, and allows early ankle motion may optimize the potential results in these complicated fractures.

Complications

Complications are frequently encountered with both the injury and the treatment of pilon fractures. Some complications are universally associated with the injury itself and include ankle joint stiffness, soft tissue breakdown, deep infection, chronic osteomyelitis, and posttraumatic ankle joint arthritis. Other complications that may be related to treatment include subtalar joint stiffness, pin tract infections, wound complications, nonunion, and malunion. The selected treatment strategy should include consideration of injury-related complications in an attempt to minimize any additional surgical complications.

In an attempt to minimize additional surgical trauma to the already compromised soft tissue envelope, methods of external fixation have been recommended in the hope of avoiding deep infection and wound breakdown.[16,20,21,23,24,26,30–32] All methods of external fixation have the potential for pin tract infections, which usually respond to oral or intravenous antibiotic therapies. Ankle-spanning external fixation has the disadvantage of associated subtalar joint stiffness but avoids placement of wires close to the injury zone and any associated fracture lines. Hybrid or circular wire fixators have improved control of the distal tibial articular segments but have the theoretical potential for transmission of bacterial infections from the pins to the fracture planes, and hence to the ankle joint. Deep infection has been reported as a complication in patients treated with hybrid fixators, even more frequently than in patients treated with open reduction.[20] The combination of limited open reduction and circular fixation has been successfully applied to patients with open or high-energy closed injuries and may represent a good overall treatment approach in these difficult injuries.[16] Nonunion and malunion remain problematic after external fixation, especially in high-energy injuries.[20,31,32] The long-term outcomes after external fixation of pilon fractures remain largely unknown. The majority of patients followed for a minimum of 5 years after their injury demonstrated radiographic evidence of ankle arthritis combined with activity limitations despite reasonable outcomes scores in one study.[29] However, secondary reconstructive procedures were rarely required and patients improved for several years after their injury.[29]

The early reports after open reduction of pilon fractures were plagued by unacceptably high rates of superficial and deep wound infections.[18,33] However, staged reconstructive procedures have minimized these complications, with soft tissue complication rates of less than 5% reported.[6,7,27,34] Allowing resolution of the associated soft tissue swelling prior to any attempts at open reduction has been important in decreasing skin slough, wound infection, and chronic osteomyelitis in these patients.[6,7] Malunion can certainly occur after open reduction, but this usually indicates a failure to initially and accurately reconstruct the alignment of the distal tibia. Nonunion occurs infrequently and can usually be managed with bone grafting prior to catastrophic failure of the distal tibial fixation. Ankle joint arthritis remains problematic despite attempts at accurately reconstructing the articular surface. However, there is very little literature reviewing long-term outcomes after an accurate open reduction of pilon fractures using a staged protocol.

Pearls

- The position of the foot at the time of impact combined with the direction of the applied force will determine the resultant fracture pattern and articular impaction.
- In displaced, complete articular fractures (type 43C), closed methods are ineffective in accurately reducing the articular segments.
- In the case of an intact fibula associated with a complete articular distal tibial fracture, varus angulation commonly occurs.
- In similar complete articular distal tibial fractures *with* an associated fibular fracture, shortening is expected with associated widening of the joint.
- The anterior compartment of the leg contains, from medial to lateral, the tibialis anterior, the EHL, the EDC, and the peroneus tertius. These muscles are all innervated by branches from the peroneal nerve proximally in the leg. The deep peroneal nerve and the anterior tibial vessels are located between the EHL and EDC distally, requiring direct identification and protection in the direct anterior approach. The superficial peroneal nerve is purely

sensory and travels from posterior to anterior, crossing the anterolateral surgical incision **(Fig. 31–3).**
- The peroneal muscles (longus and brevis) occupy the lateral compartment of the leg, have a distal muscle belly posteriorly, and are firmly attached at the distal fibula by the peroneal sheath.
- The deep posterior compartment muscles are largely tendinous at the level of the ankle joint and include the posterior tibial, the flexor digitorum communis, and the FHL. The FHL has a very distal muscle belly, and its identification is especially useful in the posterolateral approach to the distal tibia.
- The gastrocnemius and soleus muscles have a common tendinous insertion at the level of the ankle joint, and their tendon sheath requires protection in any posterior approaches. The tibial nerve and the associated vascular supply posteriorly require protection and identification during posteromedial surgical exposures..

On the DVDs

Video 31–1 (Disk 4) Application of an Ankle-Spanning External Fixator This video shows the application of a spanning fixator across the ankle for the initial management of a distal tibia fracture.

Video 31–2 (Disk 4) ORIF of a Partial Articular (Type B) Pilon Fracture This video shows the delayed reduction and internal fixation of a partial articular tibial plafond fracture in a patient that had been initially managed in an ankle-spanning external fixator. A medial periarticular plate (ACE-DePuy, Warsaw, Indiana) was applied through an anteromedial incision, with percutaneous screw fixation of the distal fibula.

Video 31–3 (Disk 4) ORIF of a Pilon Fracture with a Periarticular Non-locking Plate This video demonstrates the use of a periarticular plate through minimal incisions to treat a Type 43B frac-

ture. We review the approaches for treating pilon fractures, as well as key principles used in the successful treatment of these difficult fractures.

Video 31–4 (Same as Video 4–6, Disk 1) Locked Plating of a Pilon Fracture This video demonstrates ORIF of a pilon fracture using locked plating. The benefits of stabilization of the fibula as part of the treatment strategy are reviewed. We also discuss the importance of planning the location of incisions to keep all options open.

Video 31–5 (Disk 4) ORIF of a Pilon Fracture Using a Posterior Approach This video demonstrates ORIF a pilon fracture with a severe soft tissue injury anteriorly. The posteromedial approach is used to avoid the damaged soft tissue envelope. Potential posterior approaches and the intervals the surgeon utilizes are discussed.

References

1. Tornetta P, Gorup J. Axial computed tomography of pilon fractures. Clin Orthop Relat Res 1996;323:273–276

2. Rüedi T, Matter P, Allgower M. Die intraartikul-aren Frakturen des distalen Unterschenkelendes. Helv Chir Acta 1968;35:556–582

3. Orthopaedic Trauma Association Committee for Coding and Classification. Fracture and dislocation compendium. J Orthop Trauma 1996;10(Suppl 1):319–323

4. Martin JS, Marsh JL, Bonar SK, De Coster TA, Found EM, Brandser EA. Assessment of the AO/ASIF fracture classification for the distal tibia. J Orthop Trauma 1997;11:477–483

5. Swiontkowski MF, Sands AK, Agel J, Diab M, Schwappach JR, Kreder HJ. Interobserver variation in the AO/OTA fracture classification system for pilon fractures: is there a problem? J Orthop Trauma 1997;11:467–470

6. Patterson MJ, Cole JD. Two-staged delayed open reduction and internal fixation of severe pilon fractures. J Orthop Trauma 1999;13:85–91

7. Sirkin M, Sanders R, Di Pasquale T, Herscovici D. A staged protocol for soft tissue management in the treatment of complex pilon fractures. J Orthop Trauma 1999;13:78–84

8. Rüedi T, Allgower M. Spatresultate nach operativer Behandlung der Gelenkbruche am distalen Tibiaende (sog. Pilon-Frakturen). [Late results after operative treatment of fractures of the distal tibia (pilon tibial fractures)] Unfallheilkunde 1978;81(4):319323

9. Topliss CJ, Jackson M, Atkins RM. Anatomy of pilon fractures of the distal tibia. J Bone Joint Surg Br 2005;87:692–697

10. Cole PA, Mehrle RK, Bhandari M, Zlowodzki M. The pilon map: assessment of fracture lines and comminution zones in AO C3 type pilon fractures. Poster, 2004 Orthopaedic Trauma Association Annual Meeting. Available at http://www.hwbf.org/ota/am/ota04/otapo/OTP04005.htm

11. Ostrum RF. Posterior plating of displaced Weber B fibula fractures. J Orthop Trauma 1996;10:199–203

12. Wissing JC, van Laarhoven CJ, van der Werken C. The posterior antiglide plate for fixation of fractures of the lateral malleolus. Injury 1992;23:94–96

13. Mast J, Jakob R, Ganz R. Planning and Reduction Technique in Fracture Surgery. Berlin: Springer-Verlag; 1989:48–80

14. Rubinstein RA, Green JM, Duwelius PJ. Intramedullary interlocked tibial nailing: a new technique. J Orthop Trauma 1992;6:90–95

15. Vives MJ, Abidi NA, Ishikawa SN, Taliwal RV, Sharkey PF. Soft tissue injuries with the use of safe corridors for transfixion wire placement during external fixation of distal tibia fractures: an anatomic study. J Orthop Trauma 2001;15:555–559

16. Watson JT, Moed BR, Karges DE, Cramer KE. Pilon fractures: treatment protocol based on severity of soft tissue injury. Clin Orthop Relat Res 2000;375:78–90

17. Rüedi T. Frakturen des pilon Tibial: Ergebnisse nach 9 Jahren [Intraarticular fractures of distal tibia: results after 9 years]. Arch Orthop Unfallchir 1973;76:248–254

18. Teeny SM, Wiss DA. Open reduction and internal fixation of tibial plafond fractures: variables contributing to poor results and complications. Clin Orthop Relat Res 1993;292:108–117

19. Wyrsch B, McFerran MA, McAndrew M, et al. Operative treatment of fractures of the tibial plafond: a randomized, prospective study. J Bone Joint Surg Am 1996;78:1646–1657

20. Anglen JO. Early outcome of hybrid external fixation for fracture of the distal tibia. J Orthop Trauma 1999;13:92–97

21. Bone L, Stegemann P, McNamara K, Seibel R. External fixation of severely comminuted and open tibial pilon fractures. Clin Orthop Relat Res 1993;292:101–107

22. Marsh JL. External fixation is the treatment of choice for fractures of the tibial plafond. J Orthop Trauma 1999;13:583–585

23. Marsh JL, Bonar S, Nepola JV, Decoster TA, Hurwitz SR. Use of an articulated external fixator for fractures of the tibial plafond. J Bone Joint Surg Am 1995;77:1498–1509

24. Murphy CP, D'Ambrosia R, Dabezies EJ. The small pin circular fixator for distal tibial pilon fractures with soft tissue compromise. Orthopedics 1991;14:283–290

25. Rommens PM, Claes P, Broos PL. Therapeutic strategy in pilon fractures type C2 and C3: soft tissue damage changes treatment protocol. Acta Chir Belg 1996;96:85–92

26. Tornetta P, Weiner L, Bergman M, et al. Pilon fractures: treatment with combined internal and external fixation. J Orthop Trauma 1993;7:489–496

27. Blauth M, Bastian L, Krettek C, Knop C, Evans S. Surgical options for the treatment of severe tibial pilon fractures: a study of three techniques. J Orthop Trauma 2001;15:153–160

28. Pollak AN, McCarthy ML, Bess RS, Agel J, Swiontkowski MF. Outcomes after treatment of high-energy tibial plafond injuries. J Bone Joint Surg Am 2003;85:1893–1900

29. Marsh JL, Weigel DP, Dirschl DR. Tibial plafond fractures: how do these ankles function over time? J Bone Joint Surg Am 2003;85:287–295

30. Bonar SK, Marsh JL. Unilateral external fixation for severe pilon fractures. Foot Ankle 1993;14:57–64

31. McDonald MG, Burgess RC, Bolano LE, Nicholls PJ. Ilizarov treatment of pilon fractures. Clin Orthop Relat Res 1996;325:232–238

32. Williams TM, Marsh JL, Nepola JV, De Coster TA, Hurwitz SR, Bonar SB. External fixation of tibial plafond fractures: is routine plating of the fibula necessary? J Orthop Trauma 1998;12:16–20

33. McFerran MA, Smith SW, Boulas HJ, Schwartz HS. Complications encountered in the treatment of pilon fractures. J Orthop Trauma 1992;6:195–200

34. Dickson KF, Montgomery S, Field J. High energy plafond fractures treated by a spanning external fixator initially and followed by a second stage open reduction internal fixation of the articular surface: preliminary report. Injury 2001;32(Suppl 4):SD92–98

32 Ankle Fractures and Dislocations

Cory A. Collinge and Keith Heier

Because the ankle is the most commonly injured weight-bearing joint of the body,[1] most orthopaedic surgeons routinely treat ankle injuries. A great deal has been written regarding the diagnosis and treatment of ankle fractures, although controversy persists regarding some aspects of their treatment.[2–5] The ankle joint may be injured as the result of direct, or more often, indirect trauma (rotational, translational, or axial forces). These injuries often result in variable amounts of subluxation or dislocation of the talus from the mortise of the distal tibia and fibula. It was originally shown by Ramsey and Hamilton[6] that even mild malalignment of the ankle joint leads to abnormal pressure distribution and subsequent arthritis. Generally, a good outcome might be expected if a congruent reduction, through closed or open means, can be obtained and maintained. Mont and associates[7] showed that residual radiographic abnormalities after ankle fracture surgery, especially if multiple, correlated with poorer clinical outcomes. Thus the goals of treatment for ankle fractures and disloca-tions are a stable congruent joint that allows for early joint mobility, fracture healing, and, ultimately, the prevention of arthritis. The decision for operative or nonoperative treatment of these injuries depends on whether the risks and benefits of open treatment are expected to provide improved results compared with closed treatment.

This chapter focuses on the practical operative management of ankle fractures, including surgical indications, operative methods and technical pearls, and pre- and post-operative management, based on the available literature and the authors' experiences.

Functional and Surgical Anatomy

The ankle joint consists of the articulation of three bones (tibia, talus, and fibula) that move relative to one another and are restrained by three ligament complexes **(Fig. 32–1).** The ankle joint relies on these bony and soft tissues to

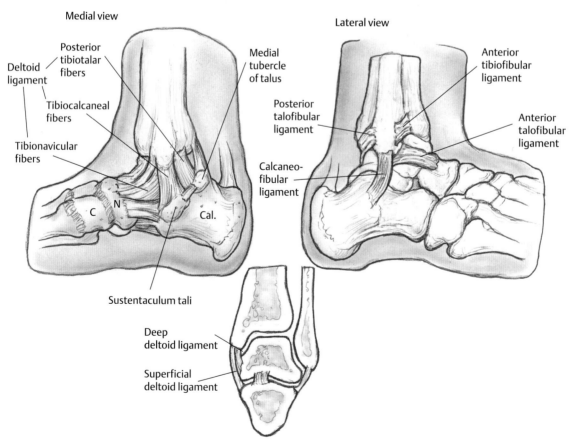

Figure 32–1 The bony and ligamentous anatomy of the ankle. C, medial cuneiform; Cal, calceneous; N, navicular.

maintain stability and alignment while allowing the motion necessary for gait. Normally, the talus sits in the ankle "mortise" articulating with the weight-bearing tibial plafond, as well as the articular facets of the medial and lateral malleoli. In the neutral position, 90% of the weight borne across the ankle joint passes through the tibial plafond.[8] Most of the ankle's motion involves dorsiflexion and plantar flexion of the foot relative to the leg. However, when viewed from above, the talus is trapezoidal in shape; thus with ankle dorsiflexion there is also widening of the mortise and external rotation of the fibula.[9] The ankle might best be regarded as a complicated hinge.

The bony ankle is maintained by three sets of ligaments: the tibiofibular "syndesmosis" and lateral and medial ankle ligament complexes **(Fig. 32–1)**. The distal tibia and fibula are held together by the syndesmosis or inferior distal tibiofibular ligament complex. The syndesmosis maintains the ankle mortise and consists of four ligaments: the anterior and posterior-inferior tibiofibular ligaments, the inferior transverse tibiofibular ligament, and the interosseous ligament. The lateral ankle ligament complex includes three distinct elements that fan out from the lateral fibula to attach to the lateral hindfoot: the anterior talofibular ligament, the calcaneofibular ligament, and the posterior talofibular ligament. Medially, the major ligament is the deltoid, which originates from the medial malleolus and includes a superficial component that inserts on the calcaneus and a deep component that inserts on the talus.[10] An injury to any of the three ligament complexes of the ankle, as well as the bony structures, can result in an unstable ankle joint. It is important to understand the anatomy because it is usually a combination of bony and ligamentous injury that will render an ankle unstable and require surgical stabilization.[9,11,12]

There is a relatively thin soft tissue envelope around the ankle, which may be quite fragile in some patients. Additionally, many tendons and neurovascular structures cross the ankle joint to supply the foot. Due to the paucity of protective soft tissues and local blood supply to these tissues, soft tissue problems or wound complications are not uncommon after an ankle injury or subsequent surgery. Considerations regarding the timing of surgery and soft tissue management are therefore critical in minimizing the risks for perioperative complications and are discussed at length in this chapter.

Classification

Optimally, a classification system should guide treatment decisions and provide insight into prognosis. The two most commonly used classification systems for ankle fractures are the Danis-Weber[13] and Lauge-Hansen[14] systems **(Fig. 32–2)**. Although orthopaedic surgeons commonly use both systems, neither is perfect and their interobserver reliability is unsatisfactory.[15] The Danis-Weber system is based on the level of the fibula fracture and is divided into three types. Type A fibula fractures occur below the level of the tibial plafond, type B fractures typically rise obliquely from the level of the plafond, and type C fractures are centered well above the plafond and typically have an associated syndesmotic injury. Although this system is relatively straightforward, it does not provide any guidance regarding treatment of a medial injury, options for fixation (except for the syndesmosis), or prognosis. The Lauge-Hansen system is based on the mechanism of injury and is more encompassing than the Danis-Weber system. It describes the typical medial injuries and proposes likely reduction maneuvers, which are of prime importance for nonoperative management of ankle fractures. The Lauge-Hansen system has been criticized for having less relevance to the surgical treatment of these injuries. The Lauge-Hansen system is based on two terms: the first describes the position of the foot at the time of injury, and the second describes the direction of the force causing the injury. The position of the foot at the time of injury dictates which structures are taut and thus likely to fail at the onset of deformation. According to this system, there are four types of ankle fractures: supination-external rotation injury (S-ER), supination-adduction (S-AD), pronation-external rotation (P-ER), and pronation-abduction (P-AB). S-ER is the most common type of ankle fracture (up to 85% of fractures) and includes an oblique or spiral fracture of the fibula along with a variable medial injury. This chapter discusses the operative treatment of ankle fractures and dislocations based on anatomical location (medial, lateral, posterior, and syndesmosis), but includes and integrates both ankle fracture classification systems into the discussion. Dislocations of the ankle are typically described by the direction of the dislocated talus. Using this system, though, little useful direction as to operative tactics or prognosis is attainable.

Fracture Assessment and Decision Making

The standard radiographic assessment of the ankle includes three views: the anteroposterior (AP), mortise (15 to 20 degrees internal rotation), and lateral views **(Fig. 32–3)**. With significant injury to the ankle, a consistent pattern of instability occurs: lateral translation and external rotation of the talus relative to the tibial plafond. Radiographic findings of obvious ankle instability may include significant fracture displacement, subluxation, or dislocation of the talus under the plafond, and widening of the medial joint space. Sometimes, radiographic findings may be more subtle. Other radiographic clues that significant injury has occurred

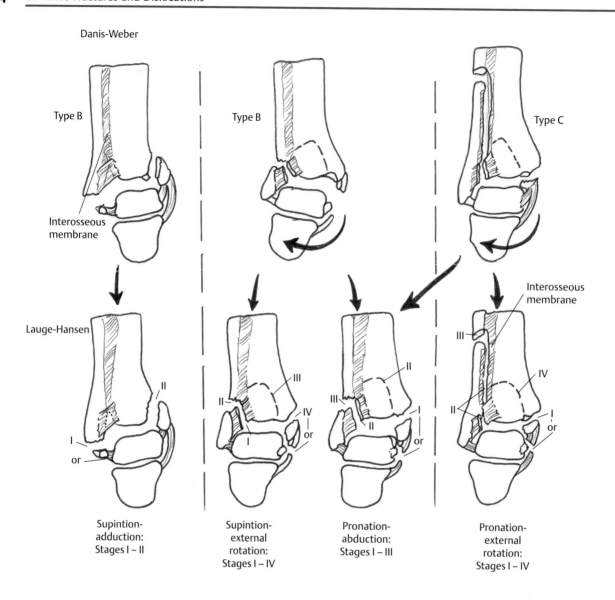

Figure 32–2 The ankle fracture classifications of Danis-Weber[13] and Lauge-Hansen.[14]

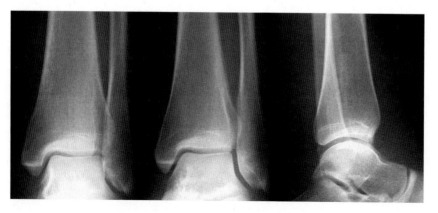

Figure 32–3 Standard ankle radiographs. From left: anteroposterior, 15 to 20 degrees internal rotation "mortise," and lateral views.

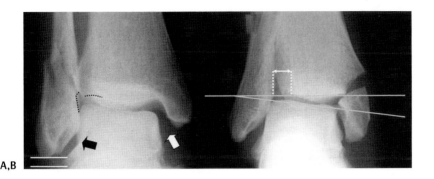

A,B

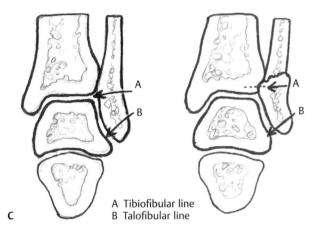

A Tibiofibular line
B Talofibular line

C

Figure 32–4 (A) Anteroposterior (AP) ankle radiograph of a displaced distal fibula fracture with an incompetent deltoid ligament ("SE-4 deltoid"). Signs of significant injury seen here include shortening of the fibula (white lines), loss of parallelism of the subchondral lines of lateral malleolus and that of the lateral talus (black arrow), loss of normal tibiofibular line (hatched black lines), and widened medial joint space (white arrow). **(B)** AP ankle radiograph demonstrating increased tibiofibular clear space (white dotted lines) and talar tilt (gray lines). **(C)** Drawing of the normal relationship of the medial fibula and lateral aspect of the talus (left) and another of how these relationships change with shortening of the distal fibula.

(Fig. 32–4A–C) include increased widened clear space, alterations in the talocrural angle, talar tilt, widened tibiofibular clear space, loss of alignment of the subchondral plates at the tibiofibular line, and shortening of the fibula by loss of parallelism of the subchondral lines of lateral malleolus and that of the lateral talus.[16–18]

At times, a fracture of the lateral malleolus may be accompanied by an injury to the deltoid ligament. Recent work has demonstrated that soft tissue indicators such as medial pain and swelling are not reliable predictors of ankle instability associated with a supination/external rotation fracture of the distal fibula.[19,20] Radiographic findings may also not clearly demonstrate the instability of this injury, and an AP or mortise stress view of the ankle taken with external rotation force may be helpful in revealing lateral talar subluxation and associated medial joint space widening.[19,20] Michelson and associates[21] advocated a "gravity stress test" as effective and less painful for the patient compared with other dynamic tests **(Fig. 32–5A,B)**. Using this method, the lateral side of the ankle is placed down on

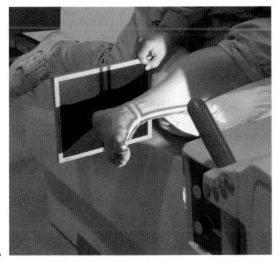

A

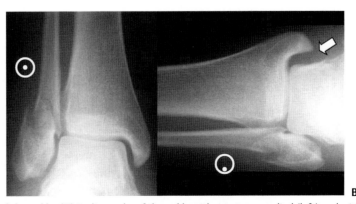

B

Figure 32–5 (A) Technique for obtaining gravity stress views of the ankle. **(B)** Radiographs of the ankle without stress applied (left) and with stress applied using gravity (right).

the table with the majority of the ankle off the edge of the table. A cross-table mortise view radiograph is performed. A positive stress test shows medial clear space widening relative to the nonstressed radiograph.

Similarly, syndesmosis injuries may be identified by obvious widening of the distal tibiofibular joint, or they may be very subtle. Although the level of the fibular fracture may be used to assess the likelihood of syndesmosis injury,[22] it has been recently emphasized that syndesmosis instability can accompany more distal Weber B fractures.[23] A few methods may accomplish the goal of demonstrating radiographically subtle syndesmosis instability. Many orthopaedic surgeons use the external rotation stress test as just described to evaluate competency of the syndesmosis. Candal-Couto and associates[24] demonstrated that disruption of the syndesmosis causes even more displacement in the anteroposterior (sagittal) plane than in the coronal plane, and suggested that stress views evaluating anteroposterior displacement of the fibula relative to the tibia may be an even more sensitive indicator of syndesmosis injury. In the case of a more proximal fibula fracture without a medial fracture, a positive stress test likely shows a deltoid *and* syndesmosis injury.

The treatment of ankle fractures with special circumstances, including open fractures and those in patients with diabetes mellitus or osteoporosis, will be discussed later in this chapter.

Indications for Surgical Treatment

As noted, the goals of treatment for ankle fractures and dislocations are the maintenance of a stable, congruent joint that allows for early joint mobility, fracture healing, and ultimately the prevention of arthritis. Fortunately, many minor ankle fractures are functionally equivalent to lateral ankle sprains, consisting of a stable, isolated lateral malleolus fracture that will lead to a good outcome if treated nonoperatively. Traditionally, closed reductions have been deemed unsatisfactory if radiographs showed a medial clear space greater than 2 mm or more than the opposite side or a displacement of the medial or lateral malleolus greater than 2 mm.[1] If a closed reduction is determined to be adequate, the patient may be treated with cast or splint immobilization and serial examinations. However, it may be very difficult to maintain the ankle in a reduced position with casting. First of all, radiographic criteria can be misleading because they are based on two-dimensional static representation of a three-dimensional dynamic joint. Second, the ability of a cast to hold the reduction is reduced as limb swelling diminishes with time; thus reduction may be lost even if diligent care is provided. Fractures that are often stable enough for nonoperative treatment include most of the Weber A fractures, as well

as some of the Weber B fractures, including low-grade Lauge-Hansen S-AD or S-ER fractures (types 1 and 2).

If closed reduction is inadequate or expected to be inadequate in accomplishing the desired goals, surgical treatment should be considered. General guidelines for the surgical treatment of ankle fractures[3,5,14,25–27] and the authors' recommendations include:

1. Weber A and S-AD fractures associated with a medial injury
2. Weber B or S-ER and P-AB fractures that occur as part of a more complex bimalleolar, trimalleolar, or bimalleolar equivalent fracture (fibular fracture with incompetent deltoid ligament)
3. Weber C and P-ER 2 and 3 fractures require surgery because of the syndesmosis injury and associated instability.
4. Open ankle fractures (see **Video 32–1, Disk 4**)
5. Ankle fracture-dislocations with more extensive bone and soft tissue injury

Surgical Treatment

Timing of Surgery

The timing of surgery is somewhat controversial but ultimately depends on the condition of the soft tissues. Several authors have suggested that surgery is best performed within 6 to 8 hours of injury, before significant edema develops.[28,29] However, the logistics of performing early surgery may be difficult. Generally, most experts agree that swelling and edema should be controlled before surgery is undertaken to minimize the risk of soft tissue complications. Marked swelling, the presence of fracture blisters, or other skin changes should delay surgery until the soft tissues have had time to recover. If this is the case, the fracture must be reduced and held in a well-padded splint, cast, or even external fixator, and the limb placed at elevation. Most ankle fractures can undergo surgical treatment with no change in technique or complication rates even up to 3 weeks after the injury.

Examination

Assessment of the soft tissues and the decision regarding timing of ankle fracture surgery are among the most important decisions a surgeon makes in these cases. Blisters, considerable swelling, or other signs of soft tissue trauma should alert the surgeon, and surgery should be delayed until these issues resolve. The "wrinkle" sign has been used in other areas of the lower extremity and may be helpful for deciding when the soft tissues are ready for ankle fracture surgery. Deformity from an ankle fracture dislocation may cause pressure necrosis of the skin over the supramalleolar area. For this reason, if surgery is not to be performed immediately, a closed reduction should be performed and a splint applied that will maintain reduction of the talus beneath the plafond and decompress the skin at risk. The patient needs a thorough lower-extremity exam despite the obvious ankle fracture. The limb should always be checked proximally for tenderness over the fibula (Maisonneuve fracture), along with examination of the Achilles' tendon and foot for associated injuries. Medial tenderness in the ankle with no fracture should alert the surgeon to the likelihood of a deltoid injury and the possibility of an unstable ankle.

Implants

In most cases, we use a small fragment set with a one-third tubular plate laterally, and 4.0 or 4.5 mm partially threaded cancellous screws (cannulated or solid) medially. The one-third tubular plate has been a "workhorse" plate for distal fibula and other ankle fractures because it easily contours to the local anatomy, is low profile, and allows ample mechanical strength for most fractures. Newer plates, however, may be beneficial in some particular cases. "Composite" plates that are one-third tubular distally and 3.5 mm proximally (DePuy, Warsaw, Indiana) may be useful in patients with poor bone quality or in cases with proximal fracture extension. Locking plate technology may also be useful in some difficult ankle fractures. These plate–screw devices create a fixed-angle construct and may be beneficial in patients with poor bone quality and fracture comminution. Care must be taken when using locking plates around the ankle, however; if they are not placed in a lag fashion like traditional nonlocked plates, they are not useful for aiding in reduction. Rarely, intramedullary devices are used to control fractures of the distal fibula, and tension-band wire techniques are sometimes useful medially or laterally for very comminuted, distal fractures that require fixation.

Preoperative Care and Planning

Fracture dislocations or subluxations must be reduced because excess pressure on the skin may cause necrosis or convert a closed fracture to an open one. A well-padded posterior and U splint is then applied to maintain reduction. The supramalleolar skin over the distal tibia is most often at risk because subluxation of the talus and malleoli typically occurs laterally. Loss of reduction may occur relatively early as swelling resolves and the splint no longer fits well.

The importance of preoperative planning cannot be overemphasized. This may be especially true for injuries around the ankle where multiple surgical incisions are often required and the injuries and soft tissues allow little leeway for surgical mistakes. Forethought as to which injury may need surgical treatment and what approaches may optimally allow access to each injury is typically time well spent.

Planning of reduction and implants begins with high-quality radiographs. On occasion comparison views of the contralateral ankle may be helpful. Rarely, computed tomography (CT) may be indicated to judge the size and position of a posterior malleolar fragment, or involvement of the distal tibiofibular joint.

Operative Setup

Patients undergoing ankle fracture surgery are typically administered general or spinal anesthesia. Local anesthesia and sedation may be used on occasion, although incomplete muscle relaxation will occur that may make fracture reduction difficult. For patients being treated for injuries of the medial and/ or lateral ankle, positioning is usually supine on a radiolucent operating table. It is often helpful to place a padded bump behind the buttock on the injured side to internally rotate the leg and allow comfortable access to the lateral malleolus. A well-padded thigh tourniquet is used to provide a dry surgical field. Place two pillows or a foam base (or later a sterile towel roll) under the fractured leg to elevate it above the contralateral leg: this assists in the surgical approaches and in obtaining lateral radiographs. A surgical prep of the limb is performed and a preoperative dose of antibiotic is administered prior to exsanguination of the leg and insufflation of the tourniquet.

Postoperatively, wound closure is performed in a multilayer fashion. Obtaining soft tissue coverage over the lateral fibular plate with a full-thickness layer of soft tissue is desired. The subcutaneous tissues and skin are closed with atraumatic technique. Again, these tissues may have little physiological reserve, and wound problems around the ankle are rarely easily treated. The authors prefer not to use staples on the skin around the foot or ankle, but instead use 4–0 nylon sutures that can be carefully tensioned.

Isolated Lateral Malleolus Fractures

The importance of reduction of the lateral malleolus and its impact on the overall ankle joint congruency and mechanics has been well recognized.[6,30] Yablon and associates[30] concluded that the lateral malleolus was the key to the anatomical reduction of bimalleolar ankle fractures because the displacement of the talus faithfully followed the displaced distal fibular fragment (this concept has recently been challenged by Tornetta,[31] who demonstrated that medial-only fixation may be sufficient in many bimalleolar injuries).

Good results are typically achieved with nonoperative treatment of isolated lateral malleolus fractures when not accompanied by a medial injury.[25] These clinical results are supported by cadaveric studies, which have shown that isolated displacement of the lateral malleolus does not cause ankle instability.[8,32] The literature supports nonoperative treatment for less than 2 mm of displacement of the lateral malleolus and a normal medial clear space.[6,33] For patients who have a closed, isolated lateral malleolus fracture with minimal displacement, the authors recommend nonoperative treatment with close follow-up.

Diagnosis of an associated deltoid ligament injury is not always easy. Medial tenderness and swelling may indicate a deltoid ligament injury, but clinical findings of a medial injury are occasionally quite subtle. Initial radiographs must be carefully scrutinized for widening of the medial joint space, which indicates incompetence of the deltoid ligament. Other methods of diagnosis include a variety of stress tests (described earlier in this chapter) and magnetic resonance imaging (MRI).

Technique of Fibular Plating

A direct lateral approach using a longitudinal incision is commonly used for the reduction and plating of fibula fractures **(Fig. 32–6)** (see **Video 32–1, Disk 4**). The fibula is usually palpable beneath the subcutaneous tissues and its borders can be defined fairly easily. At times, the skin incision may be moved posteriorly (or anteriorly) depending on the soft tissues, site of plate placement, desire to access the postero- and anterolateral tibia, or other reasons. The skin incision for posterior application of an antiglide plate is probably best modified by moving it 1 cm posteriorly to prevent soft tissue impingement during surgery. Additionally, the path of the superficial peroneal nerve is not always consistent, and meticulous dissection is required to assess whether the nerve is crossing through the operative wound, especially as the incision is carried proximally **(Fig. 32–6)**.

Most lateral malleolar fractures that require open reduction and internal fixation (ORIF) are repaired with a prebent one-third tubular plate with or without lag screws. The plate can be applied directly laterally **(Fig. 32–7A)** or posteriorly **(Fig. 32–7B)**. A laterally applied plate may result in occasional problems with implant prominence, but this position does allow for more direct access for plate application. The authors prefer to apply a posterior antiglide plate for oblique fractures whenever possible. This technique may be more mechanically effective than lateral plating and minimizes risks of implant problems.[34,35] If the first screw placed is just above the apex of the fracture, the plate can aid in the reduction by pushing the fracture into position **(Fig. 32–8A)**. A lag screw can then usually be placed through the plate to further increase fixation strength **(Fig. 32–8B)**.

Simple fibular fracture patterns, such as the typical oblique or spiral fracture of an SE-4 injury, are relatively easy to reduce. The fracture can be "freshened" by pushing the organized fracture hematoma from the fracture line that may prevent interdigitation of the fracture's bony interstices.

One or two small, pointed reduction or "lion-jaw" clamps can be used to restore length, translation, and rotation. Fracture reduction can be judged by visualizing the proximal fracture spike and ensuring that it is keyed in at the fracture's apex. As noted, a one-third tubular plate can be applied laterally or posteriorly for fixation. A lag screw can be applied before plating if a lateral plate is used, or through the plate if an antiglide plate is placed posteriorly.

Comminuted or "crushed" lateral malleolus fractures may be much more difficult to properly reduce and fix. Attention must be made to restoring proper length and rotation across the fracture. These deformities are restored when the subchondral contour of the lateral talus matches

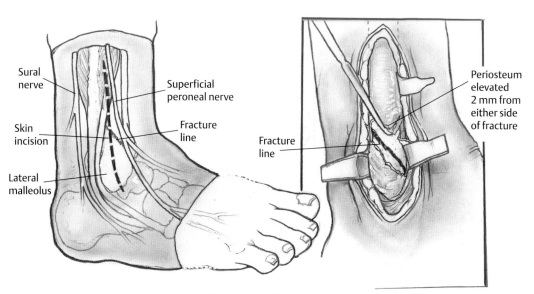

Figure 32–6 Surgical approach to the distal fibula and applied anatomy. The incision can be moved posteriorly to accommodate positioning of the plate on the posterior surface of the fibula or to allow for a posterolateral approach to the distal tibia (posterior malleolus).

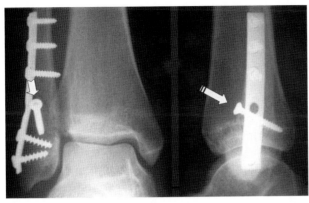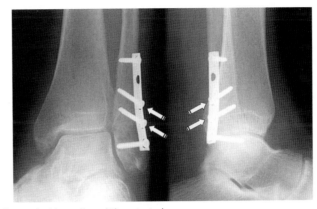

A

B

Figure 32–7 Positioning of plates for the distal fibula. **(A)** The plate can be applied laterally or **(B)** posteriorly.

that of the medial distal fibula, and the tibiofibular line is restored on the mortise view **(Figs. 32–3** and **32–4A–C).** Useful techniques for gaining reduction include indirect reduction methods. For example, the plate can be used as an indirect reduction tool.[36] Using this technique, the plate is initially applied to one side of the fracture (usually distal) and then length and rotation may be obtained using manual traction/manipulation, a mini distractor, or lamina spreaders against a "push-pull" screw. The plate is then temporarily secured to the bone proximally with a Verbrugge or other clamp and the ankle imaged. The construct can be manipulated as necessary until an acceptable alignment is achieved, and then the plate may be secured proximally with screws. An alternative method[27] is to use a pointed reduction clamp to carefully correct rotation and

bring the fibula out to length. One or two small K-wires can then be used to pin the fibula to the talus or distal tibia. A plate can then be applied and the K-wires removed. Radiographs are then checked, and if an acceptable reduction is confirmed, a plate can be definitively fixed to the bone with screws. The authors typically use a stiffer plate, such as a well-contoured 3.5 mm dynamic compression plate (Synthes USA, Paoli, PA) or "hybrid" plate (DePuy Orthopaedics, Warsaw, Indiana) in cases where there is considerable fracture shortening, comminution, or a more proximal diaphyseal injury. These more rigid plates must be carefully precontoured to include the anatomical rotation of the distal fibular shaft **(Fig. 32–4A–C),** or they may tend to malreduce the fracture as the bone moves to the plate during screw insertion.

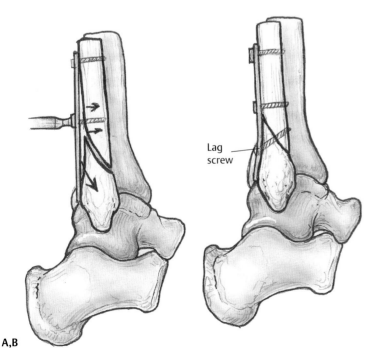

Lag
screw

A,B

Figure 32–8 An antiglide plate applied posteriorly over the fracture spike of an oblique distal fibula fracture may aid in fracture reduction, apply excellent fixation strength, and prevent implant-related problems. **(A)** Reduction is aided by the plate "pushing" the fracture spike into place. **(B)** Lag screws can then be applied for additional fixation.

Tips and Tricks

- After fixation of most unstable ankle fractures, stress views of the ankle should be performed to assess for syndesmosis injuries.
- A fracture of the fibula cannot be reduced with the aid of a locked plate and all locking screws. The fracture must be reduced prior to applying locked screws.
- A small fragment posterior to the distal fibula may represent an avulsion of the superficial peroneal retinaculum. If not addressed, this injury may lead to peroneal subluxation.

Medial Malleolus Fractures

Medial malleolus fractures usually occur in conjunction with lateral malleolus fractures, but occasionally occur as an isolated injury in P-ER or P-AB injuries (**Fig. 32–2**). It is important to obtain radiographs of the entire tibia and fibula because an "isolated" medial malleolus may be part of a more complex Maisonneuve fracture with a proximal fibula fracture and injury to the syndesmosis. Medial malleolar fractures may be transverse, oblique, or nearly vertical in orientation. Transverse or oblique fractures represent avulsion injuries and may involve the entire medial malleolus or just the anterior colliculus. This distinction is made by careful review of the lateral radiograph. Because the deep deltoid ligament attaches to the posterior colliculus, injury to the deep deltoid ligament can coexist with an anterior collicular fracture. In this case, repair of the anterior malleolar fragment will not restore competence of the medial ligament and the ankle may remain potentially unstable. In contrast, transverse fractures of the entire malleolus are not associated with ligament injury, and fixation of complete malleolar fractures restores stability.[31]

Currently, there are no long-term studies on outcomes of isolated medial malleolus fractures. The authors recommend that nondisplaced or very minimally displaced fractures be treated with immobilization, but fractures displaced more than 2 mm should be treated with ORIF.[1] Plain radiographs provide limited accuracy for imaging the medial malleolus, and even small amounts of residual radiographic displacement of medial malleolus fractures may in reality correlate to much larger amounts of true malreduction. One should carefully scrutinize all three radiographic views of the ankle in assessing these injuries, and even then, they may be better visualized with a CT scan. It has been noted that a sizable malreduced fracture may behave as a deltoid ligament injury and lead to dynamic ankle instability,[8] and painful nonunions of displaced medial malleolus fractures are not uncommon after closed treatment.[37] Strong consideration should also be given to open reduction for fractures where small osseous or osteochondral fragments are in the joint because

these can lead to mechanical wear or impingement.[38] When the fractured medial malleolus is exposed, the joint should be carefully inspected for free fragments and chondral injuries, which may indicate a more guarded prognosis for the ankle.

Technique of Medial Malleolar Fixation

The authors use a curvilinear incision extending from above the anteromedial aspect of the ankle joint superiorly and curving distally around the tip of the medial malleolus (**Fig. 32–9A,B**) (see **Video 32–1, Disk 4**). The advantage of this approach is the excellent visualization of the medial ankle joint and fracture reduction proximally. Partially threaded lag screws are then typically placed through the incision more distally. The disadvantage of this approach is that the surgeon necessarily encounters the saphenous vein and nerve, which must be carefully preserved. Some surgeons prefer a straight longitudinal medial incision extending over the fracture and the tip of the medial malleolus or a curved incision that extends around the posterior aspect of the medial malleolus.[39] A major limitation of these approaches is impaired visualization of the articular reduction and any articular injury. Furthermore, making an incision of the skin directly over the fracture could lead to potentially catastrophic wound problems.

Reduction of the medial malleolus is typically straightforward, but the authors have found a few "technical tricks" helpful. First, a somewhat thick flap of periosteum is often present medially, which may incarcerate in the fracture preventing accurate reduction or make fracture visualization more difficult. This periosteal flap may be amputated as it extends off the bone of the malleolar fragment. Second, manipulation of the malleolar fragment may be aided by insertion of one or two K-wires placed through its tip. Once reduction is achieved, these may be inserted across the fracture into the distal tibial metaphysis for provisional fixation. Other potentially useful instruments for this manipulation include the dental pick and the small, pointed reduction clamp (a drill hole can be made on the distal tibia's cortex proximally). Third, assessment of reduction is accomplished by assessing the extra-articular fracture line medially and anteriorly, as well as the anteromedial corner of the ankle joint. Finally, maintaining two points of fixation is recommended (provisionally and definitively) to prevent rotational displacement. Ideally then, if cannulated screws are to be used, three K-wires should be placed so that when a screw's pilot hole is drilled and that K-wire's stabilizing effect is lost, reduction will be maintained.

Most medial malleolus fractures are well fixed with two partially threaded cancellous lag screws (**Fig. 32–10A,B**), either cannulated (3.5 or 4.5 mm) or noncannulated (4.0 mm). Depending on the fracture configuration, smaller fragments may be fixed with a screw and a Kirschner wire (cut short and bent) placed for rotational stability. Comminuted

Figure 32–9 **(A)** Surgical approach to the medial malleolus and **(B)** applied anatomy.

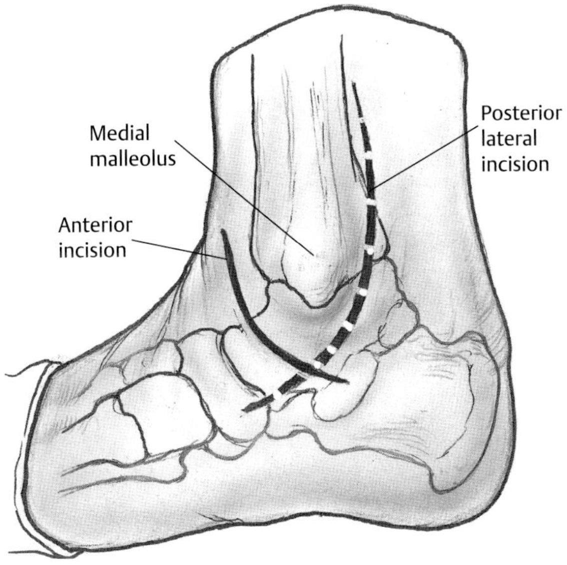

fractures may require a tension-band construct or even supplemental fixation with mini-fragment screws. S-AD type fractures **(Fig. 32–2)** or other more vertically oriented fractures that extend farther into the tibia should be fixed with an antiglide plate (with or without lag screws) to prevent vertical migration **(Fig. 32–11)**.

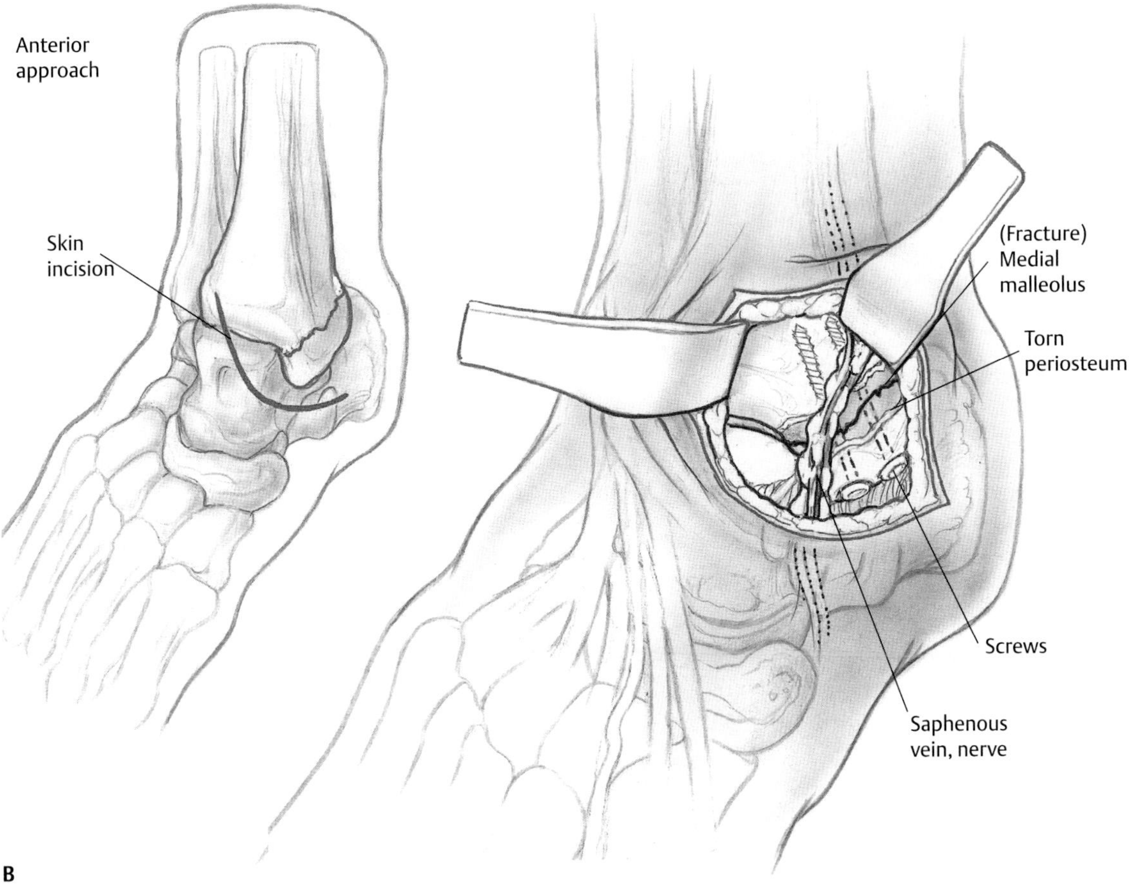

Bimalleolar Fractures

Bimalleolar ankle fractures refer to bony injuries typically involving the medial and lateral malleoli, and may include the Weber A, B, C and Lauge-Hansen S-AD 2, S-ER 3 and 4, P-ER 3 and 4, and P-AB 2 type fractures. The vast majority

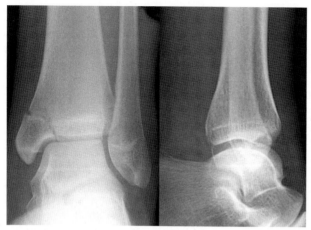
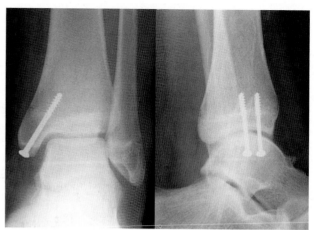

A   B

Figure 32–10 Medial malleolus fractures are most often fixed with two partially threaded lag screws from the small fragment set. **(A)** Preoperative radiographs. **(B)** Postoperative radiographs.

of injuries that involve the medial and lateral malleolus are mechanically unstable and need to be reduced and internally fixed if a good outcome is to be expected.[1] Classically, fixation of both malleoli is recommended. The methods of fixation for each injured side are discussed individually elsewhere in this chapter. The potential for syndesmosis injury must also be considered for almost all of these injuries but is most common with Weber C fibular fractures more than 4.5 cm above the plafond.[22,23,40] Recently, Ebraheim and associates[23] demonstrated that syndesmosis injury may also be present with more distal fibular fractures that are not typically considered at risk for such injury. They recommended routine intraoperative stress views of the syndesmosis after fixation of all ankle fractures.

Recent work by Tornetta[31] has demonstrated that many bimalleolar fractures are successfully stabilized by reduction and fixation of the medial malleolus alone. This is clinically relevant when fracture blisters, fasciotomy, or other considerations preclude a lateral incision. However, one potential pitfall with medial fixation alone is the isolated

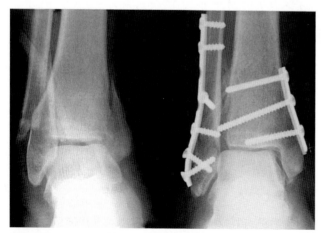

Figure 32–11 Vertical fractures (S-AD injury) of the medial malleolus may be stabilized with an antiglide plate to prevent proximal displacement.

fracture of the anterior colliculus. Fracture of the anterior colliculus of the medial malleolus may or may not be associated with deep deltoid ligament disruption. If one repairs an anterior collicular fracture and is considering medial fixation alone, a stress exam should be done after fixation to determine if medial stability has been restored. If the deep deltoid is disrupted, fixation of the anterior colliculus of the medial malleolus does not stabilize the ankle because the associated ligament injury and lateral repair is also necessary.

The "bimalleolar-equivalent injury" refers to a fibula fracture that is associated with a complete deltoid ligament injury, instead of a medial malleolus fracture. This injury merits further discussion because the misdiagnosis or mistreatment of these injuries may result in a poor outcome. The deltoid ligament originates on the medial malleolus and inserts on the talus and calcaneus. The superficial portion resists eversion, and the deep component resists external rotation of the talus and is the critical portion that maintains a stable ankle. The diagnosis of a deltoid injury is often made clinically with swelling and tenderness at or below the medial malleolus. Plain radiographs at rest, or stress views (discussed further in Fracture Assessment and Decision Making) may be needed to confirm the diagnosis, and some have even suggested MRI.

Patients with fibula fractures and an injury to the deltoid ligament rendering the ankle unstable should be treated surgically with an anatomical reduction of the fibula. It is unnecessary to repair the deltoid ligament, provided an anatomical reduction is obtained of the fibula and the medial clear space.[41] Even if the medial clear space appears reduced, it is still important to check for an associated syndesmosis injury by doing intraoperative stress views. These patients should then be treated with immobilization without early motion to allow the deltoid ligament to heal at its original length.[8] Rarely, a portion of the torn deltoid ligament may block complete reduction of the joint and the medial clear space may remain wide; when this occurs, medial exploration is indicated.[42]

Posterior Malleolus Fractures

Fracture of the ankle's posterior malleolus is caused by external rotation or abduction (Lauge-Hansen P-ER, S-ER 4, and P-AB types) with avulsion of the bone by the posterior-inferior tibiofibular ligament. Previous authors have advocated internal fixation for fractures that comprise 20 to 33% of the distal tibial articular surface to prevent posterior subluxation of the talus and articular incongruity.[43–46] Raasch and associates[47] demonstrated that stabilization of the fibula could prevent posterior subluxation of the ankle because the fibula and anterior tibiofibular ligament are the primary restraint to posterior instability of the ankle. Other studies, however, have shown that patients with posterior malleolar fragments consisting of greater than 25 to 33% of the articular surface had better clinical results with internal fixation.[45,46] One potential pitfall is the assessment of the true size of the posterior malleolar fragment: CT or MRI may be needed to truly assess the proportion of the articular surface that is involved. If the surgeon chooses not to fix the posterior malleolar fracture, Scheidt and associates[48] have recommended immobilization in the early healing period to protect against rotational and translational forces.

Technique of Posterior Malleolar Fixation

The authors recommend surgical treatment of the posterior malleolus when the fragment is greater than 25% of the tibial articular surface, when there is posterior subluxation and/or dynamic posterior instability of the ankle, or when there is an articular step-off greater than 2 mm, especially if a nonanatomical reduction of the fibula is present. The rationale for choosing between surgical treatment methods for fractures of the posterior malleolus are presented well elsewhere by Tornetta et al.[49]

The authors have adopted the following tactics to treating fractures of the posterior malleolus that require surgery. Harper and Hardin[50] showed that displacement of the posterior malleolus frequently reduces indirectly when the fibula was reduced (**Fig. 32–12A,B**). If the fracture is anatomically reduced via indirect methods, the posterior malleolus can be fixed with one or two lag screws placed anterior to posterolateral. These lag screws can be inserted percutaneously using cannulated or standard screws (**Fig. 32–12B,C**). High-quality fluoroscopic views

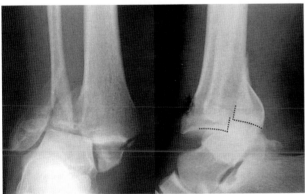
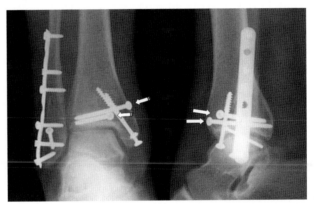
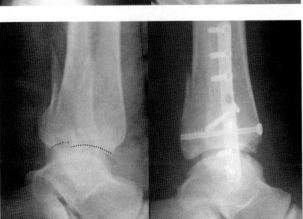

Figure 32–12 (A) If a high-quality reduction of the posterior malleolus fracture is achieved via indirect means, fixation may be percutaneously applied using **(B)** standard or **(C)** cannulated screws placed in an anterior-posterior direction.

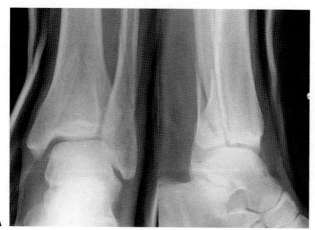
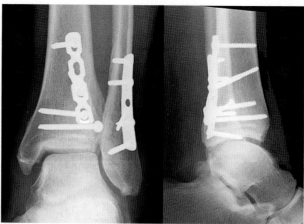

Figure 32–13 (A) Trimalleolar fracture with large posterior malleolus fracture treated with posterolateral approach and **(B)** fixation using antiglide plate and lag screws.

must be obtained of the fracture reduction and implant position if this method is used. If the posterior malleolus fracture is still displaced after the fibula is reduced, it can be reduced and fixed via an open posterolateral approach using the fibular incision with additional posterior exposure **(Fig. 32–13A,B)**.[39] If this open posterolateral approach is anticipated, the patient can be positioned laterally on a bean bag (secured with a seatbelt, but without being taped to the table) and can be gently rolled to a more supine position by deflating the bean bag once the medial side is to be addressed. Exposure is gained by opening the superficial interval between the peroneal tendons anteriorly and the Achilles' tendon posteriorly, then passing lateral to the flexor hallucis longus (FHL) **(Fig. 32–14A,B)**. The neurovascular bundle of the posteromedial leg is safely protected by the FHL, and wide exposure of the posterior aspect of the distal tibia can be achieved. The fracture typically includes an apical fracture spike that can be keyed in to achieve reduction. A buttress plate can then be placed with lag screws to achieve excellent fixation of the posterior malleolar fragment.

Syndesmosis Injury

The treatment of syndesmosis injuries associated with fractures of the ankle continues to provoke controversy among surgeons. Despite multiple anatomical and biomechanical studies addressing the mechanism of injury and diagnosis, there is no consensus regarding specific treatment guidelines, such as the type of fixation needed and postoperative management. This chapter addresses only syndesmosis injuries associated with ankle fractures; Wuest[51] and Amendola[2] provide excellent comprehensive review articles of isolated syndesmosis injuries.

The syndesmosis is composed of four ligaments: the anterior-inferior and posterior-inferior tibiofibular ligaments, the inferior transverse tibiofibular ligament, and the interosseous ligament and membrane **(Fig. 32–1)**. Disruption of the syndesmosis usually occurs as the result of an external rotation force and typically involves "high" distal fibula fractures (i.e., Weber C and Lauge-Hansen P-ER and S-ER 4 fractures). The diagnosis is usually made radiographically, although a syndesmosis injury may be obvious or quite subtle and may be revealed only by stress radiographs. Common diagnostic imaging clues include a tibia–fibula clear space of greater than 6 mm on AP and mortise films, and a tibia–fibula overlap less than 6 mm on AP radiographs and less than 1 mm on the mortise view. Additionally, the medial clear space (the space between the talus and medial malleolus) should be equal to the space superior and lateral to the talus.[52] Ebraheim and associates[23] report that CT scans comparing the injured to the normal ankle are helpful; signs of syndesmosis injury include tibiofibular diastasis, anterior subluxation of the distal fibula, and a shallow incisura fibularis. Sometimes injuries are diagnosed intraoperatively by the Cotton test, which is done by pulling the distal fibula with a towel clip to determine if it separates from the tibia.[53] More recently, it has been suggested that AP subluxation may be easier to elicit and may be a more sensitive test of syndesmosis instability.[24]

The work of Boden and associates[22] is commonly quoted during discussions regarding stabilization of the ankle syndesmosis. They found that if the deltoid ligament was intact (no medial injury), no amount of syndesmosis disruption altered ankle stability. They recommended syndesmosis fixation for patients with fibula fractures

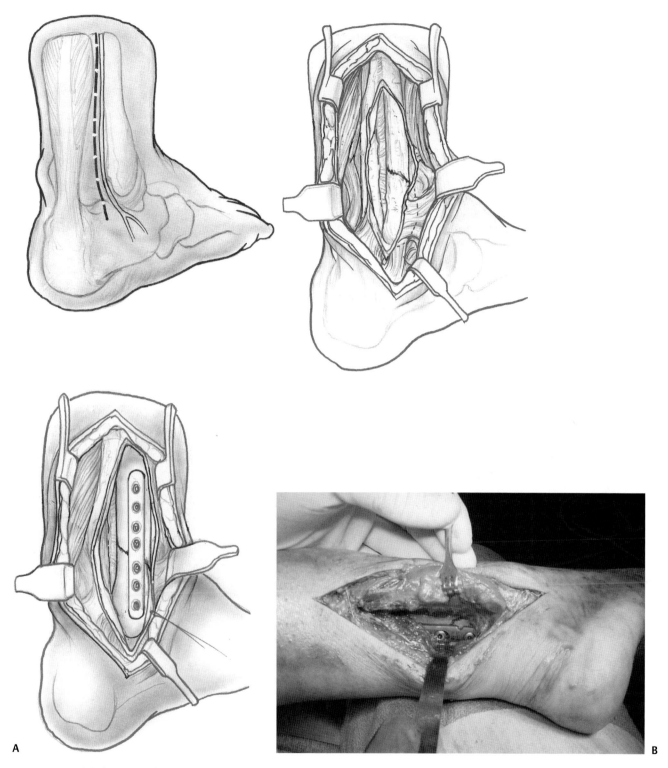

Figure 32–14 (A) The posterolateral approach to the distal tibia for access to the posterior malleolus. **(B)** Corresponding clinical photograph demonstrates wide exposure and plate fixation.

occurring greater than 4.5 cm proximal to the mortise (the "critical zone"), provided that they also had a medial injury. The degree of ankle instability in patients who had fractures of the fibula from 3.0 to 4.5 cm proximal to the mortise was not definitive in the study. Many surgeons have recommended placing a syndesmosis screw for uncertain injuries because the morbidity of a missed injury may be much greater than that of a syndesmosis screw.[54] If in doubt, the surgeon should get intraoperative external rotation or other stress radiographs, such as the Cotton test.

In many cases, both the fibular fracture and the syndesmosis injury are addressed simultaneously by repair of the fibula with a plate and screw fixation (often through the plate) of the syndesmosis. However, in some cases, syndesmosis fixation only is appropriate. In these cases, the distal fibular fragment is reduced to the talus, and two syndesmosis screws are placed. The rationale for this approach is that the fibula fracture itself is unimportant; rather, it is the reduction of the distal fibula and stabilization of the distal tibiofibular joint that is important. One advantage is that percutaneous fixation is possible. A significant disadvantage is the possibility of malreduction.

Technique of Syndesmosis Screw Fixation

The lateral and/or medial fractures should first be anatomically reduced and fixed. If the medial clear space is still wide (with or without stress test), a large tenaculum or reduction clamp can be placed from the fibula to the distal tibia. Intraoperative fluoroscopy allows for assessment of fibular alignment and length, and later helps to ensure that the screw is placed parallel to the joint. Once the joint is reduced, a syndesmosis screw should be directed parallel to the plafond and aimed slightly anteriorly from the fibula to the tibia at a level 1.5 to 2.0 cm proximal to the mortise, above the distal tibia–fibular joint (**Fig. 32–15A–C**). It is helpful to tap the pilot hole prior to screw insertion, even if self-tapping screws are used, because the screw may tend to push the tibia away from the fibula when its first few threads engage the tibial cortex. A second screw may be added slightly more superiorly, if desired. Many surgeons prefer to place syndesmosis screws with the ankle positioned in maximal dorsiflexion "to preserve ankle motion," although Tornetta and associates[55] have discredited this thinking. A fixation screw (not a lag screw) should be placed to prevent overtightening of the syndesmosis.

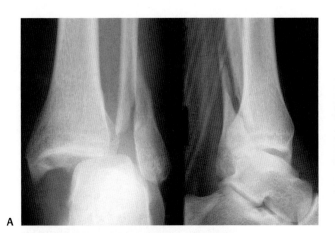

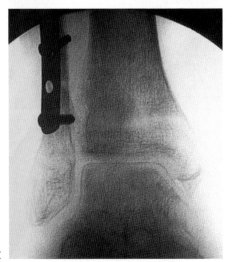

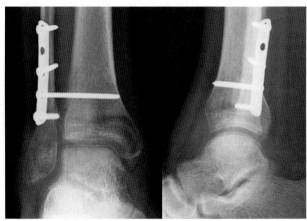

Figure 32–15 **(A)** Bimalleolar equivalent injury with syndesmosis disruption (confirmed intraoperatively) treated **(B)** with screw fixation. **(C)** The authors removed the screw in the office at 12 weeks to avoid screw breakage.

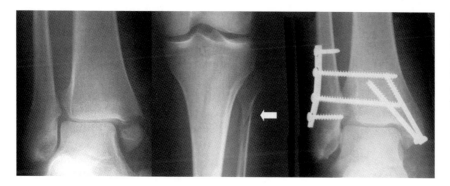

Figure 32–16 Maisonneuve injury combines a medial malleolus fracture, proximal fibula fracture, and syndesmosis injury. Fibular length and rotation must be restored before placement of the distal syndesmotic fixation. In this case, the authors inserted two syndesmosis screws through a short plate to provide stronger fixation.

Surgeons typically choose either 3.5 or 4.5 mm screws with three or four cortices of screw purchase, but these points remain controversial. No definitive biomechanical or clinical studies demonstrate an advantage of either screw size or number of cortices. Hoiness and Stromsoe[56] recently compared one 4.5 mm screw placed through four cortices (removed at 8 weeks) with two 3.5 mm screws that engaged only three cortices (not removed). At 1 year, there were no differences between the two groups in pain, functional score, or dorsiflexion. Recent articles have demonstrated that good results can also be obtained in the treatment of syndesmosis injuries with 4.5 mm polyl-L lactic acid (PLLA) bioabsorbable screws.[57] The potential benefit of the absorbable screw is that an additional procedure to remove the screw can be avoided. Although this technique is promising, the gold standard still remains metal implants for the syndesmosis.

Whether or not to remove the syndesmosis screw before weight bearing may be the most debated of all syndesmosis topics. Needleman and associates[58] showed that syndesmosis screws cause a decrease in the tibiotalar external rotation. Advocates of screw removal point out that leaving the screw in place results in abnormal ankle motion or at least screw breakage. Other studies, however, have shown that patients can be fully weight bearing with the screw in place, and that the screws eventually loosen or break with little morbidity.[59,60] Proponents of leaving the screw in place point out that the screw's loosening or breaking allow patients to have near normal ankle motion again.

The authors typically use a single 3.5 mm cortical screw, placed 1.5 to 2.0 cm above the mortise, with the ankle positioned in dorsiflexion and placed through four cortices (**Fig. 32–15B**). If the patient is large or obese, or compliance is in question, a second parallel screw may be added. The postoperative protocol is as follows: the patient is kept non–weight bearing for 6 to 7 weeks in a cast or boot, then weight bearing as tolerated in a boot for 6 weeks. Screw removal is typically performed between 12 and 14 weeks as an office procedure with postremoval radiographs obtained to verify a reduced mortise.

The previously mentioned Maisonneuve injury combines a proximal fibula fracture with a medial ankle ligamentous injury and includes a syndesmosis injury. The proximal fibula does not require operative treatment, but the syndesmosis injury should be recognized and addressed. To restore normal joint congruity, fibular length and rotation must be restored before placement of the distal syndesmotic screw(s). In this case, the authors typically place two syndesmosis screws, sometimes placing them through a two- or three-hole, one-third tubular plate to provide a stronger construct (**Fig. 32–16**).

Tips and Tricks

- A syndesmosis injury is common in cases with a fibula fracture > 4.5 mm above the mortise but may be present with more distal fractures as well.
- There is no evidence that syndesmosis screws placed in dorsiflexion cause a loss of ankle motion.
- An alternative to standard syndesmosis screw fixation that appears to provide adequate stability and may make secondary surgeries unnecessary is the use of bioabsorbable implants.

Open Fractures

Open fractures and injuries of the ankle require all of the considerations of closed injuries, as well as additional concerns about the severity of soft tissue injury and bacterial contamination. Open injuries, including ankle fractures, have been shown to be at increased risk for complications and poor outcomes when compared with closed injuries.[61,62]

The treatment of patients who have open ankle fractures begins upon arrival to the emergency room with the administration of intravenous antibiotics and tetanus prophylaxis. The wound should be examined and then covered with a saline-moistened sterile dressing. If the injury is grossly displaced, a reduction maneuver should be performed. If gross contamination of the wound is present, a brief irrigation of the wound may be helpful prior to reduction and application of a well-padded splint. Antibiotics should be provided according to current recommendations for open fractures. For example, patients who have Gustilo type I and II fractures should receive a cephalosporin (e.g., cefazolin) on admission, continued every 8 hours for at least 24 to 48 hours. Patients who have type III fractures should receive the same dose of a cephalosporin plus an aminoglycoside, a broad-spectrum antibiotic (Zosyn), or fluoroquinolone for gram-negative coverage. Farm injuries and grossly contaminated wounds should also receive penicillin.[63] Urgent wound debridement and lavage are mandatory. An aggressive and organized surgical debridement is performed to remove all foreign material and tissue of questionable viability.

Open type I and II[63] and IIIA fractures[63] can be treated with standard technique using stable internal fixation and wound closure once the wound is clean (see **Video 32–1, Disk 4**).[64,65] Bray and associates,[66] as well as Wiss and associates,[67] found that immediate ORIF of open ankle fractures caused no increased incidence of infection compared with those treated with delayed fixation. Both groups recommend this approach as the treatment of choice for most open ankle fractures. Type IIIB fractures may best be stabilized with either minimal internal fixation or an external fixator and delayed definitive fixation. Most authors agree that the wound should be re-debrided every 48 to 72 hours until the wound is "clean," and then may be closed more safely. The goal is for wound closure or a wound coverage procedure within 5 to 10 days.[65] Previous studies have shown mostly good results when these basic guidelines are followed.[66,67]

Ankle Fractures in Osteoporotic Bone

As our nation continues to age, orthopaedic surgeons will continue to be faced with more osteoporosis-related fractures, including those around the ankle. Although treatment goals for the majority of elderly patients are the same as for younger patients (i.e., restoration of ankle alignment, stability to allow for early motion, and the pre-

vention of posttraumatic arthritis), treatment decisions in patients with severe osteoporosis should be made on an individualized basis. Unfortunately, nonoperative treatment is usually poorly tolerated in many patients that suffer these injuries due to a variety of reasons, and there are fairly high complication rates with nonoperative treatment methods. With surgery, quality fixation strength may be difficult to achieve in elderly osteoporotic patients, and increased complication rates have been seen under these circumstances as well.[68,69] There are several techniques for maximizing fixation strength in patients with osteoporotic ankle fractures (**Fig. 32–17A,B**). These include plate fixation with all cancellous screws, plate and screw fixation supplemented with intramedullary pins,[70] use of locked small-fragment plates, and insertion of long, overdrilled lag screws for fixation of the medial malleolus (lag screw by technique) that capture the lateral tibial cortex. Recently, a technique of placing multiple long screws from the fibula into the tibia has been described.[71] Intramedullary fixation of the distal fibula with Rush rods, Kirschner wires, or other similar devices may be a consideration for the management of distal fibular fractures in the elderly patient with osteoporosis.

Ankle Fractures in Diabetic Patients

Ankle fractures in patients with diabetes mellitus are clearly associated with higher complication rates than in those that are unaffected by diabetes.[72,73] The effects of diabetes, including peripheral neuropathy, small vessel vascular disease, and skin changes, are predictable. Increased rates of surgical infections and wound problems in diabetics are paralleled by increased rates of skin breakdown and other problems in those treated nonoperatively. Surgically restoring stability to the unstable ankle in the diabetic with protective sensation, although not without

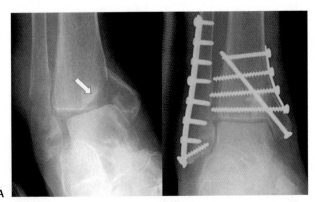

A

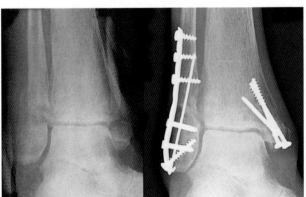

B

Figure 32–17 Techniques for increasing fixation in osteoporotic ankle fractures. **(A)** Case 1 demonstrates an osteoporotic ankle fracture with marginal impaction treated with locked plating for the fibula, calcium-phosphate cement to backfill behind the reduced marginal impaction, a buttress plate for a high medial malleolus fracture, and long lag screws (by technique) for the medial malleolus that capture the lateral tibial cortex. **(B)** Case 2 shows fixation by using a combination of cancellous and locked screws (remember, place all standard screws first) supplementing plate fixation with intramedullary K-wires,[69] and augmentation of medial malleolus fixation with mini-fragment screws.

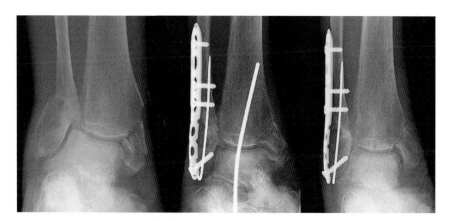

Figure 32–18 A patient with diabetes and osteoporosis presented with heavily traumatized soft tissues 4 days after this unstable bimalleolar ankle fracture. She was treated with minimally invasive plating of the fibula augmented with an intramedullary pin, a transarticular Steinmann pin to stabilize the talus under the tibial plafond, and no medial fixation.

risk, may afford the patient the best chance of a reasonable outcome and minimize the overall complication rate. Careful attention to the soft tissues must be paid both in deciding the timing of surgery as well as in operative handling of the tissues. Finally, initiation of weight bearing should be delayed until radiographic signs of healing because some of these patients may be impaired in their ability to control protected ambulation. In those patients with severe neuropathy and complete loss of protective sensation, a modified approach might be considered. Jani and associates[75] achieved relatively good results for severely neuropathic diabetic patients with ankle fractures using a protocol of transarticular pin fixation and an extended period of protected weight bearing (**Fig. 32–18**). The ankle can also be further stabilized with a unilateral fixator for a 3 to 6 week period to enhance the internal fixation stability and minimize the complications of casting in neuropathic patients.

Ankle Dislocations

Ankle dislocations that involve fractures should be treated with an urgent closed reduction to minimize the tension on the soft tissue envelope, followed by ORIF of the ankle as already described in this chapter. Dislocations that do not involve a fracture of the tibia or fibula are relatively uncommon and can usually be treated conservatively with closed reduction and casting. Ankle dislocations occur most commonly in young males as a result of motor vehicle accidents or falls. The ankle typically dislocates with the foot in plantar flexion due to the trapezoidal shape of the talus.[75] In the case of a closed dislocation, the ankle should be urgently reduced with conscious sedation or general anesthesia. It is the rare case that has a soft tissue block to reduction requiring open reduction. Once the ankle is reduced, it should be treated with 3 to 6 weeks of casting in a neutral position, depending on the degree of instability on exam. Most authors do not recommend primary repair of the ligaments, and long-term follow-up has not shown problems with instability.[76,77]

Postoperative Management

Optimizing outcome of ankle fractures requires a balance between obtaining and maintaining a reduction and restoring motion and weight bearing so the patient can return to activities without pain. For each type of ankle fracture these guidelines must be modified based on many factors: the quality of bone and the stability of the fixation, the reliability of the patient, comorbid conditions, and the need to protect the soft tissues such as the deltoid ligament and syndesmosis. Cimino and associates[78] assessed early mobilization of ankle fractures after ORIF showed that there was no loss of fixation with early motion, but that early motion resulted in the same functional outcomes as those patients that were immobilized. Previous studies have shown that there was no difference between early weight bearing in a cast and non–weight bearing in a cast so long as adequate stability was attained by surgery.[79,80] With these considerations in mind, the authors place patients in a fracture boot once sutures are removed and instruct patients on daily active range of motion exercises. The majority of patients continue non–weight bearing on the affected limb but are able to bear weight safely by 6 or 7 weeks after surgery. Guidelines for return of weight bearing though, should be individually tailored according to the stability of the reduction, the quality of the bone, and the health of the patient. Weight bearing may be further delayed for the following patients: elderly, diabetic, severe osteoporosis, wound problems, and ligament injury (syndesmosis and deltoid).

New Technology

Alternative and improved methods of fixation for ankle fractures continue to be an area of active investigation because of the uncomfortable incidence of wound-healing problems and prominent hardware about the ankle. Thordarson et al published the results of a randomized trial of a 4.5 mm polylactic acid syndesmotic screws compared with a 4.5 mm stainless steel screw in 32 patients with syndesmotic injuries.[81] There were no differences in outcome or complications in either group, and osteolysis was not seen about the bioabsorbable implants.[81] Many complications are associated with plates; investigators in Germany have developed a novel cannulated, small-diameter intramedullary device with multiple holes spaced 9 mm apart that allow for placement of cross-locking screws with an exterior jig.[82] The device was used in 194 cases, of which one third were bimalleolar injuries, and there were few soft tissue problems and only one nonunion.[82]

New "orthobiologic" agents are rapidly being introduced and are aggressively marketed to the orthopaedic surgeon. In one study, a synthetic bioglass (Cortoss, Orthovita, Malvern, Pennsylvania) was studied to determine if it could improve the fixation in osteopenic patients with ankle fractures.[83] Eighty-six "loose" screws with poor intraoperative fixation were augmented with the synthetic bone void filler, and only one loosened during follow-up. The deep infection rate after 6 months of follow-up was 5%.[96]

Complications

Wound Problems and Infection

Postoperative complications after the open treatment of ankle fractures are similar to those of other lower-extremity articular fractures. The most significant complications of operative ankle fracture treatment include postoperative infection (1 to 2%) and wound problems (4 to 5%). Many of these may be preventable with a thoughtful, cautious approach to the soft tissues, as discussed in the Preoperative Care and Planning and Exam Pearls sections of this chapter.

Marginal wound necrosis resulting in small areas of dry eschar can often be safely observed until deep tissues granulate beneath them, after which they can be removed or may spontaneously fall off. Larger areas of eschar or frank wound necrosis should prompt a consultation with a plastic surgeon, unless the orthopaedic surgeon has experience in complicated soft tissue problems. There is little redundancy to the tissues about the ankle; thus fasciocutaneous or rotation flaps are effective only for small soft tissue defects in this area. Free soft tissue transfers may be necessary for larger soft tissue voids.

Determining if an infection is a deep one may be quite difficult. Superficial cellulitis, manifest by peri-incisional redness and warmth, might be treated with antibiotics and brief observation, but certainly the presence of purulence or other signs of deep infection mandates a more aggressive approach. This typically means incision and drainage and intravenous antibiotic treatment. Methods of treatment such as local wound care, use of the whirlpool, and the Wound V.A.C. (Kinetic Concepts, Inc., San Antonio, Texas) have been effective tools for treating infected or complicated wounds. In most cases of early deep infection, the wounds can be thoroughly debrided and irrigated, and

the implants should be left in place. The infection should be treated with intravenous and then oral antibiotics. Consideration may be given to removing the implants once the fracture has healed.

Nonunion

Nonunion of the ankle is not a common problem because most of the bone in the area is metaphyseal and likely to heal. There are a few instances where ankle fractures may be prone to nonunion: medial malleolus fractures[37,84] and high-energy crush injuries of the lateral malleolus. Fractures of the medial malleolus at the level of the joint may result in residual displacement or interposed soft tissues, which may play a role in healing problems. In the authors' experience, these fracture nonunions that occur at the joint level are much more prone to be painful than tip avulsion fractures from the medial malleolus that fail to unite.

Surgical treatment of a medial malleolar nonunion typically consists of takedown of the nonunion, reapproximation of the fragments, and fixation with screws or a tension band. Both alignment and fixation may be problematic because bony resorption may be significant and the metaphyseal bone may be quite soft. Bone grafting may be necessary if tight interfragmentary compression cannot be achieved; when necessary, local tibial metaphyseal bone may be used.

Surgical treatment of lateral malleolar nonunions usually involves cases of fibular comminution with loss of length. The nonunion may also be a result of an associated syndesmosis injury. Treatment of these problems involves restoring fibular length and fixing the syndesmosis. Fibular length can be restored with a push-pull device to once again align the tip of the fibula with the lateral aspect of the talus. A bulk autograft or allograft may often need to be utilized to maintain the length.

Malunion

Malunion is now more frequently recognized since the work of Vrahas et al[85] has shown that malunion significantly alters joint contact stresses, which may lead to arthritis. Malunion may involve any portion of the ankle injury. Knowledge of the "normal" anatomy and preoperative planning allow the surgeon to minimize this risk. Also, comparison views both pre- and intraoperatively (the unprepped leg may usually be easily rotated through the draping to allow for C-arm radiography) may be useful to demonstrate the desired anatomy of the surgical reconstruction.

Malunion leading to subluxation or incongruity of the joint is likely the most important type because the risks for degeneration of the joint with loss of function can be expected.[86] If malunion appears likely to cause these problems, consideration should be given to corrective osteotomy or other operative reconstruction.[36,87–90] Simply, the goal of surgical treatment is to restore normal anatomy and kinematics to the injured ankle. A thoughtful description of the operative care of fibular malunion is given by Geissler and associates.[27]

Arthritis

Ankle arthritis is usually the result of a malreduction, an osteochondral defect (OCD), or a diffuse cartilage injury at the time of the initial fracture. Great effort should be taken to avoid a malreduction, as previously discussed in this chapter. For patients who are still having unexpected pain 3 to 6 months after the initial treatment with unremarkable radiographs, an MRI or CT scan may be performed to inspect the joint for an OCD or signs of chondrolysis. A complete discussion of the treatment of ankle arthritis is beyond the scope of this chapter, but options for mild cases include activity modification, nonsteroidal antiinflam-matories, and steroid injections. In some cases ankle arthroscopy may be useful as a diagnostic tool, as well as a therapeutic intervention. Finally, severe ankle arthritis may be treated with an ankle fusion or, in some cases, total ankle replacement.

Stiffness

Stiffness is a commonly discussed complication of ankle fracture and its treatment. Early mobilization and a course of physical therapy may improve motion after these injuries. Most patients will lose some plantar flexion and dorsiflexion relative to the uninvolved leg, but this is typically not activity limiting. Manipulation under anesthesia and formal open releases are very rarely required for ankle arthrofibrosis.

Symptomatic Hardware

Lateral plates with angled distal screws are often symptomatic, as are large medial screws. Placing the fibular plate posteriorly as an antiglide plate is a useful technique to minimize the risks of symptomatic hardware in patients with a thin soft tissue envelope. Most ankle implants can be safely removed after 1 year in those patients with symptomatic hardware.

Neuropraxia or Neuroma

Neuropraxia is the result of a stretch injury to a nerve at the time of the fracture. This most commonly occurs with the laterally based superficial peroneal nerve. In this case, sensation will almost always return to normal without intervention. In cases of slow improvement of neurological function, electromyography or a nerve conduction study can be performed between 6 and 12 weeks to document the degree of injury and the likelihood of recovery of the involved nerve. A neuroma can develop in a nerve that is compressed or lacerated. Nerves that are at risk with open reduction of the ankle are the saphenous nerve medially and the superficial peroneal nerve laterally. Close attention should be paid to the location of these nerves at the time of the incision and dissection. Both of these nerves are sensory at this level of the ankle, and in cases of refractory pain, these injured nerves can be treated with resection and burying of the free nerve ends deep in muscle or fat.

Osteochondral Fracture

It appears that chondral and osteochondral injuries occur more commonly with unstable ankle fractures than previously appreciated. Loren and Ferkel[91] performed ankle arthroscopy on 48 patients with unstable ankle fractures and found that 30 (63%) had traumatic articular surface lesions in the ankle of greater than 5 mm, including nine of 12 syndesmosis injuries. Similarly, Ono and associates[92] performed ankle arthroscopy on 105 patients treated operatively for ankle fractures and found significant cartilage injury in 21 patients (20%), including eight that had free articular fragments. The radiographs should be closely inspected preoperatively and intraoperatively for evidence of a possible OCD. CT scans can be performed prior to surgery when the presence of an OCD is expected, although only displaced OCDs are likely to be visible on initial radiographs. A portion of the articular cartilage can be seen during some approaches (e.g., medial malleolus), and if accessible, the joint should be visualized for evidence of an injury.

Many OCDs are diagnosed during the postoperative period. Osteochondral injuries may develop many months after an ankle fracture due to an initial injury to the cartilage at the time of the ankle fracture. Again, these injuries are difficult to detect on plain radiographs. A CT scan should be performed in patients who have had ORIF of their ankle with an apparent anatomical reduction, but are still having persistent pain. A stable, nondisplaced OCD should heal with a prolonged period of limited weight bearing in a boot that allows range of motion. An unstable OCD requires either excision (minimal or no bone on fragment) or ORIF with absorbable or headless screws.

Outcomes

Most patients with ankle fractures that are operatively treated can expect a return of nearly full function, although studies have demonstrated that 17 to 24% of patients may have a less than satisfactory outcome. Recent studies have demonstrated that initial impairment after ankle fracture may show improvement over longer periods of time than previously recognized, even up to 2 years.[93,94] Nonetheless, SF-36 physical function scores remain below population norms even after 2 years.[93] Negative predictors may include fracture type (syndesmosis injury, medial malleolus, posterior malleolus).[1,95] Social factors such as smoking, alcohol consumption, and level of education also affect outcomes after unstable ankle fracture.[93]

Pearls

- The medial anatomical structure maintaining the talus beneath the tibial plafond, preventing lateral displacement and external rotation, is the deep component of the deltoid ligament.
- Of the four syndesmosis ligaments, the interosseous ligament is the primary restraint to transverse motion at the tibiofibular articulation.
- For less than 2 mm of displacement of the lateral malleolus and a normal medial clear space, the treatment of choice is nonoperative treatment.
- Closed treatment of medial malleolus fractures results in a nonunion rate of 5 to 15%.
- The injury involving a fracture off the anterolateral aspect of the tibia at the insertion of the anterior-inferior tibiofibular ligament is called a Chaput fracture.

- In unstable ankle fractures, there have been osteochondral injuries noted in 20 to 50% of cases.
- Traumatic osteochondral injuries of the talus are more common on the lateral dome due to impingement of the talus with the fibula in an inversion injury.
- Open ankle fractures can routinely be treated with antibiotics, urgent irrigation and debridement, and primary ORIF (unless the wound is extremely contaminated).
- Potentially correctable social factors such as smoking and alcohol usage in patients with ankle fractures correlate with poorer outcomes.

On the DVDs

Video 32–1 (Disk 4) ORIF of an Open Ankle Fracture This video demonstrates ORIF of a Weber B ankle fracture with an open medial malleolus fracture. Soft tissue handling, extension of the fibula fracture proximally, and fixation of the medial malleolus are discussed.

References

1. Phillips WA, Schwartz HS, Keller CS, et al. A prospective, randomized study of the management of severe ankle fractures. J Bone Joint Surg Am 1985;67:67–78
2. Amendola A. Controversies in diagnosis and management of syndesmosis injuries of the ankle. Foot Ankle 1992;13:44–50
3. Heim U, Pfeiffer KM. The ankle joint. In: Heim U, Pfeiffer KM, eds. Internal Fixation of Small Fractures. Technique Recommended by the ASIF Group. 3rd ed. Berlin: Springer-Verlag; 1988:261–335
4. Michelson JD. Fractures about the ankle. J Bone Joint Surg Am 1995;77:142–152
5. Weber BG, Colton C. Malleolar fractures. In: Müller ME, Allgöwer M, Schneider R, Willenegger H, eds. Manual of Internal Fixation. 3rd ed. Berlin: Springer-Verlag; 1991:595–612
6. Ramsey PL, Hamilton W. Changes in tibiotalar area of contact caused by lateral talar shift. J Bone Joint Surg Am 1976;58:356–357
7. Mont MA, Sedlin ED, Weiner LS, Miller AR. Postoperative radiographs as predictors of clinical outcome in unstable ankle fractures. J Orthop Trauma 1992;6:352–357
8. Clarke HJ, Michelson JD, Cox QG, Jinnah RH. Tibiotalar stability in bimalleolar ankle fractures: a dynamic in vitro contact area study. Foot Ankle 1991;11:222–227
9. Grath GB. Widening of the ankle mortise: a clinical and experimental study. Acta Chir Scand Suppl 1960;263:1–88
10. Pankovich AM, Shivaram MS. Anatomical basis of variability in injuries of the medial malleolus and the deltoid ligament, I: Anatomical studies. Acta Orthop Scand 1979;50:217–223
11. Close JR. Some applications of the functional anatomy of the ankle joint. J Bone Joint Surg Am 1956;38:761–781
12. Lindsjo U. Operative treatment of ankle fracture-dislocations: a follow-up study of 306/321 consecutive cases. Clin Orthop Relat Res 1985;199:28–38
13. Weber BG. Die Verletzungen des Oberen Sprunggelenkes. In: Aktuelle Probleme in der Chirurgie. 3rd ed. Bern: Verlag Hans Huber; 1977
14. Lauge-Hansen N. Fractures of the ankle: analytic historic survey as the basis of new experimental, roentgenologic, and clinical investigations. Arch Surg 1948;56:259–317
15. Thomsen NO, Overgaard S, Olsen LH, Hansen H, Nielsen ST. Observer variation in the radiographic classification of ankle fractures. J Bone Joint Surg Br 1991;73:676–678
16. Cox FJ, Laxson WW. Fractures about the ankle joint. Am J Surg 1952;83:674–679
17. Joy G, Patzakis MJ, Harvey JP Jr. Precise evaluation of the reduction of severe ankle fractures. J Bone Joint Surg Am 1974;56:979–993
18. Katcherian D. Soft-tissue injuries of the ankle. In: Lutter LD, Mizel MS, Pfeffer GB, eds. Orthopaedic Knowledge Update: Foot and Ankle. Rosemont, IL: American Academy of Orthopaedic Surgeons; 1994:241–253
19. Egol KA, Amirtharage M, Tejwani NC, Capla EL, Koval KJ. Ankle stress test for predicting the need for surgical fixation of isolated fibular fractures. J Bone Joint Surg Am 2004;86:2393–2398
20. McConnell T, Creevy W, Tornetta P. Stress examination of supination external rotation-type fibular fractures. J Bone Joint Surg Am 2004;86:2171–2178
21. Michelson JD, Varner KE, Checcone M. Diagnosing deltoid injury in ankle fractures: the gravity stress view. Clin Orthop Relat Res 2001;387:178–182
22. Boden S, Labropoulos PA, McCowin P, Lestini WF, Hurwitz SR. Mechanical considerations for the syndesmosis screw: a cadaver study. J Bone Joint Surg Am 1989;71:1548–1555
23. Ebraheim NA, Elgafy H, Padanilam T. Syndesmotic disruption in low fibular fractures associated with deltoid ligament injury. Clin Orthop Relat Res 2003;409:260–267

24. Candal-Couto JJ, Burrow D, Bromage S, Briggs PJ. Instability of the tibio-fibular syndesmosis: have we been pulling in the wrong direction? Injury 2004;35:814–818

25. Bauer M, Bergstrom B, Hemborg A, Sandegard J. Malleolar fractures: nonoperative versus operative treatment: a controlled study. Clin Orthop Relat Res 1985;199:17–27

26. Carr JB. Malleolar fractures and soft tissue injuries of the ankle. In: Browner BD, Jupiter JB, Levine AM, Trafton PG, eds. Skeletal Trauma. 3rd ed. Philadelphia: WB Saunders; 2003:2307–2374

27. Geissler WB, Tsao AK, Hughes JL. Fractures and injuries of the ankle. In: Rockwood CA, Jr., Green DP, Bucholz RW, Heckman JD, eds. Fractures in Adults. 4th ed. Philadelphia: Lippincott-Raven; 1996: 2242–2244

28. Hoiness P, Stromsoe K. The influence of the timing of surgery on soft tissue complications and hospital stay: a review of 84 closed ankle fractures. Ann Chir Gynaecol 2000;89:6–9

29. Hahn DM, Colton CL. Malleolar fractures. In: Rüedi TP, Murphy WM, eds. AO Principles of Fracture Management. Stuttgart: Thieme; 2000:559–581

30. Yablon IG, Heller FG, Shouse L. The key role of the lateral malleolus in displaced fractures of the ankle. J Bone Joint Surg Am 1977;59:169–173

31. Tornetta P 3rd. Competence of the deltoid ligament in bimalleolar ankle fractures after medial malleolar fixation. J Bone Joint Surg Am 2000;82:843–848

32. Michelsen JD, Ahn UM, Helgemo SL. Motion of the ankle in a simulated supination-external rotation fracture model. J Bone Joint Surg Am 1996;78:1024–1031

33. Riede UN, Schenk RK, Willenegger H. Joint mechanical studies on post-traumatic arthrosis in the ankle joint, I: The intra-articular model fracture [in German]. Langenbecks Arch Chir 1971;328: 258–271

34. Schaffer JJ, Manoli A II. The antiglide plate for distal fibular fixation: a biomechanical comparison with fixation with a lateral plate. J Bone Joint Surg Am 1987;69:596–604

35. Brunner CF, Weber BG. Anti-glide plate. In: Brunner CF, Weber BG, eds. Special Techniques in Internal Fixation. Berlin: Springer-Verlag; 1982:115–127

36. Mast J, Jakob R, Ganz R. Reduction with plates. In: Mast J, Jakob R, Ganz R, eds. Planning and Reduction Technique in Fracture Surgery. Berlin: Springer-Verlag; 1989:53–54

37. Herscovici D, Sucaduto JM, Sanders RW, Infante A, DiPasquale T. Non-operative treatment of isolated medial malleolus fractures. Paper # 23, 17th Annual Meeting of the Orthopaedic Trauma Association, San Diego, CA, 2001

38. Hughes J. The medial malleolus in ankle fractures. Orthop Clin North Am 1980;11:649–660

39. Hoppenfeld S, deBoer P. The ankle and foot. In: Hoppenfeld S, deBoer P, eds. Surgical Exposures in Orthopaedics: The Anatomic Approach. 3rd ed. Philadelphia: JB Lippincott; 1984:613–626

40. Ebraheim NA, Mekhail AO, Gargasz SS. Ankle fractures involving the fibula proximal to the distal tibiotalar syndesmosis. Foot Ankle 1997;18:513–521

41. Harper MC. The deltoid ligament: an evaluation of need for surgical repair. Clin Orthop Relat Res 1988;226:156–168

42. Morris M, Chandler RW. Fractures of the ankle. Tech Orthop 1987;2:10–19

43. Jaskulka RA, Ittner G, Schedl R. Fractures of the posterior tibial margin: their role in the prognosis of malleolar fractures. J Trauma 1989;29:1565–1570

44. McDaniel WJ, Wilson FC. Trimalleolar fractures of the ankle: an end result study. Clin Orthop Relat Res 1977;122:37–45

45. Nelson MC, Jensen NK. The treatment of trimalleolar fractures of the ankle. Surg Gynecol Obstet 1940;71:509–514

46. Hartford JM, Gorczyca JT, McNamara JL, Mayor MB. Tibiotalar contact area: contribution of posterior malleolus and deltoid ligament. Clin Orthop Relat Res 1995;320:182–187

47. Raasch WG, Larkin JL, Dragovich LF. Assessment of the posterior malleolus as a restraint to posterior subluxation of the ankle. J Bone Joint Surg Am 1992;74:1201–1206

48. Scheidt KB, Stiehl JB, Skrade DA, Barnhardt T. Posterior malleolar ankle fractures: an in vitro biomechanical analysis of stability in the loaded and unloaded states. J Orthop Trauma 1992;6:96–101

49. Tornetta P 3rd, Collinge C, Karges DE. Ankle fracture: anti-glide plate of the fibula with direct open reduction internal fixation of the posterior malleolar fracture. J Orthop Trauma 2001;15: 304–305

50. Harper MC, Hardin G. Posterior malleolus fractures of the ankle associated with external rotation-abduction injuries: results with and without internal fixation. J Bone Joint Surg Am 1988;70: 1348–1356

51. Wuest TK. Injuries to the distal lower extremity syndesmosis. J Am Acad Orthop Surg 1997;5:172–181

52. Harper MC, Keller TS. A radiographic evaluation of the tibiofibular syndesmosis. Foot Ankle 1989;10:156–160

53. Mizel M. Technique tip: a revised method of the Cotton test for intra-operative evaluation of syndesmotic injuries. Foot Ankle Int 2003;24:86–87

54. Chissell HR, Jones J. The influence of a diastasis screw on the outcome of Weber type-C ankle fractures. J Bone Joint Surg Br 1995; 77:435–438

55. Tornetta P III, Spoo JE, Reynolds FA, Lee C. Overtightening of the ankle syndesmosis: is it really possible? J Bone Joint Surg Am 2001; 83:489–492

56. Hoiness P, Stromsoe K. Tricortical versus quadricortical syndesmosis fixation in ankle fractures: a prospective, randomized study comparing two methods of syndesmosis fixation. J Orthop Trauma 2004;18:331–337

57. Hovis WD, Kaiser BW, Watson JT, Bucholz RW. Treatment of syndesmotic disruptions of the ankle with bioabsorbable screw fixation. J Bone Joint Surg Am 2002;84:26–31

58. Needleman RL, Skrade DA, Stiehl JB. Effect of syndesmotic screw on ankle motion. Foot Ankle 1989;10:17–24

59. de Souza LJ, Gustilo RB, Meyer TJ. Results of operative treatment of displaced external rotation-abduction fractures on the ankle. J Bone Joint Surg Am 1985;67:1066–1074

60. Kaye RA. Stabilization of ankle syndesmosis injuries with a syndesmosis screw. Foot Ankle 1989;9:290–293

61. Gustilo RB. Current concepts in the management of open fractures. Instr Course Lect 1987;36:359–366

62. Gustilo RB, Anderson JT. Prevention of infection in the treatment of one thousand and twenty-five open fractures of long bones. J Bone Joint Surg Am 1976;58:453–458

63. Gustilo RB, Mendoza RM, Williams DN. Problems in the management of type III open fractures: a new classification of type III open fractures. J Trauma 1984;24:742–746

64. Franklin JL, Johnson KD, Hansen ST. Immediate internal fixation of open ankle fractures: report of thirty-eight cases treated with a standard protocol. J Bone Joint Surg Am 1984;66:1349–1356

65. Stiehl JB. Open fractures of the ankle joint. Instr Course Lect 1990;39:113–117

66. Bray TJ, Endicott M, Capra SE. Treatment of open ankle fractures: immediate internal fixation versus closed immobilization and delayed fixation. Clin Orthop Relat Res 1989;240:47–52

67. Wiss DA, Gilbert P, Merritt PO, Sarmiento A. Immediate internal fixation of open ankle fractures. J Orthop Trauma 1988;2:265–271

68. Beauchamp CG, Clay NR, Thexton PW. Displaced ankle fractures in patients over 50 years of age. J Bone Joint Surg Br 1983;65:329–332

69. Litchfield JC. The treatment of unstable fractures of the ankle in the elderly. Injury 1987;18:128–132

70. Koval KJ, Petraco DM, Kummer FJ, Bharam S. A new technique for complex fibula fracture fixation in the elderly: a clinical and biomechanical evaluation. J Orthop Trauma 1997;11:28–33

71. Perry M, Taranow WS, Manoli A. Multiple syndesmotic fixation for neuropathic ankle fractures with failed traditional fixation. Presented at the American Foot and Ankle Society's Winter Meeting, Dallas, TX, 2002

72. Blotter RH, Connolly E, Wasan A, Chapman MW. Acute complications in the operative treatment of isolated ankle fractures in patients with diabetes mellitus. Foot Ankle Int 1999;20:687–694

73. Flynn JM, Rodriguez-del Rio F, Piza PA. Closed ankle fractures in the diabetic patient. Foot Ankle Int 2000;21:311–319

74. Jani MM, Ricci WM, Borrelli J, Barrett SE, Johnson JE. A protocol for treatment of unstable ankle fractures using transarticular fixation in patients with diabetes mellitus and loss of protective sensibility. Foot Ankle Int 2003;24:838–844

75. Colville MR, Colville JM, Manoli A. Posteromedial dislocation of the ankle without fracture. J Bone Joint Surg Am 1987;69:706–711

76. Rivera F, Bertone C, De Martino M, Pietrobono D, Ghisellini F. Pure dislocation of the ankle: three case reports and literature review. Clin Orthop Relat Res 2001;382:179–184

77. Wroble RR, Nepola JV, Malvitz TA. Ankle dislocation without fracture. Foot Ankle 1988;9:64–74

78. Cimino W, Ichterz D, Slabaugh P. Early mobilization of ankle fractures after open reduction and internal fixation. Clin Orthop Relat Res 1991;267:152–156

79. Ahl T, Dalen N, Holmberg S, Selvik G. Early weightbearing of malleolar fractures. Acta Orthop Scand 1986;57:526–529

80. Finsen V, Saetermo R, Kibsgaard L, et al. Early postoperative weightbearing and muscle activity in patients who have a fracture of the ankle. J Bone Joint Surg Am 1989;71:23–26

81. Thordarson DB, Samuelson M, Shepherd LE, Merkle PF, Lee J. Bioabsorbable versus stainless steel screw fixation of the syndesmosis in pronation-lateral rotation ankle fractures: a prospective randomized trial. Foot Ankle Int 2001;22:335–338

82. Gehr J, Neber W, Hilsenbeck F, Friedl W. New concepts in the treatment of ankle joint fractures: the IP-XS (XSL) and IP-XXS (XXSL) nail in the treatment of ankle joint fractures. Arch Orthop Trauma Surg 2004;124:96–103

83. Andreassen GS, Høiness PR, Skraamm I, Granlund O, Engebretsen L. Use of a synthetic bone void filler to augment screws in osteopenic ankle fracture fixation. Arch Orthop Trauma Surg 2004;124: 161–165

84. Mendelsohn MA. Nonunion of malleolar fractures of the ankle. Clin Orthop Relat Res 1965;42:103–118

85. Vrahas M, Fu F, Veenis B. Intraarticular contact stresses with simulated ankle malunions. J Orthop Trauma 1994;8:159–166

86. Brodie IA, Denham RA. The treatment of unstable ankle fractures. J Bone Joint Surg Br 1974;56:256–262

87. Yablon IG, Leach RE. Reconstruction of malunited fractures of the lateral malleolus. J Bone Joint Surg Am 1989;71:521–527

88. Marti RK, Raaymakers E, Nolte PA. Malunited ankle fractures: the late results of reconstruction. J Bone Joint Surg Br 1990;72:709–713

89. Roberts C, Sherman O, Bauer D, Lusskin R. Ankle reconstruction for malunion by fibular osteotomy and lengthening with direct control of the distal fragment: a report of three cases and review of the literature. Foot Ankle 1992;13:7–13

90. Ward AJ, Ackroyd CE, Baker AS. Late lengthening of the fibula for malaligned ankle fractures. J Bone Joint Surg Br 1990;72:714–717

91. Loren GJ, Ferkel RD. Arthroscopic assessment of occult intra-articular injury in acute ankle fractures. Arthroscopy 2002;18:412–421

92. Ono A, Nishikawa S, Nagao A, Irie T, Sasaki M, Kouno T. Arthroscopically assisted treatment of ankle fractures: arthroscopic findings and surgical outcomes. Arthroscopy 2004;20:627–631

93. Bhandari M, Sprague S, Hanson B, et al. Health-related quality of life following operative treatment of unstable ankle fractures: a prospective observational study. J Orthop Trauma 2004;18: 338–345

94. Ponzer S, Nasell H, Bergman B, Tornkvist H. Functional outcome and quality of life in patients with Type B ankle fractures: a two-year follow-up study. J Orthop Trauma 1999;13:363–368

95. Bauer M, Jonsson K, Nilsson B. Thirty-year follow-up of ankle fractures. Acta Orthop Scand 1985;56:103–106

33 Foot Fractures

Timothy G. Weber, David S. Brokaw, Angela Scharfenberger, and J. Scott Broderick

Complex fractures of the hindfoot, midfoot, and forefoot are common in victims of trauma and are increasingly recognized as an important determinant of outcome. As in other areas of orthopaedic trauma, improved understanding of associated soft tissue injuries, as well as the development of specific implants and sophisticated operative techniques, have led to increased indications for operative management of foot fractures. This chapter considers the surgical management of fractures of the talus, calcaneus, midfoot, and forefoot.

Talus Fractures

Talus fractures are classified into six types: talar neck fractures, talar body fractures, talar head fractures, lateral process fractures, posterior process fractures, and osteochondral fractures. Each type requires a different approach to management.

Anatomy

The talus has a unique surgical anatomy. The bone is divided into three parts: body, neck, and head. It articulates with four bones: the fibula, tibia, navicular, and calcaneus. It also has no tendon attachments. With more than 60% of its surface area being articular, the blood supply to the talus is significantly limited. The surgeon must have a firm understanding of the vasculature so as to limit iatrogenic injury to the talar blood supply. Vascular contributions arise from the anterior tibial (AT), posterior tibial (PT), and peroneal arteries (PA). The tarsal canal artery (a branch of the PT as the deltoid artery) and the tarsal sinus artery (AT, PA) form an extraosseous vascular ring. The deltoid artery enters the deltoid ligament and provides contributions to the tarsal canal (extraosseous) and directly to the medial talar body.[1–4] Often, this is the only remaining blood supply postinjury; therefore, care must be taken to preserve this contribution. The talar head receives the most comprehensive blood supply, with the vascularity of the medial body more tenuous and the lateral body and posterior tubercles being left relatively avascular. Despite its large articular area, there is a sizeable nonarticular surface on the lateral aspect of the neck and anterior aspect of the body. Both areas are quite useful with regard to placement of fixation.

Biomechanics

The subtalar joint acts as the link between the foot distally and the leg proximally. At heel strike, the subtalar joint collapses into valgus, with the calcaneus in eversion. Distally this results in "unlocking" of the transverse tarsal joint. This unlocking gives flexibility to the longitudinal arch and aids in the passive absorption of the energy imparted to the foot at heel strike. In the movement of the foot from foot flat to toe off, the subtalar joint undergoes inversion as the calcaneus moves to a position of varus. Distally this imparts stability at the transtarsal articulation and transforms the midfoot into a rigid structure able to accept body weight.[5] There is a direct correlation between varus malalignment of the talus and loss of subtalar motion. With varus position of the talus as seen in the typical varus malunion, the subtalar joint is locked in an inverted position and the arc of eversion is restricted. This results in a rigid foot that loses its shock-absorbing capabilities at heel strike.[6,7]

Talar Neck Fractures

Classification

Talar neck fractures are classified by Hawkins into three types.[8] A type I fracture is undisplaced, type II fractures are displaced with subluxation of the subtalar joint, and in type III fractures there is subluxation or dislocation of both the tibiotalar and the subtalar joints **(Fig. 33–1A,B)**. Canale and Kelly added a type IV, which is a type III injury with an associated talonavicular dislocation.[9] Hawkins's classification has been related to the risk of avascular necrosis (AVN). More recent results, in patients managed with better fixation and treatment methods, have demonstrated improved outcomes compared with the results reported by Hawkins.

Nonoperative Treatment

Nonoperative treatment of talar neck fractures is often suboptimal and fraught with pitfalls. It can be considered for nondisplaced Hawkins type I talus fractures. Rarely, in polytrauma patients or fractures with severe soft tissue damage, closed reduction (described later in the section on percutaneous treatment in surgical techniques) of a displaced talar fracture is necessary and preferable. Because talar neck

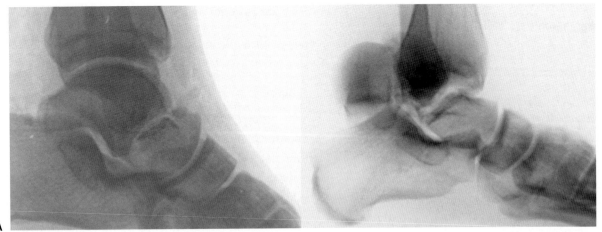

A   B

Figure 33–1 Talar neck fractures. **(A)** Hawkins II talar neck fracture. **(B)** Hawkins III talar neck fracture.

fractures often result from a dorsiflexion injury, plantar flexion is advocated for application of the cast so as not to displace the talar neck fracture.[10] Casting therefore predisposes the patient to an equinus contracture and limited motion, particularly of the subtalar joint. When closed treatment is utilized, the equinus position should be gradually eliminated by 4 weeks and the cast removed and motion started by 8 weeks. Non–weight bearing is usually recommended for 12 weeks, although limited weight bearing maybe started during weeks 8 through 12 in true type I fractures.

Indications for Surgical Treatment

Operative treatment should be considered for most all talar neck fractures, even in patients with a Hawkins type I injury. Without internal fixation, early range of motion is precluded. There is a risk of the talar neck fracture displacing when moving the tibiotalar joint into a neutral position for casting.[11–13] Furthermore, the actual displacement of the talar neck is very difficult to judge from plain radiographs and computed tomography (CT), and during open reduction many fractures are found to be more displaced than they appeared preoperatively. Lastly, even a slight degree of malunion causes significant loss of motion at the subtalar joint.[14] For these reasons operative treatment should be considered for all talus fractures.

Surgical Treatment

Operating Room Setup and Patient Positioning

The operating room (OR) table should be radiolucent with no pedestal at the foot of the bed. The patient should be positioned at the foot of the bed with the feet level with the end of the bed. A tourniquet should be placed on the thigh. A sandbag should be placed beneath the ipsilateral buttock and torso, rotating the affected extremity so that the patella is pointing straight up. This aids intraoperative imaging. A fluoroscope should be placed on the opposite

side of the table from the injury. The patient is prepped and draped above the knee. An occlusive dressing should be used to cover the toes. Prophylactic intravenous antibiotics are routinely provided.

Operative Approach

Most talus fractures are managed through a dual-incision approach (see **Video 33–1, Disk 4**). Rarely, such as when the condition of the soft tissues prohibits incisions on the dorsum of the foot, posterior to anterior fixation is necessary through a posterior approach. All talus approaches are described in this chapter.

Dual-Incision Approach

The *medial incision* is midway between the anterior tibial and posterior tibial tendons, beginning a few centimeters proximal to the medial malleolus and ending just slightly distal to the navicular (see **Video 33–1, Disk 4**). This incision is deepened through the subcutaneous tissue and with care to preserve the saphenous vein. Injury to the saphenous vein can lead to significant postoperative swelling. Where necessary, the ankle joint capsule is opened with a scalpel as opposed to electrocautery, so as not to injure the articular cartilage. Exposure is then extended from the tibia to the navicular, minimizing soft tissue dissection superior and inferior on the talar neck so as to maintain soft tissue attachments and the blood supply that they provide. The *anterolateral incision* should be centered between the peroneus tertius tendon and the extensor digitorum longus tendon, starting above the ankle joint and extending distally to the midfoot region **(Fig. 33–2)** (see **Video 33–1, Disk 4**). One should identify and protect the superficial peroneal nerve as it crosses the field. The medial border of the extensor digitorum brevis should be identified. It is common to have debris within the subtalar joint, and the exposure should continue to the inferior aspect of the talus to allow visualization and debridement of the subtalar joint. These two incisions will

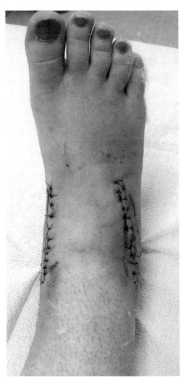

Figure 33–2 Postoperative dual incision exposure of talus fracture with nylon closure.

be used alternately to achieve an anatomical reduction and to place the appropriate fixation to stabilize the fracture.

Medial Malleolus Osteotomy

On occasion, particularly with Hawkins type III fractures, a medial malleolar osteotomy is necessary. A chevron osteotomy is depicted in **Fig. 33–3A–C.** This is created by making a saw cut parallel to the dome of the talus roughly 1 cm proximal to the plafond and then utilizing a chisel to make the vertical cut and allowing the bone to fracture into the articular surface. This creates a very stable construct when repairing the medial malleolar osteotomy and also provides better visualization of a talar body fracture. Alternatively, the osteotomy can be done obliquely, running superior-medially 45 degrees from the articular surface. With either technique, the completion of the osteotomy into the articular surface should be by way of fracture rather than by saw. This allows for more accurate reduction of the medial malleolus at the end of the procedure. Predrilling the medial malleolus prior to the osteotomy is not necessary or significantly helpful with fixation because it is often difficult to find the pilot hole in the deltoid ligament. The osteotomy is fixed with 3.5 mm cortical screws (author's preference) or 4.0 mm partially threaded screws.

Posterior Approach

This approach is not helpful for fracture reduction and is only necessary for placement of posterior to anterior fixation.

For the posterior approach, an incision is made slightly posterior to the midway point between the Achilles' tendon and the lateral malleolus. One should identify and protect the sural nerve. The approach is deepened, and the interval between the peroneal tendons and flexor hallucis longus is identified and developed. This allows access to the posterior talus.

Surgical Techniques

Percutaneous Treatment

Percutaneous treatment of talar neck fractures is rarely appropriate. It implies that a closed reduction can be accomplished, which is exceedingly difficult. Therefore, percutaneous fixation is generally limited to situations in which the soft tissues, or the patient's overall condition, preclude definitive surgical stabilization for a significant period of time. The technique of closed fracture reduction should be determined based on the plain films and CT scan and tailored to the direction of displacement. Most commonly, the talar neck will be displaced dorsally and requires distraction and plantar flexion to correct the deformity. Inversion or eversion of the hindfoot may be necessary to correct a varus or valgus deformity (i.e., a medial or lateral translation). This is followed by axial loading and extension of the foot back to a neutral position. Fracture reduction should be performed in the OR because it may take more than one attempt before a satisfactory reduction is achieved. Temporary fixation may be considered when permanent fixation must be delayed. Under fluoroscopic control, K-wires can be placed lateral to the Achilles' tendon from the posterior aspect of the talus, aimed anteromedially through the central portion of the talar neck and into the central part of the talar head. K-wires may be advanced through the talar head into the navicular for added stability and bone purchase if required. Posterior to anterior placement of wires allows the portal for entry of the K-wires to be away from the definitive surgical site and it allows the pins to be left outside the skin or buried just underneath the skin. Alternatively, definitive treatment with percutaneous cannulated screws can be considered if later open reduction and internal fixation (ORIF) is deemed impossible. A small incision is placed on the posterior-lateral aspect of the ankle, and a guide pin from the 6.5 or 7.3 mm cannulated screw set is placed in the same manner. The guide pin should be placed as inferior as possible on the posterior talar body. This decreases impingement of the screw head on the posterior malleolus during plantar flexion, which can interfere with range of motion. Because the central bone in the talar body is quite dense, overdrilling is required to form a gliding hole through the body of the talus. Prior to drilling, at least one other K-wire needs to be placed so that the reduction is not lost during screw insertion. After placement of the screw, the great toe should be flexed and extended to verify that

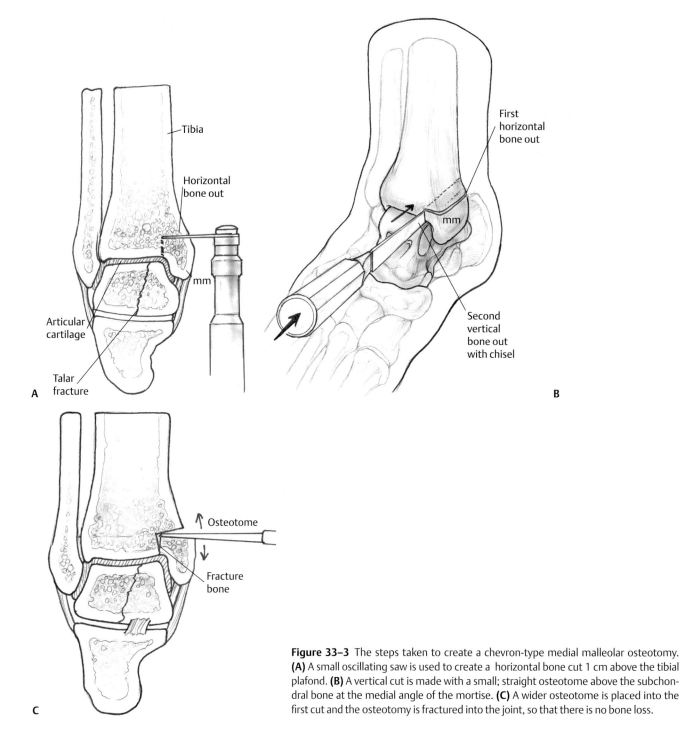

Figure 33–3 The steps taken to create a chevron-type medial malleolar osteotomy. **(A)** A small oscillating saw is used to create a horizontal bone cut 1 cm above the tibial plafond. **(B)** A vertical cut is made with a small; straight osteotome above the subchondral bone at the medial angle of the mortise. **(C)** A wider osteotome is placed into the first cut and the osteotomy is fractured into the joint, so that there is no bone loss.

the screw is not interfering with the excursion of the flexor hallucis longus tendon.

Open Treatment

Reduction Because the mechanism of talar neck fractures is usually an extension injury, the dorsal aspect of the talus is usually comminuted. Although anatomical reduction of the talar neck is the goal, reduction becomes more challenging as the dorsal comminution increases. Because

the inferior surface of the talus fails in tension, it is rarely comminuted and may be used to judge the quality of reduction **(Fig. 33–4)**. It is critical to assess the reduction of the talar neck both on the medial side and on the lateral side utilizing both incisions (see **Video 33–1, Disk 4**). It is common for the reduction to appear anatomical on the medial side and to be several millimeters off on the lateral side due to rotation. The only way to predictably reduce the talus fracture is to visualize the reduction both medially and laterally. Either 0.062 in. K wires or 2.5 mm terminally

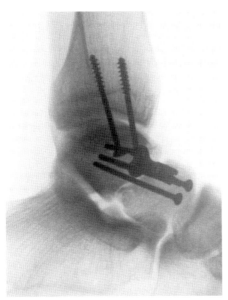

Figure 33–4 Postoperative talus with dorsal defect. Note that the inferior talus was used for reduction.

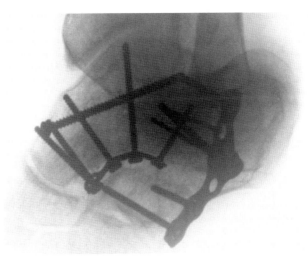

Figure 33–5 Canale view of the standard construct for talus fractures with medial positional screws and a lateral plate.

threaded Schanz pins are useful as joysticks in reducing the fragments. Because the talus is dislocated from both the ankle and subtalar joints, Hawkins type III fractures provide unique challenges. To facilitate reduction of the talus in these severe injuries, it is helpful to open the tibiocalcaneal space by some method. Use of a large lamina spreader between the tibial plafond and the posterior facet of the calcaneus is ideal because it provides distraction while allowing free flexion, extension, inversion, and eversion. Freedom of motion in these directions is often necessary to reduce the talus back into the mortise. A sponge or gauze protects the articular surfaces from the laminar spreader. Alternatively, a centrally threaded calcaneal traction pin with a traction bow, or a T-handle chuck can be used to apply traction.

Often, a medial malleolar osteotomy is required before reduction can be achieved. The posteromedial tendons and neurovascular bundle frequently block reduction and are accessible through this approach in most situations. Rarely, reduction cannot be accomplished through a medial incision with a medial malleolar osteotomy, and a direct posterior approach is required. If a posterior medial incision is necessary, it is imperative to identify and protect the neurovascular structures that are no longer in their anatomical position.

Fixation After anatomical reduction has been accomplished, preliminary fixation can be provided with K-wires. Definitive fixation is then inserted, most frequently utilizing screws alone or in combination with plates (see **Video 33–1, Disk 4**). On the medial aspect of the talus, a 2.7 or 3.5 mm cortical screw is usually used and is placed from the distal medial aspect of the talus in a retrograde fashion back into the talar body. Most often the screws are placed through the talar head and countersunk into the cartilage.

To do so, abduction of the forefoot is required through the transtarsal joint. One should verify that the screw does not impinge on talonavicular motion by checking the transtarsal motion. When there is comminution of either or both the superior and medial aspects of the talus, the screw is placed as a positioning screw rather than as a lag screw (**Fig. 33–5**). If needed, a second parallel screw can be placed directly inferior to this. If two screws are utilized, the inferior screw should be placed first along the subchondral bone of the subtalar joint. After placement of the medial screws, lateral fixation can be placed.

When screws are placed from posterior to anterior in the talus, it is mandatory to countersink these screws below the articular surface so as not to block the ankle range of motion, particularly with plantar flexion. Although 4.5 and 6.5 mm screws have been advocated, it is easier to countersink smaller 3.5 mm screws. The trajectory of the screws should take into account the concavity of the subtalar joint and the convexity of the talonavicular joint. Hardware penetrating either of these joints would be disastrous (**Fig. 33–6A,B**). It is also important to note that the neck and head of the talus occupy only the medial two thirds of the talar body. Therefore, any hardware placed from posterior to anterior must be directed from lateral to medial in the coronal plan, aiming for the great toe, so as not to violate the lateral wall of the talus and the sinus tarsi region. Mandatory imaging studies include an ankle mortise, lateral talus, anteroposterior (AP) foot, and oblique Canale view and will increase the odds of the screws being safely placed.

If the fracture line extends into the shoulder (transition area between the talar neck and body) of the talus, screw fixation alone is often adequate for stability. However, as the fracture line exists more distally along the neck of the talus, or as the dorsal comminution increases, a plate is quite useful for definitive stabilization. A 2.0 mm T-plate from the mini-fragment set is ideal for this purpose. A hole

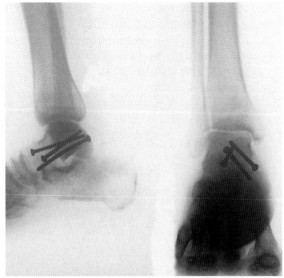

A,B

Figure 33–6 (A) Postoperative anteroposterior and **(B)** lateral radiographs of the talus showing one posterior to anterior screw and two anterior to posterior screws. Notice that the screws are 3.5 mm small-fragment screws and are countersunk

is either trimmed off or converted to a hook. The hook is placed on the shoulder of the talus and the T-portion is placed toward the head of the talus. Alternatively, mini blade plates from the handsets can be used. Care should be taken when placing these screws, particularly the distal-most screws through the T-portion of the plate, to avoid penetrating the talonavicular joint on the medial side. The distal screw should angle anteriorly to stay extra-articular at the talar head. A plate can also be used on the medial aspect of the talus. This risks injuring the blood supply to the talar body from the deltoid ligament. A medial plate is placed inferior to the articular surface of the talar body proximally and should extend distally to the edge of the articular surface of the head of the talus.

Wound Closure After the wound is irrigated, a drain is placed. Deep fascial sutures can be utilized. Subcutaneous sutures are avoided because they can injure cutaneous

nerves or strangulate the cutaneous blood supply as it travels through the subcutaneous tissue to perfuse the skin edges at the incision. The wound is closed using Allgöwer-Donati stitches using 4–0 nylon. The wound is covered with Xeroform (Kendall, Mansfield, Massachusetts) alone or Adaptic (Ethicon, Johnson & Johnson, Somerville, New Jersey) soaked in Betadine (Purdue, Stamford, Connecticut). The ankle is immobilized using a well-padded splint.

Tips and Tricks

- Because the inferior surface of the talus is usually not comminuted, use the subtalar portion of the talus as an indicator of the quality of reduction.
- Remember to debride the subtalar joint.
- With Hawkins III talus fractures, medial malleolus osteotomy is of great assistance. Plating should be considered more often to provide more stable fixation. The lateral aspect of the neck and shoulder of the body provide an excellent nonarticular surface area for placement of a plate.

Rehabilitation

The patient is placed into a well-padded, short leg splint immediately postop. If there is no concern with the skin closure the patient is allowed to begin crutch training the following day. Weight bearing on the injured leg is not allowed for at least 8 to 12 weeks. The patient is maintained in the splint until suture removal in 10 to 14 days. Then the injured foot is placed into a removable splint and an elastic stocking **(Fig. 33–7)**, and the patient is allowed to begin working on range of motion of the ankle and subtalar joints. If the fracture pattern is stable, after 8 weeks a graduated weight-bearing program starting at 50 lb and increasing by 20 lb per week can be initiated. If there is dorsal comminution or any other concern about fixation, one should delay weight bearing for 3 months. Pool therapy

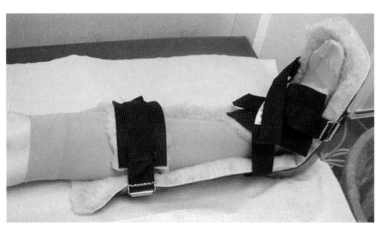

Figure 33–7 Postoperatively, a removable foot splint and an elastic stocking are utilized during the rehabilitation phase.

can be quite valuable in the time period between 8 and 12 weeks postoperatively.

New Techniques

Talar neck fractures have traditionally been treated with screws alone. The use of plates, as already described, is a newer technique that is of value for comminuted fractures and in those associated with osteopenia.

Outcomes

The mid- to long-term outcome after fracture of the talar neck is poorly documented. Vallier et al recently reported the results of surgical treatment of 102 such fractures; 60 were evaluated at an average of 3 years after surgery.[15] Functional outcome was assessed with the Foot Function Index (FFI) and Musculoskeletal Function Assessment (MFA) surveys. With both scales, significant functional impairment was observed. According to both scales, fracture comminution was associated with a worse outcome, whereas factors such as age, Hawkins's classification, or associated talar body fractures did not affect outcome.[15] Based on normative scores for the MFA, patients with talar neck fractures in this series had worse outcomes than patients with hindfoot injuries and ankle or leg injuries.[15]

Complications

Complications of talar neck fractures include osteonecrosis or AVN of the talar body, delayed union, nonunion, malunion, and arthritis of the subtalar or tibiotalar joints.[6,12,16–23] Of these, osteonecrosis has received the most attention. The so-called Hawkins sign is a radiolucent area immediately beneath the articular surface of the talar dome noted on the AP or mortise view typically evident at 6 to 8 weeks. It is evidence of revascularization of the talar dome and indicates a good prognosis. When the Hawkins sign is not present, one must be concerned about AVN. The overall incidence of AVN ranges between 13 and 69%,[8,9,11,16,18,24–28] with the two largest series quoting 21%[18] and 58%.[8] Grob et al attributed their low incidence of AVN (13%) to rigid internal fixation.[25] The Hawkins classification correlates with the incidence of AVN. For Hawkins type I fractures, it has been reported that up to 13% will develop AVN. For Hawkins type II, 20 to 50%, and for Hawkins type III, 69 to 100% have been reported to develop AVN. There does not seem to be a correlation between the time to surgery and the risk of AVN.[15] When AVN occurs, there is no consensus on the amount of weight bearing that should be allowed. In the absence of evidence that weight bearing is harmful, weight bearing should be based on fracture union and not on the presence or absence of AVN. However, it is prudent that impact activities be avoided when AVN is present. In the authors' experience, AVN occurring after talar neck fractures rarely involves the whole body, but rather, is

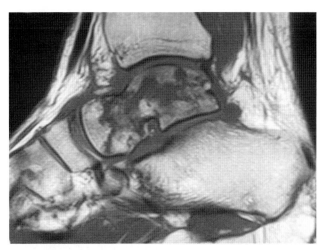

Figure 33–8 Magnetic resonance imaging of the talus showing avascular necrosis.

more localized.[29] Most often, these patients are asymptomatic and can even be seen with an excellent result.[17,24,26,28] When talar collapse occurs or AVN is symptomatic, further treatment may be required (**Fig. 33–8**).

Subtalar and ankle arthritis is a common complication after talar neck fractures, with an incidence ranging from 47 to 97%.[18,28] Subtalar arthritis has been reported in up to 50% of cases, and ankle arthritis in 33% of cases. Both joints may be involved in up to 25% of patients. Selective injections are helpful in evaluating hindfoot pain after talus fractures. Subtalar arthritis can often be successfully treated nonoperatively with a University of California at Berkeley Laboratory (UCBL) orthosis. Occasionally, pain due to ankle arthritis can be improved with an AFO. Nonsteroidal anti-inflammatories and decreased activity level are helpful to decrease pain and preserve these two major hindfoot joints. If conservative treatment fails, an attempt to salvage at least one of the two hindfoot joints (ankle or subtalar) is quite valuable to the overall function of the patient.

Delayed union, nonunion, and malunion of the talus are relatively rare. Delayed union is reported in 13%,[28] and nonunion is noted in 4%.[18] Nonunions are usually associated with a short talar neck and an adduction deformity of the forefoot.[16] Surgical reconstruction of a talar neck nonunion will usually require a tricortical bone graft to regain length and bone stock and ultimately to achieve union. Malunions are most commonly due to a missed fracture. Another cause of malunion is malreduction at the time of surgery or loss of reduction during the postop period. Both of the latter causes are directly under our control and should be exceedingly rare as causes of malunion.

Talar Body Fractures

Talar body fractures can occur in several different fracture patterns. The orientation of the primary fracture line may be coronal, sagittal, or horizontal. Standard plain radiography is

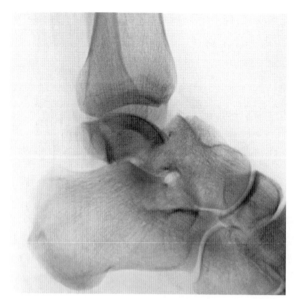

Figure 33–9 Lateral radiograph of a talar body fracture. This is not a neck fracture because of the distinction that the fracture line goes through the lateral process. Note that the subtalar joint is dislocated.

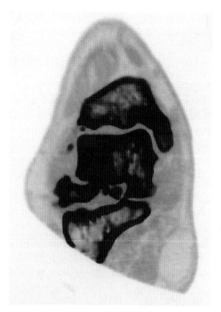

Figure 33–10 Computed tomography transverse cut showing a malunion/nonunion of a lateral process talus fracture with subtalar debris.

necessary for the initial assessment of the fracture. Whenever possible, a CT scan should be performed because it provides an overall understanding of the fracture lines and what will be required to accomplish reduction at the time of surgery.

Classification

Classification schemes for the talar body exist but are not commonly known due to the rarity of this injury. The easiest system is to separate them into three groups: group I are fractures involving the body proper regardless of the direction of the fracture line, group II are fractures of the lateral or posterior process, and group III are compression or impaction fractures. Sneppen et al classified these injuries based on anatomical location: type A, transchondral or osteochondral; type B, coronal shear; type C, sagittal shear; type D, posterior tubercle; type E, lateral process; and type F, crush fractures.[5,30] Inokuchi et al made an important contribution to distinguishing between talar neck fractures and talar body fractures.[31] If the inferior fracture line exits anterior to the lateral process, then it is considered a neck fracture, and posterior to this landmark, it becomes a talar body fracture (**Fig. 33–9**).[31] This is the point where the talus transitions to the articular surface of the posterior facet of the subtalar joint; therefore, by definition, the fracture involves both the tibiotalar and the subtalar joints.

Nonoperative Treatment

These injuries are often displaced and rarely treated nonoperatively. Unfortunately, the most common reason these injuries are treated nonoperatively is failure to diagnose the injury. The most commonly missed talar body fracture

is the lateral process fracture (**Fig. 33–10**). If displacement is 1 mm or less, then 4 to 6 weeks of short leg casting and 8 to 12 weeks of non–weight bearing are appropriate. Once the cast is removed, range of motion should be pursued aggressively.

Surgery Treatment

Most talar body fractures are treated operatively, including any fracture with greater than 1 mm of displacement, all open fractures, and any shear injury that results in a loose body within the ankle (**Fig. 33–11**).

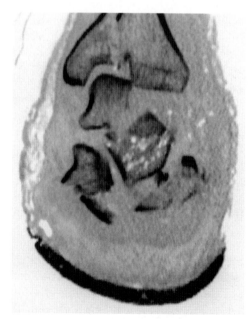

Figure 33–11 Coronal computed tomography (CT) reconstruction showing a pilon, talar body, and calcaneus fracture.

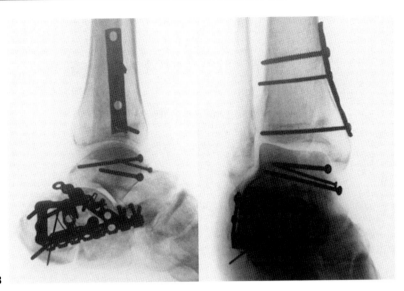

Figure 33–12 (A) Postoperative anteroposterior and **(B)** lateral radiographs showing stabilization of a pilon, talar body, and calcaneus fracture.

A,B

Surgical Techniques

Operative stabilization may require either the anteromedial or the anterolateral approaches already described. Medial malleolar osteotomy is frequently needed to be able to visualize and anatomically reduce talar body fractures. Often these injuries are associated with pilon fractures and one can use these fracture lines for visualization of the talar body fracture. On occasion, a fibular osteotomy is useful. Fibular osteotomy is performed as a segmental osteotomy, with the first cut being at the level of the joint and the second cut above the syndesmotic notch. The intercalary segment is then rolled posteriorly, leaving the peroneal tendon attachments intact. This provides good exposure for a very lateral talar body fracture.

Most talar body fractures can be fixed with screws (2.0, 2.7, and 3.5 mm), placed perpendicular to the fracture lines and countersunk into the articular surface **(Fig. 33–12A,B).** Chondral flaps are often encountered. Though the majority of these chondral injuries are not salvageable and will require debridement, some can be repaired with absorbable pins. If debrided, these areas heal with fibrocartilage and can provide a potential opportunity for placement of hardware without any further injury to the articular cartilage.

> **Tips and Tricks**
>
> - Osteotomy of the medial or lateral malleoli is often necessary to improve exposure of the talar body.
> - Use of titanium screws in this area may facilitate magnetic resonance imaging (MRI) evaluation of the talus and ankle at a later date.

Complications and Outcomes

Talar body fractures are a devastating injury, and although the outcome can be improved with operative fixation, the expectations need to be guarded at best. The most common complication of talar body fracture is posttraumatic arthrosis. The reported incidence of ankle arthrosis ranges from 50 to 90% and subtalar arthrosis was from 48 to 90%.[21,26,30,32–35] In the largest series in the literature of cases treated by open reduction and internal fixation, Vallier et al recently reported arthritis of the ankle joint in 65% and of the subtalar joint in 35%.[36] Outcomes as assessed by both general (MFA) and specific (FFI) scales demonstrate significant impairment, with worse scores in patients with AVN and collapse or posttraumatic arthritis.[36]

Osteonecrosis occurs in 35 to 40% of all talar body fractures. Open talar fractures and associated talar neck fractures are more likely to have this complication.[37] This may be improved with early anatomical reduction and rigid stabilization.[33,36]

Talar Head Fractures

Talar head fractures account for ~5 to 10% of all talus fractures.[26,32,35,38] They are usually caused by a shearing mechanism (severe abduction/adduction of the forefoot) but can also be due to an axial load injury. One needs to be alert to other injuries around the hindfoot and midfoot, particularly of the subtalar and calcaneocuboid joint. Preoperatively, a CT scan is very helpful to define the fracture pattern. It is also important to evaluate the CT scan for additional fracture lines of the talar neck that may not be seen on plain films.

Nonoperative Treatment

Most talar head fractures require operative fixation. If the displacement is 1 mm or less as verified by CT, nonoperative treatment can be considered. Immobilization with either a short leg cast or removable Velcro boot can be used. Initiating motion as early as possible is critical with this

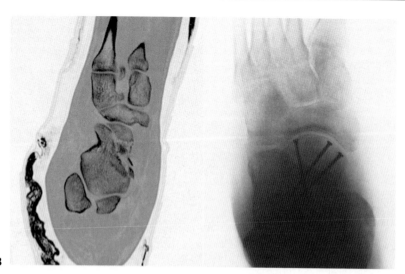

A,B

Figure 33–13 Talar head fracture. **(A)** Coronal computed tomographic scan of a talar head fracture. **(B)** Postoperative anteroposterior hindfoot view of a stabilized talar head fracture.

particular joint because of the importance that it plays in overall foot mechanics during gait. Full weight bearing can be initiated 8 to 12 weeks after injury as determined by fracture healing on radiographs.

Surgical Treatment

Talar head fractures are rarely nondisplaced and therefore the majority do need operative treatment. The surgical approach is determined by the location of the fracture: either anterior, medial, or anterolateral. Occasionally two approaches are necessary. It has been reported that a fragment up to 50% of the head can be excised,[38] but the author suggests not excising more than 30%. The goal of surgery is anatomical reduction and rigid fixation. Fixation is achieved with countersunk mini-fragment screws placed through the articular surface **(Fig. 33–13A,B).** If the articular fragment is impacted from axial loading, disimpacting the fragment is mandatory to regain the length of the medial column. Bone graft may be needed to place beneath the disimpacted fragment. If fixation with screws does not provide sufficient stability, the fragment needs to be unloaded with a medial external fixator. The fixator should be constructed in a triangular arrangement with a pin in the medial calcaneus, the medial distal tibia, and the first metatarsal. This spans the talonavicular joint and allows the appropriate distraction in all planes to unload the talar head. The patient should be placed into a posterior foot splint to maintain the foot in neutral dorsiflexion and take the tension off the distal tibia pin.

Tips and Tricks

- The medial distal tibia is a convenient site for obtaining bone graft, which may be necessary if there is an impacted fragment.

Complications and Outcomes

AVN of the talar head occurs in less than 10% of cases. Other complications include midtarsal instability and talonavicular arthritis. Malunion secondary to a missed fracture or malreduction contributes to the development of talonavicular arthritis.[5,38]

Posterior Process Talus Fractures

The posterior process of the talus is divided into lateral and medial segments by the tendon of the flexor hallucis longus. The lateral process provides the attachment of the posterior talofibular ligament. The medial process has the attachment of the posterior third of the deltoid ligament. The blood supply to the posterior process is poor, particularly the lateral portion.[39] Posterior process fractures account for 20% of talar body fractures. Lateral process fractures are more common than medial process fractures and can be confused with an ankle sprain **(Fig. 33–14A,B).** Lateral process fractures are increasingly recognized in snowboarders.

Nonoperative Treatment

Nonoperative treatment is utilized more frequently for this type of talus injury in comparison with all other talus fractures. Displacement should be less than 2 mm or the fragment should be small to consider cast treatment. This injury is associated with a higher incidence of nonunion due to the poor vascularity of this portion of the bone. Therefore, prolonged immobilization of the foot may be appropriate. Often, weight bearing can be initiated by 6 to 8 weeks.

Surgical Treatment

Most posterior process fractures require surgical intervention, either for anatomical reduction and stabilization or

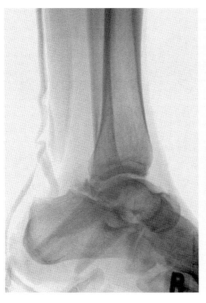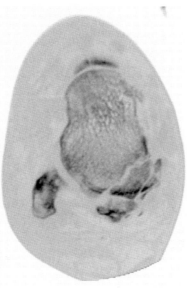

A,B

Figure 33–14 A fracture of the posterior process of the talus. **(A)** Preoperative lateral radiograph showing the posterior process fracture with talonavicular and subtalar dislocation. **(B)** Preoperative computed tomographic scan showing the fracture to involve both the medial and lateral posterior process.

for excision. The decision to fix or excise should be based on the patient's activity level, bone stock, and overall general health and the size of the fragment. People with vascular disease should be treated with excision of the fragment because of the risk of nonunion. A preoperative CT scan helps to identify the fracture lines relative to the tendons and neurovascular structures, demonstrates any articular step-off in the subtalar joint, and helps to determine the most effective interval to develop to minimize soft tissue dissection.

The lateral process is approached through a posterolateral incision. The interval between the peroneal tendons and the flexor hallucis longus tendon is utilized. This allows direct exposure of the posterior lateral corner of the talus. Dorsiflexion of the tibial talar joint allows greater exposure of the superior articular surface of the talus and helps with visualization of the reduction. Medial posterior process fractures are approached through a posteromedial incision, with care to avoid the nearby neurovascular structures. For those fractures that are repairable, fixation is performed with small- and mini-fragment screws.

> **Tips and Tricks**
>
> - To protect the medial neurovascular bundle, do the approach without the tourniquet inflated. After identifying the fracture and ensuring the protection of the neurovascular structures, inflating the tourniquet provides a bloodless field for articular reduction.
> - For both types of fracture, stabilization is usually provided by mini-fragment screws that are countersunk into the articular surface. Alternatively, when the fracture cannot be stabilized, it can be excised.

Complications and Outcomes

The posterior process is poorly vascularized, in particular, the lateral process. Therefore, nonunion is the most common complication. Parsons reviewed the literature and found that the incidence of nonunion is 60% with conservative treatment and 5% with aggressive management (ORIF or closed reduction). Larger fragments should be fixed and smaller fragments may be excised.[39,40] It should be emphasized that the lateral process fracture involves the subtalar joint. Persistent malreduction could lead to subtalar stiffness and pain.[40]

Calcaneus Fractures

The management of calcaneus fractures is controversial. Compared with other fractures of the appendicular skeleton, these occur infrequently, yet calcaneus fractures account for over 60% of all fractures occurring in the tarsal bones.[41] They occur as the result of severe forces imparted upon the hindfoot during falls from heights, motor vehicle accidents, or direct trauma. Complex articular and bony anatomy along with a vulnerable soft tissue envelope makes the operative fixation of these fractures technically demanding. Previously, nonoperative management was generally recommended, but reports of poor outcomes led Böhler and others toward advancing the science of operative intervention.[42,43] The principles of ORIF are now well established.[41,44–53] Currently, the scientific literature supports the acute surgical management of displaced fractures of the calcaneus by surgeons who have dedicated the time to master the challenging technical aspects of both the soft tissue and osseous structures associated with this fracture.

Initial Evaluation

The initial evaluation of patients with calcaneus fractures includes a careful physical exam of the axial and appendicular skeleton with emphasis on examining for other injuries commonly associated with axial loading. Pain noted on palpation of the thoracolumbar spine, pelvis, ipsilateral or contralateral hip, knee, foot, or ankle should warrant appropriate plain radiographs. There is a 20 to 25% incidence of lumbar, pelvis, hip, and/or knee bony injuries in patients with concomitant calcaneus fractures.[54]

At the same time, the injured foot should be examined for swelling, lacerations, or blisters (either hemorrhagic or nonhemorrhagic). Most open fractures have medial wounds. Open wounds should be dressed with a Betadine dressing, and appropriate parenteral antibiotics should be given. The specific management of open fractures is discussed later in this chapter. Early signs of pressure necrosis of the skin heralded by either blanching or tenting by underlying displaced bone fragments must be noticed. Severe pain and pain with passive stretching of the short toe flexors should alert the surgeon to the possibility of compartment syndrome.[55]

Initial radiographs include a lateral view of the hind foot, an AP view of the foot, a tangential Harris view of the calcaneal tuberosity, and an oblique Broden's view of the subtalar joint. CT scans are mandatory for assessment of the posterior facet and for classification. Treatment decisions should not be made without complete imaging, including both radiographs and CT.

Management of the Soft Tissues

The soft tissue envelope of the hindfoot is so important in the management of calcaneal fractures that it deserves special consideration. The periosteocutaneous sleeve of the hindfoot should be considered an organ unto itself and demands immediate and aggressive treatment regardless of the definitive fracture treatment. Prior to any surgical procedure, soft tissue edema must be controlled and diminished. In the absence of open wounds or impending pressure-related skin necrosis, a bulky compressive Jones splint can be applied. Alternatively, cast padding and an elastic wrap can be used with cryotherapy devices, such as the Cryo/Cuff (Aircast, Summit, New Jersey). These rapidly decrease edema and pain. A removable, padded, posterior foot splint should be added to prevent equinus contracture. The foot is kept elevated above the level of the heart for edema control. Some authors advocate pneumatic compression devices to enhance the diminution of swelling, although many patients find them to be too uncomfortable to use.[56,57]

There are two aspects of the soft tissue injury that should be watched for and may demand immediate attention. First of all, displaced bone fragments may compromise the overlying skin. In particular, displacement of the calcaneal tuberosity in tongue-type or tuberosity avulsion fractures

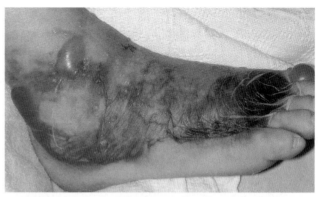

Figure 33–15 Clinical photograph of severe soft tissue injury, which would significantly alter the standard course of treatment for calcaneus fracture.

can compromise the skin of the posterior heel. Early signs of skin blanching on the posterior heel in tongue-type fractures mandate early reduction and fixation to relieve pressure on the skin. Loss of soft tissue of the posterior heel is disastrous with no simple salvage options.

The second aspect of the soft tissue injury that must be watched for is the development of fracture blisters. Their formation is dependent upon the magnitude of energy imparted to the hindfoot. Higher-energy fractures and delays of more than 4 to 8 hours in the application of a compressive splint increase the chances of blisters. Hemorrhagic blisters indicate a deeper soft tissue injury and should be avoided when incisions are planned. Nonhemorrhagic blisters denote some viable epidermal cells attached to the dermis and represent a more superficial injury. Regardless of their appearance, fracture blisters herald injury to the soft tissue envelope of the hindfoot and should be respected **(Fig. 33–15)**.[58–60] They should be covered with nonadherent gauze dressings and allowed to decompress on their own as the swelling diminishes. Blisters generally resolve by the time the foot edema allows surgical intervention. If the blisters rupture and expose the dermis, the roof should be debrided, and an antibacterial cream such as Silvadene (Monarch Pharmaceuticals, Inc., Bristol, Tennessee) can be used to prevent secondary bacterial colonization until the bed reepithelializes. If extensive areas of hemorrhagic fracture blisters remain on the lateral heel in patients 3 to 4 weeks after injury, consideration should be given for nonoperative care. Malunited fractures can be treated at a later date through a healthier soft tissue envelope utilizing a reconstructive procedure.

Soft tissue edema usually begins decreasing between the third and seventh postinjury days **(Fig. 33–16)**. The first splint is changed at 2 to 5 days to reevaluate the skin. Gentle range of motion of the forefoot and midfoot can be started to help alleviate swelling.

These treatment algorithms apply to all calcaneus fractures regardless of whether they are to be treated operatively or nonoperatively. Acute and aggressive management of the soft tissue sleeve preserves treatment options. Conversely, if one does not fully evaluate, appreciate,

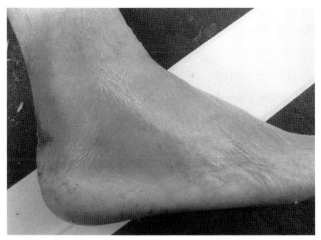

Figure 33–16 Clinical photograph of a calcaneus fracture immediately preoperative. Note the dissipation of swelling depicted by the obvious wrinkles throughout the lateral aspect of the soft tissue.

and aggressively treat the soft tissue injuries associated with this fracture, treatment options will become limited, very quickly!

Classification

Classification of calcaneus fractures requires a thorough understanding of the relevant osseous anatomy. The anterior process connects the distal lateral portion of the calcaneus to the cuboid. The superior portion of this serves as the base for the anterior facet, which supports the undersurface of the inferior talar head. The middle facet is upon the sustentaculum tali, which is also important in supporting the centromedial portion of the talar neck and body. The posterior facet is the largest articular surface and is juxtaposed beneath the inferior articular surface of the talar body. It transmits weight-bearing forces from the axial skeleton to the midfoot and forefoot via the calcaneocuboid and talonavicular joints as well as to the calcaneal tuberosity and therefore the ground. The lateral wall is relatively flat except for the peroneal tubercle. The neurovascular structures and extrinsic flexors course medially beneath the sustentaculum tali. The large tuberosity supports the posterior facet and serves as the attachment point for the gastrocsoleus mechanism. A thorough description of the pertinent anatomy is well represented in various texts of clinical anatomy.[61]

Calcaneal fractures can be described as nondisplaced or displaced, and either intra-articular or extra-articular. Experimental work by Carr demonstrated the fracture pathoanatomy previously described clinically by others.[62] Reproducible primary fracture lines occur that divide the calcaneus longitudinally into medial and lateral components. These can also extend into the calcaneocuboid joint further affecting the lateral column of the foot. A second fracture line originating at the angle of Gissane results from impaction of the lateral process of the talus and divides the calcaneus into anterior and posterior portions (**Fig. 33–17**).

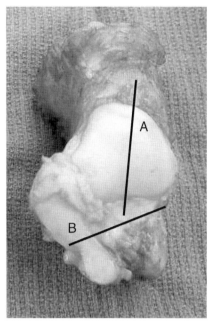

Figure 33–17 Dorsal view of gross calcaneus with typical fracture lines included. Note the posterior facet, medial facet, and anterior facet. The posterior facet is split by the first fracture line that runs longitudinally. The second fracture line divides the calcaneus into an anterior and posterior portion.

Böhler's and Gissane's angles are universally used in the description of altered radiographic anatomy in displaced calcaneus fractures. Böhler's angle is defined as the intersection of two lines at the posterior margin of the posterior facet on a lateral calcaneal radiograph (**Fig. 33–18**). One line is formed between the posterior-superior point of the tuberosity and the posterior-superior margin of the posterior facet. The second line is formed between the anterior-superior margin of the anterior process heading posteriorly to the same posterior-superior margin of the posterior facet. Böhler's angle varies between 20 and 40 degrees in normal

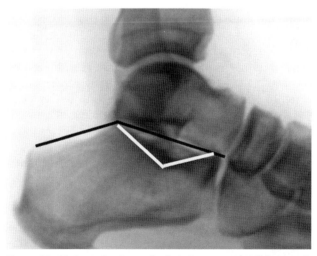

Figure 33–18 Lateral radiograph of a calcaneus with Böhler's angle (black line) and Gissane's angle (white line) superimposed over the radiograph.

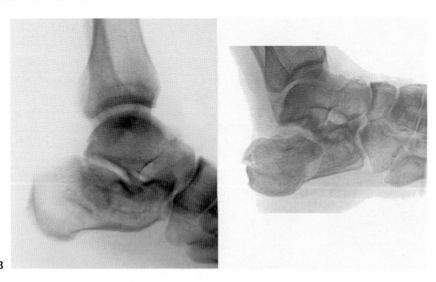

A,B

Figure 33–19 Calcaneus fractures. **(A)** Lateral radiograph of a joint compression–type calcaneus fracture. **(B)** Lateral radiograph showing a tongue-type calcaneus fracture.

subjects. The patient's normal value is ascertained from the uninjured, contralateral calcaneal radiograph. This angle decreases in displaced fractures because the posterior facet is impacted and rotated forward while the tuberosity is elevated. A decreased angle indicates a more displaced intraarticular fracture and possibly a worse prognosis with nonoperative care.[63]

The angle of Gissane is formed by the intersection of a line parallel to the superior surface of the posterior facet with a line originating at the uppermost portion of the anterior process extending downward to the most anteriorinferior portion of the posterior facet (**Fig. 33–18**). It parallels the outline of the lateral process of the talus. A normal value is obtained by measuring from the patient's contralateral uninjured calcaneus. The angle lessens as the displacement increases.

The Essex-Lopresti classification differentiates two fracture types based on the relationship of the posterior facet to that of the tuberosity. The joint depression fracture is the more common intra-articular variant, in which the posterior facet is displaced varying amounts from the tuberosity fragment. It is rotated anteriorly and downward and entrapped within the impacted cancellous bone. It usually separates from the lateral wall at a point just at or superior to the attachment of the calcaneofibular ligament and parallel with the inferior margin of the angle of Gissane (**Fig. 33–19A,B**). The less frequent tongue-type variant has a portion of the posterior facet still attached to the tuberosity fragment. There is a vertical fracture line extending downward through the sinus tarsi at the angle of Gissane. This intersects a more horizontal fracture line exiting posteriorly in the body of the tuberosity. The posterior facet is rotated downward and anteriorly, and the tuberosity portion is displaced upward at its posterior extent (**Fig. 33–19A,B**).

CT has greatly aided our understanding of fracture patterns and allows more accurate description of the intraarticular displacement. Identifying the degree of intraarticular comminution allows prognostic information to be gathered.[64,65] The Sanders classification describes the

articular displacement and comminution of the posterior facet based on the coronal CT scan.[50] The Sanders classification is based on the coronal CT image at the widest portion of the inferior-posterior facet of the talus. This anatomical landmark is divided into thirds, or columns, by two vertically oriented lines within the posterior facet. An additional line at the medial aspect of the posterior facet separates the most medial sustentacular fragment. Therefore, four potential fragments of the posterior facet can be described. Nondisplaced fractures are classified as type I regardless of the quantity of fracture lines. Type II fractures have two-part fractures of the posterior facet with subtypes IIA, IIB, IIC that describe a more medial fracture line in ascending alphabetical order (**Fig. 33–20**). Type III fractures are three-part variants with a centrally depressed

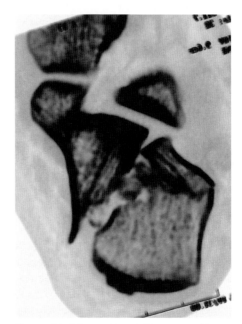

Figure 33–20 A computed tomographic scan of the calcaneus showing a joint depression–type calcaneus fracture that would be classified as a Sanders IIA.

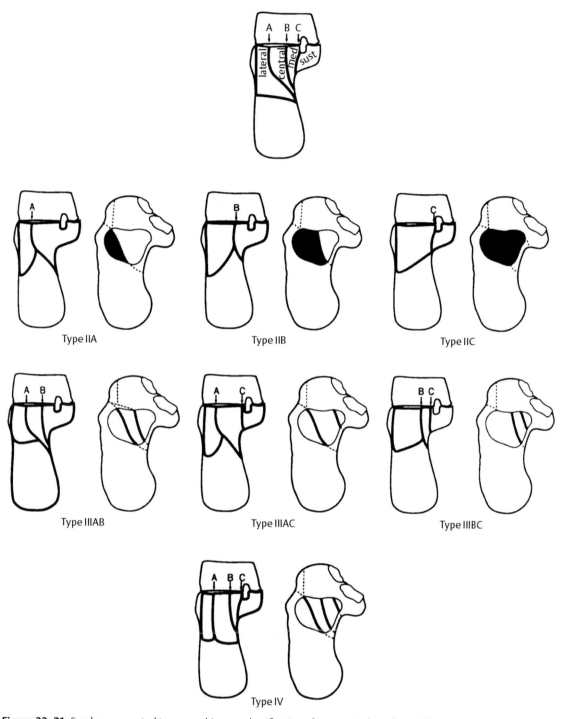

Figure 33–21 Sanders computed tomographic scan classification of intra-articular calcaneal fractures. (With permission from Sanders R. Intra-articular fractures of the calcaneus: present state of the art. J Orthop Trauma 1992;6:254, Figure 2.)

segment that is also further subtyped into IIIAB, IIIAC, or IIIBC as the depressed segment propagates medially. Type IV fractures are highly displaced and comminuted. They have at least four separate articular fragments of the posterior facet.

The Sanders classification provides prognostic information. There is a more favorable prognosis with Sanders type I and II fractures as compared with types III and IV

(Fig. 33–21).[50] This is intuitive because one would expect the function of the posterior facet to decrease as the comminution increases.

Nonoperative Treatment

The indications for nonoperative treatment of calcaneus fractures include truly nondisplaced fractures (i.e., Sanders type I) or patients with extensive medical comorbidities. These include, but are not limited to, tobacco use, peripheral vascular disease, type I diabetes (especially with neuropathy), steroid dependency, age, current soft tissue or bony infection of the hindfoot, or systemic diseases that increase the overall risk of anesthesia and operative care. Smoking cessation is demanded in all patients with calcaneal fractures.

The initial focus of nonoperative care is pain and edema control. Initially, these patients often require inpatient parenteral narcotics to manage their pain. Because of the potential development of acute compartment syndrome of the hindfoot, regional anesthesia is not recommended.

Edema control is outlined in the section on management of the soft tissue envelope. When the swelling has decreased to a point where a removable splint can be applied, hindfoot motion, including inversion, eversion, dorsiflexion, and plantar flexion is instituted. The foot is checked weekly until the swelling subsides. The patient is kept on low molecular weight heparin while an inpatient. Outpatient thromboprophylaxis is individualized. When using anticoagulation, the risk of deep vein thrombosis (DVT) must be balanced against the risk of expanding hematoma that may compromise the soft tissue envelope.

Radiographs of the hindfoot are obtained 2 weeks postfracture, and every 4 weeks thereafter. Patients are kept non–weight bearing initially and progressed to foot-flat, followed by progressive weight bearing as tolerated as the fracture heals in 8 to 12 weeks. A commercial short leg fracture brace is utilized until the patient is able to tolerate normal cushioned shoe wear, and to prevent an equinus contracture. Soft neoprene heel cups can be used as necessary when full weight bearing is achieved and normal shoe wear can be accommodated.

Indications for Surgical Treatment

There are numerous studies regarding the surgical treatment of acute displaced calcaneus fractures.[41,45–53,66–68] Traditionally, operative intervention is reserved for fractures with articular displacement of more than 2 mm. It has been demonstrated that joint contact forces within articular surface of the subtalar joint increase as displacement exceeds 2 mm.[69] This can be interpreted as analogous to the contact forces in the subtalar joint. The diminutive size of the posterior facet means that a large percentage of the weight-bearing joint may be affected by only a small displacement. A Sanders IIB or IIC injury will involve a greater percentage of the posterior facet than a type IIA fracture.

Radiographic criteria for operative intervention include the degree of comminution and displacement of the posterior facet as well as loss of the height, width, and varus position of the tuberosity. One should evaluate the integrity of the anterior process as well as its articulation with the cuboid. Restoration of these portions of the

calcaneus is critical to the functioning of the reconstructed posterior facet. Some fracture patterns (i.e., Sanders type IV) might be better suited for later reconstruction than acute repair. Some authors have recommended primary subtalar arthrodesis in these comminuted variants. Incisions used during heroic attempts to reconstruct a nonreducible posterior facet may preclude later surgical incisions needed for reconstruction. Finally, the patient must be a reasonable candidate for surgery.

Surgical Treatment

The goals of surgical correction of an acute calcaneal fracture are

1. Restore the normal orientation of the anterior process with its attached anterior and middle facets to the cuboid and lateral column of the foot.
2. Reconstruct the articular portion of the posterior facet and reattach it to the anterior process at the inferior portion of the angle of Gissane.
3. Correct shortening, varus, and excess width of the tuberosity.
4. Reattach the tuberosity to the posterior facet and inferior margin of the anterior process.
5. Fill cancellous bone voids, as necessary, and rigidly stabilize with internal fixation.
6. Close the incision without tension.

Surgical Anatomy

The vast majority of calcaneus fractures are approached surgically through an extensile lateral, L-shaped incision as described by Benirschke and colleagues (see **Video 33–2, Disk 4**).[41,48] The placement of the incision is critical; small deviations from the correct position increase the possibility of flap necrosis or neurological injury. The vertical limb is parallel to the Achilles' tendon and approximately 1 cm behind the posterior border of the fibula, and continues below the path of the peroneal tendons, curving horizontally in line with the plantar surface just above the glabral heel pad skin where it continues distally toward the calcaneocuboid joint. Care must be taken to prevent injury to the terminal branches of the sural nerve and the peroneal tendons and their sheaths.[70] This approach maximizes the exposure of the tuberosity and minimizes possible iatrogenic injury to the sural nerve.

The surgeon should understand the osteology of the calcaneus before contemplating surgical fixation. The lateral wall is relatively flat except for the peroneal tubercle. The calcaneocuboid joint is a saddle joint at its distal portion that inclines posteriorly as it courses medially. This anatomical fact is important to remember when inserting screws. The peroneus brevis tendon runs lateral to and in front of the calcaneocuboid joint. Often, the incision must be elevated superiorly to fully visualize the calcaneocuboid joint. There are cortical condensations on the lateral wall of the calcaneus for attachment of the peroneal retinaculum and the calcaneofibular ligaments. The upper surface of the tuberosity is visible through this incision, including the Achilles' tendon insertion. The posterior facet is obvious coursing downward toward the intersection with the anterior process at the angle of Gissane. This important joint slopes inferomedially as it progresses toward the middle facet and the sustentacular segment. Knowledge of this anatomical feature helps direct screws into the sustentaculum without violating the medial joint surface of the posterior facet.[71]

The lateral process and portions of the posteroinferior articular surface of the talus can also be viewed through this surgical window. The normal position of the sustentaculum tali is important to know because it is usually not visible unless a large fragment of the calcaneal posterior facet can be removed for later reconstruction. The portion of the calcaneus containing the sustentaculum tali is known as the "constant fragment" and extends anteromedially from the posterior facet. This fragment can also be more superior than the most medial portion of the posterior facet. This knowledge allows safe placement of screws into the dense sustentaculum tali from the lateral wall. These screws placed through a lateral plate tie the anterior process to the posterior facet and the tuberosity fragment. Therefore, it is vital to incorporate the sustentaculum fragment into the hardware construct. The extrinsic foot and toe flexor tendons as well as the posterior tibial nerve and vessels course below the sustentaculum tali and can be injured by inadvertent screw placement.[72,73] Obviously, screws must not exit the medial calcaneal cortex nor the most medial extent of the sustentacular tali. The position of the medial structures must be known indirectly when operating from the lateral side. When traumatic open wounds are present medially, access to the sustentaculum tali or medial wall fracture may allow debridement and limited manipulative reduction of widely displaced fragments.

Surgical Technique

After induction of general anesthesia, prophylactic cephalosporin antibiotics are given and a Foley catheter is inserted. The patient is placed in a lateral decubitus position on a radiolucent table with care to pad all potential neurovascular compression points (see **Video 33–2, Disk 4**). A pneumatic beanbag is used to support the thoracoabdominal area and pelvic ring. The downside leg is supported and a "blanket table" is constructed on top of the downside leg to support the operative leg. Both hips and knees are slightly flexed. The lateral knee is shaved to permit access to the distal lateral femoral condyle or proximal tibia for bone graft harvesting. The lateral foot and ankle are also shaved if necessary. A padded tourniquet is applied to the thigh. The entire leg from toes to groin is prepped accord-

ing to the surgeon's preference. Standard extremity draping goes up to the tourniquet so as to allow free movement of the extremity for fluoroscopy and access to the bone graft harvest sites. The extremity is elevated and exsanguinated with an elastic wrap and the tourniquet is inflated appropriately.

The incision is marked upon the skin based on anatomical landmarks previously described. A full-thickness periosteocutaneus flap is fashioned beginning at either the vertical or horizontal limb depending on the operative side and handedness of the surgeon. During the dissection, care of the soft tissues is the foremost consideration. The surgeon should make a single deliberate incision into the periosteum in line with the marked skin incision as soon as the tuberosity is encountered (i.e., at the corner of the incision). A full-thickness flap should be elevated subperiosteally with a no. 15 scalpel. The free edge of the periosteal flap can be grasped with a Senn or Ragnell retractor for exposure. Gentle traction by a skilled assistant facilitates a single-layer exposure. The thick calcaneofibular ligament is elevated off the lateral wall of the calcaneus as well as the peroneal retinaculum and tendon sheaths. Care is taken to not violate the peroneal tendon sheath and to avoid injury to the sural nerve. Following exposure of the lateral wall of the calcaneus, the dissection is continued toward the lateral portion of the posterior facet and then anteriorly until the calcaneocuboid joint is visualized. If preop CT scans do not demonstrate involvement of the calcaneocuboid joint, the distal dissection can be limited to lessen possible iatrogenic injury to the peroneal tendons or branches of the sural nerve.

If the posterior facet is obscured by displaced fragments, the comminuted lateral wall may need to be disassembled. Care is taken to leave soft tissue attachments still present at the inferior border of the fracture lateral wall, if possible. A cautery mark or skin marker can inscribe reference points on cortical fragments for later reassembly if needed. Any comminuted lateral wall fragments are kept in a moistened sponge until needed for the final reduction.

At this point, the posterior facet should be visible as well as the lateral process of the talus. Careful, deliberate dissection with a dental pick or periosteal elevator helps define the fracture planes and allow planning for reconstruction. Impacted portions of the posterior facet are elevated and removed; care is taken not to cause further chondral damage. These are cleaned with dental picks and sterile toothbrushes and placed in a moist saline sponge for later reconstruction.

At this point, a 4.0 or 5.0 mm Schanz pin is inserted into the calcaneal tuberosity to facilitate reduction via distraction at the fracture. If there is a tongue-type variant, the Schanz pin is placed in the upper tuberosity portion with its attached posterior facet. It is placed through a stab wound posteriorly through the skin and Achilles' tendon inferior and parallel to the posterior facet. A downward vector can effect reduction followed by provisional K-wire fixation.

A joint depression variant is associated with a tuberosity that is shortened and in varus position. A percutaneous posteroanterior Schanz pin in the tuberosity can impact a lengthening vector as described earlier. An additional lateral to medial Schanz pin can be used to affect an additional translational vector, pulling the heel into valgus or neutral. Reduction of the tuberosity may be difficult in older fractures that have some early consolidation. In these instances, a small, curved, periosteal elevator may be useful when used in the manner of a shoehorn. The surgeon carefully hooks the elevator under the inferomedial portion of the sustentaculum fragment and uses it as a fulcrum point to lever the tuberosity portion inferiorly and laterally. Utilizing these techniques, either solely or in tandem, restoration of length and valgus to the tuberosity fragment is achieved. This fragment is then provisionally connected to the medial portion of the anterior process with 0.054 or 0.062 in. K-wires. Reduction is checked with lateral, tangential, and Broden's fluoroscopic views.

Attention is now focused on the reduction of the anterior process. It is best to begin the reduction of the articular surfaces here and work posteriorly. Sagittal and coronal fracture lines of the calcaneocuboid portion are reduced and provisionally fixed with long 0.045 or 0.052 in. K-wires. One should identify the very dense cortical bone where the anterior process attaches to the distalmost portion of the angle of Gissane. This area usually withstands extensive comminution and is useful as a reduction aid and for screw purchase.

Next, the posterior facet is reduced to the residual "constant" sustentacular fragment as well as to the anterior process. Large, single fragments are generally easily reduced to these two landmarks. Comminuted posterior facet fractures may require reassembly on the back table prior to reduction, and the difficulty is proportional to the amount of comminution. Multifragmentary variants can have significant chondral loss, especially at the angle of Gissane, making anatomical reduction difficult. Even though the dense thalamic portion of the anterior process can be a useful cortical landmark, it can also act to shear off chondral surfaces of the posterior facet as these fragments displace as a result of the fracture. Provisional fixation with short 0.045 or 0.052 in. K-wires is used to reduce the posterior facet component to the sustentacular component. The surgeon's view of the posterior facet reduction is easier when the primary fracture line in the posterior facet is more lateral. Provisional reduction at the intersection of the anterior process and the distal portion of the posterior facet is also generally done with 0.045 or 0.052 -in. K-wires. Lateral hindfoot and Broden's fluoroscopic views are used at this point to confirm the articular reduction.

Following the articular reduction the position of the tuberosity portion needs to be "fine tuned." The superolateral portion of the tuberosity should reduce to the posterolateral corner of the posterior facet. The inferior cortex of the tuberosity should align with the inferior portion of the anterior process. These landmarks can usually be confirmed both visually and fluoroscopically utilizing lateral hindfoot, Broden's, and tangential Harris views. Long percutaneous 0.054 or 0.062 in. K-wires now connect the tuberosity to both the posterior facet and the anterior process.

Previously removed portions of the lateral wall are reassembled utilizing the reference marks to get a final confirmation of the reduction. Long K-wires can be advanced into the lesser tarsals for additional provisional fixation until the surgeon is satisfied that the reduction is acceptable. Radiographic copies of this construct are saved for the medical record.

Attention is now focused on the cancellous bone void left after provisional reduction and fixation. Autogenous cancellous bone can be retrieved in sufficient quantities from the lateral distal femur or proximal tibia. These two sources are the authors' favorite for calcaneus fracture. Others feel that no bone graft is necessary. Other options are freeze-dried or irradiated allograft cancellous bone or newer bone graft substitutes (see **Video 33–2, Disk 4**).

Definitive internal fixation is now inserted. There are several commercially available implants manufactured specifically for calcaneal fractures. All have the common features of low profile, enough flexibility to allow contouring yet sufficient rigidity to resist deformation when attached to the bone, and acceptance of multiple screws at varying angles, and all can be modified by cutting off unneeded sections. Although these prefabricated plates function well in many instances, they may limit flexibility in choices of screw placement, may require significant precontouring, and may require more extensive incisions for removal at a later date than would be needed to remove mini- and small-fragment hardware.

Small- and mini-fragment plates and screws as well as 2.7 mm reconstruction plates and cervical H-shaped plates from Synthes (Paoli, Pennsylvania) can be used. These simple plates can be customized to accommodate any fracture pattern. Long 2.0, 2.7, and 3.5 mm screws allow interfragmentary compression across larger areas, and smaller fragments that are important to fracture reduction and stability can be incorporated directly into the implant construct. Intimate knowledge of the interplay of fracture fragments is required to tie the anterior process to the posterior facet and tuberosity.

Definitive fixation begins by achieving interfragmentary compression between the articular fracture components of the calcaneocuboid joint and the posterior facet. This is usually accomplished with 2.0, 2.7, and/or 3.5 mm interfragmentary cortical screws. Occasionally 1.5 mm screws are needed in comminuted posterior facet fragments. Experience guides the placement of provisional K-wires in places that don't hinder later definitive screw placement. If preformed calcaneal plates are used, they need to be custom cut and contoured as necessary. Cortical screws are then placed divergently into the anterior

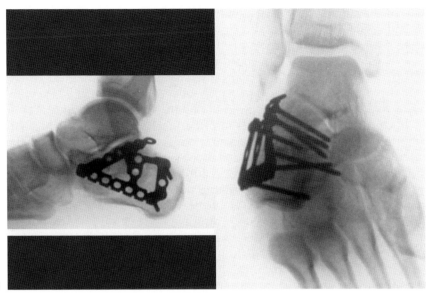

Figure 33–22 Postoperative views after repair of a calcaneal fracture with a lateral plate and screws. **(A)** Lateral view. **(B)** A Broden's view of the same patient showing the posterior facet reduction.

A,B

process, tuberosity, and posterior facet, and all are tied to the sustentacular fragment **(Fig. 33–22A,B).** Finally, all provisional K-wires are removed and final fluoroscopic views are taken. Lateral, tangential, and Broden's oblique fluoroscopic views are obtained to document definitive reduction and screw position. Tangential fluoroscopic views are mandatory to confirm that screws haven't violated the medial calcaneal wall. If screw lengths or positions are adjusted, new fluoroscopic views are needed.

After definitive fixation and bone grafting are completed, the tourniquet is deflated. A moist sponge is compressed with an elastic wrap over the lateral calcaneal wound as well as any bone graft harvest site for 5 to 10 minutes to assist with hemostasis. After this is removed, bipolar electrocautery is used to control cutaneous bleeders. Thrombostatic agents or bone wax can be used if cancellous bleeding is excessive. Often, this can be controlled by an additional 5 to 10 minutes of elastic compression. Good hemostasis is mandatory to prevent a postoperative hematoma that could put the flap at risk.

A small silicone drain, such as the TLS Surgical Drainage System (Porex Surgical Inc., Newman, Georgia) or a $\frac{1}{8}$ in. Hemovac (Zimmer, Warsaw, Indiana) is inserted and exits the foot dorsal to the flap. Wound closure is performed in two layers. The periosteal layer is closed using 0 or 2–0 absorbable sutures in an inverted mattress fashion. All of the sutures should be placed and tagged with a hemostat prior to tying. An assistant reduces the flap with gentle pressure while the operating surgeon sequentially ties the sutures starting at one corner of the incision and progressing from there. A correctly done deep closure should oppose the cutaneous edges. The cutaneous layer is closed with Allgöwer-Donati 4–0 nylon sutures with the knots at the posterior and inferior margins. Extreme care must be used in the wound closure.

Once the wound is completely sealed, the drain is checked for inadvertent capture and the perfusion of the

wound edges is reevaluated. If the skin edges are blanched between sutures, the Allgöwer-Donati knots are loosened with a microhemostat or dental pick until perfusion is assured. If the skin perfusion is in doubt, one should remove and replace the sutures. A sterile, nonadherent dressing is applied followed by a compressive, well-padded splint. Care is taken to secure the drain.

Postoperative Management

Regional anesthesia is very beneficial for pain management. If there is no contraindication, an intrathecal or a peripheral sciatic nerve block can be administered. Anticoagulation with heparin can be started immediately with peripheral nerve blocks but must be held for 12 to 24 hours if intrathecal anesthesia is used, to limit the rare chance of an epidural hematoma.

The patient is admitted to the hospital and the extremity is elevated. The patient is kept on bed rest for 36 hours. Range of motion exercises of the forefoot are begun immediately. The splint is changed before discharge (usually at 48 to 72 hours) and a new splint or a Cryo Cuff (Aircast, Summit, New Jersey) and Ace wrap with a removable posterior foot splint is added. The wound is inspected prior to discharge from the hospital. The patient is kept non–weight bearing.

The wound is examined in the office in 5 to 7 days, but sutures are not removed for 3 weeks. Subtalar motion is started as soon as the wound is sealed. X-rays, including lateral, Harris tangential, and Broden's oblique views are obtained when the sutures are removed and every 4 weeks thereafter. Fracture healing is generally noted in 8 to 12 weeks depending on the host. Progressive weight bearing is instituted until full weight bearing is obtained. Pool exercises or hydrotherapy is often very useful during the first few months. Aggressive physical therapy for dorsiflexion and plantar flexion, inversion, and eversion and ankle proprioception are continued until the patient achieves the final expected range of motion. Normal shoe wear is started when the patient is full weight bearing and augmented with custom orthotics or neoprene heel cups if needed.

Open Calcaneus Fractures

Open calcaneal fractures pose an entirely different treatment problem compared with closed fractures. Most commonly, the wound occurs medially due to lacerations by sharp cortical fragments of the sustentaculum fragment or by excessive shear forces placed upon the medial soft tissue envelope. Rarely, open wounds are due to extensive crushing or degloving injuries caused by external forces such as lawn mowers or farm and industrial machinery. The presence of the open wound mandates immediate surgical intervention.

The Gustilo-Anderson open fracture grade is determined and the neurovascular status of the limb documented.[74,75] It is important to carefully evaluate the neurovascular status because open calcaneus fractures have a higher percentage of neurovascular involvement. The status of these structures will play a large role in determining the definitive treatment. As with all open fractures, emergent debridement is mandatory. As for any open fracture, patients are given tetanus prophylaxis and appropriate intravenous antibiotics in the emergency department.

The next priority is to irrigate and debride all wounds in the OR as soon as possible, preferably within 4 to 6 hours of injury. Gross organic contamination, massive crushing or degloving injuries, or fractures originally delayed to the OR require a "second look" debridement within 24 hours. The use of meticulous soft tissue technique is mandatory for extending and exploring these wounds. The medial neurovascular bundle is almost always exposed in the depths of the wound, and it is important to identify and protect it. On occasion, the neurovascular structures can be interposed in the fracture site between the sustentaculum fragment and the tuberosity fragment.

Copious amounts of sterile irrigation are used after sharp debridement of nonviable tissue and foreign material is accomplished.

The open calcaneus fracture offers a unique opportunity in comparison to the closed calcaneus fracture with regard to management of the bony injury. One of the key problems in the reconstruction of calcaneal fractures is how to reduce the tuberosity to the sustentaculum. In closed fractures, the reduction must be done indirectly when a lateral approach is used. In contrast, in open fractures with a medial wound one may have the ability to directly visualize the cortical reduction, which can often be made anatomical (**Fig. 33–23A,B**). Anatomical reduction of the tuberosity decreases the tension on the medial wound closure that is imparted by the lateral translation of the tuberosity. Second, it returns the neurovascular structures to their original position and length, thereby improving their overall function and most importantly the venous drainage of the foot. Finally, the most difficult part of reconstructing a calcaneus fracture 2 to 3 weeks after injury is reestablishing calcaneal length and obtaining wound closure. This is due to the soft tissue envelope contracting during the time since the injury. By reestablishing the relationship of the tuberosity to the sustentaculum during the first debridement, the length of the calcaneus is restored, making later reconstruction much easier and allowing the opportunity to delay definitive reconstruction much longer if necessary.

One can maintain provisional reduction either with a mini-fragment T-plate (if the wound is deemed clean enough) or with longitudinal 9 in. K-wires placed from the tuberosity up into the sustentaculum, staying close to the medial wall of the calcaneus. These K-wires must be converted to internal fixation at the time that the traumatic wound is closed; otherwise the pin sites can increase the potential for contamination in the operative field during the definitive reconstruction. Alternatively, a fully threaded, tibiocalcaneal Steinmann pin can be utilized. This is placed

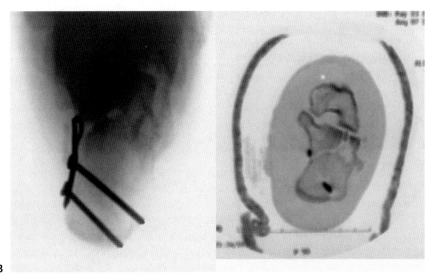

Figure 33–23 An open calcaneal fracture with a medial wound. **(A)** Axial radiograph showing the reduction of the tuberosity to the sustentaculum of the calcaneus through the open wound. **(B)** Computed tomographic scan of the same patient again showing the tuberosity reduction to the sustentaculum. Note that the lateral articular surface of the posterior facet is not yet reduced because this is staged when the soft tissues can tolerate definitive stabilization of the articular surface.

A,B

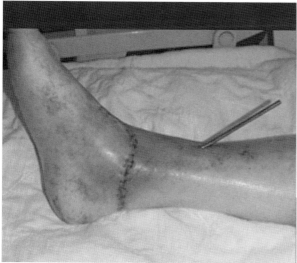

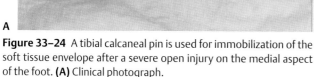

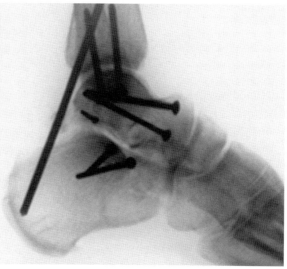

A

B

Figure 33–24 A tibial calcaneal pin is used for immobilization of the soft tissue envelope after a severe open injury on the medial aspect of the foot. **(A)** Clinical photograph.

(B) Lateral radiograph. This particular patient underwent open reduction and internal fixation of calcaneus and talus fractures.

from the anterior tibia and directed inferior and posterior to exit the tibia out the posterior malleolus. The pin is then advanced into the tuberosity after its relationship to the sustentaculum is reduced. One major advantage of this technique is that the pin site is significantly distant from the later definitive incision, which avoids the problems of later contamination of the operative field **(Fig. 33–24A,B).**

The open wounds can be managed by conventional dressings or with the newer negative pressure wound dressings. If the wound is not closed with the initial debridement, the patient is returned every 48 to 72 hours until the wound is free of obvious necrosis or infection. Atraumatic skin closure is done utilizing the Allgöwer-Donati suture technique.

Once the wound is closed, the surgical treatment is identical to that of closed fractures. Definitive treatment can be performed when the soft tissue edema has subsided and skin wrinkles have reappeared. This can take from 7 to 10 days. Edema control measurers can be utilized perioperatively as described for closed fractures. In most cases the standard lateral L incision is utilized, as already described. Standard fixation constructs can be utilized laterally.

Outcomes

The outcome after calcaneal fracture is dependent on the severity of the initial injury as well as on the method of treatment. Sanders showed that the degree of comminution of the posterior facet as demonstrated by preoperative CT scan was associated with surgical outcomes.[50] In essence, surgical outcomes are inversely proportional to the amount of comminution of the articular facets and directly proportional to the surgeon's ability to reconstruct them. Dr. Sigvard Hansen teaches that "if you make

it look like a foot, it will function like a foot." That can also be said for the calcaneus; anatomical reconstruction of the anterior, middle, and posterior facets with a neutral or slightly valgus tuberosity with restoration of the heel height and width will lead to optimum surgical outcomes. Studies previously listed in the text support this except in a subset of patients associated with workers' compensation where they have been shown to be more likely to have a secondary subtalar fusion due to continued sinus tarsi pain as compared with the non–workers' compensation patient.[76]

The operative management of calcaneus fractures can lead to good or excellent clinical results in the hands of a skilled fracture surgeon. Strict adherence to patient selection, soft tissue handling, rigid anatomical fixation, and supervised rehabilitation is mandatory. Barring any of the infrequent complications previously listed, a patient with a displaced calcaneus fracture can expect the following:

1. Two to 3 days inpatient hospitalization
2. Wound healing at 2 to 3 weeks
3. Bony union at 6 to 12 weeks
4. Partial weight bearing at 2 to 3 months
5. Full weight bearing at 3 to 4 months
6. Discontinuation of weight-bearing assistance at 4 to 6 months
7. Return to normal preinjury occupation at 6 to 9 months
8. Return of near full dorsiflexion and plantar flexion, and between 50 and 75% of inversion and eversion
9. Return of near full dorsiflexion and plantar flexion, and between 50 and 75% of inversion and eversion
10. Ability to accommodate normal shoe wear with occasional orthotic usage

- Calcaneus fractures that appear to be minimally displaced on plain radiographs can have a significantly displaced posterior facet on CT scan.
- Use a stable, radiolucent OR support for the affected leg. With the patient in the lateral position, multiple folded blankets can be made into a supportive, flat, and soft OR support. The folded blankets are placed in the popliteal fossa, anterior to the tibia, and anterior to the femur, with the knee in a flexed position. The downside leg is bent slightly less than the affected leg. Once the level is appropriate, unfolded bed blankets are placed like a tablecloth on top of the downside leg, giving a level and well-padded working surface.
- It is much easier to develop the periosteocutaneous layer during dissection of the lateral wall while using multiple no. 15 blades. These dull very quickly and should be changed every few passes. It is not unusual to use 15 to 20 no. 15 blades during this procedure.
- A transcutaneous tibiocalcaneal pin can be used to provide temporary distraction for both tongue-type and joint decompression calcaneus fractures with severe swelling. This is inserted through a predrilled anterior hole in the distal, central tibia angling downward to the posterior malleolus. After closed reduction, a fully threaded Steinmann pin is inserted with fluoroscopic control into the upper portion of the posterior calcaneal tuberosity just anterior to the Achilles' insertion. This imparts a distraction vector pushing the tuberosity inferiorly and helps maintain the integrity of the external soft tissue envelope by indirect reduction.
- When K-wires are inserted for provisional fixation, copious saline irrigation should be used because the bone is dense in some and excessive heat can cause thermal necrosis of bone.
- Modular, mini-, and small-fragment plates and screws work best for calcaneus fracture fixation. Mini-fragment plates can be "piggy-backed" over each other with screws through both plates simultaneously, thereby locking their positions. Condylar and reconstruction plates (2.7 mm) can be placed longitudinally to maintain the lateral wall and resist varus collapse of the tuberosity. Mini-fragment T plates or 2.7 mm condylar plates placed in an I-beam fashion support the posterior facet and tuberosity. Percutaneous 2.7 or 3.5 mm screws can be used longitudinally along either or both the medial and lateral cortical walls to act as an artificial cortex that resists shorting or varus collapse.
- Certain tongue-type or tuberosity avulsion variants can be managed utilizing percutaneous or limited open techniques with interfragmentary screws and small plates.
- Tourniquet time should be monitored during surgery. One should be able to deflate the tourniquet before 2 hours of elapsed time. If more time is required, the tourniquet should be left down for 15 to 30 minutes before reinflation.
- It is important to limit the tensile and shear stresses on the cutaneous wound edges during reduction and subsequent fixation. Some suggest placing K-wires in the talus to assist with flap retraction, but this maneuver potentially places very high, localized pressures on the skin and subcutaneous tissues that may lead to arteriolar and capillary occlusion and thus soft tissue complications. Similarly, overzealous retraction of the skin edge instead of the subperiosteal margin can cause permanent microvascular occlusion and limit skin profusion after the tourniquet is deflated. When not needed, such as while the posterior facet is being reconstructed on the back table or when bone graft is being harvested, the assistant-held retractors can be removed from the wound. Deliberate hydration of the wound edges with saline is also warranted throughout the case.

Complications

Complications in the surgical management of calcaneus fractures can be related to the soft tissue, osseous, articular, or tendinous structures. Surgeons skilled in this technique can minimize those risks, but these high-velocity injuries can be associated with complications themselves requiring surgical intervention.[76–78]

Soft tissues dehiscence or necrosis is a catastrophic failure. In the hands of skilled fracture surgeons, the rate of soft tissue breakdown and deep infection is less than 2% in closed fractures and 8% in open fractures.[79] Risk factors of tobacco use, diabetes, or open fractures all increase complications.[80] In Benirschke and Kramer's recent review, all soft tissue wound problems healed with debridements, antibiotics, and delayed wound closure.[79]

When soft tissue complications occur, they should be managed with staged debridements, negative pressure wound therapy, intravenous and/or oral antibiotics, and delayed closure. In the rare case where soft tissue loss is significant and secondary closure is not possible, local fasciocutaneous and microvascular free flaps can be utilized.[81,82]

Bony malunions can predispose to overloaded articular surfaces and secondary posttraumatic arthritis of the hindfoot.[83] Anatomical reduction of the anterior, medial, and posterior facets as well as the tuberosity and the anterior process is mandatory to minimize posttraumatic arthritis of a subtalar joint. Malunions can often be managed with a distraction bone block arthrodesis of the subtalar joints, augmented with calcaneal tuberosity osteotomies, if necessary.[84]

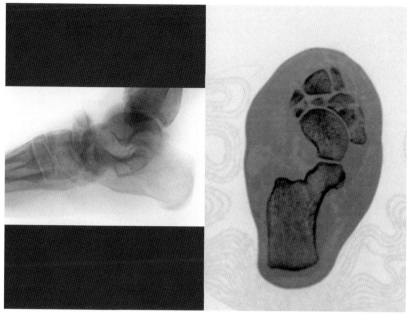

Figure 33–25 (A) Preoperative lateral foot radiograph and **(B)** computed tomographic scan of a comminuted Sangeorzan type III navicular fracture.

Neurological sequelae of injury to the sural nerve are generally limited. Patients tolerate anesthesia routinely well. Infrequent dysesthetic pain can be treated by oral, neurogenic pain medication, local steroid injections, and/or decompression. Delayed tarsal tunnel syndrome can be seen once the plantar medial soft tissues have scarred between 8 and 12 weeks postoperatively. This is managed by orthotics, antiinflammatories, and proper shoe modification. If the symptoms are progressive, appropriate neural testing can evaluate the status of the nerve and whether tarsal tunnel decompression is warranted.

Residual malunions and exostoses of the lateral wall or the sustentacular area can lead to impingement upon the peroneal posterior tendon sheaths. In general, these are treatable with antiinflammatory medications, physical therapy, and orthotics. Rarely, tendon decompression or exostectomy can be utilized to alleviate these problems.

Navicular Fractures

Tarsal navicular fractures are quite rare but can be quite disabling if they result in loss of motion or arthrosis of the talonavicular joint. The talonavicular joint provides most of the motion of the transverse tarsal articulation. It has been likened to the os-acetabulum of the foot. At the distal articulation with the three cuneiforms, there is very little motion.

Classification of Navicular Fractures

Navicular fractures are classified into three categories: fractures of the tuberosity; fractures of the dorsal edge; and fractures of the body. Sangeorzan et al further subcategorized fractures of the body into types I through III.[85]

The type I fracture has a coronal plane fracture line with a large dorsal fragment. A type II fracture has an oblique dorsal plantar fracture line with a large medial fragment, and the type III fracture has central comminution and talonavicular disruption **(Fig. 33–25A,B).**

Nonoperative Treatment

Nonoperative treatment can be considered for truly nondisplaced fractures. This **(Fig. 33–26A,B)** should be verified with a CT scan and such injuries should be observed over the first 2 weeks to verify that the fracture does not displace during treatment. Closed treatment requires 6 to 8 weeks of casting and non–weight bearing. After casting, the patient is placed into an orthotic with an arch support in an effort to protect the midfoot region of the foot. Only a small number of the fractures can be treated in this manner. The great majority will require operative stabilization.

Indications for Surgical Treatment

Indications for surgery are greater than 2 mm of gap or greater than 1 mm of step-off or any evidence of talonavicular subluxation or naviculocuneiform subluxation.

Surgical Treatment

Surgical Anatomy

The tarsal navicular provides the insertion of the posterior tibial tendon. The navicular is well vascularized, with the exception of the central portion.[86] The navicular is approached via a medial incision or a combination of

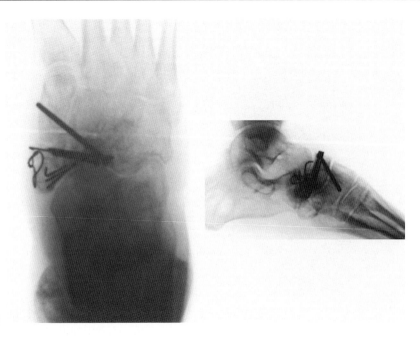

Figure 33–26 (A) Postoperative anteroposterior and **(B)** lateral radiographs demonstrating a typical fixation construct for a navicular fracture. Notice fixation extending into the cuneiforms for bone stock and also the use of a medial tension-band wire.

A,B

medial and dorsolateral incisions. Rarely will one use only an anteromedial approach.

The medial approach starts with a low medial incision that is parallel and slightly superior to the posterior tibial tendon. This is quite a bit lower than the standard anterior medial incision and allows better access to the navicular. In the great majority of navicular fractures there is a fracture line that exits in the inferior-medial portion of the navicular. This fragment can be reflected inferiorly and used as a window to the articular reduction of the remainder of the navicular fracture.

For the dorsolateral approach, the incision is centered over the navicular in line with the third metatarsal. The incision is carried down just medial to the extensor digitorum longus tendons and then medial to the muscle belly of the extensor digitorum brevis. Care must be taken to protect the neurovascular structures that lie just medial to this plane. This exposes the anterolateral talus, the dorsal aspect of the navicular, and the lateral cuneiforms.

The incision for the anteromedial approach is in the interval between the anterior tibial tendon and the extensor hallucis longus (EHL) tendon. The approach is deepened between these two tendons, exposing the dorsal aspect of the navicular.

Surgical Technique

When reviewing preoperative imaging studies, one should note whether there is lateral subluxation of the talonavicular or the naviculocuneiform joint. If not, a small medial distractor helps to distract and visualize the articular surfaces. The pins are placed in the talar neck and the first metatarsal shaft. If the lateral disruption is significant, the medial distractor actually hinders the reduction, causing even greater displacement. In this

situation, one must reconstruct the lateral navicular first, providing a lateral pillar to allow for medial distraction and to provide a foundation onto which to build the remainder of the joint. When this is necessary, a second lateral approach to the navicular is quite useful. This approach should always be considered with comminuted fractures, dorsally subluxated navicular-cuneiform fragments, or a laterally subluxated talonavicular joint. One often finds a large dorsally displaced navicular fragment; until this fragment is reduced, the talonavicular joint will remain subluxated. Alternatively, dual distractors can be used, one medial from the talar neck to the first metatarsal and one lateral from the lateral talar neck to the third metatarsal.

Joysticks, dental picks, and small elevators are useful for manipulating the articular fragments back into their anatomical position. The reduction is held temporarily with K-wires, and intraoperative fluoroscopy or plain radiography is utilized to verify the reduction. Stabilization of comminution fractures can be difficult. Small- and mini-fragment screws are used to stabilize most navicular fractures. On occasion, mini-fragment plates and tension-band wires (particularly, for the medial inferior tuberosity fragment where the posterior tibial tendon attachment is intimately in contact) can be useful. With severe comminution, fixation can be extended to the cuneiforms (**Fig. 33–26A,B**). Because there is minimal motion between the navicular and cuneiforms, the cuneiforms can provide good, stable bone stock to affix the navicular fragments to without compromising the mobility of the foot. Screws from the proximal medial aspect of the navicular can extend diagonally out into the third cuneiform. Likewise, a screw from the medial or first cuneiform can be aimed in a retrograde trajectory back into the lateral aspect of the navicular. In addition a spawning external fix-

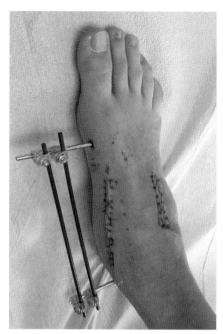

Figure 33–27 Photograph of the dorsal medial aspect of the foot showing a two-incision approach, medial and anterolateral, for a navicular fracture. Note the external fixator to help maintain medial column length and the nylon closure.

ation can be added to maintain medial column length with severe impaction (**Fig. 33–27**).

Rehabilitation

Postoperatively, the patient is maintained non–weight bearing for 8 to 12 weeks. During the last 4 weeks, pool therapy may be utilized. Weight bearing is initiated only after the patient has obtained an orthotic with medial arch support. The patient is maintained for the first 6 months in a knee-high elastic anti-embolism stockings.

> **Tips and Tricks**
>
> - It is important to evaluate the lateral column of the foot so as not to miss any concomitant injuries.

Complications and Outcomes

Complications of navicular fractures include malunion, posttraumatic arthritis and AVN, and late progressive hindfoot varus deformity. Very few articles exist on navicular fractures; therefore, outcome data are rare for this injury. Sangeorzan reported AVN in 29%, only one patient with AVN developed collapse of the navicular.[85] The adequacy of reduction seemed to correlate with outcome. Because the navicular is rarely an isolated fracture (only six of 21 in the Sangeorzan article), it is difficult to interpret outcomes.[86]

Fractures of the Cuboid

The cuboid has five articulations, all supported by strong intertarsal and tarsometatarsal ligaments. It has separate articular facets for the fourth and fifth metatarsal, and forms a saddle-shaped joint with the calcaneus. Medially, it articulates with the lateral cuneiform, and posteromedially it articulates with the navicular.[87] The plantar surface of the cuboid has a prominent ridge that receives the long plantar ligament; this ligament supports the calcaneocuboid articulation. A tuberosity on the plantar lateral aspect of the ridge articulates with the peroneus longus tendon.[88] The cuboid functions as a lateral column spacer. Loss of length in the lateral column can result in flatfoot deformity.[89] Also, its articulation with the fourth and fifth metatarsals provides nearly all the dorsal and plantar motion of the lateral column of the foot.[90]

Fractures of the cuboid and the true incidence of these fractures are unknown. The injury occurs either with a direct blow to the lateral foot, or more commonly with an applied plantar flexion and abduction force on the foot causing the cuboid to be compressed between the anterior process of the calcaneus and the fourth and fifth metatarsals. This injury should not be considered an isolated fracture but rather the lateral component of an injury that usually affects both the medial and lateral columns. This injury has been named the "nutcracker fracture."[91] In the largest series to date, 10 of 12 patients had associated medial-sided foot injuries, including fractures of the navicular, tarsometatarsal joint complex, or medial metatarsals.[89] Cuboid fractures can also be associated with fractures of the calcaneus and intermetatarsal disruption of the fourth and fifth metatarsal.

Classification

There is no accepted classification for cuboid fractures. From the literature, fractures include extra-articular shear-type fractures and intra-articular compression-type fractures. Intra-articular fractures may involve the calcaneal–cuboid articulation or the cuboid–metatarsal articulation. There may be a crush or burst fracture of the body of the cuboid superimposed on the articular impaction, with resulting loss of lateral column length.[89,92]

Nonoperative Treatment

Undisplaced fractures of the cuboid can be treated in a non–weight bearing below-knee cast for 6 weeks.

Indications for Surgical Treatment

If there is intra-articular displacement of more than 1.5 mm, or if the length of the cuboid (length of the lateral column) has been lost, ORIF with bone grafting is desired.

Surgical Treatment

Because cuboid fractures are rarely isolated, treatment of the injury needs to take all midfoot fractures into account. All injuries must be considered in the planning of surgical incisions. Usually, the medial column injury will be stabilized first because it will often effect an indirect reduction of the cuboid.

The cuboid is exposed through a 4 to 5 cm incision on the lateral aspect of the foot, dorsal to the peroneal tendons and the sural nerve, in line with the fourth metatarsal. Deep to the skin the extensor digitorum brevis (EDB) is identified and retracted dorsally, and the peroneal tendons are retracted plantarly. The periosteum over the lateral wall of the cuboid is incised and the lateral wall is opened like a trap door to access the fracture and the articular surface of the cuboid. A small external fixator with 2 mm pins is then placed on the lateral aspect of the foot, with a proximal pin in the anterior process of the calcaneus and a distal pin in each of the fourth and fifth metatarsals. Because the fixator is used to distract the cuboid back out to length (see **Video 33–3, Disk 4**), one must first assess the stability of the intertarsal joint of metatarsals four and five. If these joints are unstable, they must be stabilized to the remaining metatarsals prior to placing the external fixator.

An x-ray of the uninjured foot is obtained to judge the appropriate length of the cuboid. Reduction begins with the articular surface of the cuboid. The depressed fragments are elevated and the articular surface reduced and held with small temporary K-wires (0.035 to 0.054 in.). In the case of a crush fracture, the void in the cuboid is filled with bone graft. Tricortical iliac crest graft may be necessary if the subchondral bone that remains is not adequate for stable fixation. The tricortical graft is placed and held with K-wires. Permanent fixation is then achieved using the "cuboid plate" from Synthes (Modular Foot Set, Synthes, Paoli, Pennsylvania) (**Fig. 33–28A,B**). This 2.4 mm plate accepts both 2.0 and 2.4 mm cortical screws. Alternately, two mini-fragment (2.0 mm) plates can be utilized. Plates are placed on the dorsal to dorsolateral surface of the cuboid. The fixator is then released and the cuboid is checked for stability. If the bone graft and plates are unable to maintain the length of the cuboid, the fixator is left in place for 6 to 8 weeks.

Postoperatively, the foot is placed in a well-padded posterior splint. With the first postoperative visit the patient is placed in a removable splint and range of motion exercises are begun. The patient remains non–weight bearing for 8 weeks (12 weeks if a large graft was utilized). Formal physiotherapy is usually not required.

Complications

With conservative treatment, loss of lateral column length has been described with resultant flatfoot deformity. Although lateral column shortening of > 5% was noted in 40% in the series by Weber and Locher, none resulted in a flatfoot deformity as defined by the talo–first metatarsal angle.[89] The minimal shortening also did not interfere with functional outcome. Arthritis can occur at either the calcaneal–cuboid joint or the cuboid–metatarsal joints, but specific incidence is not known. Compartment syndrome requiring fasciotomy has been reported in up to 50% of cases.[89]

Outcomes

Main and Jowett reported poor outcome with fractures treated conservatively with plaster.[93] All four patients in their series had continued pain and were salvaged with triple arthrodesis. Jahn and Freund's series of two patients treated in plaster alone also reported poor results, with one patient requiring arthrodesis of the calcaneocuboid joint and the other requiring arthroplasty of the cubometatarsal joints.[94]

More favorable results have been reported with ORIF, with attention to joint congruity and lateral column length. Sangeorzan and Swiontkowski's series of four

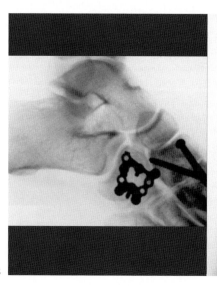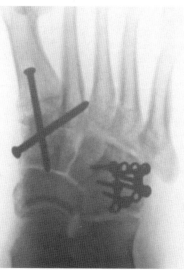

Figure 33–28 (A) Postoperative anteroposterior and **(B)** lateral radiographs showing plate fixation of the cuboid.

A,B

patients reported three patients with full pain-free range of motion with no functional limitations at 1 year follow-up.[92] Two studies used the American Orthopaedic Foot and Ankle Society (AOFAS) scores to assess patient function.[88,95] Fifty-six percent of patients had good to very good results and only 6% had poor results. Although 60% of patients had some residual pain and stiffness, the pain was often on the medial side of the foot and secondary to associated midfoot injuries.

Pearls

- The incidence of cuboid fractures is unknown but is associated with midfoot injury 80% of the time.
- ORIF is indicated for displacements of 1 to 2 mm and for any loss of length of the cuboid.
- Residual symptoms in the foot are often from associated midfoot injury.

Tarsometatarsal Joint Injuries

Injuries of the tarsometatarsal, or Lisfranc joints constitute 31% of midfoot fracture-dislocations.[96–99] Because the outcome of this injury has been shown to be dependent upon anatomical reduction,[100–102] a more aggressive surgical approach has evolved, including operative fixation for displaced "sprain"-type injuries.[103]

Subtle injuries of the tarsometatarsal joints are common, with 20% of these injuries being missed on initial presentation.[102] Injury to the tarsometatarsal joint should be suspected if there is pain and swelling of the midfoot, even if the mechanism of injury is insignificant. Plain radiographs including AP, lateral, and 30 degree oblique views of the foot reveal most injuries. The AP and oblique views should be taken with the x-ray beam parallel to the tarsometatarsal joint to minimize overlap of the bones. In all views, a line drawn along the outer cortical edge of the shaft of a metatarsal should *not* intersect with its corresponding tarsal bone. Widening of greater than 1 to 2 mm of the first interspace, between either the metatarsals or the cuneiforms, is also abnormal.[104] If there is any doubt, simulated-weight-bearing AP views should be obtained, with both feet on one cassette and as much weight as tolerated placed through the injured foot.[105] CT in the plane of the first metatarsal is also invaluable; displacement in the plane of the first metatarsal of 1 to 2 mm that is not evident on plain radiographs can be detected by CT, and the overlap seen on plain films is eliminated, revealing the true intraosseous relationships.[106] Alternatively, stress views under anesthesia can be performed (**Fig. 33–29A,B**).

Classification

The descriptive classification of tarsometatarsal injuries by Hardcastle et al is widely recognized and commonly used in the literature.[97] It describes the direction of displacement of the tarsal bones as seen on radiographs. Type A involves total incongruity of the tarsometatarsal joint, type B consists of partial incongruity at the tarsometatarsal joint, and type C consists of divergent displacement that may be either partial (a) or total (b). Although the classification allows communication between clinicians or researchers, it has not been found to have prognostic value. Earlier classifications based on mechanism of injury (direct and indirect) do have some prognostic value, however. Direct (crush) injuries tend to have a worse prognosis than indirect (rotational force) injuries.[101] This is primarily due to the associated soft tissue trauma, skin loss, and vascular injury associated with severe crush injuries.

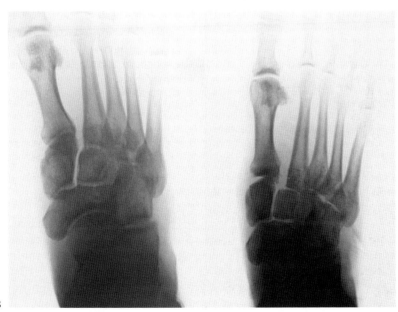

Figure 33–29 A Lisfranc injury. **(A)** Anteroposterior view of the foot showing a subtle Lisfranc injury, as indicated by apparent widening between the bases of the first and second metatarsals. **(B)** Stress view of the same foot with the x-ray beam more tangential to the tarsal metatarsal joint.

A,B

Indications for Surgical Treatment

It is the authors' opinion that *any* displacement of the tarsometatarsal joint found on x-ray or CT is an indication for operative fixation. Nonoperative treatment such as casting is reserved only for completely undisplaced "sprains." Stability of the tarsometatarsal joints must be documented with stress views before commencing with nonoperative treatment. A period of 6 weeks non–weight bearing in a cast followed by 6 weeks of protected weight bearing in a removable castboot or supportive shoe with a polydensity orthosis containing a medial arch support and metatarsal pad would be appropriate treatment.

Surgical Treatment

Surgical Anatomy

Two components of the bony anatomy contribute to the stability of the tarsometatarsal joint complex. First, the cuneiforms and corresponding metatarsal bases are dorsally based trapezoids in cross section and constitute a "Roman arch." This prevents the plantar displacement of the metatarsal bases. Second, in the coronal plane, the second metatarsal is recessed and dovetailed into the mortise formed by the medial and lateral cuneiforms, thus limiting medial and lateral translation. Thus the "keystone" for stability for the whole transverse arch of the foot is the triangular base of the second metatarsal.[107] It is imperative in the treatment of this injury to reestablish the relationship of the metatarsals with their corresponding tarsal bones.

Three sets of ligaments support the tarsometatarsal articulation: dorsal, plantar, and intraosseous. The dorsal and plantar ligaments follow a longitudinal, oblique and transverse course, uniting tarsals to metatarsals. The plantar ligaments are stronger than their dorsal counterparts. The intraosseous ligaments are the strongest of the capsuloligamentous restraints. Connections exist between the lateral four metatarsals but there is no ligament between the first and second metatarsal. Instead, the base of the second metatarsal is connected to the medial cuneiform via the named Lisfranc ligament, which is 8 to 10 mm long and 5 to 6 mm in width.[108]

Surgical Technique

In the current literature, there is consensus that anatomical reduction is required to obtain the best clinical result.[97,100-102,109,110] Controversy exists regarding the need for open reduction for all injuries, but in our opinion, open reduction gives the patient the best chance for an anatomical reduction. Differing opinion also exists as to the best form of fixation, with some authors preferring K-wire fixation whereas others strongly advocate fixation with screws.[100,101,104] Anatomical studies have shown minimal movement of the medial and middle column but

physiological movement of over 1 cm in the lateral two rays of the foot.[92] We follow the anatomical template by fixing the medial three metatarsals with rigid fixation and the lateral two with K-wire fixation. It is important for the medial and middle column to allow the foot to become rigid during the end-of-stance phase, and for lateral column to maintain its inherent mobility.[105]

Preoperatively, the soft tissue envelope of the foot must be carefully examined. If it is compromised, consideration should be given to temporary K-wire stabilization with delayed definitive surgical intervention. It is best to place the K-wires through the plantar aspect of the foot so the pin tracts are well away from the operative field. The K-wires are placed in a retrograde fashion up the metatarsal and across the metatarsal–cuneiform joint.

The patient is placed supine on the operating table, with the injured limb draped free. Use of a bump under the hip places the foot in neutral rotation, and a radiolucent triangle is placed under the knee to allow better access to the dorsum of the foot. The image intensifier should be brought in from the lateral aspect of the injured foot; this allows easier access to the medial side of the foot for K-wire and screw placement (**Fig. 33–30**).

Two incisions allow adequate access to all the tarsometatarsal joints (see **Video 33–4, Disk 4**). *The first incision* is made over the interspace between the first and second metatarsals, at the level of the tarsometatarsal joint (**Fig. 33–31A,B**). Two intervals are utilized through this one incision, one medial to the EHL, and one lateral to the extensor hallucis brevis (EHB). One begins by dividing the fascia medial to the EHL and retracting the tendon laterally. The neurovascular bundle is located lateral to the tendon and is protected by the tendon and the use of subperiosteal dissection. There is no need to isolate the neurovascular bundle, and the dissection generally stays proximal to the area of the first perforating artery. The first interval allows access to the first metatarsal and medial cuneiform. The second interval is lateral to the EHB tendon. The fascia lateral to the EHB is released and the tendon and the neurovascular bundle are retracted medially. This interval allows access to the second metatarsal and middle cuneiform. By making the skin incision longer, and with more medial retraction, the third metatarsal and lateral cuneiform can also be visualized through this interval. *The second incision* is made between the fourth and fifth metatarsals and allows access to their articulations with the cuboid. The tendons of the extensor digitorum longus and brevis will be encountered and can easily be retracted either medially or laterally to allow access to the lateral two joints.

The reconstructive procedure begins with the first metatarsal and medial cuneiform. One begins by visualizing the joints to be reduced and assessing intercuneiform stability. The joint capsule is usually disrupted but needs to be reflected for adequate visualization. Soft tissue as well as bony or cartilaginous fragments often impede reduction and need to be cleared from the joint. A small

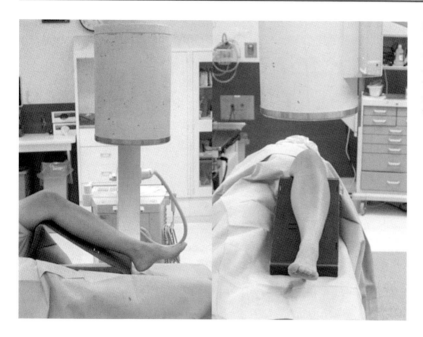

Figure 33–30 Room setup for surgical treatment of a Lisfranc fracture. Note the triangle under the knee or a bump to position the foot appropriately for both surgical approach and x-ray evaluation. For this particular injury, fluoroscopy is brought in from the injured side. This makes it easier for placement of the diagonal screw from the first cuneiform to the second metatarsal.

lamina spreader is useful in exposing the depths of individual joints.[105] The reduction is assessed by the position of the bones, with the medial, lateral, and dorsal cortices of the first metatarsal and medial cuneiform aligning in all planes. The reduction is held with a piercing reduction clamp or dental pick, followed by temporary K-wire fixation. A 4.0 mm cortical screw is then placed from the first metatarsal into the medial cuneiform along the axis of the shaft in a retrograde fashion. The screw is started 1.5 to 2.0 cm distal to the joint, aiming parallel to the floor or slightly plantarward. A recess for the screw head is created with a 4 mm bur to prevent fracture of the MT (**Fig. 33–32A,B**).

After stabilization of the medial column, one proceeds to the second metatarsal and middle cuneiform. Once the medial column is reduced, the second and third metatarsals are easier to reduce. Again, the reduction is assessed from the medial, lateral, and dorsal cortices of the second metatarsal and middle cuneiform. For the purposes of reduction, a pointed reduction clamp is placed diagonally from the distal lateral base of the second metatarsal to the proximal medial aspect of the medial cuneiform (**Fig. 33–33A,B**). The vector applied by the clamp is essential for reestablishing the keystone position of the second MT. Care must be taken not to malreduce the second metatarsal inferiorly. The reduction is held provisionally with K-wires. A screw is placed from the medial cuneiform to second metatarsal on a diagonal, re-creating the position of the Lisfranc ligament. The screw should be started

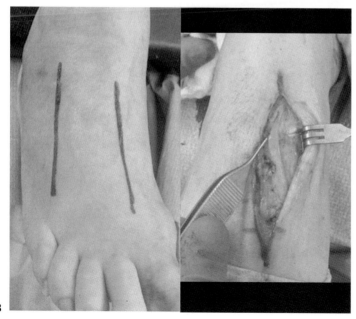

Figure 33–31 The incisions for a Lisfranc fracture. **(A)** Typically only the medial incision will be utilized. **(B)** The medial incision is extended deep medial to the extensor longus tendon allowing exposure of the first cuneiform–first metatarsal joint.

A,B

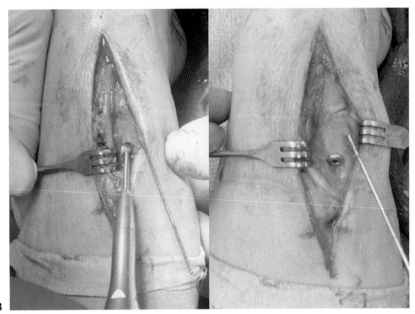

A,B

Figure 33–32 Steps in the screw fixation of the first metatarsal. **(A)** A bur is used to create a recess for the head of the retrograde screw placed from the first metatarsal to the first cuneiform. **(B)** The screw in place. Note the K-wire holding the preliminary reduction while the screw path is prepared and the screw is placed.

in the proximal dorsal corner of the medial cuneiform and aimed just below the dorsal cortex of the second metatarsal. The screw should engage four cortices to ensure bicortical fixation in the second metatarsal. Image intensification along with palpation with the depth gauge ensures the screw is in bone throughout its course. A second screw can be placed from the medial to the middle cuneiform for added stability of the medial and middle columns. When planning to use a second screw, the diagonal screw should be started more distal in the cuneiform.

Often there is enough stability of the third metatarsal after fixing the first two metatarsals. If the third metatarsal does not reduce, a similar reduction maneuver is performed

with a pointed reduction clamp and provisional K-wire fixation. A screw is then placed from the third metatarsal to the lateral cuneiform, again starting 1.5 to 2.0 cm from the joint and creating a recess with a 4 mm bur so as not to crack the cortex of the metatarsal.

Lastly, fixation of the fourth and fifth metatarsals to the cuboid is performed. These are accessed through the second incision. Again, the joint is visualized by reflecting the torn capsule. The reduction is assessed at the dorsal and medial cortices of the fourth MT and its alignment with the dorsomedial cortex of the cuboid. The fourth and fifth metatarsals tend to reduce easily and are held with percutaneous 0.062 –in. K-wires that are left out of the skin.

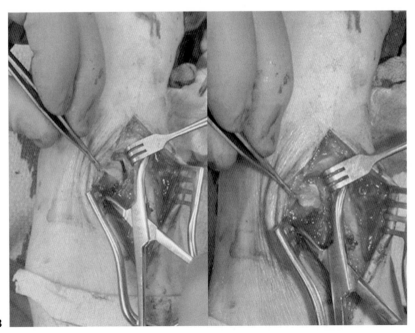

A,B

Figure 33–33 Steps in the open reduction of the tarsometatarsal joint. **(A)** The Lisfranc joint, the second metatarsal, and the corner of the first metatarsal–second cuneiform are visible. A forceps is holding onto the dorsal ligament structure and a Weber clamp or pointed reduction clamp is being positioned for reduction of this subluxation. **(B)** The effect of the clamp reducing the subluxation is depicted.

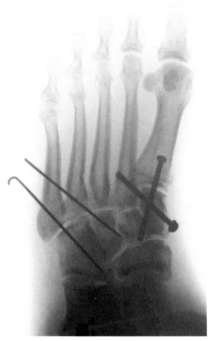

Figure 33–34 Standard Lisfranc fixation construct with a retrograde screw for the first metatarsal–first cuneiform joint. A diagonal screw from the first cuneiform to the second metatarsal is also shown, and K-wires are used for the lateral column of the foot.

Alternatively, the fourth and fifth metatarsal may be treated with closed reduction and percutaneous pinning (**Fig. 33–34**).

Tips and Tricks

- If the metatarsals are segmentally fractured, a 0.062 –in. K-wire can be used as an intramedullary device to align the metatarsal and fix it to its corresponding tarsal bone. The K-wires are placed through the plantar aspect of the foot into the metatarsal.
- With severe comminution of the medial column or first ray, a bridging plate can be placed from the first MT to the navicular.
- If the first ray is highly unstable, as in a divergent injury, an additional screw can be placed to secure the medial and middle cuneiform.
- If skin closure is too tight, a vessel loop secured to the sides of the incision with staples and crossing the wound in a Roman sandal fashion helps reapproximate the wound. Alternatively the Wound V.A.C. (Kinetic Concepts Inc., San Antonio, Texas) may be used as a temporary dressing until closure is possible.

Rehabilitation

Postoperatively, the limb is immobilized in a well-padded posterior plaster slab, followed by a below-knee non-weight-

bearing removable splint once the swelling has subsided. The patient remains non–weight bearing until the lateral K-wires are removed at 6 weeks. At that time, the patient is progressed to weight bearing in a supportive shoe with an orthotic. A polydensity orthosis with medial arch support and metatarsal pad is recommended. The screws are removed between 16 and 24 weeks, and the patient continues with a supportive shoe and orthotic for 1 year. There is usually no need for formal physical therapy.

Complications

Early complications reported in the literature include compartment syndrome (5%),[101] vascular compromise (10%),[102] need for skin grafting or flap coverage (5 to 6%),[101,110] and superficial infection (2.5%).[101] Intermediate complications include loss of reduction, screw breakage (25%),[110] and complex regional pain syndrome (25%).[102,111] The latter is seen more commonly with closed reduction without stable fixation. The most common late complication is posttraumatic osteoarthrosis (25 to 30%)[97,110] resulting in the need for arthrodesis (13%).[110] Even with anatomical reduction, a high proportion of arthrosis still occurs. This is felt to be secondary to the damage of the joint surfaces at the time of injury. Not all radiographic arthrosis is symptomatic. With poor reduction the incidence of arthrosis is significantly higher (60 vs 16%),[110] and bothersome exostosis and foot malposition can lead to problems with shoewear.[109]

Outcomes

The outcome after tarsometatarsal joint injury depends on anatomical reduction and is also negatively affected by workers' compensation status.[100] Fifty percent of patients with nonanatomical reduction are unable to return to work compared with less than 25% of patients with anatomical reduction.[100,101] The more recent literature has reported on AOFAS scores, and found significantly better scores with anatomical reduction (82 vs 70).[110] Teng et al have examined gait in patients with anatomical reduction. Although patients still had subjective complaints, objective measures of the gait cycle failed to show significant abnormality.[112] No similar study has been done in patients with nonanatomical reduction.

Pearls

- 20% missed on initial presentation
- Radiographic indices of Myerson:
  - < 2 mm between the first and second metatarsals and the medial and middle cuneiform
  - Talometatarsal angle < 15 degrees
  - No displacement of the MT in the dorsal–plantar plane
- Anatomical reduction is the key, leading to the best clinical results.

Metatarsal Fractures

Metatarsal fractures, although extremely common, receive only a limited amount of attention in the literature. In general, the vast majority of these injuries (not involving the tarsometatarsal joint complex) can be treated nonoperatively. However, certain injuries or injury patterns require operative intervention to obtain an acceptable outcome. In general, fractures of the second to fourth metatarsals are addressed similarly, whereas the approach to treatment of the first and fifth metatarsals is unique to each of those bones.

First Metatarsal

The first metatarsal is unique in a number of ways, which is why fractures of it require special consideration. The first metatarsal serves as the distal insertion of both the anterior tibialis and the peroneus longus; these tendon insertions contribute forces that are not seen in other metatarsals. Anatomically, the first metatarsal is shorter and broader, and shares its load requirements (one third to one half of body weight) with the two sesamoids.

Nonoperative treatment is appropriate for any nondisplaced fracture, which can be treated with restricted weight bearing.

More aggressive intervention is indicated whenever there is any displacement or malalignment of the first ray. The primary goal is anatomical restoration, whether it is an articular displacement or any change in length or alignment of a shaft fracture. DeLee recommends attempted closed reduction and nonoperative treatment for any fracture of the first metatarsal.[5] When this technique is employed, it must be watched closely in the weeks that follow due to the propensity of the fracture to redisplace secondary to the pull of the tendons that attach to the first metatarsal.

Open reduction and internal fixation should be considered for all first metatarsal fractures. The soft tissue envelope determines the most appropriate mode of stabilization. As with any surgical approach in the foot, strict attention to soft tissue management is mandatory. Longitudinal incisions are preferred. Awareness of the sensory nerves and protection of the paratenon are essential. While leaving the paratenon intact, the deep incision is made medial to the anterior tibialis tendon and all the way to the bone. A full-thickness flap (cutaneous to the periosteum) is then raised to the extent that is needed for reduction and placement of fixation.

Many recommendations for fixation of metatarsal fractures can be found in the literature. Depending on the fracture pattern, interfragmentary screws alone (2.7 or 2.0 mm) or plates (2.7 mm reconstruction or compression plates, semitubular, 2.0 mm/2.7 mm mini-fragment condylar blade plates) can be used **(Fig. 33–35)**. Others have recommended percutaneous cross-pinning for fractures that can be reduced with closed methods or have significant soft tissue damage. Several techniques are avail-

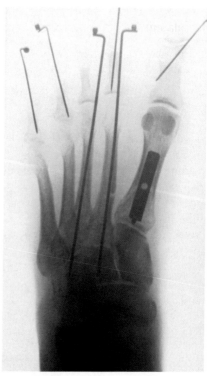

Figure 33–35 Postoperative anteroposterior view of the foot showing both plate and K-wire fixation of metatarsal and phalangeal fractures.

able to manage first metatarsal fractures that are not reconstructible.[113] One involves transfixion pins to the second metatarsal and the other is a spanning external fixator along the medial side of the first ray.

Most first MT fractures are treated with non–weight bearing for 4 to 6 weeks in some form of protection. Some of the more complex injuries need a more extended period before weight bearing is allowed, based on their radiographic and clinic healing.

Second through Fourth Metatarsals

The central metatarsals are not affected by the same forces as are the border metatarsals. Also, they share some inherent stability distally through the intermetatarsal ligaments, minimizing the shortening that may occur. Most isolated fractures of the central metatarsals can be treated in a nonoperative fashion.

The primary concern with multiple fractures is the loss of the normal weight-bearing relationship of the metatarsal heads. Deformity in the frontal plane is much better tolerated than that in the sagittal. Some have agreed that any angulation in the sagittal plane or 2 to 4 mm of shortening indicates operative fixation. In general, no other specific indications are given in the literature. The basic concept with these fractures is to correct any deformity that may lead to an imbalance in the weight distribution of the metatarsal heads.

Multiple methods of fixation of the central metatarsals have been described. The most common is longitudinal pin fixation with either open or closed reduction of the fracture. If percutaneous placement of the pin is attempted, the surgeon must do so in the first few days following injury because closed reduction of the fracture is extremely difficult after 4 to 5 days. For shaft fractures, K-wire fixation can be accomplished in either a retrograde or an antegrade/retrograde fashion. For the retrograde technique, the K-wire is started on the plantar surface in the metatarsal head. The starting point is critical to the success of this procedure; therefore, great care must be taken to start the pin in the center of the metatarsal head on the AP view and in line with the distal shaft on the lateral. It is common with the first attempt to place the pin in the apparent correct position, but to find that the pin is on the base of the proximal phalanx. This can be remedied by dorsiflexing the toe, allowing more exposure of the metatarsal head. The pin can then be advanced in a retrograde fashion to the level of the fracture, and then using it as a joystick, a reduction is affected and the pin is driven across the fracture into the proximal fragment not unlike the nailing of any other shaft fracture. Pins should be driven into the proximalmost aspect of the metatarsal base for the best purchase. This is the preferred technique for metatarsal head fractures that require reduction and fixation.

Antegrade/retrograde pinning with a K-wire is another option for reduction and stabilization of the fracture. The distal fragment should be identified and the K-wire is passed through it in an antegrade fashion. Once the K-wire exits the plantar surface, the distal end of the K-wire can then be grasped and it can be retracted to the proximal fracture edge of the distal fragment. The fracture is then reduced and the K-wire is driven across the fracture to the base of the metatarsal (**Fig. 33–35**).

If the injury is more than 5 days old, or a closed reduction cannot be obtained, an open reduction is often required. Longitudinal incisions should be made in the intermetatarsal space. This approach allows access to adjacent metatarsals if necessary. No dissection should occur between the metatarsals because this endangers the neurovascular bundles. Fixation is then obtained by either the antegrade/retrograde technique or with a quarter-tubular plate and screws.

When used, the pin should remain in place for 4 to 6 weeks, and the patient should remain non–weight bearing for that time. If the fracture pattern is stable and treated nonoperatively, the patient may be placed in a weight-bearing cast or hard-sole shoe depending on comfort level.

Fifth Metatarsal

Fractures of the fifth metatarsal constitute two distinct injury patterns, the styloid avulsion and the so-called Jones fracture. Styloid avulsions occur as a result of an inversion injury, in which the peroneus brevis insertion is avulsed from the base of the fifth metatarsal. Often the fracture includes part of the articular surface.[114] These

fractures are treated with a soft bandage in a stiff-soled shoe, with partial weight bearing allowed. Average radiographic healing occurs by 44 days, with full return to all activities by 3 months.[115]

Fractures of the base of the fifth metatarsal shaft, or Jones fractures, represent a separate entity and must be distinguished from the simple avulsion fracture because their treatment is more complex. By definition, Jones fractures are a fracture of the fifth metatarsal that occurs 1.5 cm distal to the styloid. The nutrient artery for the fifth metatarsal enters at the midshaft area, and the base of the metatarsal is supplied by a small retrograde branch.[115] As seen in other bones with retrograde blood flow, healing problems often occur for this fracture.

Jones fractures are subcategorized into acute and chronic fractures. Acute fractures occur as a result of distinct trauma, where a load is placed at the plantar aspect of the lateral border of the foot, imparting a bending moment at the shaft metaphyseal interface. On x-ray evaluation, the fracture edges look sharp and "fresh."[116] Acute fractures may be treated conservatively in a non-weight-bearing cast. The time to union is variable, with average healing in 21 weeks.[117] Failure of conservative treatment ranges from 12 to 28%.[117,118]

Chronic Jones fractures represent a stress fracture of the fifth metatarsal. These most often occur in young male athletes involved in take-off jumping sports (high jump, basketball) or in sports with ball of the foot weight bearing combined with cutting activities.[109] Lateral foot tenderness will often precede radiographic evidence of fracture, and often a bone scan or MRI is required for definitive diagnosis. X-ray findings range from the thin radiolucency of a fresh fracture to the cortical thickening and intramedullary narrowing associated with a chronic stress fracture. Because the stress fractures occur predominantly in young athletes, and because the nonunion rate averages 50%, surgical intervention is indicated.[117]

Both acute and chronic Jones fractures may be treated in the same way; namely, with the use of an intramedullary screw, placed antegrade from the tip of the fifth metatarsal styloid. The patient is placed in the lateral position on a radiolucent table. A percutaneous technique is utilized. A small incision is placed proximal to the tip of the styloid, and a hemostat is used to dissect down to the tip of the styloid. Image intensification is utilized to localize the start point. A 2.5 mm drill is placed at the tip of the styloid and passed across the fracture site, with the use of orthogonal C-arm image. The canal is then widened using a 3.2 mm and ultimately a 4.5 mm drill bit. A fully threaded 4.5 mm cortical screw is then placed with the threads across the fracture site (**Fig. 33–36**). In the cases of chronic fractures, the fracture site may be opened and the intramedullary canal reestablished under direct vision, prior to placement of the screw from the tip of the styloid. The nonunion site may be augmented with autogenous bone graft from the proximal tibia or distal femur.

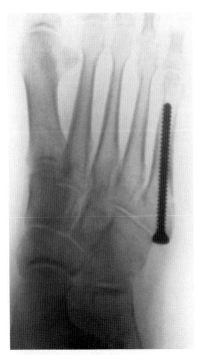

Figure 33–36 A postoperative oblique radiograph showing an intramedullary screw for fixation of the base of the fifth metatarsal fracture (Jones fracture).

Postoperatively, the foot is placed in a below-knee non-weight-bearing cast until stitches are removed. Full weight bearing may be commenced at 2 weeks, but athletic activities should be restricted. Success of this technique has been reported at 100% after 8 weeks.[119]

Metatarsal–Phalangeal Joint Injuries

First Metatarsal–Phalangeal Joint

Because of its plantar anatomy, dislocation of the first metatarsal–phalangeal joint (MTP) joint is unusual. When it does occur it is due to a hyperextension injury with failure of proximal plantar plates. The metatarsal head usually buttonholes through the plantar structure, which makes closed reduction difficult. Multiple approaches have been recommended for open reduction, each with its specific risks and benefits. Once reduced, the joint is usually stable and can be treated with weight bearing as tolerated in a short leg cast or hard-sole shoe.

Second through Fifth Metatarsal–Phalangeal Joints

Dislocations of the lesser MTP joints are uncommon. When they do occur, however, they usually present as dorsolateral dislocations. Most can be reduced in a closed fashion and are stable after reduction, although reports of complex dislocations exist in the literature. As with the first MTP, the plantar plate is the usual interposed structure. Open reduction through a dorsal longitudinal incision should be performed. After reduction, even complex dislocations are usually stable. If instability persists, a longitudinal K-wire should be placed across the joint and removed at approximately 4 weeks.

Stable reductions can be treated with buddy taping and a hard-soled shoe for 4 to 6 weeks. Dislocations that require pinning can be weight bearing as tolerated in a hard-soled shoe after the pin is removed at 4 to 6 weeks.

Phalangeal Fractures

Great Toe

As with other injuries, fractures of the great toe proximal phalanx are treated more aggressively than those of the other toes. Because of the unequal forces across the proximal phalanx, unreduced fractures will heal in a plantar-flexed position. This malreduction can lead to pressure problems after healing. For this reason, displaced or unstable fractures should be reduced and fixed with either crossed K-wires or mini-fragmentary implants. Both nonoperatively and operatively treated fractures are then buddy taped and placed in a hard-soled shoe for 3 to 4 weeks.

Lesser Toes

Fractures of the lesser toe phalanges can usually be treated with buddy taping and protection in a hard-soled or open-toed shoe. Even fractures that need closed reduction can be successfully treated in this manner. The only fractures that require more aggressive treatment are those that clinically present with "overlapping" toes. These can be treated with closed reduction and longitudinal pinning. Postoperative treatment is identical to the foregoing.

On the DVDs

Video 33–1 (Disk 4) ORIF of a Talus Fracture This video demonstrates open reduction and internal fixation of a talus fracture using a lag screw combined with a small plate. The two incision technique is used to allow full visualization of the reduction.

Video 33–2 (Disk 4) ORIF of a Calcaneus Fracture This video demonstrates open reduction and internal fixation of a comminuted intraarticular calcaneus fracture with the addition of Norion cement to supplement the fixation.

Video 33–3 (Disk 4) Closed Reduction and External Fixation of a Cuboid (Lateral Column) Fracture This patient sustained a "nutcracker" comminuted cuboid fracture. He was treated with external fixation to maintain the length of the lateral column and allow healing.

Video 33–4 (Disk 4) ORIF of a Lisfranc Fracture Dislocation This video demonstrates oRIF of a Lisfranc fracture, taking care to obtain a reduction of the keystone of the base of the second metatarsal against the middle and medial cuneiforms.

References

1. Haliburton RA, Sullivan CR, Kelly PJ, Peterson LFA. The extra-osseous and intra-osseous blood supply of the talus. J Bone Joint Surg Am 1958;40-A:1115–1120
2. Kelly PJ, Sullivan CR. Blood supply of the talus. Clin Orthop Relat Res 1963;30:37–44
3. Mulfinger GL, Trueta J. The blood supply of the talus. J Bone Joint Surg Br 1970;52:160–167
4. Schatzker J, Tile M. The management of fractures and dislocations of the talus. In: Tscherne H, Schatzker J, eds. Major Fractures of the Pilon, the Talus and the Calcaneus: Current Concepts of Treatment. Berlin: Springer-Verlag; 1993:87–104
5. DeLee JC. Fractures and dislocations of the foot. In: Mann RA, Coughlin MJ, eds. Surgery of the Foot Ankle. 6th ed. St. Louis: Mosby; 1993:1539–1600
6. Daniels TR, Smith JW. Talar neck fractures. Foot Ankle 1993;14:225–234
7. Hansen ST Jr. Functional Reconstruction of the Foot and Ankle. Philadelphia: Lippincott, Williams and Wilkins; 2000:65–104
8. Hawkins LG. Fractures of the neck of the talus. J Bone Joint Surg Am 1970;52:991–1002
9. Canale ST, Kelly FB. Fractures of the neck of the talus: long term evaluation of seventy-one cases. J Bone Joint Surg Am 1978;60:143–156
10. Heckman JD. Fractures and dislocations of the foot. In: Rockwood CA Jr, Green DP, Bucholz RW, eds. Fractures in Adults. 3rd ed. Vol 2. Philadelphia: JB Lippincott; 1991:2071–2085
11. Penny JN, Davis LA. Fractures and fracture-dislocations of the neck of the talus. J Trauma 1980;20:1029–1037
12. Szyszkowitz R, Reschauer R, Seggl W. Eighty-five talus fractures treated by ORIF with five to eight years of follow-up study in 69 patients. Clin Orthop Relat Res 1985;199:97–107
13. McKeever FM. Treatment of complications of fractures and dislocations of the talus. Clin Orthop Relat Res 1963;30:45–52
14. Sangeorzan BJ, Wagner UA, Harrington RM, Tencer AF. Contact characteristics of the subtalar joint: the effect of talar neck misalignment. J Orthop Res 1992;10:544–551
15. Vallier HA, Nork SE, Barei DP, Benirschke SK, Sangeorzan BJ. Talar neck fractures: results and outcomes. J Bone Joint Surg Am 2004;86-A:1616–1624
16. Behrens F. Long-term results of displaced talar neck fractures. In: Tscherne H, Schatzker J, eds. Major Fractures of the Pilon, the Talus, and the Calcaneus: Current Concepts of Treatment. Berlin: Springer-Verlag; 1993:113–121
17. Gilquist J, Oretop N, Strenstrom A, Rieger A, Wennberg E. Late results after vertical fracture of the talus. Injury 1974;6:173–179
18. Lorentzen JE, Christensen SB, Krogsoe O, Sneppen O. Fractures of the neck of the talus. Acta Orthop Scand 1977;48:115–120
19. Szyskowitz R, Seggl W, Wildburger R. Late results of fractures and fracture-dislocation after ORIF. In: Tscherne H, Schatzker J, eds. Major Fractures of the Pilon, the Talus, and the Calcaneus: Current Concepts of Treatment. Berlin: Springer-Verlag; 1993:105–112
20. Pantazopoulos T, Galanos P, Vayanos E, Mitsou A, Hartofilakidis-Garofalidis G. Fractures of the neck of the talus. Acta Orthop Scand 1974;45:296–306
21. Mindell ER, Cisek EE, Kartalian G, Dziob JM. Late results of injuries to the talus. J Bone Joint Surg Am 1963;45:221–245
22. Baumhauer JF, Alvarez RG. Controversies in treating talus fractures. Orthop Clin North Am 1995;26:335–351
23. Boyd HB, Knight RA. Fractures of the astragalus. South Med J 1942;35:160–167
24. Dunn AR, Bernard J, Campbell RD. Fractures of the talus. J Trauma 1966;6:443–468
25. Grob D, Simpson LA, Weber BG, Bray T. Operative treatment of displaced talus fractures. Clin Orthop Relat Res 1985;199:88–96
26. Kenwright J, Taylor RG. Major injuries of the talus. J Bone Joint Surg Br 1970;52:36–48
27. Miller WE. Operative intervention for fracture of the talus. In: Bateman J, Trott A, eds. The Foot and Ankle. Miami: Thieme; 1980:52
28. Peterson L, Goldie IF, Irstam L. Fracture of the neck of the talus: a clinical study. Acta Orthop Scand 1977;48:696–706

29. Richardson EG, Graves SC. Fracture and dislocations of the foot. In: Campbells Operative Orthopaedics. 8th ed. St. Louis: CV Mosby; 1992:2896

30. Sneppen O, Christensen SB, Krogsoe O, Lorentzen J. Fracture of the body of the talus. Acta Orthop Scand 1977;48:317–324

31. Inokuchi S, Ogawa K, Usami N. Classification of fractures of the talus: clear differentiation between neck and body fractures. Foot Ankle Int 1996;17:748–750

32. Coltart WD. Aviator's astragalus. J Bone Joint Surg Br 1952;34:545–566

33. Elgafy H, Ebraheim NA, Tile M, Stephen D, Kase J. Fractures of the talus: experience of two level 1 trauma centers. Foot Ankle Int 2000;21:1023–1029

34. Kleiger B. Fractures of the talus. J Bone Joint Surg Am 1948;30:735–744

35. Pennal GF. Fractures of the talus. Clin Orthop Relat Res 1963;30:53–63

36. Vallier HA, Nork SE, Benirschke SK, Sangeorzan BJ. Surgical treatment of talar body fractures. J Bone Joint Surg Am 2003;85:1716–1724

37. Thordarson DB, Triffon MJ, Terk MR. Magnetic resonance imaging to detect avascular necrosis after open reduction and internal fixation of talar neck fractures. Foot Ankle Int 1996;17:742–747

38. Adelaar RS. The treatment of complex fractures of the talus. Orthop Clin North Am 1989;20:691–707

39. Adelaar RS. Occult injuries of the talus. In: Adelaar RS, ed. Complex Foot and Ankle Trauma. Philadelphia: Lippincott-Raven; 1999:95–107

40. Parsons SJ. Relation between the occurrence of bony union and outcome for fractures of the lateral process of the talus: a case report and analysis of published reports. Br J Sports Med 2003;37:274–276

41. Sangeorzan BJ, Benirschke SK, Carr JB. Surgical management of fractures of the os calcis. Instr Course Lect 1995;44:359–370

42. Böhler L. Diagnosis, pathology and treatment of fractures of the os calcis. J Bone Joint Surg Am 1931;13:75–89

43. Essex-Lopresti P. The mechanism, reduction technique, and results in fractures of the os calcis. Clin Orthop Relat Res 1993; 290:3–16

44. Aldridge JM III, Easley M, Nunley JA. Open calcaneal fractures: results of operative treatment. J Orthop Trauma 2004;18:7–11

45. Sanders R. Intra-articular fractures of the calcaneus: present state of the art. J Orthop Trauma 1992;6:252–265

46. Buckley RE, Meek RN. Comparison of open versus closed reduction of intraarticular calcaneal fractures: a matched cohort in workmen. J Orthop Trauma 1992;6:216–222

47. Crosby LA, Fitzgibbons T. Intraarticular calcaneal fractures: results of closed treatment. Clin Orthop Relat Res 1993;290:47–54

48. Benirschke SK, Sangeorzan BJ. Extensive intraarticular fractures of the foot: surgical management of calcaneal fractures. Clin Orthop Relat Res 1993;292:128–134

49. Letournel E. Open treatment of acute calcaneal fractures. Clin Orthop Relat Res 1993;290:60–67

50. Sanders R, Fortin P, Dipasquale T, Walling A. Operative treatment in 120 displaced intraarticular calcaneal fractures. Clin Orthop Relat Res 1993;290:87–95

51. Zwipp H, Tscherne H, Thermann H, Weber T. Osteosynthesis of displaced intraarticular fractures of the calcaneus: results in 123 cases. Clin Orthop Relat Res 1993;290:76–86

52. Sanders R, Gregory P. Operative treatment of intra-articular fractures of the calcaneus. Orthop Clin North Am 1995;26:203–214

53. Sanders R. Current concepts review: displaced intra-articular fractures of the calcaneus. J Bone Joint Surg Am 2000;82:225–250

54. Sangeorzan BJ. Foot and ankle joint. In: Hansen ST and Swiontkowski MF, eds. Orthopaedic Trauma Protocols. New York: Raven; 1993:339–368

55. Myerson M, Manoli A. Compartment syndrome of the foot after calcaneal fractures. Clin Orthop Relat Res 1993;290:142–150

56. Garner AMN, Fox RH, Lawrence C, Bunker TD, Ling RSM, MacEachern AG. Reduction of post-traumatic swelling and compartment pressure by impulse compression of the foot. J Bone Joint Surg Br 1990;72-B:810–815

57. Thordarson DB, Greene N, Shepherd L, Perlman M. Facilitating edema resolution with a foot pump after calcaneus fracture. J Orthop Trauma. 1999;13:43–46

58. Giordano CP, Koval KJ. Treatment of fracture blisters: a prospective study of 53 cases. J Orthop Trauma 1995;9:171–176

59. Giordano CP, Koval KJ, Zuckerman JD, Desai P. Fracture blisters. Clin Orthop Relat Res 1994;307:214–221

60. Giordano CP, Scott D, Koval KJ, et al. Fracture blister formation: a laboratory study. J Trauma 1995;38:907–909

61. Hollinshead WH. Anatomy for Surgeons: The Back and Limbs. Knee, Leg, Ankle and Foot. Vol 3. Philadelphia: Harper & Row; 1982:791–793

62. Carr JB. Mechanism and pathoanatomy of the intraarticular calcaneal fracture. Clin Orthop Relat Res 1993;290:36–40

63. Loucks C, Buckley R. Bohler's angle: correlation with outcome in displaced intra-articular calcaneal fractures. J Orthop Trauma 1999;13:554–558

64. Gilmer PW, Herzenberg J, Frank JL, Silverman P, Martinez S, Goldner JL. Computerized tomographic analysis of acute calcaneal fractures. Foot Ankle 1986;6:184–193

65. Crosby LA, Fitzgibbons T. Computerized tomography scanning of acute intra-articular fractures of the calcaneus. J Bone Joint Surg Am 1990;72:852–859

66. Fernandez DL, Koella C. Combined percutaneous and "minimal" internal fixation for displaced articular fractures of the calcaneus. Clin Orthop Relat Res 1993;290:108–116

67. Tornetta P III. Open reduction and internal fixation of the calcaneus using minifragment plates. J Orthop Trauma 1996;10:63–67

68. Tornetta P III. The Essex-Lopresti reduction for calcaneal fractures revisited. J Orthop Trauma 1998;12:469–473

69. Sangeorzan BJ, Ananthakrishan D, Tencer AF. Contact characteristics of the subtalar joint after a simulated calcaneus fracture. J Orthop Trauma 1995;9:251–258

70. Lawrence SJ, Botte MJ. The sural nerve in the foot and ankle: an anatomic study with clinical and surgical implications. Foot Ankle Int 1994;15:490–494

71. Jordan C, Mirzabeigi E, Williams S. Determining the angle of screw placement for internal fixation of calcaneal fractures. J Orthop Trauma 1999;13:47–50

72. Albert MJ, Waggoner SM, Smith JW. Internal fixation of calcaneus fractures: an anatomical study of structures at risk. J Orthop Trauma 1995;9:107–112

73. Mekhail AO, Ebraheim NA, Heck BE, Yeasting RA. Anatomic considerations for safe placement of calcaneal pins. Clin Orthop Relat Res 1996;332:254–259

74. Gustilo RB, Anderson JT. Prevention of infection in the treatment of one thousand and twenty-five open fractures of long bones: retrospective and prospective analyses. J Bone Joint Surg Am 1976;58: 453–458

75. Csizy M, Buckley R, Tough S, et al. Displaced intra-articular calcaneal fractures. Variables predicting late subtalar fusion. J Orthop Trauma 2003;17:106–112

76. Gustilo RB, Mendoza RM, Williams DN. Problems in the management of type III (severe) open fractures: a new classification of type III open fractures. J Trauma 1984;24:742–746

77. Myerson M, Quill GE Jr. Late complications of fractures of the calcaneus. J Bone Joint Surg Am 1993;75:331–341

78. Howard JL, Buckley R, McCormack R, et al. Complications following management of displaced intra-articular calcaneal fractures: a prospective randomized trial comparing open reduction internal fixation with nonoperative management. J Orthop Trauma 2003;17:241–249

79. Benirschke SK, Kramer PA. Wound healing complications in closed and open calcaneal fractures. J Orthop Trauma 2004;18:1–6

80. Folk JW, Starr AJ, Early JS. Early wound complications of operative treatment of calcaneus fractures: analysis of 190 fractures. J Orthop Trauma 1999;13:369–372

81. Masquelet AC, Gilbert A. Transfers from the lower limb. In: Masquelet AC and Gilbert A, eds. An Atlas of Flaps in Limb Reconstruction. Philadelphia: JB Lippincott; 1995:95–202

82. Masquelet AC, Gilbert A. Indications for pedicled island flaps. In: Masquelet AC and Gilbert A, eds. An Atlas of Flaps in Limb Reconstruction. Philadelphia: JB Lippincott; 1995:241–260

83. Borrelli J Jr, Torzilli PA, Grigiene R, Helfet DL. Effect of impact load on articular cartilage: development of an intra-articular fracture model. J Orthop Trauma 1997;11:319–326

84. Carr JB, Hansen ST, Benirschke SK. Subtalar distraction bone block fusion for late complications of os calcis fractures. Foot Ankle 1988;9:81–86

85. Sangeorzan BJ, Benirschke SK, Mosca V, Mayo KA, Hansen ST. Displaced intra-articular fractures of the tarsal navicular. J Bone Joint Surg Am 1989;71:1504–1510

86. Torg JS, Pavlov H, Cooley LH, et al. Stress fracture of the tarsal navicular: a retrospective review of twenty-one cases. J Bone Joint Surg Am 1982;64:700–712

87. Heckman JD. Fractures and dislocations of the foot. In: Rockwood CA Jr, Green DP, eds. Fractures in Adults. 4th ed. Vol 2. Philadelphia: JB Lippincott; 1996:2267–2405

88. Buscemi MJ, Page BJ II. Transcuneiform fracture: cuboid dislocation of the midfoot. J Trauma 1986;26:290–292

89. Weber M, Locher S. Reconstruction of the cuboid in compression fractures: short to midterm results in 12 patients. Foot Ankle Int 2002;23:1008–1013

90. Ouzounian TJ, Shereff MJ. In vitro determination of midfoot motion. Foot Ankle 1989;10:140–146

91. Hermel M, Gershon-Cohen J. The nutcracker fracture of the cuboid by indirect violence. Radiology 1953;60:850–856

92. Sangeorzan B, Swiontkowski M. Displaced fractures of the cuboid. J Bone Joint Surg Br. 1990;72:376–378

93. Main B, Jowett R. Injuries of the midtarsal joint. J Bone Joint Surg Br 1975;57:89–97

94. Jahn H, Freund KG. Isolated fractures of the cuboid bone: two case reports with review of the literature. J Foot Surg 1989;28:512–515

95. Holbein O, Bauer G, Kinzl L. Die Dislozierte Kuboidfraktur: Klinik und Therapie einer seltenen Fussverletzung. Unfallchirurg. 1998;101:214–221

96. Richter M, Wippermann B, Krettek C, Schratt E, Hufner T, Thermann H. Fractures and fracture dislocations of the midfoot: occurrence, causes and long-term results. Foot Ankle Int 2001;22: 392–398

97. Hardcastle PH, Reschauer R, Kutscha-Lissberg E, Schoffmann W. Injuries to the tarsometatarsal joint. J Bone Joint Surg Br 1982;64:349–356

98. Aitken AP, Poulson D. Dislocations of the tarsometatarsal joint. J Bone Joint Surg Am 1963;45-A:246–260

99. English TA. Dislocations of the metatarsal bone and adjacent toe. J Bone Joint Surg Br 1964;46:700–704

100. Resch S, Stenstrom A. The treatment of tarsometatarsal injuries. Foot Ankle 1990;11:117–123

101. Arntz CT, Veith RG, Hansen ST Jr. Fracture and fracture-dislocations of the tarsometatarsal joint. J Bone Joint Surg Am 1988; 70:173–181

102. Goossens M, De Stoop N. Lisfranc's fracture-dislocations: etiology, radiology, and results of treatment. Clin Orthop Relat Res 1983;176:154–162

103. Faciszewski T, Burks RT, Manaster BJ. Subtle injuries of the Lisfranc joint. J Bone Joint Surg Am 1990;72:1519–1522

104. Myerson MS. The diagnosis and treatment of injury to the tarsometatarsal joint complex. J Bone Joint Surg Br 1999; 81:756–763

105. Trevino SG, Kodros S. Controversies in tarsometatarsal injuries. Orthop Clin North Am 1995;26:229–238

106. Lu J, Ebraheim NA, Skie M, Porshinsky B, Yeasting RA. Radiographic and computed tomographic evaluation of Lisfranc dislocation: a cadaver study. Foot Ankle Int 1997;18:351–355

107. Preidler KW, Yung-Cheng W, Brossmann J, Trudell D, Daenen B, Resnick D. Tarsometatarsal joint: anatomic details on MR images. Radiology 1996;199:733–736

108. De Palma L, Santucci A, Sabetta SP, Rapali S. Anatomy of the Lisfranc joint complex. Foot Ankle Int 1997;18:356–364

109. Buzzard BM, Briggs PJ. Surgical management of acute tarsometatarsal fracture dislocation in the adult. Clin Orthop Relat Res 1998;353:125–133

110. Kuo RS, Tejwani NC, Digiovanni CW, et al. Outcome after open reduction and internal fixation of Lisfranc joint injuries. J Bone Joint Surg Am 2000;82-A:1609–1618

111. Mulier T, Reynders P, Dereymaeker G, Broos P. Severe Lisfrancs injuries: primary arthrodesis or ORIF. Foot Ankle Int 2002;23:902–905

112. Teng AL, Pinzur MS, Lomasney L, Mohoney L, Havey R. Functional outcome following anatomic restoration of tarsal-metatarsal fracture dislocation. Foot Ankle Int 2002;23:922–926

113. Schildhaur TA, Nork SE, Sangeorzan BJ. Temporary bridge plating of the medial column in severe foot injuries. J Orthop Trauma 2003;17:513–552

114. Sammarco GJ. The Jones fracture. Instr Course Lect 1993; 42:201–205

115. Wiener BD, Linder F, Giattini JFG. Treatment of fractures of the fifth metatarsal: a prospective study. Foot Ankle Int 1997;18: 267–269

116. Shereff M, Yang QM, Kummer FJ, Frey CC, Greenidge N. Vascular anatomy of the fifth metatarsal. Foot Ankle 1991;11:350–353

117. Clapper MF, O'Brien TJ, Lyons PM. Fractures of the fifth metatarsal: analysis of a fracture registry. Clin Orthop Relat Res 1995;315:238–241

118. Josefsson PO, Karlsson M, Redlund-Johnell I, Wendeberg B. Jones fracture: surgical versus nonsurgical treatment. Clin Orthop Relat Res 1994;299:252–255

119. Portland G, Kelikian A, Kodros S. Acute surgical management of Jones' fractures. Foot Ankle Int 2003;24:829–833

34 The Polytrauma Patient

Erika J. Mitchell, Philip J. Kregor, and Andrew H. Schmidt

Many patients with musculoskeletal injury have multiple fractures and/or other injuries of the head, chest, or abdomen. In such patients, there is a complex interplay between the effects of their systemic injuries on their fractures and the effects of their fractures (and the treatment of those fractures) on their systemic injuries. Paradoxically, some patients with severe trauma survive their initial injuries only to succumb to complications of multiorgan failure and sepsis later. Appropriate initial management of fractures in multiply injured patients has a profound influence on their overall recovery and prognosis and reduces the rate of serious complications, including acute respiratory distress syndrome (ARDS), multiorgan failure, fat embolism, and thromboembolic disease. This final chapter summarizes our rapidly advancing understanding of the physiological response to trauma, describes the systemic effects of musculoskeletal injury, and uses this information to describe a rational approach to prioritizing and managing musculoskeletal trauma in the multiply injured patient. Case histories are presented that illustrate these points.

Evaluation of the Polytrauma Patient

The care and treatment of the polytraumatized patient require a team approach and attention to detail in the setting of an emergent situation. Although the general surgery trauma service typically coordinates the patient's care, multiple services are often involved, including orthopaedic surgery, vascular surgery, neurosurgery, and anesthesia. These various services must communicate regarding their efforts and requirements to ensure that the patient receives the most efficient care.[1]

Evaluation begins with the principles of advanced trauma life support (ATLS), issued by the American College of Surgeons, Chicago, Illinois. Thorough assessment of the patient includes an understanding of the patient's medical history and the events leading to the injuries. The mechanism of injury can lead to suspicion of particular types of injuries that may not be obvious on primary or secondary survey. Prolonged extrication times may predispose the patient to hypothermia and may raise suspicion of soft tissue crush injuries despite a negative fracture workup. These patients as well as those with high-energy fractures or large transfusion requirements should be closely monitored for compartment syndrome. Transfusion requirements prior to arrival at the hospital in addition to what is charted in the hospital may indicate a need for platelets or fresh frozen plasma prior to or during any immediate operative procedures.

Skin integrity and soft tissue injury should be assessed for all fractures. Closed injuries can still be associated with significant soft tissue injury or a closed degloving (Morel-Lavallée) lesion. Displaced or unstable pelvic ring injuries warrant rectal and vaginal examination for open injuries. Appropriate antibiotics should be given for open injuries, and history once again becomes important. Wounds contaminated by soil should receive penicillin G and tetanus immunoglobulin if necessary. Wounds exposed to water sources may require coverage with ciprofloxacin for waterborne bacteria.

All fractures and dislocations need to be assessed for neurovascular abnormalities. When found, appropriate studies and consultations should ensue prior to surgical treatment. Vascular injuries may be identified on clinical exam alone or by diagnostic measures such as an ankle-brachial index (ABI) less than 0.9.[2,3] Computed tomographic (CT) angiography may be used to further assess the need for vascular intervention. Communication with the vascular surgeons regarding timing of surgeries and placement of incisions is extremely important. Generally, bony stabilization should be performed prior to revascularization to enable the vascular surgeon to assess the need for length of the vessel repair and prevent stresses on the repair. This can be done in a rapid manner with external fixation in cases of limb-threatening injuries or with definitive fixation if the warm ischemia time is short. Incisions can usually be made in a manner that is not detrimental to either service if planned cooperatively. Fasciotomy should be considered in cases of prolonged ischemia to prevent compartment syndrome secondary to reperfusion. Once again, incision placement for compartment release needs to be planned if further procedures are to be performed.

Angiography should be considered in patients with pelvic injuries requiring transfusion of more than four units of packed red blood cells (PRBCs) in less than 24 hours or more than six units of PRBCs in less than 48 hours despite temporary stabilization efforts or sheeting.[4] Persistent hemodynamic instability in the face of a negative peritoneal lavage may indicate a possible retroperitoneal bleed where other sources (e.g., bilateral femur fractures) have been ruled out and may benefit from angiography.

Although the orthopaedic focus is on care of the fracture(s), attention needs to be given to injuries of other body systems to appropriately plan surgical approaches and patient positioning. Patients with intra-abdominal injuries requiring emergent/urgent laparotomy need special consideration if there are associated pelvic ring injuries. Incisions for laparotomy can be problematic if there is a pelvic ring injury that will require an anterior approach. Similarly, placement of suprapubic catheters in patients with bladder or urethral disruption should be coordinated between services to prevent placement in the region of a future incision or within a pelvic hematoma predisposing the patient to infection. Long intra-abdominal or thoracic procedures can also lead to hypothermia and coagulopathy, which may require a delay in orthopaedic intervention or conversion to damage-control techniques.[5]

Spine injuries can also affect the priority of orthopaedic intervention. Unstable injuries may require bracing or surgery prior to treatment of other fractures. Such injuries also need to be kept in mind when planning the operative approach and patient positioning in the operating room.

Assessment of the patient does not stop in the trauma bay. Ongoing survey of the patient should occur throughout the hospital course for missed injuries, evolution of compartment syndrome, early signs of infection, and so forth. The incidence of missed injuries in the first 24 hours of admission is as high as 12% in the multiply injured patient.[6,7] Patients who are intubated and sedated are at particularly high risk, and surveillance must be vigilant.[7]

The Physiological Response to Trauma

Injuries, whether simple or complex, cause pain, bleeding, and activation of the systemic inflammatory response. Although inflammation has long been characterized as the first stage of healing, we are only beginning to gain an understanding of the diverse metabolic, physiological, and immunologic changes that occur after injury. For example, numerous investigators have documented changes in the levels of circulating proinflammatory and anti-inflammatory cytokines following injury.[8–17] These alterations of the biochemical milieu cause widespread secondary changes in organ function, involving the immunologic, cardiovascular, pulmonary, and gastrointestinal systems, among

others.[8,9] Skeletal injuries, especially long-bone fractures, have been shown to contribute to such problems.[13] In a murine model, closed femoral fractures were shown to cause immunosuppression and altered gastrointestinal permeability.[18]

Our current understanding of the pathophysiology of trauma divides injuries and their effects into "first hits" and "second hits." So-called first hits are the initial injury and its immediate effects, including organ, skeletal, and soft tissue injury, hypotension, and hypoxemia. The second hits are subsequent complications or interventions that cause a reactivation or exaggeration of the initial response to injury, and by so doing, cause further morbidity and mortality.[19] Examples of second hits are compartment syndrome, sepsis, hypotension, and invasive surgery. Femoral nailing is one of the best characterized examples of a second hit.[12,13] Avoiding iatrogenic exacerbation of the systemic inflammatory response is the primary focus of the concept of "damage-control orthopaedics," discussed later in this chapter.

Systemic Inflammatory Response Syndrome

Both severe injury and major surgery (including orthopaedic surgery) cause the release of numerous cytokines, arachidonic acid metabolites, complement factors, acute-phase reactants, and hormones. Taken together, these changes represent the systemic inflammatory response. The clinical manifestations of these metabolic changes are multiple and include fever, tachycardia, hyperventilation, and leukocytosis. Although these changes occur in predictable patterns, the magnitude of the response to a given level of injury is variable and may be genetically determined.[20] Coincidently, anti-inflammatory mediators are also produced; this is known as the compensatory anti-inflammatory response syndrome (CARS).[10] Any imbalance between the normal systemic inflammatory and anti-inflammatory responses to injury can contribute to multiorgan dysfunction syndrome (MODS), ARDS, and/or sepsis.[10]

In 1991, a consensus conference established specific criteria for the diagnosis of systemic inflammatory response syndrome (SIRS) **(Table 34–1)**.[21] The presence of SIRS can be

Table 34–1 Definition of SIRS and SIRS Score

SIRS score, as defined by the Consensus Conference of the American College of Chest Physicians/Society of Critical Care Medicine (ACCP/SCCM): At least two of the four clinical parameters must be fulfilled to make the diagnosis of SIRS.[21]	SIRS score: Four variables are used, scored at 0 or 1, to give a total score from 0 to 4. A SIRS score above 1, in the absence of systemic sepsis, is evidence of a systemic inflammatory response.[17]
Heart rate > 90/min	Pulse > 90 beats/min
Leukocytes < 4000/mm³, > 12,000/mm³, or ≥ 10% juvenile neutrophil granulocytes	Leukocyte count < 4000/mm³ or > 12,000/mm³
Breathing rate > 20/min, with $PaCO_2$ < 32 mm Hg	Respiratory rate > 20 breaths/min (or $PaCO_2$ < 33 mm Hg)
Temperature < 36°C or > 38°C	Core temperature > 34°C or < 38°C

SIRS, systemic inflammatory response syndrome.

easily quantified by the SIRS score[17] and is predictive of several complications, including ARDS, disseminated intravascular coagulation, acute renal failure, and shock.[14]

The systemic inflammatory response is mediated by the release of numerous cytokines from injured tissues or in response to tissue and/or end-organ hypoxia and hypoperfusion. Cytokines are polypeptides that act in an autocrine or paracrine manner to induce changes in cellular function. Proinflammatory cytokines are numerous and include tumor necrosis factor-α (TNF-α), interleukin-1β (IL-1β), IL-6, and IL-8, also known as neutrophil activating peptide (NAP). Increased serum levels of these cytokines are found in patients with evidence of systemic inflammation, as well as in the bronchoalveolar lavage of patients with thoracic trauma or ARDS.[9] Serum levels of IL-6 correlate with the amount of overall soft tissue trauma and chest trauma,[16] the injury severity score (ISS); and the incidence of MODS, ARDS, and sepsis, as well as with outcome.[8]

High levels of circulating proinflammatory cytokines induce many physiological changes. Polymorphonuclear leukocytes (PMNs) are recruited to the site of injury and are stimulated to release proteases and oxygen free radicals. The coagulation and complement cascades are activated as well as the kallikrein-kinin system. The liver is stimulated to produce acute-phase reactants such as C-reactive protein (CRP), α1-antitrypsin, α2-macroglobulin, ceruloplasmin, lipopolysaccharide (LPS)-binding protein (LBP), fibrinogen, and prothrombin. A more thorough review of this topic can be found elsewhere.[10,22]

As mentioned, the accumulation and stimulation of PMNs at the site of injury is one of the first events of the host response to injury. Although the recruitment and activation of PMNs at the site of injury is crucial for the killing and phagocytosis of bacteria and the removal of dead tissue, this same early host response has a paradoxically detrimental effect as well, both locally and systemically. Activated PMNs, in the presence of proinflammatory cytokines and toxins such as LPS, upregulate adhesion molecules (adhesins) and adhere to endothelial tissue. Increased levels of adhesins can be measured in trauma patients and are predictive of complications.[11]

The accumulation of activated PMNs at the site of injury is thought to be one of the primary causes of secondary tissue injury.[23] When stimulated, activated PMNs and macrophages release proteolytic enzymes such as elastase and metalloproteinase, as well as generate reactive oxygen species.[23,24] These enzymes degrade most proteins in the extracellular matrix as well as important plasma proteins. In addition, neutrophil elastase induces the further release of proinflammatory cytokines, potentially exacerbating the problem. Increased levels of elastase and elastase-α1-protease-inhibitor complex are detectable in trauma patients depending on the injury severity and the posttraumatic course.[15]

Multiorgan Dysfunction Syndrome

Occasionally, multiply injured patients develop progressive failure of their host-defense mechanisms, manifested by sepsis and progressive cerebral, cardiovascular, pulmonary, hepatic, gastrointestinal, renal, and circulatory dysfunction and collapse.[25] This clinical phenomenon has been called by many names, including multiorgan failure and MODS. Although MODS was initially thought to be the end result of sepsis, it is now known to occur in nonseptic patients as well (although sepsis may develop later). Current thinking attributes delayed-onset MODS to an imbalance between the pro- and anti-inflammatory mechanisms.[17,26] There are many proposed theories about the etiology of MODS. At the most basic cellular level, many different abnormalities occur as a part of MODS, including endothelial cell damage, increased vascular permeability with capillary leakage, and microcirculatory failure with cellular hypoxia and apoptosis of parenchymal cells.[25] Virtually all major organ systems can be affected individually or in combination (**Table 34–2**), and patients that develop MODS often succumb despite intensive care unit (ICU) support.

Fracture Care and the Systemic Inflammatory Response—The Second Hit

The treatment of musculoskeletal trauma can influence the development of SIRS and MODS. For many trauma victims, appropriate resuscitation restores homeostasis, the SIRS scores remain low, and the patient benefits from early fracture care, which prevents the complications that follow from prolonged immobilization (**Fig. 34–1A–G**). Fixa-

Table 34–2 Organ Systems Involved in Multiorgan Dysfunction Syndrome (MODS)

Organ System	Functional Disturbances in MODS
Cerebral	Cerebral edema
Cardiovascular	Hypotension, shock
Pulmonary	Acute lung injury or acute respiratory distress syndrome
Hepatic	Abnormal synthesis of acute phase reactants and cytokines, decreased hepatocyte function/jaundice
Gastrointestinal	Increased mucosal permeability and bacterial translocation
Renal	Renal tubular necrosis, acute renal failure
Hematologic	Disseminated intravascular coagulation

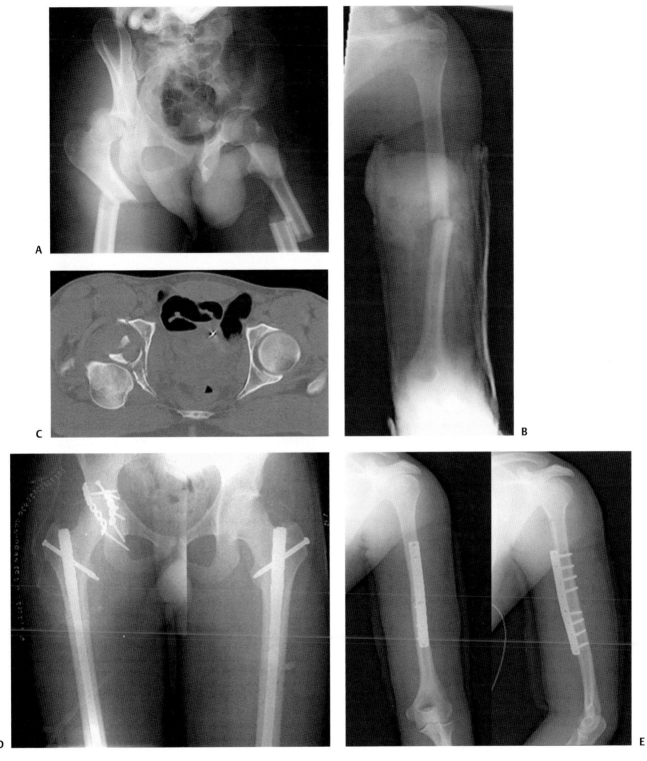

Figure 34–1 A patient with multiple fractures who underwent immediate fixation of all fractures without complication. **(A)** Anteroposterior (AP) view of the pelvis showing a right hip dislocation with an associated transverse and posterior wall acetabular fracture as well as bilateral femoral shaft fractures. **(B)** AP view of the left humerus showing a transverse fracture. **(C)** Computed tomographic cut of the right hip showing the fracture/dislocation. The patient was young and without head, chest, spinal, or abdominal trauma. He was taken urgently to surgery and underwent open reduction of his hip, right femoral nailing, repair of his right acetabulum, and left femoral nailing. **(D)** Postoperative x-rays of this legs after repair of his pelvic and femoral fractures. **(E)** Postoperative x-rays of his left arm after later plating of his humerus. *(Continued on page 856)*

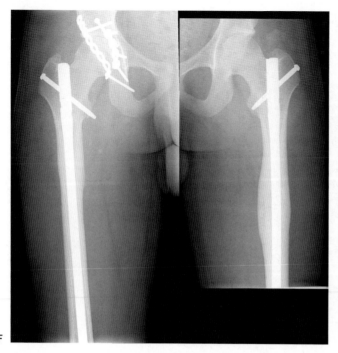
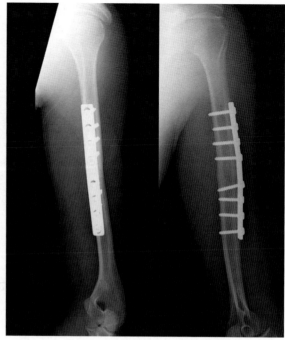

Figure 34–1 *(Continued)* A patient with multiple fractures who underwent immediate fixation of all fractures without complication. **(F)** X-rays of his pelvis and legs 1 year later showing that his fractures were nicely healed and his hip was without signs of osteonecrosis or arthrosis. **(G)** Final x-rays of his humerus.

tion of long-bone fractures in particular, however, has been shown to represent a second hit to the patient and may exacerbate the systemic inflammatory response and precipitate the development of any or all of the components of SIRS and MODS **(Fig. 34–2A–D).**[12,13,19] Giannoudis et al studied the level of inflammatory markers IL-6 and elastase in femoral shaft fractures treated with reamed and unreamed nailing. Both markers were significantly elevated compared with controls at the time of admission. Intramedullary nailing caused a further elevation in both markers, demonstrating a systemic inflammatory response to nailing. Although there was a trend toward a greater response in patients treated with reamed nailing, these data did not reach statistical significance.[19] It has been proposed that extensive surgery should be avoided in the "borderline" patient.[5]

Currently, research efforts are being directed at characterizing the biochemical and physiological parameters that define a borderline patient, so that treatment may be better individualized and matched to what the patient is capable of withstanding physiologically **(Table 34–3).** For example, Pape and colleagues looked at multiply injured but clinically stable patients with femur fractures and divided them into three groups based on management of their femur fracture: primary femoral nailing, primary external fixation, and delayed femoral nailing.[13] Both clinical parameters and serum levels of IL-1, IL-6, and IL-8 were followed. These investigators found that levels of IL-6 and IL-8 were higher after primary femoral nailing than after primary external fixation or after secondary (delayed) in-

tramedullary nailing, although no significant clinical differences were found.[13] In a more recent study from the same center, a similar population of patients was studied; however, the SIRS score and the Marshall multiorgan dysfunction score[27] were used as outcome parameters.[28] Once again, patients undergoing immediate femoral nailing were compared with a second group of patients undergoing primary external fixation and later conversion to a femoral nail. Despite having lower injury severity scores, the mean SIRS score was significantly higher in the primary nailing group from 12 hours until 72 hours postoperatively compared with the external fixation group. When

Table 34–3 Parameters Used to Define the "Borderline" Patient

Multiple injuries (ISS > 20) and chest trauma (chest AIS > 2)

Multiple injuries, including abdominal/pelvic trauma and shock (initial BP < 90 mm Hg)

Severe polytrauma (ISS > 40), without chest trauma

Bilateral pulmonary contusion

Initial mean pulmonary arterial pressure > 24 mm Hg

Increase of pulmonary artery pressure during femoral nailing > 6 mm Hg

AIS, Abbreviated Injury Scale; BP, blood pressure; ISS, injury severity score.
Adapted with permission from Pape HC, Tscherne H. Early definitive fracture fixation, pulmonary function and systemic effects. In: Baue AE, Faist E, Fry M, eds. Multiple Organ Failure. New York: Springer Verlag; 2000:279–290.

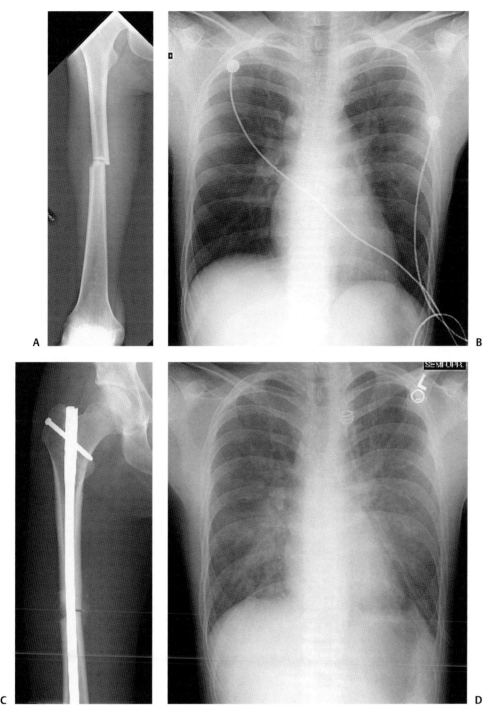

Figure 34–2 A patient with an isolated femur fracture that developed pulmonary infiltrates after undergoing uncomplicated primary reamed femoral nailing. The patient required prolonged ventilator support, although he ultimately made a full recovery. **(A)** X-ray of his simple, isolated right femur fracture. **(B)** His admission chest radi-ograph was normal. **(C)** He underwent immediate intramedullary nailing of his femur, as seen in this postoperative x-ray. He developed progressive respiratory distress postoperatively and required admission to the medical intensive care unit. **(D)** Follow-up chest films showed bilateral pulmonary infiltrates.

the patients initially undergoing external fixation later underwent intramedullary nailing, the SIRS scores remained lower than those in the primary nailing group.[28] These studies provide strong evidence that choices made during the clinical management of femur fractures in multiply injured patients may influence the risk of SIRS and MODS.

Prioritization of Injury Treatment

In the 1970s, acute fracture treatment was rarely performed due to the commonly held concept that trauma patients were "too sick for surgery." These patients were typically left in traction for prolonged periods of time and underwent definitive fixation (if fixation was performed at all) on a delayed basis. In the late 1980s, with improvements in clinical care and monitoring, a push began to treat fractures on a more urgent basis with the understanding that this could decrease the incidence of fat embolism syndrome and allow more rapid mobilization of the patient. Early retrospective studies demonstrated the benefits of such an approach, showing a decrease in ARDS, pneumonia, and length of hospital stay.[29] Bone et al performed a prospective, randomized study examining delayed (< 48 h) versus early fixation (> 24 h) of femoral shaft fractures and found that early stabilization had a decreased rate of ARDS, a shorter period of assisted ventilation, and a shorter hospital stay.[30]

As early stabilization became more common, it became recognized that some patients with multiple injuries had a higher incidence of complications with early intramedullary nailing of femoral shaft fractures (see **Video 34–1, Disk 4**).[31] This was particularly concerning in patients who had preoperative evidence of pulmonary trauma, in whom immediate femoral nailing appeared to be associated with the development of ARDS postoperatively.[31] Although femoral nailing has demonstrable effects on pulmonary physiology,[32] later work has shown that the incidence of ARDS and other pulmonary complications is more likely to be the result of the severity of chest trauma than the method of fracture fixation.[33]

Furthermore, as described in the section "The Physiological Response to Trauma," we now have a better understanding of the inflammatory response to severe injury, and recent evidence suggests that urgent provisional stabi-

Table 34–4 Guidelines for the Timing of Operative Intervention in the Trauma Patient

Emergent (within 1–2 h maximum)

- Compartment syndrome
- Closed or open reduction of dislocation or fracture/dislocation where vascularity of limb, vascularity/integrity of overlying skin, or nerves are compromised due to the deformity of the dislocation or fracture (e.g., lateral subtalar joint dislocation that is not reducible and where the patient has numbness on the plantar aspect of foot with blanching over the medial skin of the ankle; tongue-type calcaneus fracture where the tuber is blanching the skin in the Achilles' tendon region)
- Stabilization of fractures associated with vascular injuries
- Closed reduction of joint dislocations (e.g., hip, knee)
- Mechanical stabilization of unstable pelvic injuries in hemodynamically unstable patients

Urgent (within 6–12 h maximum)

- Stabilization of long-bone (e.g., femur, tibia) fractures in the polytrauma patient
- Open reduction and internal fixation of a femoral neck fracture in a young adult
- Open reduction and internal fixation of displaced talar neck fracture
- Debridement and stabilization of open fractures
- Reduction and stabilization of unstable spine injuries with evolving neurological deficits

Expedient (< 24 h maximum)

- Stabilization of femur fractures in the nonpolytraumatized patient (i.e., isolated injury)
- Stabilization (e.g., external fixation) across axially unstable articular injuries (e.g., tibial plateau and pilon fractures)
- Hip fractures (e.g., high-energy intertrochanteric femur fractures)

Semielective (1–10 days maximum)

- Foot and ankle fractures excluding pilon and calcaneus fractures
- Acetabular fractures
- Definitive management of unstable pelvic ring injuries
- Closed upper extremity trauma (e.g., supracondylar-intercondylar distal humerus fracture, both-bone forearm fracture)
- Reduction and stabilization of unstable spine injuries with complete neurological deficit or without neurological deficit

Elective (1–4 weeks)

- Articular fractures about the lower extremity where soft tissues dictate the timing of surgery (e.g., calcaneus, pilon, tibial plateau fractures)

lization of fractures with delayed definitive fixation may improve patient outcomes. This method has been termed damage-control orthopaedics (DCO).

Timing of Surgical Interventions

Prolonged operative treatment in the acute setting can lead to hypothermia and coagulopathy. A core body temperature of 34°C is associated with increased mortality, decreased platelet activity, and altered fibrinolysis. Traumatized patients often receive large volumes of intravenous fluids at ambient temperature and may undergo abdominal or thoracic surgical procedures predisposing them to hypothermia. Patients requiring blood transfusion will be depleted of platelets, factor V, and factor VIII. These factors add to the systemic stressors of the initial traumatic event and need to be considered in the timing of surgical treatment of orthopaedic injuries.

The orthopaedic surgeon plays a key role in the management of the polytrauma patient by assessing the musculoskeletal injuries and deciding which injuries need to be treated emergently (i.e., within 1 to 2 hours), urgently (within 6 to 12 hours), expediently (within 24 hours), semielectively (between 1 and 7 days), and electively (in 1 to 4 weeks). In this realm, **Table 34–4** outlines a schema for the timing of orthopaedic injuries in the trauma patient. Clearly, this is not meant to be a strict mandate because the exact timing of treatment of injuries should be determined by the particular characteristics of the injuries themselves, the stability of the patient, and the availability of an appropriate surgical team.

Damage-Control Orthopaedics

DCO entails staged treatment of fractures in patients with multiple injuries requiring resuscitation efforts. The first stage is temporary stabilization and includes control of hemorrhage, debridement of open wounds, and external fixation. In the patient who is in extremis, these procedures may need to be performed in the trauma room or the ICU. The second stage is resuscitation, during which the patient returns to the ICU for close monitoring, repletion of blood products, and further hemodynamic stabilization. The third stage consists of definitive fixation of the fracture once the patient is optimized for orthopaedic intervention.

DCO provides enough fracture stabilization to allow the patient to be mobilized and to decrease local inflammation that can contribute to systemic changes, while at the same time avoiding major surgery that would constitute a second hit to the patient after the initial trauma. Although external fixation is the primary method used during damage control, unreamed femoral nailing may also fall into this category. Studies have shown that unreamed femoral nailing may cause less additional operative burden than reamed nailing,[19] and potentially less embolic burden on the lungs, although

Table 34–5 Parameters for Definitive Fracture Care

Systolic blood pressure	> 90 mm Hg
Core temperature	> 34°C
Urine output	> 150 mL/h
Cerebral perfusion pressure	> 70 mm Hg
Systemic inflammatory response syndrome score	< 2
$PaO_2:FiO_2$ ratio	> 280
Lactate	< 2.0 mmol/L
Platelet count	> 100,000/μL
C-reactive protein	< 11 mg/dL
Interleukin-6	< 500 pg/dL

this remains somewhat controversial.[34] Furthermore, at least for some patients who are in the operating room already, unreamed femoral nailing may be expeditiously performed.

Pape et al categorized the polytraumatized patient into having four potential conditions: stable, borderline, unstable, and in extremis.[35] Stable patients are hemodynamically stable and normothermic, with a lactate less than 2.0 mmol/L and no respiratory difficulties or coagulopathy (**Table 34–5**). Stable patients can have definitive management of their injuries in the early time period (> 24 h), but this is not imperative. Borderline patients require resuscitation before going to the operating room; they potentially may have definitive early management of their orthopaedic injuries but remain at high risk for rapid deterioration. These patients are defined as those with an ISS greater than 40, or greater than 20 if there is an associated thoracic injury, hypothermia (colder than 35°C), multiple injuries associated with severe abdominal/pelvic injury and systolic blood pressure less than 90 mm Hg, evidence of pulmonary contusion, bilateral femur fractures, or moderate/severe head injuries (**Table 34–3**). These patients fall into a "gray zone" and can be considered for early total care but with caution and a low threshold for conversion to DCO if the patient worsens or proves unstable during the first operative intervention. The unstable patient should undergo damage-control stabilization with further resuscitation. Patients who are in extremis are those who are failing resuscitative measures and may need to have external fixation placed at the bedside in the ICU setting.[35,36]

Although monitoring IL-6 levels may be clinically relevant to assess patient readiness for surgery, it is not a standard laboratory procedure, which makes its utility difficult in the hospital setting. Serum lactate levels are routinely used because of the ease and speed of obtaining the information. Lactate is a measure of tissue perfusion. In cases of trauma, inadequate tissue perfusion secondary to hypoxia, blood loss, or cardiogenic shock results in elevated blood lactate levels. Normal values range from 0.8 to 2.0 mmol/L.

Studies have shown that the degree of elevated lactate on admission and the number of days of elevation above normal correlate with multiorgan dysfunction.[37,38] Other markers used are platelet counts greater than 100,000 per μL, CRP less than 11 mg/dL, and PO_2:FiO_2 ratio greater than 280.[39] The SIRS score as described earlier in this chapter has been shown to be predictive of mortality and infection risk and may also be used as a marker for adequate resuscitation for surgery (**Table 34–5**).[40–42]

Techniques of Damage-Control Orthopaedics

The primary surgical interventions in DCO are irrigation and debridement of open wounds, reduction of dislocations, and external fixation of the lower extremities and/or pelvis. External fixators may be applied to individual bones, such as the tibia or femur, or applied across joints such as the knee or ankle (see **Video 34–2, Disk 4**). The concept is very similar to the techniques of spanning external fixation discussed for the management of tibial plateau fractures in Chapter 29 and tibial plafond fractures in Chapter 31. External fixation can be performed rapidly, and occasionally in conjunction with other emergent procedures. In one study, the average surgical time for external fixation was 35 minutes compared with the 135 minutes for intramedullary nailing as a secondary procedure.[43]

Newer reaming techniques that decrease the intramedullary pressure can also be employed if intramedullary nailing is to be performed on a borderline patient or on the patient with multiple long-bone fractures. This technique involves use of a specialized reamer that irrigates and suctions the medullary canal throughout reaming (see **Video 34–3, Disk 4**). Animal model studies have demonstrated significantly reduced intramedullary pressure and degree of fat embolization with use of this technique.[44,45] This may reduce the incidence of fat embolism and help prevent pulmonary complications, although clinical studies are pending.

Spanning External Fixation (see **Video 34–1, Disk 4**)
The patient is typically positioned supine on a radiolucent operating room table. The injured limb is prepped and draped. A tourniquet may or may not be used depending on the clinical situation; it is not needed solely for external fixation but may be useful if any open procedures are necessary. Typically, 5.0 mm Schanz pins are used. Pins are predrilled and inserted manually. Placement of the pins is important because one must consider that the pin sites will become contaminated. Therefore, pin sites should be placed far away from potential incisions or areas where later internal fixation might be performed. After each pin is placed, the skin should be inspected and released if it is tented by the pin.

For knee-spanning fixators, the proximal pins are placed in an anterolateral location to avoid "spearing" the quadriceps muscles. For the tibia, pins are usually placed into the crest or into the medial subcutaneous border. Two

pins are sufficient in each bone. The two femoral and two tibial pins are typically connected to each other with one bar. Because the tibial and femoral bars are usually in different planes, the two bars may need to be connected with a third bar (**Fig. 34–3A**). Occasionally, if there are associated fractures or soft tissue injuries of the lower leg, it may be necessary to span to the ankle (**Fig. 34–3B**).

For ankle-spanning fixators, three pins are typically used (**Fig. 34–4**). Two pins are placed into the proximal anterior crest of the tibia, above the anticipated extent of later internal fixation. A centrally threaded pin is placed in the calcaneal tuberosity. This pin is started medially on the hindfoot so that the neurovascular bundle remains safe. Fluoroscopy may be used if desired, but x-rays of the foot and ankle should always be done before fixator application so that inadvertent insertion of a pin into a fractured calcaneus can be avoided. The two proximal pins are connected together with a short bar, and two longer bars are connected to the calcaneal pin. One should note that this imparts a posteriorly directed force on the ankle joint. If posterior ankle subluxation exists, such a configuration may exacerbate it. In this case, a more rectangular frame may be used.

Conversion of External Fixation to Intramedullary Nailing
Conversion from provisional external fixation to definitive intramedullary nailing is done whenever the patient's physiology and clinical status allow. Delayed conversion after 2 weeks has caused concern due to the increased risk of infection arising from pin site contamination. Rates of infection have been reported to be 1.7 to 3%. Increased rates are seen if fixation is delayed more than 2 weeks.[43,46,47]

Special Considerations in the Head-Injured Patient

Although no conclusive evidence has been obtained regarding the timing of fracture fixation in the polytraumatized patient with head injury, this topic merits consideration. Surgical procedures can cause hypotension and hypoxia associated with operative blood loss and general anesthesia. A large volume of fluids is also generally given intraoperatively. These factors can combine to cause significant alterations in cerebral perfusion, which may affect the long-term cognitive outcome of the patient with a head injury.

It has been shown that negative or minimal head CT findings in polytraumatized patients do not rule out the possibility of progression or new lesions during the hospital course.[48,49] Stein et al found that 48% of polytraumatized head-injured patients had new or progressive lesions on serial CT scans. Fifty-five percent of these patients had coagulopathies compared with 9% of those with stable lesions. They determined that there is an 85% risk of progressive or secondary head injury if there is at least one abnormal clotting parameter.[48]

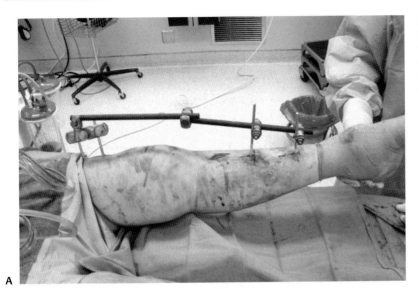

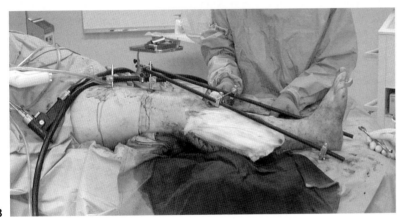

Figure 34–3 Photographs of a knee-spanning external fixator. **(A)** Knee-spanning fixator in a patient with a tibial plateau fracture. **(B)** A femur-calcaneus fixator in a woman with a left femur fracture, right tibial plateau fracture, and right distal tibial pilon fracture. In this case, the fixator spans both her proximal and distal tibial fractures.

The literature is split between early fixation versus delayed fixation in head-injured patients. Multiple studies report no difference in neurological outcome when fixation is performed in the first 24 hour period. Kalb et al reviewed 123 patients treated for femoral shaft fractures with concomitant head injury.[50] Eighty-four were treated

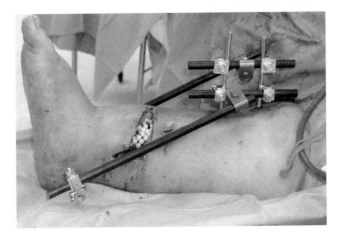

Figure 34–4 Photograph of an ankle-spanning external fixator.

within the first 24 hours. There was no significant difference in the volume of fluids given in the early resuscitative period, but there was a significantly greater blood loss and volume of fluid given intraoperatively to those patients treated early. Despite this, there were no differences found in postoperative neurological or nonneurological complications. The early treatment group actually had higher cerebral perfusion pressures intraoperatively than the late treatment group, indicating that the increased volume of intraoperative fluid and blood product was adequate to keep up with the greater losses.[50] Brundage et al also found no significant difference in postoperative Glasgow coma scores (GCSs) of patients treated at different time intervals.[51] In this study, however, the authors note that the patients treated in the early group were fully resuscitated prior to operative intervention, and this represented only 65% of the total cohort. Poole et al also demonstrated no adverse neurological effects of early fixation of femoral shaft fractures if the systolic blood pressure is maintained greater than 90 mm Hg and hypoxia is avoided with oxygen saturations kept above 90%. Pulmonary complications were associated with head injury regardless of timing, however.[52] Unfortunately, in most of these studies the neurological outcome measure is the GCS, which is not a good predictor of cognitive function.[49]

Townsend et al found that hypotension in head-injured patients undergoing femoral nailing correlated with timing of fixation. Of patients treated in the first 2 hours, 68.2% had intraoperative hypotension compared with 8.3% of those taken to the operating room after more than 24 hours. Despite this, however, they were unable to show a relationship between intraoperative hypotension and neurological outcome.[53] Jaicks et al showed that patients with significant closed head injuries treated with early femoral fixation had a similar neurological complication rate but had a lower GCS on discharge despite preoperative GCS scores that were similar to the late fixation group.[54]

In both cases, however, all authors seem to agree that avoidance of hypoxia and hypothermia with maintenance of cerebral perfusion is critical. Coordination with the neurosurgical team and anesthesia with appropriate preoperative resuscitation and reversal of coagulopathy are key factors in avoiding adverse neurological outcomes secondary to fracture fixation.

Outcomes

The influence of various factors such as intramedullary reaming, thoracic trauma, timing of intramedullary nailing and damage-control techniques on pulmonary complications, length of ICU and hospital stay, and mortality have been evaluated in numerous studies. Furthermore, several scoring systems have been developed to aid in predicting such outcomes in polytraumatized patients. These instruments enable a relatively rapid assessment of the multiply injured patient for assistance in decision making for surgical timing and possible events during the hospital course.

The ISS has been a standard tool for outcome measurements; however, this is perhaps being replaced by the new injury severity score (NISS), which has been shown to be more predictive of MODS, sepsis, and ICU and hospital length of stay.[55-57] The NISS takes the three worst Abbreviated Injury Scale (AIS) scores, regardless of body region, which may give a more accurate picture of the additive severity of injuries. A NISS of 20 correlates with an ISS of 16 defining mild trauma, with moderate trauma defined as a NISS of 30 (ISS 25) and severe trauma having a NISS of 55 (ISS 50).[55] Kilgo et al described the AIS$_{max}$, which simply used the worst AIS score as a predictor. This was found to be more predictive of mortality in multiply injured patients compared with the ISS or NISS.[58] Harwood et al also analyzed the AIS$_{max}$ and found it to be a better predictor of mortality in penetrating trauma only.[55] The SIRS score described earlier in this chapter can also be a predictor of outcome in trauma patients. Napolitano et al demonstrated that a SIRS score $\geq$ 2 was associated with a higher rate of mortality (6.9% compared with 1.1%) and increased length of hospital stay.[41]

ARDS and pulmonary complications are of significant concern in multiply injured patients, particularly in the presence of long-bone fractures. Timing of fracture treatment as well as the use of reaming has been examined in multiple studies. Bone et al performed a prospective, randomized trial of early versus delayed femoral nailing in multiply injured patients with an ISS greater than 18. They found that isolated femur fractures had no difference in pulmonary complications when treated definitively within 24 hours or after 24 hours. However, there was a significantly higher incidence of ARDS in patients treated in the delayed fixation group. The early fixation group also required fewer days of ventilatory support (1.4 d vs 9.9 d).[30] Seibel et al found similar results with patients treated with definitive fixation at > 24 hours requiring 3.4 days of ventilatory support compared with 9.4 days in the late group as well as shorter ICU stays (7.5 d vs 15 d) and shorter hospital stays (23 d vs 45 d).[29] Johnson et al found a fivefold increase in ARDS in patients with an ISS greater than 18 treated in delayed fashion compared with within 24 hours. If the ISS was greater than 40, ARDS was present in 75% of patients treated with delayed fixation compared with 17% of the early fixation group.[59]

Femoral reaming for intramedullary nailing has been thought to contribute to pulmonary complications, particularly in patients with lung contusions. The means by which reaming causes pulmonary dysfunction is multifactorial. First, by creating and disseminating fat emboli that are trapped by the pulmonary circulation, reaming directly affects cardiopulmonary function. Second, by further stimulating the systemic inflammatory response (second hit), reaming contributes to acute lung injury as part of SIRS/MODS.[12,13,19] It has been shown in a sheep model that there is increased pulmonary capillary permeability and increased activation of polymorphonuclear lymphocytes with reamed intramedullary nailing in the presence of a lung contusion. This suggests that the inflammatory response to reaming contributes to the development of ARDS.[32] A large retrospective study by Pape et al investigated early intramedullary nailing in patients with and without thoracic trauma. Those without pulmonary injuries benefited from early fixation with decreased ICU stays and number of days requiring ventilatory support. However, those with severe chest trauma (AIS < 2) had a higher incidence of ARDS (33% compared with 7.7%) and mortality (21% compared with 4%).[31]

To the contrary, multiple studies have shown that early (> 24 h) intramedullary nailing of femoral shaft fractures does not increase the risk of ARDS in cases of thoracic trauma in stable patients. Bosse et al found no difference in ARDS, length of stay, days requiring ventilator support, pneumonia, or MODS in patients treated with nailing compared with plating performed in the first 24 hours in patients with thoracic injuries, suggesting that reaming is not a contributing factor to pulmonary compromise in femoral fixation in this patient population.[33] Handolin et al had similar findings in a retrospective review of patients with pulmonary contusion treated with reamed femoral nailing within 24 hours of injury.[60] A recent study by the Canadian Orthopaedic Trauma Society analyzed data from seven level I trauma centers and found no difference in the incidence of ARDS in patients treated with reamed intramedullary nailing versus unreamed nailing. Chest AIS $\geq$ 2 and ISS $\geq$ 18 were not found to be predictive of development of ARDS.[61]

Intramedullary nailing of multiple long-bone fractures may create an additive effect, increasing the risk of pulmonary complications, particularly in patients with thoracic trauma. Zalavras et al prospectively observed patients with unilateral and bilateral femur fractures and determined that multiple intramedullary nailings and thoracic trauma were independent risk factors for the development of pulmonary complications.[62] Specialized reamers with the ability to irrigate and aspirate the medullary canal may be of particular use in these situations to decrease the embolic load. Pulmonary permeability and polymorphonuclear lymphocyte activation as well as volume of fat embolization have been shown to be decreased compared with traditional reaming in animal models.[44,45,63]

Pape et al analyzed data from three different time periods during which different protocols of prioritization were used in the treatment of femoral shaft fractures in polytraumatized patients. The three groups encompassed a period of early total care (intramedullary nailing in the first 24 h), intermediate treatment (shift toward external fixation in high-risk patients), and damage-control orthopaedics (external fixation in the first 24 h followed by definitive fixation). A significant decrease in multiorgan failure and ARDS was found in patients treated with early external fixation compared with those treated with primary intramedullary nailing. The authors admit that there were concurrent changes in overall critical care management of patients in the different time periods that may confound the data. However, in the damage-control group, patients treated with primary external fixation had no significant differences in complications compared with those treated with early intramedullary nailing despite a higher ISS in the former group.[64]

This correlates with a prospective study by the same author evaluating the levels of inflammatory markers and timing of the secondary procedure after temporary stabilization for damage-control purposes. Patients receiving definitive fixation on days 2 to 4 had a higher incidence of MODS and ARDS than those treated with secondary procedures on days 5 to 8. The combination of IL-6 levels greater than 500 pg/dL on admission and definitive treatment performed on days 2 to 4 was very strongly associated with MODS.[65] In a study by Brundage et al ARDS was highest in patients definitively treated with primary intramedullary nailing for femoral shaft fracture in 2 to 5 days, correlating with these findings.[51]

Outcomes in the polytraumatized patient are dependent on multiple variables. The key to maximizing good outcomes in this patient population is to recognize the complex interaction of local and systemic inflammation in the setting of thoracic and intracranial injuries, and the potential effects of iatrogenic insults such as orthopaedic surgical intervention. The surgeon needs to use clinical and laboratory markers of these physiological parameters to best determine the timing and type of intervention in concert with the efforts of other members of the trauma team.

Case Studies

Case 1 This 21-year-old male was involved in a motor vehicle collision at approximately 3 A.M. His initial evaluation in the emergency room revealed the following injuries: small subdural hematoma, complex facial fractures, a closed left subtrochanteric femur fracture, a complex left tibial/talar body/calcaneus fracture with a stellate open fracture wound of 6 cm on the plantar aspect of the foot, and a right open type II (4 cm) tibial fracture (**Fig. 34–5A–D**). The patient underwent aggressive resuscitation with warm intravenous fluids, warm blankets, and intubation and sedation. His laboratory numbers at individual time periods are shown in **Table 34–6**. The laboratory values therefore were indicative of a coagulopathic, underresuscitated patient.

The left lower extremity was felt to be a severe injury with regard to the displacement of his tibia, the accompanying soft tissue (muscle, tendon, nerve) injury, and the plantar wound associated with the exposed tibial articular surface.

Table 34–6 Case 1: Laboratory Values Indicating Acidosis and Coagulopathy

	Hematocrit (%) (nL 42–50)	Platelets (10^{-6}/L) (nL 135–370)	Prothrombin Time (sec) (nL 13–15)	Partial Thromboplastin Time (sec) (nL 25–34)	Calcium (mg/dL) (nL 8.5–10.5)	pH (nL 7.35–7.45)	Lactate (mEq/L) (nL 0.5–2.2)
3:00 A.M.	36	223					
5:00 A.M.	27	144				7.20	2.8
7:00 A.M.	23	121	21.5	35	5.0	7.25	2.1
11:40 A.M.	30	91	16.7	30.3	7.6	7.28	3.4

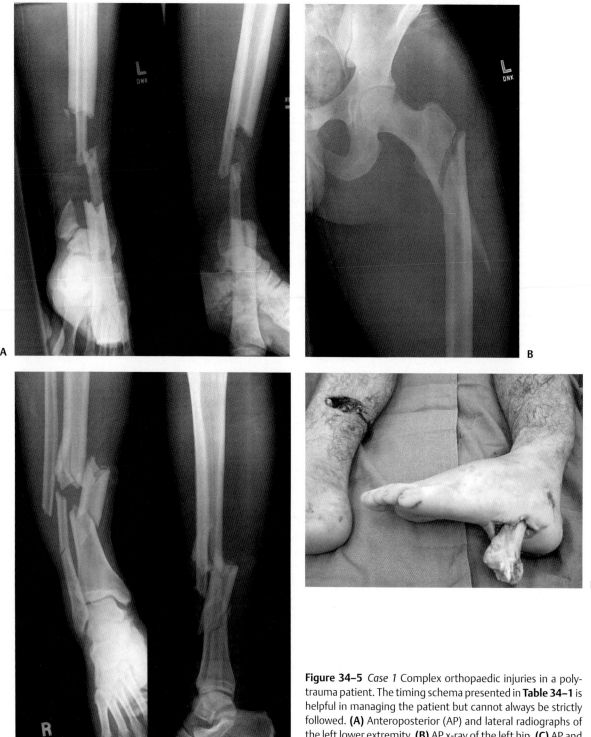

Figure 34–5 *Case 1* Complex orthopaedic injuries in a polytrauma patient. The timing schema presented in **Table 34–1** is helpful in managing the patient but cannot always be strictly followed. **(A)** Anteroposterior (AP) and lateral radiographs of the left lower extremity. **(B)** AP x-ray of the left hip. **(C)** AP and lateral radiographs of the right tibia. **(D)** Photograph of the injuries on his bilateral lower extremities. *(Continued)*

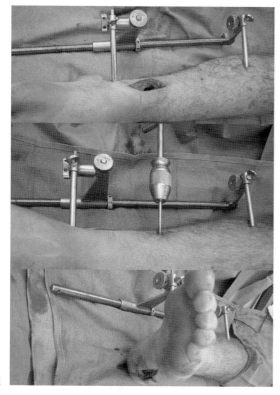
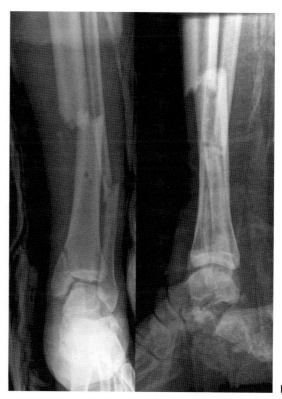

E   F

Figure 34–5 *(Continued) Case 1* **(E)** Intraoperative view of reduction of the left tibial shaft, which had imploded through the ankle syndesmosis, talus, and calcaneus. This was not easy. A femoral distractor was used from the intact medial talar body and the proximal tibial shaft, and a Schanz pin was used in the distal tibial shaft to aid the re- duction. Additionally, an open incision was made on the anteromedial aspect of the ankle to help restore alignment. **(F)** AP and lateral radiographs of the left lower extremity after tibial shaft reduction and splinting. *(Continued on page 866)*

Because of the severity of his left lower extremity injuries, this case was placed in the emergent/urgent category, with plans for initial debridement and stabilization within the next several hours. Close communication with the general surgery and anesthesia teams was maintained, and the severity of the injury was explained. A short operative intervention was planned, with the goal of debridement of the open wounds, possible intramedullary nailing of the right tibia, and reduction of the left tibial shaft fracture. Because the patient was not well resuscitated, the plan was not to address the left proximal femur in the first surgical intervention but to come back to the operating room in the next 24 hours for definitive repair of his left proximal femur fracture and possibly the left tibia. Additionally, if the patient had any significant deterioration in the operating room, we were prepared to perform DCO by external fixation of all injuries. The initial operative intervention lasted 2 hours beginning at ~7:30 A.M., during which time several procedures were accomplished: (1) irrigation and debridement of the right tibial wound, (2) intramedullary nailing of the right tibial fracture, (3) irrigation and debridement of the left plantar wound, (4) open reduction to the tibial shaft displacement on the left, and (5) splinting of the left lower extremity **(Fig. 34–5E–G)**.

Two surgical teams worked on the left and right lower extremities at the same time. No intervention was made on his left proximal femur fracture, although external fixation of this injury (pelvis to proximal femur) was a consideration. Additionally, external fixation of the left lower extremity was also a consideration (rather than splinting) but was difficult because of the calcaneus and talus fracture. The patient underwent ongoing resuscitation during the operating room intervention, with fluid resuscitation, fresh frozen plasma, packed red blood cells, platelets, and calcium replacement. His laboratory values after the surgical intervention indicated the need for further resuscitation, but we had not "lost ground" and had accomplished our initial urgent orthopaedic trauma goals. If the patient had significantly deteriorated intraoperatively, consideration of immediate left below-knee amputation would have been reasonable.

The patient stabilized over the next 18 hours, and his coagulopathy and acidosis improved. He was therefore taken back to the operating room on postinjury day 1 and had (1) repeat irrigation and debridement with closure of his left plantar wound, (2) open reduction and internal fixation of his left subtrochanteric femur fracture, (3) provisional fixation of the medial malleolar ankle fracture to

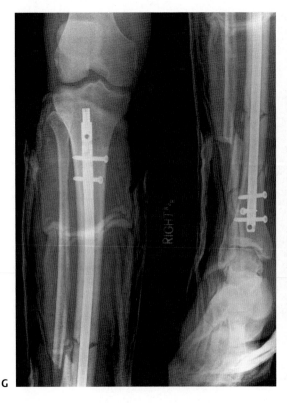

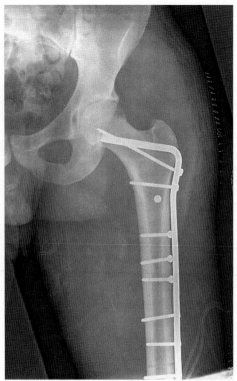

G

H

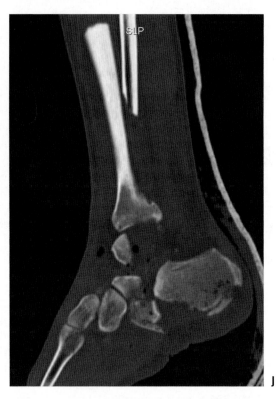

I

J

Figure 34–5 *(Continued) Case 1* **(G)** AP and lateral radiographs of the right tibia after intramedullary nailing. **(H)** AP of the left hip after open reduction and internal fixation of the left proximal femur fracture. **(I)** AP and lateral radiographs of the left tibia after intramedullary nailing and provisional fixation of his medial malleolus to maintain some ankle stability. **(J)** Computed tomographic scan reconstruction views of the calcaneus and talus fractures. Given the complexity of these injuries, soft tissue swelling, and his initial instability, this is staged for 1.5 to 2 weeks later.

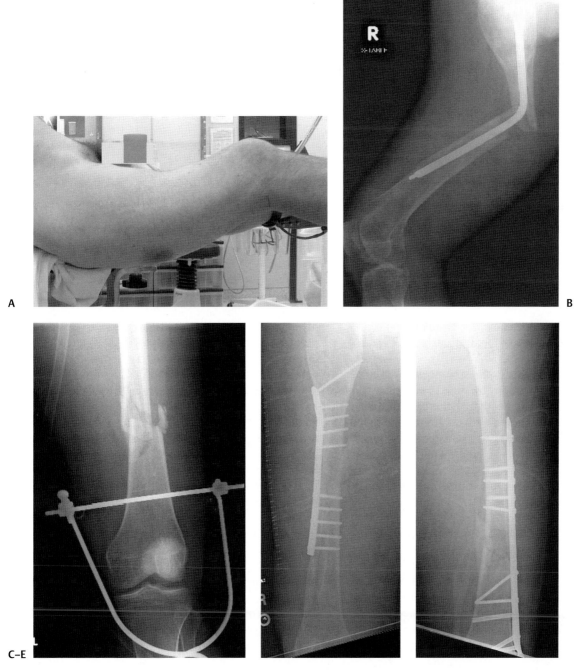

A

B

C–E

Figure 34–6 *Case 2* **(A)** Clinical photograph of the patient's right thigh, with a stable deformity. **(B)** Lateral x-ray of the right femur, showing a bent nail and abnormal bone consistent with fibrous dysplasia. **(C)** Traction x-ray of the opposite left femur fracture. Postoperative x-rays of the **(D)** right and **(E)** left femurs following plating.

gain ankle stability, and (4) splinting of his left lower extremity (**Fig. 34–5H,I**).

The patient slowly stabilized over the next 3 days and had his facial fractures fixed on postinjury day 7. Definitive fixation of his ankle, talus, and calcaneus fractures was deferred until postinjury day 15 (**Fig. 34–5J**). The delay was to allow time for him to recover from his initial trauma and to allow time for the swelling about his lower extremity to decrease.

Case 2 A 34-year-old motorcyclist presented with bilateral femoral shaft fractures but no other injuries. He was healthy but had a history of fibrous dysplasia affecting his right pelvis and right femur. He had undergone previous intramedullary nailing of the right femur as a child. The patient knew no details of that surgery. The patient was alert and oriented and initially described himself as completely healthy. However, the anesthetist noted a loud heart murmur, and the patient then recalled that he had a ventricular septal defect (VSD) and had recently been told that he should have it repaired.

On examination, the patient was alert with stable vital signs. He had a stable but deformed right thigh with a fixed apex-posterior angulation (**Fig. 34–6A**). His left femur was deformed and unstable. Radiographs showed bilateral femur fractures, marked abnormalities of the right femur and right hemipelvis, and a bent nail in the right femur (**Fig. 34–6B,C**).

This patient was at risk for intracerebral fat embolism if he were to develop a left to right shunt during surgery due to transient elevations of pulmonary artery pressure as a consequence of pulmonary fat embolism. Intramedullary instrumentation of either femur was therefore felt to be too dangerous because it would cause further pulmonary embolization. The patient underwent bilateral femoral plating with removal of his bent nail, which had to be sectioned and removed in two pieces (**Fig. 34–6D,E**). He underwent elective closure of his VSD at a later date.

Case 3 This case illustrates how the overall stability of a patient will influence the orthopaedic surgeon's decision regarding amputation versus limb salvage of a lower extremity injury. The patient is a healthy 21-year-old male who was involved in a waterskiing accident where his right thigh and calf were injured by the boat propeller (**Fig. 34–7A,B**). He was noted to have significant blood loss at the scene. The patient was evaluated in the emergency room, and a provisional tourniquet was placed about his leg. The patient had ongoing resuscitation with warm intravenous fluids and warm blankets. His laboratory values were hematocrit 25% (nL 42 to 50), prothrombin time 22.7 sec (nL 13 to 15), and lactate 0.7 mEq/L (nL 0.5 to 2.2). He therefore received fresh frozen plasma because his laboratories were indicative of a coagulopathy. He was, however, otherwise stable with no other injuries and a blood pressure of 110/70.

The patient was taken emergently to the operating room for irrigation and debridement of his leg wounds, where the peroneal artery was ligated after it was found to be a major source of blood loss. The tibial nerve was intact (**Fig. 34–7C**). There was a 90% transection of the Achilles' tendon, and 100% transection of the peroneus longus tendon. Both were felt to be repairable, however. The operative team consisted of both the orthopaedic surgeon and the plastic surgeon, with the general surgery trauma attending physician directing the resuscitation. All three surgeons were present in the operating room in the middle of the night. The patient underwent provisional closure of the wounds in the subcutaneous layers and splint application.

The patient underwent repeat irrigation and debridement on postinjury day 2, and again on postinjury day 4,

when the fibula was plated (**Fig. 34–7D**), the thigh wound was closed, the lower leg was definitively closed where possible, and a Wound V.A.C. (Kinetic Concepts Inc., San Antonio, Texas) was applied to the areas that later need to be skin grafted. The overall functional result will not be perfect, but will be reasonable (**Fig. 34–7E**). *The key point of this case is that if the patient was in extremis with other injuries, then consideration to initial amputation would be advisable in looking at the "big picture" of the patient. In this case, the patient was stable and without other injuries, and the patient could withstand multiple surgeries in the first several days to salvage his leg.*

Case 4 The patient was a 26-year-old male who was a helmeted rider in a high-speed motorcycle crash. He presented via helicopter, awake and alert with a Glasgow coma score (GCS) of 14. His medical history was unremarkable with the exception of tobacco use. There was obvious gross deformity of bilateral lower extremities with open wounds over the right and left thighs. His vital signs were stable. Laboratories were drawn but returned hemolyzed. The nursing staff had difficulty obtaining repeat blood work, and during this time the patient also lost IV access. A CT of the head, chest, spine, abdomen, and pelvis was negative for any intra-abdominal or thoracic injuries. Radiographs demonstrated a right femoral neck fracture, right femoral shaft fracture, left supracondylar femur fracture, displaced right clavicle fracture, and left distal radius fracture (**Fig. 34–8A–E**). Dressings were placed over the open wounds, and the distal radius fracture was splinted in the trauma bay.

The general surgery trauma service evaluated the patient and "cleared" him for operative treatment. An IV was finally restarted, and fluids were bolused. The patient remained hemodynamically stable, but it was recognized that despite this he was compensating for significant blood loss given his bilateral femur fractures. The decision was made to proceed to the operating room with the plan to perform an irrigation and debridement of both thigh wounds with possible open reduction and internal fixation of the right femoral neck, possible retrograde nailing of both femurs, and delayed treatment of the upper extremity injuries.

Laboratories were obtained in the preoperative holding area by anesthesia. A discussion was held with the anesthesia staff that the decision of how far to proceed with the plan was dependent on laboratory findings that were pending.

On induction of anesthesia, the patient became hypotensive and had a drop in oxygen saturation. He responded well to a small dose of vasopressors. The first laboratory value to come back was a K+ of 7.0. Given the hypotension, elevated potassium, and unclear resuscitation, the deci-

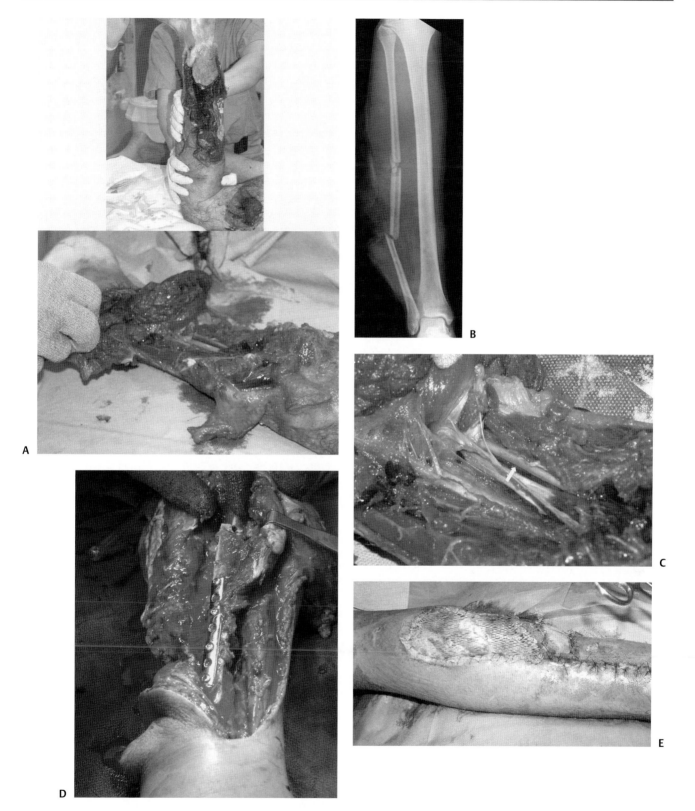

Figure 34–7 *Case 3* Severe soft tissue injury produced by a boat propeller in a healthy 21-year-old male. Because the patient had no other injuries and responded well to resuscitation, the operative team had the luxury of "definitive" management with four surgical procedures in the 10 days after the accident. This might not be possible in a polytrauma patient. Thus the management of the same injury in a polytrauma patient would likely be different. **(A)** Intraoperative photo of the soft tissue injury to the posterior aspect of the right calf and pos-

terolateral right thigh. **(B)** Anteroposterior radiograph of the osseous injury to the right leg. The tibia is not fractured. **(C)** The tibial nerve was intact (arrow). **(D)** Intraoperative view of the proximal aspect of the fibula fracture being plated on postinjury day 4. At the same time the Achilles' tendon and peroneus longus were repaired, which necessitated leaving the ankle in some plantar flexion to protect the repair. **(E)** The posterior closure of the leg seen at postinjury day 10 at the time of split-thickness skin grafting.

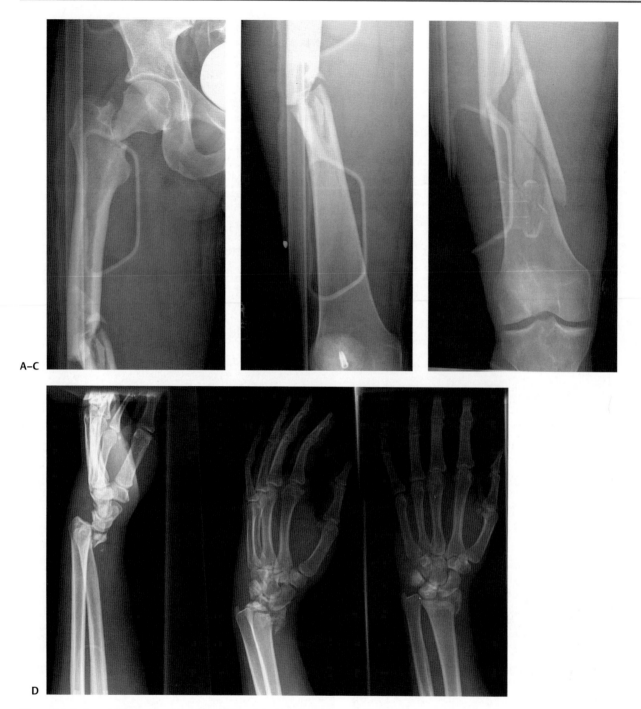

A–C

D

Figure 34–8 *Case 4* **(A)** Preoperative radiographs of the right femoral neck, **(B)** right femoral shaft, **(C)** left femoral shaft, **(D)** left distal radius. (*Continued*)

sion was made to convert to DCO, and a right femoral external fixator was placed, followed by a spanning left external fixator (**Fig. 34–8F,G**). Complete laboratories followed demonstrating a lactate of 4.7 and a hematocrit of 32.

The patient was returned to the trauma ICU. He had been weaned off vasopressors during the operative procedure and was resuscitated overnight. Lactate in the morning was 1.4. He was hemodynamically stable through the night, and the decision was made to proceed with fixation

of the femoral neck with retrograde intramedullary nailing of the bilateral femur fractures if he tolerated the first procedure.

The patient underwent open reduction and internal fixation of the femoral neck fracture without any difficulties; his vital signs and laboratories remained normal with a lactate of 0.8 and hematocrit of 40. Bilateral retrograde femoral nailing was then performed using a specialized reamer that irrigates and suctions the canal during ream-

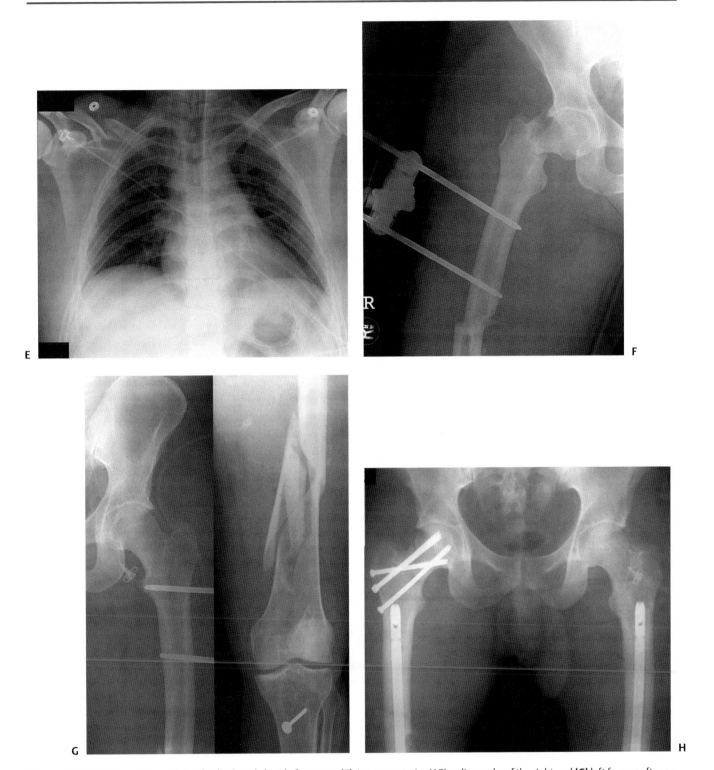

Figure 34–8 *(Continued) Case 4* **(E)** right displaced clavicle fractures. **(F)** Anteroposterior (AP) radiographs of the right and **(G)** left femurs after external fixation. The following are all postoperative films showing definitive fixation of all fractures. **(H)** AP radiograph of the pelvis demonstrating screw fixation of the right femoral neck. *(Continued on page 872)*

ing to reduce the risk of fat embolism. Although the patient remained stable throughout the procedure, the decision was made to repair the left distal radius and right clavicle fractures on a separate day to allow the patient to have further resuscitation after this second operative procedure (**Fig. 34–8H–L**).

The patient had no sequelae of this second operative event, and he returned to the operating room for simultaneous fixation of his right clavicle and left distal radius. He was extubated on postoperative day 2 of his last procedure.

Although appropriate preoperative laboratory values were not available prior to going to the operating room, the case

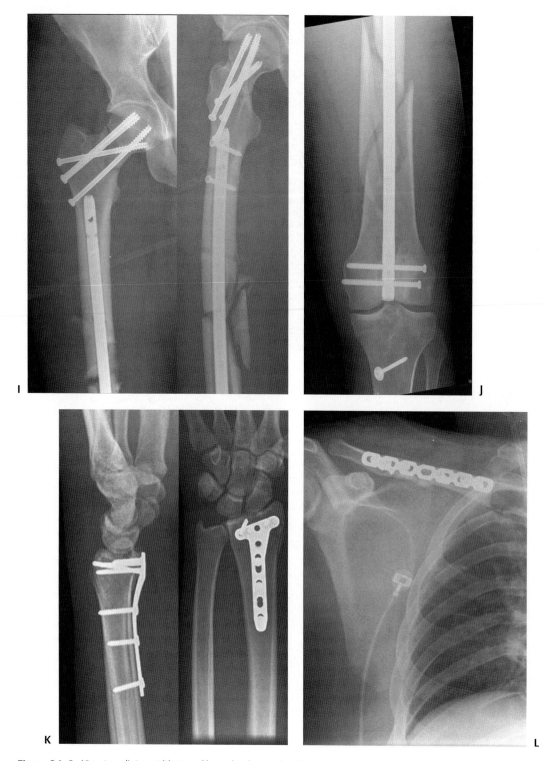

Figure 34–8 *(Continued) Case 4* **(I)** AP and lateral radiographs of the right femur. **(J)** AP radiograph of the left femur. **(K)** AP and lateral radiographs of the right wrist. **(L)** AP of the right clavicle.

proceeded with the full understanding of all services involved that this patient clearly had significant blood loss from bilateral femur fractures, and was likely underresuscitated given the lack of IV access for a period of time in the trauma bay. The operating room was prepared for external fixation at the start of the case, causing no delay in conversion to DCO.

Case 5 This was a 31-year-old female who was a restrained driver in a rollover motor vehicle accident. She had no significant medical history and was not taking any medications at the time of admission. She arrived at the trauma bay awake and alert with a GCS of 15. There was obvious gross deformity of bilateral lower extremities

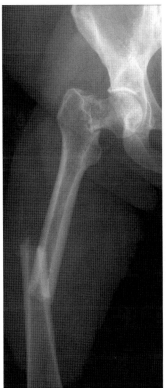
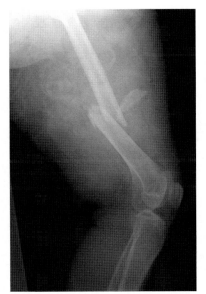
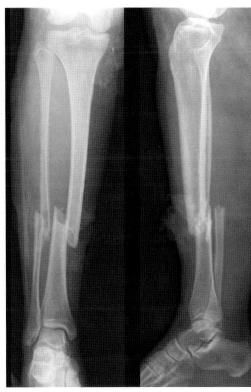

A–C

Figure 34–9 *Case 5* Preoperative radiographs of the bilateral lower extremity injuries. The right tibia, right knee, and left femur were all open injuries. **(A)** Anteroposterior (AP) radiographs of the right femur demonstrating the femoral neck and ipsilateral shaft fractures.

(B) Radiograph of the left femur with a type 2 open femoral shaft fracture. **(C)** AP and lateral radiographs of the type 3A open right tibia fracture. *(Continued on page 874)*

with large open wounds over the right knee and right tibia and a smaller 2 cm wound over the left femur. Her vital signs were remarkably stable with a blood pressure of 130/80, heart rate 110s to 120s, and O₂Sat 99%. Her laboratory results revealed a low hematocrit of 19 with a platelet count of 171. Coagulation screen was normal. Lactate measured 1.5.

A CT scan of the head, chest, spine, abdomen, and pelvis was negative with the exception of a right femoral neck fracture. Radiographic evaluation revealed a displaced right femoral neck fracture, right femoral shaft fracture, right tibial shaft fracture, and left femoral shaft fracture **(Fig. 34–9A–C)**. After discussion with the general surgery trauma service, blood products were started in anticipation of irrigation and debridement of her open fractures with temporizing versus definitive treatment of her fractures depending on her intraoperative course.

The surgical plan consisted of irrigation and debridement of the right-sided wounds followed by intramedullary nailing of the right tibia to enable some traction for reduction of the femoral neck fracture. An open reduction of the femoral neck would then follow with retrograde intramedullary nailing of the right femur as the final procedure on the right side. The left side would then be treated with irrigation and de-

bridement followed by antegrade femoral nailing. A discussion was held with anesthesia preoperatively to inform them that laboratories should be drawn frequently (30 to 60 minute intervals) and that, if there were any signs of decompensation, damage-control techniques could be undertaken at any of the outlined stages.

The patient underwent induction of general anesthesia without any complications. Her hematocrit remained between 28 and 31 at each time point with transfusion of blood products pre- and intraoperatively. Her vital signs all remained stable. At the end of each stage a discussion was held with anesthesia to determine if we should continue with the next procedure. At the end of all orthopaedic procedures, the patient continued to do well physiologically, and vascular surgery proceeded with placement of an inferior vena cava filter **(Fig. 34–9D–G)**.

The patient was kept intubated after surgery secondary to the long operative course and the volume of fluids given intraoperatively. She was alert immediately postoperatively and was extubated 24 hours later and tolerated this without difficulty. The patient was discharged home on postoperative day 5.

Key points in this case include the constant communication that occurred with the anesthesia team regarding

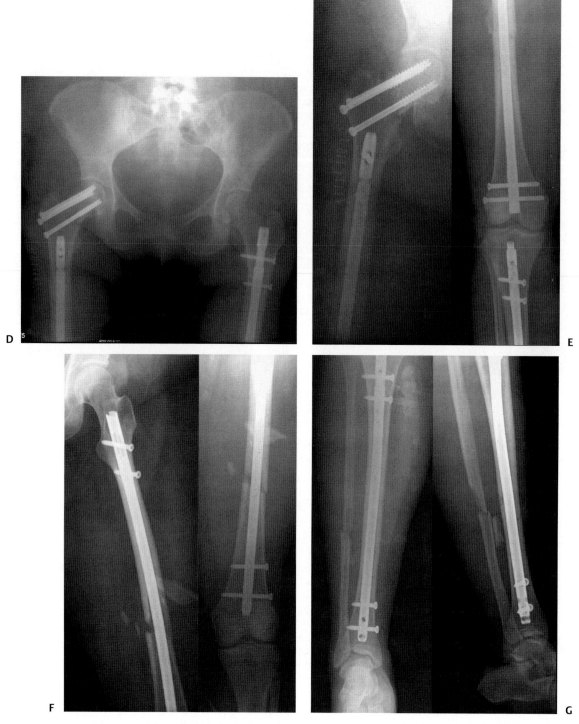

Figure 34–9 *(Continued) Case 5* Preoperative radiographs of the bilateral lower extremity injuries. The right tibia, right knee, and left femur were all open injuries. **(D)** AP pelvis radiograph demonstrating screw fixation after open reduction and internal fixation of the femoral neck. **(E,F)** AP and lateral radiographs of the right and left femurs after retrograde intramedullary nailing. **(G)** AP and lateral radiographs of the right tibia after intramedullary nailing.

the plan and frequency of laboratories with the ability to abort at various intervals if necessary. It should also be recognized that this patient's young age and preinjury health contributed to her ability to tolerate a long surgery with multiple procedures. All staff in the room were also made aware of the possibility of converting to DCO if necessary, and external fixation instrumentation was available in the room.

Summary

Patients with high ISSs, thoracic trauma, head injuries, and significant resuscitation requirements need to be evaluated on a case-by-case basis for timing of fracture fixation. Factors such as patient age and medical comorbidities should also fall into the equation. A summary of parameters to consider is provided in **Table 34–5**. Although early total care of fractures has been shown to decrease hospital and ICU length of stay and enable earlier patient mobility, prolonged surgical procedures in the first 24 hours can predispose a polytraumatized patient to hypoxia and hypoperfusion, leading to multiorgan dysfunction. Caution should be taken in borderline patients undergoing early operative procedures, with particular attention to intraoperative monitoring of resuscitative needs with serial hematocrits, coagulation panels, lactate levels, core body temperatures, and ICP where indicated.

Pearls

- Vascular injuries may be identified on clinical exam alone or by diagnostic measures, such as an ABI less than 0.9.
- Angiography should be considered in patients with pelvic injuries requiring transfusion of more than four units of packed red blood cells (PRBCs) in less than 24 hours or more than six units of PRBCs in less than 48 hours despite temporary stabilization efforts or sheeting.
- The incidence of missed injuries in the first 24 hours of admission is as high as 12% in the multiply injured patient.

- Serum levels of IL-6 correlate the amount of overall soft tissue trauma and chest trauma. IL-6 is one of the best characterized cytokines associated with the acute inflammatory response.
- The NISS may be more predictive of outcome than the ISS in the multiply injured patient with orthopaedic involvement.
- A SIRS score ≥ 2 is associated with a higher rate of mortality (6.9%).

On the DVDs

Video 34–1 (Same as **Video 24–1, Disk 3**) **Unreamed Femoral Nailing to Treat Bilateral Femur Fractures in a Multitrauma Patient** This video shows the use of unreamed nails in a multitrauma patient with a pulmonary injury and bilateral femur fractures. Decision-making and the steps to treat this patient are reviewed.

Video 34–2 (Same as **Video 31–1, Disk 4**) **Application of an Ankle-Spanning External Fixator** This video shows the application of a spanning fixator across the ankle for the initial management of a distal tibia fracture.

Video 34–3 (Same as **Video 5–3, Disk 1**) **The Use of a Reamer-Irrigator-Aspirator** This video demonstrates a new reamer that reams long bones in a single pass while aspirating the medullary contents. Animal data and tran-esophageal echocardiography demonstrate that this system decreases the volume of pulmonary emboli during reaming of long bones.

References

1. Dutton RP, Cooper C, Jones A, Leone S, Kramer ME, Scalea TM. Daily multidisciplinary rounds shorten length of stay for trauma patients. J Trauma 2003;55:913–919
2. Mills WJ, Barei DP, McNair P. The value of the ankle-brachial index for diagnosing arterial injury after knee dislocation: a prospective study. J Trauma 2004;56:1261–1265
3. Miranda FE, Dennis JW, Veldenz HC, Dovgan PS, Frykberg ER. Confirmation of the safety and accuracy of physical examination in the evaluation of knee dislocation for injury of the popliteal artery: a prospective study. J Trauma 2002;52:247–251
4. Giannoudis PV, Pape HC. Damage control orthopaedics in unstable pelvic ring injuries. Injury 2004;35:671–677
5. Pape H, Stalp M, Dahlweid M, Regel G, Tscherne H. Optimal duration of primary surgery with regards to a "borderline" situation in polytrauma patients [in German]. Arbeitsgemeinschaft "Polytrauma" der Deutschen Gesellschaft für Unfallchirurgie. Unfallchirurg 1999; 102:861–869
6. Chan RN, Ainscow D, Sikorski JM. Diagnostic failures in the multiple injured. J Trauma 1980;20:684–687
7. Buduhan G, McRitchie DI. Missed injuries in patients with multiple trauma. J Trauma 2000;49:600–605
8. Bhatia M, Moochhala S. Role of inflammatory mediators in the pathophysiology of acute respiratory distress syndrome. J Pathol 2004;202:145–156
9. Donnelly TJ, Meade P, Jagels M, et al. Cytokine, complement, and endotoxin profiles associated with the development of the adult respiratory distress syndrome after severe injury. Crit Care Med 1994;22:768–776

10. Keel M, Trentz O. Pathophysiology of polytrauma. Injury 2005;36: 691–709

11. Law MM, Cryer HG, Abraham E. Elevated levels of soluble ICAM-1 correlate with the development of multiple organ failure in severely injured trauma patients. J Trauma 1994;37:100–109

12. Pape H-C, Schmidt RE, Rice J, et al. Biochemical changes after trauma and skeletal surgery of the lower extremity: quantification of the operative burden. Crit Care Med 2000;28:3441–3448

13. Pape H-C, Grimme K, van Griensven M, et al. Impact of intramedullary instrumentation versus damage control for femoral fractures on immunoinflammatory parameters: prospective randomized analysis by the EPOFF Study Group. J Trauma 2003;55:7–13

14. Rangel-Frausto MS, Pittet D, Costigan M, Hwang T, Davis CS, Wenzel RP. The natural history of the systemic inflammatory response syndrome (SIRS): a prospective study. JAMA 1995;273:117–123

15. Roumen RM, Redl H, Schlag G, et al. Inflammatory mediators in relation to the development of multiple organ failure in patients after severe blunt trauma. Crit Care Med 1995;23:474–480

16. Strecker W, Gebhard F, Perl M, et al. Biochemical characterization of individual injury pattern and injury severity. Injury 2003;34: 879–887

17. Talmor M, Hydo L, Barie PS. Relationship of systemic inflammatory response syndrome to organ dysfunction, length of stay, and mortality in critical surgical illness: effect of intensive care unit resuscitation. Arch Surg 1999;134:81–87

18. Napolitano LM, Koruda MJ, Meyer AA, Baker CC. The impact of femur fracture with associated soft tissue injury on immune function and intestinal permeability. Shock 1996;5:202–207

19. Giannoudis PV, Smith RM, Bellamy MC, Morrison JF, Dickson RA, Guillou PJ. Stimulation of the inflammatory system by reamed and unreamed nailing of femoral fractures: an analysis of the second hit. J Bone Joint Surg Br 1999;81:356–361

20. Hildebrand F, Pape H-C, Griensven M, et al. Genetic predisposition for a compromised immune system after multiple trauma. Shock 2005;24:518–522

21. American College of Chest Physicians/Society of Critical Care Medicine Consensus Conference: definitions for sepsis and organ failure and guidelines for the use of innovative therapies in sepsis. Crit Care Med 1992;20:864–874

22. Giannoudis PV. Current concepts of the inflammatory response after major trauma: an update. Injury 2003;34:397–404

23. Fujishima S, Aikawa N. Neutrophil-mediated tissue injury and its modulation. Intensive Care Med 1995;21:277–285

24. Smith JA. Neutrophils, host defense, and inflammation: a double-edged sword. J Leukoc Biol 1994;56:672–686

25. Rensing H, Bauer M. Multiple organ failure: mechanisms, clinical manifestations and treatment strategies [in German]. Anaesthesist 2001;50:819–841

26. Singer M, De Santis V, Vitale D, Jeffcoate W. Multiorgan failure is an adaptive, endocrine-mediated, metabolic response to overwhelming systemic inflammation. Lancet 2004;364:545–548

27. Marshall JC, Cook DJ, Christou NV, Bernard GR, Sprung CL, Sibbald WJ. Multiple organ dysfunction score: a reliable descriptor of a complex clinical outcome. Crit Care Med 1995;23:1638–1652

28. Harwood PJ, Giannoudis PV, van Griensven M, Krettek C, Pape H-C. Alterations in the systemic inflammatory response after early total care and damage control procedures for femoral shaft fracture in severely injured patients. J Trauma 2005;58:446–452

29. Seibel R, LaDuca J, Hassett JM, et al. Blunt multiple trauma (ISS 36), femur traction, and the pulmonary failure-septic state. Ann Surg 1985;202:283–295

30. Bone LB, Johnson KD, Weigelt J, Scheinberg R. Early versus delayed stabilization of femoral fractures: a prospective randomized study. J Bone Joint Surg Am 1989;71:336–340

31. Pape HC, Auf'm'Kolk M, Paffrath T, Regel G, Sturm JA, Tscherne H. Primary intramedullary femur fixation in multiple trauma patients with associated lung contusion: a cause of posttraumatic ARDS? J Trauma 1993;34:540–547

32. Hildebrand F, Giannoudis P, van Griensven M, et al. Secondary effects of femoral instrumentation on pulmonary physiology in a standardised sheep model: what is the effect of lung contusion and reaming? Injury 2005;36:544–555

33. Bosse MJ, MacKenzie EJ, Riemer BL, et al. Adult respiratory distress syndrome, pneumonia, and mortality following thoracic injury and a femoral fracture treated either with intramedullary nailing with reaming of with a plate: a comparative study. J Bone Joint Surg Am 1997;79:799–809

34. Wolinsky PR, Banit D, Parker RE, et al. Reamed intramedullary femoral nailing after induction of an "ARDS-like" state in sheep: effect on clinically applicable markers of pulmonary function. J Orthop Trauma 1998;12:169–175

35. Pape HC, Giannoudis P, Krettek C. The timing of fracture treatment in polytrauma patients: relevance of damage control orthopedic surgery. Am J Surg 2002;183:622–629

36. Hildebrand F, Giannoudis P, Kretteck C, Pape HC. Damage control: extremities. Injury 2004;35:678–689

37. Cerovic O, Golubovic V, Spec-Marn A, Kremzar B, Vidmar G. Relationship between injury severity and lactate levels in severely injured patients. Intensive Care Med 2003;29:1300–1305

38. Manikis P, Jankowski S, Zhang H, Kahn RJ, Vincent JL. Correlation of serial blood lactate levels to organ failure and mortality after trauma. Am J Emerg Med 1995;13:619–622

39. Waydhas C, Nast-Kolb D, Jochum M, et al. Inflammatory mediators, infection, sepsis, and multiple organ failure after severe trauma. Arch Surg 1992;127:460–467

40. Malone DL, Kuhls D, Napolitano LM, McCarter R, Scalea T. Back to basics: validation of the admission systemic inflammatory response syndrome score in predicting outcome in trauma. J Trauma 2001;51:458–463

41. Napolitano LM, Ferrer T, McCarter RJ Jr, Scalea TM. Systemic inflammatory response syndrome score at admission independently predicts mortality and length of stay in trauma patients. J Trauma 2000;49:647–652

42. Bochicchio GV, Napolitano LM, Joshi M, McCarter RJ Jr, Scalea TM. Systemic inflammatory response syndrome score at admission independently predicts infection in blunt trauma patients. J Trauma 2001;50:817–820

43. Scalea TM, Boswell SA, Scott JD, Mitchell KA, Kramer ME, Pollak AN. External fixation as a bridge to intramedullary nailing for patients with multiple injuries and with femur fractures: damage control orthopedics. J Trauma 2000;48:613–621

44. Joist A, Schult M, Ortmann C, et al. Rinsing-suction reamer attenuates intramedullary pressure increase and fat intravasation in a sheep model. J Trauma 2004;57:146–151

45. Schult M, Kuchle R, Hofmann A, et al. Pathophysiological advantages of rinsing-suction-reaming (RSR) in a pig model for intramedullary nailing. J Orthop Res 2006;24:1186–1192

46. Nowotarski PJ, Turen CH, Brumback RJ, Scarboro JM. Conversion of external fixation to intramedullary nailing for fractures of the shaft of the femur in multiply injured patients. J Bone Joint Surg Am 2000;82:781–788

47. Harwood PJ, Giannoudis PV, Probst C, Krettek C, Pape HC. The risk of local infective complications after damage control procedures for femoral shaft fracture. J Orthop Trauma 2006;20:181–189

48. Stein SC, Young GS, Talucci RC, Greenbaum BH, Ross SE. Delayed brain injury after head trauma: significance of coagulopathy. Neurosurgery 1992;30:160–165

49. Zafonte RD, Hammond FM, Mann NR, Wood DL, Black KL, Millis SR. Relationship between Glasgow coma scale and functional outcome. Am J Phys Med Rehabil 1996;75:364–369

50. Kalb DC, Ney AL, Rodriguez JL, et al. Assessment of the relationship between timing of fixation of the fracture and secondary brain injury in patients with multiple trauma. Surgery 1998;124:739–744

51. Brundage SI, McGhan R, Jurkovich GJ, Mack CD, Maier RV. Timing of femur fracture fixation: effect on outcome in patients with thoracic and head injuries. J Trauma 2002;52:299–307

52. Poole GV, Miller JD, Agnew SG, Griswold JA. Lower extremity fracture fixation in head-injured patients. J Trauma 1992;32:654–659

53. Townsend RN, Lheureau T, Protech J, Riemer B, Simon D. Timing fracture repair in patients with severe brain injury (Glasgow coma scale score < 9). J Trauma 1998;44:977–982

54. Jaicks RR, Cohn SM, Moller BA. Early fracture fixation may be deleterious after head injury. J Trauma 1997;42:1–5

55. Harwood PJ, Giannoudis PV, Probst C, van Griensven M, Krettek C, Pape H-C. Which AIS based scoring system is the best predictor of outcome in orthopaedic blunt trauma patients? J Trauma 2006; 60:334–340

56. Balogh ZJ, Varga E, Tomka J, Suveges G, Toth L, Simonka JA. The new injury severity score is a better predictor of extended hospitalization and intensive care unit admission than the injury severity score in patients with multiple orthopaedic injuries. J Orthop Trauma 2003;17:508–512

57. Osler T, Baker SP, Long W. A modification of the injury severity score that both improves accuracy and simplifies scoring. J Trauma 1997;43:922–925

58. Kilgo PD, Osler TM, Meredith W. The worst injury predicts mortality outcome the best: rethinking the role of multiple injuries in trauma outcome scoring. J Trauma 2003;55:599–606

59. Johnson KD, Cadambi A, Seibert GB. Incidence of adult respiratory distress syndrome in patients with multiple musculoskeletal injuries: effect of early operative stabilization of fractures. J Trauma 1985;25:375–384

60. Handolin L, Pajarinen J, Lassus J, Tulikoura I. Early intramedullary nailing of lower extremity fracture and respiratory function in polytraumatized patients with a chest injury: a retrospective study of 61 patients. Acta Orthop Scand 2004;75:477–480

61. Reamed versus unreamed intramedullary nailing of the femur: comparison of the rate of ARDS in multiple injured patients. J Orthop Trauma 2006;20:384–387

62. Zalavras C, Velmahos GC, Chan L, Demetriades D, Patzakis MJ. Risk factors for respiratory failure following femoral fractures: the role of multiple intramedullary nailing. Injury 2005;36:751–757

63. Pape H-C, Zelle BA, Hildebrand F, Giannoudis PV, Krettek C, van Griensven M. Reamed femoral nailing in sheep: does irrigation and aspiration of intramedullary contents alter the systemic response? J Bone Joint Surg Am 2005;87:2515–2522

64. Pape H-C, Hildebrand F, Pertschy S, et al. Changes in the management of femoral shaft fractures in polytrauma patients: from early total care to damage control orthopedic surgery. J Trauma 2002; 53:452–461

65. Pape H-C, van Griensven M, Rice J, et al. Major secondary surgery in blunt trauma patients and perioperative cytokine liberation: determination of the clinical relevance of biochemical markers. J Trauma 2001;50:989–1000

Index

Page numbers followed an italic *f* or *t* indicate entries in figures or tables, respectively.

quadriceps tendon disruption in, 678, 681–682,
683*f*, 684
rehabilitation for
postoperative, 682
as treatment, 679
surgical treatment of, 679–685
anatomical considerations in, 679
techniques for, 679–682
patella function in, 664, 664*f*
Kocher-Langenbeck approach
for acetabular fractures, 479–483, 488–496
advantages of, 480
closure in, 483
fracture reduction in, 483
gluteus maximus in, 480–482, 480*f*
iliotibial band in, 480–481, 480*f*
incision and exposure in, 480–483, 480*f*–482*f*
indications for, 479
patient positioning for, 479–480, 482*f*
for posterior column fractures, 490–491
for posterior wall fractures, 488–490, 488*f*–491*f*
sciatic nerve in, 481*f*, 482–483, 482*f*
for transverse fractures, 491, 492*f*
for transverse with posterior wall fractures,
492–495, 493*f*–495*f*
for T-type fractures, 495–496, 496*f*–497*f*
for femoral head fractures, 528–529, 531, 536
Kocher method, of shoulder reduction, 258
Kyle classification, of intertrochanteric femur fractures,
567–568
Kyphoplasty
for thoracic spine fracture, 170–171, 170*f*, 176
for thoracolumbar spine fracture, 202

L

Lactate levels, in polytrauma patients, 859–860, 866*t*, 867
Laminectomy, for thoracic spine fracture, 169*f*
Lateral collateral ligament, 306–307
in elbow dislocations, 309*f*, 312, 313*f*, 315, 315*f*, 323,
328
in radial head fracture, 309–310, 309*f*, 323
Lateral femoral circumflex artery, in femoral neck
fractures, 548
Lateral malleolus fractures
comminuted or crushed, 798–799
deltoid ligament injury with, 793–795, 795*f*, 798
fibular plating for, 798–800, 799*f*
freshening of, 798
isolated, 797–800
with medial malleolus fracture, 801–803
nonoperative treatment of, 797–798
surgical approach to, 798, 798*f*
tips and tricks, 800
Lateral mass fractures, 142–143
fusion for, 155
posterior stabilization of, 154–155, 155*f*
screw fixation of, 155, 156*f*

surgical treatment of, 154–155
indications for, 146
Lateral mass screw fixation
in atlantoaxial fusion, 122–125, 124*f*–125*f*
outcomes and complications of, 133
of atlas fracture, 105, 106*f*
of facet joint fracture-dislocation, 149*f*, 150
of lateral mass fracture, 155, 156*f*
in occipitocervical fusion, 121, 121*f*
Lateral meniscus tears, with tibial plateau fractures, 713,
716, 717*t*
Lateral parapatellar approach, 719–720
Lateral process talus fractures, 824–825
Lauge-Hansen classification, of ankle fractures, 793, 794*f*
Lavage, high-pressure pulsatile, for soft-tissue injury, 4
Leg fasciotomy
single-incision, 50–52, 52*f*
two-incision, 48*f*, 49–50, 49*f*–51*f*
Lesser arc injuries, 390–391, 391*f*
Lesser trochanteric shape sign, for femoral rotational
determination, 68, 69*f*
Lesser tuberosity, in proximal humeral fracture,
239–240
Less Invasive Stabilization System (LISS), 1, 62–71, 64*f*
advantages of, 64
disadvantages of, 64
for femur, 64–68, 649, 651–654
anterolateral approach for, 64, 65*f*
articular reduction for, 64–65
Blumensaat's line in, 65, 68*f*
cable technique in, 65, 67*f*
lateral approach for, 64, 65*f*
lesser trochanteric shape sign in, 68, 69*f*
limb alignment for, 65–68, 67*f*–69*f*
meter stick technique in, 65–68, 69*f*
notch sign in, 65, 68*f*
positioning of, 64–65, 652*f*
reduction for, 64–65
screw fixation of, 65, 66*f*–67*f*
submuscular insertion of, 64, 66*f*, 651–654
surgical sequence for, 651–654, 653*f*–656*f*
flexibility of, 64
surgical technique for, 63–71
for tibia, 70–71
articular reduction for, 70
limb alignment for, 70
meter-stick technique in, 71
outcomes of, 74
positioning of, 70
screw fixation of, 70
submuscular insertion of, 70, 70*f*
for tibial plateau fractures, 724–728
fixator placement in, 726–727, 726*f*
forceps removal in, 727, 727*f*
ideal construct in, 727, 727*f*
indications for, 725
patient positioning for, 725–726

in occipitocervical fusion, 121, 121*f*
of odontoid fracture, 110–113
of olecranon fracture, 333–334, 333*f*
in olecranon osteotomy, 295, 295*f*
of patellar fractures, 668–669
of phalangeal shaft fractures (hand), 419, 419*f*
of posterior malleolus fractures, 803–804
of proximal humeral fracture, 242, 244, 248
of pubic ramus fractures, 453
of radial styloid fractures, 398–399, 399*f*–400*f*
of Rolando's fracture, 432, 432*f*
of sacral fractures, 465
of sacroiliac joint dislocation, 454–455,
    457–461
of scaphoid fractures, 405–409
of syndesmosis injuries, 806–807, 806*f*
of talar body fractures, 823
of talar head fractures, 824
of talar neck fractures, 817–820
of tarsometatarsal joint injuries, 843–845
of thoracic spine fracture, 171, 172*f*, 174, 174*f*, 176
of thoracolumbar fracture-dislocation, 197
of thoracolumbar spine fractures, 189–190, 190*f*,
    192–194, 193*f*–194*f*
of tibial plateau fractures, 720–722
of trapezium fractures, 409–410
of trapezoid fractures, 410
of ulna fracture, 350–352, 351*f*
Scuderi technique, of quadriceps tendon repair, 682
Seat-belt injuries, 165, 169, 179–181, 180*f*
    nonoperative treatment of, 184–185
    surgical indications in, 185–186
    surgical techniques for, 194–197
Second hit phenomenon, 611, 626–627, 853–856, 857*f*
Second metatarsal fractures, 846–847
    deformity with, 846
    fixation options for, 846–847, 846*f*
Second metatarsal-phalangeal joint injuries, 848
Selective arteriography, 708
Self-compression plates, 58, 58*f*
Serratus anterior, in scapula fracture, 217
720 degree approach, for facet joint fracture-dislocation,
    151
Seventh American College of Chest Physicians
    Conference on Antithrombotic and
    Thrombolytic Therapy: Evidence-Based
    Guidelines, 586
Short radiolunate ligament, 387, 387*f*
Shoulder dislocation, 238, 256–260
    anterior-inferior, 257
    arthroscopic-assisted capsulorrhaphy for, 260
    arthroscopy for, 260
    classic Bankart (Perthes) lesion with, 260
    classification of, 256–257
    complications of, 260
    inferior (luxatio erecta), 257
    magnetic resonance imaging of, 257
    natural history of, 238, 260

neurological injury with, 260
nonoperative treatment of, 257–259
    indications for, 258
    techniques of, 258–259
outcomes of, 260
pathology of, 260
pearls about, 260
posterior, 257
    locked, 259–260
recurrent, risk factors for, 257, 260
reduction techniques for, 258–259
    analgesia for, 259
    atraumatic, 258
    external rotation, 259
    Hippocratic, 258
    Kocher, 258
    Milch, 258
    muscle relaxants for, 259
    Stimson, 259
    traditional, 258
rehabilitation for, as treatment, 259
reverse Hill-Sachs lesion with, 259
rotator cuff tear with, 257
surgical treatment of, 259–260
    anatomical considerations in, 260
    definitive repair of injured structures in, 259
    indications for, 259–260
    management of acute injury in, 259
    techniques for, 260
treatment goals in, 238
in young *versus* elderly patients, 238
Shoulder girdle injuries, 207–236. *See also*
    specific types
Shoulder spica casting, for humeral shaft
    fractures, 266
Shoulder stability, 256
Sigmoid notch of distal radius, 364
Single-bundle reconstruction, of posterior cruciate
    ligament, 694–697
    femoral tunnel preparation in, 695
    femur-sided graft fixation in, 696–697
    graft preparation for, 696
    patient positioning for, 695
    steps in, 694
    tibial-inlay site preparation in, 696
    tibial-sided graft fixation in, 696, 697*f*
Single-incision leg fasciotomy, 50–52, 52*f*
SIRS. *See* Systemic inflammatory response syndrome
Skeletal traction. *See* Traction
Skin
    assessment of, in soft tissue injury, 4
    integrity, in polytrauma patient, 852
    vasculature of, 2–3, 3*f*
Skin graft
    for soft tissue injury, 5, 13
    split-thickness, 13
Skin graft substitutes, 14
Skin traction, 14

The complete, annotated contents for the DVDs is found on page xxi, following the contents. Also, at the end of each chapter, before references, is a boxed listing of the videos that demonstrate techniques described in that chapter. See inside front cover for DVDs 1 and 2 and their contents.